Postsurgical Orthopedic

SPORTS REHABILITATION

Knee & Shoulder

Postsurgical Orthopedic

SPORTS REHABILITATION

Knee & Shoulder

ROBERT C. MANSKE
DPT, MED, MPT, SCS, ATC, CSCS

Assistant Professor, Department of Physical Therapy
Wichita State University
Physical Therapist
Via Christi Orthopedic and Sports Physical Therapy
Athletic Trainer, Via Christi Sports Medicine
Teaching Associate
Department of Family Medicine
University of Kansas Medical School
Via Christi Sports Medicine Fellowship Residency Program
Wichita, KS

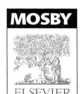

MOSBY

ELSEVIER

11830 Westline Industrial Drive
St. Louis, Missouri 63146

POSTSURGICAL ORTHOPEDIC SPORTS REHABILITATION: ISBN-13: 978-0-323-02702-1
KNEE AND SHOULDER   ISBN-10:   0-323-02702-4

Notice

ISBN-13: 978-0-323-02702-1
ISBN-10: 0-323-02702-4

Acquisitions Editor: Kathy Falk
Publishing Services Manager: Peggy Fagen
Design Direction: Amy Buxton
Cover Designer: Bill Smith Studio
Text Designer: Valerie Brewster

Printed in the United States

Last digit is the print number: 9 8 7 6 5 4 3 2 1

I would like to dedicate this book, my first, to my grandmother, Dorothy Kimbell. She is unknowingly one of the most influential persons who have helped shape and mold my life. My grandmother has quietly demonstrated numerous personal values for our family such as faith, fairness, caring, honesty, independence, integrity, and honor, to name just a few. She rarely raises her voice, leading by actions and example rather than by the spoken word. Often before making important decisions to life's questions that appear exceedingly cloudy, I ponder one simple question: What would Grandma think is the right choice? Suddenly, these difficult, cloudy decisions become very clear! If we can pass on to others, and continue to demonstrate, the values you have shown us all, the world will be a much better place!

Preface

My initial goal in editing *Postsurgical Orthopedic Sports Rehabilitation: Knee and Shoulder* was to provide an invaluable resource for those clinicians or students practicing in orthopedic sports rehabilitation, and in particular those who primarily treat in the niche of knee and shoulder patient populations. In my practice in orthopedic sports rehabilitation, I have felt the frustration of not fully understanding surgical procedures or the rehabilitation that follows any of those given procedures. In many cases, surgery for any single disorder may be done by a variety of procedures, all of which have their own unique rehabilitation nuances. Because many surgeons believe that rehabilitation has as much, if not a greater, impact on postsurgical outcomes than does the actual surgery, proper postsurgical care is critical.

This text is divided into three basic sections. The first, *Concepts in Postsurgical Management*, lays the foundation for the subsequent chapters. This first section describes the soft tissue healing process, the effects of immobilization and mobilization, the pre- and postoperative knee and shoulder evaluation, and training for strength and neuromuscular control. The second section, *The Knee*, is broken into chapters for ligament injuries, meniscus injuries, and cartilage injuries. The knee section also has several special chapters related to complications following ACL reconstruction, the implications of strain gauge studies, prevention of ACL rupture, and complications following meniscus surgery. The third section, *The Shoulder*, is broken into chapters related to AC joint injuries, shoulder capsular and ligament stabilization procedures, labral repairs, rotator cuff repairs, and biceps tendon disorders.

Each of the chapters in this book begins with a detailed description of the history behind the given surgical procedure and follows with details regarding exactly how the surgery has been performed. Most chapters have teamed one or more rehabilitation clinicians with an orthopedic surgeon so that both the critical aspects of the surgical procedure and the postoperative rehabilitation that soon ensues can be discussed in thorough detail.

With that in mind I have had the opportunity to collect and compile postsurgical protocols written by some of the most well known authors in our field of orthopedic sports rehabilitation. Because rehabilitation and the field of medicine in general are dynamic entities, these protocols and surgical descriptions have been developed and shaped by clinical and biomechanical research, yet also contain empirically based opinion and evidence-based guidelines where appropriate. The challenge of this text is to bring readers the most up-to-date rehabilitation techniques and treatment methods in an area of medicine that changes literally on a daily basis.

May this book offer anyone working in the extremely rewarding field of rehabilitation a look into the latest surgical and postsurgical treatment methods for two of the most fascinating and complex joints in our musculoskeletal system, the knee and shoulder.

Robert C. Manske

Acknowledgments

How does one acknowledge so many people? There are so many individuals that knowingly or unknowingly have helped or given support during the production of this book.

Special thanks to Marion Waldman, for giving me this wonderful and challenging opportunity, and to Marge Fraser, Cynthia and David Mondgock, and Meghan Ziegler, all of whom I could not have done without.

Thanks to my colleagues at Wichita State University College of Health Professions and Department of Physical Therapy for their support in all of my endeavors. Special thanks to Dale Barb for all the deep discussions, Ken Pitetti for giving me something to aim for and providing constant encouragement for a job well done, Barb Smith for her tutelage in the academe process, and Cam Wilson for letting me do what I love to do!

Thanks to all the Via Christi Medical Center staff and professional colleagues for allowing me the pleasure of practicing in such a fun environment. Yes, this does include you, Janice Lam! I especially want to thank Kim Yearout and Cyndia LaFleur for allowing me the flexibility to wear many hats, including physical therapy clinician, athletic trainer, and researcher.

I thank Doctors Dan Prohaska and Mark Stovak for their friendship, their respect, and their trust in me to treat their patients. Thank you both for being inquisitive, like me, and helping to find the answers that may someday solve some of sports medicines confusion and unknown!

I also owe a thank you to all of the past students at Wichita State University Department of Physical Therapy, whom I have had the pleasure of instructing in our fascinating field of rehabilitation.

Although numerous therapists have given guidance to me through the last 12 years, I would like to acknowledge two who have counseled me the most. I have nothing but respect for and gratitude to George J. Davies, who has been like a second father for me. George has not only been a teacher, mentor, and colleague but has also become a very close friend. George, I look forward to learning from you for years to come. Todd Ellenbecker has given me his superb advice, friendship, and continued support throughout the production of this book.

I want to thank Mike Reiman, JW Matheson, and Chris Durall for encouragement and friendship. You guys are the best! Thanks to the staff at Gundersen Lutheran Sports Medicine Department and to all the Fellows who have succeeded following Schulte and myself. I am indebted to the expert contributors who have made this book possible. Without all of you, this book could not have been produced. Thanks to family who have supported me throughout this book.

Last but not least, I want thank my three favorite girls—Julie, Racheal, and Halle—for their love and support.

Contributors

Chris Alford, PT, SCS, ATC, CSCS
Twin Lakes Physical Therapy, Inc.
Milledgeville, GA

David W. Altchek, MD
Associate Professor of Clinical Surgery
Weill Medical College of Cornell University
Attending Orthopedic Surgeon
Hospital for Special Surgery
New York, NY

Annunziato Amendola, MD
Professor, Department of Orthopaedics & Rehabilitation
Medical Director, Center for Sports Medicine
University of Iowa
Iowa City, IA

James R. Andrews, MD
Medical Director
Alabama Sports Medicine Institute
Birmingham, Alabama
Clinical Professor of Surgery
Department of Orthopaedic Surgery
University of Alabama at Birmingham School of Medicine
Birmingham, AL

Kelly Ashton, PT
Staff Physical Therapist
NovaCare Rehabilitation
Milton, FL

David S. Bailie, MD
Chief of Orthopaedic Surgery, Scottsdale Healthcare Shea
    Hospital
Scottsdale, AZ

Lori A. Bolgla, PhD, PT, ATC
Assistant Professor
Department of Physical Therapy
Medical College of Georgia
Augusta, GA

Kristen F. Brinks, MS, PT, ATC
Gundersen Lutheran Department of Sports Medicine
Onalaska, WI

E. Lyle Cain, MD
Orthopedic Surgeon
Alabama Sports Medicine and Orthopedic Center
American Sports Medicine Institute
Birmingham, AL

John T. Cavanaugh, MEd, PT, ATC
Adjunct Professor
Department of Sports Sciences and Physical Education
Hofstra University
Hempstead, New York
Team Physical Therapist
Athletic Department
United States Merchant Marine Academy
Kings Point, NY

Angelo J. Colosimo, MD
Assistant Professor of Orthopedics
Director, Division of Sports Medicine
Department of Orthopaedics and Sports Medicine
University of Cincinnati
Cincinnati, OH

**George J. Davies, DPT, MEd, PT, SCS, ATC,
LAT, CSCS, FAPTA**
Professor, Department of Physical Therapy Armstrong
    Atlantic State University
Savannah, GA
Sports Physical Therapist and Consultant
Gundersen Lutheran Sports Medicine
LaCrosse, WI

Mark S. DeCarlo, PT, ATC
Methodist Sports Medicine Center
Indianapolis, IN

Patrick Denton, MD
Pee Dee Orthopaedic Associates, PC
Florence, SC

Jeffrey R. Dugas, MD
Orthopedic Surgeon
Alabama Sports Medicine and Orthopedic Center
Clinical Instructor
American Sports Medicine Institute
Birmingham, AL

Christopher J. Durall, DPT, SCS, ATC, CSCS
Director of Physical Therapy Unit
Student Health Center
University of Wisconsin—La Crosse
La Crosse, WI

Marsha Eifert-Mangine, EdD(c), PT, ATC
Assistant Professor
Department of Health Sciences
Program in Physical Therapy
College of Mount St. Joseph
Associate Director of Research
Nova Care Rehabilitation
Cincinnati, OH

Todd S. Ellenbecker, PT, DPT, MS, SCS, OCS, CSCS
Clinic Director
Physiotherapy Associates Scottsdale Sports Clinic
Scottsdale, AZ
National Director of Clinical Research
Physiotherapy Associates
Memphis, TN

John H. Fernandez, PT, ATC, OCS, CSCS
Acelera Physiotherapy Associates
Andover, KS

Bradley L. Fowler, MD
Gundersen Lutheran Department of Sports Medicine
Onalaska, WI

Travis L. Francis, MS, LAT, ATC
Manager Sports Medicine
Via Christi Rehabilitation Center
Wichita, KS

Charles E. Giangarra, MD
Associate Professor Department of Orthopedic Surgery
Chief, Department of Athletics and Orthopedic Sports
    Medicine
Marshall University
Huntington, WV

W. Bays Gibson, MPT, DPT
Lucas Therapies
Salem, VA

Karl R. Glick, BS, PT
Physical Therapy Services at Cypress
Wichita, KS

Christopher D. Harner, MD
Medical Director and Professor
Department of Orthopaedic Surgery
Center for Sports Medicine
University of Pittsburgh Medical Center
Pittsburgh, PA

Bryan C. Heiderscheit, PhD, PT
Director, Assistant Professor
Neuromuscular Biomechanics Laboratory
Department of Orthopedics and Rehabilitation
Division of Physical Therapy
University of Wisconsin—Madison
Madison, WI

Timothy D. Henne, MD
River Valley Orthopedics
Grand Rapids, MI

Timothy E. Hewett, PhD
Director
Sports Medicine Biodynamics Center
Children's Hospital Research Foundation
Assistant Professor
University of Cincinnati College of Medicine
Cincinnati, OH

C. Scott Humphrey, MD
Shoulder and Upper Extremity Fellow
Department of Orthopaedics
California Pacific Medical Center
San Francisco, CA

James J. Irrgang, PhD, PT, ATC
Associate Professor, Departments of Orthopaedic Surgery
    and Physical Therapy
School of Health and Rehabilitation Services
University of Pittsburgh
Pittsburgh, PA

Jason Jennings, DPT, SCS, ATC, MTC, CSCS
Physical Therapist/Athletic Trainer
Gundersen Lutheran Department of Sports Medicine
Onalaska, WI

Laura E. Keller, MPT
Physical Therapist
Director of Rehabilitation
The Stone Clinic
Orthopaedic Surgery, Sports Medicine, and Rehabilitation
San Francisco, CA

W. Benjamin Kibler, MD, FACSM
Medical Director
Lexington Clinic Sports Medicine Center
Lexington, KY

Daniel J.R. Krauschaar, MPT, CSCS
Director of Outpatient Physical Therapy, Director of
    Rehabilitation Education
Hughston Rehabilitation
The Houghston Clinic
Columbus, GA

Pieter Kroon, PT, OCS, FAAOMPT
Program Director
The Manual Therapy Institute
Cedar Park, TX

Darin T. Leetun, MD
Department of Orthopaedic Surgery
Portage Rehabilitation & Sports Medicine
Hancock, MI

Michelle M. Lesperance, MS, LAT, ATC
Program Director
Athletic Training Program
Assistant Professor of Kinesiology
Greensboro College
Greensboro, NC

Michael Levinson, PT
Clinical Supervisor
Sports Medicine
Rehabilitation Department
Hospital for Special Surgery
New York, NY

Ryan Livermore, MD
Department of Orthopedic Surgery
University of Kansas
Wichita School of Medicine
Wichita, KS

Janice K. Loudon, PT, PhD, ATC
Associate Professor
Department of Physical Therapy and Rehabilitation
    Science
University of Kansas Medical Center
Kansas City, KS

Leonard C. Macrina, MSPT, CSCS
Physical Therapist
Champion Sports Medicine
Birmingham, AL

Scott D. Mair, MD
Associate Professor of Orthopaedic Surgery
University of Kentucky
Lexington, KY

Terry R. Malone, PT, EdD, ATC, FAPTA
Professor of Physical Therapy
University of Kentucky
Lexington, KY

Robert E. Mangine, MEd, PT, ATC
Director of Rehabilitation, Head Football Trainer
Department of Athletics
Clinical Instructor
Department of Orthopaedics/Division of Sports Medicine
University of Cincinnati
Director of Research and Clinical Education
NovaCare Rehabilitation
Cincinnati, OH

Robert C. Manske, DPT, MEd, MPT, SCS, ATC, CSCS
Assistant Professor, Department of Physical Therapy
Wichita State University
Physical Therapist
Via Christi Orthopedic and Sports Physical Therapy
Athletic Trainer, Via Christi Sports Medicine
Teaching Associate
Department of Family Medicine
University of Kansas Medical School
Via Christi Sports Medicine Fellowship Residency
    Program
Wichita, KS

James W. Matheson, PT, DPT, MS, SCS, CSCS
Physical Therapist
Therapy Partners, Inc.
Minnesota Sport and Spine Rehabilitation
Minneapolis, MN

David S. Miers, PT, OCS, FAAOMPT, CSCS
Muscle and Spine Rehabilitation Center
St. Augusta, MI

Stephen J. Minning, MPT
Center Manager
Department of Physical Therapy
NovaCare Rehabilitation
Cincinnati, Ohio
Associate Director of Research
Department of Sports Medicine
University of Cincinnati
Cincinnati, OH

Stephen J. Nicholas, MD
Director
Nicholas Institute of Sports Medicine and Athletic Trauma
New York, NY

Brian Norton, MS, ATC
Head Athletic Trainer
Athletic Training Services
Eastern Washington University
Cheney, WA

Roger V. Ostrander, MD
Andrews Institute for Orthopaedic and Sports Medicine
Gulf Breeze, FL

Christopher R. Price, MD
Department of Orthopedic Surgery
Missoula Bone and Joint
Missoula, MT

Daniel Prohaska, MD
Advanced Orthopedic Associates
Wichita, KS

Michael P. Reiman, PT, MEd, ATC, CSCS
Assistant Professor
Department of Physical Therapy
Wichita State University
Wichita, Kansas
Clinical Physical Therapist
Via Christi Outpatient Orthopedic and Sports Physical
    Therapy
Wichita, KS

Michael M. Reinold, PT, DPT, ATC, CSCS
Assistant Athletic Director
Boston Red Sox
Boston, MA

Richard L. Romeyn, MD
Southeast Minnesota Sports Medicine and Orthopedic
    Surgery Specialists
Winona, MN

Amit Sahasrabudhe, MD
Orthopaedic Resident
Department of Orthopaedic Surgery
University of Pittsburgh School of Medicine
Pittsburgh, PA

Robert A. Schulte, PT, DSc, SCS, ACSM-ES, MBA
Associate Professor
Department of Physical Therapy
University of Mary
Bismark, ND
CEO, University Associates Sports and Orthopedic
  Specialists, PC
Mandan, ND

Aruna M. Seneviratne, MD
Assistant Attending Orthopedic Surgeon
Department of Orthopaedic Surgery
Lenox Hill Hospital
New York, NY

Nicholas A. Sgaglione, MD
Associate Clinical Professor of Orthopaedics
Department of Orthopaedics
Albert Einstein College of Medicine
Bronx, NY
Chief, Division of Sports Medicine
Associate Chairman, Department of Orthopaedics
North Shore University Hospital
Manhasset, NY

K. Donald Shelbourne, MD
The Shelbourne Clinic at Methodist Hospital
Associate Clinical Professor
Indiana University School of Medicine
Methodist Sports Medicine Center
Indianapolis, IN

Naomi N. Shields, MD
Clinical Assistant Professor
Department of Surgery—Orthopedics
University of Kansas School of Medicine—Wichita
Wichita, KS

Brandon Smetana
The Stone Clinic
San Francisco, CA

Julious P. Smith III, MD
Instructor
Department of Orthopaedic Surgery
Medical College of Virginia Campus
Virginia Commonwealth University
Richmond, VA

Kevin R. Stone, MD
The Stone Clinic
San Francisco, CA

Mark Stovak, MD
Medical Director, Via Christi Sports Medicine
Program Director, Sports Medicine Fellowship Program at
  Via Christi
Associate Director
Via Christi Family Medicine Residency Program
Director, Kansas University School of Medicine—Wichita
Clinical Assistant Professor, Family and Community
  Medicine
Kansas University School of Medicine—Wichita
Wichita, KS

Gary Sutton, PT, MS, SCS, OCS, ATC, CSCS
Out-patient Orthopaedics Manager
Sports and Occupational Rehabilitation Center
Henrico Doctors' Hospital
Adjunct Clinical Associate Professor
Department of Physical Therapy
Medical College of Virginia Campus
Virginia Commonwealth University
Richmond, VA

Suzanne M. Tanner, MD
Gundersen Lutheran Department of Sports Medicine
Onalaska, WI

Kimberly Turman, MD
Orthopaedic Surgery Resident
Department of Orthopaedic Surgery and Rehabilitation
University of Nebraska Medical Center
Omaha, NE

Timothy F. Tyler, MS, PT, ATC
Clinical Research Associate
Nicholas Institute of Sports Medicine and Athletic Trauma
Lenox Hill Hospital
New York, NY
Director
Pro Sports of Westchester
Scarsdale, NY

Ann W. Walgenbach, RNC, FNP, MSC
Clinical Research Coordinator
The Stone Clinic
San Francisco, CA

Cory Warner, MPT, CSCS
Athlete Enhancement Director
Sports Physical Therapy
University Associates—Sports and Orthopedic Specialists,
  PC
Mandan, ND

Robin West, MD
Assistant Professor
Department of Orthopaedic Surgery
University of Pittsburgh School of Medicine
Pittsburgh, PA

Kevin E. Wilk, DPT, PT
National Director of Research and Clinical Education
Champion Sports Medicine
Birmingham, AL

Glenn N. Williams, PT, PhD, ATC, SCS
Assistant Professor
Graduate Program in Physical Therapy & Rehabilitation
Assistant Professor
Department of Orthopaedics & Rehabilitation
Carver College of Medicine

Director of Research
Sports Medicine Center
University of Iowa
Iowa City, IA

Kim Yearout, PT, BS
Director of Outpatient Occupational Therapy and Physical
   Therapy Services
Via Christi Regional Medical Center
Our Lady of Lourdes Rehabilitation Center
Wichita, KS

Contents

Concepts in Postsurgical Management

CHAPTER 1

Postsurgical Soft Tissue Healing

Michelle M. Lesperance, MS, LAT, ATC
Travis L. Francis, MS, LAT, ATC
Brian Norton, MS, ATC

CHAPTER OUTLINE

TO DEVELOP REHABILITATION PRO-GRAMS enabling patients to achieve their goals in the most efficient manner, physical therapists and athletic trainers must have a thorough understanding of the healing process. The purpose of this chapter is to describe the inflammatory process in general, as well as define soft tissue classifications and characteristics. Following these definitions, healing will be defined in terms of primary and secondary intent. Finally, the healing process with regard to each type of connective tissue will be differentiated so that clinicians can more clearly understand how to develop individual rehabilitation programs for specific sports and orthopedic injuries.

INTRODUCTION TO POSTSURGICAL SOFT TISSUE HEALING

During postsurgical soft tissue healing, the inflammatory response initially begins when blood vessels are torn, causing bleeding to occur into the interstitial spaces. This bleeding causes a series of vascular and cellular reactions, including the activation of blood platelets that function to control bleeding. Activation of blood platelets is a primary hemostatic response that triggers various chemical mediators such as serotonin and adenosine diphosphate (ADP), ultimately leading to the formation of a clot. These chemical mediators activate vasoconstriction of the arterioles, which leads to the accumulation of activated platelets forming a temporary hemostatic clot. The formation of this clot is considered a secondary hemostatic response that subsequently initiates the accumulation of a fibrin network that functions to provide stability to the newly formed clot. This fibrin network provides the structural framework for accumulation of blood elements (red and white blood cells) and connective tissue cells (fibroblasts). White blood cells are necessary to resolve inflammation during the primary stages of the healing process, and fibroblasts are needed for the formation of fibrous connective tissue and collagen synthesis during the secondary stages of soft tissue healing. Thus the fibrin network that results during clot formation establishes a direct link between hemostasis and the subsequent tissue repair and maturation process.

PHASES OF HEALING

Injuries to the musculoskeletal system commonly involve tendons, ligaments, and joint capsules. These structures heal through a series of events occurring in vascular tissues in response to injury or surgical trauma, secondary to infection and other related disease. Although bone is considered a connective tissue, the process of bone healing differs from other soft connective tissue healing. This process will be discussed later in this chapter. The body's response to injury or trauma is immediate and direct.

Connective tissue that has been damaged or injured heals with fibrous scar formation, termed *repair*, rather than by

regeneration of tissue, which will restore normal tissue function and structure. The series of events occurring in the vascular system and at the cellular level for soft tissue healing is essentially the same in all soft connective tissues. The repair process is not specific to any one particular connective tissue primarily because each tissue has a different structural makeup. This process will be expanded on later in the chapter. Soft connective tissue healing involves three basic processes. Many authors using differing descriptive language have defined them. The phases of soft tissue healing were described by Bryant[1] as (1) inflammation, (2) fibroplasia, and (3) scar maturation. Daly[2] described the process as (1) inflammation, (2) granulation tissue formation, and (3) matrix and remodeling. Martinez-Hernandez and Amenta[3] described it similarly using the terminology (1) inflammation, (2) proliferation, and (3) maturation. It should be noted that the only difference is in the terminology, not the process for which it occurs. It is important to understand that these events in soft connective tissue healing are sequential and each stage overlaps the preceding stage. The duration of each stage is dependent on various factors including, but not limited to, extent of injured tissue, vascularity to injured tissue, and type of tissue injured. Factors that impede healing of connective soft tissue are discussed later in this chapter.

INFLAMMATION

The first stage of connective tissue repair is inflammation. Inflammation is a normal, broad response to vascular changes in injured connective tissue. Inflammation is essential for tissue repair; without it, healing or repair of injured tissue will not occur. There are five characteristics of inflammation: swelling (tumor), redness (rubor), heat (calor), pain (dolor), and loss of function or motion (functio laesa). The inflammatory process is essentially the same whether it is from acute trauma to tissue or repetitive microtrauma (overuse) injury to connective tissue. Inflammation can be categorized in three overlapping stages: (1) acute, (2) subacute, and (3) chronic. The acute inflammation stage lasts for approximately 3 to 4 days; the subacute stage lasts for approximately 10 days to 2 weeks; and the chronic stage essentially begins at the end of the subacute stage and can continue for months or longer (Figure 1-1). Chronic inflammation does not occur with all injuries, and some injuries avoid this phase altogether. Kloth and Miller[4] have described chronic inflammation as unresolved acute inflammation responses, recurrent or repetitive microtrauma, or persistent irritation from foreign material in the tissues.

Acute Inflammation

Acute inflammation is activated by a series of chemical mediators that primarily affect the vascular system and cells of the injured tissues. It is the initial response to trauma or injury to tissue and functions to localize and/or destroy foreign material or agents. As stated before, this is a normal response

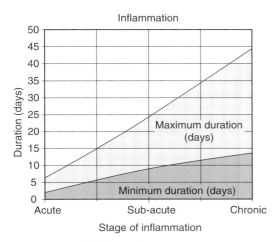

Figure 1-1: Stages of inflammation.

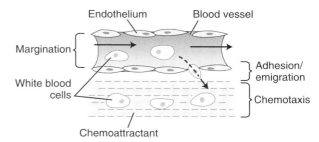

Figure 1-2: Transudation process.

to trauma and is essential for tissue repair. If the vascular and cellular reactions of acute inflammation are successful in eradicating necrotic tissue, foreign material, and other agents, which will depend on the nature of the injured tissue, a favorable environment for an unproblematic tissue repair will be created.

Acute inflammation has a comparatively short duration with regard to the other categories of inflammation. Acute inflammatory responses peak within a few hours of injury and may last for 2 to 4 days. During this period, acute inflammation is characterized by vascular responses that result in excess fluid accumulation in the affected tissue(s) (edema) and cellular responses that include proliferation of white blood cells and phagocytosis. It is important to note that many of these physiologic occurrences at the vascular and cellular levels are interrelated in acute inflammation. They will be discussed separately so as to better understand their important qualities within the acute inflammation stage.

Vascular Changes

With acute inflammation, there is a sequence of vascular responses; vasoconstriction occurs, immediately followed by vasodilation and increased blood flow, increased vascular permeability, and increased blood viscosity with slowing of blood flow.[5] These vascular responses result in an accumulation of interstitial fluid in the injured area, termed *edema*. Along with vascular changes occurring in blood vessels, impediment of local lymph vessels with a decline in lymphatic drainage of interstitial fluid also contributes to edema. Despite these apparent negative effects, vascular changes are necessary for the phagocytotic functions of white blood cells.

Pursuant to the initial transient vasoconstriction of damaged blood vessels within a few minutes after injury, blood vessels will vasodilate, increasing blood flow to the injured area. Coinciding with these vascular changes, increased vascular permeability also occurs. Histamine is

released at the time of injury by mast cells, as well as basophils and platelets, initiating vasodilation and vascular permeability. Contraction of endothelial cells in the wall of small blood vessels caused by the histamine release will account for the initial increase in vascular permeability. As cellular contraction occurs, the endothelial cells separate, creating intercellular gaps in the vascular wall. Enhanced by an increase in intravascular hydrostatic pressure, fluid filtrates through these gaps into interstitial spaces, a process called *transudation* (Figure 1-2). The histamine response in the vascular tissues is short in duration, lasting roughly an hour. Other chemicals that have been associated with increased vascular permeability include prostaglandins, bradykinin, leukotrienes, and complement proteins.[6]

Dorland's Illustrated Medical Dictionary[7] defines *transudate* as "a plasma derived fluid substance which has passed through a membrane or been extruded from a tissue, sometimes as a result of inflammation." The fluid accumulates in tissue and causes edema and is the result of increased venous and capillary pressure, rather than altered vascular permeability (which leads to cellular exudate formation). Exudate, on the other hand, is material such as fluid, cells, or cellular debris that has escaped from blood vessels and has been deposited in tissues or on tissue surfaces, usually as a result of inflammation. An exudate, in contrast to a transudate, is characterized by a high content of protein, cells, or solid materials derived from cells.[7] Transudate is the fluid that escapes through the permeable vascular wall. This fluid is composed mainly of water and contains very few blood cells and has very low protein content. Exudation occurs as vascular permeability increases, allowing blood cells and plasma proteins to escape, which causes extravascular fluid to become more viscous. Exudate is the result of this excess interstitial fluid, the trademark of acute inflammatory edema. With exudation of fluids into the interstitial spaces, red blood cells become concentrated in small blood vessels, the viscosity of the blood increases, and a slowing of blood flow occurs.[5] As this "stasis" of blood flow develops, circulating white blood cells are allowed to come into contact with the inner lining of the vascular wall and are positioned for migration through the intercellular gaps in the vascular wall. As stated before, increased vascular permeability causes edema, but it also allows for the migration of phagocytotic white blood cells (neutrophils) into the injured tissues. At this stage an important link has been established between the vascular responses in acute inflammation and the phagocytic activities associated with white blood cells.

Under normal physiologic conditions, intravascular fluid moves through the vascular wall and into the interstitial space and is drained into the lymphatic system through lymph vessels so as not to allow edema to occur. With injury to tissue, the lymphatic system is slowed to localize the inflammatory response. This permits phagocytosis of white blood cells to eradicate pathogenic microorganisms and bacteria, thus preventing transportation into other body parts.

Vascular responses occurring in acute inflammation result in three of the five cardinal signs of inflammation (Table 1-1). Vasodilation and increased blood flow contribute to increased tissue temperature (hyperthermia) and redness (erythema), while vascular permeability with exudation of fluids into the interstitial spaces causes swelling (edema). In addition to these vascular responses to acute inflammation, cellular necrosis may occur as a complication of early vascular response to injury. If local circulation is impaired (ischemia) and a diminished oxygen supply (hypoxia) occurs due to increased interstitial pressure and formation of edema in injured tissues, ischemic cellular necrosis can occur. This is referred to as *secondary hypoxic injury*.[8] The degree of necessary tissue repair increases due to the secondary hypoxic injury and related tissue destruction caused by the initial trauma.

The fourth cardinal sign of inflammation is pain. Pain can be caused by circulatory impairment (i.e., ischemic pain) or the formation of edema with increased pressure on nociceptive nerve endings (pain receptors) in injured tissues. Pain is intensified by and is most commonly associated with protective muscle spasm. The fifth cardinal sign of inflammation, loss of function and decreased ability to contract the muscle, may be attributed to the injury itself, resulting in the pain-spasm-pain cycle, the mass effect of edema, or both. *Autogenic inhibition* is when the muscle shuts down because of the pain-spasm-pain cycle.

Cellular Response

The white blood cells' response to inflammation provides both nonspecific and specific defenses against invading path-

ogenic microorganisms. The innate defense system, the non-specific defense, provides general protection against a wide variety of pathogenic agents. Physical barriers (skin), as well as mechanical and chemical barriers, provide an initial non-specific defense. The adaptive defense system is a specific immunologic response to persistent pathogens. The adaptive defense system will be discussed as it relates to chronic inflammation later in this chapter.

Cellular responses of the innate defense system occur during acute inflammation and are characterized by proliferation of white blood cells (leukocytes) and phagocytosis of pathogenic microorganisms. Increased production of leukocytes by red bone marrow is the initial cellular response, which is defined as *hemopoiesis*. An increase in the accumulation of white blood cells in the blood is called *leukocytosis* and results from a release of leukocytes in bone marrow. A vast number of leukocytes accumulate in the blood within a few hours of initial trauma. Neutrophils, eosinophils, and basophils (granular leukocytes), along with monocytes and lymphocytes (nongranular leukocytes), are attracted to the affected tissues. Neutrophils are the most numerous type of leukocytes in whole blood; thus they represent the vast majority of white blood cells at the site of injury during the early phase of acute inflammation. Following proliferation at the site of injury, the sequence of leukocyte activity includes the following: margination, adhesion, emigration or diapedesis, chemotaxis, and phagocytosis (see Figure 1-2).

As earlier indicated, the slowing of the blood flow in the damaged vessels allows contact of the leukocytes, which are circulating in the blood, to the endothelial lining of the vascular wall. Margination is the process by which leukocytes move from the central portion of the blood vessel and accumulate along the endothelial surface. Adhesion occurs as leukocytes attach to the vascular wall following margination. A few hours after injury, the endothelial surface of the vascular wall is covered with leukocytes as a result of margination and adhesion.

Increased vascular permeability following margination and adhesion allows leukocytes to move through the intercellular gaps in the vascular wall into the interstitial spaces where they migrate to the damaged tissues. This movement

---

TABLE 1-1

Cardinal Signs of Inflammation and Their Physiologic Causes

CARDINAL SIGN OF INFLAMMATION	PHYSIOLOGIC CAUSE
Tumor (swelling)	Vascular permeability with exudate fluids in interstitial spaces
Rubor (redness)	Vasodilation; increased blood flow
Color (heat)	Vasodilation; increased blood flow
Dolor (pain)	Circulatory impairment (ischemic pain); formation of edema with pressure on nociceptive nerve endings
Functio laeso (loss of function)	Decreased ability to contract muscle; pain-spasm-pain cycle

of leukocytes through the vascular wall is called *emigration* or *diapedesis*. It should be noted that since this fluid now contains blood cells and plasma proteins, the fluid is termed exudate. After emigration/diapedesis, leukocytes are attracted to the damaged tissues by various chemicals called *chemotactic factors*, which prepare the area for phagocytosis. This process is called *chemotaxis*. Neutrophils are the most active phagocytic cell during the first 24 hours following acute inflammation. Neutrophils are short-lived in comparison to other leukocytes. They appear to reach their maximum potential within 6 to 12 hours and disintegrate within 24 to 48 hours. Within 48 hours, monocytes replace the neutrophils as the primary phagocytic cells during the late acute and subacute stages of inflammation.[5,9]

Phagocytosis is the process by which neutrophils proliferate in damaged tissues. Phagocytosis is the nonspecific cellular response to tissue debris, pathogenic microorganisms, and foreign material, which are disposed of in preparation for fibroplasia, the next phase in connective tissue repair. The primary mechanisms of phagocytosis are described by Cotran, Kumar, and Robbins[5] as the recognition of invading pathogenic microorganisms and adherence of the phagocytic cell to the surface of the pathogenic agent; engulfment (indigestion) of the pathogenic agent by the extensions of the phagocytic cell membrane; and the degradation (digestion) of the pathogenic agent. Pus is the result of exudate from an accumulation of neutrophils in response to bacterial invasion containing degenerated or dead leukocytes.

Subacute Inflammation

Successful phagocytosis normally will mark the end of the acute stage of inflammation. With favorable conditions, signs and symptoms of acute inflammation will subside within 3 to 4 days after injury. Subsequently, the subacute phase signs and symptoms will subside and eventually disappear in approximately 2 weeks. With the departure of neutrophils, the "warriors" of the acute phase of inflammation, monocytes become the primary phagocytic cells of the late acute and subacute phases. Once monocytes emigrate through the intercellular gaps in the vascular wall and into the interstitial spaces, they enlarge and mature into long-living, highly phagocytic cells called *macrophages*.[9] Macrophages represent the vast majority of the phagocytic cells beginning 3 days after injury and continue for approximately 2 weeks. They move freely in the tissues and accumulate at the site of pathogen invasion. Their task is much like those of the neutrophil phagocytic cells, but as mentioned before they have an extended "life span."

Chronic Inflammation

If phagocytosis of invading pathogenic agents by neutrophils and macrophages is successful, the early inflammatory reactions to injury are most often resolved. Chronic inflammation is motivated by unrelenting pathogenic agents and can last for several weeks or even months. Chronic inflammation occurs when damaged tissues are infected by pathogenic agents that cannot be phagocytized during the acute and subacute phases of the inflammatory response. Incidentally, chronic inflammation represents an extension of the acute inflammatory response, which may be further prolonged by recurrent injury to affected tissue.[10] In other cases, chronic inflammation may be distinguished by a steady onset that eventually becomes symptomatic. Examples of this type of inflammation are tenosynovitis, bursitis, and synovitis. In addition to the sustained presence of macrophages, an increase in the amount of lymphocytes in damaged tissues is a characteristic of cellular response in chronic inflammation. Lymphocytes, which are found in lymphatic tissues, are the primary nonphagocytic cells responsible for the specific body defenses against invading pathogens. In this regard, specific body defenses protect against (provide immunity to) specific pathogens, whereas nonspecific body defenses combat a wide scope of pathogenic agents. Antigens are those pathogens that invoke a specific immune response. As stated earlier, the defense mechanisms that respond to specific antigens are components of the adaptive defense system.[5]

Two types of lymphocytes, B cells and T cells, mediate specific immune responses. Unlike neutrophils and macrophages of the nonspecific defense system, which respond to a wide variety of pathogenic agents, each type of lymphocyte is predisposed to recognize and respond to a specific antigen. When a foreign antigen is present, lymphocytes respond through complex processes of proliferation and differentiation into various cell types. Two types of immunity are produced: humoral immunity and cellular immunity. Humoral immunity results from differentiation of B cells into plasma cells that produce antibodies and immunoglobulins that neutralize or destroy specific pathogenic agents. Cellular immunity results from differentiation of T cells into various cell types that destroy foreign antigens both directly and indirectly through B cell regulation activity. The specific immune system functions as a second line of defense against invading pathogenic agents that may take several days or longer due to the immunologic response. The immunologic response functions when nonspecific defenses do not adequately provide the needed protection to injured tissue. The specific immune response will eventually become dominant in the presence of persistent pathogens.

Fibroplastic Repair Phase

Once tissue debris, foreign agents, and other pathogenic materials are removed from the site of trauma through phagocytosis, the second stage of soft tissue healing begins.

The secondary stage, most commonly referred to as the *fibroplastic repair phase* or *fibroplasia*, initially begins with the vascular and cellular changes that take place shortly after trauma and that subsequently lead to the formation of a dense fibrous scar. The formation of this scar is facilitated with the proliferation of fibroblasts to the damaged tissues. The fibroblasts are directly responsible for collagen synthesis or fibrogenesis. The synthesis of collagen facilitates the formation of a fibrous type of connective tissue known as *granulated tissue* to develop at the trauma site. Initially this granulated tissue is less dense and immature, but through a mechanism called *wound contraction,* the newly formed tissue matures into a dense, more fibrous scar. The formation of a fibrous scar marks the beginning of the third and final stage of soft tissue healing. This final stage is known as the *maturation process* in which the scar matrix gains tensile strength through the continuation of collagen synthesis and lysis that function to remodel the scar into appropriate size and shape. The cross-linkage of collagen also functions to increase the tensile strength and stability of the scar matrix before the realignment of the collagen fibers occurs. This realignment of fibers differs among various types of tissues, but the repositioning of collagen fibers to meet the types of multidirectional forces that may be placed on the tissues is paramount among all tissues.

Fibroblasts and Collagen Formation

Fibroblasts are lured to the injury site by macrophages that release various chemicals to attract this migration. Once the fibroblasts proliferate to the area, they localize in the fibrin thread network of the clot. The accumulated fibroblasts are directly responsible for the formation of collagen at the clot. Collagen, which is the main supportive protein for all connective tissue types, functions to develop the new tissue matrix at the clot site. This new tissue matrix is formed through the synergistic process of collagen synthesis and lysis, which function to build up and break down, respectively. Because of the trauma, the synthesis of collagen formation is first and foremost, whereas lysis occurs later in the healing process.

The synthesis of collagen is an essential process that must take place in order to restore the extracellular connective tissue matrix. The type of collagen formed is determined at the cellular level by the formation of a 3 polypeptide alpha chain that develops a procollagen molecule. (Specific types of collagen that function to produce collagen fibrils are Types I, II, and III, collectively called *fibrillar collagens.*[11]) The procollagen molecules that are formed accumulate in the extracellular matrix where they are grouped together to form tropocollagen (Figure 1-3). Tropocollagen molecules are reinforced first by weak hydrogen bonds and then by joining with covalent bonds to form fibrils. This maturation of the tropocollagen molecule triggers the process of fibrogenesis, in which the collagen fibers are formed. The continuation of fibrogenesis facilitates the structural maturity and strength of the collagen fibers and enables them to group together into fasciculi (bundles) that are necessary in providing the structural foundation of various types of connective tissues, such as tendons and ligaments.

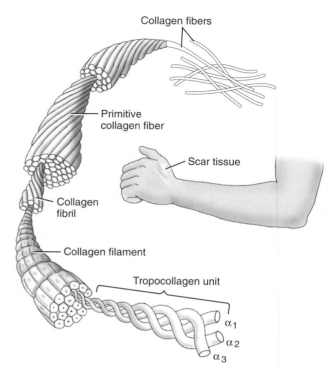

Figure 1-3: Illustration of collagen composition: tropocollagen to collagen fibers.

Granulated Tissue Formation

Through the process of collagen synthesis and fibrogenesis, a temporary fibrous type of connective tissue is formed at the trauma site. This tissue, called *granulated tissue,* is fibrous, but is relatively immature and lacks tensile strength. This type of tissue has two different characteristics: synthesis of Type III collagen formation in the tissue matrix, and formation of new vascular network, which is called *neovascularization.*

As discussed previously, the type of collagen formed during collagen synthesis depends on the chemical makeup of the procollagen molecule. Types I and II collagen are predominantly associated with musculoskeletal structures (tendons, ligaments, and joint capsules), whereas Type III collagen is normally found in blood vessels and the layers of the skin.[3] With granulated tissue being primarily vascular, it is understandable that the extracellular matrix would consist of predominantly Type III collagen fibers.[12] Eventually the synthesis of Type III collagen fibers is replaced by the synthesis of Type I collagen, leading to a dense, more fibrous scar.

Along with the formation of Type III collagen fibers, the development of a new vascular network begins to form in the granulated tissue. This formation of new blood vessels, called *angiogenesis,* occurs from new capillary extensions that are extended from the nontraumatized blood vessels in adjacent tissues. Anastomoses are formed within a few days serving to bridge and connect the extended capillaries, thus forming the new vascular matrix. In addition to the vascular development, new lymph vessel systems are also formed within the matrix.

Wound Contraction

Wound contraction is a healing response that functions to reduce the size of the tissue defect and subsequently decrease the amount of damaged tissue that needs repair. This response involves myofibroblasts, which are located in currently existing fibers and surrounding margins of the wound. These myofibroblasts function to pull newly formed collagen fibers in damaged tissues toward the center of the defect, thus reducing the size of the tissue defect.[1] This contraction is accomplished by the two proteins, actin and myosin, that make up myofibroblasts. Actin and myosin interact with the newly formed collagen fibers in the extracellular matrix, forming a weblike adhesive base for wound contraction.[2,13]

Fibrous Tissue Formation

The maturation of granulated tissue to a more dense fibrous type of connective tissue occurs due to several vascular and cellular events. Specifically, the transition from the synthesis of Type III to Type I collagen must take place for fibrous scar formation to occur. Also, the overall increase in amount of collagen deposition at the repair site accelerates. Last, the resorption of capillaries with minimal blood flow in the scar matrix occurs.[14]

The replacement of Type III with Type I collagen directly leads to the development of a dense fibrous scar. Type I collagen, as mentioned previously, is the predominant collagen type found in musculoskeletal structures such as tendons and ligaments. Type I collagen provides the mature structural elements for normal connective tissue matrix.[3] The increase in the accumulation of Type I collagen leads to the formation of bundles in damaged tissues, thus increasing the tensile strength of the scar matrix. The maturation of the scar occurs simultaneously with the continued elevation of Type I collagen synthesis and the gradual degradation of Type III collagen.

In addition to the transition from the synthesis of Type III to Type I collagen, an overall increase in the amount of collagen production and formation, unrelated to type, occurs during the formation of a fibrous scar. Thus the increase in the tensile strength of the scar results from the type of collagen, as well as the amount of collagen that is deposited in the healing tissues.

During fibrous scar formation, the established vascular network will also undergo numerous changes. The extensive vascular network is composed of capillaries functioning to provide nutrition to newly formed tissues. However, not all of these capillaries are functional and those that contain minimal blood flow are resolved during transition from granulated tissue to fibrous scar.[5]

Scar Maturation

Once fibrous scar has been formed, the scar matrix begins to undergo structural biomechanical changes that will eventually lead to an increase in scar tensile strength. This maturing process is most often referred to as *scar maturation*. Scar maturation results from several key contributing factors. The first is the process of continued collagen synthesis and lysis, which is most often referred to as the *collagen turnover rate*, as well as the overall increase in the number of mature collagen cross-links and the linear realignment of these collagen fibers (Table 1-2).

The rate of collagen turnover is the process that leads to the balancing of collagen synthesis and lysis during the later stages of soft tissue healing. In the early stages of soft tissue healing, collagen production far surpasses collagen degradation. However, this tends to balance out toward the end of the fibroplastic repair phase. Collagen production still exceeds degradation, but the lysis of collagen is a vital component in scar maturation.

Collagen lysis occurs due to a protein-degrading enzyme known as *collagenase*. Collagenase is secreted from fibroblasts and macrophages and functions to break down Type I, II, and III fibrillar collagens.[5,14] The rate of collagen lysis is strongest in the weaker Type III collagen fibers and the weakest against the stronger Type I fibers. The main reason

TABLE 1-2

Factors Contributing to Scar Maturation

FACTOR	METHOD OF INCREASING SCAR TENSILE STRENGTH
Rate of collagen turnover	Continued production of Type I fibers coupled with the breakdown of Type III collagen fibers
Increase in mature collagen cross-links	Links formed through covalent bonds function to bridge collagen molecules together, forming collagen cross-links
Linear realignment of collagen fibers	Repositioning of collagen fibers to better resemble their normal characteristics, as well as structural support against resistance

Type III fibers are more susceptible to degradation is because they are deposited early during the formation of granulated tissue, whereas Type I fibers are deposited during fibrous scar formation. Thus the degradation of Type III collagen fibers and the continued production of Type I collagen fibers lead to an increase in the overall tensile strength of the scar.

Another factor in scar maturation is the formation of collagen cross-links that form within and between collagen molecules. They are formed early during the formation of granulated tissue through a weak chemical hydrogen bond and then later in scar maturation with the formation of an intermolecular covalent bond. These bonds form cross-links that function to bridge collagen molecules together, leading to an increase in scar tensile strength.

In addition to collagen cross-links, realignment or repositioning of collagen fibers in the scar matrix contributes to an increase in scar tensile strength. During scar maturation, collagen fibers are repositioned, according to their normal tissue characteristics, to maximize the tensile strength of the scar. Collagen fiber orientation differs substantially among the various types of connective tissues and is directly related to each tissue's respective function. Tendon fibers are arranged in a parallel fashion to provide optimal resistance to unidirectional tensile forces, whereas ligaments are organized in a nonparallel fashion to provide optimal resistance to multidirectional tissue forces.[15] The reorientation of collagen fibers coupled with the development of collagen cross-links and continued synthesis of Type I collagen all function to increase the overall tensile strength, thus resulting in complete scar maturation.

PHYSIOLOGY OF TISSUES

Soft tissue is composed of cells, an intracellular matrix, and water. Groups of cells that have a common structure and work together as a unit are called *tissues*. The intracellular matrix, a nonliving material, fills gaps between cells and serves as a supportive structure of the cell. This matrix may be thicker in some tissues and minimal in others. The largest single ingredient of soft tissue is water, making up about 70% of the weight of any given soft tissue.[16] Water is of primary importance in maintaining proper cell function and acts to lubricate the joints and absorb forces.[16]

To understand the healing process that tissues undergo following microtrauma or macrotrauma, surgery, or infection, it is important to understand the types of affected tissues. Although the healing process is not specific to any one particular connective tissue, the type of soft tissue will have some impact on the length of the process, as well as the cell function in each stage. The soft tissues that are discussed in this chapter include connective, muscle, epithelial, and nervous tissues. These structural components of the body are all classified as soft tissues except bone.[17] Epithelial and nervous tissues are described briefly; however, the focus is primarily on muscle and connective tissue. In this chapter,

to simplify our understanding of the musculoskeletal anatomy, bone is classified as a type of connective tissue.

HEALING PROCESS IN TISSUES

Healing by Primary or Secondary Intent

Healing of soft tissues may occur by primary or secondary intent. Healing by primary intent means that the tissue has been surgically repaired. A laceration that is sutured heals by primary intent. Healing by secondary intent is healing that occurs on its own accord.

Connective Tissue

Connective tissue is the most predominant tissue in the body.[18] The various types of connective tissue are tendons, ligaments, joint capsules, and articular cartilage. In addition, bone, blood, and adipose are typically classified as connective tissue. Connective tissue connects and supports structures. Connective tissues also function to compartmentalize body structures (e.g., sheaths surrounding muscle). They have the ability to reproduce, but not as rapidly as epithelial cells. Some types of connective tissue have an adequate blood supply, whereas others are lacking. Articular cartilage, for example, has a limited blood supply, thus limited potential for secondary healing. Tissues with a good blood supply heal quicker (e.g., muscle), whereas tissues that have poor blood supply tend to heal slower or not at all (e.g., articular cartilage). Three types of fibers are found in connective tissues. Collagen, elastic, and reticular fibers are found in varying amounts in different connective tissues.[13] This variation accounts for the different structural makeup of connective tissues, such as ligaments, tendons, and joint capsules.

Collagen is a major structural protein forming strong, flexible, inelastic structures that hold connective tissues together.[13] Collagen gives tissues the ability to resist deformation and mechanical stresses. A higher proportion of collagen in a given tissue indicates relatively greater tensile strength but less flexibility. Elastic tissues aid in the recovery of imparted stresses by retracting when stretched. Elastic fibers are smaller than collagen fibers but also contribute to the tensile strength of connective tissue.[19] Elastic fibers are found predominantly in blood vessels, muscle, and skin because they have the ability to recoil once stretched. Tendons, on the other hand, have very little elasticity because they contain a high amount of collagen and less elastin. Collagen is also found in other inelastic tissues such as ligaments, fascia, cartilage, and bone.

Reticular fibers are similar to collagen fibers but thinner. They function to support glands and organs (e.g., lymph nodes, liver, and spleen). This is done by arising at points where connective tissues join with other tissues and assist in holding various tissue layers together. Reticular fibers, composed primarily of Type III collagen, form networks of supportive structures that allow cells to move in loosely arranged tissues.

There are several types of connective tissue. Fibrous connective tissue is composed of strong collagenous fibers that bind tissues together.[13] There are two types of fibrous tissue. Loose connective tissue provides the thin, loosely woven structural framework for organs, such as the liver, bone marrow, and lymph glands. It helps with structure and connection of nonconnective tissue layers. It is found beneath the skin and attaches the skin to the tissues underneath. Loose connective tissue consists of collagen and tissue fluid, providing an area for blood, lymphatic vessels, and nerve fibers. Collagen fibers are the predominant component of dense connective tissue. These densely packed, grouped fibers have less ground substance than loose connective tissue. A meshwork of collagen fibers makes up dense connective tissue, forming tough capsules and sheaths around organs. As parallel bundles of regularly arranged fibers, dense connective tissue also forms tendons and ligaments.

Connective tissue heals with collagen only and therefore results in tissue with decreased elasticity and decreased flexibility. The healing response to injury differs among different types of connective tissue. Connective tissue discussed here includes articular cartilage, ligaments, tendons, and bone. Some classify bone as a connective tissue and therefore the healing process of bone is also discussed.

Cartilage

Structure and Function

Cartilage is a dense connective tissue composed of chondrocytes. It provides support and structure for the skeletal system. Three types of cartilage exist: hyaline cartilage, fibrocartilage, and elastic cartilage. Hyaline cartilage, also known as articular cartilage, lines the articulating surfaces of bones and contains a high amount of collagen. Fibrocartilage is found in the intervertebral disks, as well as menisci. Elastic cartilage is found in the larynx and in the auricle of the ear, and since it has more elastin than the others, it is more flexible. Because hyaline cartilage is more frequently injured, it is discussed in greater detail.

Structural Makeup

Cartilage lacks blood vessels, nerves, and a lymphatic system. Therefore these cells must rely on receiving nutrients through the process of diffusion from the extracellular matrix of the bone that lies underneath or from the synovial fluid. Because of the lack of blood supply, partial-thickness tears of articular cartilage are repaired with scar tissue. If an individual sustains a full-thickness tear, the defect may be repaired by the regeneration of fibrocartilage.

Water contributes as much as 80% of the wet weight of articular cartilage, and its significance is its contribution to shock absorption.[20] Collagen makes up the majority of the dry weight, primarily with Type II collagen.[20]

Response to Injury

The healing response of cartilage after trauma and its potential to repair depend on the location of injury, the type of injury that has been sustained, and whether the injury involves damage to the subchondral bone (Table 1-3).[21] When damage occurs only to the articular cartilage, typically symptoms are minimal. Cartilage lacks a blood supply and therefore the inflammatory process does not occur. Buckwalter and Mow[21] describe three types of articular cartilage injuries. The first, as mentioned earlier, involves damage to the matrix without "visible disruption of the articular cartilage." If the basic structure remains intact and a significant number of undamaged cells remain, the cells can restore the normal tissue composition.[21] If the matrix or cells sustain significant damage or if the tissue is subjected to further damage, the lesion may progress. When the cartilage is disrupted during injuries such as a fracture to the articular surface, new tissue may not fill in the defect. The lesion may progress depending on the location and size of the lesion and the structural integrity of the joint. Joint stability and alignment are also factors in the healing process. Finally, when damage to the articular cartilage involves subchondral bone, the clot and repair tissue from bone can fill in the articular cartilage defect and give access to the inflammatory cells, permitting the formation of granulation tissue.[3] This type of injury is also known as an *osteochondral fracture*. If this process occurs without being hindered, healing proceeds according

---

TABLE 1-3

Time Frame for Cartilage Healing

TIME FRAME	WHAT IS OCCURRING?
Immediately	Cartilage lacks a blood supply so the inflammation process does not occur
	Initial step is formation of a fibrin clot
5-7 days	Fibroblasts infiltrate into area and combine with collagen to replace the clot
2 weeks	Fibroblasts change into chondrocytes
4 weeks	Chondrocytes are primary cells
8 weeks	Defect resembles normal cartilage
	Type I collagen fibers are predominantly present
6 months	Type I and Type II collagen fibers appear normal

From Houglum P: *Therapeutic exercise for athletic injuries*, Champaign, IL, 2001, Human Kinetics.

to schedule and differentiation of granulation tissue cells into chondrocytes occurs in approximately 2 weeks. "Two months after the injury, an apparent normal cartilage has formed, healing the original defect; however, this cartilage has a low proteoglycan content."[3] "One year after the injury, the new cartilage usually undergoes extensive fibrillar degeneration, and erosive changes occur as the tissue becomes attenuated."[3]

Ligaments

Structure and Function

Ligaments are arranged in parallel bundles of collagen composed of rows of fibroblasts. These collagen bundles may have a wave pattern that allows slight elongation of the structure without causing damage to the tissue. Ligaments function to guide the position of bone during normal motion and also contribute to joint stability by connecting adjoining bones. Ligaments also provide proprioceptive input or a sense of joint position through the function of free nerve endings and mechanoreceptors located within the ligament. Ligaments may be thickened portions of a joint capsule or may be separate from the capsule. An injury to a ligament is termed a *sprain* versus a muscular *strain*. With a Grade I ligament sprain the damage is minimal, with microscopic stretching or tearing of fibers, minimal structural loss, and minimal effusion and ecchymosis. A Grade II ligament sprain occurs as a result of moderate tearing of ligamentous collagen fibers. There is a significant structural loss and weakening of the joint. A Grade III ligament sprain occurs when the ligament fibers tear completely, resulting in a severe loss of structural integrity and joint stability. There is significant bruising, swelling, and hemarthrosis in the injured area. Functional loss for a Grade III ligament sprain is severe, and return to activity takes a minimum of 6 to 8 weeks. Surgery is often indicated for repair of the damaged ligament.

Structural Makeup

Ligaments are composed of fibroblasts surrounded by an extracellular matrix formed by collagen and water. Ligaments are composed of 90% Type I and 10% Type III collagen, resulting in greater tensile strength. Ligaments are less vascularized than tendons, so the repair process takes longer than tendons; in some ligaments, the tissue fibers may regress or disappear completely.

Response to Injury

When ligaments tear, there is significant pain and bleeding. The edema occurs as a result of the inflammatory response, which results in an infiltration of erythrocytes, leukocytes, and lymphocytes. The time frame for ligament healing is summarized in Table 1-3. If the ligament tear is extracapsular, bleeding occurs in a subcutaneous space. If a ligament tear is intracapsular, bleeding occurs within the joint capsule until clotting occurs or the pressure becomes so great that the bleeding stops.

Within 72 hours after injury, there is minimal blood flow from the damaged vessels and inflammatory cells are attracted into the area to promote vascular dilation and increased vascular permeability. The fibroblasts begin to form a new matrix consisting of a higher concentration of water, glycosaminoglycans, and type III collagen. At this point, there is little tensile strength of the ligament.[22] During the next 6 weeks, new capillary budding occurs and fibroblasts work to help form a fibrin clot.[13] Torn ends of the ligament may be reconnected by the formation of this clot. Constituents of the intracellular matrix contribute to the proliferation of the scar that is formed. Initially, the scar is soft, but eventually it becomes more elastic.[13] Collagen fibers lay down in a random fashion resulting in an irregular-shaped matrix. After approximately 6 weeks, Type I collagen replaces Type III collagen. The glycosaminoglycans and amount of water decrease, along with the inflamed cells. The fibrils increase in size and begin to form tightly packed bundles. At this point, the number of fibroblasts decreases. Matrix organization increases as fibrils align along lines of stress and blood vessels decrease. Elastin decreases as tensile strength increases.

Over the next several months, maturation of the scar occurs and collagen is aligned according to fiber realignment. Stress imparted to the tissues can also cause alignment of the scar fibers. This phase of the healing process may last as long as 12 months, but is dependent on the protection warranted the ligament and whether the ends of the ligament are connected via scar. The healing process can also be affected by lack of sufficient stress to allow proper realignment of fibers.

Ligaments that heal by primary intent typically heal with less scar tissue than ligaments that heal on their own. Initially, these tissues appear stronger than unrepaired ligaments. However, there is some debate as to whether this strength is maintained with time.[13]

Ligaments left to heal on their own do so with more scar tissue than surgically repaired ligaments. The scar tissue is not as flexible as the original tissue and may cause ligament elongation. This increase in length can lead to joint instability.[13] The medial collateral ligament can heal spontaneously without surgical intervention.[23] With intraarticular ligament tears, however, this may not happen because of the presence of synovial fluid. This synovial fluid may prevent the fibrin clot from forming and thus decreases the opportunity for healing.[13]

Studies have shown that the longer ligaments are immobilized, the less strength they will have.[20] Therefore immobilization causes a decrease in ligament tensile strength and can also cause a weakening of the insertion into bone. Hence, some therapeutic stress to the tissue is appropriate during the healing process and encourages a better-aligned and stronger scar (Table 1-4).

Tendons

Structure and Function

Tendons are cords of regularly arranged collagen fibers that connect muscle tissue to bone. They are composed of densely packed fibers arranged in a parallel fashion, giving tendons one of the highest tensile strengths of all soft tissues.

Structural Makeup

Tendons are made up of approximately 85% collagen and 15% ground substance. Therefore they are capable of resisting large stresses and transmitting those forces from muscle to bone. Ligaments and tendons are very similar in composition, although there is a slightly higher elastin content in ligaments. In ligaments, collagen fibers are arranged in a woven pattern, whereas tendon fibers are more linear.[16] This linear pattern of fibers is the reason why tendons do not resist shear and compressive forces well, and why functionally, tendons are designed to transmit loads with less energy and less deformation.

Response to Injury

Injuries to tendons can result from an acute trauma or from repetitive stress to the structure. When a tendon is strained because of an increased mechanical load beyond its tensile strength, the inflammatory phase begins (Table 1-5). Within 4 days following the injury, repair begins, with the infiltration of fibroblasts and phagocytic cells. There is a rapid decrease in tensile strength secondary to this process. Collagen synthesis begins within 7 to 8 days. Fibroblasts are the most common cell type in the second phase, called *fibroplasia*, which is typically complete in 16 days. Both cells and collagen fibers are oriented perpendicular to the long axis of the tendon. Over the next 2 months, remodeling of the injured site occurs, resulting in the alignment of the collagen fibers along the tendon's long axis.[24] Four months following the injury, maturation is complete (provided the necessary loading has occurred). If the tendon's sheath is damaged, there is a possibility that scar tissue adhesions will form.

Bone

Structure and Function

Bone is sometimes considered a type of connective tissue. Bone protects internal organs, serves as a lever for muscles, and provides a supportive framework for the body. Bone

---

TABLE 1-4

Time Frame for Ligament Healing

TIME FRAME	WHAT IS OCCURRING?
Immediately	Erythrocytes, leukocytes, and lymphocytes arrive at the injury site
24 hours	Macrophages and monocytes arrive to remove debris from injured area
72 hours	Minimal blood flow from the damaged tissues
Next 6 weeks	New capillary budding
	Fibroblasts work to help form a fibrin clot
	Collagen fibers lay down in a random fashion
6 weeks-1 year	Type I collagen replaces Type III collagen
	Fibrils increase in size and begin to form tightly packed bundles
	Number of fibroblasts decreases
Approximately 1 year	Strength is almost returned to normal (provided reinjury has not occurred during this time)

From Houglum P: *Therapeutic exercise for athletic injuries,* Champaign, IL, 2001, Human Kinetics.

TABLE 1-5

Time Frame for Tendon Healing

TIME FRAME	WHAT IS OCCURRING?
Immediately	Inflammation phase begins with the formation of a clot
4 days	Repair begins with infiltration of fibroblasts and phagocytic cells
7-8 days	Collagen synthesis begins and collagen reaches its maximum in approximately 4 weeks
16 days	Fibroplasia is typically complete
	Fibroblasts are predominant cell types and now both cells and collagen fibers are oriented perpendicular to the long axis of the tendon
2 months	Remodeling of injured site occurs, resulting in alignment of collagen fibers along the tendon's long axis
4 months	Fibroblasts change to tenocytes; Type II collagen is replaced by Type I collagen
	Maturation is typically complete
Approximately 1 year	Remodeling can continue for a year after injury; by this time, strength is returned to 85%-95% of normal

From Houglum P: *Therapeutic exercise for athletic injuries,* Champaign, IL, 2001, Human Kinetics.

consists of living cells and minerals deposited in a matrix. These cells, called *osteocytes* (analogous to phagocytes), are produced by osteoblasts (analogous to fibroblasts) and reabsorbed by osteoclasts.[25]

Structural Makeup

Bone is produced as concentric layers of calcified material laid around blood vessels. The outermost layer of a bone is called the *periosteum*. This is an innervated and vascular structure providing nutrition to the cortical (compact) bone. The cancellous bone, known as *spongy bone,* has its own vascular supply and contains bone marrow. Red marrow produces red blood cells. Bones have epiphyseal plates, which, when damaged, may result in structural abnormalities.

Response to Injury

Bone undergoes three stages of healing when damaged (Table 1-6). When a bone is initially fractured, blood vessels are damaged and a hematoma forms. This acute inflammatory phase lasts approximately 4 days. Within 5 to 7 days, the hematoma resolves and osteoblasts have already entered the area to produce a fibrin clot. During repair and regeneration, osteoclasts reabsorb damaged bone tissues and old bone cells, whereas osteoblastic activity produces new bone cells. A weak

TABLE 1-6

Time Frame for Bone Healing

TIME FRAME	WHAT IS OCCURRING?
Immediately (0-4 days)	Bone is fractured
	Acute inflammatory phase begins with damaged blood vessels and the formation of a hematoma
	Mast cells and macrophages appear
5-7 days	Hematoma resolves
	Osteoblasts arrive to help produce fibrin clot
7 days-4 weeks	Osteoblasts form soft callus
4 weeks	Hard callus forms
	Osteoclasts reabsorb damaged tissue
6-10 weeks	Circulation is reestablished
12-16 weeks	Fracture healed
	Maturation-remodeling phase continues
Approximately 12 weeks	Bone strong enough to withstand normal forces

From Houglum P: *Therapeutic exercise for athletic injuries,* Champaign, IL, 2001, Human Kinetics.

bony callus forms between the fractured bone ends, which slowly strengthens over time. This process of callus formation is called *endochondral bone healing.* Direct bone healing occurs when the fractured ends are immobilized in direct contact with one another.[19] This allows new bony tissue to be deposited at the fracture site, without the formation of a callus.

The final phase, maturation and remodeling, involves osteoblastic and osteoclastic activity. The process continues until the bone is strong enough to withstand normal forces.

Muscle Tissue

Structure and Function

Muscle tissue is composed of cells that have the unique ability to shorten or contract. Muscle tissue is essential to move the musculoskeletal system, circulate blood, and move food through the bowel.[25] Muscle tissue has the ability to contract because of its composition of actin and myosin fibers. Muscle tissue is highly cellular and has an abundant supply of blood vessels.

Structural Makeup

Three types of muscle tissue are skeletal, smooth, and cardiac. Skeletal muscle tissue is also referred to as striated muscle and is multinuclear, meaning that striated muscle has two or more nuclei. Skeletal muscle is under voluntary control and functions to move bones. Cells of skeletal muscle are long and thin and are termed *fibers* or *myofibers.* They are usually arranged in bundles that are surrounded by connective tissue. This is significant in that muscle has the ability to regenerate, but the connective tissue surrounding the muscle must heal by repair. Actin and myosin are contractile proteins that are a part of the muscle tissue. Smooth muscle cells are uninucleic and are involuntary. Smooth muscle cells are spindle shaped, have a single centrally located nucleus, and do not have the striated appearance of skeletal muscle. Smooth muscle lines blood vessels and is found in the digestive tract. Cardiac muscle is located only in the heart. It is a highly vascularized tissue that is involuntary; however, it can be initiated with stimulation and can generate an action potential. It maintains blood flow throughout the body as the heart pumps.

Response to Injury

Skeletal muscle may be damaged by trauma (injury) or infection. Injuries to muscle result when tension generated exceeds the tensile capacity of the muscle fibers.[26] Direct trauma can also create muscle dysfunction. Contusions result when muscle fibers have been damaged or partially disrupted from a direct blow. The excessive force that causes a contusion may cause internal bleeding, resulting in ecchymosis externally and edema internally. Capillary rupture increases bleeding, which may lead to the formation of a hematoma. When a hematoma forms, a slower recovery time is required to return to normal function. If this hematoma is left unresolved, compartment syndrome or myositis ossificans may result.[27]

Muscle strains are estimated to represent 50% of athletic injuries.[28] They are caused by a sudden concentric or eccentric muscular contraction. A mild muscle strain causes minimal damage to the muscle fibers. The inflammatory process results in minimal swelling and pain. With a mild muscle strain, there is minimal loss of function. A moderate or second-degree muscle strain causes a partial tear of the muscle fibers and results in damage to the musculotendinous junction.[29,30] A severe or third-degree strain is a complete tear of the muscle fibers, resulting in a large hematoma and a much longer recovery time. Healing shows muscular fibrosis at the site of injury. Complete tears may require surgical intervention.

Muscle tissue is well vascularized and can heal rather quickly. An example of this is the microtearing that occurs when a muscle is eccentrically contracted. The pain subsides within 2 to 3 days, and the muscle returns to normal. This is referred to as *delayed-onset muscle soreness*. The healing process of muscle after injury involves two competitive events: regeneration of muscle fibers and production of scar tissue to repair surrounding connective tissue (Table 1-7). Initially, hemorrhage and edema occur and degenerative changes begin. Phagocytosis clears debris from the area. Skeletal muscle cells are permanent cells with no proliferative capacity[3]; however, during muscle regeneration, trophic substances released by injured muscle activate satellite cells.[31] Once acti-vated, the satellite cells can grow and differentiate to form new skeletal muscle cells after the other muscle fibers have died. This process may take weeks to occur.

If a muscle is completely severed, the two segments heal by dense scar tissue formation.[32] Muscle does not regenerate across the scar and functional continuity is not restored.[32]

Epithelial Tissue

Structure and Function

Epithelial tissue, commonly known as skin, covers all internal and external body surfaces. However, epithelial tissue may also include tissue that lines the esophagus, which is not part of the skin. Epithelial tissue lines body cavities, as well as hollow organs, and is the predominant tissue found in exocrine glands.[25] This type of tissue performs numerous functions including protecting the body from microbes, and, by lining them, epithelial tissues help give organs shape. Additionally, they help retain fluids within tissues and function in digestive tract absorption and gland secretive physiology. Skin is nourished by blood vessels within the dermis. Because the epithelial tissue lacks a distinct blood supply, it depends on diffusion to receive nutrients and to eliminate waste products.[13] White blood cells and other cells that protect against germs are contained within the dermis. Nerve fibers and fat cells are also contained within the dermis.

Structural Makeup

Epithelial tissue is *keratinized*, meaning the surface is covered with dead cells that are filled with a water-resistant protein called *keratin*. This surface is dry and exposed to a wide range of environmental factors. This protective layer is renewed constantly by the division of cells within the deeper layers of the epidermis. In fact, the entire epidermis is replaced every 2 weeks. Epithelial cells are closely packed together with no room for blood vessels between cells; therefore the epithelium must receive nutrients from the tissue beneath, which has large intercellular spaces that contain blood and lymph vessels and nerves. These capillaries are located within the tissue fluid of the dermis. The vascularity of the dermis and the process of diffusion allow epithelial tissue to heal rather quickly, provided the healing process is allowed to proceed without interruption.

Response to Injury

Injuries that may occur to epithelial tissue include wounds, infection, inflammation, and disease. Epithelial tissues can also be traumatized during surgical procedures. Fortunately, epithelial cells can regenerate following trauma. The time frame required for healing typically occurs within a few days provided that the wound is superficial and there is an optimal environment for healing to occur[25] (Table 1-8).

TABLE 1-7

Time Frame for Muscle Healing

TIME FRAME	WHAT IS OCCURRING?
Immediately (6 hours)	Fibers are damaged, macrophages arrive
1-4 days	Fibroblasts appear; decrease in muscle tension
7 days	Scar tissue is seen in large muscle fibers
7-10 days	Tensile strength increases
10 days	Phagocytes increase in number and now macrophages are the primary phagocytes that are present
2 weeks	Myotubes appear in the area
3 weeks	Muscle fibers are seen
1.5-6 months	Contraction ability is 85%-90% of normal

From Houglum P: *Therapeutic exercise for athletic injuries,* Champaign, IL, 2001, Human Kinetics.

When a laceration or an incision occurs, it takes a few days for the body to seal the wound. A few weeks later, the tissue can typically return to its full strength, and several months later, the remodeling will be complete. The size of the scar depends on how much damage the tissue has sustained. If the injury is deep, affecting several layers, the tissue is replaced with scar tissue. This is known as *metaplasia* (transformation of cells from a normal to an abnormal state). This scar tissue can lead to the formation of adhesions, which may limit range of motion. The reason that this scar tissue is not as functional as normal tissue is that the collagen matrix forms in an unorganized and haphazard manner, leaving scar tissue less flexible. This tissue may not have the same tensile strength of the original tissue, leaving it less functional than the original tissue. This decrease in strength may also result in the tissue being reinjured.

The epidermis can also respond to environmental stimuli. For example, if constant pressure is placed on it, the rate of cell division increases. This increase in cell division causes the formation of calluses.

Nervous Tissue

Structure and Function

Nervous tissue is made up of cells called *neurons* and *neuroglia*. Each cell type has unique characteristics. Neurons are specialized to generate and conduct electrical activity, and neuroglia provide structural support to the neurons. Neuroglia function to bind neurons together and influence the nourishment and electrical activity of neurons. Each neuron consists of a cell body, dendrites, and an axon. The cell body contains the nucleus, which serves as the metabolic center for the cell. The dendrites are extensions of the cell body and receive information from other neurons or receptor cells. The axon conducts nerve impulses from the cell body to another neuron or effector (muscle or gland) cell.

Structural Makeup

Nervous tissue makes up either the central nervous system (CNS) or the peripheral nervous system (PNS). Nerve cells within the CNS (brain and spinal cord) are highly specialized, whereas nerve cells in the PNS are similar to each other.[25] Nerve cells transmit electrical signals from the CNS to the muscles and sensory organs, orchestrating all of the voluntary and involuntary bodily functions.[13] Nerve tissue does not follow the normal phases of healing, because of its unique connective tissue structure. For an axon to transmit a signal, it needs to have a viable hollow tube. A tube that is disrupted or scarred interferes with the conduction velocity of the nerve and does not allow transmission of a signal.

Response to Injury

Nerve cells are easily damaged by physical trauma, toxins, infections, and metabolic imbalances. Nerve heals in its own way depending on the amount of injury to the nerve. Nerve tissue cannot regenerate once the nerve cell dies. Peripheral nerves can regenerate provided the injury does not affect the cell body. The closer the injury is to the cell body, the harder it is for the nerve to regenerate. Neurapraxia is the mildest type of lesion that produces neurologic deficits. It results in a loss of conduction along a nerve without axon degeneration.[18] If the myelin sheath is left intact, the nerve may be able to regenerate. If there is damage to the body of the nerve cell, this damage is permanent. Neurotmesis results in a complete loss of nerve function with little apparent anatomic damage to the nerve itself. Axonometis is damage to the nerve tissue without actually severing it. This injury, caused by crushing, pinching, or prolonged pressure, may cause an interruption of the nerve axon followed by complete degeneration of the peripheral segment, without severing the supportive structure of the nerve.[18] This is what occurs with the formation of a neuroma. The axon degenerates distal to the point of injury, and then it regenerates inside the myelin sheath at a rate of approximately 0.25 inch per month.[25] Nerves in the CNS cannot regenerate, and the individual suffers permanent loss of function if these nerves are damaged.

FACTORS THAT HINDER THE HEALING PROCESS

Several factors may hinder the healing process in living tissues. The extent of the injury, the individual's diet, and swelling are a few of the factors that can have an effect on the healing process. In addition, the amount of time a structure has been immobilized, the blood flow to the area, and the medications an individual is taking can all modify the healing process. Other factors can also deter the healing process and are discussed briefly.

Extent of Injury

The first factor that can affect the healing process is the extent of the injury. When macrotears occur as a result of acute trauma, there is greater destruction of the tissue, resulting in a longer time for debridement, more clinical symptoms, and alterations in normal function. For example, an

TABLE 1-8

Time Frame for Epithelial Tissue Healing

TIME FRAME	WHAT IS OCCURRING?
0-3 days	Wound is sealed
2-3 weeks	Tissue returns to full strength
6-18 months	Remodeling phase is complete

athlete sustaining a Grade I medial collateral ligament (MCL) tear has very little swelling and instability. The athlete may be able to return to play within a single week. However, if an athlete sustains a Grade III MCL tear, there is moderate swelling and instability, and this degree of injury may take up to 6 weeks to heal.

Nutrition

An individual's diet can play a significant part in the healing process.[3] Diets that lack protein and certain vitamins can hinder the healing process. For example, lack of vitamin C has been found to increase the time required for healing. The lack of vitamin C contributes to poor vascularization and scanty collagen deposition.

Edema

Edema may limit the healing process. With increased swelling, the body takes longer to progress from the inflammatory phase to the proliferation phase. Increased pressure caused by swelling retards the healing process, causing separation of tissues and inhibiting neuromuscular control. The nutrition of the tissue may also be hindered from edema.

Immobilization

Rest can be a double-edged sword when it comes to healing tissue. Immobilization is necessary to protect the injured structures, but a lack of stress can inhibit the proper alignment of some tissues. For example, studies have shown that ligaments in particular respond favorably to an increase in tensile strength. Immobilization causes the ligament matrix to decrease in size after just a few weeks. This can have deleterious mechanical effects on the noninjured ligaments and will cause them to be weak and less stiff.[33]

Blood Supply

A lack of circulation or proper blood supply to an injured area will impede the healing process. The initial process of phagocytosis and fibroblast delivery may not occur if blood is not delivered to the area. This is the reason that ice is critical immediately following an injury. Ice causes constriction of the blood vessels and decreases the need for oxygen, thus decreasing the amount of damage to the tissues.

Nonsteroidal Antiinflammatory Drugs

Nonsteroidal antiinflammatory drugs (NSAIDs) are the most commonly prescribed antiinflammatory drugs. NSAIDs help reduce pain by decreasing inflammation and inhibiting prostaglandin production. Prostaglandins stimulate nociceptors (pain fibers) and enhance edema formation by increasing permeability of blood vessels.[13] When these factors are limited, the healing process can occur more efficiently.

Other Factors

Other factors that can cause delayed or suboptimal healing include infection, corticosteroids, and excessive scar formation. The presence of bacteria can delay the healing process and cause excessive scar formation. Large doses of corticosteroids have been found to inhibit wound healing.[28,34] Hypertrophic scars can increase the maturation phase of healing, causing a delay in the healing process.

SUMMARY

This chapter discusses the phases of healing and the healing process that occurs in different tissues. The three phases of healing are the inflammatory response, the fibroplastic repair phase, and the maturation-remodeling phase. Four types of tissues are discussed: epithelial, muscle, nervous, and connective tissues. Each type of tissue produces different responses to injury or trauma in slightly different time frames. These responses are discussed in detail, to allow a better understanding of the soft tissue healing process.

References

1. Bryant WM: *Wound healing*, Reading, MA, 1977, CIBA Pharmaceutical Co.
2. Daly TJ: The repair phase of wound healing—re-epithelialization and contraction. In Kloth LC, McCulloh JM, Feeder JA, editors: *Wound healing: alternatives in management*, Philadephia, 1990, FA Davis.
3. Martinez-Hernandez A, Amenta PS: Basic concepts in wound healing. In Leadbetter WB, Buckwalter JA, Gordon SL, editors: *Sports-induced inflammation*, Park Ridge, IL, 1990, American Academy of Orthopaedic Surgeons.
4. Kloth LC, Miller KH: The inflammatory response to wounding. In Kloth LC, McCulloh JM, Feeder JA, editors: *Wound healing: alternatives in management*, Philadephia, 1990, FA Davis.
5. Cotran RS, Kumar V, Robbins SL: *Robbins pathologic basis of disease*, ed 4, Philadephia, 1989, Saunders.
6. Stevens A, Lowe J: *Pathology*, St Louis, 1995, Mosby.
7. *Dorland's Illustrated Medical Dictionary*, ed 27, Philadelphia, 1988, Saunders.
8. Knight KL: Cold as a modifier of sports-induced inflammation. In Leadbetter WB, Buckwalter JA, Gordon SL, editors: *Sports-induced inflammation*, Park Ridge, IL, 1990, American Academy of Orthopaedic Surgeons.
9. Hettinga DL: Inflammatory response of synovial joint structures. In Gould JA III, editor: *Orthopaedic and sports physical therapy*, ed 2, St Louis, 1990, Mosby.
10. Reed B: Wound healing and the use of thermal agents. In Michlovitz SL, editor: *Thermal agents in rehabilitation*, ed 3, Philadephia, 1996, FA Davis.
11. Junqueira LC, Carneiro J, Kelly RO: *Basic histology*, ed 8, Norwalk, CT, 1995, Appleton & Lange.
12. Groner J, Weeks PM: Healing of hard and soft tissues of the hand. In Strickland JW, Rettig AC: *Hand injuries in athletes*, Philadelphia, 1992, Saunders.
13. Price H: Connective tissue in wound healing. In Kloth LC, McCulloh JM, Feeder JA, editors: *Wound healing: alternatives in management*, Philadephia, 1990, FA Davis.

14. Martinez-Hernandez A: Repair, regeneration, and fibrosis. In Rubin E, Farber JL, editors: *Pathology*, ed 2, Philadelphia, 1994, JB Lippincott.

15. Carlstedt CA, Nordin M: Biomechanics of tendons and ligaments. In Nordin M, Frankel VH, editors: *Basic biomechanics of the musculoskeletal system*, ed 2, Philadelphia, 1989, Lea & Febiger.

16. Medoff RJ: Soft tissue healing, *Ann Sports Med* 3(2):67, 1987.

17. Guyton AC: *Pocket companion of textbook of medical physiology*, Philadelphia, 1998, Saunders.

18. Starkey C: *Therapeutic modalities*, ed 3, Philadelphia, 2003, FA Davis.

19. Anderson M, Hall S, Martin M: *Sports injury management*, ed 2, Baltimore, 2000, Lippincott Williams & Wilkins.

20. Malone TR, McPoil TG, Nitz AJ: *Orthopedic and sports physical therapy*, ed 3, St Louis, 1997, Mosby.

21. Buckwalter JA, Mow VC: Cartilage repair in osteoarthritis. In Moskowitz RW, Howell DS, Goldberg VM, Mankin HJ, editors: *Osteoarthritis: diagnosis and management*, ed 2, Philadephia, 1992, Saunders.

22. Aronen JA, Chronister R, Pve P, McDevitt ER: Thigh contusions: minimizing the length of time before return to full athletic activities with early immobilization in 120 cases of knee flexion. Paper presented at 16th annual meeting of AOSSM, Sun Valley, ID, 1990.

23. Caplan A, Carlson B, Faulkner J, et al: Skeletal muscle. In Woo SLY, Buckwater JA, editors: *Injury and repair of the musculoskeletal soft tissues*, Park Ridge, IL, 1988, AAOS.

24. Leadbetter WB, Buckwalter JA, Gordon SL: *Sports induced inflammation: clinical and basic science concepts*, Park Ridge, IL, 1990, AAOS.

25. O'Connor D: *Clinical pathology for athletic trainers*, Thorofare, NJ, 2001, Slack, pp 19-29.

26. Bandy WD, Dunleavy K: Pathophysiology. In Zachazewski JE, Magee DJ, Quillen WS, editors: *Athletic injuries and rehabilitation*, Philadelphia, 1996, Saunders.

27. Widsor RE, Lox DM: *Soft tissue injuries: diagnosis and treatment*, Philadelphia, 1998, Hamley & Bellus, pp 1-8.

28. Kibler WB: Clinical aspects of muscle injury, *Med Sci Sports Exerc* 22:450-452, 1990.

29. Desmet AA, Best TM: MR imaging of the distribution and location of acute hamstring injuries in athletes, *Am J Roentgenol* 174:393-399, 2000.

30. Speer KP, Lohnes JE, Garrett WE: Radiographic imaging of muscle strain injury, *Am J Sports Med* 21:89-95, 1993.

31. Schultz E, McCormick KM: Skeletal muscle satellite cells, *Rev Physiol Biochem Pharmacol* 123:213-257, 1994.

32. Sandberg N, Steinhardt C: On the effects of cortisone on the histamine formation of skin wounds in the rat, *Acta Chir Scand* 127:574-577, 1964.

33. Zachazewski JE, Magee DJ, Quillen WS: *Athletic injuries and rehabilitation*, Philadelphia, 1996, Saunders.

34. Erlich HP, Hunt TK: Effects of cortisone and vitamin A on wound healing, *Ann Surg* 167:324, 1968.

CHAPTER 2

Mobilization of the Shoulder and Knee following Postsurgical Immobilization

David S. Miers, PT, OCS, FAAOMPT, CSCS
Pieter Kroon, PT, OCS, FAAOMPT

CHAPTER OUTLINE

THE OBJECTIVES OF THIS CHAPTER ARE

to (1) describe why immobilization is important following trauma and surgical procedures; (2) describe the effects of immobilization on the joint and surrounding soft tissue structures; (3) review basic concepts of anatomy and joint function and movement (osteokinematics and arthrokinematics); (4) describe the basic concepts of mobilization; and (5) describe specific joint mobilizations that might be performed following postsurgical immobilization of the shoulder and knee.

OVERVIEW OF THE PHYSIOLOGIC EFFECTS OF IMMOBILIZATION

During the past 20 to 30 years, the use of immobilization following trauma and surgical procedures, other than for fracture, has significantly decreased in both frequency and the length of the immobilization time frames. This has occurred as a result of a greater understanding of the negative effects of immobilization, sometimes being counterproductive to the surgical repair, and significant advances in surgical technique.

Understanding the effects of immobilization is paramount in the establishment of a comprehensive postsurgical rehabilitation program. The following is a general description of the events following immobilization. One must also consider the healing process that is occurring at the surgical site. Without joint motion, the primary process for which a joint and its components get physiologic requirements, function is severely compromised. The connective tissues contract and reorganize, effectively becoming denser. This often results in a restricted and nonfunctional joint.[1-4] Changes can occur in as few as 3 days and include laying down of collagen in a disorganized pattern. These adverse effects are "magnified when edema, trauma, or impaired circulation is also present."[1] Effects on bone, ligaments, synovium, capsule, tendons, and muscle are deleterious, and are to varying degrees dependent on a variety of factors. With non–weight-bearing status, bone may lose as much as 50% of bone density in as little as 12 weeks.[1,3] This may result in an increase in fracture rate during the postimmobilization rehabilitation period if proper consideration is not taken. In addition, with prolonged immobilization ligaments become less organized and stiff with less ability to resist tensile forces placed on them.[1,3,4] The synovial capsule depends on loading and movement for proper function. With immobilization, decreased mobility, decreased viscosity, and increased adhesive contracture may occur. With tendinous structures, decreased tensile capacity and excursion properties are limited.[1,5] Musculature structures tend to atrophy and adapt to newly lengthened or shortened positions, and have less extensibility. In the shortened position, the effects of immobilization seem to be greater because atrophy is more pronounced than while immobilized in a lengthened position. Additionally, the number of motor units in muscular structures is decreased. There may be an increase in the number of sarcomeres when immobilization occurs in a lengthened position. Furthermore, following prolonged immobilization a decrease in coordination of muscle firing, a decrease in the length/tension relationships, and a decrease in power/force production may be seen.[1,4,6-9]

BIOMECHANICS OF THE SHOULDER

To provide the correct treatment procedure, especially mobilization techniques, the clinician must have a solid understanding of joint biomechanics. A general review of the osteokinematics and arthrokinematics of the shoulder and knee is provided.

The shoulder is the most mobile of all joints, having three degrees of freedom in all three planes in space. In the sagittal plane, flexion and extension occur about a transverse axis; abduction and adduction occur in the frontal plane about an anterior-posterior axis; and internal and external rotation occur about a longitudinal axis. Axial rotation is a resultant of movement in other planes. Scapular motion and clavicular motion are essential components of a properly functioning shoulder girdle. The scapular movements generally occur in the horizontal plane and consist of medial-lateral movements, elevation and depression, and rotational movements. The sternoclavicular joint has two degrees of motion. At the sternoclavicular joint, movement occurs in a frontal plane for superior and inferior movements, and movement in the horizontal plane occurs for anterior-posterior movements. A third type of movement, axial rotation of about 30 degrees, is thought to be due to the laxity of the surrounding ligaments. The acromioclavicular joint allows for a functional axial rotation of about 30 degrees. This, combined with the sternoclavicular joint, allows for approximately 60 degrees of upward rotation of the scapula.

The head of the humerus is biconvex, facing superior/medial/posterior.[10] The glenoid cavity is found at the superior-lateral angle of the scapula and faces laterally, anteriorly, and slightly superior and is biconcave in shape.[10] The articular surfaces of the sternoclavicular joint are saddle shaped. The clavicular surface is convex superior/inferior and concave anterior/posterior. The acromioclavicular joint structure has the acromion facing anterior/medial/superior and is considered to be flat.[10] However, the configuration of the articular cartilage makes the joint surface slightly convex.[10] The clavicular surface is flat or slightly convex and faces inferior/posterior and lateral.[11]

BIOMECHANICS OF THE KNEE

The biomechanics of the knee joint are often thought of as being "simple." However, with detailed study, one will find that the knee joint is quite complex and fascinating. The knee has one degree of freedom, allowing for flexion and extension.[10] An accessory second degree of freedom allows for axial rotation. The knee is a hinge joint allowing flexion/extension about a medial/lateral axis. The femoral condyles are convex in both planes and are separated by a central groove. The tibial surfaces are essentially two surfaces separated by a ridge. The medial tibial condyle is biconcave, and the lateral condyle is concave medial/lateral and convex anterior/posterior.[10] Movements of the patella on the femur include the force of the quadriceps, which is superior/lateral. This superior/lateral force is turned vertical by the central groove of the femoral patellar surface into the intercondylar notch. With flexion and extension of the knee, the patella moves in a sagittal plane, relative to the tibia, along an arc in line with the tibial tuberosity.[11]

JOINT MOBILIZATION

It should be noted that only the physiologic motions and joint surfaces are covered in this chapter. It is paramount to understand the interrelationships of the surrounding ligamentous, capsular, and muscular anatomy of the knee complex to provide even the most basic of rehabilitation procedures. Joint structure has been covered to provide a basis of review for the mobilization procedures that follow.

When considering the various physical therapy interventions available to the clinician who is treating the postimmobilization patient, one should carefully consider all of the following factors: subjective complaints and the physical examination, reason for the immobilization (medical condition or procedure), stage of healing of the condition, and skill level of the therapist to correctly apply the intervention.

As with any physical therapy intervention, a careful subjective examination should be performed. A complete subjective examination is not the focus of this chapter; see Chapters 3 and 4 for details of a complete physical examination. However, a few key components are worth highlighting regarding the immobilization patient:

- Protocol given by physician; surgical procedure performed
- Special questions regarding contraindications relative to manual therapy
- Functional limitations or difficulties of the patient

The American Physical Therapy Association's *Guide to Physical Therapist Practice* defines *mobilization* as "a manual therapy technique comprising a continuum of skilled passive movements to the joints and or related soft tissues that are applied at varying speeds and amplitudes, including a small amplitude/high velocity therapeutic movement."[12]

Maitland[13] describes five grades of mobilization. A grade one mobilization is a small-amplitude movement near the starting position of the range, whereas a grade two mobilization is a large-amplitude movement that carries well into the range. A grade two mobilization can occupy any part of the range that is free of any stiffness or muscle spasm. A grade three mobilization is a large-amplitude movement that moves into stiffness or muscle spasm, and a grade four mobilization is a small-amplitude movement stretching into stiffness or muscle spasm. A grade five mobilization is a high-velocity, low-amplitude thrust performed at end-range.

Some of the proposed effects of joint mobilization are divided into two main categories: mechanical and neurophysiologic. These categories include, but are not limited to, the following:

- Stretching or rupturing intraarticular adhesions
- Relaxation of reflexively contracted muscles
- Activation mechanoreceptors
- Releasing impacted tissues (meniscoid inclusions)
- Altering positional relationships (i.e., protrusion to nerve root)
- Temporarily removing pressure from sensitive structures
- Stimulating the fast-conducting epicritic fibers
- Psychologic effects

Indications for mobilization include the following: presence of dysfunction; neurologic effects to reduce pain and guarding; and mechanical effects to overcome restrictions.

The likelihood of causing serious damage with extremity joint mobilization techniques is very small. Contraindications fall into several categories:

- Absence of dysfunction
- Relative to the clinician's skill and experience
- Presence of serious pathology that mobilization may affect adversely

Absolute contraindications include the following:

- Anything that can weaken bone: osteoporosis, neoplasm, infection
- Fracture
- Ligament rupture
- No working hypothesis
- Excessive pain or resistance
- Empty end feel and severe multidirectional spasm, which can be the result of various serious pathologic findings
- Acute rheumatoid arthritis episode (possibility of increased tissue damage and severe exacerbation)
- Chronic pain and fibromyalgia-type syndromes, in both of which there are inadequate signs to explain the patient's widespread symptoms
- Emotionally dependent patients; there is a chance of developing long-term dependency without much hope of benefit

Regional contraindications include the following:

- Vertebral artery syndrome
- Traumatized transverse ligament
- Cauda equina syndrome; possibility of serious damage and permanent palsy

Cautions include the following:

- Disk prolapse
- Pharmacology: steroidal drugs, anticoagulants, drugs unfamiliar to the therapist
- Hunch or feel (i.e., clinical impression)
- Pregnancy: risk of ligamentous damage due to relaxin effect and risk of coinciding with miscarriage
- Inflammation: possibility of severe exacerbation
- History of neoplastic disease: risk of recurrence
- Age
- Depleted general health
- Patient unable to relax
- Physique

Mobilization of the shoulder and knee is only one of the numerous manual techniques available to the physical therapist following immobilization. All of the available manual techniques have merit and are only as good as the skill level of the practitioner using them. Each technique must be used in the correct instance based on skill, experience, the postsurgical physical examination, and the diagnosis that has been established. A sampling of other techniques that are available includes soft tissue mobilization, neural tension testing and treatment, manipulation, muscle energy techniques, and mobilization with movement. Many of these procedures are often used before or after a traditional mobilization, with improved outcomes.

Neuromuscular reeducation following joint mobilization is necessary in order to train the muscles in the newly gained range of motion. Gains made after joint mobilization are often temporary if neuromuscular control is not restored.

Treatment should focus on restoration of physiologic movements—cardinal plane and accessory movements of both the joint in question and the joints relative to the immobilized segment. For example, following shoulder immobilization the clinician should carefully examine the elbow and wrist complex, scapula, acromioclavicular joint, sternoclavicular joint, and cervical spine. With the postimmobilized knee patient, examination of the hip and the proximal and distal fibular joints should occur.

MOVEMENT AT THE ARTICULAR SURFACES

To perform a physiologically correct mobilization to a joint, a complete knowledge of the accessory joint motions is required. The rules governing joint arthrokinematics have long been established and are worth reviewing.

Spin: Movement around an axis.

Glide: One point on one surface comes in contact with a new point on another surface (Figures 2-1 and 2-2).

Roll: A new point on one surface comes in contact with a new point on another surface (Figures 2-3 and 2-4).

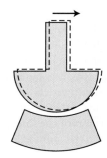

Figure 2-1: Convex on concave gliding.

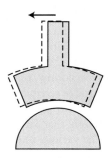

Figure 2-2: Concave on convex gliding.

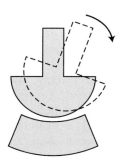

Figure 2-3: Convex on concave rolling.

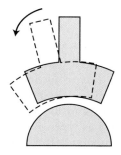

Figure 2-4: Concave on convex rolling.

The more congruent the joint surfaces, the greater the proportion of gliding to rolling movement. Therefore decreased gliding will greatly affect movement in a highly congruent joint and can lead to joint dysfunction.

Convex-concave rules are as follows:

- Rolling and gliding occur in the same direction when a concavity moves on a convexity.[10] Rolling and gliding

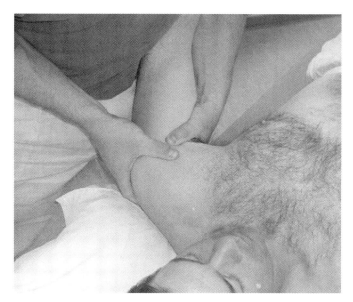

Figure 2-5: Distraction of the glenohumeral joint.

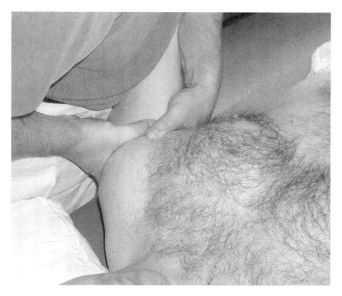

Figure 2-6: Inferior glide of the head of the humerus.

occur in the opposite direction when a convexity moves on a concavity.[1]

- Because joint hypomobility is often treated by performing gliding movements, it is important to know the direction of the restricted joint gliding.

To perform joint and soft tissue mobilizations well, a thorough understanding of the anatomy and biomechanics of the joints involved is essential. The following sections describe selected joint mobilization techniques for the postoperative shoulder and knee, respectively.

SELECTED JOINT MOBILIZATION TECHNIQUES OF THE SHOULDER

Figure 2-5 shows distraction of the glenohumeral joint.

- *Patient:* The patient lies supine with the shoulder in a resting position.
- *Clinician:* The clinician stands next to the table facing the patient. The clinician's medial hand grasps the patient's upper arm next to the patient's axilla. The clinician's lateral hand grasps the lateral aspect of the patient's upper arm. The patient's hand and forearm are supported between the therapist's arm and ribs. The clinician distracts the patient's humerus in a lateral, superior, and anterior direction. For sustained mobilization, a fixation belt can be used around the upper trunk, under both axillae and secured to the table.

Figure 2-6 shows inferior glide of the head of the humerus.

- *Patient:* The patient lies supine with the shoulder in a resting position.
- *Clinician:* The clinician stands facing the patient with the medial hand under the patient's upper arm while the lateral hand is on the superior lateral border of the humeral head. The clinician distracts the humerus lightly with the medial hand and glides the humerus inferiorly with the lateral hand. This increases abduction/flexion at the 0- to 60-degree range. For sustained mobilizations, the patient should be stabilized by placing a belt diagonally across the patient's chest and under the axilla.

Figure 2-7 shows anterior glide of the head of the humerus.

- *Patient:* The patient lies prone, with a stabilization pad under the coracoid process to block the scapula.
- *Clinician:* The clinician stands at the side of the table, placing his or her medial hand under the patient's axilla, while the lateral hand is on the posterolateral aspect of the humerus. The patient's shoulder is in a resting position with the patient's forearm between the clinician's knees. The clinician mildly distracts the humerus and then mobilizes anteriorly with both hands. This technique increases both external rotation and extension.

Figure 2-8 shows posterior glide of the head of the humerus.

- *Patient:* The patient lies supine with the shoulder in a resting position. A sandbag or towel under the scapula will help stabilize the scapula.
- *Clinician:* The clinician stands at the side of the table facing the patient. The clinician's medial hand grasps the patient's upper arm next to the patient's axilla. The clinician's lateral hand is placed on the superior-anterior aspect of the patient's humeral head. With both hands, the clinician distracts lightly, and then glides the humerus posteriorly. This technique increases internal rotation and flexion.

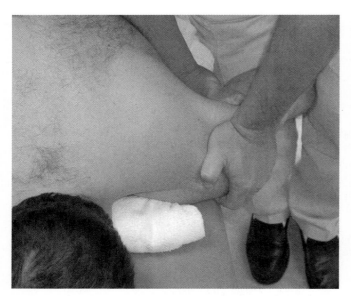

Figure 2-7: Anterior glide of the head of the humerus.

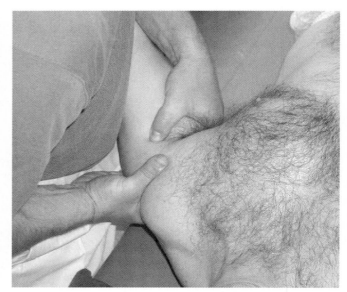

Figure 2-9: Combined planes mobilization of the head of the humerus.

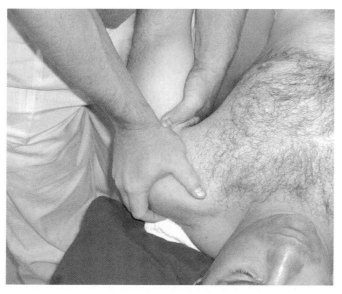

Figure 2-8: Posterior glide of the head of the humerus.

Figure 2-9 shows combined planes mobilization of the head of the humerus.

- *Patient:* The patient lies supine with the arm in position above 60 degrees of abduction.
- *Clinician:* The clinician stands at the side of the table facing the patient. The clinician grasps the humerus as close to the axilla as possible, distracting and gliding inferiorly. The clinician then adds external rotation of the humerus by using a rocking-type motion with his or her hips. Sequence: distract, distal glide, abduction, external rotation. This technique increases abduction from 80 to 180 degrees.

Figure 2-10 shows distraction of the scapulothoracic joint.

- *Patient:* The patient is in a side-lying position, facing the clinician.
- *Clinician:* The clinician stands at the side of the table, facing the patient. The clinician's abdomen is placed against the patient's to stabilize. The patient's upper arm is placed over the clinician's inferior forearm. The clinician's inferior hand cups the inferior angle of the scapula. The superior hand is placed on the patient's acromion and superior angle of the scapula. Mobilize the scapula in circumduction, protraction, retraction, cranially, and caudally. This helps to massage the subscapularis. The clinician can then hook his or her fingers under the medial border of the scapula and it can be distracted from the thorax. While distracting, move it in the direction of restriction.

Figure 2-11 shows anterior/posterior glide of the acromioclavicular joint.

- *Patient:* The patient lies supine with the upper arm on a pillow.
- *Clinician:* The clinician stands at the side of the table, facing the patient. The clinician's lateral hand grasps the patient's shoulder with the thumb and places the index finger on the patient's acromion. The thumb of the clinician's medial hand is placed on the anterior surface of the lateral end of the clavicle, with the fingers on the posterior surface of the clavicle. The clinician glides the clavicle anteriorly and posteriorly and assesses for range and end feel.

Figure 2-12 shows anterior motion and rotation of the clavicle in the acromioclavicular joint.

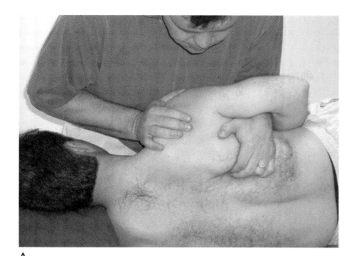

A

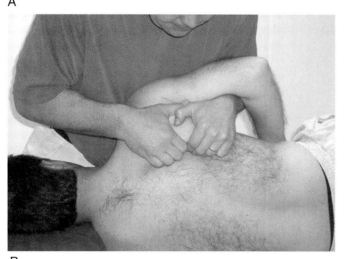

B

Figure 2-10: Distraction of the scapulothoracic joint.

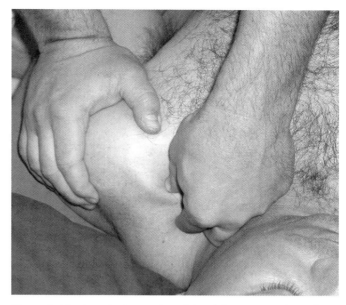

Figure 2-11: Anterior/posterior glide of the acromioclavicular joint.

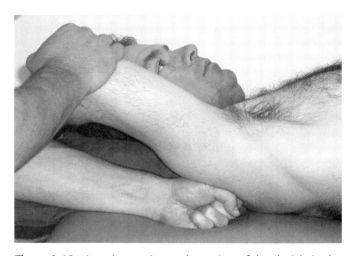

Figure 2-12: Anterior motion and rotation of the clavicle in the acromioclavicular joint.

- *Patient:* The patient lies supine with the arm abducted and elevated.
- *Clinician:* The clinician stands at the head of the table, holding the patient's arm with his or her lateral hand. The clinician makes a fist with the medial hand. The clinician's proximal interphalangeal joint rests under the posterior/lateral surface of the clavicle. The clinician's ulnar side of the hand rests on the table to block the clavicle from rotating posteriorly, while moving the patient's arm into more flexion. This technique improves flexion and abduction and restores acromioclavicular joint function.

Figure 2-13 shows test and anterior-posterior motion of the sternoclavicular joint.

- *Patient:* The patient lies supine with his or her head in slight side bending toward the side being worked on, which places the cervical spine muscles in a shortened position of rest.

- *Clinician:* The clinician stands at the side of the table facing the patient and places a pillow under the affected arm.
  - *For anterior glide:* The clinician's index and middle fingers of the lateral hand are placed behind the posterior surface of the patient's clavicle, and the clinician's thumb is placed on the anterior surface of the patient's clavicle. The clinician moves the clavicle anteriorly with the lateral hand while palpating acromioclavicular joint mobility with the thumb of his or her medial hand.
  - *For posterior glide:* The clinician places his or her thumb on the medial end of the patient's clavicle. The clinician mobilizes posteriorly and checks for

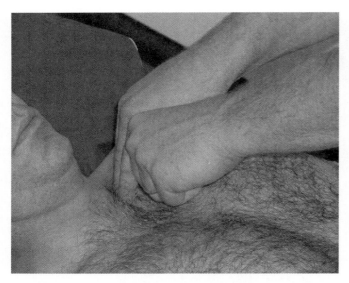

Figure 2-13: Test and anterior-posterior motion of the sternoclavicular joint.

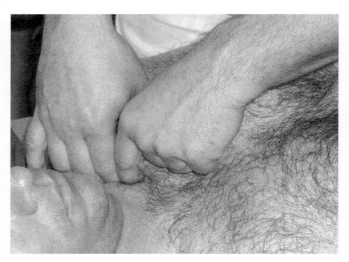

Figure 2-15: Test and superior glide of the sternoclavicular joint.

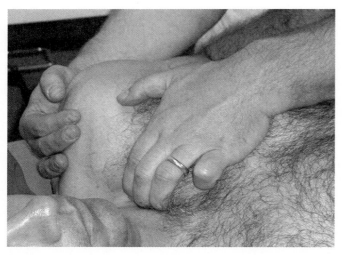

Figure 2-14: Test and inferior glide of the sternoclavicular joint.

range of motion and end feel. Test and treatment techniques are the same. Anterior mobilization improves protraction; posterior mobilization improves retraction.

Figure 2-14 shows test and inferior glide of the sternoclavicular joint.

- *Patient:* The patient lies supine.
- *Clinician:* The clinician stands at the side of the table, facing the patient. The clinician places the lateral hand on the patient's acromion, while the index and middle fingers of the medial hand are placed on the superior portion of the medial end of the patient's clavicle. The clinician assesses range of motion and end feel by moving the medial portion of the clavicle inferiorly with the

medial hand as the lateral hand elevates the shoulder. The mobilization technique is done in similar fashion. This technique increases shoulder elevation.

Figure 2-15 shows test and superior glide of the sternoclavicular joint.

- *Patient:* The patient lies supine.
- *Clinician:* The clinician stands at the side of the table, facing the patient. The clinician places the thumb of his or her medial hand on the inferior portion of the medial end of the patient's clavicle, and his or her index finger on the superior portion of the patient's clavicle. The clinician places the thumb of the lateral hand next to the other thumb, while his or her fingers are on the superior portion of the patient's clavicle. The clinician moves the clavicle superiorly/inferiorly, assessing for range of motion and end feel. The clinician can mobilize the joint in a similar fashion. Inferior glide of the proximal clavicle increases elevation of the shoulder, and superior glide improves depression of the shoulder.

Figure 2-16 shows scapular framing, a soft tissue technique for the scapular borders.

- *Patient:* The patient is placed in a side-lying position with the affected side up.
- *Clinician:* The clinician stands at the side of the table, facing the patient. (A) The medial border of the patient's scapula is stroked from cranial to caudal while keeping the scapula in mild retraction. (B) The superior border of the scapula is mobilized with fingertips working from medial to lateral and from neck to shoulder. (C) To work on the lateral border of the scapula, the clinician places the top hand on the lateral border of the scapula close to the glenohumeral joint. The palm of the clinician's other hand applies the stroke down the lateral border of the scapula. The clinician's thumb may be used to treat specific lesions.

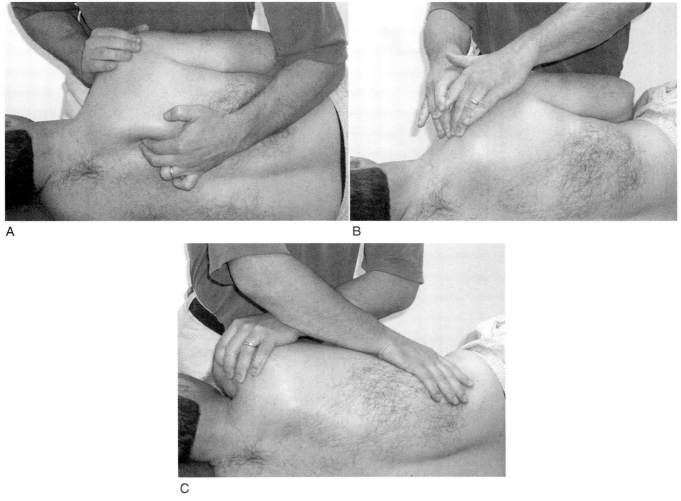

A

B

C

Figure 2-16: Scapular framing.

Figure 2-17 shows soft tissue technique to the quadrangular space.

- *Patient:* The patient is placed in a side-lying position with the affected side up, facing away from the clinician.
- *Clinician:* The clinician stands at the side of the table, facing the patient. The clinician's top hand grasps the patient's upper arm and elevates the shoulder. The tips of the clinician's third and fourth fingers are placed on the quadrangular space. The clinician identifies the soft tissue restrictions. Strumming, parallel, and perpendicular deformation techniques can be applied to the affected areas.

SELECTED JOINT MOBILIZATION TECHNIQUES OF THE KNEE

Figure 2-18 shows distraction of the knee joint while the patient is supine.

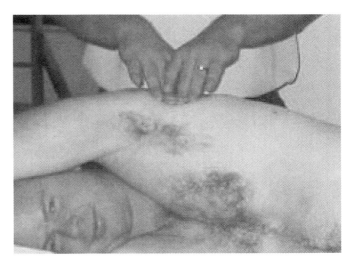

Figure 2-17: Soft tissue technique to the quadrangular space.

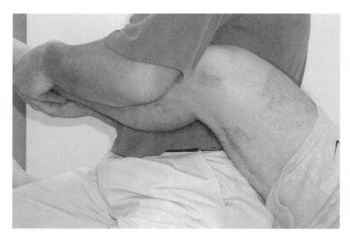

Figure 2-18: Distraction of the knee joint, supine.

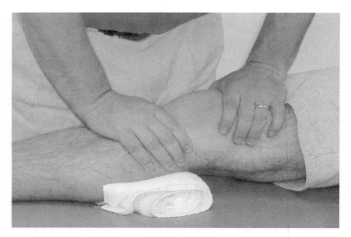

Figure 2-20: Posterior glide of the femur on the tibia.

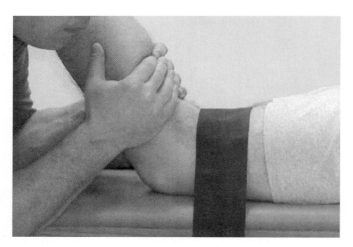

Figure 2-19: Distraction of the knee joint, prone.

- *Patient:* The patient lies supine, with the hip flexed to 90 degrees and externally rotated and the knee flexed to 90 degrees.
- *Clinician:* The clinician sits on the table facing away from the patient. The clinician's lower back is placed against the patient's posterior thigh. The patient's lower leg is placed on the clinician's abdomen, locked on the lateral rib cage with elbow and forearm. The clinician wraps his or her hands around the patient's ankle superior to the malleoli. The clinician rotates the trunk away to distract the tibia from the femur.

Figure 2-19 shows distraction of the knee joint while the patient is prone.

- *Patient:* The patient lies prone, with his or her knee flexed approximately 25 degrees and the dorsum of the foot resting on the therapist's shoulder. The patient's distal femur is stabilized with a belt.
- *Clinician:* The clinician stands at the end of the table. The clinician places both hands around the patient's

proximal calf with the hypothenar eminences of both hands on the anterior tibial plateaus. The clinician distracts the patient's knee joint by extending the clinician's knees and hips.

Figure 2-20 shows posterior glide of the femur on the tibia.

- *Patient:* The patient lies supine. The patient's knee is placed in the resting position by putting a bolster under the proximal tibia just distal to the joint line.
- *Clinician:* The clinician stands at the side of the table, facing the patient. The clinician's distal hand stabilizes the patient's tibia just below the joint line. The clinician keeps the elbow extended. The clinician's mobilizing hand is placed on the femur just above the patella. Keeping the elbow extended, the clinician mobilizes the femur in a posterior direction. This technique increases extension of the knee.

Figure 2-21 shows posterior glide of the tibia on the femur.

- *Patient:* The patient lies supine. The patient's knee is placed in the resting position by putting a bolster under the distal end of the femur just proximal to the joint line.
- *Clinician:* The clinician stands at the side of the table, facing the patient. The clinician places the proximal hand on the patient's distal femur just proximal to the patella. The clinician's mobilizing hand is placed on the proximal tibia just below the joint line. Keeping the elbow extended, the clinician mobilizes the tibia in the posterior direction. This technique increases flexion of the knee.

Figure 2-22 shows the medial/lateral mobility test and mobilization of the patellofemoral joint.

- *Patient:* The patient lies supine.
- *Clinician:* The clinician stands at the side of the table, facing the patient.

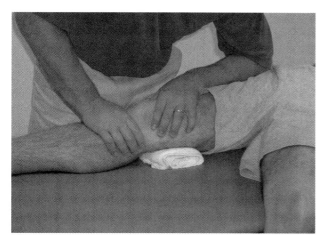

Figure 2-21: Posterior glide of the tibia on the femur.

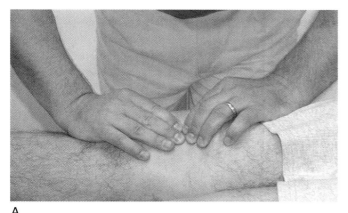

A

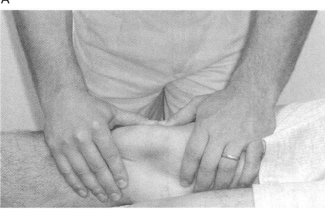

B

Figure 2-22: Medial/lateral mobility test and mobilization of the patellofemoral joint.

- *For lateral glide of the patella:* The clinician places the pads of the second and third fingers of both hands on the medial side of the patient's patella. The pads of the thumbs are placed on the tibia and femur, just below the lateral border of the patella. The clinician moves the patella in a lateral direction and assesses

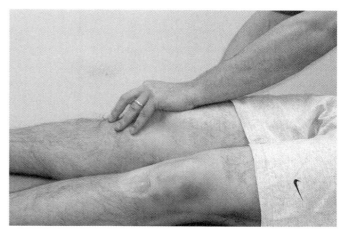

Figure 2-23: Inferior glide of the patella.

range of motion and end feel. The mobilization is done in a similar fashion. Restoring proper patellar mobility helps improve flexion and extension of the knee joint.

- *For medial glide of the patella:* The clinician places the pads of both thumbs on the lateral border of the patient's patella. The clinician moves the patella in a medial direction and assesses range of motion and end feel. The mobilization is done in a similar fashion.

Figure 2-23 shows inferior glide of the patella.

- *Patient:* The patient lies supine.
- *Clinician:* The clinician stands at the side of the table, facing the patient. The clinician places the heel of the hand on the superior border of the patient's patella. Keeping the elbow extended, the clinician moves the patella in a distal direction and assesses range of motion and end feel. The mobilization is done in similar fashion. This technique improves knee flexion.

Figure 2-24 shows the mobility test for the proximal tibiofibular joint.

- *Patient:* The patient lies supine with the knee flexed to 90 degrees.
- *Clinician:* The clinician sits on the patient's forefoot. The clinician places the medial hand over the patient's medial proximal tibia. The clinician's mobilizing hand molds all four fingertips onto the posterior surface of the patient's fibular head, taking care to avoid irritating the peroneal nerve. The clinician glides the fibular head in an anterior-lateral and posterior-medial direction, assessing range of motion and end feel, comparing with the opposite side.

Figure 2-25 shows anterior glide of the fibula at the proximal tibiofibular joint.

- *Patient:* The patient is on hands and knees with the affected foot over the edge of the table.

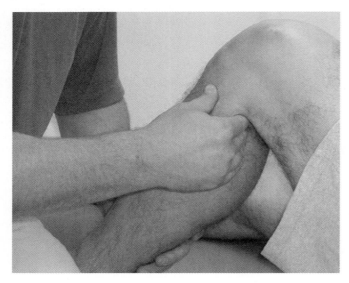

Figure 2-24: Mobility test of the proximal tibiofibular joint.

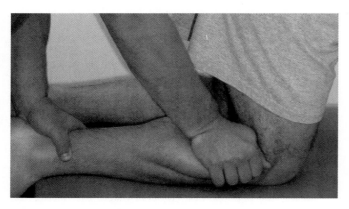

Figure 2-25: Anterior glide of the fibula at the proximal tibiofibular joint.

- *Clinician:* The clinician stands across the table from the affected leg. The patient's tibia is stabilized against the table by the patient's body weight and by the clinician's medial hand holding the lower leg. The thenar eminence of the clinician's mobilizing hand is placed on the patient's posterior-medial fibular head. Keeping the elbow extended, the clinician mobilizes in an anterior-lateral direction.

SUMMARY

This chapter on mobilization of the postsurgical knee and shoulder covered the effects of the postimmobilization on the mechanics of the knee and shoulder joints. Joint mobilization to treat the resulting loss of range of motion is presented. Basic anatomy, biomechanics, and concepts of joint mobilization are also addressed, along with selected applicable mobilization techniques for the knee and shoulder. Mobilization of the postsurgical knee and shoulder is an important component of a comprehensive rehabilitation program. A strong understanding of the physiologic process, anatomy, and biomechanics is the essential first step prior to the application of a mobilization technique. A complete review of the surgical procedure and the stage of the healing process following the surgical procedure are imperative. For optimal results with mobilization of the postsurgical knee and shoulder, proper patient position and correct application of amplitude and direction are essential to obtain a safe and effective clinical outcome.

References

1. Cry LM, Ross RG: How controlled stress affects healing tissues, *J Hand Ther* 11:125-130, 1998.
2. Kottke FJ, Pauley DL, Ptak RA: The rationale for prolonged stretching for correction of shortening connective tissue, *Arch Phys Med Rehabil* 47(3):45-52, 1966.
3. Buckwalter JA: Effects of early motion on healing of musculoskeletal tissues, *Hand Clin* 12:13-24, 1996.
4. Maxey L, Magnusson J: *Rehabilition for the postsurgical orthopedic patient,* St Louis, 2001, Mosby, pp 2-8.
5. Akeson WH, Amiel D, Abel MF, et al: Effects of immobilization on joints, *Clin Orthop* 219:28-37, 1987.
6. Warren CG, Lehmann JF, Koblanski JN: Heat and stretch procedures: an evaluation using rat tail tendon, *Arch Phys Med Rehabil* 57:122-126, 1976.
7. St-Pierre D, Gardiner PF: The effects of immobilization and exercise on muscle function: a review, *Physiol Canada* 39:24-36, 1987.
8. Gossman MR, Sahrmann SA, Rose SE: Review of length associated changes in muscle: experimental evidence and clinical implications, *Phys Ther* 62:1799-1808, 1982.
9. Williams PE, Goldspink G: Changes in sarcomere length and physiologic properties in immobilized muscle, *J Anat* 127:459-468, 1977.
10. Kaltenborn F, Evjenth O: *Manual mobilization of the extremity joints,* ed 4, Oslo, Norway, 1989, Olan Noris Bokhandel.
11. Rogers M: *Orthopaedic manual physical therapy certificate program,* Unpublished residency course workbook, 1996.
12. American Physical Therapy Association: Guide to physical therapist practice, ed 2, *Phys Ther* 81:9-744, 2001.
13. Maitland G, Hangeveld E: *Maitland's vertebral manipulation,* ed 6, Oxford, 2001, Butterworth-Heinemann.

CHAPTER 3

Preoperative and Postsurgical Musculoskeletal Examination of the Knee

Robert C. Manske, DPT, MPT, MEd, SCS, ATC, CSCS
Mark Stovak, MD, FAAFP

CHAPTER OUTLINE

AS WITH ANY MUSCULOSKELETAL IN-JURY, a comprehensive examination of the patient with a suspected knee injury allows the clinician to determine the patient's baseline status that will be used to guide the treatment and rehabilitation process. A thorough understanding of both the anatomy and biomechanics of the knee is necessary. The goal of this chapter is to provide the reader with a detailed description of the preoperative and postoperative physical examination of the patient with an injured knee.

The best time to examine a patient undergoing surgery is before his or her knee surgery, or preoperatively. This chapter describes both the preoperative and postoperative physical examination of the knee. It is during the preoperative examination that the clinician may glean valuable information regarding the status of the knee that may not be able to be assessed immediately following surgery. This baseline information may not be able to be performed postsurgically because of soft tissue healing constraints, immobilization procedures, or postoperative pain associated with the various surgical procedures. Both preoperatively and postoperatively, the clinician should use a standard, consistent, systematic approach to examine and evaluate the knee complex. A thorough physical examination will assess both the involved and the uninvolved extremity.

HISTORY

As with any musculoskeletal injury, the examination should begin with a thorough patient medical history.[1] The patient's medical history should clearly define the pathology. It was D. H. O'Donoghue who stated, "Let the patient tell his story in his own words."[2] In most cases, if allowed, the patient will guide you to the correct diagnosis with his or her description of the injury. As the clinician becomes more experienced with the subjective portion of the examination, he or she will most likely be able to recognize various descriptions of injury mechanisms, various clusters of signs and symptoms that give a general idea of the pathology at hand from the medical history alone. Following an adequate history the clinician uses the clinical examination to implicate or rule out specific structures that may be causing the pathology that is believed to be at fault.

SYSTEMS REVIEW

The presence of symptoms that are contradictory to a typical musculoskeletal injury must alert the clinician to pathologies that may have neurologic or systemic implications. During the history it is imperative to listen for "red flags" as described by Stith and colleagues.[3] While performing the systems review, the clinician needs to be aware of conditions in which the pathology may be outside his or her scope of practice. These red flag symptoms (Table 3-1) would alert the clinician to immediately refer the patient back to the physician without initiation of treatments.[3]

TABLE 3-1

"Red Flag" Findings in Patient History That Necessitate Need for Physician Referral

CAUSE	SYMPTOMS
Cancer	Persistent pain at night
	Constant pain anywhere in the body
	Unexplained weight loss—10-15 lb in 2 weeks or less
	Loss of appetite
	Unusual lumps or growths
	Unwarranted fatigue
Cardiovascular	Shortness of breath
	Dizziness
	Pain or a feeling of heaviness in chest
	Pulsating pain anywhere in the body
	Constant and severe pain in the lower leg (calf) or arm
	Discolored or painful feet
	Swelling with no history of injury
Gastrointestinal	Frequent or severe abdominal pain
	Frequent heartburn or indigestion
	Frequent nausea or vomiting
Genitourinary	Change in or problems with bladder function
	Unusual menstrual irregularities
Neurologic	Changes in hearing
	Frequent or severe headaches with no history of injury
	Problems with swallowing or changes in speech
	Changes in vision (blurriness or loss of sight)
	Problems with balance, coordination, or falling
	Fainting spells (drop attacks)
	Sudden weakness
Miscellaneous	Fever or night sweats
	Recent severe emotional disturbances
	Swelling or redness in any joint without history of injury
	Pregnancy

From Stith JS, Sahrmann SA, Dixon KK, Norton BJ: Curriculum to prepare diagnosticians in physical therapy, *J Phys Ther Educ* 9:46-53, 1995.

Additionally, the subjective examination should include details relating to the patient's age and occupation, inciting trauma, and history of the current problem, including both past and present symptoms. The patient's age can help narrow down a suspected pathology from those that have been previously determined to be doubtful for the given age-group. For instance, the odds that an adolescent would have degenerative knee osteoarthritis are low because the condition occurs much more commonly in the elderly. Meniscal and ligamentous injuries appear more commonly in the more active younger population.

MECHANISM OF INJURY

The mechanism of injury is important because it can give the clinician an idea of the involved structures. Descriptions of how the knee was injured detailing both knee and foot positions (closed kinetic chain vs. open kinetic chain) can enhance the clinician's ability to obtain an accurate diagnosis. A common mechanism of injury to the knee is flexion or hyperflexion with a posterior-directed force to the tibia, which can injure the posterior cruciate ligament (Figure 3-1). A hyperextension injury to the knee often results in rupture of the anterior cruciate ligament and, if severe enough, also the posterior cruciate ligament (Figure 3-2). A valgus force to the knee is probably the most common cause of ligament injury and will result in an isolated medial collateral ligament (MCL) injury. Although a sufficient valgus force can also injure the anterior cruciate ligament (ACL), the posterior medial capsule and the medial meniscus may also be injured concomitantly (Figure 3-3). A straight varus force will most often injure the lateral collateral ligament (LCL), whereas with enough stress the posterolateral capsule and the posterior cruciate ligament (PCL) can also be injured. The mechanism of injury can also include a rotational component involving the cruciate ligaments, the collateral ligaments, the menisci, or the patella. Medial rotation of the femur through its long axis while the foot is planted can cause a patellar dislocation or subluxation, a meniscus tear, or osteochondral injury.

DEMOGRAPHICS

In addition to the mechanism of injury, the clinician should question the patient regarding prior and present level of function. What sports does the athlete participate in presently?

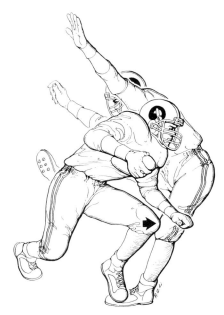

Figure 3-2: Hyperextension injury can lead to ACL or ACL/PCL disruption. *(From Scott WN, editor: Ligament and extensor mechanism injuries to the knee: diagnosis and treatment, St Louis, 1991, Mosby, p 88, Fig 7-2.)*

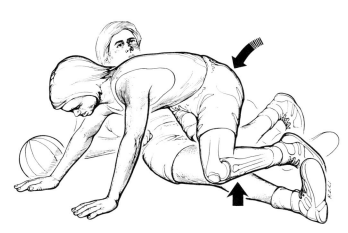

Figure 3-1: Hyperflexion with or without an anterior blow to the tibia can lead to isolated PCL injury. *(From Scott WN, editor: Ligament and extensor mechanism injuries to the knee: diagnosis and treatment, St Louis, 1991, Mosby, p 89, Fig 7-3.)*

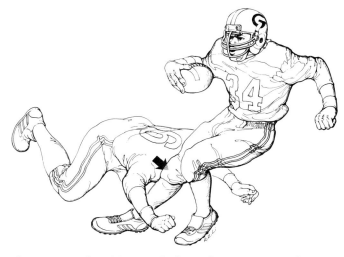

Figure 3-3: Valgus injury to the knee. *(From Scott WN, editor: Ligament and extensor mechanism injuries to the knee: diagnosis and treatment, St Louis, 1991, Mosby, p 88, Fig 7-1.)*

Certain injuries are much more probable with various athletic activities. For example, a cross-country runner is more likely to exhibit patellofemoral pain due to the repetitive nature of running, whereas the female basketball or soccer player is more likely to injure the ACL. What activities make the symptoms worse? What activities improve the symptoms?

CHRONICITY

Next the clinician ascertains the duration, location, and intensity of pain. The clinician should attempt to determine the symptoms present initially after the injury in comparison to the present symptoms. Have the symptoms improved, stayed the same, or become worse? Symptoms are acute if they have been present for up to 7 to 10 days.[4] A subacute condition is one that has been present for more than 10 days but less than 7 weeks, whereas the chronic condition has been present for more than 7 weeks.[4] In general, a complaint of instability of the knee will warrant inspection of the ligamentous structures around the knee. Both catching and locking are common symptoms in the knee. Although not as common, true locking of the knee is generally the result of a torn meniscus or a large loose body that does not allow the knee to move through its normal arthrokinematic motions. Catching of the knee is common and is often confused with locking. Catching symptoms can be the result of meniscus tears, loose bodies, an inflamed synovial fold, or patellofemoral maltracking. Momentary locking, also known as pseudolocking, may be caused by any of the aforementioned conditions or from muscle inhibitory pain. Giving way can also occur due to reflex inhibition caused by a variety of painful knee conditions.

IRRITABILITY AND BEHAVIOR OF SYMPTOMS

The intensity of the patient's pain is a relative concept. We recommend the use of a subjective visual analog pain rating scale where "0" equals no pain and progresses sequentially to "10," which equals the worst pain ever experienced. Have the symptoms worsened, stayed the same, or improved? In most cases symptoms that are already improving have a better prognosis than those that are worsening.

PHYSICAL EXAMINATION

Observation

To fully appreciate any abnormalities of bony or soft tissue structures around the knee, the patient must be properly undressed. In all cases your patient needs a gown or shorts to allow adequate visualization of both the involved and the uninvolved knee. Observation should begin by viewing total lower extremity alignment for symmetry or asymmetry. This is followed by specific observation for findings that may include ecchymosis, joint effusion, or localized soft tissue edema.

It is important to view the knee from all angles to determine symmetric versus asymmetric structures. A comprehensive knowledge of the normal variance of the size and shape of structures around the knee is beneficial. Gait and ambulatory status should be evaluated, keeping in mind that in the large variety of knee injuries gait may be normal, or with an acute injury gait may not be tolerated and may require the use of an assistive device.

Anterior Observation

The anterior observation should begin by looking for any swelling, ecchymosis, or abrasions while the patient is in the standing position. Standing posture, gait pattern, and ambulatory ability should be observed and analyzed to detect any deviation from the norm. From a position anterior to the patient, observation for either genu varum or genu valgum positions of the knee can compare the injured with the uninjured extremity. These deformities can occur unilaterally or bilaterally and can potentially cause malalignment elsewhere.[4] When measuring the angle of the leg from a line drawn on the anterior side of the knee, a normal patient's alignment should range from 180 to 195 degrees, genu valgum would be less than 180 degrees, and an angle greater than 195 degrees is described as genu varum.[5] According to Magee,[4] one way to quickly screen for these postures is by having the patient positioned so that the patellae face forward and the medial aspects of the knees and medial malleoli of both limbs are as close together as possible. If the knees touch and the ankles do not, the patient has a genu valgum knee position.[4] If two or more fingers fit between the knees when the ankles are touching, the patient has a genu varum knee deformity.[6] Q-angle measures the relationship of the quadriceps muscle line of pull to the patellofemoral joint while the knee is extended. The position of the patella, which normally faces forward, can be ascertained in the standing position. Squinting patella will be seen in the person with internal tibial or femoral torsions. Femoral anteversion will cause a relative internal rotation of the femur along its long axis, resulting in the patella being located in a more medial position.

When viewing the actual patella itself, there is a normal 1 : 1 ratio between the patellar tendon length and the patellar height.[7] A longer patellar tendon will produce a patella alta or high-riding patella, whereas a shorter patellar tendon will produce a patellar baja or patella infera. We are in agreement with Woodland and Francis,[8] who feel that the Q-angle should be measured in a weight-bearing position in order to functionally evaluate the effects of lower extremity loading and foot posture.[8] A unilaterally high-riding patella with concomitant spasm of the quadriceps muscle would be indicative of a ruptured patellar tendon.[5] A visual observation of the overall mass of the quadriceps muscle tone can be seen from the front of the patient. Methods for measuring girth are described later in this chapter. An enlargement of the tibial tuberosity commonly known as Osgood-Schlatter disease can be seen at the proximal tibia.

Medial Observation

Several key structures are located on the medial side of the knee. An acute macrotraumatic injury with a lateral valgus fall and a quick onset of intraarticular effusion that causes medial knee pain and instability should make the clinician suspicious of injury to the MCL. Injury to the MCL will cause intraarticular swelling if the injury has ruptured the deep portions of the ligament, which leads to concomitant injury to the deep capsule. Injury to the superficial portions of the ligament may only cause minor edema to the area surrounding the MCL. Consequently, in special tests for knee effusion it is important to differentiate severity and injured structures, because they will require different treatment approaches. A history of microtraumatic stress may lead to a pes anserine tendonitis or bursitis. A small area of swelling may be seen at the distal attachment of the sartorius, gracilis, and semitendinosus tendons. Last, the vastus medialis obliquus should display normal muscle tone and girth compared with that of the opposite limb.[5] The vastus medialis muscle group has been shown to be the first to atrophy after injury.[5]

Posterior Observation

Swelling in the popliteal fossa can be indicative of several problems. First, posterior capsule swelling known as a Baker cyst (Figure 3-4) is a herniation of joint fluid into a bursa in the medial gastrocnemius muscle that can cause knee pain and swelling. Ecchymosis and extracapsular edema may be indicative of a distal hamstring or proximal gastrocnemius injury.

Lateral Observation

A lateral view can reveal the amount of knee hyperextension. Additionally, the presence of a camel sign may be noted on the lateral view. The camel sign is seen with an abnormally high-riding patella (patella alta). The high-riding patella appears similar to one hump of a camel's back, and the second camel hump is seen at the infrapatellar fat pad or inflamed infrapatellar bursa, just anterior to the fat pad.[4]

Gait

Observation of gait during the evaluation is critical to fully understand functional limitations caused by the presenting pathology. A self-protected, painful gait is described as *antalgic*.[4] Usually in this case the stance time on the affected leg is of shorter duration than that of the unaffected leg. Additionally, the swing phase is often shorter, resulting in a shortened step length on the involved side. Another common orthopedic gait pattern is the arthrogenic gait, due to stiffness in the affected joints.[4] The arthrogenic gait pattern may or may not be painful and is thought to result more from stiffness or deformity. The patient with this gait pattern may ambulate with the foot in plantar flexion on the opposite side to increase clearance, while the affected leg is circumducted at the hip. In many instances the patient may require the use

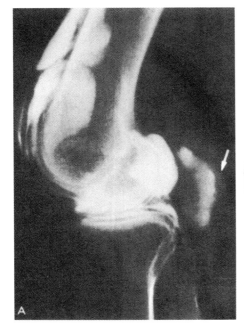
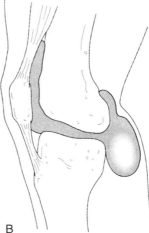

Figure 3-4: A, Popliteal (Baker's) cyst. **B,** Schematic diagram of Baker's cyst. *(A, From Reilly BM: Practical strategies in outpatient medicine, Philadelphia, 1991, Saunders, p 1179. B, From Magee DJ: Orthopedic physical assessment, ed 4, Philadelphia, 2002, Saunders, p 672.)*

of an assistive device. Adequate assessment of any ambulatory device requires assessment of sequencing, height, and actual use.

Palpation

Palpation does not generally correlate to the exact location of the patient pathology, but rather the symptom from the problem. However, Post and Fulkerson[9] determined that the area of sensitivity in the knee corresponds very closely with anterior knee pain. Post and Fulkerson[9] evaluated 90 patients with knee pain but were blinded from the patient's actual pain diagram. The physicians then filled out a pain diagram depicting where they thought the patient's pain was emanating from based on their physical examination and palpation. Based on their results, 85% of all patient complaint zones were included in the physician's diagram based on their own physical examination. Therefore, at least in the knee, areas of tenderness located on clinical examination do correspond to areas of patient complaint and may be very helpful in directing attention to specific areas during the remainder of the physical examination.

Most structures in the knee are easily palpable because of the lack of adipose tissue directly surrounding the knee. When performing the palpation portion of the examination, the therapist should assess for tissue temperature, effusion or edema, tissue thickness, or unusual nodules. When uncertain as to whether a finding is normal or abnormal, the therapist almost always can perform a bilateral comparison. Specific areas of palpation should routinely follow a methodical sequence, rather than random palpation, to ensure that critical areas are not missed. It is commonplace to palpate the area of most tenderness last so that the patient's pain is not elevated, potentially masking less involved areas or causing apprehension during the rest of the examination process.

Table 3-2 lists bony and soft tissue structures for palpation during the knee examination.

SCREENING EXAMINATION

A screening examination is always in order when examining the knee and surrounding structures. Several areas proximal to the knee can cause pain or symptoms mimicking structural knee pain. Lumbar spine radiculopathy can cause pain in or around the knee because of the primary nerve roots of L2 to L5. In children, hip pathology such as Legg-Calvé-Perthes disease may be seen by abnormalities of hip abduction with discomfort, whereas a loss of hip internal rotation could mean slipped capital femoral epiphysis. Each of these pathologies may initially cause knee pain. A screening examination of the lumbar spine; sacroiliac joint; hip, ankle, and foot range of motion (ROM); myotome testing; and neurologic assessment should be sufficient to notice pathology arising from other potential locales.

Range of Motion

Range of motion of the knee must take into account the various surrounding muscles and their propensity to become tight or of insufficient length when testing. In short, ROM must be differentiated from muscle flexibility.

To determine active range of motion (AROM) of knee flexion, the patient is generally asked to flex his or her knee actively, keeping the foot off the supporting surface. Because the patient is lying supine, the proximal hip is already stabilized. With passive range of motion (PROM) testing, the patient is allowed to scoot or pull his or her tibia back toward the buttocks. Measurement locations are the same as for AROM testing. One should notice a soft tissue end feel of passive knee flexion that is due to compression of the

---

TABLE 3-2

Bony and Soft Tissue Palpation of the Knee

BONY STRUCTURES	MUSCULAR STRUCTURES	OTHER STRUCTURES
Patella	Vastus medialis	Patellar tendon
Inferior pole	Vastus lateralis	Patellar retinaculum
Superior pole	Rectus femoris	Knee bursa
Tibial tubercle	Biceps femoris	Synovial plica
Adductor tubercle	Semitendinosus	Medial collateral ligament
Medial femoral condyle	Semimembranosus	Lateral collateral ligament
Medial tibial plateau	Gracillis	Superior capsule
Lateral femoral condyle	Sartorius	
Lateral tibial plateau	Tensor fascia lata	
Patellar facets	Iliotibial band	
Tibiofemoral joint line	Adductor muscle group	
Fibular head	Gastrocnemius	
Gerdy's tubercle		

hamstrings and the gastrocnemius and soleus with full knee flexion. Knee extension measurement landmarks remain the same. We measure knee extension passively by placing a bolster or towel roll under the heel, propping it higher than the knee in case the subject has genu recurvatum (Figure 3-5). Active knee extension is measured while the patient performs a straight leg raise. Many individuals normally exhibit up to 10 degrees of knee hyperextension. See Table 3-3 for normal knee range of motion. The end feel for knee hyperextension should be firm because of tissue in the posterior knee capsule.

Flexibility

Muscular structures of the knee commonly demonstrate insufficient length. To make most efficient use of time, these

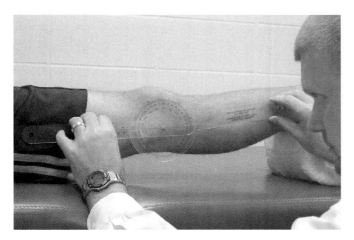

Figure 3-5: Passive knee extension goniometry.

various structures should be tested first in supine position during that portion of assessment followed by the prone position when that portion of the examination is done.

We test for hamstring flexibility in the 90/90 position (90 degrees of hip flexion and 90 degrees of knee flexion). From the 90/90 position, the knee is passively extended while the femur is maintained in the same vertical starting position (Figure 3-6, *A*).

The Thomas test measures hip flexor (iliopsoas) tightness in the supine position. With the patient supine and the lower legs off the edge of the table, the uninvolved hip is passively flexed. Once the contralateral hip is flexed to a position of approximately 125 degrees, the amount of contralateral hip flexion and contralateral knee extension is noted. This position for testing is sought for consistency with each measurement. A tight iliopsoas muscle will result in contralateral hip flexion. If the involved thigh is off the examining table, a goniometer can be used to measure the angle from table to the thigh to better allow objectivity. While in this same position, the clinician can assess the rectus femoris with the Kendall test.[4] While still supine in the same position as the end of the Thomas test, a tight rectus femoris will result in contralateral knee extension or inability to flex the knee without a greater amount of concomitant contralateral hip flexion. We believe that the knee should be able to be passively flexed in this position to about 90 to 110 degrees for adequate muscle tendon flexibility. A common compensatory pattern during the Kendall test is known as the "J" sign, which occurs when the hip falls into abduction as the contralateral limb is flexed.[4]

The presence of inflexibility of the tensor fascia latae muscle and the iliotibial tract can be assessed via the Ober's test (with knee flexed) and modified Ober's test (with knee straight). With the patient in a side-lying position, the

TABLE 3-3

Average Knee Ranges of Motion

	AMERICAN ACADEMY OF ORTHOPEDIC SURGEONS*	KENDALL, MCCREARY, AND PROVANCE†	HOPPENFELD‡	AMERICAN MEDICAL ASSOCIATION§
Flexion	0-135	0-140	0-135	0-150
Hyperextension	0-10	0	0	NA
Internal rotation	0-10			
External rotation	0-10			

Adapted from Norkin CC, White DJ: *Measurement of joint motion: a guide to goniometry,* ed 2, Philadelphia, 1995, FA Davis.
*American Academy of Orthopedic Surgeons: *Joint motion: method of measuring and recording,* Chicago, 1965, American Academy of Orthopedic Surgeons.
†Kendall FP, McCreary EK, Provance PG: *Muscle testing and function with posture and pain,* ed 4, Baltimore, 1993, Williams & Wilkins.
‡Hoppenfeld S: *Physical examination of the spine and extremities,* New York, 1976, Appleton-Century-Crofts.
§American Medical Association: *Guides to the evaluation of permanent impairment,* ed 3, Chicago, 1998, American Medical Association.

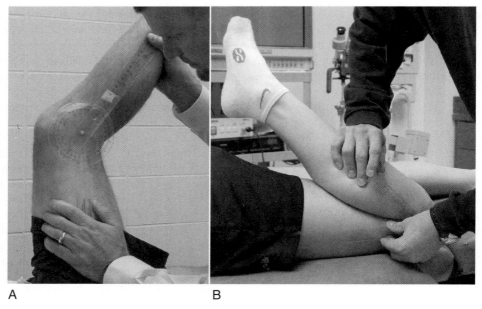

Figure 3-6: A, Hamstring flexibility testing. **B,** Rectus femoris flexibility testing.

examiner stands behind and holds the patient's uppermost knee in either full extension or partial flexion. The examiner then passively abducts and extends the patient's hip and allows the limb to drop into hip adduction. A positive test is present if the limb remains abducted with the muscles totally relaxed.[4] A critical component of this test is to extend the hip slightly so that the ITB passes over the greater trochanter of the femur.[4]

Because the rectus femoris muscle crosses both the knee and the hip joints, it can become passively insufficient. Since the hip is flexed during supine testing of knee ROM, the proximal portion of the rectus femoris is placed on slack; therefore inflexibility is rarely seen during ROM testing of knee flexion in this position. Ely's test is performed while lying prone and placing the hip in neutral or extension, which places the rectus femoris on a stretch proximally at the hip and again distally once the knee is flexed.[4] When the knee is flexed from this prone position, the rectus is dramatically lengthened and often exhibits muscular tightness (Figure 3-6, *B*). The clinician needs to be aware of the common compensatory pattern of flexing the hip while measuring rectus muscle flexibility.

NEUROLOGIC EXAMINATION

Sensation

Although not commonly a problem during the routine knee examination, problems dealing with decreased sensation are common postoperatively. Examination of sensation can be important to determine if cutaneous neurologic impairment in a dermatomal distribution is present (Figure 3-7). Light touch, pinprick, and thermal discrimination can be determined at each dermatome level if needed. This evaluation

will be compared with the uninvolved extremity to detect differences from side to side. Simple, quick examinations of sharp and dull can utilize a pinwheel or the blunt end of the reflex hammer. Running the fingers softly over the dermatomes bilaterally can assess light touch. While testing dermatomes, the patient should close his or her eyes or turn the head so that the patient does not use visual stimulation to determine sensation.

Reflexes

Reflexes for the patella (L4) and the hamstrings (L5) should be examined and compared bilaterally. Reflexes are rated on a 0 to 4 scale with 0/4 = absent reflexes, 1/4 = hyporeactive reflexes, 2/4 = normal response, 3/4 = hypertonic reflexes, and 4/4 = clonus.[4] Reflexes are best tested with the patient relaxed as much as possible. If your patient is in severe pain, reflex testing may not be accurate because of muscle guarding during the testing maneuvers. To test the patellar tendon reflex (L4), the clinician should instruct the patient to sit on the edge of the examining table with the knee flexed to 90 degrees. Using the reflex hammer, the clinician should tap the middle of the patellar tendon and assess the response (Figure 3-8). The hamstring (L5) tendon reflex is tested with the patient prone on the examining table with the knee passively flexed approximately 30 to 40 degrees. The clinician will percuss his or her own thumb with the small (sharp) end of the reflex hammer as it rests on the hamstring tendons (Figure 3-9). If reflexes are difficult to obtain with conventional testing, the patient can be asked to clench the teeth or pull the arms apart by squeezing the fingers of each hand and pulling the arms apart,[4] enlisting the Jendrassik maneuver to additionally facilitate the reflex response.[10,11] The Jendrassik maneuver activity increases the facilitative activity of the

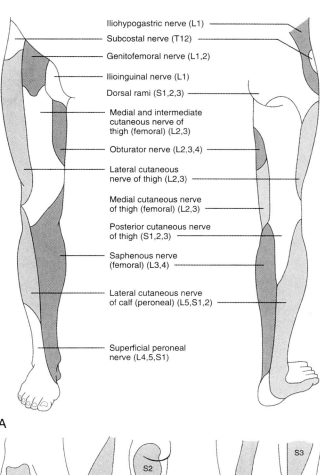

A

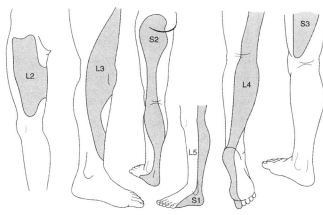

B

Figure 3-7: A, Peripheral nerve sensory distribution about the knee. **B,** Dermatomes about the knee. *(From Magee DJ: Orthopedic physical assessment, ed 4, Philadelphia, 2002, Saunders, pp 735 and 736, Figs 12-127 and 12-128.)*

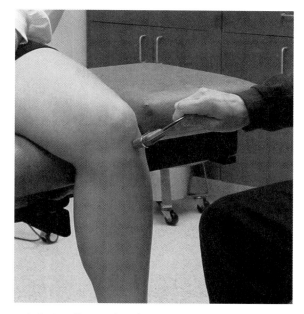

Figure 3-8: Patellar tendon deep tendon reflex.

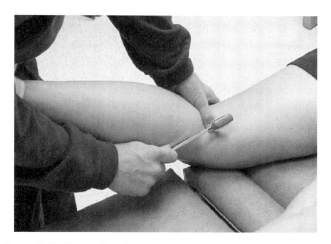

Figure 3-9: Hamstring deep tendon reflex.

spinal cord, thereby accentuating a minimally active reflex.[12] If a higher reflex is found using this technique, it should be noted that this facilitation was used.

Proprioception and Kinesthesia

Proprioception was initially described by Sherrington[13] as the afferent information from "proprioceptors" located in the "proprioceptive field" that contributes to conscious sensations, total posture, and segmental posture. Proprioceptors are those receptors located in joints, muscles, and tendons that were "adapted for excitation consonantly with changes going on in the organism itself."[13] *Kinesthesia* is defined as a submodality of proprioception sense associated with the sensation of joint movement or joint position, either from internal forces (active) or external forces (passive).[14]

There are several ways that the clinical components of joint proprioception can be measured. Kinesthesia, or perception of joint position, can be measured objectively. Reproduction either actively or passively through joint repositioning can be measured clinically. The clinician can place the patient's limb in a desired position for a duration of up to 10 seconds. This gives the blindfolded patient an adequate amount of time to focus mentally on this position. The clinician then moves the limb back to the starting position and asks the patient to actively reproduce the position. The clinician measures the amount of error, in degrees, that occurred during the joint repositioning. The uninvolved extremity can be used as a control for the injured extremity.

Balance is the body's coordinated neuromuscular response to maintain equilibrium.[15] We have found that one of the oldest ways to assess balance, the single-leg stance, is often too easy because it only assesses static balance. We have found it more beneficial to assess dynamic balance through lower extremity excursion testing. While standing on a single leg, the patient reaches as far as possible in multiple directions with the contralateral extremity. The distance from the front of the stance foot to the front of the reaching foot is recorded. The distance reached with the involved extremity is compared with that of the uninvolved extremity.[16] Manske and Anderson[17] have found the lower extremity excursion test to be very reliable, with an intraclass correlation coefficient of 0.94 to 0.98. Additionally, Hertel and colleagues[18] found intraclass correlation coefficients of 0.82 to 0.96 for the same test, which they call the star excursion balance test. Manske and Anderson[17] also found no differences between dominant and nondominant lower extremity scores with healthy subjects performing the lower extremity functional reach test. This is important so that the uninvolved extremity can be used as a reference or control limb during balance testing.

MANUAL MUSCLE TESTING

Manual muscle testing (MMT) allows the clinician to assess strength of either individual muscles or groups of muscles commonly used around the knee. During MMT, the clinician applies a manual resistance to the extremity, which is placed in a specifically designed position based on the muscle size, the length/tension relationship of the muscle, and the effects of gravity. The strength of a given muscle or group of muscles can then be compared bilaterally to determine weakness.[19,20] Manual muscle testing procedures described in this text utilize some of the standard theories described in MMT texts, although positions used may be slightly different to allow a more expedient examination. See texts such as Kendall, McCreary, and Provance[21] and Daniels and Worthingham[22] for descriptions of MMT procedures. We commonly use the "make to" test when applying resistance to the tested muscles or groups of muscles. During this form of testing, the examiner gradually increases the amount of manual resistance as the patient is increasing resistance to the maximum level that he or she can tolerate. We believe that this form of testing is more comfortable to the patient and less painful than the standard break test. We have seen on

occasion those who misuse the standard break test by not allowing adequate time for generation of muscle force production, thus giving inaccurate results. If using the standard break test, we caution the clinician to give the patient at minimum approximately 5 seconds to contract the tested muscle group before applying significant resistance to allow a more accurate assessment of strength.

Grades of strength can be determined in several ways. We most commonly use the 5-point scale, although other methods can be used, such as the 10-point scale; percentages; and wording such as normal, good, fair, poor, trace, and zero (Table 3-4).

The knee extensor group is tested in the seated position. Performing knee extension uses the quadriceps muscle, which is a summation of numerous muscles including the rectus femoris, vastus intermedius, vastus lateralis, vastus medialis longus, and oblique. None of the component muscles of the quadriceps group has the ability to be tested in isolation. The patient should be allowed to lean backward in the tripod position to relieve tension from the hamstrings. The patient should extend the knee until there is slight flexion. Testing the extensor strength in full extension or into hyperextension approximates the closed-packed position of the knee and allows maximum articular congruency and maximal ligamentous tightness. Furthermore, this extended position allows the screw home mechanism, leaving the knee in a much more stable position. The examiner's hand gives resistance over the ventral surface of the lower leg just above the ankle in the direction of knee flexion.

Testing the hamstrings is most commonly described in the prone position, but we commonly screen for weakness in the seated position. We believe that despite testing in the seated position, we can still delineate weakness between the medial and lateral hamstring muscle groups. While seated, the patient is asked to flex his or her knee to 90 degrees. The examiner places his or her hand on the dorsal surface of the patient's lower leg just proximal to the ankle joint. When testing the hamstring muscles in aggregate, the examiner applies a force to the lower leg in the direction of straight knee extension while the patient's foot is kept neutral. When testing the biceps femoris, the patient is asked to externally rotate the tibia, which preferentially recruits the biceps femoris. With the foot and ankle held in external rotation, the examiner applies an anterior-directed force. To test the semitendinosus and semimembranosus, the patient is asked to internally rotate his or her foot and ankle, preferentially recruiting those specific muscles. With any of the tests for the hamstring muscle group, watch carefully for active dorsiflexion, in an attempt by the patient to use the tenodesis effect of the gastrocnemius muscle group.

SPECIAL TESTING

Following standard tests of ROM, musculoskeletal strength assessment, sensation, and reflexes, the clinician requires further testing to determine specific causes of pathology. The clinician will use special tests to help rule out or implicate tissues or structures at fault.

An important concept worth mentioning before discussing special tests, particularly special tests for ligamentous instability, is the concept of primary versus secondary restraints. Ligaments of the knee are responsible for providing limitation of motion (restraint) in various fashions.[23] A ligament may work as a primary or a secondary restraint. For a given motion, the primary restraint is the one that provides the greatest limitation to instability. When the primary structure is disrupted, the structure that then provides the restraint to movement is considered the secondary restraint. Thus disruption of a secondary restraint while the primary is still intact results in minimal or no unusual joint laxity. Much more appreciable is the enhanced pathologic motion that can be seen when both primary and secondary restraints are disrupted. A good example in the knee can be seen with the MCL and the ACL. The MCL is the primary restraint to a valgus force at the knee, yet it is also a secondary restraint to anterior translation. A pure MCL injury, if isolated, will not cause anterior displacement of the tibia as long as the ACL is intact. However, if the ACL is disrupted, the MCL will be one of the structures that helps limit anterior translation, because it is a secondary restraint to anterior motion of the tibia with a deficient ACL. This anterior motion will be further exaggerated if both the MCL and ACL are disrupted.

This chapter uses Davies' knee special testing algorithm[24] to allow a systematic examination of the knee in a fast, efficient, and appropriate manner. This algorithm was specifically designed so that most knee structures can be evaluated in an efficient manner with minimal patient position changes.

Joint Effusion

Swelling can be either edema or effusion of the knee joint and can cause pain, muscle inhibition, and decreased ROM. A moderate to severe amount of swelling in the knee can easily be seen by the naked eye, whereas minor effusions may go unseen. Knee effusions have been commonly implicated as causing reflex inhibition to the vasti muscles of the anterior knee.[25-28] Previously it has been shown that only 50 to 60 ml of fluid in the knee joint can inhibit the rectus femoris and the vastus lateralis, and it takes only a scant 20 to 30 ml of fluid to inhibit the vastus medialis.[26] Circumferential measurements can be taken at various locations around the knee to assess objectively for joint swelling and effusion

TABLE 3-4

Manual Muscle Testing Grading Systems

FUNCTION OF MUSCLE					SYMBOLS			
No Movement								
No contraction felt in muscle	Zero	0	0	0	(0)	(0.0)	0%	0
Tendon becomes prominent or feeble contraction felt in muscle, but no visible movement of the part	Trace	T	T	1	(1)	(1.0)	T	T
Movement in Horizontal Plane								
Moves through partial range of motion	Poor−	P−	1	2−	(1½)	(1.5)	10%	1
Moves through complete range of motion	Poor	P	2	2	(2)	(2.0)	20%	2
Moves to completion of range against resistance or moves to completion of range and holds against pressure	Poor+	P+	3	2+	(2⅓)	(2.33)	30%	3
Antigravity Position								
Moves through partial range of motion	Poor+	P+	3	2+	(2⅓)	(2.33)	30%	3
Gradual release from test position	Fair−	F−	4	3−	(2⅔)	(2.66)	40%	4
Holds test position (no added pressure)	Fair	F	5	3	(3)	(3.0)	50%	5
Holds test position against slight pressure	Fair+	F+	6	3+	(3⅓)	(3.33)	60%	6
Holds test position against slight to moderate pressure	Good−	G−	7	4−	(3⅔)	(3.66)	70%	7
Holds test position against moderate pressure	Good	G	8	4	(4)	(4.0)	80%	8
Holds test position against moderate to strong pressure	Good+	G+	9	4+	(4½)	(4.5)	90%	9
Holds test position against strong resistance	Normal	N	10	5	(5)	(5.0)	100%	10

From Kendall FP, McCreary EK, Provance PG: *Muscle testing and function with posture and pain*, ed 4, Baltimore, 1993, Williams & Wilkins.

(Table 3-5).[29,30] Measurements similar to this have been shown to be a reliable method of assessing joint effusion.[31]

Special tests used to determine effusion include the milking test and the patellar ballottement test. The milking test can be used to determine an intraarticular effusion. The patient lies supine with knees in full extension or the position of comfort. If there is significant effusion, the knee will seek the position of maximum volume of approximately 30 degrees of knee flexion. This position will cause the patient to keep the knee in a slightly flexed position because of pain when tension is placed on the already tight capsule. The clinician gives pressure with one hand along the tibial plateau at the location of the inferior portion of the joint capsule. With his or her other hand, the clinician gives pressure both medially and laterally running proximal to distal along the distal thigh in an attempt to push any intraarticular fluid out of the superior capsule into the inferior portion of the capsule. The clinician then brushes one side of the joint, looking for a fluid wave along the other side of the joint (Figure 3-10). Even a small joint effusion can become much more apparent using this test.

In the patellar ballottement test,[4] the knee is placed in full extension or in a position of comfort. The clinician stands alongside the extremity to be tested and applies gentle pressure to the anterior patella to attempt to cause a posterior displacement (Figure 3-11). The patella is then released. If a significant effusion is present, the patella will "bob" anteriorly after pressure is released. This test will feel very similar to pushing down with fingers on a full water balloon and feeling the balloon push back once pressure is released.

Static Patellofemoral Position, Mobility, and Subluxation

While the patient is still in the supine position, the next set of tests in the algorithm, which are specific for the patellofemoral joint, are performed. To begin, the patella can be assessed for its resting position relative to the femoral condyles. Both orientation and mobility are best described by the patella's four components of motion: patellar glide, medial

and lateral tilt, rotation, and anterior and posterior tilt. One of the more common abnormalities is the resting position of lateral glide. With the patella resting in this position, the distance from the medial epicondyle of the femur to the center of the patella is greater than the distance from the

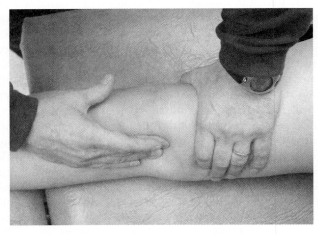

Figure 3-10: Milking test for joint effusion.

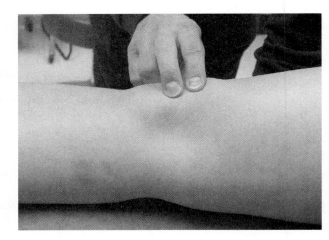

Figure 3-11: Patellar ballottement test.

TABLE 3-5

Circumferential Location and Clinical Rationale

LOCATION OF MEASUREMENT	CLINICAL RATIONALE
20 cm proximal to joint line	Quadriceps atrophy (generalized)
10 cm proximal to joint line	Quadriceps atrophy (more specific to vastus medialis obliquus) or suprapatellar pouch for effusion
Joint line	General effusion
15 cm distal to joint line	Gastrocnemius/soleus atrophy or lower leg edema

From Manske RC, Davies GJ: A nonsurgical approach to examination and treatment of the patellofemoral joint, part I: examination of the patellofemoral joint, *Crit Rev Phys Rehabil Med* 15(2):141-166, 2003.

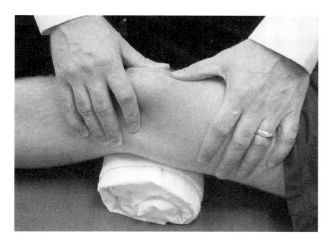

Figure 3-12: Passive patellar glide test.

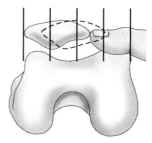

Figure 3-13: Assessment of patellar mobility medially and laterally. The patellofemoral joint can be mentally divided into quadrants and patellar mobility assessed in both directions. *(From Walsh WM: Recurrent dislocation of the knee in adolescents. In DeLee JC, Drez D, Miller MD, editors: DeLee and Drez's orthopedic sports medicine principles and practice, vol 2, Philadelphia, 2003, Saunders, p 1722.)*

lateral epicondyle of the femur to the center of the patella. A resting position of medial patellar glide is a very rare case, reserved for those patients who might have received an overzealous lateral-release surgical procedure.

Although we commonly use the procedure described previously to assess static patellar position, we also concede that this method of testing is problematic. Tomsich and colleagues[32] assessed the reliability of visual assessment of patellar orientation. Testing order of both the subjects and the therapists was randomized during this study. Intratester kappa coefficients ranged from 0.40 to 0.57, demonstrating questionable reliability. Even lower were scores for intertester reliability, ranging from 0.01 to 0.30.

Both passive medial and lateral glide positions of the patella are performed to assess the superficial retinacular fibers.[33] This test is performed with the patient supine and knee flexed to about 20 to 30 degrees. The patient's involved extremity has the quadriceps relaxed while the clinician glides the patella both medially and laterally with a cupping position of the fingers while preventing a patellar tilt (Figure 3-12). By dividing the patella into four quadrants, objective descriptions of the amount of translation can be measured (Figure 3-13). In a normal individual without pathology the patella should glide a distance of about two quadrants, or one half the width of the patella. A lateral glide of three or more quadrants is considered hypermobile and indicative of incompetent medial restraints such as the medial retinaculum and medial patellofemoral ligament. A medial glide of one quadrant or less is consistent with a tight lateral superficial retinaculum. A displacement medially of three or more quadrants is considered a hypermobile patella.[33]

A straight lateral glide test is also known as the patellar apprehension test of Fairbank.[34] This test is performed in the same position and technique as the prior test for lateral passive patellar glide. If the patient senses instability in the knee, he or she will actively contract the quadriceps muscle in an attempt to prevent the patella from subluxing or dislocating laterally. A positive test is an indication of

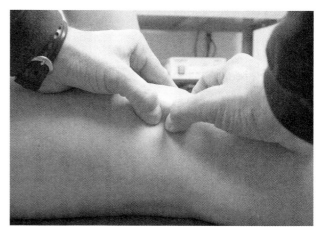

Figure 3-14: Medial tilt of patella to check for tight deep lateral retinaculum.

"apprehension" from the passive lateral translation of the patella and is commonly pathognomonic for patellar instability.

A patellar position of a medial and lateral tilt can also cause pathology. The passive medial and lateral patellar tilt test is commonly used to assess the deep fibers of the patellar retinaculum. In this test the patient lies supine with his or her knees fully extended and the quadriceps relaxed. The clinician attempts to gently lift the lateral border of the patella away from the lateral femoral condyle (Figure 3-14). Normal mobility of the deep portion of the patellar retinaculum will allow up to 15 degrees of medial tilt (Figure 3-15). A patella that can only be tilted medially to neutral (i.e., with the patella's anterior surface parallel to the floor) or less would be consistent with restricted deep lateral retinacular fibers and further classified as hypomobile. Greater than 15 degrees of medial tilt would be considered hypermobile.

To prevent unnecessary moving of the patient, patellar tracking can be performed next while still in the seated position. When assessing whether patellar tracking is

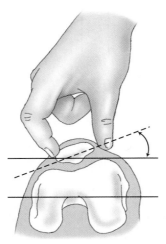

Figure 3-15: Passive patellar tilt test. In this left knee, the patella can be tilted so that the lateral edge is well anterior to the medial edge. *(From Walsh WM: Recurrent dislocation of the knee in adolescents. In DeLee JC, Drez D, Miller MD, editors: DeLee and Drez's orthopedic sports medicine principles and practice, vol 2, Philadelphia, 2003, Saunders, p 1721.)*

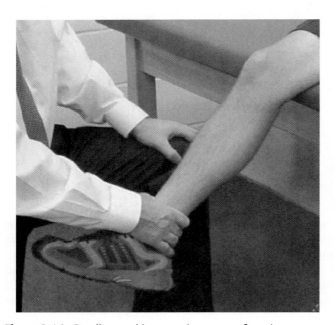

Figure 3-16: Patellar tracking: passive range of motion.

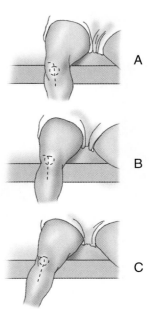

Figure 3-17: J sign. As the knee is extended from a 90-degree flexed position **(A)** to a fully extended position **(C)**, the patella describes an exaggerated inverted J-shaped course, indicating predominance of laterally directed forces. *(From Walsh WM: Recurrent dislocation of the knee in adolescents. In DeLee JC, Drez D, Miller MD, editors: DeLee and Drez's orthopedic sports medicine principles and practice, vol 2, Philadelphia, 2003, Saunders, p 1718.)*

position at 90 degrees of knee flexion. As the knee is passively extended, the patella will follow the trochlear groove of the femur and move in a slightly medial direction until full terminal extension, at which time the patella tracks back slightly laterally because of the attachment of the tibial tubercle. The quality and quantity of motion should be assessed and compared with the uninvolved extremity. An abrupt lateral jump at the end of terminal extension is commonly called a *pathologic J sign.*[35] The term *J sign* refers to the inverted J-shaped course of the patella as it follows the trochlear groove (Figure 3-17). Passive patellar tracking assesses status of the noncontractile tissue around the knee.

Active patellar tracking assesses the contractile tissue and can be performed by having the patient actively extend the knee from a position of 90 degrees of flexion to full knee extension (Figure 3-18). While still in the tripod position, a sharp lateral deviation toward the end of knee extension while testing actively may be indicative of an inadequate vastus medialis obliquus (VMO) muscle. This may particularly be the case when the clinician assesses passive patellar tracking as normal, followed by active tracking in which the patella moves laterally at terminal extension.

Further testing of patellar tracking can be performed in the closed kinetic chain position during a mini-squat. As with the other tests of patellar tracking, the patella should engage the sulcus at about 20 to 30 degrees of knee flexion. Pain during the closed chain mini-squat may indicate chondral changes to the posterior patella. Additionally,

dysfunctional, the clinician should assess both passive and active tracking to determine if the tracking pathology is caused by either contractile or noncontractile components. To assess noncontractile components, the patient is seated comfortably in the tripod position. The clinician grasps the patient's foot and passively extends the knee from a position of 90 degrees of knee flexion to full knee extension (Figure 3-16). Generally, the patella engages the femoral condyles at about 20 to 30 degrees of knee flexion. In a normally functioning knee, the patella should rest in a slightly lateral

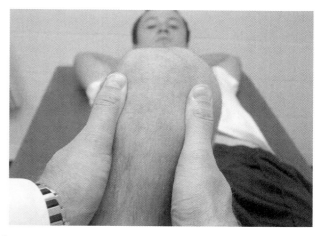

Figure 3-20: Step-up test for posterior cruciate ligament deficiency. Thumbs are parallel to the patellar tendon so that the proximal phalanx is on the tibial plateau, interphalangeal joint at the joint line, and thumb pads placed on distal end of the femur.

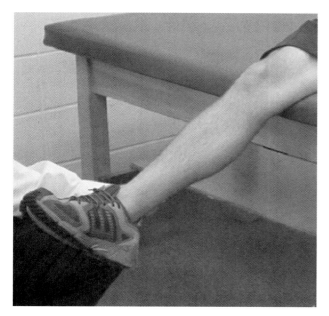

Figure 3-18: Patellar tracking: active range of motion.

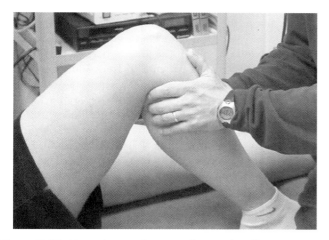

Figure 3-19: Posterior sag for posterior cruciate ligament deficiency at 80 degrees of knee flexion to prevent "chock-block" effect of meniscus.

peripatellar crepitus may be noted with this test. Pain during this test could also cause quadriceps shutdown, resulting in abnormal tracking patterns.

Cruciate Ligament Testing

The tibial sag sign can be performed in several variations. The first method can be tested in 80 degrees of knee flexion and 45 degrees of hip flexion while the patient lies supine with quadriceps and hamstring muscles relaxed (Figure 3-19). If a PCL is ruptured, the tibia will appear to sag posteriorly, creating a concave appearance to the patellar tendon. The Clancy step-up test is one way to quickly assess for this injury and is performed by placing thumb pads on the femoral

condyles while the interphalangeal joints of the thumb are at the knee joint line and the tibial plateau. In a stable knee, the anterior portion of the tibial plateau is located approximately 1 cm anterior to the distal femoral condyles with the knee in 80 degrees of flexion. Therefore a slight step-up exists from the patient's femoral condyle to the anterior tibia (Figure 3-20). Absence of this step-up is indicative of a PCL tear. This injury may also include pathology to the posterior capsular structures, including the posterior medial oblique ligament and the arcuate complex.[36]

The posterior drawer test is performed with the patient supine and the involved hip flexed 45 degrees and the knee flexed 80 degrees while the clinician holds the involved tibia in a neutral position. The position of 80 degrees of knee flexion is used to prevent the meniscus' ability to act as a "chock block" during this test. While using his or her thumbs to palpate the proximal tibial plateau, the clinician gives a posteriorly directed force onto the proximal tibia while feeling for both quantity of movement and quality of the end feel (Figure 3-21). A positive test result would be indicated if the involved tibia moves further posteriorly on the femur than does the uninvolved tibia.

The next several tests are used to assess the ACL. The anterior drawer (AD) test is a common test to determine ACL function. Katz and Fingeroth[37] report sensitivity of the AD test to be 40.9%, whereas it is 96.8% specific. Sung-Jae Kim and Hyun-Kon Kim[38] report that the AD test was positive in 79.6% of patients with a confirmed arthroscopic diagnosis of ACL rupture. Several conditions can cause a false-positive finding when performing the AD test. Problems include hamstring muscle spasm, presence of a tense hemarthrosis, or the "chock-block" action of the meniscus.[39] In addition, when the knee is flexed to 80 to 90 degrees, secondary structures that restrain anterior tibial translation may become taut, not allowing as much anterior excursion.

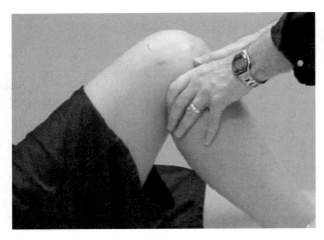

Figure 3-21: Posterior glide at 80 degrees of knee flexion to prevent the meniscus' ability to act as a "chock block."

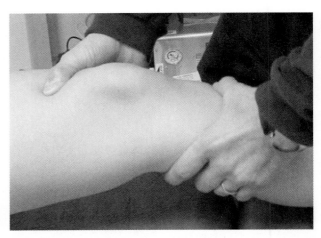

Figure 3-23: Lachman test for anterior cruciate ligament deficiency.

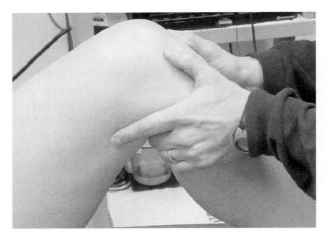

Figure 3-22: Anterior drawer test for anterior cruciate ligament deficiency.

In this position of knee flexion, the anterior medial band of the ACL is selectively taut, so the AD test more specifically examines that portion.

To perform the AD test, the patient lies supine with the knee flexed 80 to 90 degrees and the hip flexed 45 degrees. The clinician sits at the foot of the examining table while sitting atop the patient's affected neutral forefoot, stabilizing the distal end of the extremity (Figure 3-22). The clinician's hands are placed around the proximal tibia in such a way that the fingers are on the dorsal surface of the proximal tibia, palpating the hamstring muscles to ensure relaxation. The clinician's thumbs fall along the medial and lateral joint lines to enable an objective assessment of tibial excursion. The clinician then draws the proximal tibia forward on the stable femur. The clinician assesses both the amount of anterior excursion and the end feel. A positive result on an AD test could implicate injury to noncontractile structures, including the ACL anteromedial bundle, middle and posterior one-third medial and lateral capsule, MCL deep fibers, iliotibial

band, posterior oblique ligament, arcuate complex, and PCL.[4,36,40]

Probably the most recognized test for one-plane anterior instability is the Lachman test. Being the "gold standard" test for anterior instability, the Lachman test has been reported to better assess the integrity of both bands of the ACL because of the knee position. The accuracy of this test in experienced hands is 85% in the unanesthetized patient and 100% in the anesthetized patient.[41,42] Katz and Fingeroth[37] found the Lachman test to be 81.8% sensitive and 96.8% specific, and Flemming and colleagues[43] report up to 95% sensitivity. Lack of patient relaxation, difficulty with testing a large extremity, and control of knee flexion are several of the disadvantages of using the Lachman test. Torg and colleagues[44] also report several factors that may cause problems with interpreting the Lachman test. These include a tear of the posterior horn of the medial meniscus, hamstring spasm, and increased knee capsular tension from a hemarthrosis.[44]

To perform the Lachman test, the patient lies supine on the examination table with the clinician holding the injured extremity in approximately 30 degrees of knee flexion. The clinician's outside hand will hold the patient's femur firmly, while the inside hand grasps the proximal portion of the tibia (Figure 3-23). A clinical pearl is to place the elbow of the outside arm on the examiner's iliac crest to assist in stabilization of the femur. The clinician should very slightly rotate the tibia externally while applying an anterior tibial translation force to the posterior medial portion of the tibia. A positive test occurs if the translation ends in a soft end feel and the amount of laxity found is greater than that when testing the contralateral, noninjured knee. It must be noted that a false-positive result with this test can easily occur in the patient with a torn PCL. With a torn PCL, the tibia will be resting in a position posterior to its normal. When performing the Lachman test in the patient with a PCL tear, the tibia will have a greater amount of anterior translation because it is resting in a more posterior position than the uninjured extremity. This is one reason that testing for the PCL is done before testing for the ACL when using the knee special testing algorithm.

The Lachman and AD tests are both used to test the ACL for straight anterior (single-plane) laxity caused by ligament rupture. Because other secondary structures may become involved, it is important to assess for rotary (multiplane) instability. Numerous tests have been devised with this in mind. Galway and colleagues[45] first described the classic pivot shift test as a forward subluxation of the lateral tibial plateau on the femoral condyle in extension and the spontaneous reduction in flexion. Now this classic description has become the name of the test used to replicate this movement of the tibia on the femur. Several authors have described other structures that would be injured when a pivot shift is positive, including the mid-third lateral capsular ligaments,[46] the posterolateral capsule,[47] and the iliotibial band.[48]

The first test described will be the hyperextension recurvatum test[49], which is performed with the knee in a position of full extension. Standing at the foot of the examining table, the clinician assesses the amount of passive hyperextension of the injured knee in comparison with the uninjured knee. The clinician grasps the hallux of each foot and, with the quadriceps completely relaxed, allows the knee to fully hyperextend (Figure 3-24). A knee with a torn PCL or posterolateral capsule will demonstrate a greater amount of passive knee hyperextension on the lateral aspect of the joint than on the uninjured knee. If a posterolateral rotation instability also exists, a lateral or external rotation of the tibia may be seen.

To perform the pivot shift test, the clinician grasps the patient's lower leg with the distal hand around the foot and the proximal hand at the knee joint with the thumb behind the fibular head. While the knee is fully extended, the distal hand applies an internal rotation force to the tibia distally via the foot and ankle, while the proximally placed hand is used to exert a valgus stress to the tibia. The knee is slowly flexed.

When the test is positive, the tibia will subluxate anteriorly and then reduce as the knee is flexed (Figure 3-25). This reduction generally occurs at around 20 to 40 degrees of knee flexion as the iliotibial (IT) band suddenly reduces the tibia posteriorly, as it moves from a knee extensor to a knee flexor, thereby pulling the tibia into its correct position. To have a positive pivot shift test, the subluxation must first occur, followed by a relocation of the lateral tibia. When the result is positive, this test can cause a significant "clunk."[47] The Hughston jerk test is a modification of the pivot shift test.[23] Still in the supine position, the clinician supports the lower extremity with the knee flexed approximately 90 degrees with the tibia internally rotated. A valgus stress again is exerted on the proximal tibia while the knee is slowly extended. A subluxation of the tibia becomes evident at approximately 30 degrees of flexion and is perceived as a "jerk" by the patient and clinician. As the clinician further extends the knee, the tibia will eventually become reduced.

A normally functioning IT band is required to have a true positive pivot shift or jerk test. An intact IT band prohibits tibial subluxation in full extension and after about 40 degrees of knee flexion.[23] In between those ROMs, a pivot shift can occur. The posterior pull of the IT band is responsible for reducing the tibia at greater than 40 degrees of knee flexion. As the knee is flexed beyond 40 degrees, the IT band becomes tightened as it moves from a position more anterior to the knee axis of flexion to a position more posterior to the knee axis of flexion, causing the internally rotated tibia to reduce.[23] With the jerk test the sequence is just reversed.

The flexion-rotation drawer test[48,49] is more comfortable for the patient. The clinician grasps the knee with both hands while the patient's ankle is held between the clinician's arm and trunk. Initially the clinician will hold the patient's knee in approximately 15 degrees of knee flexion, which is the position from which the tibia is subluxed (Figure 3-26). In this position the ACL is lax and the patient's femur drops backward and rotates externally relative to the tibia. The

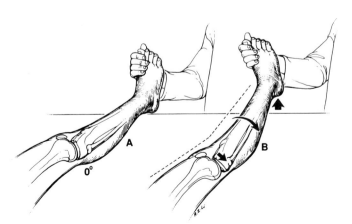

Figure 3-24: Hyperextension recurvatum test. (From Tria AJ, editor: Ligaments of the knee. In Klein KS: *An illustrated guide to the knee,* New York, 1992, Churchill Livingstone, p 63, Fig 4-17.)

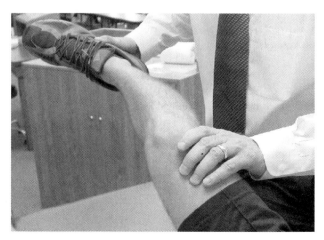

Figure 3-25: Pivot shift test for anterior cruciate ligament deficiency.

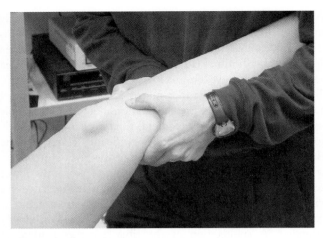

Figure 3-26: Flexion rotation drawer test for anterior cruciate ligament deficiency.

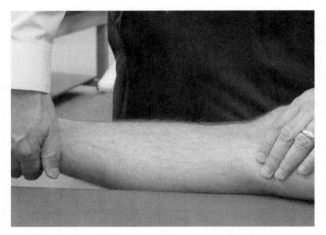

Figure 3-27: Valgus stress test for medial collateral ligament deficiency.

clinician then holds the tibia in neutral rotation as he or she flexes the knee to 20 to 30 degrees. While flexing the knee slightly, the clinician also pushes the patient's tibia in a posterior direction, which reduces tibial subluxation, indicating a positive test.

Collateral Ligament Testing

Medial and lateral stability tests are performed using single-plane tests. The valgus stress test is the most common physical examination test to determine medial joint stability. This test is performed in both full knee extension and approximately 20 to 30 degrees of knee flexion. The clinician uses his or her leg as a fulcrum at the joint while palpating the medial joint line and MCL with the proximal hand. The clinician then exerts a valgus force to the tibiofemoral joint by pushing medially while at the same time moving the foot in a lateral direction (Figure 3-27). A clinical pearl is to close the joint first to enable palpation of the amount of true joint

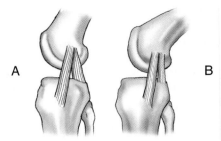

Figure 3-28: Medial view of knee showing superficial medial collateral ligament and posterior oblique ligament. **A,** Knee in extension with posterior fibers of the medial ligament tight. **B,** Knee in flexion with posterior fibers of the medial ligament loose. *(From Indelicato PA, Linton RC: Medial ligament injuries in the adult. In DeLee JC, Drez D, Miller MD, editors: DeLee and Drez's orthopedic sports medicine principles and practice, vol 2, Philadelphia, 2003, Saunders.)*

opening, giving the examiner the ability to kinesthetically feel the medial joint opening, rather than beginning the test at any arbitrary starting point. A positive test is indicated by either laxity when comparing the involved with the uninvolved knee, pain along the MCL, or both. Again, with most ligament testing both the quality and quantity of joint opening, as well as end feel, are noted and compared with the uninvolved side. When testing the MCL in full extension, several structures could be involved, including the MCL, the posterior oblique ligament, the ACL, the PCL, and the medial middle one-third of the joint capsule. When testing in full extension, all of these structures could potentially stabilize the knee. Joint laxity with a valgus stress test at 25 degrees that was not found at 0 degrees indicates an isolated MCL tear. The other medial knee secondary stabilizers will be lax at this angle of knee flexion, which places more stress isolated to the MCL (Figure 3-28). Grood and colleagues[50] report that the MCL accounts for 57% of restraint against valgus stress at 5 degrees of knee flexion and 78% at 25 degrees of knee flexion.

The varus stress test is used to evaluate the integrity of the LCL. This test is very similar to the valgus stress test for the MCL. With the knee in full extension, and then in 30 degrees of flexion, the examiner applies a varus stress to the tibiofemoral joint using similar techniques (Figure 3-29). Substantial laxity in full extension could mean a tear to the LCL, the ACL, or the PCL, whereas laxity at 30 degrees of flexion would indicate an isolated tear of the LCL. The LCL and the PCL are commonly injured when there is excessive lateral laxity; other structures that could be injured include the mid-third lateral capsule, the arcuate-popliteus complex, and the IT band.[50]

Meniscus Tests

Because there are no less than 17 tests to implicate a torn meniscus, several are included in the knee special testing algorithm. The first of these is the recurvatum test. We find

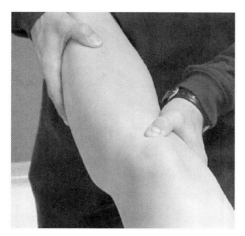

Figure 3-29: Varus stress test for lateral collateral ligament deficiency.

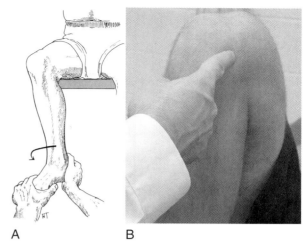

A   B

Figure 3-31: A, Steinmann's point tenderness test. **B,** Modification of the Steinmann test to implicate posterior horn of meniscus. *(A, From Insall JN, Scott WN: Surgery of the knee, ed 3, New York, 2001, Churchill Livingstone, p 490, Fig 24-27.)*

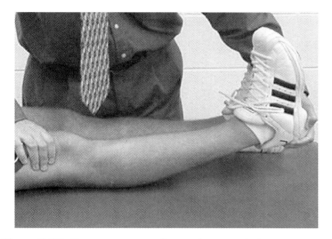

Figure 3-30: Recurvatum test for meniscus pathology.

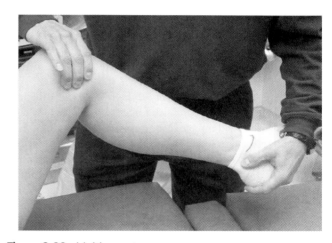

Figure 3-32: McMurray test.

this most commonly positive for a radial tear that extends into the anterior lateral meniscus. The patient is supine with the knee in full extension. The clinician takes the patient's knee into passive extension, and overpressure is then given at the end ROM (Figure 3-30). A positive test is indicated by joint line pain with this maneuver.

The Steinmann test is performed with the patient seated, hanging the knee over the edge of the examining table at 90 degrees of knee flexion.[51] The clinician then grasps the foot and sharply rotates the tibia first internally, then externally (Figure 3-31, *A*). A sharp pain in either the medial or lateral joint line suggests a positive test result. Andrews and colleagues[52] have previously shown that the posterior horn of the meniscus is most often torn when the medial meniscus is injured; therefore we perform a supine modification of the Steinmann test in which the knee is fully flexed with passive overpressure at end ROM in an attempt to more accurately assess the posterior horn of the meniscus. A positive test is indicated by pain along one of the joint lines (Figure 3-31, *B*). Performance of this test in supine position at this time in

the knee special testing algorithm is done to prevent unnecessary changes in patient position.

The McMurray test[53] is the classic test done for meniscus tears. With the patient supine, the clinician grasps the patient's knee with the proximal hand while the distal hand grasps the foot and ankle. The clinician then internally rotates the tibia on the femur using the foot as a handhold. The knee is taken into full flexion. While palpating the knee and applying a valgus stress with the proximal hand, the knee is then moved into a varus, internally rotated position while the knee is extended. As the knee is flexed a second time, external tibial rotation with a valgus force can be used to implicate a tear (Figure 3-32). A click, a snap, locking, pseudolocking, or pain in either the lateral or medial joint line is indicative of a positive test for a meniscus tear.

The final test used for meniscus pathology is the Apley compression test.[54] This test is done toward the end of the

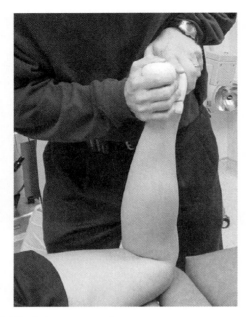

Figure 3-33: Apley compression test.

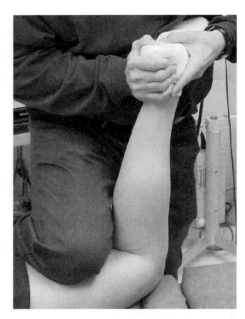

Figure 3-34: Apley distraction test for collateral ligament deficiency.

knee special testing algorithm and is the first test to place the patient in the prone position in an attempt to minimize unnecessary patient movements. With the thigh stabilized and the knee positioned prone at 90 degrees of knee flexion, the clinician applies a compressive force through the long axis of the tibia in an attempt to compress the meniscus. While compressing through the long axis of the tibial shaft, the clinician internally and externally rotates the tibia, attempting to compress a torn meniscus of the posterior horn (Figure 3-33). A positive test is indicated by pain in the respective medial or lateral joint line. During times of acute significant swelling, the Apley test is more easily tolerated because of the limited knee flexion required (only 90 degrees). Davies[24] has described a dynamic version of the Apley compression test in which the clinician compresses the tibiofemoral joint while simultaneously moving the knee from flexion to extension, thus allowing assessment of the meniscus from posterior horn to anterior.

All of the meniscus tests are used in an attempt to entrap an excessively mobile meniscus or a torn meniscal fragment. The clinician must remember that in patients with concomitant injuries, the pain with these meniscal tests may be due to these other injuries. For example, a swollen knee will not allow deep knee flexion to test the posterior horns of the meniscus. Additionally, a patient with an injured MCL will most likely have pain from the injured collateral while performing the external tibial rotation component of the McMurray test. Being aware of comorbidities is important so that the clinician is able to accurately interpret test results.

A final test to implicate the collateral ligaments, also performed in the prone position, is the Apley distraction test.[54]

With the patient still in the prone position, the clinician flexes the knee to 90 degrees. The clinician holds the patient's thigh tight onto the table with either the examiner's knee or one of the examiner's hands. The clinician then distracts the patient's tibia along the long axis of the tibia (Figure 3-34). To more provocatively stress the collateral ligaments, while distracting the knee, the clinician can also either internally rotate the tibia or apply a varus moment to the knee to stress the LCL more, whereas externally rotating and applying a valgus moment will stress the MCL more. When performing this additional varus or valgus movement, the clinician must ensure that the thigh is stable, so that concomitant hip internal or external rotation does not take place.

KT-1000 Arthrometer Testing

A highly objective instrument to evaluate ACL laxity is the KT-1000 (MEDmetric Corp., San Diego, CA). In 1983, Daniel and colleagues introduced the commercially available KT-1000. Numerous investigators have found the KT-1000 to be valid and reliable.[55-67] The KT-1000 is an easy-to-use, portable ligament arthrometer that can be used with patients who have incurred an acute injury or those with more chronic forms of instability. Testing can be performed at various time frames throughout the rehabilitation process, depending on physician preferences.

The KT-1000 is placed on the proximal tibia and stabilized with two straps. Each of these straps surrounds the tibia and lower leg. Two sensor pads, one located on the patella and the other at the tibial tubercle, move freely to measure the relative motion between the two pads. Through a force handle located slightly distal to the tibial pad, various forces are placed through the tibia, while the patella is stabilized to limit any motion from the femur, which rests underneath. We generally use four passive displacement measurements: 15 lb anterior displacement, 20 lb anterior displacement, 30 lb anterior displacement, and the manual maximum anterior displacement.[68]

According to Daniel and Stone,[68] in a unilaterally injured patient, a right-left difference of less than 3 mm is classified as normal motion, and a right-left difference on any test of 3 mm or greater is classified as pathologic.

If the patient is able to tolerate higher-level physical performance tests, he or she will be taken through what we call a functional testing algorithm, which is described in Chapter 10.

POSTOPERATIVE EXAMINATION

Because postoperatively the clinician should know the extent of the pathology and the repaired tissue, the postoperative evaluation is usually much more abbreviated than the evaluation of the patient preoperatively. The postoperative knee evaluation begins with inspection and observation of the knee and surrounding structures. With most surgeries there is some degree of soft tissue trauma. This trauma will usually result in joint effusion and soft tissue edema. Anthropometric measurements of limb girth can be made as described earlier in this chapter. Although historically one was able to tell what surgical procedure was performed by the surgical incisions, this is no longer the case with the extensive use of arthroscopy or arthroscopically aided procedures. When the patient exhibits extensive postoperative swelling, it is imperative to check the neurovascular status of the rest of the limb. A simple check of superficial sensation, blanching of the toes to assess peripheral blood flow, or dorsalis pedis (absent in approximately 15% of the general population) or posterior tibial pulse is generally sufficient to rule out lack of perfusion to the distal extremities. Skin color and temperature should also be assessed. Although some slight superficial warmness may remain for up to a week, a red and hot knee is most often a sign of infection. The incision should be checked daily for any signs of infection, which include purulent drainage, swelling, redness, and increased temperature. Incision healing should be adequate for bathing and showering by 2 weeks after surgery. Edema is commonly present in the postsurgical knee. Edema is a leakage of fluid into the superficial dermal tissues. Use of a compression wrap can keep edema to a minimum.

Assessing knee ROM following knee surgery always is dependent on the surgical procedure performed and the rehabilitation philosophy of the surgeon. Although full knee extension is usually warranted immediately following surgeries such as ACL reconstruction, there are times when full knee extension may not be warranted. The patient with a combined ACL reconstruction and MCL repair may be potentially harmed if the knee is taken to full passive extension too soon, because in this position a significant strain is placed on the MCL, leading to ligament attenuation. Although beneficial for the isolated ACL reconstruction patient, full knee extension should not be performed unless the clinician understands the surgery performed, due to possible ROM restrictions and soft tissue healing time frames.

Similar circumstances can be seen when measuring passive knee flexion following surgical repair. It is not uncommon to have limited knee flexion ROM after knee surgery. As will be seen in the chapters that follow, hamstring ACL reconstruction, meniscus repair, MCL repair, and articular cartilage transplant surgeries often limit knee flexion motion to no greater than 60 to 90 degrees for several weeks. Moreover, the patient with a severely effused knee will demonstrate substantially less ROM than the patient with limited knee swelling.

The ability to contract the quadriceps is an important functional activity and provides the clinician with a way to ensure adequate neuromuscular control. Without a strong quadriceps contraction, safe ambulation without an assistive device or brace is usually not allowed. Several tests can be used to determine quadriceps contractile state, also known as quadriceps tone. One way to determine quadriceps function is the patient's ability or inability to perform a straight leg raise without a quadriceps lag. If unable to perform a straight leg raise properly, the quadriceps is not fully functioning. A bent leg raise is generally contraindicated in those following ACL reconstruction, because a quadriceps contraction with the knee slightly flexed is thought to substantially increase strain on the ACL. If unable to perform a straight leg raise, the patient should remain in the postoperative knee brace locked at 0 degrees until the patient can maintain this position independently. Techniques to facilitate a quadriceps contraction are described in later chapters. One method of assessing quadriceps tone is by palpating the patella while the patient attempts to contract the quadriceps muscle. If you are unable to passively translate the patella medially or laterally while the patient is attempting to contract the quadriceps, there is adequate "tone." If the patella is easily passively moved while the patient is attempting to contract, the ability to contract the quadriceps is limited.

Finally, all patients should have their gait and their ability to use their respective assistive devices analyzed. Gait assessment and training should at minimum include ambulation with devices on level ground and traversing steps or stairs appropriately. Use of a gait belt is a must during any assessment of gait training regardless of your initial impression of the patient's ability. Quadriceps shutdown, or reflexive giving way of the knee, is not uncommon following knee surgery and can happen when least expected. Preventive safety measures such as the standard use of a gait belt are a necessity with any postoperative lower extremity patient. In cases of large patients, even with the use of a gait belt, potentially more than one therapist may be required to assist with ambulation training to ensure adequate safety.

SUMMARY

A systematic and thorough history, subjective examination, systems review, and physical examination should be used during routine preoperative and postoperative evaluation. This chapter describes an efficient manner in which to evaluate both the preoperative and postoperative knee.

References

1. Gould JA, Davies GJ: Orthopedic and sports rehabilitation concepts. In Gould JA, Davies GJ, editors: *Orthopedic and sports physical therapy,* St Louis, 1985, Mosby.

2. O'Donoghue DH: Treatment of acute ligament injuries of the knee, *Orthop Clin* 4:617-645, 1973.

3. Stith JS, Sahrmann SA, Dixon KK, Norton BJ: Curriculum to prepare diagnosticians in physical therapy, *J Phys Ther Educ* 9:46-53, 1995.

4. Magee DJ: *Orthopedic physical assessment,* ed 4, Philadelphia, 2002, Saunders.

5. Starkey C, Ryan J: *Evaluation of orthopedic and athletic injuries,* ed 2, Philadelphia, 2002, FA Davis.

6. Hawkins RJ: *Musculoskeletal examination,* St Louis, 1995, Mosby.

7. Insall R, Salvati I: Patellar position in the normal knee joint, *Radiology* 101:101-104, 1971.

8. Woodland LH, Francis RS: Parameters and comparisons of the quadriceps angle of college-aged men and women in the supine and standing positions, *Am J Sports Med* 20:208-211, 1992.

9. Post WR, Fulkerson J: Knee pain diagrams: correlation with physical examination findings in patients with anterior knee pain, *Arthroscopy* 10(6):618-623, 1984.

10. Davies GJ, DeCarlo MS: Examining the shoulder complex. In Bandy W, editor: *Current concepts in rehabilitation of the shoulder,* LaCrosse, WI. 1995, Sports Physical Therapy Section.

11. Davies GJ et al: Functional examination of the shoulder complex, *Phys Sports Med* 9:82, 1981.

12. Hagbarth KE, Wallen G, Burke D, Lofstedt L: Effects of the Jendrassik maneuver on muscle spindle activity in man, *J Neurol Neurosurg Psych* 38:1143-1153, 1975.

13. Sherrington CS: *The integrative action of the nervous system,* New Haven, CT, 1906, Yale University Press.

14. Lephart SM, Riemann BL, Fu FH: Introduction to the sensorimotor system. In Lephart SM, Fu FH, editors: *Proprioception and neuromuscular control in joint stability,* Champaign, IL, 2000, Human Kinetics.

15. Baker CL: *The Hughston Clinic sports medicine field manual,* Baltimore, MD, 1996, Williams & Wilkins.

16. Kinzey SH, Armstrong CW: Reliability of star excursion tests in assessing dynamic balance, *J Orthop Sports Ther* 27:356-360, 1998.

17. Manske RC, Anderson J: Test-retest reliability of the functional reach test, *J Orthop Sports Phys Ther (Abst)* 34(1):A52, 2004.

18. Hertel J, Miller SJ, Denegar CR: Intratester and intertester reliability during the star excursion balance tests, *J Sport Rehabil* 9:104-116, 2000.

19. Hoppenfeld S: *Physical examination of the spine and extremities,* New York, 1976, Appleton-Century-Crofts.

20. Hislop HJ, Montgomery J: *Muscle testing,* ed 6, Philadelphia, 1995, Saunders.

21. Kendall FP, McCreary EK, Provance PG: *Muscle testing and function with posture and pain,* ed 4, Baltimore, 1993, Williams & Wilkins.

22. Daniels L, Worthingham C: *Muscle testing. Techniques of manual examination,* ed 7, Philadelphia, 2002, Saunders.

23. Ritchie JR, Miller MD, Harner CD: History and physical evaluation. In Fu FH, Harner CD, Vince KG, Miller MD, editors: *Knee surgery,* vol 1, Baltimore, 1994, Williams & Wilkins.

24. Davies GJ: Personal communications, 2004.

25. DeAndrade JR, Grant C, Dixon A: Joint distention and reflex muscle inhibition in the knee, *J Bone Joint Surg* 47A:313-322, 1965.

26. Spencer JD, Hayes KC, Alexander IJ: Knee joint effusion and quadriceps reflex inhibition in man, *Arch Phys Med Rehabil* 65:171-177, 1984.

27. Stokes M, Young A: Investigations of quadriceps inhibition: implications for clinical practice, *Physiotherapy* 70:425-428, 1984.

28. Stratford P: Electromyography of the quadriceps femoris muscle in subjects with normal knees and acutely effused knees, *Phys Ther* 62:279-283, 1981.

29. Davies GJ, Larsen R: Examining the knee, *Phys Sports Med* 7:48-73, 1978.

30. Manske RC, Davies GJ: A nonsurgical approach to examination and treatment of the patellofemoral joint, part I: examination of the patellofemoral joint, *Crit Rev Phys Rehabil Med* 15(2):141-166, 2003.

31. Soderberg GL, Ballantyne BT, Kestel LL: Reliability of lower extremity girth measurements after anterior cruciate ligament reconstruction, *Physiother Res Int* 1(1):7-16, 1996.

32. Tomsich DA, Nitz AJ, Threlkeld AJ, Sharpiro R: Patellofemoral alignment: reliability, *J Orthop Sports Phys Ther* 23:200-208, 1996.

33. Kolwich PA, Paulos LE, Rosenberg TD, Farnsworth S: Lateral release of the patella: indications and contraindications, *Am J Sports Med* 18:359-365, 1990.

34. Fairbank KA: Internal derangement of the knee in children, *Proc R Soc London* 3:11, 1937.

35. Scurdi GR, editor: *The patella,* New York, 1995, Springer-Verlag.

36. Ellenbecker TS: Clinical examination. In Ellenbecker TS, editor: *Knee ligament rehabilitation,* New York, 2000, Churchill Livingstone.

37. Katz JW, Fingeroth RJ: The diagnostic accuracy of ruptures of the anterior cruciate ligament comparing the Lachman's test, the anterior drawer sign, and the pivot-shift test in acute and chronic knee injuries, *Am J Sports Med* 14:88-91, 1986.

38. Sung-Jae Kim, Hyun-Kon Kim: Reliability of the anterior drawer test, the pivot shift test and the Lachman test, *Clin Orthop* 317:237-242, 1995.

39. Malone T, McPoil T, Nitz AJ: *Orthopedic and sports physical therapy,* ed 3, St Louis, 1997, Mosby.

40. Wallace LA, Mangine RE, Malone T: The knee. In Gould JA, Davies GJ, editors: *Orthopedic and sports physical therapy,* St Louis, 1985, Mosby.

41. Dehaven K: Arthroscopy in the diagnosis and management of the anterior cruciate ligament deficient knee, *Clin Orthop* 172:52-56, 1983.

42. Donaldson WF, Warren RF, Wickiewicz T: A comparison of acute anterior cruciate ligament examinations. Initial vs. examination under anesthesia, *Am J Sports Med* 13:5-10, 1985.

43. Flemming BC, Johnson RJ, Shapiro E, et al: Clinical versus uninstrumented knee testing on autopsy specimens, *Clin Orthop Rel Res* 282:196-207, 1992.

44. Torg JS, Conrad W, Kalen V: Clinical diagnosis of anterior cruciate ligament instability in the athlete, *Am J Sports Med* 4:84-93, 1976.

45. Galway RD, Beauprea A, Macintosh DL: The pivot shift syndrome. A clinical study of symptomatic ACL insufficiency (abstract), *J Bone Joint Surg* 54B:558, 1972.

46. Hughston JC, Andrews JR, Cross MJ, Moschi A: Classification of knee ligament instabilities. Part II. The lateral compartment, *J Bone Joint Surg* 58A:173-179, 1976.

47. Noyes FR, Grood ES, Suntay WJ, Butler DL: The three dimensional laxity of the anterior cruciate deficient knee as determined by clinical laxity tests, *Iowa Orthop J* 3:32-44, 1983.

48. Noyes FR, Butler D, Grood ES, et al: Clinical paradoxes of anterior cruciate instability and a new test to detect its instability, *Orthop Trans* 2:36, 1978.

49. Tria AJ, Hosea TM: Diagnosis of knee ligament injuries: clinical. In Scott WN, editor: *Ligament and extensor mechanism injuries of the knee,* St Louis, 1991, Mosby.

50. Grood ES, Noyes FR, Butler DL, Suntay WJ: Ligamentous and capsular restraints preventing medial and lateral laxity in intact human cadaver knees, *J Bone Joint Surg* 63A(8):1257-1269, 1981.

51. Ricklin P, Ruttiman A, del Buono MS: *Meniscal lesions: practical problems of clinical diagnosis, arthrography, and therapy,* Orlando, FL, 1971, Grune & Stratton.

52. Andrews JR, Norwood LA Jr, Cross MJ: The double bucket handle tear of the medial meniscus, *Am J Sports Med* 3:232, 1975.

53. McMurray TP: The semilunar cartilages, *Br J Surg* 29:407, 1941.

54. Apley AG: The diagnosis of meniscus injuries: some new clinical methods, *J Bone Joint Surg* 29B:78-84, 1946.

55. Daniel DM, Malcom LL, Losse G, et al: An instrumented measurement of anterior laxity of the knee, *J Bone Joint Surg* 67A:720-725, 1985.

56. Anderson AF, Snyder RB, Federspielo CF, Lipscomb AB: Instrumented evaluation of knee laxity: a comparison of five arthrometers, *Am J Sports Med* 20(2):135-140, 1992.

57. Anderson AF, Lipscomb AB: Preoperative instrumented testing of anterior and posterior knee laxity, *Am J Sports Med* 17(3):387-392, 1989.

58. Fiebert I, Gresley J, Hoffman S, et al: Comparative measurements of anterior tibial translation using the KT-1000 knee arthrometer with the leg in neutral, internal rotation, and external rotation, *J Orthop Sports Phys Ther* 19:331-334, 1994.

59. Hanten WP, Pace MB: Reliability of measuring anterior laxity of the knee joint using a knee ligament arthrometer, *Phys Ther* 57:357-359, 1987.

60. Highgenboten CL, Jackson AW, Jansson KA, Meske NB: KT-1000 arthrometer: conscious and unconscious test results using 15, 20, and 30 pounds of force, *Am J Sports Med* 20(4):450-454, 1992.

61. Highgenboten CL, Jackson A, Meske NB: Genucom, KT-1000, and Stryker knee laxity measuring device comparisons. Device reproducibility and interdevice comparison in asymptomatic subjects, *Am J Sports Med* 17(6):743-746, 1989.

62. Kolwalk DL, Wojtys EM, Disher J, Loubert P: Quantitative analysis of the measuring capabilities of the KT-1000 knee ligament arthrometer, *Am J Sports Med* 21(5):744-747, 1993.

63. Muneta T, Ezura Y, Sekiya I, Yamamoto H: Anterior knee laxity and loss of extension after anterior cruciate ligament injury, *Am J Sports Med* 24(5):603-607, 1996.

64. Queale WS, Snyder-Mackler L, Handling KA, et al: Instrumented examination of knee laxity in patients with anterior cruciate deficiency: a comparison of the KT-1000, Knee Signature System, and Genucom, *J Orthop Sports Phys Ther* 19:345-351, 1994.

65. Staubli HU, Jakob RP: Anterior knee motion analysis. Measurement and simultaneous radiography, *Am J Sports Med* 19(2):172-177, 1991.

66. Steiner ME, Brown C, Zarins B, et al: Measurement of anterior-posterior displacement of the knee. A comparison of the results with instrumented devices and with clinical examination, *J Bone Joint Surg* 72A:1307-1315, 1990.

67. Wroble RR, Van Ginkel LA, Grood ES, et al: Repeatability of the KT-1000 arthrometer in a normal population, *Am J Sports Med* 18:396-399, 1990.

68. Daniel DM, Stone ML: KT-1000 anterior-posterior displacement measurements. In Daniel DM, Akeson W, O'Connor J, editors: *Knee ligaments: structure, function, and injury,* New York, 1990, Raven Press.

CHAPTER 4

Preoperative and Postsurgical Musculoskeletal Examination of the Shoulder

Robert C. Manske, DPT, MPT, MEd, SCS, ATC, CSCS
Mark Stovak, MD, FAAFP

CHAPTER OUTLINE

THE PROPER CLINICAL EXAMINATION

and evaluation of the shoulder is often a difficult challenge because of the numerous pathologies that can occur at this complex joint. Despite this challenge, the cornerstone of any treatment plan or approach relies on a proper diagnosis made by the clinical physical examination. All too often clinicians rely on the latest state-of-the-art advancements in diagnostic imaging techniques, rather than their clinical physical examination. Even the experienced clinician can be confused by the sheer complexity of the shoulder's arthrokinematic and kinesiologic interdependency. Despite this complexity, in most cases, one can reach a working medical or physical therapy diagnosis following a thorough medical history and clinical examination. The experienced clinician displays advanced knowledge of anatomy, biomechanics, kinesiology, and pathomechanics. It is on this foundation of knowledge that the clinician builds with each successive shoulder patient that he or she examines and ultimately evaluates and treats. The clinical physical examination is part skill and part art that is never fully mastered, but continually built on by increasing one's own knowledge as one continues to progress from novice to expert clinician.

According to the *Guide to Physical Therapist Practice*, evaluation is a dynamic process involving clinical decision making by the physical therapist based on data gathered during the examination.[1] The ultimate goals of the physical examination are to determine the involved structures and respective causes of dysfunction, and the current stage of the dysfunction. The clinician can then determine which intervention and treatment techniques should be used to return the patient to his or her prior level of function.

The best time to examine a patient is preoperatively. This chapter describes both the preoperative and postoperative physical examinations. During the preoperative examination the clinician may glean valuable information regarding the status of the shoulder that may not be able to be assessed immediately following surgery. This baseline information may not be testable postsurgically because of soft tissue healing constraints, immobilization procedures, or postoperative pain associated with the various surgical procedures. Both preoperatively and postoperatively, the clinician should use a standard, consistent, systematic approach to examination and evaluation of the shoulder and related structures. Examination of the shoulder can be highly complex and confusing because of the numerous tissues within the shoulder girdle that may potentially be a source of pain. Furthermore, the cervical spine, diaphragm, spleen, heart, and lungs have the capacity to refer pain to the shoulders. Once pain referred from these visceral-type structures has been ruled out as a cause of pathology, a thorough musculoskeletal examination is performed to examine both the involved and the uninvolved entire upper quadrant and the cervical spine.

DEMOGRAPHICS

Questions to be asked during the history-taking portion of the examination for a shoulder patient require determining the patient's previous and present level of function. With regard to occupation and previous activity, is the patient a laborer, a recreational athlete, or a competitive athlete? Is the patient required to use his or her arm overhead and, if so, how often during the normal day? What activities appear to aggravate the condition? Does the patient have a prior history of injury or surgery? Is the injury to the patient's dominant shoulder? Does sleeping seem to irritate the shoulder? Since many individuals sleep on their side, it is possible that pain during nighttime hours may be due to the scapula protracting, compromising the subacromial space. Although no time is probably optimal, discussions regarding workers' compensation or litigation are necessary. It has been well documented that those who are seeking financial benefit from their injury rarely respond as well or as quickly as those not having a secondary gain.[2-7]

Pain, limitation of motion, weakness, instability, and sensory changes are common complaints from the patient with shoulder pathologies. The therapist should quantify the severity and degree of the patient's complaint of pain, as well as determine to the best of his or her ability the actual offending structures. This includes determining whether the pain is localized or referred from the head, neck, or spine.

CHRONICITY AND IRRITABILITY

Initial questioning should be centered on when the symptoms began and what the state of symptoms is presently. Symptoms can be described as acute if they have been present for up to 7 to 10 days. With this form of presentation, the patient will generally remember the actual incident that caused the condition. Causes could include trauma (macrotrauma), overuse (microtrauma), or a drastic change in pattern of use of the shoulder over the last several days (e.g., increasing tennis practice from a standard 1.5 hours a day to 5 hours a day in preparation for an upcoming tournament). In the acute condition, the most common complaint is pain; secondary symptoms may include stiffness, weakness, loss of motion, functional disability, catching, and crepitus.[8] A subacute condition exists if it has persisted for a period of 10 days to 7 weeks, whereas the chronic condition is present for longer than 7 weeks.[9] With the subacute and chronic conditions, the patient may not remember the exact inciting event that caused the symptoms, thus making the diagnosis more dependent on the physical examination. Documentation of the severity of the symptoms during the physical examination needs to be determined. Are the symptoms improving, staying the same, or worsening? This detail will give the clinician an idea of the irritability of the condition and the reason why the patient is seeking treatment at this time. The patient who exhibits an irritable condition may require relative rest from the offending activity initially to begin the treatment process, whereas the patient with a less irritable or nonirritable condition may be able to begin immediate therapeutic procedures to increase joint mobility, muscular strength, endurance, and neuromuscular activation.

RED FLAGS

During the history it is imperative to listen for "red flags" as described by Stith and colleagues.[10] While performing the systems review of a particular patient, the clinician needs to be aware of conditions in which the pathology may be outside the scope of the clinician's practice. These red flag symptoms would alert the clinician to immediately refer the patient back to the referring physician.[10] Because various musculoskeletal injuries typically have histories, signs, and symptoms that can be clustered to help determine their expected pattern of recovery, those that do not fit the norm must be ruled out as severe pathology requiring referral to other medical professionals. When symptoms begin to stray from the norm, such as inability to induce pain in a typical manner with motions or postures, when pain appears to be greater at night or when resting than during activity, or even when symptoms are similar in multiple other joints of the body, the clinician must rule out internal organs or systemic disease as a possible source of pathology.

PATIENT HISTORY

The patient history often helps define the pathology. As the clinician becomes more experienced with the physical examination, he or she will most likely have a general idea of the pathology at hand after taking the initial history. Following an adequate history, the clinician uses the clinical examination to implicate or rule out specific structures that may be causing or contributing to the pathology.

PREDISPOSING FACTORS

The clinician should determine the patient's age, because it is commonly known that rotator cuff (RTC) pathology is one of the most common shoulder injuries in those age 50 to 70 years and older. While assessing cadavers that were over 50 years of age, Lehman and colleagues[11] found that 20% of RTC tears were in those older than 60 years of age, whereas those younger than age 60 had only a 6% tear rate. Despite this dramatic increase in the occurrence of RTC pathology in the elderly, the clinician must remember that younger athletes are not totally immune to these problems. Professional athletes in their twenties have been shown to have attritional defects in their tendinous cuff, as well as degenerative spurs beneath their acromions.[12] Another pathology that is potentially age related is the "frozen shoulder," otherwise known as adhesive capsulitis. This condition, whose hallmark clinical finding is a dramatic loss of both active and passive shoulder range of motion that occurs in a predictable pattern, is most commonly seen in women ages 45 to 60 years.[13,14]

The unstable shoulder is much more prevalent in the 18- to 22-year-old age range. Coincidentally, it is in these younger, more active patients that there is a dramatic increase in risk of redislocation. This recurrent dislocation rate has been previously reported at anywhere from 80% to 95% in the younger population.[15,16] Additionally, the earlier stages of RTC pathology such as tendonitis or tendinosis may be more common in the 25- to 40-year-old age-group.[17]

PAIN TYPE AND LOCATION

Shoulder pain type and location must be clearly defined. The type of pain can usually be discerned by asking key questions regarding symptoms. Pain described as deep, dull, and poorly localized may be attributed to bony structures or deep muscular and ligamentous structures, or it may potentially be visceral.[18] Some report that skin, tendon, or bursal tissue symptoms can be superficial, sharp, or burning.[19] Insults of vascular origin may be described as pulsating, throbbing pain, whereas nerve injury can cause various symptoms from severe deep pain to paresthesia, dysthesia, and numbness in the extremity.

Although the location of the patient's pain is not 100% accurate in being the exact source of pain, known pain patterns do exist. Isolating an exact location of pain in the shoulder may be challenging. For example, the supraspinatus tendon inserts into a conjoined tendon of the remaining cuff muscles along their humeral insertion. Additionally, the long head of the biceps tendon is ensheathed by the subscapularis and supraspinatus tendon; thus palpation in this area can obscure the exact pain location.[20]

OBJECTIVE PHYSICAL EXAMINATION

Cervical Screen

Because cervical spine pathology can commonly refer pain to the shoulder and periscapular area, cervical spine screening tests are a must. Pain into the proximal lateral arm can occur due to C5 or C6 nerve root compression. Irritation of these nerves can cause pain or muscle dysfunction in or around the shoulder girdle complex.

First and foremost, a routine screening of the cervical spine is necessary to rule out the possibility of pathologic conditions emanating from the spine. Radiculopathy from the cervical nerve roots can cause referred pain into and around the shoulder. A cervical spine screening should commence with active cervical motions in all planes. If these motions are full and painless, overpressure can be cautiously given at the end of the active movements. Cervical spine compression and distraction tests and Spurling's test are useful, quick tests to implicate cervical pathology. The distraction test is performed by placing one hand under the patient's chin and the other around the occiput and then slowly lifting the patient's head. A positive test result occurs if the patient's pain is relieved or decreased when the head is lifted, indicating that pressure is being released off of nerve roots.[9] Straight cervical compression attempts to compress nerve roots, cervical facet joints, or intervertebral disks and is considered the first part of Spurling's test. The next maneuver in the sequence of Spurling's test includes cervical compression with extension, followed by side bending, and ending with the head in extension and rotation. Pain that radiates into the arm with testing is considered positive. This test is not specific for any single problem and can be positive with a variety of pathologies, including stenosis, cervical spondylosis, osteophytes, trophic facet joints, or a herniated disk.[9]

Observation

To fully appreciate any abnormalities of bony or soft tissue structures around the shoulder, the patient must be properly undressed. In most cases males can be shirtless, whereas females would prefer a gown draped appropriately with a halter top or sports bra. Because some cultures do not allow those of the opposite gender to be viewed undressed, accommodations should be made as appropriate to expedite the examination.

It is important to view the shoulder from all angles to determine symmetric versus asymmetric structures. A comprehensive knowledge of the normal variance of the size and shape of structures around the shoulder is beneficial. If appropriate, the clinician may want to observe the patient remove his or her coat or shirt to determine how limitations affect even the simplest activities of daily living.

One of the first major determinations to be made during the physical examination and observation is the amount of generalized ligamentous laxity the patient is endowed with. Although the diagnostic criteria for joint hypermobility are not well defined and have been inconsistent in descriptive papers,[21-24] it is a worthwhile goal to determine if they are present in the patient at hand. Probably the most common method of determining generalized ligamentous laxity is through use of the Beighton scale. The Beighton scale is generally considered the yardstick of proposed hypermobility scales and is commonly used clinically.[25] The Beighton scale gives a patient points for each of the following characteristics: passive extension of the metacarpophalangeal joint past 90 degrees (Figure 4-1), passive opposition of the thumb to the forearm (Figure 4-2), hyperextension of the elbow past 10 degrees (Figure 4-3), hyperextension of the knee past 10 degrees (Figure 4-4), and trunk flexion allowing the palms to be placed flat on the floor. Each limb is scored separately and given a single point if positive, and being able to touch hands flat on the floor also generates a single point, for a total of up to 9 points. Although no consensus exists on the threshold for hypermobility, scores of 5/9 to 6/9 are generally considered positive.

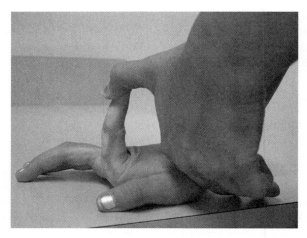

Figure 4-1: Passive extension of the fifth finger past 90 degrees indicating generalized ligamentous laxity.

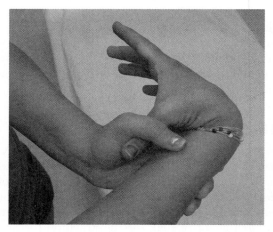

Figure 4-2: Thumb to forearm indicating generalized ligamentous laxity.

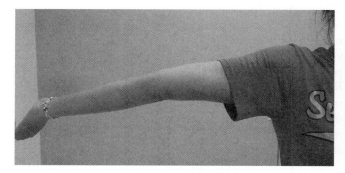

Figure 4-3: Elbow hyperextension greater than 10 degrees indicating generalized ligamentous laxity.

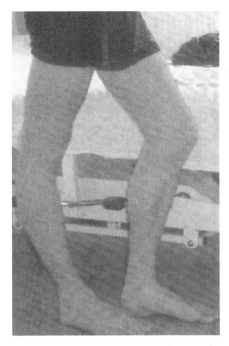

Figure 4-4: Knee hyperextension greater than 10 degrees indicating generalized ligamentous laxity. *(From Keer R, Grahame R:* Hypermobility syndrome, *London, 2003, Butterworth Heinemann.)*

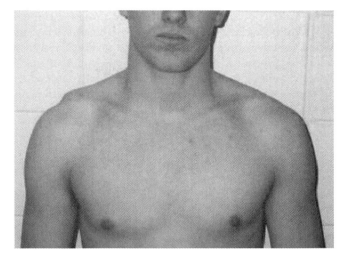

Figure 4-5: Right shoulder step-off deformity in high school football player indicating grade II acromioclavicular joint injury.

Anterior Observation

From the anterior view, the clinician initially scans from the top of the head to the shoulders. The head and neck should remain in the midline of the body with little or no lateral deviation. Muscular spasm resulting from overuse or from cervical spine pathology may cause a lateral tilting of the cervical spine to the contralateral side of injury. As with each of the views, any decrease in muscle tone or atrophy should be noted. In addition, the clinician should note any malalignment of bony structures. A common area to see bony malalignment in the shoulder would be with the anterior view of the clavicle. Patients with an anteriorly rounded protracted shoulder often demonstrate a clavicle that protrudes anteriorly on the ipsilateral side. Additionally, the clavicle, when fractured, can heal with a callus formation that can be visualized and palpated. Greater than a grade I ligament sprain to the acromioclavicular (AC) joint would cause the distal end of the clavicle to be in an elevated position in comparison with the acromion. With a grade II or III injury to the AC joint, this elevation will be greater, indicating a more severe sprain involving the coracoclavicular ligaments as well. This deformity is commonly known as a step-off deformity (Figure 4-5). A static sulcus sign might be seen if there is a loss of muscle tone caused by neurovascular compromise or injury such as a stroke. Normally the deltoid muscle exhibits a rounded appearance; however, it may look flattened with paralysis of the C5 nerve root or following an anteriorly dislocated glenohumeral joint. An anteriorly dislocated glenohumeral joint would probably be rarely seen acutely in an outpatient physical therapy clinic, yet may be common in athletic training and emergency care. This form of dislocation will generally be very painful, and the patient will seek medical attention immediately. *Handedness* is a common finding and means that the dominant shoulder will normally hang slightly lower than the nondominant because of increased muscle mass, hypermobility of the joint capsule and ligaments surrounding the shoulder, and increased flexibility of the musculotendinous structures.[9]

Posterior Observation

When viewing the patient from the dorsal side of the body, the clinician notes any soft tissue or bony abnormalities. The muscular contours of the deltoids should appear normal. The upper portion of the trapezius may be hypertonic or appear in spasm because of overuse pathology or injury to the cervical spine. Atrophy of the trapezius and sternocleidomastoid may be seen in the individual with a spinal accessory nerve injury. When the supraspinatus and infraspinatus fossae appear hollowed, one would suspect dysfunction of the cervical nerve roots, peripheral nerves (e.g., suprascapular nerve), or upper plexus or injury to the muscular portion of the given muscles.[26] The scapula normally sits on the dorsal thoracic cage from approximately T2 to T7. There should be minimal scapular tipping or winging. Tipping of the scapula occurs when the inferior scapular angle moves posteriorly while the superior border moves anteriorly.[27] Tipping can be the result of several problems, including a tight pectoralis minor or lower trapezius weakness. A certain amount of scapular tipping is normal, and without any tipping the superior border of the scapula would be raised off the rib cage when the scapula is elevated.[27] Winging of the scapula occurs when the medial border of the scapula is displaced posteriorly. Winging of the scapula most often results from weakness of the rhomboid muscles, a long thoracic nerve palsy, dorsal scapular nerve injury, or a weak serratus anterior (Figure 4-6). Magee[9] has described both static and dynamic winging. Static winging is present at rest and is usually caused by a structural deformity of the scapula, clavicle, spine, or ribs.[28] Dynamic winging occurs during movement of the shoulder and upper extremity. Dynamic winging can have numerous causes, including but not limited to long thoracic nerve palsy, trapezius palsy or weakness, rhomboid weakness, multidirec-

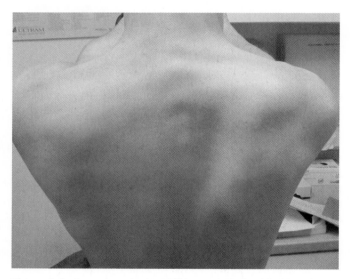

Figure 4-6: Scapular winging. Kibler type II classification due to long thoracic nerve palsy. *(From Manske RC, Reiman MP, Stovak M: Nonoperative and operative management of snapping scapula, Am J Sports Med 32[6]:1554-1565, 2004.)*

tional instability, or a painful shoulder limiting motion at the glenohumeral joint.[9]

Kibler and McMullen[29] have described scapular dyskinesis as an alteration in the normal position or motion of the scapula during coupled scapulohumeral movements. Kibler and colleagues[30] recently reported a moderate level of intertester and intratester reliability during visual estimation of scapular dysfunction movement patterns. Alterations in scapular motion are common with shoulder injuries and have been shown to occur in 68% to 100% of patients with shoulder pathology.[31] Four types of dyskinesis have been categorized by observing the patient's arm at rest and during elevation and depression of the arm in the scapular plane.[29] The type I scapular dyskinesis is characterized by a prominence of the inferior medial scapular border (tipping). This aberrant position of the scapula is primarily due to abnormal motion around the transverse axis.[29] A type II dyskinesis is characterized by a prominence of the entire medial scapular border and represents abnormal scapular rotation around a vertical axis (winging).[29] A type III dyskinesis is characterized by superior translation of the entire scapula and prominence of the superior medial scapular border.[29] The type IV scapula is symmetric bilaterally and is considered normal (Table 4-1).

In addition to describing scapular dyskinesis, Kibler[32,33] also has developed a manner in which dynamic measurement of scapular motion can be objectified. The lateral scapular slide test (LSST) was developed to evaluate scapular position and the scapular muscles' ability to stabilize at varying degrees of shoulder abduction. Because the test measurements are taken at several static positions, it is not truly a dynamic test.

TABLE 4-1

Scapular Dyskinesis System Used to Describe Abnormal Scapular Motion

PATTERN	DEFINITION
Inferior angle (type I)	At rest, the inferior medial scapular border may be prominent dorsally. During arm motion, the inferior angle tilts dorsally and the acromion tilts ventrally over the top of the thorax. The axis of the rotation is in the horizontal plane.
Medial border (type II)	At rest, the entire medial border may be prominent dorsally. During arm motion, the medial scapular border tilts dorsally off the thorax. The axis of the rotation is vertical in the frontal plane.
Superior border (type III)	At rest, the superior border of the scapula may be elevated and the scapula can also be anteriorly displaced. During arm motion, a shoulder shrug initiates movement without significant winging of the scapula occurring. The axis of motion is in the sagittal plane.
Symmetric scapulohumeral (type IV)	At rest, the position of both scapulae are relatively symmetric, taking into account that the dominant arm may be slightly lower. During arm motion, the scapulae rotate symmetrically upward such that the inferior angles translate laterally away from the midline and the scapular medial border remains flush against the thoracic wall. The reverse occurs during lowering of the arm.

From Kibler BW, Uhl TL, Maddux JWQ, et al: Qualitative clinical evaluation of scapular dysfunction: a reliability study, *J Shoulder Elbow Surg* 11:550-560, 2002.

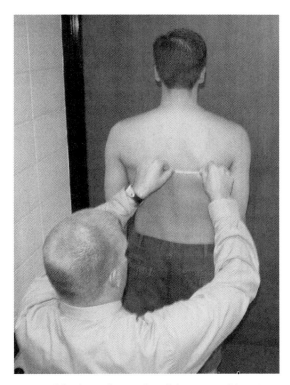

Figure 4-7: Kibler lateral scapular slide test position 1.

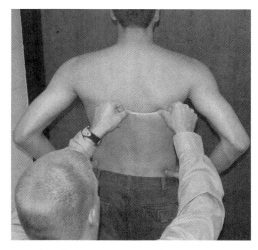

Figure 4-8: Kibler lateral scapular slide test position 2.

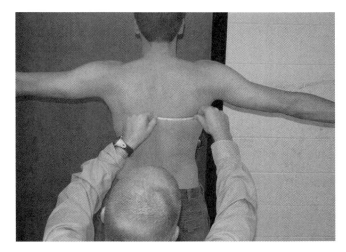

Figure 4-9: Kibler lateral scapular slide test position 3.

To begin, the clinician stands behind the patient so that the clinician can take three measurements on both the affected and the unaffected extremities. The measurement is taken from the inferior angle of the scapula to the most adjacent thoracic vertebral spinous process. The distance should be measured in centimeters and recorded for both extremities. In LSST position 1, the arms are relaxed at the patient's sides (Figure 4-7); LSST position 2 is that of hands-on-hips (iliac crest), with thumbs pointing posteriorly (Figure 4-8). The final measurement is taken with the glenohumeral joint at 90 degrees of abduction in the frontal plane with full glenohumeral internal rotation (Figure 4-9). This position is probably the hardest of the three to take because of muscle tension hiding the inferior angle.

Kibler[32] originally thought that differences between sides of greater than 1 cm indicated decreased shoulder function. Since then, Kibler has conceded that a positive finding of the LSST is probably closer to a difference in measurement of 1.5 cm between sides. The reliability of the LSST has been questioned in the past (Table 4-2).

A common finding with those who display multidirectional instability (MDI) is the protuberance of the posterolateral inferior edge of the acromion when viewed from the rear. With MDI patients there is commonly a small dimple along the posterolateral shoulder, possibly indicative of the increased laxity causing a partial sulcus sign with the arm hanging at the side.

Lateral Observation

When viewed from the lateral side, the head and neck should be lined so that the external auditory meatus is directly over the tip of the shoulder. The cervical spine should have some lordosis to its habitus, and the thoracic spine should demonstrate slight kyphosis. Most clinicians will probably agree that optimal alignment is generally the exception rather than the rule, and most patients exhibit some degree of forward head position. Also, the shoulders should be along the mid-axillary line of the torso. The shoulders are often rounded in an anterior fashion.

Supine Observation

Viewing from the head of the table can allow visualization of pec minor tightness. This is a simple sign that often goes unrecognized; however, it can be used to find muscle tightness that can contribute significantly to numerous shoulder etiologies. When lying supine, the posterior region of the acromion should sit off the table equidistant bilaterally. When the affected shoulder rests higher than the unaffected, pec minor tightness must be suspected (Figure 4-10).

Range of Motion

Because mobility of the shoulder is a prerequisite for function of the entire upper extremity, examination of range of motion (ROM) is important. Assessment of ROM always examines active range of motion (AROM) before passive range of motion (PROM). Assessment in this fashion allows the clinician to determine exactly what ROM the patient is able to volitionally perform actively. In most cases, patients will stop their ROM when they start to feel discomfort. This gives the clinician a good idea of where he or she may meet resistance or reach the patient's pain barrier when PROM is assessed. Average ROM for the shoulders has been described by Norkin and White[34] (Table 4-3). These AROMs must be clearly visualized and analyzed to detect faulty shoulder movement patterns. It is agreed that all the component joints of the shoulder assist with elevation. These joints include not only the glenohumeral joint, but also the sternoclavicular

TABLE 4-2

Lateral Scapular Slide Reliability Interclass and Intraclass Correlation Coefficients (ICCs)

AUTHORS	INTRATESTER	INTERTESTER
Kibler et al*	0.84-0.88	0.77-0.85
Gibson et al†	0.81-0.88	0.18-0.92
T'Jonck et al‡	0.69-0.96	0.72-0.90
Odem et al§	0.52-0.80	0.43-0.79

*Kibler WB, Uhl TL, Maddux JWQ, et al: Qualitative clinical evaluation of scapular dysfunction: a reliability study, *J Shoulder Elbow Surg* 11:550-556, 2002.
†Gibson MH, Goebel GV, Jordon TM, et al: A reliability study of measurement techniques to determine static scapular position, *J Orthop Sports Phys Ther* 21(2):100-106, 1995.
‡T'Jonck L, Lysens R, Gunther G: Measurement of scapular position and rotation: a reliability study, *Physiother Res Int* 1(3):148-158, 1996.
§Odem CJ, Taylor AB, Hurd CE, et al: Measurement of scapular asymmetry and assessment of shoulder dysfunction using the lateral scapular slide test: a reliability and validity study, *Phys Ther* 18(2):799-809, 2001.

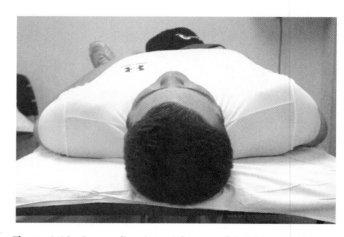

Figure 4-10: Pectoralis minor tightness of the right shoulder. *(From Manske RC, Reiman MP, Stovak M: Nonoperative and operative management of snapping scapula, Am J Sports Med 32[6]:1554-1565, 2004.)*

TABLE 4-3

Average Shoulder Ranges of Motion

	AMERICAN ACADEMY OF ORTHOPEDIC SURGEONS*	KENDALL, MCCREARY, AND PROVANCE†	HOPPENFELD‡	AMERICAN MEDICAL ASSOCIATION§
Flexion	0-180	0-180	0-90	0-150
Extension	0-60	0-45	0-45	0-50
Abduction	0-180	0-180	0-180	0-180
Medial rotation	0-70	0-70	0-55	0-90
Lateral rotation	0-90	0-90	0-45	0-90

Adapted from Norkin CC, White DJ: *Measurement of joint motion: a guide to goniometry*, ed 2, Philadelphia, 1995, FA Davis.
*American Academy of Orthopedic Surgeons: *Joint motion: method of measuring and recording*, Chicago, 1965, American Academy of Orthopedic Surgeons.
†Kendall FP, McCreary EK, Provance PG: *Muscle testing and function with posture and pain*, ed 4, Baltimore, 1993, Williams & Wilkins.
‡Hoppenfeld S: *Physical examination of the spine and extremities*, New York, 1976, Appleton-Century-Crofts.
§American Medical Association: *Guides to the evaluation of permanent impairment*, ed 3, Chicago, 1988, American Medical Association.

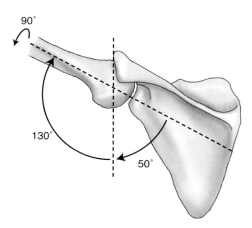

Figure 4-11: Scapulohumeral rhythm. *(From Magee DJ: Orthopedic physical assessment, ed 4, Philadelphia, 2002, Saunders.)*

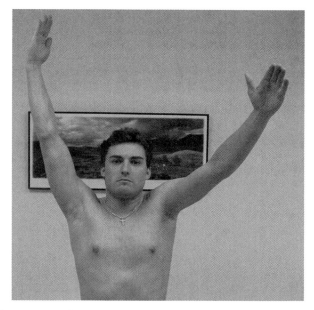

Figure 4-12: Shrug sign indicative of rotator cuff dysfunction in throwing shoulder of professional baseball pitcher.

joint, the AC joint, and the scapulothoracic joint. During approximately the first 60 degrees of elevation, the scapula is described as in the "setting phase" when the scapula seeks a position of stability on the thoracic wall.[20,35,36] Following this first phase there is a 2 : 1 ratio of glenohumeral motion to scapulothoracic motion. Simply stated, for every 2 degrees of glenohumeral motion there is 1 degree of scapulothoracic motion to fully elevate the shoulder 180 degrees (Figure 4-11). Therefore, 120 degrees of elevation occurs at the glenohumeral joint, whereas only 60 degrees occurs as the result of scapular upward rotation, protraction, and elevation.

This motion is termed *scapulohumeral rhythm*. When dysfunction occurs, this smoothly coordinated movement between the scapula and the humerus may be altered. Pathologies such as an adhesive capsulitis, RTC impingement, and RTC tear cause excessive scapular elevation, lateral rotation, or shoulder shrugging, which may run the gamut of being dramatic to subtle. The *reverse scapulohumeral rhythm* occurs when the scapula is shrugging, causing a greater amount of scapular movement than glenohumeral movement, leading to a 1 : 1 scapulohumeral ratio (Figure 4-12).[9]

Numerous authors have presented the concept of the painful arc.[37-40] The painful arc syndrome usually occurs during active abduction between 60 and 120 degrees of motion. Numerous structures can be compressed when one has a painful arc. These structures can include the supraspinatus muscle, the long head of the biceps, the coracoacromial arch, and the subacromial bursa. Weakness of the scapular upward rotators can also cause a painful arc, due to the scapula not rotating upwardly or laterally. The upward rotation and protraction move the lateral acromion superiorly, allowing more room for the soft tissue structures in the subacromial space. Another cause of painful arc is decreased mobility of the inferior and posterior capsule. With this clinical problem, as the humerus is elevated, the dynamic inferior translatory force of the RTC group is unable to oppose the superior-directed force that the restricted inferior or posterior capsule places on the humerus (Figure 4-13).

Harryman and colleagues[41] have shown that passive translations of the glenohumeral joint are accompanied by an obligate translation of the humeral head opposite the side of the tight capsule. These obligate translations are a departure from the normal arthrokinematics of shoulder joint motion. In this example, a tight inferior or posterior capsule has been shown to cause an anterior-superior humeral translation with shoulder flexion passive movements. This superior translation abuts the underlying musculature into the coracoacromial arch, resulting in impingement. Another common problem resulting in subacromial impingement is the result of a relative weakness of the lower RTC muscles. This weakness adversely affects the dynamic caudal glide of glenohumeral motion. The deltoid muscles' superior force vector results in a superior migration of the humeral head during overhead elevation.

Assessment of these motions can occur in several positions. Active range of motion of the shoulder is commonly assessed with the patient in a seated or standing position, whereas PROM of the shoulder can be assessed with the patient in a seated, standing, or supine position. Active range of motion predominantly assesses the contractile structures around the shoulder, whereas PROM primarily assesses the noncontractile structures or static stabilizers. Noncontractile structures include joint capsules, ligaments, bursae, blood vessels, and cartilage (both hyaline and fibrous).[9] It must be understood that even though AROM assessment is used to determine function of the contractile components, the noncontractile structures are still stressed during these types of motion. With overpressure of all motions, the clinician can assess the end feel of tissues that maintain end-range structural stability. The end feels for shoulder motions are listed in Table 4-4.

Several key principles exist that will assist the examiner in measuring and recording an accurate ROM of the shoulder. For all motions, a zero starting position should be used as described by the American Academy of Orthopedic Surgeons.[42] In this way, ROM is added as the joint is moved away from the zero starting position. The joint motion of the shoulder should be compared with that of the contralateral extremity. Any differences in ROM can be described in degrees or percentages of loss or increase, comparatively. The ROM achieved should be compared not only with the uninvolved shoulder, but also with norms of individuals of similar age, sex, and somatotype. Last, when measured in the position of greatest comfort, the patient usually demonstrates a greater amount of motion.[42]

Elevation of the shoulder can be measured in either abduction (frontal plane) or flexion (sagittal plane). Posterior shoulder capsular tightness can limit forward flexion, and inferior capsular tightness can limit both forward flexion and abduction. A final plane of shoulder elevation is known as scaption. Motion in the scapular plane, or *scaption*, generally occurs in a plane approximately 30 to 45 degrees anterior to the frontal plane.[27] This plane is generally the most comfortable to elevate the arm for several reasons. Because this plane is located between both the frontal and the sagittal planes,

there is less posterior and inferior capsular tightness restricting glenohumeral motion as the humerus is elevated throughout its full ROM. Others have proposed that the plane of the scapula does not require the humerus to laterally rotate as much during elevation as compared with classic abduction in the sagittal plane.[27] Shoulder flexion is measured in the sagittal plane centering the fulcrum of the goniometer near the acromion process. The stationary arm of the goniometer is aligned along the midaxillary line, and the movable arm is aligned with the lateral midline of the humerus[32] (Figure 4-14). Shoulder abduction is measured in the frontal plane with the fulcrum located close to the posterior aspect of the acromion process. The stationary arm is aligned parallel to the spinous process of the vertebral column, and the movable arm is located at the posterior midline of the humerus[32] (Figure 4-15).

It is worth noting that following surgical repair of the shoulder joint, glenohumeral ROM is measured from the position of 0 degrees of shoulder abduction. Preoperatively, glenohumeral internal and external rotation ROM is most often measured with the patient in a supine position and the shoulder abducted 90 degrees and the elbow flexed 90 degrees. The forearm should be perpendicular to the measuring surface with the forearm in neutral. A pad can be placed

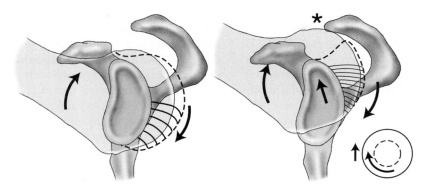

Figure 4-13: Inferior capsular tightness resulting in impingement. *(From Matsen FA, Arnts CT: Subacromial impingement. In Rockwood CA, Matsen FA, editors: The shoulder, ed 2, vol 2, Philadelphia, 1990, Saunders.)*

TABLE 4-4

End Feels for Passive Range of Motion of the Glenohumeral Joint

MOTION	END FEEL
Flexion	Tissue stretch
Extension	Tissue stretch
Abduction	Bone-to-bone or tissue stretch
Medial rotation	Tissue stretch
Lateral rotation	Tissue stretch

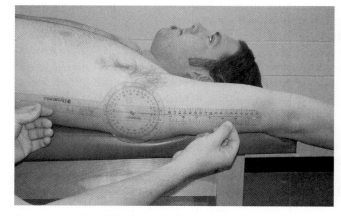

Figure 4-14: Shoulder forward flexion goniometry.

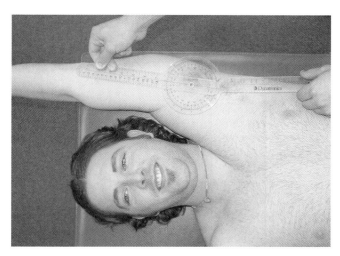

Figure 4-15: Shoulder abduction goniometry.

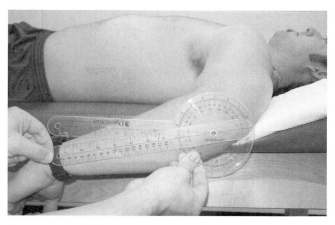

Figure 4-17: Full shoulder range of motion without scapular stabilization (glenohumeral and scapulothoracic).

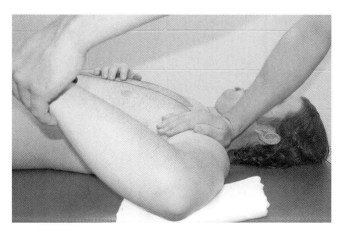

Figure 4-16: Shoulder internal rotation range of motion with scapula stabilized (glenohumeral only).

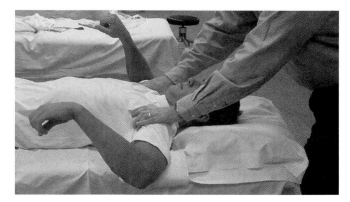

Figure 4-18: Glenohumeral internal rotation deficit (GIRD).

under the elbow if the humerus is resting in a horizontally extended/abducted position to decrease tightness in the anterior capsule and shoulder musculature.

To measure glenohumeral internal rotation, the humerus is kept in 90 degrees of abduction while the scapula is prevented from elevating or tilting anteriorly. The forearm, with the palm facing toward the examining table, should be taken toward the supporting surface, moving the extremity into internal rotation. The goniometer is placed directly over the olecranon and the distal arm aligned parallel to the ulnar styloid process. Once a firm end point is felt because of tension from the posterior capsule or cuff muscles, the ROM measurement should be taken. At this point the clinician has measured the isolated amount of internal rotation ROM available at the glenohumeral joint alone (Figure 4-16). Another measurement can be taken of composite shoulder internal rotation ROM. Composite internal rotation ROM can be measured by allowing the scapula to protract as needed to gain as much ROM as possible when taking the measurement. Because the scapula is not normally stabilized when

the shoulder is commonly used in everyday life, this measurement appears to be much more functional. The measurement of isolated glenohumeral internal rotation ROM is still very important because it provides the exact amount of ROM isolated at only the glenohumeral joint. This allows the clinician to determine posterior capsular/cuff mobility or tightness (Figure 4-17).

Glenohumeral internal rotation deficit (GIRD) is a common finding seen in athletes who use overhead motions.[43] Some report that GIRD may be one of the most important pathologic processes that occur in a throwing athlete's shoulder.[43] GIRD is defined as the loss in degrees of glenohumeral internal rotation of the throwing shoulder compared with the nonthrowing shoulder (Figure 4-18). Using the internal shoulder rotation measurement method described previously, the clinician compares the amount of glenohumeral internal rotation ROM bilaterally. An unacceptable level of GIRD is a decrease of internal rotation ROM either greater than 20 degrees or greater than 10% of the total rotation seen in the nonthrowing shoulder.

External rotation ROM is taken from the same starting position as described for the internal rotation ROM measurement. In this measurement the forearm is taken posteriorly so that the extensor surface of the forearm is moved toward the head of the examining table (Figure 4-19).

NEUROLOGIC EXAMINATION

Sensation

Assessment of sensation is important to determine cutaneous neurologic impairment in dermatomal distribution. Semmes Weinstein sensation kits utilize various diameters of mono-filaments to assess sensation at each dermatomal level. In addition, light touch, pin-prick, and thermal discrimination can be determined at each level. This evaluation is compared with the uninvolved extremity to detect differences from side to side. Simple, quick examinations of sharp and dull can use a pinwheel or the blunt end of the reflex hammer. Running the fingers softly over the dermatomes bilaterally can assess light touch (Figure 4-20). While testing dermatomes, the patient should close his or her eyes or turn the head so that the patient does not use visual stimulation to determine sensation.

Reflexes

Reflexes for the biceps (C5), the brachioradialis (C5 to C6), and the triceps (C7) should be examined and compared bilat-erally. Reflexes are rated on a 0 to 4 scale with 0/4 = absent reflexes, 1/4 = hypotonic reflexes, 2/4 = normal response, 3/4 = hypertonic reflexes, and 4/4 = clonus. Reflexes are best tested with the patient as relaxed as possible. If the patient is in severe pain, reflex testing may not be as accurate because of muscle guarding during the testing maneuvers. To test the biceps tendon reflex (C5), the clinician should cradle the

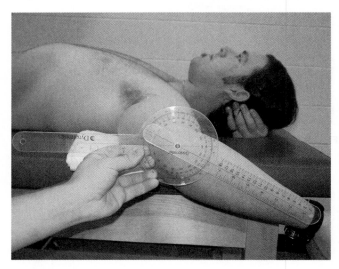

Figure 4-19: Shoulder external rotation goniometry.

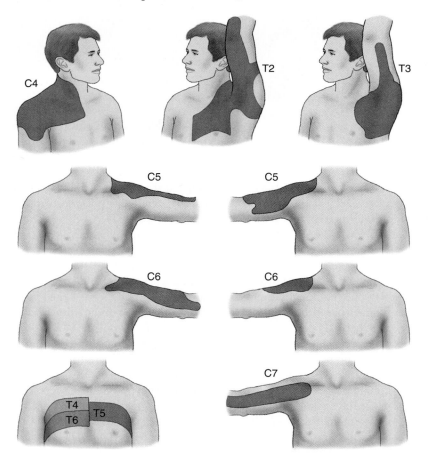

Figure 4-20: Shoulder dermatomes. *(From Magee DJ:* Orthopedic physical assessment, *ed 4, Philadelphia, 2002, Saunders.)*

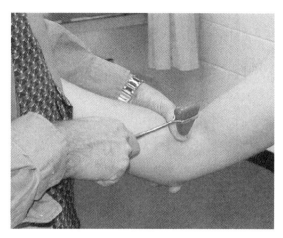

Figure 4-21: Biceps brachii deep tendon reflex.

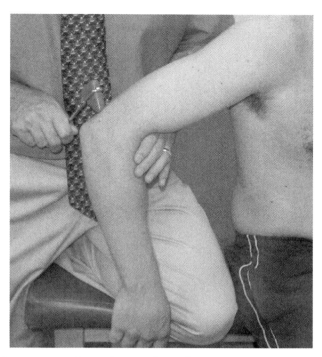

Figure 4-22: Triceps deep tendon reflex.

patient's elbow flexed approximately 70 degrees while palpating the biceps distal tendon with his or her thumb. With the other hand the clinician percusses his or her own thumb with the small (sharp) end of the reflex hammer to assess the reflex ability of the biceps tendon (Figure 4-21). The brachioradialis tendon (C5 to C6) can be tested by either cradling the patient's arm as during testing the biceps reflex or by resting the patient's forearm on his or her lap. Using the flat end of the reflex hammer, the brachioradialis tendon is percussed just proximal to the distal end of the radius. The triceps (C7) tendon reflex is tested with the shoulder internally rotated and the shoulder abducted so that the dorsal surface of the elbow faces superiorly. The hammer is percussed directly to the triceps tendon and the reflex determined (Figure 4-22). If reflexes are difficult to obtain with conventional testing, the patient can be asked to clench his or her teeth or squeeze his or her legs together,[9] enlisting the Jendrassik's maneuver to additionally facilitate the reflex response.[44,45] The Jendrassik maneuver facilitates activity of the spinal cord, accentuating a minimally active reflex.[46]

MANUAL MUSCLE TESTING

Manual muscle testing (MMT) allows the clinician to assess strength of either individual muscles or groups of muscles commonly used in and around the shoulder. During MMT, the clinician applies a manual resistance to the extremity, which is placed in a specifically designed position based on the muscle size, the length/tension relationship of the muscle, and the effects of gravity. The strength of a given muscle or group of muscles can then be compared bilaterally to determine weakness.[47,48]

Several problems exist when manually testing the shoulder complex. Pain can create a reflexive inhibition to muscle firing patterns, making the patient appear to have a weakness, when in fact the muscle still has full strength.[27] Another common problem with standard MMT procedures listed in various texts occurs with positioning. Evaluating strength of

a patient with a chronic frozen shoulder may not allow testing at standard positions because of decreased capsular mobility. For example, testing of the serratus anterior, middle, and lower trapezius may be impossible because of the ROM needed to properly test these crucial muscles. Because MMT is a basic skill required of all rehabilitation specialists, details regarding specific tests for muscular strength are not discussed in this chapter. See texts such as Kendall, McCreary, and Provance[49] and Daniels and Worthingham[50] for descriptions of MMT procedures. At minimum, MMT of the shoulder should include assessment of the shoulder, elbow, forearm, wrist, and hand. Myotomes can be assessed to quickly rule out cervical neurologic involvement. C1: cervical rotation; C2, C3, and C4: scapular elevation; C4: diaphragm; C5: shoulder abduction; C6: wrist extension; C7: wrist flexion; C8: thumb extension; T1: abductor digiti minimi. Specific motions at the shoulder should be tested for strength and include shoulder flexion, shoulder abduction, shoulder extension, shoulder adduction, horizontal abduction and adduction, internal and external shoulder rotation, and all scapular motions, including protraction, retraction, elevation, and depression.

Grades of strength can be determined in several ways. We most commonly use the 5-point scale, although other methods can be used such as the 10-point scale; percentages; and wording such as normal, good, fair, poor, trace, and zero (Table 4-5).

In addition to standard MMT, the sequence of pain to resistance can garner significant information related to muscle-tendon unit function. The pain-resistance sequence as described by Cyriax[19] should be used along with standard

MMT. This method of assessment can be used to help determine the acuteness or chronicity of the patient's symptoms (Table 4-6).

PALPATION

Palpation of soft tissue and bony structures is done not only in an attempt to elicit tenderness, but also to assess tissue texture, firmness, temperature, thickness, and abnormal prominences. Table 4-7 lists bony, muscular, and other soft tissue structures. We have developed a test that empirically appears to be sensitive for scapular fractures that we call the *scapular percussion test*. Applying a firm tapping-type strike to the spine of the scapula has often reproduced the patient's symptoms in those with scapular fractures. This firm tapping probably elicits a painful response from free nerve endings at the fracture site causing symptoms of deep bone pain. Although this procedure has not been researched for validity or reliability, we have found it to be useful in our hands.

SPECIAL TESTING

Special testing of the shoulder is paramount to determine the exact pathology and to corroborate the cluster of signs and symptoms from the entire examination. The clinician uses special tests to rule out or implicate tissues or structures that may be at fault.

Using Davies' shoulder special testing algorithm,[51] one can systematically examine the shoulder in a fast, efficient, and appropriate manner. This algorithm was specifically designed so that all shoulder structures can be evaluated efficiently with a minimum number of patient position changes. The algorithm is also based on the corroboration of various tests to implicate specific tissue structures. Initially, when beginning the special testing sequence of events the clinician must determine the tissue status in and around the glenohumeral joint. Static restraint of glenohumeral motion can be achieved with assistance from the glenoid fossa, the glenoid labrum, and the glenohumeral ligaments and capsule. Special tests to determine the status of the glenoid fossa and labrum are discussed later. The clinician can test the glenohumeral ligaments and capsule with the sulcus signs and the anterior and posterior load and shift.

Capsular Stability

The sulcus sign with the arm positioned at 0 degrees of abduction tests the superior capsule, the superior gleno-

---

TABLE 4-5

Manual Muscle Testing Grading Systems

FUNCTION OF MUSCLE					SYMBOLS				
No Movement									
No contraction felt in muscle	Zero	0	0	0	(0)	(0.0)	0%	0
Tendon becomes prominent or feeble contraction felt in muscle, but no visible movement of the part	Trace	T	T	1	(1)	(1.0)	T	T
Movement in Horizontal Plane									
Moves through partial range of motion	Poor−	P−	1	2−	$(1\frac{1}{2})$	(1.5)	10%	1
Moves through complete range of motion	Poor	P	2	2	(2)	(2.0)	20%	2
Moves to completion of range against resistance or moves to completion of range and holds against pressure	Poor+	P+	3	2+	$(2\frac{1}{3})$	(2.33)	30%	3
Antigravity Position									
Moves through partial range of motion	Poor+	P+	3	2+	$(2\frac{1}{3})$	(2.33)	30%	3
Gradual release from test position	Fair−	F−	4	3−	$(2\frac{2}{3})$	(2.66)	40%	4
Holds test position (no added pressure)	Fair	F	5	3	(3)	(3.0)	50%	5
Holds test position against slight pressure	Fair+	F+	6	3+	$(3\frac{1}{3})$	(3.33)	60%	6
Holds test position against slight to moderate pressure	Good−	G−	7	4−	$(3\frac{2}{3})$	(3.66)	70%	7
Holds test position against moderate pressure	Good	G	8	4	(4)	(4.0)	80%	8
Holds test position against moderate to strong pressure	Good+	G+	9	4+	$(4\frac{1}{2})$	(4.5)	90%	9
Holds test position against strong resistance	Normal	N	10	5	(5)	(5.0)	100%	10

From Kendall FP, McCreary EK, Provance PG: *Muscle testing and function with posture and pain*, ed 4, Baltimore, 1993, Williams & Wilkins.

TABLE 4-6

Cyriax Pain Resistance Sequence

ONSET OF PAIN	LESION	DESCRIPTION
Pain before resistance	Acute	Onset of pain before reaching end ROM. Any additional resistance felt is usually attributed to muscle guarding.
Pain with resistance	Subacute	Pain and resistance that occur at the same time.
Pain after resistance	Chronic	Minimal to no pain, if any, after the examiner reaches resistance.

Adapted from Cyriax J: *Textbook of orthopaedic medicine*, vol I, *Diagnosis of soft tissue lesions*, London, 1982, Bailliere Tindall.

humeral ligaments, and the rotator interval. This area of the shoulder includes the coracohumeral ligaments and the rotator interval. The rotator interval is described as a triangular-shaped region between the inferior border of the supraspinatus tendon and the superior border of the sub-scapularis tendon.[52] The clinician grasps the patient's relaxed arm just distal to the elbow on the dorsal surface of the forearm. The clinician then applies a gentle, inferiorly directed force (181.4 N)[53] parallel to the long axis of the humerus (Figure 4-23). In the patient with increased glenohumeral laxity, a sulcus sign will appear just inferior to the acromion. If the patient exhibits a positive sulcus sign, this is thought to demonstrate MDI. This description of instability (MDI) is somewhat of a misnomer because the patient may not actually have clinical instability; however, the patient does demonstrate a great degree of shoulder laxity. Most often this simple test is used to assess overall shoulder laxity. Those who demonstrate generalized ligamentous laxity may exhibit a positive sulcus sign bilaterally. The sulcus sign should be considered pathologic if the patient feels unstable or as though the shoulder is about to sublux when testing is performed. A sulcus sign can be graded by measuring the distance from the inferior acromion to the head of the humerus (Table 4-8). The interpretation of a sulcus sign

TABLE 4-7

Bony and Soft Tissue Palpation

BONY STRUCTURES	MUSCULAR STRUCTURES	OTHER
Clavicle	Deltoid	Joint capsule
Acromion	Anterior	Transverse humeral ligament
First rib	Medial	Subdeltoid bursa
Acromioclavicular joint	Posterior	Subacromial bursa
Coracoid process	Trapezius	Sternoclavicular ligaments
Greater tubercle	Upper third	Acromioclavicular ligaments
Lesser tubercle	Middle third	Coracoacromial ligament
Bicipital groove	Lower third	Coracoclavicular ligaments
Humerus	Pectoralis major	
Sternoclavicular joint	Pectoralis minor	
Manubrium	Serratus anterior	
Ribs	Rhomboid major	
Sternum	Rhomboid minor	
Scapula	Latissimus dorsi	
Scapular spine	Supraspinatus	
Medial border of scapula	Infraspinatus	
Lateral border of scapula	Teres major and minor	
	Subscapularis	
	Biceps brachii	
	Triceps	
	Levator scapula	

being pathologic should be reserved for examination grades of 2+ or greater.[54] A pathologic sulcus (2+ or greater) at 0 degrees of abduction that persists on externally rotating the humerus is highly suggestive of an RTC interval lesion.[54]

The Feagin test is the follow-up test after the sulcus sign at 0 degrees and when positive is more indicative of selective laxity of the inferior glenohumeral ligament complex.[55] The patient is tested best when relaxed in the sitting position beside the clinician. The clinician holds the patient's upper extremity at 90 degrees of abduction, with the patient's forearm over the clinician's shoulder and elbow extended. The clinician uses one hand to apply an inferiorly and slightly anteriorly directed force while the other hand palpates the edge of the acromion and the humeral head to feel for

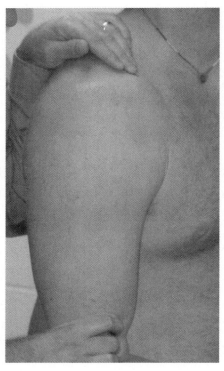

Figure 4-23: Sulcus sign at 0 degrees (arm at side) for superior capsule laxity.

TABLE 4-8
Grading of Sulcus Sign

ACROMIOHUMERAL INTERVAL	GRADE
Up to 1 cm	1+
1 to 2 cm	2+
Greater than 2 cm	3+

Adapted from Norris TR: Diagnostic techniques of shoulder instability, *AAOS Course Lectures* 34:239, 1985.

displacement anteriorly and inferiorly (Figure 4-24). A sense of apprehension, pain, or an increased amount of translation in the inferior direction as compared with the uninvolved side is considered a positive sign.

The next test to be performed for instability is the anterior and posterior load and shift.[56-58] The patient should be sitting in a relaxed position with his or her arm resting comfortably in the lap, while maintaining good posture to ensure accurate results with this testing maneuver. The clinician uses his or her stabilizing hand to grasp the patient's shoulder by holding the clavicle and acromion with the fingers while the forearm and elbow are placed along the scapula, posteriorly stabilizing it. With the other hand, the clinician grasps the patient's proximal humerus with the thumb over the posterior humeral head and the fingers around the anterior humeral head. The clinician should attempt to determine the actual resting position of the humeral head before translation. Often the humeral head rests in an anterior position. This position will allow the fingers to feel a slight depression anterior and medial to the humeral head. The clinician gently pushes the humeral head medially to seat the humerus in the glenoid fossa.[59] This is considered the load portion of the test and allows the humeral head to be placed in a neutral or centered position. The shift portion of the test is the actual translation made anteriorly (203.1 N in normal subjects)[53] or posteriorly (191.8 N in normal subjects)[53] from this neutral position and depends on the resting position found. The clinician notes the amount of anterior and posterior translation and compares this amount with the noninvolved extremity (Figure 4-25).

Without performing the load portion of the test, it is common to feel that the posterior translation is greater than anterior, leading one to incorrectly assume that the patient exhibits an isolated posterior laxity. This is generally not the case. The average amount of passive humeral head translation is 14.5 mm anteriorly and 14.0 mm posteriorly in normal human subjects.[53] Because many patients' shoulders are

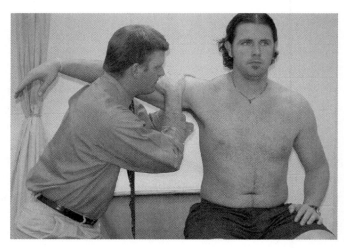

Figure 4-24: Sulcus sign at 90 degrees of abduction for inferior capsular laxity.

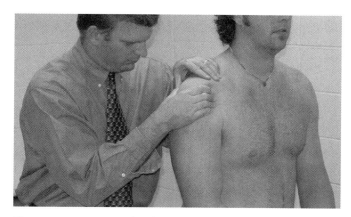

Figure 4-25: Posterior load and shift for posterior capsular laxity.

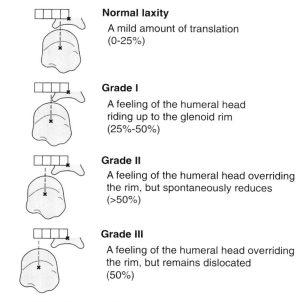

Normal laxity
A mild amount of translation (0-25%)

Grade I
A feeling of the humeral head riding up to the glenoid rim (25%-50%)

Grade II
A feeling of the humeral head overriding the rim, but spontaneously reduces (>50%)

Grade III
A feeling of the humeral head overriding the rim, but remains dislocated (50%)

Figure 4-26: Grades of anterior glenohumeral translation. *(From Magee DJ: Orthopedic physical assessment, ed 4, Philadelphia, 2002, Saunders.)*

protracted and anteriorly rounded, the humeral head may naturally rest in an anteriorly displaced position. With the head in this location, a selected anteromedial translation (shift) may be minimal, because the humeral head's resting position has already placed the anterior capsule on tension. With this same scenario, the posterior shift will appear to be through a greater distance, thus yielding a false indication that a posterior laxity is present. Regardless of the resting position of the shoulder, the amount of anterior and posterior motion should be compared bilaterally, and a unilateral increase in passive mobility is considered a positive test. Silliman and Hawkins,[58] Hawkins and Mohtadi,[59] and Altchek and colleagues[60] have described grading of humeral translation (Figure 4-26). The clinician must realize that authors cannot seem to agree as to which translation is normally greatest, whether translation is equal in both direc-

tions, or whether shoulder dominance affects humeral head translations.[61-63] Numerous authors report finding capsular restraint symmetry in the glenohumeral joint.[53,61,64] These findings substantiate the circle concept of shoulder stability, which states that shoulder laxity is equal in all directions because of the unique arrangement of the shoulder joint capsule.[61,65,66]

These first several tests for capsular stability should be performed on everyone regardless of pathology and will give the clinician an idea of the patient's soft tissue restraint status. This will allow the clinician to determine whether the patient has a hypomobile or hypermobile shoulder. It will be valuable throughout the rest of the rehabilitation progression in determining which types of exercises should be performed and how quickly the patient can be progressed.

Seated Labral Testing

Continuing in the seated position, the next progression of special tests would include several tests to evaluate integrity of the biceps-labral complex. These tests should be performed if your patient describes a macrotraumatic type of injury, complains of "deep" shoulder pain, or describes locking or pseudolocking with active and passive shoulder movements. The compression rotation test was initially described by Guidi and Suckerman[67] and Snyder and colleagues.[68] We commonly perform it slightly differently than the initial description. The glenohumeral joint is placed at 45 degrees of abduction as the clinician stabilizes the superior portion of the shoulder with one hand and grasps the elbow in the other. The distal hand applies a compressive force up the long axis of the humerus toward the superior labrum. While compressing the humerus cranially, a concurrently produced clockwise and counterclockwise circumduction is performed in an attempt to entrap a piece of labrum between the humeral head and the glenoid fossa. The patient's complaint of pain, snapping, or catching sensations is considered a positive test for a superior labral tear, or "superior labrum anterior to posterior" (SLAP).

Another seated test to determine a SLAP lesion is the anterior slide test. In the same position as that described for the compression rotation test, the clinician grasps the elbow flexed 90 degrees while the patient has his or her hands on hips with the thumbs pointing posteriorly. Holding at the elbow, the clinician supplies a forward and compressive (superior) force to the arm. The patient is asked to push back against this force (Figure 4-27). A sensation of painful popping, catching, or locking indicates a positive test. This specific test has been reported to have approximately 80% sensitivity for detection of superior labrum tears.[69] Another version of this test is performed with the patient's arm at 0 degrees of abduction, while compressive force is again applied cranially up the long axis of the humerus while the shoulder is moved through an arc of 0 to 45 degrees of flexion or extension. Similar to the compression rotation, the clinician is attempting to compress a torn or irritated portion of the

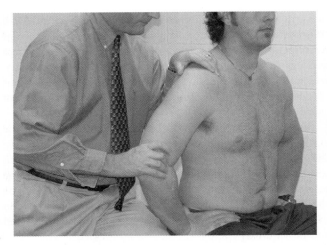

Figure 4-27: Anterior slide (labral tear test).

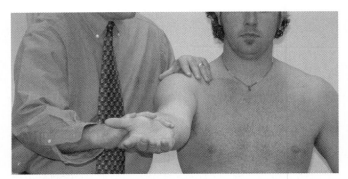

Figure 4-28: Speed's test.

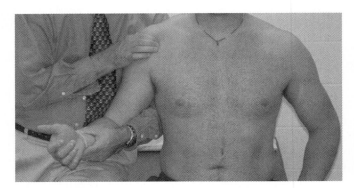

Figure 4-29: Yeargason's test for long head of biceps tendinopathy or biceps tendon instability.

superior labrum against the humeral head. We also call the maneuver in which the humerus is extended while the humeral head is compressed into the superior joint the anterior slide, because it compresses the anterior portion of the labrum, indicating a possible eccentric deceleration traction injury. When the humerus is flexed we call it the posterior slide, which attempts to compress a torn or irritated posterior portion of the labrum, indicating a possible "peel back" mechanism of injury.

While still in the seated position, several tests should be performed to assess the integrity and function of the long head of the biceps. Some believe that through its compressive force at the humeral head, the long head of the biceps can actually function as a humeral head depressor during shoulder movements.[70-72] It is commonly known that the long head of the biceps can assist with the motion of shoulder flexion because its origin and insertion cross both the elbow and glenohumeral joints.

One of the most common tests for biceps tendon pathology is Speed's test. The clinician asks the patient to flex the shoulder to 90 degrees with the elbow extended and the forearm fully supinated. The clinician provides resistance to the distal forearm in the direction of shoulder and elbow extension. This resistance given distal across the two joints creates a forceful recruitment of the biceps muscle-tendon unit (Figure 4-28). Depending on the location and type of pain, several injuries can be implicated. A positive test with complaints of anterior superficial pain would indicate biceps tendonitis, paratendinitis, or tendinosis.[73] We have commonly seen patients with SLAP lesions who have a positive result on Speed's test. In this pathology, the complaint of pain will be deep in the shoulder. This is understandable because the long head of the biceps attaches to the superior portion of the labrum. Any pathology to that area could potentially contribute to pain in the long head of the biceps during provocation testing. Bennett[74] found Speed's test to be only 13.8% specific but 90% sensitive. Bennett found that Speed's test could be positive for a variety of shoulder pathol-

ogies, including impingement of supraspinatus and acromion or into the subacromial bursae, secondary instability due to shoulder instability, a tight posterior capsule or a coracoacromial ligament spur, or even a Bankart lesion. Bennett had one patient who had a negative Speed's test despite having a complete avulsion of the biceps tendon. Bennett speculates that when the biceps tendon becomes completely avulsed out of the bicipital groove, it will usually scar to other surrounding structures. Thus with no forces transmitted to the proximal shoulder, Speed's test was negative.

Yeargason's test is another commonly used test for assessing pathology of the long head of the biceps. Yeargason's test was initially described as early as 1931.[75] As in the previous test, the patient is seated with his or her elbow flexed at 90 degrees. The clinician grasps the patient's distal forearm with the hand closest to the patient, while the outer hand palpates the bicipital groove. The patient is instructed to simultaneously flex the elbow, supinate the forearm, and laterally rotate the shoulder against resistance given by the examiner (Figure 4-29). The clinician's palpating hand will feel for a subluxation of the long head of the biceps tendon, which can occur if there is pathology of the transverse humeral ligament that restrains excessive movement of the long head. When the transverse humeral ligament is torn, a popping or snapping sensation may be felt along the bicipital groove. Pain or tenderness on palpation of the long head may indicate tendinopathy or possibly the SLAP lesion mentioned previously.

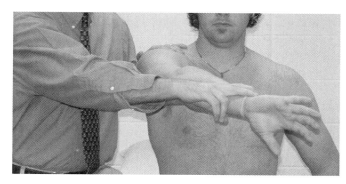

Figure 4-30: O'Brien active compression part I.

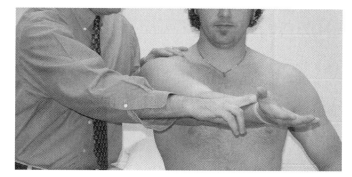

Figure 4-31: O'Brien active compression part II.

Using a sequence of several testing procedures for a given pathology is an example of using corroborative special testing to implicate, in this case, the long head of the biceps.

Acromioclavicular Joint Testing

The active compression test of O'Brien is a test that can be used to implicate a SLAP lesion or an AC joint injury.[76,77] This test, which is becoming more mainstream in diagnosing SLAP lesions and AC joint pathology, has been proven to be accurate almost 100% of the time.[77] Standing next to the affected extremity, the clinician asks the patient to flex the shoulder to 90 degrees, followed by horizontally adducting the shoulder 10 to 15 degrees medial to the sagittal plane. From this position, the clinician maximally internally rotates the patient's shoulder and applies an inferiorly directed force to the distal forearm and ascertains whether this maneuver causes pain (Figure 4-30). If no pain occurs, the test is negative. Pain that does occur will generally be in one of two locales: superiorly at the AC joint or deep in the shoulder to implicate a SLAP lesion. Once the location of pain has been determined, the clinician externally rotates the patient's shoulder and supinates the forearm, maintaining the position of 10 to 15 degrees of horizontal adduction. Resistance is given to the distal forearm, and the patient is again queried regarding pain (Figure 4-31). If deep pain is reduced or eliminated, a SLAP lesion is probable. If the pain that is located superiorly is reduced or eliminated, the probable

cause is AC joint pathology (either ligament sprain or degenerative joint disease). No change in pain or worsening of symptoms would indicate some other form of pathology rather than the two discussed.

With the patient still sitting, several simple tests can be performed to implicate pathology at the AC joint. Acromioclavicular joint pathology should normally be expected in patients over age 40, especially if their history describes a traumatic fall onto the superior portion of the shoulder or a fall onto an outstretched hand. With AC joint ligament sprains greater than grade I, a step-off deformity is normally present. Most commonly, the AC joint itself is tender to palpate, whereas pain is located superiorly on the shoulder. Acromioclavicular joint arthralgia has also been shown to be a common source of pain in weightlifters who have performed heavy pressing lifts. The AC posterior shear test[45] is performed next. The clinician's anterior hand is placed slightly medial to the distalmost portion of the clavicle, and the posterior hand is placed at the posterolateral aspect of the acromion. A compressive force is given along the anterior clavicle in a posterior direction, shearing the AC joint posteriorly. A positive test is indicated by pain in the AC joint or by hypermobility or hypomobility when compared with the uninvolved shoulder.

The active compression test of O'Brien and the AC posterior shear test are two corroborative tests for the AC joint. These tests implicate or rule out AC involvement before the arm is taken into an overhead position during clinical examination.

Impingement Tests

Because RTC pathology is so prevalent, there is critical need to differentiate various forms of impairment such as tendonitis, bursitis, and partial- to full-thickness RTC tears. Impingement tests can help differentiate RTC tendonitis from a tear. The patient with an acute impingement syndrome will generally improve significantly with proper physical therapy treatments, but the patient with a significant RTC tear may not.

Impingement syndromes can be due to several problems, including primary impingement (described as primary cuff disease associated with a humeral head that does not depress normally because of RTC weakness); the presence of a tight posterior capsule; or narrowing of the subacromial space, due to either a type III (hooked) acromion,[78] degenerative spurs, os acromiale, a congenitally thick coracoacromial ligament,[79] or an inflamed bursa or cuff. Impingement can also occur secondary to another cause, such as glenohumeral instability.[80] With instability the RTC muscles are fatigued from attempting to maintain dynamic stability of the glenohumeral joint; therefore they are unable to perform their role as humeral head depressors.

The Neer's impingement sign is used to compress the patient's supraspinatus or long head of the biceps into the undersurface of the acromion or the coracoacromial arch,

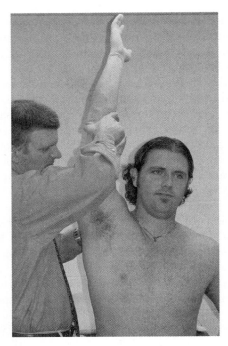

Figure 4-32: Neer's impingement test.

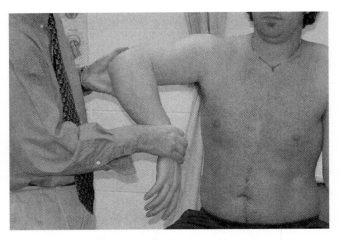

Figure 4-33: Hawkins-Kennedy impingement test.

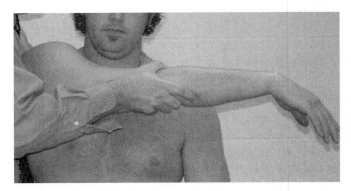

Figure 4-34: Crossover acromioclavicular joint impingement test.

respectively, in an attempt to replicate the patient's pain during overhead lifting or reaching. The clinician grasps the patient's arm at the level of the elbow, keeping the arm in the neutral position, and passively elevates the arm through a full range of forward flexion. Once end ROM is felt, a passive overpressure is given to compress the supraspinatus or long head of the biceps underneath the anterior-inferior portion of the acromion or coracoacromial arch (Figure 4-32). A positive test is indicated by pain during the test.

Another common impingement test is that described by Hawkins and Kennedy.[81] In this procedure the arm is elevated to 90 degrees in the plane of the scapula with the elbow flexed 90 degrees. From this position the clinician gently internally rotates the shoulder in an attempt to compress the greater tuberosity and the supraspinatus tendon underneath the coracoacromial arch (Figure 4-33). A positive test is the patient's complaint of pain. Valadie and colleagues[82] found that when using the Hawkins-Kennedy impingement test on cadavers, all specimens demonstrated contact between the RTC and the coracoacromial ligament and between the undersurface of the RTC and the glenoid rim.

The corocoid impingement test is used to elicit a compressive force on structures surrounding the shoulder. The clinician stands directly in front of the patient and passively flexes the patient's arm to 90 degrees in the sagittal plane with the elbow flexed to 90 degrees. From this position the clinician gently internally rotates the shoulder as in the Hawkins-Kennedy test. With the corocoid impingement test, several locations of pathology can be determined. A complaint of pain medially would indicate long head of the biceps or subscapularis dysfunction, and lateral pain would implicate the supraspinatus.

In the crossover impingement test, the clinician passively flexes the patient's arm to 90 degrees, and then horizontally adducts the arm across his or her body to end ROM. The clinician must place a stabilizing hand behind the patient's contralateral shoulder for stabilization because the patient will commonly rotate the trunk in the direction to avoid pain (Figure 4-34). Pain can be felt in several locations and is only indicative of AC joint pathology if superior pain is located at the actual joint itself.[83-85] Medial shoulder pain with the crossover test may be from a bicipital tendinopathy or subscapularis pathology; lateral pain implicates subacromial structures; and posterior pain could implicate the infraspinatus, teres minor, or a posterior capsulitis or internal impingement.

Rotator Cuff Tear Testing

There are numerous tests to determine integrity of the RTC. One such test is the drop arm test. While standing behind the patient, the clinician passively takes the patient's shoulder to 90 degrees of abduction in the scapular plane and asks the patient to hold that position. One of the clinician's hands should be placed under the patient's arm so that the injured extremity can be caught if the patient is unable to hold this position. If the patient is able to hold the position, the clinician gently taps the superior portion of the distal forearm in an attempt to break the held position. If the patient is unable to hold this position, an RTC tear is probable. A modification of this test is performed by passively elevating the patient's arm to end ROM. The clinician then releases the patient's arm and asks him or her to slowly lower the arm to 0 degrees in the frontal plane. As with the original drop arm test, the clinician should follow with his or her hand under the patient's arm as it is eccentrically lowered in case of a break or drop of the arm. The inability to lower the arm into adduction would indicate an RTC tear.

Lag signs have been described by Hertel and colleagues[86] to determine RTC pathology. To perform the external rotation lag sign, the patient sits in front of the clinician with the elbow passively flexed to 90 degrees, while the shoulder is taken to 20 degrees of elevation in the scapular plane and near maximal external rotation minus 5 degrees to avoid elastic recoil in the shoulder. The patient is asked to actively maintain the position of external rotation in elevation as the clinician releases the wrist, while still maintaining hold of the elbow (Figure 4-35). A lag at the wrist will indicate a tear or rupture of the infraspinatus muscle. The magnitude of the lag is measured to the nearest 5 degrees, with small tears measuring less than a 5-degree lag and complete tears measuring greater than a 5-degree lag. This portion of the test implicates the infraspinatus; the second portion tests the supraspinatus tendon.

In the second portion, the extremity is in the same position as previously described. From this position the clinician asks the patient to hold the affected arm as the clinician releases the elbow (Figure 4-36). The amount of lag or drop of the elbow is recorded to the nearest 5 degrees. A 5-degree lag would indicate a small tear of the supraspinatus, whereas a complete rupture of the supraspinatus would cause a lag greater than 5 degrees. A modification of this test has been described by Davies and is performed in the exact manner as the previous test except that it is performed in the position

of 90 degrees of elbow and shoulder abduction. This test places much greater stress on the RTC and places the shoulder in a much more functional position. With all lag tests, interpretation may be difficult following pathologic changes in ROM. When PROM is reduced because of capsular contracture or increased because of subscapularis rupture, for instance, a false-negative or a false-positive result must be expected.[87]

The internal rotation lag sign[86] has been described to assess function of the subscapularis. The clinician stands beside the patient's involved extremity. The affected arm is held by the clinician in almost maximal internal rotation. The elbow is flexed to 90 degrees while the shoulder is abducted approximately 20 degrees and extended about 20 degrees. The dorsum of the patient's hand is lifted away from the lumbar region until almost full internal rotation is reached. The patient is then asked to actively maintain this position as the clinician releases the wrist while still maintaining support at the elbow. The sign is positive when a lag occurs (Figure 4-37). The magnitude of the lag is recorded to the nearest 5 degrees. An obvious lag will occur with large tears, whereas a small lag may suggest a partial tear of the

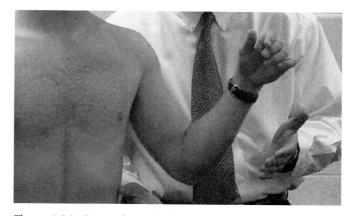

Figure 4-36: External rotation lag sign test part II.

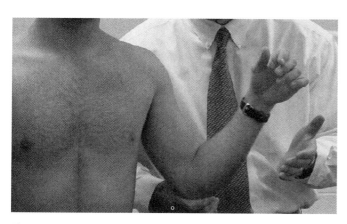

Figure 4-35: External rotation lag sign test part I.

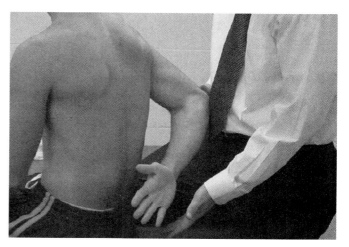

Figure 4-37: Internal rotation lag sign.

subscapularis muscle. This test may be difficult if not impossible for patients who have moderate to severe limitation in shoulder internal rotation ROM, such as those who have been in prolonged immobilization or those suffering from an adhesive capsulitis. The main difference between this test and the classic lift off test of Gerber and Krushell[88] is that in the latter the patient actively attempts to lift the dorsum of the hand off the lower back area. Inability to lift the dorsum of the hand off the lumbar region would indicate a subscapularis tear.

Recent evidence by Hurschler and colleagues[89] finds the external rotation lag sign to be highly sensitive (100%) for the infraspinatus–teres minor muscles at 20, 40, and 60 degrees of elevation. The same study found much lower sensitivity, peaking at 60% sensitive at 90 degrees of elevation, for the supraspinatus muscle. Therefore the lag sign appears to be highly sensitive only for the infraspinatus–teres minor muscles, especially at higher elevations, where the supraspinatus cannot compensate. Lag signs have little or no power to diagnose isolated supraspinatus defects in the presence of a functioning infraspinatus–teres minor unit.

Thoracic Outlet Testing

Several important tests done while in the seated position are not commonly a part of the Davies special testing algorithm. The last tests performed while sitting are to determine the presence or absence of thoracic outlet syndrome (TOS). TOS is a collection of signs and symptoms that can be exacerbated by abnormal compression of the neurovascular bundle by bony, ligamentous, or muscular occlusions that occur between the cervical spine and the lower border of the axilla. Structures that make up the neurovascular bundle include the brachial plexus, the subclavian artery, and the subclavian vein. Compression of the neurovascular bundle in or around the cervicoaxillary canal can cause both vascular and neurologic symptoms, including the following: swelling in the arm or hand; discoloration of the arm or hand; a feeling of heaviness in the arm; deep, toothache-like pain in the neck, shoulder, arm, or hand; fatigue in the arms and hands; superficial vein distention in the extremity; paresthesia (loss of sensation) and numbness and tingling in the upper extremity; muscle weakness in the upper extremity; difficulty with fine motor skills; and pain in the upper extremity.

Three major areas appear to be most problematic and contribute to TOS. The first location is the cervical spine, where compression of the interscalene space between the anterior and middle scalenes can cause compression. The second location, slightly distal to the scalenes, is the space below the clavicle, where compression of the structures with the first rib can occur. This may be due to muscle inflexibility, an elevated first rib, or poor posture. The third location of compression is under and behind the tendon of the pectoralis minor muscle.

Determination of TOS can be simple if the clinician has knowledge of special tests to use for each of the three most

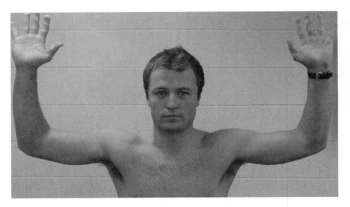

Figure 4-38: Roos test for thoracic outlet syndrome.

common areas of compression. It makes perfect sense that treatment for TOS by stretching the scalenes will not result in positive outcomes if the actual location of compression is behind the pectoralis minor. The clinician should have at minimum one special test for each of the three locations of compression to adequately determine the cause of the TOS.

In the Roos test (also called the positive abduction and external rotation position test and the elevated arm stress test), the patient abducts the shoulder to 90 degrees, flexes the elbow 90 degrees slightly posterior to the frontal plane, and then laterally rotates the shoulders.[90-92] Once in this position, the patient is asked to slowly open and close his or her hands for up to 3 minutes (Figure 4-38). Some minor fatigue that may occur bilaterally is considered negative. A positive test happens when the patient reports a return of the symptoms. This most likely indicates neurovascular compression behind the tendon of the pectoralis minor.

Two other tests that we believe most commonly implicate the costoclavicular region are the Wright test,[93] or Wright maneuver, also known as the hyperabduction test, and the Allen test, which may also indicate compression at the scalenes. In the Wright test, the patient's arm is taken into full passive elevation and lateral rotation by the clinician. While palpating for a pulse at the radial artery, the clinician asks the patient to take a deep breath, then rotate or extend the neck to add additional effects (Figure 4-39). A difference in pulse during these various maneuvers, and a return of the patient's symptoms, can be considered a positive test. A slight modification of this test is known as the Allen maneuver. In the Allen maneuver, the shoulder is abducted approximately 100 degrees and the elbow flexed approximately 90 degrees. In this position the patient is asked to rotate the head away from the side being tested (Figure 4-40). A diminished pulse or return of symptoms is considered positive. In this position the test may be positive because of scalenes or the pectoralis minor region.

Compression between the clavicle and the first rib is known as the costoclavicular sign or test.[9] In the test to implicate TOS at this locale, the clinician palpates the radial pulse while the patient is asked to draw his or her shoulders

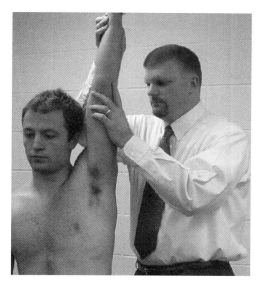

Figure 4-39: Wright test for thoracic outlet syndrome.

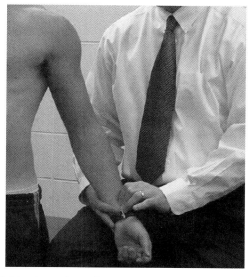

Figure 4-41: Costoclavicular sign for thoracic outlet syndrome.

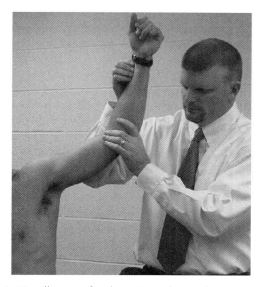

Figure 4-40: Allen test for thoracic outlet syndrome.

down and posterior similar to the military "at attention" position (Figure 4-41). A diminished pulse or return of the patient's symptoms is a positive test.

Last, several tests are used to implicate the scalenes as a site of entrapment of the neurovascular bundle. In the classic Adson maneuver, the patient is asked to actively rotate his or her head toward the examined side, take a breath, and hold it, while the clinician extends and laterally rotates the shoulder while looking for a decrease in pulse (Figure 4-42, *A*).[94] This appears to implicate a compression that is due to active contraction of the scalenes while rotating toward the tested side, and it also elevates the ribs and may cause compression between the clavicle and first rib. A modification of this test described in Magee[9] (Figure 4-42, *B*) finds the patient rotating the head to the opposite side of the tested extremity. As

with all TOS testing, a diminished pulse or return of symptoms is considered a positive test.

Several things must be pointed out regarding TOS testing. First and foremost, no single test can give the clinician all the information needed to be obtained. A series of tests musts be used to implicate or rule out all of the common areas of entrapment. It is not uncommon to see compression at more than one locale. Treatment of one location when in fact the pathology exists at multiple areas will result in less than optimal results. Second, not everyone who demonstrates a decrease in pulse is considered to have a positive test. Many individuals without TOS may have a diminished pulse with these tests, and many with a positive test will have a diminution bilaterally. A positive test in our minds includes either a return of symptoms or a diminished pulse with return of symptoms. We have seen many patients with a diminution of pulse but no symptoms.

Supine Instability Tests

Following the seated portion of the physical examination, the remainder of the algorithm includes supine testing procedures. Macrotraumatic instability is a problem that is seen clinically in sports medicine and orthopedic practice. The anterior apprehension test described initially by Rowe and Zarins[95] is used to test for overt anterior instability at the glenohumeral joint. This test should be performed on any patient with a history of macrotrauma to the shoulder, a history of recurrent subluxations, or a complaint of "dead arm" syndrome. In our experience, this test is best done with the patient lying supine on the examining table. In the supine position the scapula is stabilized and the patient is able to relax. The clinician stands along the patient's affected side and abducts the patient's arm to 90 degrees, flexes the elbow to 90 degrees, and externally rotates the shoulder slowly. A

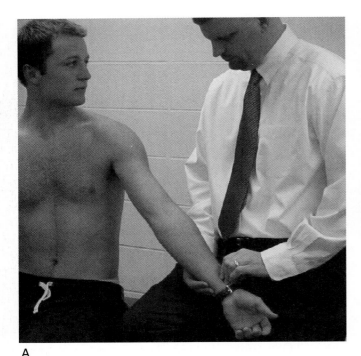

A

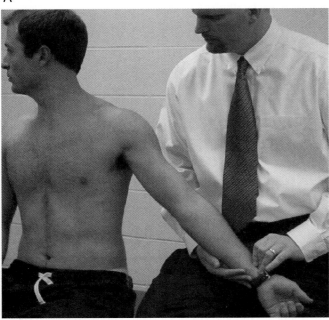

B

Figure 4-42: Adson test for thoracic outlet syndrome. **A,** Head rotated toward side being tested. **B,** Magee modification with head rotated away from side being tested.

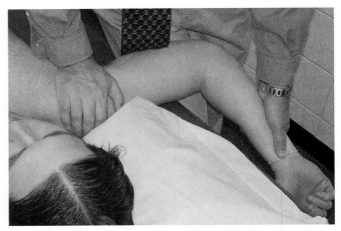

Figure 4-43: Jobe subluxation relocation test.

positive test is indicated by a look or feeling of apprehension or alarm on the patient's face and the patient's resistance to further motion at the glenohumeral joint. Pain is not necessarily an indication that this test is positive (Figure 4-43). The patient may report that this maneuver feels much like the offending incident when the shoulder was previously subluxated or dislocated. With this test, it is best to proceed

cautiously because too fast of a movement into external rotation may cause another dislocation. If this test is positive, there is no need to perform tests for microinstability.

The Jobe subluxation relocation test[96] is used primarily for anterior microinstability or internal impingement. Anterior microinstability is undetectable with previous instability tests. Therefore, during performance of the anterior load and shift and the apprehension sign, instability may not be noted. Microinstability may only occur when the patient's shoulder is stressed at the extremes of ROM (e.g., in the late cocking phase of throwing). For the Jobe subluxation relocation test to be positive, the patient must complain of anterior shoulder pain with this maneuver. The complaint this time is of anterior shoulder pain, not apprehension. In a patient with recurrent dislocations the maneuver will produce pain and apprehension, whereas a normal shoulder will be asymptomatic. If the patient describes anterior pain, the clinician then applies posterior stress to the anterior shoulder with the other hand. The relocation test relocates the humeral head into the glenoid fossa, which should relieve the patient's pain. Therefore a Jobe subluxation relocation test is positive with subluxation pain and decreased or no pain with the relocation portion of the test. In most cases, after reduction the patient will allow further external rotation of the shoulder before the return of anterior shoulder pain. Magee[9] reports several interpretations to this test. If pain predominated when doing the Jobe test and disappears with the relocation portion of the examination, the diagnosis is microanterior instability, either at the glenohumeral joint or caused by a secondary impingement from pathology at the scapulothoracic joint. If apprehension predominated during the Jobe test yet decreased with the relocation maneuver, the diagnosis is purely glenohumeral instability, subluxation, or dislocation. A patient with primary impingement will not demonstrate a change in pain with the relocation component of the test.[96-98]

If the patient complains of posterior shoulder pain with the subluxation component of the Jobe subluxation relocation

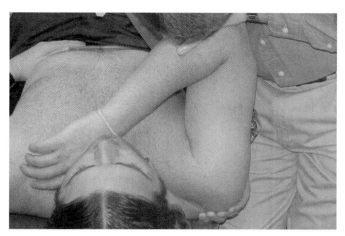

Figure 4-44: Posterior glide at 90 degrees of shoulder flexion for posterior instability.

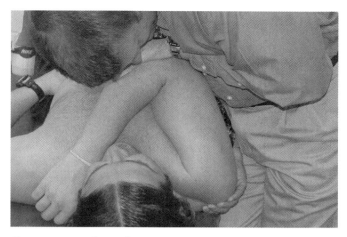

Figure 4-45: Jerk test for posterior instability.

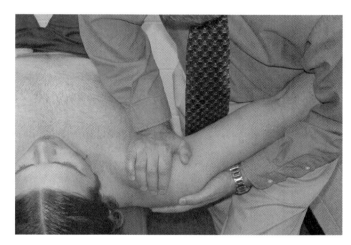

Figure 4-46: Posterior glide at 90 degrees of shoulder abduction and neutral rotation for posterior instability.

test, but the pain is relieved by the relocation phase, posterior impingement is the cause.[99]

Posterior Capsule Stability

Several tests can be used to determine pure posterior instability. Posterior instability tests should be used when the patient relates a macrotraumatic injury caused by a posteriorly directed force, a history of posterior subluxation, complaint of posterior shoulder pain, or complaints of clicking, popping, or clunking. One such test is the posterior glide, tested initially with the posterior capsule taut from a position of stability.[100] The clinician stands alongside the patient, holding the affected extremity in glenohumeral flexion and internal rotation. With the patient in a supine position, the clinician palpates the posterior head of the humerus while the top hand applies a posteriorly directed force with an axial compression load along the long axis of the humerus. The clinician's index and middle fingers of the palpating hand locate the posterior glenoid fossa, while the ring and little fingers of the same hand palpate the posterior humeral head (Figure 4-44). If the humeral head is translated posteriorly more than 50% of its diameter, posterior instability is considered evident.

During the jerk test, the clinician applies a posteriorly directed force through the long axis of the humerus.[101] As the clinician applies this force, he or she also horizontally adducts the shoulder in a direction medial to the sagittal plane (Figure 4-45). In a positive test the clinician will feel a quick "jerk" as the humeral head is subluxed off the posterior glenoid fossa and another possible "jerk" as the humeral head is relocated as the humerus is moved back to the starting position.

With the posterior glide II, the patient's arm is abducted passively to 90 degrees and the elbow remains in full extension.[100] The patient's distal hand and forearm should be held comfortably between the clinician's elbow and trunk. The clinician uses one hand along the posterior glenoid fossa and

posterior humeral head to attempt to feel for posterior translation during the maneuver. The clinician uses the other hand to apply a posteriorly directed force along the anterior humeral head (Figure 4-46). An increased amount of translation as compared with the uninvolved extremity is considered a positive test. It must be remembered that in this position the posterior capsule is slack, similar to the posterior load and shift test; therefore significant translation may be available. This test should be done cautiously and slowly so as not to impart an iatrogenic posterior subluxation or dislocation.

Supine Labral Tests

Bankart lesion tests should be used if the patient describes a history of macrotrauma, recurrent subluxations, pain anteriorly or deep in the shoulder, clicking, clunking, or sensations of locking or pseudolocking. During the clunk test the clinician takes the patient's shoulder into full elevation and grasps the patient's proximal humerus as close to the glenohumeral joint as possible.[102] A circumduction motion is performed both clockwise and counterclockwise in an attempt to scour the glenoid fossa (Figure 4-47). A positive finding is any of the complaints listed previously. It is imperative to remember the locations of different lesions to more accurately determine which lesion may be causing symptoms. For instance, using the right shoulder as a guide, a SLAP lesion would be located in the 10 to 2 o'clock position (see Figure 4-48), whereas a Bankart lesion would be located at the 6 to 9 o'clock position (Figure 4-49). A variation of the clunk test (the clunk test II) is used to determine the stability of the glenoid labrum. With the clunk test II the clinician places one hand at the patient's elbow, which is flexed 90 degrees, while the other hand is placed on the posterior shoulder, acting as a fulcrum. The clinician abducts the patient's arm over the patient's head in the frontal plane while simultaneously horizontally adducting and abducting the humerus back and forth anterior and posterior to the frontal plane (Figure 4-50). A slight compressive force is given along the long axis of the humerus in an attempt to entrap a torn piece of labrum, thus implicating a Bankart lesion. A positive finding would be any of the positive findings described for the clunk test I.

The last labral test to be described in the algorithm is the crank test.[103,104] The crank test assesses the shoulder complex for a Bankart lesion or a SLAP lesion. The examiner stands at the patient's head facing the foot of the examining table, alongside the extremity to be examined. The clinician takes the patient's arm into 150 to 160 degrees of elevation in the scapular plane. Once the clinician finds this position, one of his or her hands gives a compressive force along the long axis of the humerus, while the other hand internally and externally rotates the upper extremity (Figure 4-51). A positive finding is clicking, clunking, pain, pseudolocking, or any combination of these symptoms.

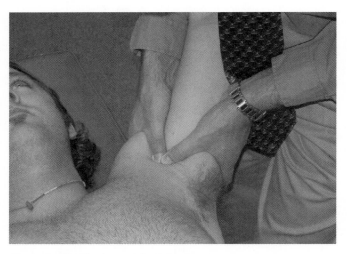

Figure 4-47: Clunk test I for labral tears.

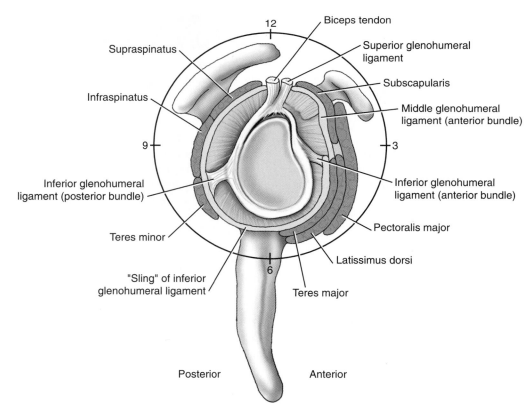

Figure 4-48: SLAP lesion. *(From Magee DJ:* Orthopedic physical assessment, *ed 4, Philadelphia, 2002, Saunders.)*

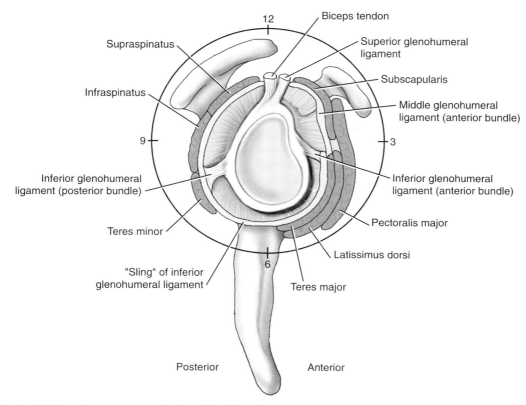

Figure 4-49: Bankart lesion. *(From Magee DJ: Orthopedic physical assessment, ed 4, Philadelphia, 2002, Saunders.)*

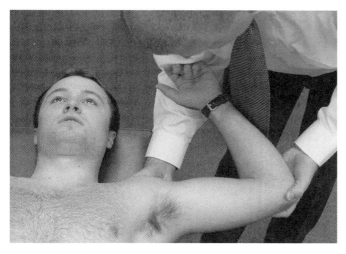

Figure 4-50: Clunk test II for labral tears.

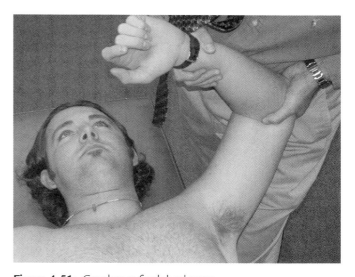

Figure 4-51: Crank test for labral tears.

Posterior Capsule Elongation

The final test to be described in this chapter is to assess for posterior shoulder capsule tightness. This is imperative because of the assumption that a tight posterior capsule may cause increased anterior-superior migration of the humeral head during shoulder elevation.[105] Described by Tyler and colleagues,[106] this test measures the amount of horizontal adduction of the glenohumeral joint while the patient is in a side-lying position. To perform this test, the patient is placed in the side-lying position with the affected shoulder up. The hips are flexed 45 degrees while the knees are flexed 90 degrees for proper trunk stabilization. Facing the patient, the clinician grasps the affected elbow near the epicondyles and passively moves the shoulder to 90 degrees of abduction in neutral rotation (Figure 4-52). Using the other hand, the clinician stabilizes the patient's scapula in a position of retraction. With the scapula held in the retracted position, the

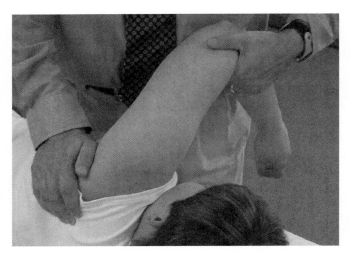

Figure 4-52: Beginning position for posterior capsule tightness assessment.

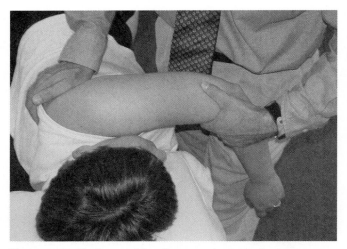

Figure 4-53: Ending position for posterior capsule tightness assessment.

humerus is then allowed to passively adduct across the body, until motion has ceased or rotation of the humerus occurs, indicating capsular or muscular tension (Figures 4-52 and 4-53). The distance from the top of the treatment table to the patient's elbow can be measured and compared with the unaffected shoulder. A greater distance would indicate a tighter posterior capsule and less posterior shoulder flexibility. Tyler and colleagues[107] have shown intratester reliability using Interclass and Intraclass Coefficients (ICCs) from 0.92 to 0.95 and an intertester reliability of 0.80. If positive, this test may indicate the need for passive stretching or joint mobilizations to increase posterior capsule/muscle mobility.

POSTOPERATIVE EVALUATION

The postoperative evaluation of the shoulder joint is similar to the preoperative evaluation with the exceptions of limitations related to surgical procedures, immobilization, and soft tissue healing constraints. To perform a safe and effective postoperative evaluation of the shoulder complex, it is of primary importance that the clinician thoroughly understands the operative procedure performed and possible common complications or associated problems that occur with the surgical interventions. It is difficult to perform excellent postoperative rehabilitation without having clear communication between the physician and therapist. There are too many nuances, not to mention individual patient anatomic, physiologic, and psychologic variances, that may require slight alterations in the standard surgical procedure or postoperative protocol and that may have a profound effect on the patient's eventual outcome. It is not uncommon to receive a referral for an RTC repair in which the referring physician has not mentioned tissue status, repair size, or the fact that the physician also performed a Bankart repair for a chronically torn labrum. Without these and other important pieces of information, the therapist may jeopardize the healing process by not fully understanding the extent of the surgical procedure performed. Any therapist treating postoperative shoulder patients must keep up to date with the latest surgical procedures and how those procedures may affect the rehabilitation that follows.

The postoperative examination is based on the surgical procedures performed and the time frame from surgery. An examination 2 days after type II RTC arthroscopic repair will obviously be different than an examination of that same patient 6 weeks after the same repair.

To begin, observation of the shoulder following surgical repair is similar to the preoperative examination, yet the clinician should be keener in looking for soft tissue swelling, areas of redness around incisions or portal sites, and the presence of any ecchymosis or discoloration in or around the shoulder region. Incision and portal sites are common locations of infection and must be thoroughly assessed. A slight redness and warmth around the incision site for several days following surgery is expected, due to the acute inflammatory process. This initial period of redness should be brief, and areas of redness should resolve if proper healing is occurring. If the size of the reddened area is increasing, an infection may be present. Usually this process also involves a significantly increased superficial skin temperature and occasionally some drainage from the incision or portal sites. If this condition occurs, a referral immediately back to the supervising physician is crucial. In many cases a simple course of antibiotics prescribed by the physician will take care of an infection. Swelling is very hard to objectively quantify in the shoulder because of muscle contours, as well as the size and shape of the joint. We do not normally recommend direct measurement of joint swelling as we do in other areas of the body, yet it is common to make note of any noticeable fullness or swelling of the soft tissues in the shoulder joint.

Immediately following shoulder surgery, many surgeons supply the patient with a shoulder sling or immobilizer. Careful attention should be made to how the patient is wearing this device. Even the basic immobilizer can be quite frustrating to the average patient. The length of time that the immobilizer will need to be used is usually determined by physician preference. Again, clear communication between physician and clinician is beneficial regarding this situation.

Range-of-motion testing is determined by the surgical procedures performed. For example, because of the peel-back mechanism following repair of a posterior type-II SLAP lesion, external rotation is contraindicated past neutral for the first 4 to 6 weeks.[108] Following a massive RTC tear repair in which the deltoid was taken down, AROM may not be initiated for 6 to 8 weeks. Consequently, understanding various surgical procedures is extremely important. Knowledge of postsurgical time frames and the degree of ROM that is appropriate following a given surgical procedure is paramount. The following chapters detail each surgical procedure with emphasis on various ROM, strength, or other pertinent limitations to be followed during the postoperative care of each surgical patient.

Just as ROM may be initially limited, so will muscle strengthening. In most cases immediately following surgery, pain is going to inhibit strength directly around the shoulder. ROM limitations will supercede strength assessment. For example, the massive RTC tear patient cannot even actively lift his or her arm into abduction for 6 to 8 weeks; therefore there is no need to worry about middle deltoid and supraspinatus strength initially. If the surgical procedure does not involve the remaining upper extremity musculature, strength assessment of those muscles can be performed carefully. Elbow flexion and extension, wrist flexion and extension, supination, pronation, and grip strength can give the clinician an assessment of the overall strength of the upper extremity. Furthermore, strength testing of the remaining myotome levels may detect an early neuropathy. A complete strength assessment of the shoulder requires adequate integrity of the involved tissues.

In most instances a sensory and reflex examination can be performed as indicated preoperatively. Loss of cutaneous innervation may be noticed with decrease in sensation to light touch, dull touch, or hot or cold sensation in a given dermatomal distribution. Reflex integrity should normally not change presurgically to postsurgically.

In most cases special testing of the shoulder joint immediately following surgery is not necessary. Special tests may be used periodically throughout the postoperative rehabilitation phase to determine tissue status. For instance, approximately 8 weeks following subacromial decompression the clinician may assess subacromial impingement of soft tissues by using the Neer's test or Hawkins-Kennedy test. At an appropriate time frame, dictated by size and quality of tissue repair, the drop arm test or lag signs may be performed on the patient after RTC repair. Caution must be used when performing special testing following surgical procedures so that repaired tissues are not stressed too early in the postoperative phase.

The objective data that are gained from this initial postoperative evaluation are used to guide the patient safely through the rehabilitation phase. Data gained in the postoperative evaluation are required to enable the clinician to set realistic patient goals in an effort to return the patient to his or her prior functional status.

SUMMARY

This chapter provides the clinician with a thorough understanding of tests and measures to be performed on a preoperative or postoperative patient. It is common for the preoperative evaluation to be much more detailed than the postoperative evaluation because many times the full extent of the evaluated pathology is not yet known. The postoperative evaluation presents its own challenges, which require the clinician to fully understand the surgical procedures involved. The remainder of this text describes in detail many common orthopedic sports surgical procedures for the knee and shoulder.

References

1. *Guide to Physical Therapist Practice*, ed 2, *Phys Ther* 81:9-744, 2001.
2. Nicholson GP: Arthroscopic acromioplasty: a comparison between workers' compensation and non-workers' compensation populations, *J Bone Joint Surg* 85A:682-689, 2003.
3. Harryman DT, Hettrich BS, Smith KL, et al: A prospective multipractice investigation of patients with full-thickness rotator cuff tears: the importance of comorbidities, practice, and other covariables on self-assessed shoulder function and health status, *J Bone Joint Surg* 85A:690-696, 2003.
4. Viola RW, Boatright KC, Smith KL, et al: Do shoulder patients insured by workers' compensation present with worse self-assessed function and health status? *J Shoulder Elbow Surg* 9:368-372, 2000.
5. Misamore GW, Ziegler DW, Rushton JL: Repair of the rotator cuff. A comparison of results in two populations of patients, *J Bone Joint Surg* 77A:1335-1339, 1995.
6. Gupta R, Leggin BG, Iannotti JP: Results of surgical repair of full-thickness tears of the rotator cuff, *Orthop Clin North Am* 28:241-248, 1997.
7. Iannotti JP, Bernot MP, Kuhlman JR, et al: Postoperative assessment of shoulder function: a prospective study of full-thickness rotator cuff tears, *J Shoulder Elbow Surg* 5:449-457, 1996.
8. Hawkins RJ, Bokor DJ: Clinical evaluation of shoulder problems. In Rockwook CA, Matsen FA, editors: *The shoulder*, ed 2, Philadelphia, 1990, Saunders.
9. Magee DJ: *Orthopedic physical assessment*, ed 4, Philadelphia, 2002, Saunders.
10. Stith JS, Sahrmann SA, Dixon KK, Norton BJ: Curriculum to prepare diagnosticians in physical therapy, *J Phys Ther Educ* 9(2):46-53, 1995.
11. Lehman C, Cuomo F, Kummar FJ, Zuckerman JD: The incidence of full thickness rotator cuff tears in a large cadaver population, *Bull Hosp Jt Dis* 54:30-31, 1995.
12. Yocum LA: Assessing the shoulder: history, physical examination, differential diagnosis, and special tests used, *Clin Sports Med* 2(2):281-289, 1983.

13. Hawkins RJ, Kennedy JC: Impingement syndrome in the athletic shoulder, *Am J Sports Med* 8(3):151-158, 1980.

14. Hulstyn MJ, Weiss AP: Adhesive capsulitis of the shoulder, *Orthop Rev* 22:425-433, 1993.

15. Calandra J, Baker C, Uribe J: The incidence of Hill-Sachs lesion in initial anterior shoulder dislocations, *Arthroscopy* 5(4):254-257, 1989.

16. Rowe C: Acute and recurrent anterior dislocation of the shoulder, *Orthop Clin North Am* 11(2):253-270, 1980.

17. Neer CS: Impingement lesions, *Clin Orthop* 173:70-77, 1983.

18. Boissonnault WG. *Examination in physical therapy practice: screening for medical disease,* New York, 1991, Churchill Livingstone.

19. Cyriax J: *Textbook of orthopaedic medicine,* ed 8, London, 1982, Bailliere Tindall.

20. Clark JM, Harryman DT: Tendons, ligaments and capsule of the rotator cuff, *J Bone Joint Surg* 74A:713-725, 1992.

21. Bulbena A, Duro JC, Porta M, et al: Clinical assessment of hypermobility of joints: assembling criteria, *J Rheumatol* 19:115-122, 1992.

22. Beighton P, Solomon L, Soskolne CL: Articular mobility in an African population, *Ann Rheum Dis* 32:413-418, 1973.

23. Carter C, Wilkinson J: Persistent joint laxity and congenital dislocation of the hip, *J Bone Joint Surg* 46B:40-45, 1964.

24. Rotes J: *Rheumatologia clinica,* Barcelona, Spain, 1983, Espaxs.

25. Grahame R: The hypermobility syndrome, *Ann Rheum Dis* 49:190-200, 1990.

26. Kelley MJ: Evaluation of the shoulder. In Kelley MJ, Clark WA: *Orthopedic therapy of the shoulder,* Philadelphia, 1994, JB Lippincott.

27. Levangie PK, Norkin CC: *Joint structure and function: a comprehensive analysis,* ed 3, Philadelphia, 2001, FA Davis, p 215.

28. Fiddian NJ, King RJ: The winged scapula, *Clin Orthop* 185:228-236, 1984.

29. Kibler WB, McMullen J: Scapular dyskinesis and its relation to shoulder pain, *J Am Acad Orthop Surg* 11:142-151, 2003.

30. Kibler WB, Uhl TL, Maddux JWQ, et al: Qualitative clinical evaluation of scapular dysfunction: a reliability study, *J Shoulder Elbow Surg* 11:550-556, 2002.

31. Warner JJ, Micheli LJ, Arslanian LE, et al: Scapulothoracic motion in normal shoulders and shoulders with glenohumeral instability and impingement syndrome: a study using moire topographic analysis, *Clin Orthop* 285:191-199, 1992.

32. Kibler WB: The role of the scapula in the overhead throwing motion, *Contemp Orthop* 22(5):525-532, 1991.

33. Kibler WB: The role of the scapula in athletic shoulder function, *Am J Sports Med* 26(2):325-337, 1998.

34. Norkin CC, White DJ: *Measurement of joint motion. A guide to goniometry,* Philadelphia, 1995, FA Davis.

35. Inman VT, Saunders JB: Referred pain from skeletal structures, *J Nerv Ment Dis* 99:660-667, 1944.

36. Codman EA: *The shoulder,* Boston, 1934, Thomas Todd.

37. DePalma AF: *Surgery of the shoulder,* Philadelphia, 1973, JB Lippincott.

38. Kessell L, Watson M: The painful arc syndrome: clinical classification as a guide to management, *J Bone Joint Surg* 59B:166-172, 1977.

39. Neer CS: Anterior acromioplasty for the chronic impingement syndrome in the shoulder: a preliminary report, *J Bone Joint Surg* 54A(1):41-50, 1972.

40. Thein LA, Greenfield BH: Impingement syndrome and impingement-related instability. In Donatelli RA, editor: *Physical therapy of the shoulder,* ed 3, Philadelphia, 1997, Churchill Livingstone.

41. Harryman DT, Sidles JA, Clark JM, et al: Translation of the humeral head on the glenoid with passive glenohumeral motion, *J Bone Joint Surg* 72A:1334-1343, 1990.

42. American Academy of Orthopedic Surgeons: *Joint motion: method of measuring and recording,* Chicago, 1965, American Academy of Orthopedic Surgeons.

43. Burkhart SS, Morgan CD, Kibler WB: The disabled throwing shoulder: spectrum of pathology part I: pathoanatomy and biomechanics, *Arthroscopy* 19(4):404-420, 2004.

44. Davies GJ, DeCarlo MS: Examining the shoulder complex. In Bandy W, editor: *Current concepts in rehabilitation of the shoulder,* La Crosse, WI, 1995, Sports Physical Therapy Section.

45. Davies GJ, Gould J, Larsen R: Functional examination of the shoulder complex, *Phys Sports Med* 9:82-97, 1981.

46. Hagbarth KE, Wallen G, Burke D, Lofstedt L: Effects of the Jendrassik maneuver on muscle spindle activity in man, *J Neurol Neurosurg Psych* 38:1143-1153, 1975.

47. Hoppenfeld S: *Physical examination of the spine and extremities,* New York, 1976, Appleton-Century-Crofts.

48. Hislop HJ, Montgomery J: *Muscle testing,* ed 6, Philadelphia, 1995, Saunders.

49. Kendall FP, McCreary EK, Provance PG: *Muscle testing and function with posture and pain,* ed 4, Baltimore, 1993, Williams & Wilkins.

50. Daniels L, Worthingham C: *Muscle testing. Techniques of manual examination,* ed 7, Philadelphia, 2002, Saunders.

51. Cappel K, Clark MA, Davies GJ, Ellenbecker TS: Clinical exam of the shoulder. In Tovin B, Greenfield BH: *Evaluation of the shoulder: an integrated guide to physical therapy practice,* Philadelphia, 2001, FA Davis.

52. Warner JP: The gross anatomy of the joint surfaces, ligaments, labrum, and capsule. In Matson FA, Fu FH, Hawkins RJ, editors: *The shoulder: a balance of mobility and stability,* Rosemont, IL, 1993, American Academy of Orthopedic Surgeons.

53. Borsa PA, Saukers EL, Herling DE, Manzour WF: In vivo quantification of capsular end-point in the nonimpaired glenohumeral joint using an instrumented measurement system, *J Orthop Sports Phys Ther* 31(8):419-431, 2001.

54. Doukas WC, Speer KP: Anatomy, pathology, and biomechanics of shoulder instability, *Op Tech Sports Med* 8:179-187, 2000.

55. Rockwood CA: Subluxations and dislocations about the shoulder. In Rockwood CA, Green DP, editors: *Fractures in adults,* Philadelphia, 1984, JB Lippincott.

56. Cofield RH, Irving JF: Evaluation and classification of shoulder instability: with special reference to examination under anesthesia, *Clin Orthop* 223:32-43, 1987.

57. Baker CL, Uribe JW, Whitman C: Arthroscopic evaluation of acute initial shoulder dislocations, *Am J Sports Med* 18:25-28, 1990.

58. Silliman JF, Hawkins RJ: Classification and physical diagnosis of instability of the shoulder, *Clin Orthop* 291:7-19, 1993.

59. Hawkins RJ, Mohtadi NG: Clinical evaluation of shoulder instability, *Clin J Sports Med* 1:59-64, 1991.

60. Altchek DA, Warren RF, Sdyhar MJ, Ortiz T: T-plasty: a technique for treating multidirectional instability in the athlete, *J Bone Joint Surg* 73A:105-112, 1991.

61. Sauers EL, Borsa PA, Herling DE, Stanley RD: Instrumental measurement of glenohumeral joint laxity and its relationship to passive range of motion and generalized joint laxity, *Am J Sports Med* 29:142-150, 2001.

62. Sauers EL, Borsa PA, Herling DE, Stanley RD: Instrumental measurement of glenohumeral joint laxity: reliability and normative data, *Knee Surg Sports Traumatol Arthros* 9:34-41, 2001.

63. Ellenbecker TS, Matalino AJ, Elam E, Caplinger R: Quantification of anterior translation of the humeral head in the throwing shoulder—manual assessment vs. stress radiography, *Am J Sports Med* 28:161-167, 2000.

64. Harryman DT, Sidles JA, Harris BS, Matsen FA: Laxity of normal glenohumeral joint: a quantitative in vivo assessment, *J Shoulder Elbow Surg* 1:66-76, 1992.

65. Maki NJ: Cineradiographic studies with shoulder instabilities, *Am J Sports Med* 16:362-364, 1988.

66. Speer KP: Anatomy and pathomechanics of shoulder instability, *Clin Sports Med* 14:751-760, 1995.

67. Guidi EJ, Suckerman JD: Glenoid labral lesions. In Andrews JR, Wilk KE, editors: *The athlete's shoulder,* New York, 1994, Churchill Livingstone.

68. Snyder SJ, Karzel RP, Del Pizzo W, et al: SLAP lesions of the shoulder, *Arthroscopy* 6:274-279, 1990.

69. Kibler WB: Specificity and sensitivity of the anterior slide test in throwing athletes with superior glenoid labral tears, *Arthroscopy* 11:296-300, 1995.

70. Itoi E, Hsu HS, An KN: Biomechanical investigation of the glenohumeral joint, *J Shoulder Elbow Surg* 5:407-424, 1996.

71. Itoi E, Motzkin NE, Morrey BF, An KN: Stabilizing function of the long head of the biceps in the hanging arm position, *J Shoulder Elbow Surg* 3:135-142, 1994.

72. Itoi E, Neuman SR, Kuechle DK, Morrey BF: Dynamic anterior stabilizers of the shoulder with the arm in abduction, *J Bone Joint Surg* 76B:834-836, 1994.

73. Khan KM, Cook JL, Taunton JE, Bonar F: Overuse tendinosis, not tendonitis. Part 1: a new paradigm for a difficult clinical problem, *Phys Sportsmed* 28:38-48, 2000.

74. Bennett WF: Specificity of the Speed's test: arthroscopic technique for evaluating the biceps tendon at the level of the bicipital groove, *Arthroscopy* 14(8):789-796, 1998.

75. Yeargason RM: Supination sign, *J Bone Joint Surg* 13:160, 1931.

76. Meister K: Injuries to the throwing athlete. Part II: evaluation/treatment, *Am J Sports Med* 28:587-601, 2000.

77. O'Brien SJ, Pagnoni MJ, Fealy S, et al: The active compression test: a new and effective test for diagnosing labral tears and acromioclavicular (AC) joint abnormality, *Am J Sports Med* 26:610-613, 1998.

78. Bigliani LU, Morrison DS, April EW: The morphology of the acromion and its relationship to rotator cuff tears, *Orthop Trans* 10:228, 1986.

79. Bramhall JP, Scarpinato DF, Andrews JR: Operative arthroscopy of the shoulder. In Andrews JR, Wilk KE, editors: *The athlete's shoulder,* New York, 1994, Churchill Livingstone.

80. Jobe FW, Glousman RE: Rotator cuff dysfunction and associated glenohumeral instability in the throwing athlete. In Paulos LE, Tibone JE, editors: *Operative techniques in shoulder surgery,* Rockville, MD, 1991, Aspen Publishers.

81. Hawkins RJ, Kennedy JC: Impingement syndrome in athletes, *Am J Sports Med* 8:151-158, 1980.

82. Valadie AL, Jobe CM, Pink MM, et al: Anatomy of provocative tests for impingement syndrome of the shoulder, *J Shoulder Elbow Surg* 9:36-46, 2000.

83. Axe MJ: Acromioclavicular joint injuries in the athlete, *Sports Med Arthroscopy Rev* 8:182-191, 2000.

84. Clark HD, McCann PD: Acromioclavicular joint injuries, *Orthop Clin North Am* 31:177-187, 2000.

85. Shaffer BS: Painful conditions of the acromioclavicular joint, *J Am Acad Orthop Surg* 7:176-188, 1990.

86. Hertel R, Ballmer FT, Lombert SM, Gerber CH: Lag signs in the diagnosis of rotator cuff rupture, *J Shoulder Elbow Surg* 5:307-313, 1996.

87. Tennent TD, Beach WR, Meyers JF: A review of the special tests associated with shoulder examination. Part I: the rotator cuff tests, *Am J Sports Med* 31(1):154-160, 2003.

88. Gerber C, Krushell RJ: Isolated ruptures of the subscapularis muscle, *J Bone Joint Surg* 73B:389-394, 1991.

89. Hurschler C, Wulker N, Windhagen H, et al: Evaluation of the lag sign tests for external rotator function of the shoulder, *J Shoulder Elbow Surg* 13:298-304, 2004.

90. Roos DB: Congenital anomalies associated with thoracic outlet syndrome, *J Surg* 132:771-778, 1976.

91. Liebenson CS: Thoracic outlet syndrome: diagnosis and conservative management, *J Manip Physiol Ther* 11:493-499, 1988.

92. Ribbe EB, Lindgren SH, Norgren NE: Clinical diagnosis of thoracic outlet syndrome: evaluation of patients with cervicobrachial symptoms, *Manual Med* 2:82-85, 1984.

93. Wright IS: The neurovascular syndrome produced by hyperabduction of the arms, *Am Heart J* 29:1-19, 1945.

94. Adson AW, Coffey: Cervical rib: a method of anterior approach for relief of symptoms by division of the scalenus anticus, *Ann Surg* 85:839-857, 1927.

95. Rowe CR, Zarins B: Recurrent transient subluxation of the shoulder, *J Bone Joint Surg* 63A:863-872, 1981.

96. Kvitne RS, Jobe FW: The diagnosis and treatment of anterior instability in the throwing athlete, *Clin Orthop* 291:107-123, 1993.

97. Jobe FW, Kvitne RS, Giangarra CE: Shoulder pain in the overhand or throwing athlete: the relationship of anterior instability and rotator cuff impingement, *Orthop Rev* 18:963-975, 1989.

98. Speer KP, Hannafin JA, Alteck DW, Warren RF: An evaluation of the shoulder relocation test, *Am J Sports Med* 22:177-183, 1994.

99. Jobe CM: Superior glenoid impingement, *Orthop Clin North Am* 28:137-143, 1997.

100. Gerber C, Ganz R: Clinical assessment of instability of the shoulder, *J Bone Joint Surg* 66B:551-556, 1984.

101. Matsen FA, Thomas SC, Rockwood CA, Wirth MA: Glenohumeral instability. In Rockwood CA, Matsen FA, editors: *The shoulder,* ed 2, Philadelphia, 1998, Saunders.

102. Andrews JR, Gillogly S: Physical examination of the shoulder in throwing athletes. In Zarins B, Andrews JR, Carson WG, editors: *Injuries to the throwing arm,* Philadelphia, 1985, Saunders.

103. Lui SH, Henry MH, Nuccion SL: A prospective evaluation of a new physical examination in predicting glenoid labral tears, *Am J Sports Med* 24:721-725, 1996.

104. Lui SH, Henry MH, Nuccion SL, et al: Diagnosis of glenoid labral tears: a comparison between magnetic resonance imaging and clinical examinations, *Am J Sports Med* 24:149-154, 1996.

105. Matsen FA, Artnz CT: Subacromial impingement. In Rockwood CA, Matsen FA, editors: *The shoulder,* Philadelphia, 1998, Saunders.

106. Tyler TF, Roy T, Nicholas SJ, et al: Reliability and validity of a new method of measuring posterior shoulder tightness, *J Orthop Sports Phys Ther* 29(5):262-274, 1999.

107. Tyler TF, Nicholas SJ, Roy T, et al: Quantification of posterior capsular tightness and motion loss in patients with shoulder impingement, *Am J Sports Med* 28(5):262-274, 1999.

108. Burkhart SS, Morgan CD: The peel-back mechanism: its role in producing and extending posterior type II SLAP lesions and its effect on SLAP repair rehabilitation, *Arthroscopy* 14(6):637-640, 1998.

CHAPTER 5

Training for Strength, Power, and Endurance

Michael P. Reiman, MEd, PT, ATC, CSCS

USA Weightlifting Level 1 Coach
USA Track-and-Field Level 1 Coach

CHAPTER OUTLINE

REHABILITATION FOLLOWING A SURGI-CAL procedure is especially imperative for the athletic participant. A multifactorial rehabilitation program for the athletic population must be well planned and thought out. Thought must be given to the various skills that the athlete must possess to be successful at his or her sport. The rehabilitation specialist needs to take into account that particular athlete and ask several crucial questions. What are the athlete's particular strengths and weaknesses? Will these weaknesses be detrimental to the athlete's successful return to the playing field? How must these weaknesses be best addressed to ensure success of the athlete, as well as complementing the postoperative rehabilitation plan?

It is beyond the scope of this chapter to completely and accurately summarize strength, power, and endurance training for the athlete. This is especially true in regard to the athlete who has undergone surgical intervention and is training to return to sport. The rehabilitative process in that regard is multidimensional and beyond summarization. This chapter is, though, an attempt to familiarize rehabilitation specialists with factors and variables regarding strength, power, and endurance, in order that they may make informed decisions that are based on recent and relevant scientific literature. The principles and information can be presented and applied to each individual athlete with respect to each athlete's situation.

The main objective of this chapter is to outline principles and key points to be evaluated when training for strength, power, and endurance in the postsurgical knee and shoulder athletic population. The emphasis is on training parameters that apply to the end stages of the rehabilitation process, the return to the playing field, and beyond. For step-by-step protocols, see the remainder of this text.

Specific training principles should be closely followed to allow the proper program design and ensure the athlete's successful return to the playing field. Following these principles will allow the rehabilitation specialist to more accurately control any risk factors for future injury potential. Proper training methods are essential in allowing athletes to meet their goals on returning to their sport following injury and subsequent surgical intervention.

BASIC TRAINING PRINCIPLES

Principle of Individuality

Every athlete is a unique individual and should be treated accordingly. An athlete's genetic makeup plays a major role in determining how and to what degree he or she responds to a training stimulus. Several factors should be considered when designing a resistance training program, including age, sex, medical history, previous training background, injury history, overall health, training goals, motivation, and any healing restraints related to the injury or surgery. Any specific needs and abilities of that particular athlete must be addressed.

Principle of Specificity

The principle of specificity states that the body makes gains from exercise and training according to the manner in which the body trains. The way the athlete trains is how he or she will function. An efficient, effective program will lead to the desired goals. Incorrectly applying this principle will result in wasted energy and time with less than optimal results. When developing a training program using this principle, one should consider the following:

- Energy-source specificity
- Muscle action specificity
- Muscle group specificity
- Velocity specificity

Energy-source specificity involves training the correct energy source. The rehabilitation specialist determines which metabolic systems are predominant in the athlete's sport and trains them accordingly. There are aerobic and anaerobic sources of energy for muscle actions (Table 5-1). Anaerobic energy sources are predominant in shorter duration, more intense activities. Therefore, when the training goal is to increase the anaerobic energy sources, training should be of short duration and high intensity. In comparison, the aerobic energy source is more predominant, and therefore more efficient, with training bouts of longer duration and lower intensity. Resistance training is most commonly used to elicit adaptations in the anaerobic energy sources.

Variables of the training program such as intensity, volume, and rest periods are driven by the energy system that is being trained. Performance in a sport or training session can often be limited by the energy system being used. Correct training of the proper energy system involves critically looking at the sport involved and determining work-to-rest ratios. Does the sport involve continuous activity, or are there short periods of very high intensity with rest periods between? Determining which energy system is dominant in a particular sport will determine the training intensity, the training volume, and the amount of recovery time.

Metabolism is highly specific to the intensity and duration of the sporting event, to the extent that excessive development of one type of fitness may have a profoundly detrimental effect on another type of fitness. For instance, regular, in-season aerobic training can significantly decrease the strength and power of weightlifters and track-and-field athletes.[1]

Muscle action or *testing specificity* indicates that gains in strength are in part specific to the type of muscle action used in training (e.g., isometric, concentric/eccentric, isokinetic). This specificity of strength gains is caused by neural adaptations resulting in the ability to recruit the muscles to perform a particular type of muscle action.[2] Different sports have different and sometimes unique movements. The training program should reflect this. Training the specific movements of that sport allows the athlete to perform more efficiently in that sport. Sports often involve more than one type of muscle action. An offensive lineman in football, for example, can perform an isometric muscle action, while simultaneously performing a concentric and eccentric action, all while being engaged with an opponent. Different muscle groups can and will also have different muscle actions.

Muscle group and joint action specificity means training the muscle group(s) and joint(s) that are involved in the sport. This can involve training agonistic muscle groups one way and antagonistic muscle groups another way. Training both sets of muscle groups to perform the same function is counterproductive if they are not asked to do the same movements. Synergistic and stabilization muscle actions should also be taken into consideration. Isolating single muscle groups during resistance training can be less effective for transferring strength to multijoint or complex movements than performing such movements under loaded conditions.[3] Key points noted by Harman[4] in regard to specificity of training include the following:

1. Training is most effective when resistance exercises are similar to the sport movement (or movements) in which improvement is sought (target activity).

2. Select exercises similar to the target activity with regard to joint movements and the directions of those movements.

3. Joint ranges of motion in the training exercises should be at least as large as those of the target activity.

In skeletal muscle, different muscle fiber types (slow and fast twitch) are recruited with different intensities and duration of load and stimulus.[2,4-7] During moderate-intensity, prolonged exercise, slow-twitch (ST) muscle fibers are primarily recruited. High-intensity, short-duration exercise recruits primarily the fast-twitch (FT) muscle fibers. The preferential recruitment of muscle fibers is predicted by the intensity of the exercise performed.[5-7] It has been generally accepted that during voluntary muscle contractions there is an orderly recruitment of motor units according to the size principle.[8] This implies that ST fiber involvement is obligatory, regardless of the power and velocity being generated by the FT fibers that are recruited once higher intensities are generated.[9] Figure 5-1 summarizes this preferential recruitment. Type I (red, ST, slow oxidative) fibers have different metabolic and contractile properties compared with type II (white, FT, fast oxidative glycolitic, fast glycolitic) fibers (Table 5-2). Type II fibers are better adapted to perform anaerobic work, whereas type I fibers are better adapted to perform aerobic work.[2] Type II fibers are more predominant in short-duration, explosive activities compared with longer-duration activities of less intensity (type I fibers). The force per unit area of fast and slow motor fibers is similar, but the FT motor units typically possess larger cross-sectional areas and produce greater force per single motor unit.[10]

All human muscles contain both ST and FT motor units.[10] The proportion of fast and slow motor fibers in mixed muscles varies among athletes, often depending on such factors as genetics and type of training. Endurance athletes have a high percentage of ST motor units, whereas FT motor units are predominant among strength and power athletes. Untrained people cannot recruit all their FT motor units.[10] Athletes engaged in strength and power training show increased motor unit activation.[10]

Although FT fibers are used in shorter, faster activities, it is not the speed of contraction but rather the force intensity of the muscle that causes the motor nerves to recruit the FT fibers.[5-7] This explains why athletes in speed-related sports have to increase power. The high-power movements performed by these athletes activate the FT fibers, making them capable of performing explosive and fast actions. The intensity, duration, and pattern of loading imposed on the muscle determine the proportion of involvement by the different fiber types and the degree to which each is conditioned by a given regimen of training.[1]

Velocity specificity concerns the velocity of movement that the sport requires of different parts of the athlete's body.

TABLE 5-1

Major Characteristics of Primary Energy Systems

PRIMARY SOURCE OF ENERGY	DURATION	WORK TO REST RATIOS
ATP-PC (Phosphagen)	First 20 to 30 seconds of exercise	1. 1:12 to 1:20 for work at 90%-100% of maximum power (0-10 seconds)
		2. 1:3 to 1:5 for work at 75%-90% of maximum power (15-30 seconds)
Phosphagens and anaerobic glycolysis	Major source of energy from 30 to 90 seconds of exercise	1:3 to 1:4
Anaerobic glycolysis and aerobic metabolism	From 90 to approximately 180 seconds of exercise	1:1 to 1:3
Oxygen (aerobic metabolism)	Predominates over other energy systems after the second minute of exercise	1:1 (longer duration, less intensity) to 1:3 (shorter duration, higher intensity)

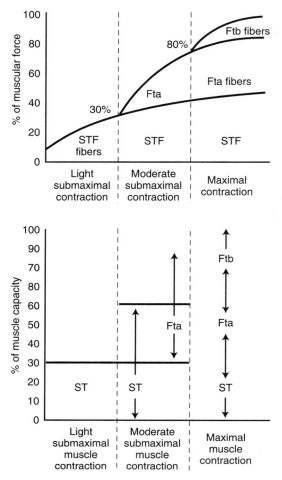

Figure 5-1: Preferential muscle fiber recruitment is predicated on the intensity of the muscle contraction. *STF,* Slow-twitch fiber; *FTA* or *Fta,* fast-twitch A; *FTB* or *Ftb,* fast-twitch B. *(From Davies G: A compendium of isokinetics in clinical usage and rehabilitation techniques, ed 4, Onalaska, WI, 1992, S & S Publishers.)*

Training gains are specific to the velocities at which exercises are performed. In other words, training-induced strength gains in a resistance exercise program primarily occur at the training speeds, with very limited physiologic overflow to other speeds of movement.[1,2,5,11,12] Training at slower speeds improves efficiency of movement at slower speeds, but there is little transfer to faster speeds. Training at faster speeds is essential to improving speed and power in athletics because few sports are performed at slow speeds. Transfer of training from one speed to another is not completely clear, yet it has been shown that high-velocity training provides more improvement at low velocity than vice versa.[2] The neural mechanism behind this has yet to be determined.[3] To achieve maximum benefit in performance that involves speed- or velocity-specific requirements, the training stimulus should be applied at or above the required velocity.[3]

Principle of Progressive Overload

The *principle of progressive overload* states that in order to continue making gains in an exercise program, stress to the muscle must be progressively overloaded as it becomes capable of producing greater force, power, or endurance. Once a body adapts to an exercise program workload, it will not continue to progress unless the workload is increased in some manner. Therefore, to continually improve physiologic function, progressive increases in load must be applied, to which adaptations will again occur.[3] If the athlete does not continue to adapt, eventually he or she will plateau and regress. Resistive exercises should be performed with enough frequency, intensity, and duration to produce overload without producing fatigue.[13] Occasionally it is necessary to train an athlete in some state of fatigue to replicate game situations. This concept is discussed later in the section on endurance training.

TABLE 5-2

Muscle Fiber Type Characteristics

CHARACTERISTIC	SLOW TWITCH (ST), TYPE I	FAST TWITCH A (FTA), TYPE IIA	FAST TWITCH B (FTB), TYPE IIB
Nerve conduction velocity	Slow	Fast	Fast
Motor neuron size	Small	Large	Large
Aerobic capacity	High	Moderate	Low
Anaerobic capacity	Low	High	High
Power output	Low	Moderate-high	High
Contraction speed	Slow	Fast	Fast
Fatigue resistance	High	Reasonably resistant	Low
Recovery after exercise	Rapid	Fairly rapid	Slow
Recruitment order	First	Second	Last (usually only when very intense and rapid effort required)

There are several methods to progressively overload the muscle.[14] Some methods that have been used include increasing the resistance; increasing the training volume by increasing the number of repetitions, sets, or exercises performed; altering rest periods; and increasing repetition velocity during submaximal resistances. The most common method is to increase the resistance.[2] Progressive overloading should be gradually adapted to the athlete's program. The athlete should have sufficient time to adapt to the present program before making significant changes. The American College of Sports Medicine[14] recommends that changes in total training volume should be made in small increments of 2.5% to 5% to avoid the possibility of overtraining.

When loads are applied, they should be specific to the desired effect (specificity principle), be appropriate to the individual (individualization principle), consider the time in the seasonal calendar (periodization), and be appropriate in terms of the type of stimulus (frequency, intensity, and duration).

Principle of Variety

To reach high performance, the volume of training must surpass a threshold of 1,000 hours per year.[6] Any athlete serious about training must dedicate 4 to 6 hours to strength training each week, in addition to technical, tactical, and other elements of general and specific conditioning.[6]

With these high demands to succeed, this repetitive training could lead to monotony and result in the athlete losing interest in the sport altogether. The training program must therefore include variety. Ways to vary a training program without losing the ultimate goal include the following:

- Vary types of resistance—free weights, machine resistance, elastic tubing, isokinetics, aquatic resistance, and so on.
- Vary the type of muscle contraction.
- Vary the speed of contraction (if appropriate).
- Vary the order of exercises performed (if applicable to program design goals).
- Vary the training environment—location, type of surface, team versus individual training, and so on.
- Vary between training cycles or phases (see Periodization of Athlete Training later in this chapter).
- Train in other sports or in a wide variety of skills (depending on stage of athletic development).

There are other ways to vary the training program, depending on the goals of the program and the athlete involved. As an example, training programs for Olympic athletes need to vary from year to year because of the nature of the competition. These athletes need to have different levels of peak phases in their programs, with the ultimate goal to peak at the Olympic competition in their respective sport. Varying their training will not only ensure timeliness of their peak effort, but will also prevent stagnant training.

It is therefore important to keep the athlete interested in the training program. Giving the athlete input into planning the training program can help maintain interest and excitement in his or her training regimen.

SPORT ANALYSIS

Training an athlete after an operative procedure requires an analysis of the specific needs of that particular athlete and the sport in which he or she participates. Table 5-3 is a list of some specific sport characteristics that need to be properly addressed throughout the athlete's program.

A biomechanical analysis of the sport determines which particular muscles are involved in the sport and to what degree they are involved. Prime movers, synergists, antagonists, and so on can be determined by keenly observing the movements required by the sport. Determining the muscle involvement, and the extent of that involvement, allows the rehabilitation specialist to choose specific exercises that use those muscles and types of muscular actions in a manner specific to the sport for which the athlete is training.

The amount of movement of a joint and the specific type of muscular contraction (concentric, eccentric, isometric), as well as the percentage of open versus closed kinetic chain characteristics that are involved, can also be determined via biomechanical analysis (Table 5-4). It is also important to know the relationship of force and velocity with concentric versus eccentric muscle actions (Figure 5-2). As the velocity of muscle shortening increases, the force that the muscle can

TABLE 5-3

Sport Analysis Characteristics to Consider with Injured Athletes in Returning to Athletic Competition

Specific movements performed in sport	Specific muscles involved and in what manner
	Joint angles/range of movement in the sport
	Type of muscle contraction
	Open vs. closed kinetic chain movements
	Load requirements of the sport
	Velocity/speed requirements of sport
Metabolic systems primarily involved	ATP-PC source
	Lactic acid source
	Oxygen source
Injury history and prevention	Site of present injury
	Sites of previous injury/injury history
	Most common sites of injury in that sport
	Anatomic/biomechanical factors of each athlete

generate decreases. During an eccentric contraction, it is generally believed that as the velocity of active muscle lengthening increases, force production in the muscle increases but then quickly levels off.[15,16] It is hypothesized that this may be an important aspect for shock absorption or rapid deceleration of a limb during quick changes of direction.[16] The rehabilitation specialist can use this information to train the respective concentric and eccentric components of movement appropriate to the demands of the sport in respect to the velocity of muscle contraction.

The specific load requirement of the sport is an important consideration. Most sport skill cannot be loaded without changing the movement pattern or technique.[2] The use of too heavy of a weight or implement risks altering the specific movement pattern required for that sport. In fact, it has been shown that if a runner trains on a surface with more than a 2% incline, running technique will be altered significantly.[17]

Performance of every activity or sport derives a percentage of needed energy from all energy sources.[18] Most sports are one energy system dominant.[2,18] The program design must determine the extent of each energy system's involvement and

be outlined accordingly. Anaerobic energy system–dominant sports are trained significantly different than those sports that derive the majority of their metabolism from the oxygen energy source. The different anaerobic sources, adenosine triphosphate–phosphocreatine (ATP-PC) and anaerobic glycolysis, are also trained differently due, in large part, to the amount of time the athlete is active in the sport.

The prevention of reinjury is an important goal for an athlete's training program. Well-planned rehabilitation and training programs should take into account several factors, including past injury history, past medical history, and the primary sites of injury of the sport to which the athlete will be returning. *Prehabilitation* is a recent term used in the literature that refers to the use of training methods as a means of preventing initial injury by training the joints and muscles that are most susceptible to injury in an activity.[2] Knowing that the shoulder, knee, and abdominal regions are the most frequently injured in volleyball,[19] for example, the strength and conditioning professional could specifically train these areas in terms of muscle imbalances, joint range-of-motion deficits, proprioceptive deficits, and so on. Understanding a sport's typical injury profile and the athlete's previous medical and injury history can assist in designing a proper training program for return to play. Continually educating the athlete as he or she progresses along the rehabilitation continuum will help prevent further injury.

DETRAINING

Cessation from training following injury or surgery can have profound, lasting effects. The athlete has to recover from the trauma of the injury/surgery, as well as the effects of detraining. Trauma following surgery is compounded by the athlete's state of detraining. Minimizing the effects of detraining is of fundamental importance. Complete cessation of all forms of training is not desirable for the competitive athlete. The athlete can continue to do leg and arm conditioning/strengthening, as well as core strengthening/conditioning and either

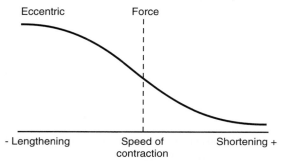

Figure 5-2: Force-velocity curve comparisons for concentric and eccentric contractions. *(From Davies G: A compendium of isokinetics in clinical usage and rehabilitation techniques, ed 4, Onalaska, WI, 1992, S & S Publishers.)*

TABLE 5-4

Open and Closed Kinetic Chain Characteristics

OPEN KINETIC CHAIN	CLOSED KINETIC CHAIN
Distal segment moves in space	Distal segment remains fixed in place
Only segments distal to moving joint move	Movement may occur distal and/or proximal to moving joint
Single muscle group involvement	Multiple muscle group involvement
Single plane of movement	Multiplanar movement
Concentric *or* eccentric muscle contraction	Eccentric/concentric co-contraction
Non–weight bearing	Weight bearing
"Isolated" movement	"Functional" movement
Low proprioceptive demand	High proprioceptive demand
Low joint compression forces	Higher joint compression forces

anaerobic or aerobic modified training (dependent, of course, on surgical protocol and restrictions, etc.). It is important to maintain some semblance of the athlete's prior physical condition by whatever means are appropriate.

As noted by Nicholas and colleagues,[20] the rehabilitation specialist must be concerned with the fact that the strength of the lower body is an integrated unit, which can be affected in many different areas, some quite remote from the site of pathology. The concept of totaled leg strength was established to include the sum strength of the quadriceps, hamstring, hip abductors, hip adductors, and hip flexors as measured isokinetically.[20] This concept can further be generalized to include not only the rest of the lower extremity strengths, but also the totaled arm strength measurements with respect to involved and noninvolved sides. Injury and subsequent surgical follow-up can cause weakness not only to the involved shoulder or knee but also to the proximal and distal joints of the respective limb. Rehabilitation of the athlete should account for the entire kinetic chain. Rehabilitation can initially focus on the joint proximal and distal to the injury/surgical site if this is appropriate.

Complete cessation of training will, in most instances, result in an immediate decline of strength.[2] Early studies indicate that when training ceases completely or is drastically reduced, strength gains decline at a slower rate than the rate at which strength increased.[21-25] After only 2 weeks of detraining, significant reductions in work capacity can be measured, and improvements can be lost within several months.[26] Postoperative trauma may further compound this strength loss initially. After the first month of detraining, loss of strength occurs at a greater rate than the loss of muscle size.[27]

Cardiovascular fitness may be lost more quickly than high force and power production.[2] Endurance adaptations are most sensitive to periods of inactivity because of their enzymatic basis.[28] Strength may be maintained for up to 2 weeks in power athletes,[29] whereas strength loss in recreationally trained individuals has been shown to take longer (i.e., 6 weeks) because of lower initial strength levels than those who were highly trained before detraining.[30] Eccentric force and power does, however, seem to be more sensitive to detraining effects over a few weeks, especially in trained athletes.[30,31] Thorstensson[32] has suggested that the ability to perform complex skills involving strength components (e.g., the vertical jump) may be lost if not included in the training program. Wilmore and Costill[7] noted that sport-specific strength or power decreases significantly with 4 weeks of rest or reduced workout frequency. It is therefore plausible that motor performance deficits would occur, due to the fact that sport-specific strength or power may be delayed until later rehabilitative stages for reasons such as soft tissue healing constraints or fracture healing time frames. Maintaining some semblance of these types of motor performance activities, as per appropriate postoperative restrictions, could help reduce their detraining effects.

Electromyogram information by Hakkinen and Komi[33] indicates that the initial strength loss that occurs as a result of detraining is due to neural mechanisms, with muscle atrophy contributing to further strength loss as the detraining duration continues. The general trend toward muscle fiber degeneration is partly due to degeneration of the motor units, in which ST (type I) fibers are usually the first to lose their ability to produce force. FT (type II) fibers are generally least affected by inactivity.[6] As has been previously discussed, type II fibers require a higher recruiting stimulus. Also previously noted is the fact that the type I fibers have a higher enzymatic basis. The combination of these two factors most likely explains this discrepancy in order of force production. Strength increases both because of adaptations within the nervous system (learning and improved coordination) and muscle hypertrophy.[34,35] Strength gains from hypertrophy show slower losses compared with strength gains from nervous system adaptations.[1] This is an important aspect for the rehabilitation specialist to consider. The athlete requiring mostly strength or endurance in his or her respective sport will be less affected by detraining than the athlete relying to a greater degree on power because the power aspect of a sport has a higher neural component. Emphasizing training of the nervous system component of strength and power as early as possible, by whatever means possible, is an important consideration in the rehabilitation of the postinjury/postsurgical athlete.

TYPES OF TRAINING RESISTANCE

Some of the most common types of resistance used in sports medicine and athletic conditioning/reconditioning are machine-designed resistance, free weights, elastic resistance, fluid resistance, and isokinetics.

Machine resistance is common in the athletic environment. The large majority of weight rooms are equipped with several types of weight-stacked machines for the purpose of athletic rehabilitation and performance enhancement. The main source of resistance for machines is via pulleys, cams, cables, and gears. These different mechanisms of machine resistance provide increased control over the direction and pattern of resistance. Advantages of machines include the following:[2,4]

- Safety—less skill is required to maintain control of a weight stack than free weights. The machine provides an artificial means of support while lifting the weight. Machine stabilization allows the athlete to isolate a muscle group, such as early in the rehabilitation process.
- Design flexibility—machines can be designed to resist some motions that are difficult to resist with free weights (e.g., hip adduction and abduction).
- Ease of use—it is quicker and easier to select weight on a weight-stacked machine than it is to load a barbell with various amounts of weight.

Advantages of free weights include the following:[4,36]

- Whole body training—the movement of the free weight is constrained by the athlete lifting the weight rather than the machine itself. Muscles are required to work in stabilization as well as support. The athlete uses greater muscle synergistic actions.

- Bilateral strength imbalances are minimized because of the inability to shift or compensate with one side. With free weights, the athlete is most often required to use bilateral extremities to successfully complete the maneuver because no external stabilization is provided.

- Greater range of motion is afforded with free weights. The athlete's range of motion is not restricted by the design limitations of a particular machine.

- Free weights require the athlete to work in all three planes of motion. The athlete is more likely to be able to simulate the specific aspects of a sport if movement is allowed in all three planes (Figure 5-3). Machines tend to isolate single muscle groups; the lifting of free weights involves the more natural coordination of several muscle groups.

With all of the advantages listed for free weights, there is a notable disadvantage that needs to be addressed (as well as for machine resistance) during the athlete's training. A considerable amount of time is spent on the deceleration phase of an athlete's lift. The deceleration phase of a repetition occurs when the resistance's movement slows even though there is an attempt to increase or maintain movement speed.[2] This is an unavoidable component of lifting with free weights and weight-stacked machines. The bar is decelerating for a considerable proportion (24%) of the concentric movement.[37] This deceleration phase inflates to 52% when the athlete performs the lift with lighter resistance (e.g., 81% of 1 repetition maximum [RM]).[37] If an athlete attempts to lift at a faster velocity to simulate the sporting activity, the duration of the deceleration phase will increase because the athlete must slow the bar to a complete stop at the end of the range of movement.[38]

The deceleration results from a decreased activation of the agonists during the later phase of the lift and may be accompanied by a considerable activation of the antagonists, particularly when using lighter resistances and trying to lift the weight quickly.[2,39] Decelerating the resistive force is not a common parameter in sports, especially in sports in which an implement is released or involves a projectile (track-and-field throws, soccer, volleyball, basketball, etc.). This deceleration is unwanted when the athlete is attempting to maximize his or her power.

Minimizing the deceleration phase can be accomplished if the athlete actually throws or jumps with the weight. This has been previously referred to as "dynamic" or "explosive" resistance training, but is probably best described as "ballistic" resistance training.[2,40] Ballistic implies acceleration, high velocity, and actual projection into free space.[2,40] Medicine balls are valuable tools to accomplish ballistic training. Medicine ball training can be performed with the lower

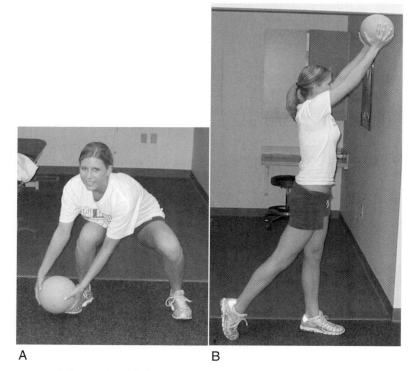

A   B

Figure 5-3: A, Multiplanar squat and diagonal reach (start position). **B,** Multiplanar squat and diagonal reach (end position). Emphasis should be placed on unlocking opposite side hip to avoid excessive trunk rotation.

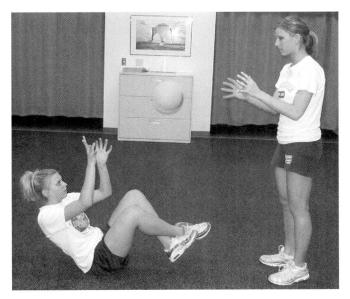

Figure 5-4: Medicine ball partner toss with upper trunk emphasis.

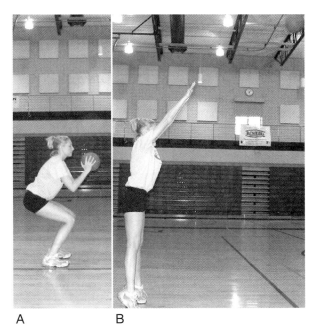

A   B

Figure 5-6: A, Set position for medicine ball toss with full body extension and jump. **B,** Medicine ball full extension and jump with ball release end position.

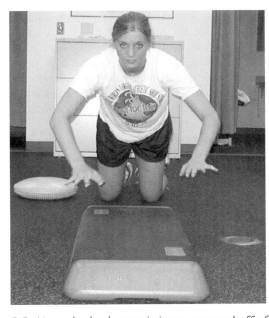

Figure 5-5: Upper body plyometric jump onto and off of step.

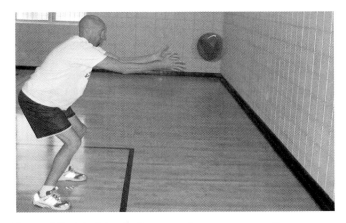

Figure 5-7: Medicine ball toss against concrete wall.

body, upper body, trunk, and whole body movements (Figures 5-4 to 5-6). The use of a solid wall or surface allows a rebound or plyometric capability with training (Figure 5-7). Additional advantages of medicine ball training include the following:[41] ability to work in a sports-general position or pattern, teaching summation of force from ground through the entire kinetic chain, allowing the muscles to contract at a speed similar to that encountered in sports, convenience (medicine ball training can be done alone), and total body conditioning. Disadvantages include a large space requirement with a masonry wall to throw against and the need for numerous medicine balls ranging in size and weight.[41]

Elastic resistance is becoming more popular, especially in the rehabilitation environment. Elastic resistance force is roughly proportional to the product of the distance the elastic component is stretched beyond its resting length and a constant that reflects the physical characteristics of the elastic component.[4] The use of elastic resistance is popular because of its low cost, ease of use, and variable degrees of resistance; it also allows functional patterns of movement, has multiple uses, and requires little space.

One major disadvantage of elastic resistance is the fact that it is contrary to the force capability patterns of virtually all human muscle groups.[4] Elastic resistance starts with low resistance and ends with its highest resistance at the end of the range of motion (ROM). The vast majority of all human muscle groups demonstrate a substantial decrease of force capability at end ranges. This concept must be taken into consideration, especially in the early phases of postoperative rehabilitation when muscle isolation–type exercises may be favored, because it is generally during this stage of training that the muscle tolerates the least amount of resistance. Using elastic resistance at end ranges of muscle contraction would be contradictory to the length/tension curve capabilities of normal muscle and could potentially overload an already susceptible muscle. The majority of human muscle, according to the length/tension curve, generates the greatest amount of force at or near midrange sarcomere length[7,13] or near resting length.[4]

Fluid resistance is the resistive force encountered by an object moving through a fluid (liquid or gas) or by a fluid moving past or around an object.[4] Fluid resistance is a significant factor in many sports activities, including swimming, golf, sprint running, discus throwing, and baseball pitching.[4]

Unlike free weights or weight machines, fluid resistance machines lack eccentric muscle actions. Fluid resistance machines involve alternate concentric actions of antagonistic muscle groups, allowing each muscle group to rest while its antagonist works.[4] This is a significant disadvantage in most sporting events because there is frequently an eccentric component to the movement performed. Baseball pitching, for example, has a significant eccentric component involved in the deceleration phase. This cannot be replicated with these types of resistance machines. Any sporting movement that involves running, jumping, or throwing a projectile cannot be accurately replicated with this type of resistance. Another factor to consider is that fluid resistance has different forms, including air and water, which can be difficult to specifically replicate.

Isokinetic resistance refers to muscular action performed at a constant angular velocity.[2] The preset velocity of movement is controlled by the machine dynamometer.

Three phases have been associated with each isokinetic effort: an acceleration phase, in which the machine makes adjustments for the preset limb velocity; a constant velocity phase, in which torque measurement occurs; and a deceleration phase.[42,43] Some repetitive training is required to adjust to the accommodating resistance, especially on the athlete who is used to variable resistance with the traditional weight-lifting–type devices and movements.

Advantages of isokinetic training include the following:[2,5]

- Accommodates dynamic loading of a muscle throughout the range of motion
- High validity and reliability of the equipment
- Ability to train over a wide range of movement velocities
- Minimal muscle and joint soreness
- Resistance is accommodating to pain and fatigue

- Feedback is often provided instantaneously to the athlete
- Large amount of objective data available
- High inherent safety factor (therefore minimal risk to the athlete)

Disadvantages of isokinetic training include the following:[2,5]

- Affordability of the equipment
- Inconvenience of adjustment of equipment for various joints and ease of various setups
- Time consumption if more than one joint is exercised
- Some artificial parameters until the limb actually moves at the velocity of the dynamometer
- Isokinetic muscle actions do not exist in daily life and sport activity

STRENGTH

Strength is the ability of the muscle to exert maximum force or torque at a specified or determined velocity.[44] Strength is an essential component of all rehabilitation and performance enhancement programs. Strength varies for different muscle actions such as eccentric, concentric, and isometric.[45] Because all muscles function eccentrically, isometrically, and concentrically in all three planes of motion, an integrated training program should utilize a multidimensional/multiplanar training approach using the entire muscle contraction spectrum and velocity contraction spectrum.[1,2,10,46,47]

The biomechanical factors of human strength include the following:[4]

1. Neural control—muscle strength generally increases as more motor units are involved in the contraction, the motor units are greater in size, or the rate of firing is faster. Much of the improvement in strength evidenced in the first few weeks of resistance training is attributable to neural adaptations.[48]

2. Muscle cross-sectional area—all else being equal, the force a muscle can exert is related to its cross-sectional area rather than its volume.[49]

3. Muscle fiber arrangement—pennation appears to enhance force during high-speed concentric muscle action, particularly at ROM extremes, but may reduce force capability for eccentric, isometric, or low-speed muscle actions.[50]

4. Muscle length—a muscle can generate most force at about resting length and less force when in an elongated or a shortened state.

5. Joint angle—changes in strength throughout the joint ROM affect force capability. The amount of torque exerted about a given joint varies throughout the joint's ROM because of the force versus muscle length relationship, as well as the geometric arrangement of muscles, tendons, and joint structures.

6. Force-velocity relationship—greater velocity is generally associated with a lower force capability.

    a. Eccentric muscle actions produce greater force with the advantage of requiring less energy per unit of muscle force.[51-53]

    b. Concentric muscle contraction velocity—as depicted in the force-velocity curve, the faster a muscle contracts, the less force it can exert.

7. Strength-to-mass ratio—according to Newton's second law,[54] force equals mass times acceleration ($F = M \times A$); therefore acceleration equals force divided by mass ($A = F/M$). Thus the strength-to-mass ratio directly reflects an athlete's ability to accelerate his or her body.

8. Body size—as body size increases, body mass increases more rapidly than does muscle strength. Given constant body proportions, the smaller athlete has a higher strength-to-mass ratio than the larger athlete.[55]

One of the primary steps in the rehabilitation/training progression is the redevelopment and improvement of the athlete's strength. When developing the training program for the athlete's return to sport, the entire athlete must be considered, not just the primary area of injury. The specificity principle is paramount in respect to training for that particular sport and athletic injury.

Maximum strength can be improved, at least partially, through neuromuscular training. This type of training improves intramuscular and intermuscular coordination. Intramuscular coordination is the ability of the neuromuscular system to allow optimal levels of motor unit recruitment and motor unit synchronization. This allows for high levels of force production, stabilization, and force reduction. Intermuscular coordination is the ability of the neuromuscular system to allow agonists, antagonists, stabilizers, and neutralizers to work synergistically in an integrated, multiplanar environment. This leads to decreased Golgi tendon organ and antagonistic muscle inhibition, as well as increased joint stabilization dynamically. Cumulatively, this leads to increased neuromuscular efficiency.[1,2,10,46,47]

Types of Strength

Every athlete requires strength to be successful, but different types of strength exist. Categorization of strength capabilities into discrete types (absolute strength, relative strength, speed-strength, explosive strength, strength-endurance, etc.) can be somewhat restrictive, because all are interrelated in their production and development, despite their inherent specificity. Strength types are rarely, if ever, displayed separately, but are components of every movement.[1]

Strength can be expressed in terms of absolute and relative. *Absolute strength* is a measure of the maximum amount of strength or force generated in a movement or exercise. This would indicate the maximum amount of weight that an athlete could lift once (1 RM). Absolute strength is limited by neuromuscular inhibition. Lack of intramuscular and intermuscular coordination decreases motor unit recruitment and synchronization, decreasing force production.[12,56] Absolute strength is paramount in interior linemen in football, athletes in combative sports, power lifters, and shot-putters.

Relative strength is the maximum amount of force generated per unit of body weight. In other words,

$$\text{Relative strength} = \text{Absolute strength}/ \text{Total body weight of athlete}$$

Optimal levels of relative strength are required for sports that require an athlete to control his or her body weight against gravity or external resistance (e.g., wrestling, gymnastics, figure skating, rock climbing, running, boxing).[1,46,47] Achieving a high level of relative strength in any sport requiring weight classes is an advantage for that athlete over competitors with lower relative strength.

Differentiation between absolute and relative strength is not only important in a specific sport, but also between genders. A woman's upper body strength averages 55% of a man's, and her lower body strength averages 72% of a man's.[57-61] These measurements were taken in absolute terms. However, if expressed relative to total body weight and fat-free mass, women's strengths were often more equivalent to men's.[62] Generally, data indicate that women's upper body strength is less than that of men's in absolute terms and relative to total body weight or fat-free mass.[2] Women's absolute lower body strength is less than that of men's, but may be equivalent relative to fat-free mass. This may indicate that women's weight training programs for many sports and activities should emphasize upper body training in an attempt to improve performance.[2]

In sports disciplines where absolute muscular strength is important (shot put, heaviest weight class of weightlifting), strength training should lead to an increase of muscle mass. In disciplines where either an athlete's whole body has to be moved (gymnastics, pole vault, jumps), or the athlete's weight has to remain within certain limits (boxing and wrestling), the relative muscular strength is of greatest importance. With the same level of training, heavier athletes have a greater absolute muscular strength and a lower relative muscular strength than their lighter counterparts.[11]

Both absolute and relative strength are irrespective of the time required to produce the force, or rate of force development (RFD).[11] Time is not a parameter accounted for in either absolute or relative strength. RFD is an important aspect in athletics and is discussed further in the section on power.

Static or isometric strength is used when the tension of a muscle increases while its length remains constant. Early in the rehabilitation program, isometric exercises are initiated in the involved extremity to regain lost strength. Because of joint angle specificity of isometric strengthening, multiple-angle isometric contractions every 20 degrees may be used to achieve strength throughout the range of motion.[63] The transfer of strength gain to other angles varies from 10% to over 50%, and is greater for muscles lengthened during isometric tension than for muscles shortened.[10,64] Nevertheless, because of the highly specific conditions of applying strength in sports, it is best to perform sport-specific exercises in the exact positions used in that particular sport.[11]

Dynamic strength is that strength exhibited when the length of the muscle changes while the muscle contracts. Dynamic strength is divided into slow strength, speed strength, amortizing strength (slow and fast), reactive strength, explosive strength, and starting strength.[11]

- Slow strength is used when near maximal mass is given minimal acceleration. Lifting a heavy barbell slowly is an example.

- Slow amortizing strength is a slow eccentric action such as slowly lowering a heavy weight. The force values shown in eccentric tensions are greater than in any other type of muscle actions[10] (see Figure 5-2).

- Fast amortizing strength is used in fast eccentric actions such as landings or catching a hard-thrown object.

- Reactive strength is used for fast switching from eccentric to concentric actions such as landing and immediately jumping up. The faster a muscle is loaded eccentrically, the greater the concentric force production.[65] Reactive strength is used in all jumps other than those done from standing still. Track-and-field jumps commonly require reactive strength.

- Speed strength denotes the result of dividing the athlete's maximum strength value in a given movement by the time it takes to reach that value.[66] It can also be expressed as the ability to exert maximum force during high-speed movement.[67]

- Explosive strength is the ability to rapidly increase force.[66] It can also be defined as the ability to apply as much force as possible in the shortest time[67] and is useful in all situations where a considerable mass has to be moved quickly, for example, in sprinting starts and in wrestling throws.

- Starting strength is the maximum amount of force a person can develop at the beginning of a movement (in the first 30 milliseconds after beginning the contraction).

Many sporting activities take place so rapidly that it is virtually impossible to recruit an adequate number of muscle fibers. Therefore many sporting performances do not depend solely on the ability to produce maximum strength. Presuming technical skill is adequate, performance may also be limited by the inability to produce the optimal level of strength at any given instant.[1] This ability to produce power is an extremely valuable tool in the athletic environment.

POWER

Power is defined as work per unit of time (force times distance divided by time). Because the definition of velocity is distance divided by time, power can further be defined as force times velocity. Therefore time is an essential element when training for power. How fast force is developed is a key component in the training program designed to develop power. RFD can be defined as the rate at which strength is developed or increases.[1] It is advantageous for a muscle to develop as much force as possible in as little time as possible because force is required almost instantly in many sporting activities. Rate of force production is the single most important neural adaptation for the majority of athletic individuals.[12] In other words, rate of force development in the muscles is another factor vital to sporting prowess.[1]

Training programs dedicated to the development of power require both high-force training and high-quality power movements in which time and the rapidity of movements play a vital role in the quality of the exercise.[2] Training for absolute strength is important for the development of power. When an individual athlete plateaus in strength development, or is required to produce strength more quickly, specialized power training appears to be even more important to optimize power development.[68,69] It has been suggested that one cannot have a high degree of power without first being relatively strong.[70] Adequate baseline strength is not only appropriate for advancing the training plan, but also for injury prevention. Preventing any further or additional injury in the athlete returning to his or her sport is of paramount importance.

Movement time during most explosive activities is typically less than 300 milliseconds, and most of the maximal force increases cannot be realized over such a short period of time.[2] Typically, the athlete does not have the time necessary to use his or her maximum strength. Slow-velocity strength is beneficial to explosive power development, however, because all movement starts at zero or very slow velocity. It is at these very slow velocities that strength, or force (as depicted in the power equation), is beneficial to the development of power. As higher velocities are achieved, the capacity of slow-velocity strength to produce high force at rapidly shortening velocities diminishes.[71-74]

Power is the functional application of both strength and speed. Power results from the integration of maximum strength and speed.[6] It is the key component for most athletic performances.[75] If two individuals have the same strength but the first individual is able to move an identical resistance force more quickly, the first individual has the ability to generate more power.

It has been demonstrated that individuals must train with heavy loads (85% to 100%) and light loads (30%) at high speeds to develop optimal levels of speed strength (starting, explosive, and reactive).[76] Even though lifting heavy loads (85% to 100% of 1 RM) looks slow, it is applied as fast as possible in order to recruit and synchronize as many motor units as possible.

Training with relatively light loads of approximately 30% of maximum performed at high speeds was investigated by Wilson and colleagues.[77] This load level was found to be superior to plyometric training and traditional weight training (80% to 90% of 1 RM) in developing dynamic athletic performance.

Plyometric training is beneficial in developing dynamic athletic power and performance. Plyometrics are exercises that enable a muscle to reach its maximum strength in as short a time as possible.[78,79] Plyometrics are a method of developing explosive power, an important component of most athletic performances.[79]

Plyometric exercises are based on the stretch-reflex properties of the muscle.[78,79] The rapid stretching (loading) of the muscle activates the muscle spindle reflex, which sends a strong stimulus through the spinal cord to the muscles.[79] This stimulus causes the muscle fibers to contract powerfully in the opposite direction. A rapid deceleration (eccentric action) of a mass followed by a rapid acceleration (concentric contraction) of mass in another direction is the basis of plyometric training.[80] This so-called amortization phase should be kept as short as possible to maximize force in a minimum amount of time. The amount of elastic energy stored in eccentric (negative) work determines the recoil of elastic energy during the concentric (positive) work component. This rapid eccentric movement evokes the stretch reflex, or stretch-shortening cycle, which results in greater concentric contraction of the same muscles.[67] Eccentric muscle actions produce greater force with the advantage of requiring less energy (see Figure 5-2).

Plyometrics can be done with upper body, trunk, and lower body. These are often total body movements. A baseline level of strength should be achieved before successful implementation of plyometric training.[67,78,79] An often-prescribed recommendation in layman's literature is the once-used Russian suggestion of the ability to perform a maximum squat of 1.5 to 2 times the body's weight before attempting depth jumps and similar shock training.[79] However, because plyometric principles are incorporated in activities as basic as walking and running, it is proposed that plyometrics should be included in all resistance training programs for both athletes and patients.[81] It is important to note that the 1.5 to 2 times body weight guideline was actually suggested as a guideline to begin high-level plyometrics, but has been incorrectly applied to all forms of plyometric training.[41] The position statement from the National Strength and Conditioning Association (NSCA)[80] is that athletes weighing over 220 pounds should not depth jump from platforms higher than 18 inches.

Because of the high physical demands of plyometric training, it is recommended that it be performed only one to three times per week.[67,78,79] Only appropriate personnel should implement plyometric training, due to its high intensity requirement. Special care must be taken to correctly implement proper technique and appropriate load and rest intervals. Load is measured in number of foot contacts and depths jumped. As with any other form of resistance training, plyometrics should start with low-intensity exercises and progress, as appropriate, to higher-intensity exercises. An athlete's progression should be based on his or her competence and suc-

cessful achievement at that level of training. Rest intervals should be long enough to allow maximum effort on the next set (from 5 to 10 seconds to 2 to 4 minutes), and recovery between training sessions should be at least 2 days, and most often as long as 4 days.[67] Time for complete recovery should be allowed between plyometric exercise sets. It has been emphasized that planning of all plyometric training dosages be done on the continuum of progressive development as dictated by stress and exercise complexity.[79] As the complexity and intensity of the training increases, the volume decreases, and vice versa.

Upper body plyometrics consist primarily of medicine ball training. The key to medicine ball training is velocity, and the emphasis should be on speed of movement. Any time an athlete struggles to throw the medicine ball, the ball is too heavy.[41] Recommendations on proper ball weight depend on the athlete's control, and can be found in Boyle.[41] Medicine ball training also has the advantage of unilateral training (Figure 5-8).

Other forms of plyometric training for the upper body include push-ups with explosion off the wall or floor and drills with a stability ball. These are also complex drills that should be properly progressed.

As with other forms of training, plyometrics should be performed in all three planes of movement. Progression from single-plane movements to multiplanar movement should be gradual and closely monitored. Because most injuries occur

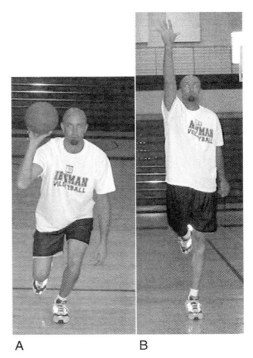

A   B

Figure 5-8: A, Unilateral medicine ball throw start position. **B,** Unilateral medicine ball throw end position.

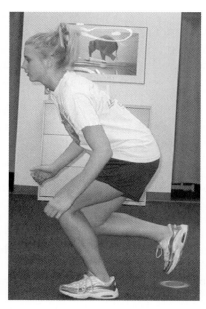

Figure 5-9: Step and hold maneuver correctly performed.

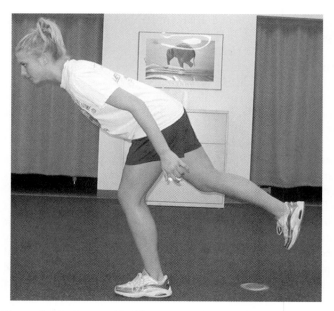

Figure 5-10: Step and hold maneuver incorrectly performed (excessive hip dominance).

in the transverse plane,[12,56] all forms of training should incorporate this plane of movement—not only to determine an athlete's readiness to return to sport, but also as a form of future injury prevention.

Another mechanism of injury prevention in regard to plyometric training is muscle coactivation. This is especially relevant in the case of muscle coactivation of quadriceps and hamstrings for anterior cruciate ligament (ACL) injury prevention strategies. It has been suggested that individuals with hypertrophied quadriceps muscles have less coactivation of the hamstring muscle group because of reciprocal inhibition.[82] This decreased muscle coactivation can have a deleterious effect on the ACL and predispose athletes to noncontact injuries.[83,84] Plyometric training may produce neuromuscular adaptations that develop a more symmetric quadriceps/hamstring coactivation for balanced dynamic restraint.[85] Improved muscle coactivation allows the athlete to more successfully decelerate his or her body, allowing the athlete to more efficiently use the stored potential energy in the form of acceleration.

The plyometric progression can consist of many levels, from eccentric control to depth or shock jumps. Eccentric control can consist of drills as simple as step and hold, in which the athlete takes off from one leg and lands on the opposite leg and holds for isometric/static contraction (Figure 5-9). The athlete must be able to control this position without excessive compensatory movement in the frontal or transverse planes. The athlete should also have adequate quadriceps strength and quadriceps/hamstring muscle coactivation to limit compensatory hip dominance (Figure 5-10). These controlled landings and jumps onto a low-level platform are level 1 plyometric activities. These activities are the basis of further progression with plyometric training.

Level 2 plyometrics involves low-intensity jumping. This involves jumping rope or low-level, small-amplitude jumps over a line. These jumps should be initiated bilaterally and progressed to unilateral or alternating jumps as appropriate.

Level 3 is in-place jumping. The athlete initially performs static holds (as in the first level) for up to 5 seconds. Progression to faster jumps and quicker amortization occurs as the athlete is ready.

Level 4 consists of bounding-type activities. This level initially consists of double leg jumps and progresses to hops, skipping, and eventually bounding. Again the progression is to shorter ground reaction time and explosive concentric action after controlled landing.

Level 5 is depth jumps. These are recommended for elite athletes only. Depth jumps include jumping down from a stable base (box, etc.) and immediately jumping back up. The athlete must have excellent body control and have successfully completed the previous levels without any compensations, injury, and so on. Depth jump contacts should be limited to 20 to 30 foot contacts per session initially and progressed as appropriate.

Power is often classified as either aerobic or anaerobic. Aerobic power is the amount of work a person can perform. It is normally determined by the rate at which oxygen is used during exercise.[86] Anaerobic power is the amount of work performed using primarily anaerobic energy systems. Anaerobic power is strongly related to explosive movements,[86] and is often measured via vertical jump testing.

Unloaded training has been shown to improve the explosive qualities of athletes when used as a peaking cycle late in the season.[87] The athlete is "unloaded" using large rubber cords suspended from the ceiling or stable overhead apparatus with a harness around the athlete, while the athlete performs various types of jumping maneuvers. Concurrent strength training is also used to maintain strength levels. This form of training can be used by athletes who jump frequently (volleyball, basketball, etc.) during the peaking, late in-season cycle. The lowered impact and loading during such training may reduce injury and limit overtraining at a time in the competitive season when such problems tend to occur.[87]

Another form of training used by the rehabilitation specialist to improve power and subsequent athletic performance is Olympic weightlifting. This form of lifting requires very explosive power. The RFD required in Olympic lifts is extremely fast. The two Olympic lifts are the snatch, in which the barbell is lifted from the floor to an overhead position in one complete movement, and the clean and jerk, in which the barbell is first lifted from the floor to the level of the shoulders in one movement, and then pressed overhead in a second movement. The Olympic lifts require whole body participation for successful completion.

Variations of these two main lifts are often used by breaking down the lifts into their component parts or by using dumbbells to perform more unilateral training. These multiple variations can be used not only to improve the Olympic lifts themselves, but also to make the training more applicable to the athlete's sport.

The Olympic lifts and their variations require a significant amount of supervision and training from a qualified professional. A great deal of technical training is involved in learning the proper performance of these lifts. Another disadvantage of these lifts is that they are single plane in nature unless dumbbells are used to involve more than one plane of movement (Figure 5-11).

ENDURANCE

Endurance is the ability to work for prolonged periods of time and the ability to resist fatigue.[18,88] Endurance for an athlete can be either local muscle endurance or the more commonly described cardiovascular endurance. Muscle endurance is the ability of a local, isolated muscle group to perform repeated contractions over a period of time, whereas cardiovascular endurance is defined as the ability of the body to sustain prolonged exercise.[75] Activities requiring cardiovascular endurance require concurrent muscular endurance, although tasks requiring muscular endurance do not always necessitate cardiovascular endurance. Muscular endurance training has a positive transfer to cardiovascular endurance.[13]

A fundamental adaptive response to endurance training is an increase in the aerobic capacity of the trained musculature.[27] This allows the athlete to continue training or sporting competition at a given intensity for a longer period of time compared with pretraining status. This adaptation is the result of glycogen sparing (less glycogen is used during the exercise). Increased fat utilization during this type of activity also contributes to glycogen sparing. The combina-

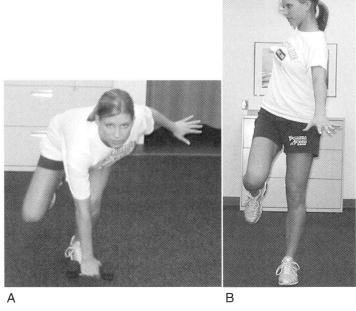

A   B

Figure 5-11: A, Unilateral (alternate)—dumbbell snatch maneuver start position. (avoid excessive trunk flexion). **B,** Unilateral (alternate)—dumbbell snatch maneuver (end position) with emphasis on transverse plane movement. Special consideration should be given to hip rotation versus excessive trunk rotation (as shown).

tion of these events allows the athlete to be more aerobically efficient, enabling the athlete to prolong his or her training or performance. The athlete also produces less lactic acid.

Training for muscular endurance involves using aerobic exercise of very low relative intensity and an overall volume that is high. This type of program involves submaximal muscle contractions extended over a large number of repetitions with little recovery between each set.

During endurance training there is a selective hypertrophy of type I muscle fibers because of their increased recruitment during endurance activities.[89] Relatively little evidence exists to suggest a conversion of type II fibers to type I fibers as a result of chronic endurance training, but there may be a gradual conversion of type IIb fibers to type IIa fibers.[90] This type of conversion is significant, in that type IIa fibers possess a greater oxidative capacity than type IIb fibers, as well as functional characteristics more similar to type I fibers. The result of this conversion is a greater number of muscle fibers that can contribute to endurance performance.[91]

The physiologic causes of fatigue have been reported in the literature as either peripheral or central mechanisms. Peripheral mechanisms are associated with sites outside of the central nervous system, whereas central mechanisms are associated with sites found within the central nervous system.[92] The differences can be summarized as failure occurring because of electrical excitation (i.e., central) or failure within the contractile mechanism itself (i.e., peripherally).[13] Endurance adaptations are most likely to occur at the peripheral level, and more specifically, at the specific limb or muscle group level, reinforcing the need for specificity of exercise.[93]

The ability to fully activate a muscle by electrical stimulation when fatigued provides support for central fatigue mechanisms, even though debate continues regarding this mechanism's contribution to physiologic fatigue.[13] There is, however, surprisingly little correlation between the onset of fatigue and the exhaustion of local reserves of CP and ATP.[94] Perhaps the central mechanism does play a significant role.

The rehabilitation specialists' major focus lies with the peripheral mechanism and how it can be improved. Both muscular endurance and cardiovascular endurance are necessary for the successful participation in athletic performances requiring an endurance component. Muscular endurance is required to complete cardiovascular endurance training activities. Endurance training can be performed using a variety of exercise modes and techniques, as well as varying program variables, and generally involves low-intensity, long-duration activities.

Lactate threshold (LT) is an important factor in determining fitness level in a conditioning program. LT has been termed the *exercise intensity* or *relative intensity* at which blood lactate begins an abrupt increase above the baseline concentration.[95] LT delineates an increasing dependence on anaerobic mechanisms and typically begins at 50% to 60% of maximum oxygen uptake in untrained subjects and at 70% to 80% in trained subjects.[96,97] LT is also the best single predictor of performance in long-distance running over distances from 5 km to the marathon.[98]

VO_2max is an influential determinant of fitness level in regard to conditioning. It is referred to as *aerobic capacity,* or *maximum oxygen uptake.* It is the amount of oxygen that is being consumed. VO_2max is regarded by most as the best single measurement of cardiovascular endurance and fitness. It has been suggested, though, that a good performance requires more than a high VO_2max.[99] VO_2max has been criticized as being significantly overrated as a measurement of endurance ability, especially for game sports.[100]

Another major determinant of successful endurance performance is the percentage of VO_2max that an athlete can maintain for a prolonged period. This percentage of VO_2max is probably related to the LT, which is likely the major determinant of the pace tolerated during a long-term endurance event. Therefore the ability to perform at a higher percentage of VO_2max probably reflects a higher LT. There is some evidence that highly trained athletes, who have reached their genetic ceiling for VO_2max, can still improve performance by augmenting their LT.[101] Neither the time course nor the optimum training stimulus for improvement of LT is known.[101]

Economy of movement is also an important determinant of successful endurance performance. In distance runners with similar VO_2max values, running economy correlates well with performance.[102] During running, the submaximum oxygen intake of an individual is directly and linearly related to his or her running velocity.[98] Maximizing strength-endurance and technique allows the athlete to improve his or her economy of movement. With improved strength-endurance and technique, the athlete functions more efficiently, requiring less energy expenditure. This allows the athlete to more easily reach his or her athletic potential. This is true for strength- and power-dominated sports, as it appears that very fast sprinters are distinguished by more efficient organization of the locomotor system.[1] Rehabilitation specialists also need to critically look at sport technique in endurance athletes. Economical movement in these athletes is essential to successful athletic participation. Training athletes in different technical movements while in a semifatigued state is beneficial in terms of endurance, especially if appropriate personnel critically assess the technique. The athlete learns to maintain technique in gamelike situations. This is also beneficial in terms of injury prevention and prehabilitation training. The rehabilitation specialist must be careful not to push the athlete too far in this realm. This is true not only from an injury prevention standpoint, but also in relation to the specificity of training principle. The work-to-rest ratios should be kept similar to those of game situations.

Circuit training is a popular method of training to simultaneously build both strength and endurance. Circuit training is essentially interval strength training, consisting of a group of exercises (usually six to nine or more) that are completed sequentially.[100] Occasionally, fewer exercises are performed if a special emphasis is needed. In these cases the duration can be extended with more completions of the circuit. The circuit duration can be either time based or repetition based. The training circuit should be designed with specific goals in mind, depending on the type of athlete and training objectives. Rest periods can be planned after each exercise and after each circuit or can be eliminated after the exercises if necessary, depending on the objectives of the circuit. Circuit training can be done for upper body, lower body, core/trunk, or whole body emphasis.

To increase muscular endurance, high-volume circuit training is preferable to moderate long-distance running or cycling.[103,104] Running as little as 4 km per day has been shown to decrease vertical jump ability (one of the best indicators of explosive power).[103,104] Circuit training is the primary method for the development of strength and power endurance.[100,104] Primary goals of circuit training are to develop muscular endurance, increase work capacity, enable large numbers of athletes to train at one time, and target specific areas or physical qualities.[100,104]

Training the "core" of the body should emphasize endurance. The core is an integrated functional unit consisting of the lumbo-pelvic-hip complex, thoracic spine, and cervical spine.[100,104] Most of the major core muscles are postural muscles.[12,105] These are mostly tonic, type I endurance muscles that need to be trained accordingly. *Core strength* is defined as the ability of the lumbo-pelvic-hip musculature to maintain the athlete's center of gravity over his or her base of support during dynamic movements.[100,104] Having strong extremity muscles, yet a weak core stabilization system, equates to a lack of adequate force transfer for efficient movement. Much of the energy that these athletes produce by the lower extremities will be lost in the transfer up the kinetic chain.

Functional activities are multiplanar and require acceleration, deceleration, and dynamic stabilization.[105] The core performs all of these functions during functional movements.[100,104] This dynamic stabilization component is often critical for allowing appropriate deceleration and subsequent acceleration to occur. Because the intensity of endurance exercises tends to be low,[13] and core musculature is constantly active, endurance training for this area of the body can be performed daily.

As with training other body parts, training the core should be progressively challenged to include more functional positions. Initially, exercises may need to be initiated in supine and prone positions. Progression would include standing and more challenging exercises in the supine and prone positions (Figure 5-12).

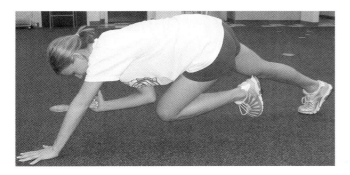

Figure 5-12: Trunk stabilization in hands and knees position—opposite elbow to opposite knee.

Generally, endurance training is of lower intensity and higher volume in comparison to training for strength and power. It has even been suggested that for muscle endurance activities of medium to long duration, as many as 30 to greater than 150 repetitions be performed (depending on load percent of 1 RM).[6] A 30% load repetition range would be greater than 100 to 150, whereas a 50% load repetition range would be 40 to 50.

Table 5-5 gives a general outline of the different training variables in relation to strength, power, and endurance training. This information is a compilation of sources meant to be used as a general outline to assist with more advanced program design by the rehabilitation specialist in regard to each specific athlete.*

The rehabilitation specialist should evaluate all of these factors when implementing a training program for the endurance athlete. Training simply with longer time duration without respect to other factors, such as core stability/endurance and economy of movement, is capricious planning.

CONCURRENT TRAINING

It has been suggested that athletes involved in sports that are primarily anaerobic should add aerobic training to enhance their recovery mechanisms. Aerobic training, however, may reduce anaerobic performance capabilities, particularly high-strength, high-power performance.[106] Combining these two types of training can reduce maximum strength,[106,107] and especially speed- and power-related performance,[108] although the exact mechanism is not known.[109]

Frequency of training seems to be a relevant training variable. Concurrent strength and endurance training 5 or 6 days per week impairs strength development,[106,108,110-113] but

---

*References 1, 2, 6, 11, 12, 100, and 104.

TABLE 5-5

Comparison of Training Characteristics/Variables

VARIABLE	STRENGTH	POWER	STRENGTH-ENDURANCE	ENDURANCE
Load/Intensity (% of 1 RM)	80%-100%	Strength/force (70%-100%), velocity (30%-45%), or up to 10% body weight	50%-70%	Circuit training (40%-60%)
Repetitions	Very low to low (1-6)	1-5 (strength) 5-10 (power)	12-25	Moderate to high (15-30[+])
Sets	3-5	4-6	2-3	2-5
Rest Period	3-6 minutes	2-6 minutes	30-60 seconds	45-90 seconds (1 : 1 work : rest ratio)
Speed of Performance	Slow to medium (speed of effort is as fast as possible)	Fast/explosive	Slow to medium (emphasize stabilization)	Medium
Primary Energy Source	(1) Phosphagen (2) Anaerobic glycolysis	Phosphagen	Anaerobic glycolysis/ aerobic	Aerobic

limiting training the same muscle groups to 3 days per week on alternate days does not seem to cause any significant detriment.[107,114-119] It has even been recommended that both strength and endurance training for the same muscle group can be performed on the same day, but not more than 3 days per week.[120]

Limiting the duration of endurance training may help prevent strength development impairment.[120] Periodization of the training program would allocate the duration of such an endurance phase or microcycle. Careful planning should consider the athlete's needs for such an endurance phase and its pertinent length. This duration should take into account several factors, not the least of which is the athlete's sport and position in that sport. Athletes on the same team may not need to train in the same manner, as in the case of a baseball pitcher versus an outfielder. The outfielder will, at points in the game, be required to run full speed in multiple directions to catch a ball. His or her training should reflect this requirement.

Evidence indicates that strength training enhances endurance through improvement of structural strength. It also retards muscle breakdown caused by impact forces in running.[103,104] Strength training does not interfere with the development of maximal aerobic power.[120] It has not been determined whether any significant difference occurs in performance adaptations by performing either strength or endurance training first in a concurrent workout.[120]

Concurrent strength and plyometric training have shown greater changes in motor performance tests than with either type of training by itself.[121] Motor performance tasks generally include vertical jump, long jump, sprint performance, and so on. It has been concluded that both types of training should be included in resistance training programs when gains in motor performance are desired.[2]

Strength, power, and endurance are all important abilities for successful athletic performance. The dominant ability is the one in which that particular sport requires the highest contribution. Most sports require peak performance in at least two abilities.[6] Therefore there is often interdependence on at least two of these abilities in most sports.[6] Combining strength and endurance creates muscular endurance. The combination of speed and endurance is called speed-endurance. Agility is the complex combination of speed, coordination, flexibility, and power. This is often demonstrated in sports such as gymnastics, wrestling, football, soccer, volleyball, baseball, boxing, diving, and figure skating.[6] The goal of the rehabilitation process is to determine this combination and to eliminate any deficiencies in these areas, and improve on the dominant abilities required of the athlete.

PERIODIZATION OF ATHLETE TRAINING

Periodization is a year-round training concept developed by Vorobyev[122] and Matveyev.[123] It is the gradual cycling of specificity, intensity, and volume of training to achieve optimal development of performance capacities.[124] Periodiza-

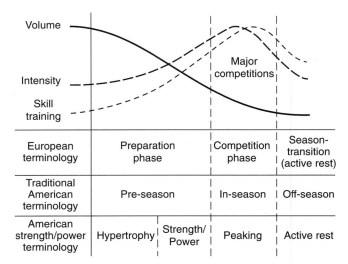

Figure 5-13: Periodization training phases. *(From Sanders M, Sanders B: Principles of resistance training. In Bandy WD, Sanders B, editors: Therapeutic exercise: techniques for intervention, Baltimore, 2001, Lippincott Williams & Wilkins.)*

tion is the planning of the athlete's yearly training program in order to meet the athlete's performance goals. It is designed to gear an athlete's training program to allow the athlete to achieve peak performance at a specified time of the year. Periodization is also advantageous in preventing a plateau in training from occurring during a prolonged training regimen by providing manipulation of the different variables and continual stimulation to the athlete in phases or cycles.[6]

The periodization model is made up of various cycles. A microcycle is the smallest period in the model, and usually consists of 1 week of training. Multiple microcycles make up a mesocycle. Several distinct mesocycles make up a macrocycle. Macrocycle is the largest cycle and usually refers to the entire training year.

The hypertrophy phase occurs during the early stages of the off-season preparation. As noted in Figure 5-13, this phase is characterized by high volume and low intensity. The goal of this stage is to develop a base on which to build the training plan. The volume is high to allow the athlete to make the appropriate physiologic adaptations necessary in preparation for the upcoming season.

The strength/power phase is a transition stage between the preparation and competition phases of the training cycle. The volume is decreased and the intensity is increased from the previous phase. This phase is a transition from an emphasis on volume to an emphasis on developing power; therefore the volume of work performed is decreased to avoid undue fatigue. Intensity is increased to more closely replicate the needs of power training.

Emphasis in the competition or peaking phase is on peaking for the major competitions during the athletic season. The volume is low to avoid fatigue and injury, whereas the intensity and skill training are very high to allow the athlete to be at his or her optimal level at the appropriate competitions.

The phase after the major competition season is the active rest phase. It is during this time when volume, skill training, and intensity are significantly diminished to allow the athlete to continue to maintain some form of conditioning not directly involving that particular sport. This phase is often used to give athletes a reprieve from the constant rigors of their sport. The athlete performs some type of conditioning to avoid the detrimental effects of detraining.

Periodization models can be classified as either the traditional strength/power periodization or undulating periodization. The strength/power model follows a general trend of decreasing training volume and increasing training intensity as training progresses (see Figure 5-13). Undulating periodization is a more recent model of periodization.[2]

With undulating periodization, typically training intensity and volume are varied using different training zones. This type of periodization model is often developed to maintain variation in the training stimulus. The variation in the training is much greater within a mesocycle as compared with the traditional model. Three training zones are typically used, such as 4 to 6 RM, 8 to 10 RM, and 12 to 15 RM zones.[2] The training zones are varied on a training session, weekly, or biweekly manner. The training zones are not necessarily sequentially performed, however, so training intensity or volume follows a pattern of consistently increasing or decreasing over time.[2] This variance in intensity and volume allows fitness gains to occur over long training seasons. Athletes who could benefit from this model include multisport athletes and athletes who are participating not only in school teams, but club teams as well. The goal of this type of periodization is to alternate volume and intensity to create both cellular and neural changes.[100,104]

FUNCTIONAL TRAINING

There has been a more recent shift in training methods to include "functional training," or training specific movements involved in athletics. Functional strength in a given movement involves skilled neuromuscular coordination of many participating muscle groups.[1] Increased recognition of the importance of movement-specific resistance training programs (e.g., functional training) over the past decade has led to the development of specific equipment designed to improve core stability, rotational strength and power, balance, reaction time, speed, acceleration, and agility.[125]

With this increased emphasis on functional training, there is a need for a heightened awareness to be certain athletes are appropriate for some of the more advanced methods. The rehabilitation strength and conditioning specialist should make certain that the athlete does not have any significant isolated muscle or synergistic weaknesses that would further be neglected by training patterns of movement, instead of concentrating on the isolated weaknesses and then

progressing to the functional patterns of movement. Overlooking isolated weaknesses could lead to further muscle imbalances and potentially further injury. Traditional forms of weightlifting and isolated muscle/muscle synergistic contractions have their place in the rehabilitation realm, especially in regard to correction of imbalances and weaknesses in the kinetic chain.

As mentioned previously, function varies throughout the body. Different joints are often required to perform different functions. A specific joint may be required to produce acceleration, deceleration, stabilization, or some combination of each. Functional training of stabilization muscles involves training them to stabilize better, often by performing simple exercises through small ranges of motion.[41] In the pursuit of functionally training an athlete, the stabilization concept is often neglected. The three key groups in need of stabilization training are as follows:[41]

- The deep abdominal muscles (transversus abdominis and internal oblique)
- The hip abductors and rotators (Figure 5-14)
- The scapula stabilizers (Figures 5-15 to 5-17)

It is often thought that these muscle groups need to be isolated to improve their function.[41] In these situations, it has often been suggested that single-joint isolation exercises be implemented to specifically recruit these muscles. These muscles have been implicated as often being neglected in traditional forms of strength training, hence the more recent return to emphasis on isolation exercises.[12,41,105]

However, this concept requires careful consideration. If large loads are imposed on a given muscle group by intense resistance, isolation becomes virtually impossible.[1] Muscles used for static stabilization immediately become involved. If

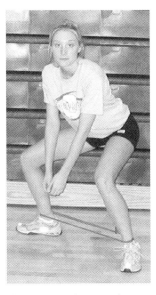

Figure 5-14: Hip abductor and external rotator functional volleyball position strengthening with resistive band.

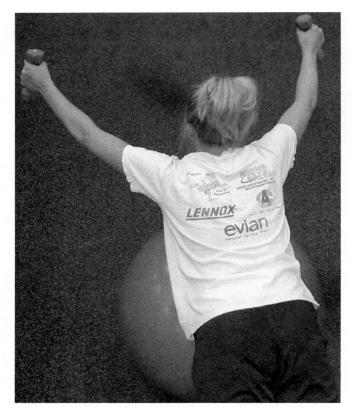

Figure 5-15: Open chain scapular stabilization strengthening on stability ball.

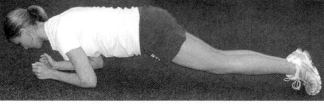

A

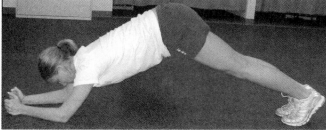

B

Figure 5-16: A, Shoulder girdle and trunk stabilization (shoulders forward over hands position with scapula retracted). **B,** Shoulder girdle and trunk stabilization (pike position with scapula protracted).

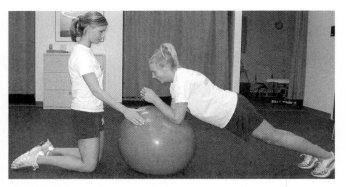

Figure 5-17: Shoulder girdle and trunk stabilization with perturbation.

the prime movers are unable to meet the demands of the load, several other muscle groups, including stabilizers, synergists, and antagonists, may all be recruited by the nervous system to augment the action of the prime movers.[1] Giannakopoulos and colleagues[126] determined that complex exercise strengthening of the rotator cuff significantly improved muscular performance over isolated muscle strengthening, indicating that isolated exercises are only effective when the training goal is to strengthen the weaker muscle group, but these isolated exercises must be replaced by more complex and closed chain exercises in order to obtain considerable improvement of the rotator cuff strength. It was proposed that a strengthening program should start with isolated movements for better stimulation of the weaker muscles and then continue with complex exercise for greater strengthening.

The rehabilitation specialist should closely monitor the athlete and his or her patterns of movement during the performance of the required task to ensure elimination of compensatory movements.

There have been two opposing theories of supplementary strength training in sport.[1] One theory proposes that strength training should simulate the sporting movements as closely as possible with regard to movement pattern, velocity, force-time curve, type of muscle contraction, and so forth; the other theory maintains that it is sufficient to train the relevant muscles with no regard to specificity. Separate practice of technical skills should permit one to utilize in sporting movements the strength gained in nonspecific training. Although both approaches to training will improve performance, current scientific research strongly supports the superiority of the specificity principle in at least 10 respects:[1]

- Type of muscle contraction
- Movement pattern
- Region of movement
- Velocity of movement
- Force of contraction
- Muscle fiber recruitment
- Metabolism
- Biomechanical adaptation

- Flexibility
- Fatigue

Exercises should be selected to mimic the skills of the particular sport; to maximize strengthening of the prime movers; and, in some cases, to produce "motor memory," consolidating the technical skills involved.[6] Strength exercises that resemble the technical pattern repeat similar motions, giving the exercises a learning component.[6] This is especially important for the postoperative patient attempting to return to his or her respective sport. This athlete is relearning component movement patterns of his or her position in the sport not only from being out of the sport for recovery, but also from the negative effects of injury and postoperative trauma. The athlete, depending on his or her respective condition, may not have performed these movements for several weeks or even months. Having the athlete perform at least component movements of his or her position in the sport is necessary to the athlete's successful completion of the rehabilitation process. Also, as noted by Estlander and colleagues,[127] one of the main reasons for poor results of exercise programs is failure to adequately train the patient in functional activities.

Misuse of specificity results in asymmetric body development and neglects the antagonistic and stabilizer muscles. Overemphasizing specificity can result in poor development of prime movers; one-sided, specialized muscle function; and injuries.[6] Laying a foundation of general strength, especially with the athlete recovering from injury, will help the athlete avoid additional injury and improve future performance potential.

PROGRAM DESIGN

The athlete's training plan should be systematically devised, especially in the case of the athlete returning from injury or surgical intervention. The variables that need careful consideration include the muscle groups to train and in what manner, the type of muscle contraction required, the type of resistance and equipment required, open versus closed kinetic chain, the volume and intensity required, the work/rest ratios to train to replicate the sport, the order in which to perform the selected exercises, injury site training, correction of any residual deficits, and how the injury will affect the athlete's return to his or her respective sport.

Proper program design necessitates the use of an appropriate training plan to allow the athlete to peak at the opportune time. The appropriate time must be in agreement with return-to-sport protocols and proper conditioning principles and time frames. Training should be used as a means of returning to sports participation; sports participation should not be used as a means of training (i.e., "Train to play, don't play to train").

Multiple variables must be considered when designing a training program. Some program variables include frequency of training, intensity or load used in training, number of repetitions and sets, number and length of rest periods, types of exercises and muscle contractions, type of resistance used, periodization stage in the training cycle, and the order in which the exercises are performed.

Some general parameters have been suggested for both within a daily training session and within a training cycle progression:[*]

- Large muscle group before small muscle group exercises (if training all major muscle groups in a workout or training lower and upper body exercises on alternating days)
- Multiple-joint before single-joint exercises (if training all major muscle groups in a workout, if training lower and upper body exercises on alternating days, or, in some situations, if training isolation muscle exercises)
- Alternating of push and pull exercises for total body sessions (if training all major muscle groups in a workout or training lower and upper body exercises on alternating days)
- Exercises for weak points (priority) performed before exercises for strong points of an individual
- Olympic lifts before basic strength and single-joint exercises in a single training session

General progressions for training plans/cycles include the following:

- Develop basic joint strength and flexibility before developing power
- Power-type exercises before other exercise types in a single training session
- Most intense to least intense (particularly when performing several exercises consecutively for the same muscle group)
- Simple exercises before complex exercises (Figure 5-18)
- Core stability before extremity mobility
- Controlled environment before uncontrolled environment
- Horizontal movements before vertical movements
- Stress-free positions before stressful positions
- Slow velocity before high velocity
- Unidirectional movements before multidirectional movements
- Create stability—whether it is from contractile sources, noncontractile sources, neuromuscular (kinesthetic) sources, or any combination thereof
- Strengthen the core to be able to stabilize
- Eccentric control before eccentric to concentric energy transfer (amortization phase) with plyometrics
- Develop sport-specific strength

---

*References 1, 2, 6, 10, 11, 100, 104, 126, 128, and 129.

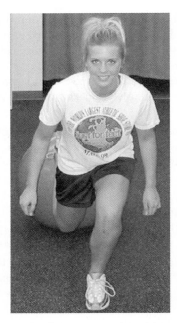

Figure 5-18: Lunge made more complex with opposite foot on stability ball.

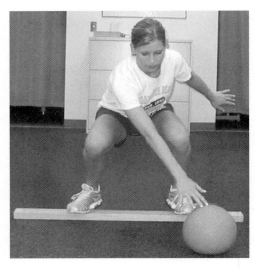

Figure 5-19: Squat on two-by-four with diagonal reach for increased proprioceptive demand.

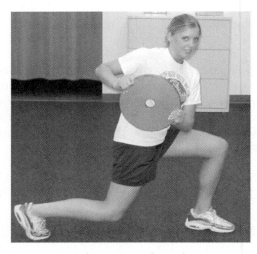

Figure 5-20: Lunge with upper trunk weight rotation to opposite side of lead leg.

- Train movements, not muscles
- Exercises should be multijoint and multiplanar as appropriate
- Exercises should incorporate appropriate sport-specific speed of movement (in relation to specific sport)
- Train core before extremity strength
- Train body weight before external resistance
- With body weight exercises, a range of 10 to 20 repetitions is necessary to force adaptation; use higher repetitions for hypertrophy development and lower repetitions with multiple sets for neural development
- Train strength before strength-endurance
- Training should be of high proprioceptive demand (Figure 5-19)

Table 5-5 (earlier in this chapter) gives a general outline of the different training variables in relation to strength, power, and endurance training. This information is meant to be used as a general outline to assist with more advanced program design by the rehabilitation specialist in regard to each specific athlete.[*]

There are several popular systems of resistance, including single- versus multiple-set systems, "superset" systems, pyramid systems, and the split routine training system. For a detailed description of these and other training systems, see Fleck and Kraemer.[2]

The training program should be planned according to the major emphasis or goals of that stage in training. Each specific training session should include an adequate warm-up that includes dynamic movements, such as those shown in Figures 5-20 to 5-22, to properly prepare the nervous system. A proper cool-down should consist of stretching of the major muscle groups trained in the session.

The training program should be systematically progressed. The athlete returning after surgery will need special monitoring. Progression should be undertaken from a standpoint of the entire training program, as well as from a day-to-day, week-to-week, and month-to-month basis. The strength and conditioning specialist should continually reevaluate the progress of the athlete to make certain the athlete is ready for the next level of progression.

---

[*]References 1, 2, 6, 11, 12, 14, 39, 47, 77, 80, 81, 100, 104, 120, and 128.

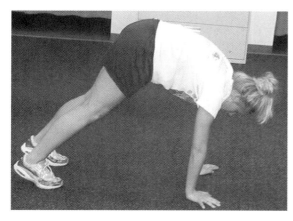

Figure 5-21: Inchworm exercise: starting in push-up position, walk hands back to feet keeping legs as straight as possible. Draw abdomen in and avoid trunk flexion compensation (as shown). Emphasis should be on hinging movement at hip.

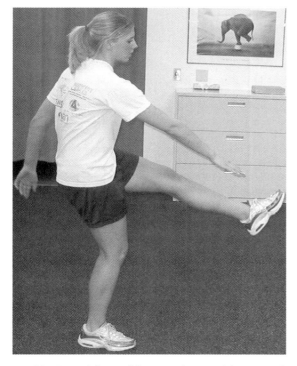

Figure 5-22: Toy soldier walking exercise: reaching opposite hand to opposite foot.

SUMMARY

Training athletes for successful athletic participation requires careful thought and planning. The athlete who is returning from an injury requires additional concerns. It is imperative to the athlete's success to design the training program according to the sport-specific demands. This chapter outlines several areas of concern that should be addressed at some point in the athlete's return to the competitive environment. The training plan should carefully consider not only the athlete's sport and other tangible factors, but also the individual athlete. Allowing the athlete to participate in his or her training plan will increase the likelihood of success.

Athletes will probably be more compliant with a training program that they can relate to their sporting activity.

Reevaluation should be a main theme of the training program, not only of the athlete but of the training program itself. The training program may need to be modified, especially in the case of an athlete returning from a surgical procedure. The training program should be functional in terms of both exercise and its relationship to the athlete's sport.

References

1. Siff MC, Verkhoshansky YV: *Supertraining,* ed 4, Denver, 1999, Supertraining International.
2. Fleck SJ, Kraemer WJ: *Designing resistance training programs,* ed 3, Champaign, IL, 2004, Human Kinetics.
3. Wenger HA, McFadyen PF, McFadyen RA: Physiological principles of conditioning. In Zachazewski JE, Magee DJ, Quillen WS, editors: *Athletic injuries and rehabilitation,* Philadelphia, 1996, Saunders.
4. Harman E: The biomechanics of resistance exercise. In Baechle TR, editor: *Essentials of strength training and conditioning,* Champaign, IL, 1994, Human Kinetics.
5. Davies GA: *Compendium of isokinetics in clinical usage and rehabilitation techniques,* ed 4, Onalaska, WI, 1992, S&S Publishers.
6. Bompa TO: *Periodization training for sports,* Champaign, IL, 1999, Human Kinetics.
7. Wilmore JH, Costill DL: *Physiology of sport and exercise,* ed 2, Champaign, IL, 1999, Human Kinetics.
8. Henneman E, Somjen G, Carpenter DO: Functional significance of cell size in spinal motorneurons, *J Neurophysiol* 28:560-580, 1965.
9. Green HJ: Muscle power: fiber type, recruitment, metabolism and fatigue. In Jones NL, McCartney N, McComas AJ, editors: *Human muscle power,* Champaign, IL, 1986, Human Kinetics.
10. Zatsiorsky VM: *Science and practice of strength training,* Champaign, IL, 1995, Human Kinetics.
11. Kurz T: *Science of sports training: how to plan and control training for peak performance,* ed 2, Island Pond, VT, 2001, Stadion.
12. Clark MA: *Integrated training for the new millennium,* Thousand Oaks, CA, 2001, National Academy of Sports Medicine.
13. Thein-Brody L: Endurance impairment. In Hall CM, Thein BL, editors: *Therapeutic exercise: moving toward function,* Philadelphia, 1999, Lippincott Williams & Wilkins.
14. American College of Sports Medicine: Position stand. Progression models in resistance training for healthy adults, *Med Sci Sports Exerc* 34:364-380, 2002.
15. Levangie PK, Norkin CC: *Joint structure and function: a comprehensive analysis,* Baltimore, 1978, FA Davis.
16. Smith LK, Weiss EL, Lehmkuhl LD: *Brunnstrom's clinical kinesiology,* Philadelphia, 1996, FA Davis.
17. Chu DA: *Explosive power and strength: complex training for maximum results,* Champaign, IL, 1996, Human Kinetics.
18. McCardle WD, Katch, FI, Katch VI: *Exercise physiology: energy, nutrition, and human performance,* ed 4, Baltimore, 1996, Lippincott Williams & Wilkins.
19. Aagard H, Scavenius M, Jorgensen U: An epidemiological analysis of the injury pattern in indoor and in beach volleyball, *Int J Sports Med* 18(3):217-221, 1997.

20. Nicholas JA, Strizak AM, Veras G: A study of thigh muscle weakness in different pathological states of the lower extremity, *Am J Sports Med* 4(6):241-248, 1976.

21. McMorris RO, Elkins EC: A study of production and evaluation of muscular hypertrophy, *Arch Phys Med Rev* 35:420-426, 1954.

22. Morehouse C: Development and maintenance of isometric strength of subjects with diverse initial strengths, *Res Quarterly* 38:449-456, 1967.

23. Rasch P: Isometric exercise and gains of muscular strength. In Shepard R, editor: *Frontiers of fitness*, Springfield, 1971, Thomas.

24. Rasch P, Morehouse L: Effect of static and dynamic exercises on muscular strength and hypertrophy, *J Appl Physiol* 11:29-34, 1957.

25. Waldman R, Stull G: Effects of various periods of inactivity on retention of newly acquired levels of muscular endurance, *Res Quarterly* 40:393-401, 1969.

26. Glenn TM, Mulcare JA: Principles of aerobic exercise. In Kisner C, Colby LA, editors: *Therapeutic exercise: foundations and techniques*, Philadelphia, 2002, FA Davis.

27. Dudley GA, Harris RT: Neuromuscular adaptations to conditioning. In Baechle TR, editor: *Essentials of strength training and conditioning*, Champaign, IL, 1994, Human Kinetics.

28. Kraemer WJ: General adaptations to resistance and endurance training programs. In Baechle TR, editor: *Essentials of strength training and conditioning*, Champaign, IL, 1994, Human Kinetics.

29. Hortobagyi T, Houmard JA, Stevenson JR, et al: The effects of detraining on power athletes, *Med Sci Sports Exerc* 25:929-935, 1993.

30. Kraemer WJ, Koziris LP, Ratamess NA, et al: Detraining produces minimal changes in physical performance and hormonal variables in recreationally strength-trained men, *J Strength Conditioning Res* 16:373-382, 2002.

31. Mujika I, Padilla S: Muscular characteristics of detraining in humans, *Med Sci Sports Exerc* 33:1297-1303, 2001.

32. Thorstensson A: Observations on strength training and detraining, *Acta Phys Scand* 100:491-493, 1977.

33. Hakkinen K, Komi PV: Changes in neuromuscular performance in voluntary and reflex contraction during strength training in man, *Int J Sports Med* 4:282-288, 1983.

34. Moritani T, DeVries HA: Neural factors versus hypertrophy in the time course of muscle strength gain, *Am J Phys Med* 82:521-524, 1979.

35. Sale DG: Neural adaptation to resistance training, *Med Sci Sports Exerc* 20:S135-S145, 1988.

36. Gambetta V: *Building the complete athlete. Seminar manual*, ed 4, Sarasota, 1997, Optimum Sports Training.

37. Elliot BC, Wilson GJ, Kerr GK: A biomechanical analysis of the sticking region in the bench press, *Med Sci Sports Exerc* 21:450-462, 1989.

38. Newton RU, Wilson GJ: The kinetics and kinematics of powerful upper body movements: the effects of load. In *Abstracts of the International Society of Biomechanics XIVth Congress*, Paris, July 4-8, 1993.

39. Kraemer WJ, Newton RU: Training for muscular power, *Phys Med Rehabil Clin North Am* 11:341-368, 2000.

40. Newton RU, Wilson GJ: Reducing the risk of injury during plyometric training: the effects of dampeners, *Sports Medicine, Training and Rehabilitation* 4:1-7, 1993.

41. Boyle M: *Functional training for sports*, Champaign, IL, 2004, Human Kinetics.

42. Osternig LR: Isokinetic dynamometry: implications for muscle testing and rehabilitation. In Pandolf KB, editor: *Exercise and sport science reviews*, New York, 1986, MacMillan.

43. Kraemer WJ, Fry AC: Strength testing: development and evaluation of methodology. In Maud PJ, Foster C, editors: *Physiological assessment of human fitness*, Champaign, IL, 1995, Human Kinetics.

44. Knuttgen HG, Kraemer WJ: Terminology and measurement in exercise performance, *J Appl Sport Sci Res* 1:1-10, 1987.

45. Kraemer WJ: Involvement of eccentric muscle action may optimize adaptations to resistance training, *Sport Sci Ex* 4:230-238, 1992.

46. Bompa TO: *Theory and methodology of training*, Dubuque, IA, 1983, Kendall/Hunt.

47. Fleck SJ, Schutt RC: Types of strength training, *Clin Sports Med* 4:159-167, 1985.

48. Morris JM, Lucas DB, Bresler B: Role of the trunk in stability of the spine, *J Bone Joint Surg* 43A:327-351, 1961.

49. Ikai M, Fukunaga T: Calculation of muscle strength per unit cross-sectional area of human muscle by means of ultrasonic measurement, *Int Z Angew Physiol Arbeitphysiol* 26:26-32, 1968.

50. Scott SH, Winter DA: A comparison of three muscle pennation assumptions and their effect on isometric and isotonic force, *J Biomech* 24(2):163-167, 1991.

51. Bonde-Peterson F, Knuttgen HG, Henriksson J: Muscle metabolism during exercise with concentric and eccentric contractions, *J Appl Physiol* 33:792-795, 1972.

52. Eloranta V, Komi PV: Function of the quadriceps femoris muscle under maximal concentric and eccentric contraction, *EMG Clin Neurophys* 20:159-174, 1980.

53. Komi PV, Kaneko M, Aura O: EMG activity of the leg extensor muscles with special reference to mechanical efficiency in concentric and eccentric exercise, *Int J Sports Med* 8:22-29, 1987.

54. Meriam J: *Engineering mechanics*, vol 2, *Dynamics*, New York, 1978, Wiley.

55. Astrand P, Rodahl K: *Textbook of work physiology*, ed 3, New York, 1986, McGraw-Hill.

56. Clark MA: The scientific and clinical rationale for the use of closed and open chain rehabilitation. In Ellenbecker TS, editor: *Knee ligament rehabilitation*, Philadelphia, 2000, Churchill Livingstone.

57. Bishop P, Cureton K, Collins M: Sex difference in muscular strength in equally trained men and women, *Ergonomics* 30:675-687, 1987.

58. Knapik JJ, Wright JE, Kowal DM, et al: The influence of U.S. Army basic initial entry training on the muscular strength of men and women, *Aviation, Space and Environmental Medicine* 51:1086-1090, 1980.

59. Laubach LL: Comparative muscular strength of men and women: a review of the literature, *Aviation, Space and Environmental Medicine* 47:534-542, 1976.

60. Sharp MA: Physical fitness and occupational performance of women in the U.S. Army, *Work* 2:80-92, 1994.

61. Wilmore JH, Parr RB, Girandola RN, et al: Physiological alterations consequent to circuit weight training, *Med Sci Sports* 10:79-84, 1978.

62. Wilmore JH: Alterations in strength, body composition, and anthropometric measurements consequent to a 10-week weight training program, *Med Sci Sports* 6:133-138, 1974.

63. Knapik JJ, Mawdsley RH, Ramos MU: Angular specificity and test mode specificity of isometric and isokinetic strength training, *J Orthop Sports Phys Ther* 5:58-65, 1983.

64. Thepaut-Mathieu C, Van Hoecke J, Maton B: Myoelectrical and mechanical changes linked to length specificity during isometric training, *J Appl Physiol* 64:1500-1505, 1988.

65. Lundin PE: A review of plyometric training, *Natl Strength Condition Assoc J* 7(3):65-70, 1985.

66. Tidow G: Aspects of strength training in athletics, *New Studies in Athletics* 5:93-110, 1990.

67. Allerheiligen WB: Speed development and plyometric training. In Baechle TR, editor: *Essentials of strength training and conditioning*, Champaign, IL, 1994, Human Kinetics.

68. Baker D: A series of studies on the training of high-intensity muscle power and rugby league football player, *J Strength Conditioning Res* 15:198-209, 2001.

69. Newton RU, Kraemer WJ, Hakkinen K: Effects of ballistic training on preseason preparation of elite volleyball players, *Med Sci Sports Exerc* 31:323-330, 1999.

70. Wilson GJ, Murphy AJ, Walshe AD: Performance benefits from weight and plyometric training: effects of initial strength levels, *Coaching and Sport Science Journal* 2:3-8, 1997.

71. Duchateau J, Hainaut K: Isometric and dynamic training: differential effects on mechanical properties of a human muscle, *J Appl Physiol* 56:296-301, 1984.

72. Kanehisa H, Miyashita M: Effect of isometric and isokinetic muscle training on static strength and dynamic power, *J Appl Physiol* 50:365-371, 1983.

73. Kaneko M, Fuchimoto T, Toji H, et al: Training effect of different loads on the force-velocity relationship and mechanical power output in human muscle, *Scand J Sports Sci* 5:50-55, 1983.

74. Moss BM, Refsnes PE, Abildgaard A, et al: Effects of maximal effort strength training with different loads on dynamic strength, cross-sectional area, load-power, and load-velocity relationships, *Eur J Appl Physiol* 75:193-199, 1997.

75. Wilmore JH, Costill DL: *Physiology of sport and exercise*, ed 2, Champaign, IL, 1999, Human Kinetics.

76. Newton RU, Kraemer WJ: Developing explosive muscular power: implications for a mixed methods training strategy, *J Strength Cond* 16:20-31, 1994.

77. Wilson GJ, Newton RU, Murphy AJ, et al: The optimal training load for the development of dynamic athletic performance, *Med Sci Sports Exerc* 25(11):1279-1286, 1993.

78. Chu DA: *Jumping into plyometrics*, Champaign, IL, 1992, Human Kinetics.

79. Radcliffe JC, Farentinos RC: *High powered plyometrics*, Champaign, IL, 1999, Human Kinetics.

80. Wathen D: NSCA position stand: plyometric exercise, *NSCA Journal* 15(3):16, 1993.

81. Falkel JE, Cipriani DL: Physiological principles of resistance training and rehabilitation. In Zachazewski JE, Magee DJ, Quillen WS, editors: *Athletic injuries and rehabilitation*, Philadelphia, 1996, Saunders.

82. Baratta R, Solomonow M, Zhou BH, et al: Muscular coactivation: the role of the antagonist musculature in maintaining knee stability, *Am J Sports Med* 16:113-122, 1988.

83. Cowling EJ, Steel JR: Is lower limb muscle synchrony during landing affected by gender? Implications for variations in ACL injury rates, *J Electromyogr Kinesiol* 11:263-268, 2001.

84. Renstrom P, Arms SW, Stanwyck TS, et al: Strain within the anterior cruciate ligament during hamstring and quadriceps activity, *Am J Sports Med* 14:83-87, 1986.

85. Solomonow M, Baratta R, Zhou BH, et al: The synergistic action of the anterior cruciate ligament and thigh muscles in maintaining joint stability, *Am J Sports Med* 15:207-213, 1987.

86. Anderson B: Flexibility testing, *NSCA Journal* 3(2):20-23, 1981.

87. Robertson KM, Newton RU, Dugan E, et al: 3-week unloading cycle in-season increases vertical jump of collegiate women volleyball players. Abstract poster presentation. In 25th Annual NSCA National Conference and Exhibition, Las Vegas, 2002.

88. Powers SK, Howley ET: *Exercise physiology: theory and application*, Boston, 2001, McGraw-Hill.

89. Costill DL, Daniels J, Evans W, et al: Skeletal muscle enzymes and fiber composition in male and female track athletes, *J Appl Physiol* 40(2):149-154, 1976.

90. Anderson P, Henriksson J: Training induced changes in the subgroups of human type II skeletal muscle fibers, *Acta Physiol Scand* 99:123-125, 1975.

91. Conroy BP, Earle RW: Bone, muscle, and connective tissue adaptations to physical activity. In Baechle TR, editor: *Essentials of strength training and conditioning*, Champaign, IL, 1994, Human Kinetics.

92. Kukukla CG: Human skeletal muscle fatigue. In Currier DP, Nelson RM, editors: *Dynamics of human biologic tissues*, Philadelphia, 1992, FA Davis.

93. Ratzin Jackson CG, Dickinson AL: Adaptations of skeletal muscle to strength or endurance training. In Grana WA, Lombardo JA, Sharkey BJ, Stone JA, editors: *Advances in sports medicine and fitness*, Chicago, 1988, Year Book Medical Publishers.

94. Thompson LV, Fitts RV: Muscle fatigue in the frog semitendinosus; role of high energy phosphate and Pi, *Am J Physiol* 263:C803-C809, 1992.

95. Yoshida I: Effect of dietary modifications on lactate threshold and onset of blood lactate accumulation during incremental exercise, *Eur J Appl Physiol* 53:200-205, 1984.

96. Cerretelli P, Ambrosoli G, Fumagalli M: Anaerobic recovery in man, *Eur J Appl Physiol* 34:141-148, 1975.

97. Farrell PA, Wilmore JH, Coyle EF, et al: Plasma lactate accumulation and distance running performance, *Med Sci Sports* 11(4):338-344, 1979.

98. Svedenhag J: Endurance conditioning. In Shephard RJ, Astrand PO: *Endurance in sport*, ed 2, Oxford, 2000, Blackwell Science.

99. Costill DL: Metabolic responses during distance running, *J Appl Physiol* 28:251-255, 1970.

100. Gambetta V: *Gambetta method: a common sense guide to functional training for athletic performance*, Sarasota, 2002, Gambetta Sports Training Systems.

101. O'Toole ML: Endurance training for women. In Shephard RJ, Astrand PO: *Endurance in sport*, ed 2, Oxford, 2000, Blackwell Science.

102. Conley DL, Krahenbuhl GS: Running economy and distance running performance of highly trained athletes, *Med Sci Sports Exerc* 12:357-360, 1980.

103. Ward PE, Ward RD: *Encyclopedia of weight training*, ed 2, Laguna Hills, CA, 1997, QPT Publications.

104. Gambetta V: *Pumping gravity: functional strength training. Course manual*, Sarasota, 2002, Optimum Sports Training.

105. Crisco J, Panjabi MM: The intersegmental and multisegmental muscles of the lumbar spine, *Spine* 16:793-799, 1991.

106. Hickson RC: Interference of strength development by simultaneously training for strength and endurance, *Eur J Appl Physiol* 215:255-263, 1980.

107. Craig BW, Lucas J, Pohlman R, et al: The effects of running, weightlifting and a combination of both on growth hormone release, *J Appl Sport Sci Res* 5(4):198-203, 1991.

108. Dudley GA, Djamil R: Incompatibility of endurance- and strength-training modes of exercise, *J Appl Physiol* 59(5): 1446-1451, 1985.

109. Stone MH, Fleck SJ, Kraemer WJ, et al: Health and performance related adaptations to resistive training, *Sports Med* 11(4): 210-231, 1991.

110. Bell GJ, Syrotuik D, Socha I, et al: Effect of strength training and concurrent strength and endurance training on strength, testosterone, and cortisol, *J Strength Conditioning Res* 11:57-64, 1997.

111. Bell GJ, Syrotuik, D, Martin TP: Effect of concurrent strength and endurance training on skeletal muscle properties and hormone concentrations in humans, *Eur J Appl Physiol* 81:418-427, 2000.

112. Hennessey LC, Watson AWS: The interference effects of training for strength and endurance simultaneously, *J Strength Conditioning Res* 8:12-19, 1994.

113. Hunter GR, Demment R, Miller D: Development of strength and maximum oxygen uptake during simultaneous training for strength and endurance, *J Sports Med Phys Fit* 27:269-275, 1987.

114. Abernathy PJ, Quigley BM: Concurrent strength and endurance training of the elbow extensors, *J Strength Conditioning Res* 7: 234-240, 1993.

115. Gravelle BL, Blessing DL: Physiological adaptation in women concurrently training for strength and endurance, *J Strength Conditioning Res* 14:5-13, 2000.

116. McCarthy JP, Agre JC, Graf BK, et al: Compatibility of adaptive responses with combining strength and endurance training, *Med Sci Sports Exerc* 27:429-436, 1995.

117. Sale DG, MacDougall JD, Jacobs I, et al: Interaction between concurrent strength and endurance training, *J Appl Physiol* 68:260-270, 1990.

118. Volpe SL, Walberg-Rankin J, Webb Rodman K, et al: The effect of endurance running on training adaptations in women partici-

pating in a weight lifting program, *J Strength Conditioning Res* 7:101-107, 1993.

119. McCarthy JP, Pozniak MA, Agre JC: Neuromuscular adaptations to concurrent strength and endurance training, *Med Sci Sports Exerc* 34:511-519, 2002.

120. McCarthy JP: Concurrent strength and endurance training: antagonism or compatibility. Seminar lecture notes. In 25th Annual NSCA National Conference and Exhibition, Las Vegas, 2002.

121. Adams K, O'Shea JP, O'Shea KL, et al: The effect of six weeks of squat, plyometric and squat-plyometric training on power production, *J Appl Sport Sci Res* 6:36-41, 1992.

122. Vorobyev AN: *Textbook of weightlifting,* Budapest, 1978, International Weightlifting Federation.

123. Matveyev L: *Fundamentals of sport training,* Moscow, 1981, Progress Press.

124. Sanders M, Sanders B: Principles of resistance training. In Bandy WD, Sanders B, editors: *Therapeutic exercise: techniques for intervention,* Baltimore, 2001, Lippincott Williams & Wilkins.

125. Santana JC: *Functional training: breaking the bonds of traditionalism,* Boca Raton, FL, 2000, Optimum Performance Systems.

126. Giannakopoulos K, Beneka A, Malliou P, et al: Isolated vs. complex exercises in strengthening the rotator cuff muscle group, *J Strength Conditioning Res* 18(1):144-148, 2004.

127. Estlander A, Mellin G, VanHaranta H, et al: Effects and follow-up of a multimodel treatment program including intensive physical training for low back patients, *Scand J Rehabil Med* 23:97, 1991.

128. Kraemer WJ, Ratamess NA: Physiology of resistance training: current issues. In *Orthopaedic physical therapy clinics of North America: exercise technologies,* Philadelphia, 2000, Saunders.

129. Noth J: Cortical and peripheral control. In Komi PV, editor: *Strength and power in sport,* London, 1992, Blackwell Scientific.

CHAPTER 6

Restoring Dynamic Stability after Knee Surgery

Glenn N. Williams, PT, PhD, ATC, SCS
Annunziato Amendola, MD

CHAPTER OUTLINE

DYNAMIC KNEE STABILITY

It is no surprise that knee joint injuries are among the most common injuries in sports because this joint lies between the human body's longest lever arms (the femur and tibia) and is surrounded by some of its most powerful muscle groups. Sports that include jumping, cutting, pivoting, or sudden deceleration are especially perilous to the knee because the loads and rate of loading experienced by the ligaments, capsule, and tendons of the knee joint are extreme. Despite these extreme loading conditions, most athletes play sports such as basketball, football, and soccer aggressively without ever seriously injuring their knees. The ability of a person to maintain knee joint stability under the rapidly changing, high-magnitude loading conditions experienced in sports and other functional activities of daily living is referred to as *dynamic knee stability*.

Dynamic knee stability is achieved through a complex interaction among articular geometry, soft tissue restraints, and the dynamic effects of weight-bearing and muscle action. The bony geometry of the femur (rounded condyles) and tibia (relatively flat condyles) provides little stability to the knee joint. The specific shape and the structural properties of the menisci improve tibiofemoral congruity and enable these functional "gaskets" to serve as a "buttress" to abnormal translation between the tibia and femur.[1,2] The knee contains a dynamic network of ligaments, the most notable being the cruciate and collateral ligaments.[3-5] The ligaments, capsule, and musculotendinous soft tissues of the knee contribute significantly to its stability. Although there is a primary ligament for each of the cardinal loading planes, the knee ligaments are oriented so that more than one ligament is usually resisting the loads placed on the knee.[3,5-7] Under mild-to-moderate loading conditions, articular geometry and the soft tissue restraints of the knee are sufficient to maintain joint stability; however, the loads involved in sports that require quick changes of direction and jumping can exceed the structural properties of the ligaments.[8,9] Consequently, further stabilizing forces are required to maintain stability and prevent knee injuries.

Compressive loads associated with weight-bearing activities promote joint approximation and thereby minimize some of the strain on the soft tissues of the knee during athletic participation. It is estimated that these compressive loads can reduce ligament strain by approximately 40%.[10,11] Although the protective benefit of the loads exhibited in weight bearing should not be trivialized, it is often not sufficient to maintain stability under aggressive loading conditions. The stabilizing forces provided by coordinated activity of the muscles surrounding the knee are critically important to the maintenance of dynamic knee stability under such conditions. The operative word here is *coordinated*, because poorly timed muscle activity can promote knee instability. Indeed, researchers have suggested that the quadriceps muscle forces alone are great enough to rupture the anterior cruciate liga-

ment (ACL) if applied in an unopposed fashion under specific conditions.[9]

The ability to produce controlled movement through coordinated muscle activity is referred to as *sensorimotor control* (neuromuscular control).[12] Although sensorimotor control is a critical factor in the maintenance of dynamic knee stability, it too is insufficient in and of itself. The forces generated by the muscles surrounding the knee must be sufficient to counterbalance the destabilizing loads placed on the knee, and these stabilizing muscle forces must be able to be recruited in a coordinated fashion throughout the duration of a grueling athletic competition. Thus dynamic knee stability is the result of an interaction among the combined effects of sensorimotor control, strength, and endurance, as well as the stabilizing contributions of articular geometry, soft tissue restraints, and joint compressive loads associated with weight bearing. It is sensorimotor control, strength, and endurance that rehabilitation specialists focus on, because these are the components of dynamic knee stability that we can improve with well-designed exercise programs. The focus of this chapter is the integration of recent scientific advances related to sensorimotor control into the treatment plans of people who have undergone knee surgery. Although some of the treatment methods that are discussed may also lead to improvements in strength and endurance, training methods centered on developing strength and endurance are not discussed in detail. For a more detailed description of the science and art of promoting knee strength and endurance, see Chapter 5.

MECHANISMS OF SENSORIMOTOR CONTROL

Sensorimotor control results from the integration of processes that take place throughout the hierarchic structure of the nervous system and requires the synergistic function of a large number of nervous and musculoskeletal system structures. Although we have learned a great deal about the neuromuscular control system in recent years, much is still unknown. Consequently, it should be noted that the following discussion of the mechanisms of sensorimotor control is a theoretic framework based on the evidence currently available in the scientific literature.

Somatosensory System

The somatosensory system includes the components of the central and peripheral nervous systems that receive, transmit, and interpret sensory information related to the mechanical conditions in the muscles and connective tissues, as well as touch, pain, and temperature. There are three categories of specialized receptors in the somatosensory system: (1) mechanoreceptors, which provide feedback related to the mechanical state of muscles, joint tissues, and the skin; (2) thermoreceptors, which provide feedback related to temperature; and (3) nociceptors, which are pain receptors. The central nervous system (CNS) is continually bombarded with impulses from each of these categories of receptors and processes them simultaneously. Although this chapter focuses on the function of the mechanoreceptors, it is important to recognize that pain and abnormal temperature may also affect dynamic knee stability. For example, patients with painful, inflamed knees often have muscle inhibition that promotes knee instability and impairs function. It is reasonable that some of this inhibition is due to the sensation of pain, increased temperature, and the chemical environment within the inflamed knee. Such factors may affect knee function even if they are not severe enough to be recognized consciously by the patient.

Mechanoreceptors are generally classified into three groups: (1) muscle receptors, (2) joint receptors, and (3) cutaneous (skin) receptors. The structure and function of these receptors is only briefly described in this chapter because detailed descriptions are available in the literature.[12-16] The idea that the CNS deals with the signals arising from these receptors separately is a common misconception in the orthopedic–sports medicine community. This misconception is understandable, because we usually discuss the function of these receptors separately and researchers often isolate or focus on the function of a single type of receptor in their studies. In reality, the current evidence suggests that the CNS processes ensembles of sensory information from many receptors simultaneously.[17-19] Ensemble processing allows thousands of impulses to be processed per second, which enables the CNS to rapidly obtain an accurate picture of the conditions at the periphery from the net feedback received. As a result, effective responses to potentially harmful disturbances are made efficiently and the system remains in relative homeostasis. Ensemble processing also leads to more appropriate responses because there is a level of redundancy within the system that allows compensation for errors in feedback.

The mechanisms by which computer users transfer data over high-speed broadband networks provides an illustrative example of the signal processing performed by the CNS (note that this example is not meant to be physiologically accurate; rather, it is simply intended to clarify the "picture"). Computer users today are able to send voice, video, and other data over a single wire (e.g., cable TV connection) in a manner that seems simultaneous to the user. The computer system and broadband network achieve this task by sending packets of data rapidly over the wire. The complex signal processing performed by the computers, servers, routers, and switches within the broadband network enables a large number of computer users working at the same time within a neighborhood or corporation to rapidly send large amounts of data over a relatively small number of wires (in comparison to the number of users). It is no surprise that terms such as *neural network* and *artificial intelligence* exist in the computer sciences.

Muscle Receptors

Two types of muscle receptors are commonly described: Golgi tendon organs and muscle spindles. Golgi tendon organs are embedded within the collagen of the musculotendinous junction. Each Golgi tendon organ is attached to a small number of extrafusal muscle fibers (25 or fewer) from a small number of motor units (15 or fewer); the exact number of fibers varies according to the muscle-tendon unit the receptor is contained within.[20-22] A single axon enters the capsule of each Golgi tendon organ and branches into a series of unmyelinated fibers that are interwoven with the collagen fibers of the tendon. When muscle contraction or other loads take up the slack within the network of collagen fibers, the nerve endings are stimulated. Golgi tendon organs are sensitive to small changes in force (sensitivity varies across receptors; it is as little as 0.1 g or less for some Golgi tendon units), which allows the nervous system to provide highly specific responses to force feedback.[21]

The second type of muscle receptors is referred to as muscle spindles. Muscle spindles are encapsulated receptors (4 to 10 mm long) that lie parallel to muscle fibers. These receptors are sensitive to changes in length (stretch) and velocity.[14,23] Muscle spindles contain three types of intrafusal muscle fibers: nuclear chain fibers and two types of nuclear bag fibers (static and dynamic). These intrafusal muscle fibers are innervated by both sensory and motor (gamma) axons. The gamma motor neurons innervating muscle spindles are known as the fusimotor system. Coactivation between the alpha motor system and the fusimotor system enables muscle spindles to remain sensitive to changes in length and velocity throughout the joint range of motion (ROM).[14] There is also evidence suggesting that fusimotor system activation is directly influenced by feedback from receptors located in the skin, ligaments/capsule, and muscles.[18,24,25] Integration of muscle spindle function with that of mechanoreceptors in other tissues may improve the accuracy and effectiveness of motor responses by creating a more redundant system and increasing the potency of responses.

Joint Receptors

There are four primary types of joint receptors: Ruffini endings, pacinian corpuscles, Golgi tendon organ–like endings, and free nerve endings (Table 6-1).[12] These receptors are described by the joint state in which they are active (static, dynamic, or both), the stimulus intensity for activation (high vs. low threshold), and whether or not they remain active with persistent stimuli (slowly vs. rapidly adapting). Each type of joint receptor relays unique sensory feedback to the CNS. Ruffini endings, pacinian corpuscles, and Golgi tendon organ–like endings are distributed relatively sparsely in the midsubstance of the ligaments and other joint connective tissues, but more densely near the structure's attachment sites. Thus it is no surprise that these receptors are most active near the limits of joint translation or rotation.[15,26] Conversely, free nerve endings are widely distributed throughout the connective tissues of the joint. Joint receptors appear to perform the primary function of protecting joints from rotation and translation beyond the physical ROM, but also provide feedback related to joint position sense and kinesthesia.[15,27,28]

Cutaneous Receptors

Historically, sensory feedback from cutaneous receptors has not been closely associated with joint stability. It is now believed that cutaneous receptors play an important role in the sensation of movement either by providing direct feedback or by facilitating feedback from other receptors (e.g., muscle receptors).[29,30] Edin[30] has provided specific evidence that indicates that cutaneous receptor feedback provides information regarding movement of the knee joint. This finding may help to explain the reported improvements in joint position sense and threshold to detection of passive movement associated with wearing braces or neoprene sleeves.[31,32] Further research is needed to establish the degree to which feedback from cutaneous receptors contributes to dynamic joint stability.

Motor Response Pathways

Somatosensory feedback is mediated at three levels of the CNS: (1) the spinal cord, (2) the brainstem and cerebellum, and (3) the cerebral cortex (Table 6-2). Although it is convenient to discuss each of these motor response pathways separately, it should be recognized that all of these pathways are functioning simultaneously in the control of human movement and dynamic knee stability. Sensorimotor control is best thought of as a complex, highly integrated process involving thousands of ensembles of sensory information

---

TABLE 6-1

Joint Receptors in the Tissues of the Knee

RECEPTOR TYPE	LOCATION	STIMULUS	ACTIVITY PROFILE	ACTIVATION THRESHOLD	RESPONSE TO PERSISTENT STIMULI
Ruffini endings (I)	Capsule and ligaments	Joint position Intraarticular pressure Amplitude of movement Velocity of movement	Static or dynamic	Low threshold	Slowly adapting
Pacinian corpuscles (II)	Capsule, ligaments, menisci, fat pads	Acceleration or deceleration	Dynamic only	Low threshold	Rapidly adapting
Golgi tendon organ–like (III)	Ligaments and menisci	Tension in ligaments, especially at end-range of motion	Dynamic only	High threshold	Slowly adapting
Free nerve endings (IV)	Widely distributed in most connective tissues of the joint	Pain from mechanical or chemical origin	Inactive except in the presence of noxious stimuli, then static or dynamic	High threshold	Slowly adapting

---

TABLE 6-2

Motor Response Pathways Used in Dynamic Knee Stability

MOTOR RESPONSE PATHWAY	LOCATION OF MEDIATION	TYPICAL LATENCY	MODIFIABLE	SLOWS WITH MORE DEGREES OF FREEDOM
Spinal reflexes	Segmental level of the spinal cord	30-50 ms	No	No
Long-loop reflexes	Brainstem and cerebellum	50-80 ms	No	No
Triggered reactions	Brainstem and cortical centers	80-120 ms	Yes	Yes
Reaction time	Cortical centers	120-180 ms	Yes	Yes

from the periphery that are processed by a network of neurons, interneurons, and CNS centers that use an equally complex system of pathways and neurons to activate muscles and produce coordinated movement.

In the spinal cord, segmental spinal reflexes are produced. Some spinal reflexes are simple monosynaptic circuits (e.g., muscle stretch reflexes); others are more complex, involving synapses with one or more interneurons. These spinal reflexes can be excitatory or inhibitory and are part of a distributed network that facilitates rapid postural adjustments and regulation of limb mechanics in movement.[33,34]

Long-loop reflexes result from sensory feedback mediated in the brainstem and cerebellum. Somatosensory signals ascend to the brainstem and cerebellum through the dorsal lateral and spinocerebellar tracts.[35] Motor responses descend from the brainstem and cerebellum via the medial and lateral pathways, which activate proximal and distal musculature, respectively.[35] The processing in the brainstem and cerebellum leads to greater flexibility in the reflexive responses, which can adapt based on visual cues, experience, and instructions given to the individual.[36-38] Researchers have described evidence of a long-loop reflex arc between the knee capsule/ligaments and hamstring muscles in people with ACL insufficiency that is activated in response to knee translation resulting from lower limb perturbations.[39] Although some have questioned a direct hamstrings-ACL reflex loop,[40,41] there is no doubt that long-loop responses are important in maintaining dynamic knee stability.

Triggered reactions are preprogrammed, coordinated responses that occur in response to feedback in the periphery.[42,43] These reactions include processing in the higher centers of the brain; however, preprogramming secondary to learning or other factors enables some of the typical processing steps in the higher centers to be bypassed, which results in faster responses than would be expected with typical voluntary reaction time responses.[42,43] Although preprogramming leads to quicker responses, this comes at the cost of response flexibility. Because triggered reactions are processed at higher levels of the CNS, they are more complex and integrated than reflexes; however, increased sensory stimuli or unanticipated conditions slow response rates because of the increased processing requirements.

Voluntary responses are mediated in the cerebral cortex. The dorsal column projections from the spinal cord synapse in the brainstem and those continuing to the primary somatosensory cortex do so primarily through the medial lemniscal system.[44] The sensory and motor cortices are somatotopically organized, as is depicted with the sensory and motor homunculi. The highest level of motor control occurs in three specialized areas of the motor cortex: the primary motor cortex, the premotor cortex, and the supplementary motor area.[45] Each of these areas projects directly to spinal cord via the corticospinal tract and indirectly through the pathways of the brainstem.[35] Voluntary responses take the longest to occur, but are also the most flexible and adaptable. As with triggered reactions, response time increases as the number of variables that need to be processed increases (Hick's law).[43,46,47]

Proprioception

Proprioception is a commonly misused term in sports medicine.[48] The term was coined by Sherrington[49] a century ago from the Latin words *proprius* (one's own) and *(re)ceptus* (the act of receiving), which when combined imply the modality of sensing one's own body position or movement. If one reviews the contemporary literature it will become apparent that the term *proprioception* means different things to different people. To some it is synonymous with sensorimotor control, whereas others refer to it as specialized sensory modality alone (the classic definition). Gandevia and coworkers[29] have recently defined proprioception as a sensory modality including (1) detection of the position and movement of joints, (2) sensation of force and contraction, and (3) sensation of the orientation of body segments, as well as the body as a whole. Because of the broad use of this term, it is best to define proprioception whenever this term is used.

Can we improve proprioception with training? It appears that with training there are improvements in the efficiency of signal processing, but it is unlikely that we significantly alter the physiologic function of the mechanoreceptors. Current theory suggests that under slowly developing or controlled conditions we can improve proprioceptive acuity; however, it is unlikely that we can have a meaningful impact under typical sports performance conditions.[50]

Regulation of Muscle Stiffness

Stiffness is defined as the change in force (tension) divided by the change in length. This concept is often conceptualized by the function of a spring. Stiff springs require a great deal of force to change their length, whereas low-stiffness springs are very compliant. The material and mechanical properties of muscles allow them to be the "springs" between a person's skeletal system and the environment. It is no surprise that muscles are often modeled as springs or a combination of springs and dashpots (i.e., dampers or pistons).[51,52] Muscle stiffness is the result of three components: (1) passive factors associated with the material properties of the musculotendinous tissues, (2) active intrinsic properties associated with the cross-bridge attachments and length/tension properties of the muscle, and (3) reflexive components associated with length and force feedback from muscle spindles and tendon organs.[53-55] The net stiffness of the muscles surrounding the knee produce a degree of joint stiffness that resists sudden translations or rotations of the joint.[33-34] Perturbations generally alter both muscle length and force, which in turn alters the feedback from the muscle spindles and tendon organs.[55] Force and length feedback from these receptors leads to changes in muscle activation, which in turn modulates muscle and joint stiffness.[33,34,55] The fusimotor system appears to play an important role in this regulation of muscle stiffness.[18,25,56] Akazawa and co-workers[56] have suggested that the fusimotor system modulates muscle spindle sensitivity and thereby reflex stiffness. Reflex stiffness appears to have its greatest impact during postural tasks or slow movements because the intensity of stretch reflexes is suppressed during movement.[57,58] Intrinsic muscle stiffness is thought to be the first line of defense against perturbations because it is always present.[53,56] In addition to being related to the material properties of the muscle, intrinsic stiffness is a function of activation and the history of reflexive muscle activity.[53,54,56] Thus intrinsic muscle stiffness, reflexive stiffness, and fusimotor activity are all interdependent.

Evidence from animal models suggests that joint afferents in the ligaments and capsule have a direct impact on fusimotor activity.[59-61] Although it remains unclear if similar direct pathways exist in humans, the results of these studies suggest that feedback from the ligaments and capsule of the knee is involved in continually modulating the stiffness of the joint. It is widely held that reactive muscle responses are unlikely to prevent joint injuries unless the rate of loading is relatively slow or there is sufficient stiffness present from preinjury event muscle activation.[12,62] The continuous process of muscle stiffness regulation described in the preceding paragraphs, though debated among neurophysiologists and still under investigation, appears to be a critical factor in dynamic knee stability and injury prevention. Of interest, recent work by Wojtys and colleagues[62,63] and Granata and colleagues[64,65] has demonstrated that females have lower active musculoskeletal stiffness at the knee joint than their male counterparts when performing the same tasks. This finding may help explain the higher incidence of noncontact knee joint injuries observed in the female athlete population.[66-68]

Control of Posture and Movement

The nervous system uses three sources of sensory information in maintaining postural stability (the ability to maintain the body's center of mass within its stability limits): (1) somatosensory feedback, (2) visual feedback, and (3) vestibular feedback.[69,70] Although these sensory systems are unique, research also suggests that these systems interact and that the CNS processes a variety of information simultaneously and responds to the net input.[69,71] Other factors that affect postural stability include the mechanical properties of the body (and its tissues) and the properties of the support surface.[69] Responses to postural perturbation vary according to the direction and intensity of the perturbation.[38,72-74] In general, when forward sway is induced, muscles on the posterior aspect of the body are recruited to provide stability, whereas muscles on the front side of the body are recruited when posterior sway is induced.[38,72] A control strategy involving muscles around the ankle is implemented with small perturbations. With larger perturbations the muscles of the thigh, hip, and trunk are recruited (hip strategy), and eventually a person must take a step to maintain postural control (stepping strategy).[70,73] Although these postural control strategies

can be modified to suit the environmental conditions one is presented with, responses to postural disturbances are usually predictable and automatic.[70]

The maintenance of dynamic knee stability during movement involves everything discussed to this point (i.e., anatomic factors, somatosensory feedback, descending control signals, stiffness regulation, postural control) and the ongoing complex neural control of gait or other movement tasks.[12] Caution is warranted when extrapolating the results from studies performed under static, controlled, or simplified conditions to typical sports participation because of the noteworthy differences in loading conditions and the increased complexity of the neural control of such movements.

EFFECTS OF KNEE LIGAMENT INJURY

Knee ligament injuries are generally marked by swelling/effusion, pain, and an antalgic gait that often requires the use of assistive devices. Consequently, most people sustaining knee ligament injuries are treated with relative rest, ice, and medications to control pain and inflammation, and they are often placed in an immobilizer or brace. Immobilization, decreased activity levels, pain, and effusion generally lead to rapid atrophy of the quadriceps and lateral gastrocnemius muscles, which appears to alter neuromuscular function.[75,76] The effects of knee ligament injury on sensorimotor function have been studied extensively, but most of this work has been done in the ACL-deficient population. For this reason, it makes sense for us to concentrate primarily on the results of work in the ACL-deficient population. These studies can be broken into the following primary categories: (1) detection of movement and joint repositioning studies, (2) analysis of muscle responses when loads are applied to the tibia, (3) assessment of specificity of muscle action (voluntary muscle control), and (4) evaluation of kinematics and kinetics in functional tasks.

Detection of Movement and Joint Repositioning

Several researchers have attempted to assess "proprioception" after knee ligament injuries using threshold to detection of passive movement (TTDPM), threshold to detection of passive movement direction (TTDPMD), or joint repositioning studies.[28,77-79] In TTDPM and TTDPMD studies, the knee is rotated at a very slow rate (0.5 to 2.0 degrees per second) in an attempt to isolate slowly adapting joint receptors.[80] During testing, subjects are blindfolded and listen to white noise in order to reduce feedback from other systems (visual and auditory) that may assist the subjects in performing the task (Figure 6-1). The two tests are similar except that in TTDPM studies subjects are asked to signal (either verbally or by pressing a button) when they first perceive that their joint is moving, whereas in TTDPMD they must also identify the direction toward which the joint segment is moving. By necessity, these tests generally require a reaction

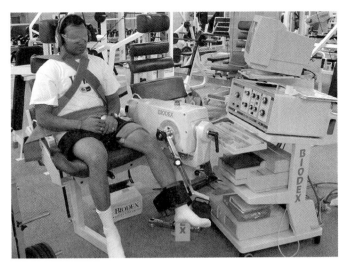

Figure 6-1: Patient setup for threshold to detection of passive movement (TTDPM) and active joint position sense testing or training on an isokinetic dynamometer.

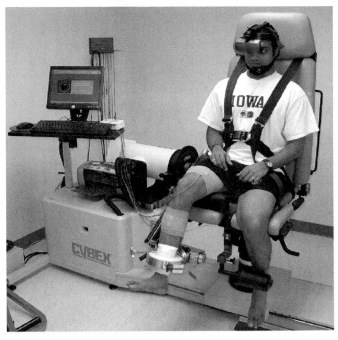

Figure 6-2: Setup for the target matching protocol used to test specificity of muscle action.

time response (pushing a button, a verbal response, or another manual signal). Such responses are mediated at the cortical level, rather than the segmental spinal level or in the brainstem where a meaningful portion of somatosensory feedback is mediated during functional activities. Furthermore, these reaction time methods have a degree of variability associated with them. In joint repositioning studies, the distal segment of the joint is rotated to a specific angle by the examiner or a testing device and the subject is instructed to signal when the joint is passively placed in that position again or actively reposition his or her joint at the specified joint angle. Active joint repositioning can be done under weight-bearing or non–weight-bearing conditions, whereas passive tests are done under non–weight-bearing conditions. It should be recognized that active joint repositioning tests assess both proprioceptive acuity and motor function. Most researchers have reported that people who have sustained knee ligaments injuries have decreased TTDPM, decreased TTDPMD, and reduced joint position sense;[28,77,79] however, this finding has not been universal.[78]

Muscle Responses to Destabilizing Loads

Researchers have observed delayed hamstring response times when sudden destabilizing loads (generally in the anterior direction) have been applied to the tibias of people with ACL-deficient knees.[81,82] Wojtys and Huston[81] also observed an altered order of recruitment such that the quadriceps muscles were recruited before the hamstrings in the subjects with acute ACL injuries, whereas the opposite order was observed in stable knees. A primary quadriceps response to loads that promote anterior instability is dysfunctional because this response further destabilizes the knee.

Specificity of Muscle Action

The muscle control strategies of people who have sustained knee ligament injuries have generally been assessed during functional tasks such as walking, running, or jumping. This approach allows the researcher to assess muscle activity during functional tasks; however, it is difficult to assess a person's fundamental muscle control strategies under these circumstances because it is hard to differentiate fundamental motor control strategies from reactive strategies that are employed to compensate for pathologic knee motion or other factors associated with the injury. Assessing fundamental strategies in such tasks is also complicated by the fact that events at the foot, ankle, and hip can all induce muscle activity about the knee. To assess the fundamental motor control strategies of people with ACL-deficient knees with relative confidence, Williams and co-workers[76,83] used a more basic design in which subjects were tested under low-load, isometric conditions (Figure 6-2) at knee angles where there is little tibial translation; therefore reactive (compensatory) muscle activity was minimized.[84-85] The experimental protocol used in these studies is an established method of assessing motor control that requires subjects to match targets projected in front of them by producing force against a load cell in many directions with fine control.[86-88]

The degree of focus observed in the muscle activity patterns of ACL-deficient subjects (i.e., their specificity of muscle action) was compared with that of age-matched and activity-level–matched people with uninjured knees by calculating a specificity index using established circular statistics methods.[89,90] People with ACL deficiency were found to have diminished specificity of muscle action in several muscles of their involved limbs.[83] The most notable findings were in the quadriceps muscles (especially the vastus lateralis) and the lateral gastrocnemius muscles.[83] In a subsequent study, these authors demonstrated that similar patterns of altered quadriceps control are observed when people with ACL deficiency perform the static muscle control testing described previously and dynamic short-arc quadriceps exercises in the terminal 30 degrees of knee extension.[76] This finding suggests that the observed quadriceps dysfunction is relatively global. Like Wojtys and Huston,[81] Williams and colleagues[76,83] observed seemingly inappropriate patterns of quadriceps activity. On the basis of this finding, the authors theorized that some of the increased hamstring activity often observed when people with ACL deficiency perform functional tasks is required to compensate for the altered quadriceps function they have observed. These findings support the need for rehabilitation methods directed at improving quadriceps muscle control in this population.

Kinematics and Kinetics in Functional Tasks

Several authors have observed altered knee joint kinematics or kinetics in the gait patterns of people who have sustained significant ligament injuries.[91-94] Others have evaluated the electromyogram activity patterns of the muscles surrounding the knee during gait and other functional tasks and have also observed altered activity patterns.[95-98] The hallmark of these studies has been a decreased knee extensor moment associated with a stiffening strategy in which there is increased hamstring activity, increased knee flexion, and often increased activity in the gastrocnemius or soleus muscles.[91,92,94,96] This stiffening strategy is apparently employed to stabilize the knee during the tasks. Although this stabilization strategy enables the injured person to perform functional activities of daily living, it results in increased loading of the articular cartilage of the knee, which could promote degenerative joint disease if present over a sufficient duration. Interestingly, a differential response to ACL injury has been described in which people who are able to cope with the injury demonstrate kinetic patterns similar to uninjured people, but kinematic patterns similar to people who are unable to cope with ACL deficiency.[92] Williams and co-workers[99] have provided further support for this differential response by demonstrating that noncopers have noteworthy atrophy of their quadriceps (especially the vastus lateralis and vastus intermedius) and lateral gastrocnemius muscles, as well as diminished specificity of muscle action in these same muscles, whereas copers have little atrophy and specificity of muscle action values that are not significantly different than those of people with uninjured knees.

RESTORATION OF DYNAMIC KNEE STABILITY

The restoration of dynamic knee stability following surgical treatment of knee ligament injuries is best achieved with a progressive approach that is patient specific and integrates traditional methods of addressing strength, joint motion, cardiovascular endurance, agility, and sport-specific skills with a variety of neuromuscular training methods. Early minimization of impairments such as pain, effusion, ROM deficits, and poor muscle activation is critical because these impairments limit the patient's ability to effectively strengthen his or her muscles and produce coordinated muscle activation. Aggressive strengthening of the muscles surrounding the knee, as well as the muscles of the lumbo-pelvic girdle (the "core"), is paramount. Because serious knee ligament injuries such as ACL injuries have an especially profound impact on the quadriceps muscle group, these muscles should receive special attention.[75] The intensity, frequency, and volume of exercise should be patient specific, but consistent with the latest evidence and strength and conditioning concepts in the literature. As stated previously, this chapter focuses on methods of neuromuscular training, rather than strength training or conditioning; however, the importance of strength and endurance cannot be overemphasized because these parameters provide the framework on which coordinated movement is built. Neuromuscular training and strength/endurance training are not exclusive, but overlap in that most neuromuscular training methods also assist with either strength or conditioning.

Neuromuscular training after knee surgery can be broken into three broad categories: (1) TTDPM and joint repositioning exercises, (2) perturbation/postural control exercises, and (3) dynamic control/agility training exercises. Each of these categories of exercise has a unique focus and theoretically makes different contributions to dynamic knee stability.

Detection of Movement and Joint Repositioning Exercises

As soon as a patient's impairments (pain, effusion, ROM deficits, and muscle inhibition) are under control, TTDPM and joint repositioning exercises usually begin. Threshold to detection of passive movement exercises are hard to perform manually because it is difficult for a rehabilitation specialist to move the limb without the patient knowing it. Consequently, isokinetic testing systems or custom-made equipment is generally required. Joint repositioning can be performed manually, although it is often easier to use testing equipment because of the mass of the lower extremity. Most training is performed in the open kinetic chain; however, active joint positioning exercises can be performed objectively in the closed kinetic chain with commercially available devices such as the SportsRAC and Core:Tx (both sold by Performance Health Technologies, Boulder, CO).

As discussed earlier in the chapter, it is very unlikely that these exercises alter the sensory ability of the mechanoreceptors surrounding the knee. Instead, these exercises most likely do one or more of the following: (1) alter the manner in which the sensory information is processed, (2) improve the efficiency with which the sensory information is processed, (3) improve muscle control in active joint repositioning, or (4) promote an increased central "consciousness" of the knee (i.e., although there is little change in the sensory feedback from the joint, the patient's repetitive focus on that sensory feedback may lead to changes in higher brain function that result in increased awareness of the knee joint and where it is in space). Although these four mechanisms are plausible, it should be clearly stated that we currently do not know the exact mechanisms of improvements in joint position sense and movement detection. It is clear, however, that patients' precision in performing these exercises does improve.

Perturbation Training and Postural Control Exercises

Most neuromuscular training exercises fall under the category of perturbation training. Perturbation training includes any treatment method in which a destabilizing load is applied to the limb or body of the patient in order to induce a specific neuromuscular response. These perturbations may be applied through unstable support surfaces; manual loads applied to the limb or body by a rehabilitation specialist; or the use of equipment such as weighted balls, resistance bands/cords, balance platforms, and other tools capable of generating destabilizing loads. Perturbation training is directed at teaching patients to respond appropriately to perturbations. The appropriateness of a response depends on several factors, including: the magnitude of the destabilizing load, the velocity at which it is given, the direction in which it is applied, and other factors such as whether or not the perturbation is anticipated. In general, the goal is for the patient to have a coordinated recruitment of muscles that produces a stabilizing load that is specific to the perturbation conditions, rather than a gross co-contraction strategy that either prevents the perturbation or stabilizes the extremity. In circumstances where the perturbation is either extremely violent or rapid, generalized co-contraction may be appropriate; however, under most training conditions the response should be specific and coordinated.

One of the most common mistakes rehabilitation specialists make when having people perform neuromuscular training is allowing them or encouraging them to perform a forceful general co-contraction of the hamstrings, quadriceps, and triceps surae musculature. Why is generalized co-contraction usually inappropriate? Because generalized co-contraction is not functional. Most destabilizing loads occur while people are moving (i.e., running, cutting, pivoting). With generalized co-contraction the patient attempts to make his or her joint rigid, which by definition is contradictory to agile movement. The training of generalized co-contraction is a product of our typical clinical environment and training methods, which primarily consist of situations in which the patient's body is relatively static in stance or another position. Although the joint may be rotating or translating in these circumstances, patients usually do not perform dynamic tasks such as running, jumping, and pivoting until late in the rehabilitation process. The degree to which exercises performed in relatively static positions translate to the sports environment is currently unclear.

In theory, progressive application of functionally challenging perturbations promotes improved neuromuscular control. Perturbation training exercises are generally progressed in the following ways: (1) transitioning from double- to single-limb support; (2) having the patient stand on a less stable surface such as foam, an air-filled disk or dome, or a piece of equipment that challenges stability (e.g., a balance platform); (3) having the patient close his or her eyes and removing verbal cues; (4) using resistive bands or cords to apply loads; (5) applying perturbations manually with the hand or by shifting the support surface; or (6) increasing the number of tasks (degrees of freedom) that the patient must deal with (e.g., having the patient catch a ball while standing in single-leg stance on an unstable surface).

When attempting to restore dynamic knee stability, the patient's knee should be flexed at least 10 degrees. This eliminates the stability provided by the screw-home mechanism and ensures that the knee muscles are targeted by the exercises. With the knee locked, the ankle is challenged to a much greater degree than the knee; however, with the knee flexed, the stability of both the knee and the ankle joint is challenged. Varying the degree of knee flexion during training is advised because this may promote effective responses throughout the range of joint motion.

Perturbation training methods after knee surgery also generally begin shortly after a patient's impairments have resolved. The first exercises employed usually include single-leg stance on a stable surface, squats, and step-up/step-down drills in the forward and lateral directions (emphasizing eccentric quadriceps muscle control). Resistance bands and cords can be used independently (Figure 6-3) or as an implement by which rehabilitation specialists apply destabilizing loads to the extremity. When control is demonstrated on a stable surface, patients are progressed to unstable surfaces. Air-filled cushions, disks, domes, balance boards, rocker boards, and roller boards are common methods of altering the support surface. Double-leg balance and squatting on disks and domes (Figure 6-4) are good exercises when transitioning from stable to unstable surfaces. These exercises can be made more difficult by having the patient close his or her eyes. Before performing exercises in single-leg stance, it may be helpful to perform neuromuscular training with the

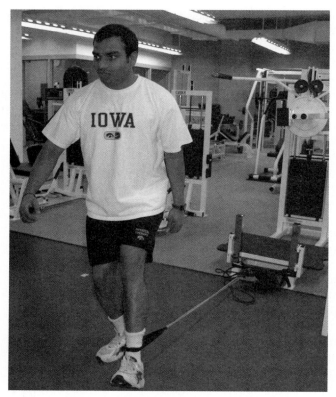

Figure 6-3: Neuromuscular training in single-leg stance using a resistance cord. In this exercise, the cord is attached to the uninvolved extremity of the patient. The patient is positioned so that all slack in the cord is taken up so that with movement (forward, backward, and off-plane) destabilizing loads are applied to the patient's involved extremity.

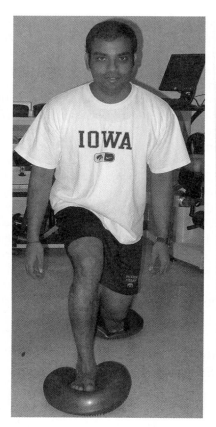

Figure 6-4: Lunge on air-filled disks.

uninjured leg on a stable surface and the surgically treated leg on an unstable surface such as a roller board (Figure 6-5). When appropriate neuromuscular responses to perturbations are observed in mixed arrangements, the patient is progressed to single-leg stance exercises.

Single-leg stance on unstable surfaces usually begins with the patient standing unilaterally on air cushions, disks, domes (Figure 6-6), or rebounders/trampolines with the eyes open. Air-filled disks are available in several color-coded levels of resistance, similar to exercise bands and cords. More compliant disks are more difficult to balance on than less compliant disks, so the difficulty associated with the disk color coding is generally the inverse of the difficulty associated with the resistance bands used in strengthening (i.e., for strengthening, red is less challenging than blue, but when balancing on disks, red is usually more difficult than blue). The difficulty associated with single-leg balance on air-filled domes can be modulated by increasing or decreasing the air pressure in the dome.

Early single-leg stance exercises on unstable surfaces are generally performed for time (e.g., 5 repetitions of balancing

for 30 seconds). They can be advanced by increasing the duration that the patient performs the task, by having the patient close his or her eyes, by having the patient perform a task such as squatting on the unstable surface, or by manually perturbing the patient (Figure 6-7). In addition to providing manual perturbations to the patient's upper body, rehabilitation specialists can apply loads to the limb using direct or indirect methods. A good example of a direct method of applying loads to the limb is the use of a resistance band to apply an anterior, anteromedial, or anterolateral load to the tibia of a patient who is recovering from ACL reconstruction (Figure 6-8). There are many indirect methods of loading the limb in single-leg stance. Patients can use oscillating resistance devices with progressive grades of resistance while performing single-leg stance on an unstable surface (Figure 6-9). The rehabilitation specialist can also have the patient perform sport-specific tasks such as catching a ball with the hands (Figure 6-10), striking a ball with a tennis racquet, or catching a ball with a lacrosse stick while the patient balances on an unstable surface. Several factors make these exercises especially good choices: They are fun, functional, challenging (the patient is forced to concentrate on something other than the knee), and easily progressed (e.g., by making the patient catch a ball in more challenging locations or by increasing ball velocity or weight). Another method of applying indirect loads to the extremity is to perturb the support

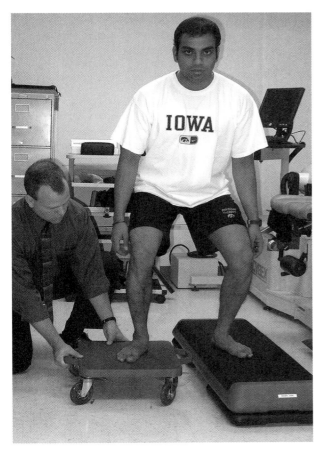

Figure 6-5: A mixed stable-unstable design in which the patient's uninvolved extremity is on a stable surface and the involved extremity is on a roller board. The rehabilitation specialist translates or rotates the roller board and the patient attempts to recruit a specific, coordinated muscle response to the perturbation.

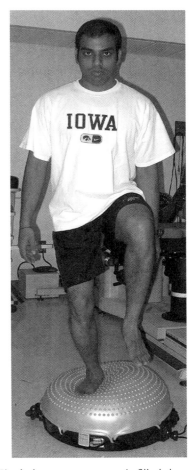

Figure 6-6: Single-leg stance on an air-filled dome.

surface. Examples of perturbation of support surfaces include the rehabilitation specialist applying loads to a rocker board as the patient stands on it (these can be oriented in anterior-posterior, medial-lateral, or diagonal directions to provide different types of perturbations), applying an indentation load to a dome, or moving a roller board under the patient as she or he stands on it (Figure 6-11).

Researchers at the University of Delaware have described a perturbation of support surfaces training program used to promote dynamic knee stability.[12,100-102] This progressive perturbation training program uses rocker boards, mixed stable-unstable surface designs, and roller boards in isolation and in combination with the sport-specific tasks such as those described previously to promote coordinated neuromuscular responses (Figure 6-12). The perturbation program is performed in conjunction with other traditional rehabilitation methods such as strengthening exercises, cardiovascular training, agility drills, and sport-skill training.[12,100] In the early stages of the program, the support surfaces are per-

turbed in the sagittal plane and the patient is given verbal cues before the perturbations. As the patient progresses the perturbations become more complicated (e.g., they are performed in other planes), more forceful and rapid, and verbal cues are removed. The University of Delaware researchers also emphasize the importance of the patient producing coordinated responses rather than rigid co-contraction.[12,100,101] Most of the work related to this approach has been performed in patients with acute ACL injuries rather than those who have undergone surgery.[100-102] In the acute injury population, a 10-session approach is generally used.[12,100] Although a similar number of sessions may be sufficient in the ACL-reconstructed population, the optimum number of sessions has not been determined for this population.

Perturbation training exercises are a fun, progressive, and challenging method for promoting dynamic knee stability. The rehabilitation specialist is encouraged to be innovative and creative, but also meticulous in the application of these exercises. Perturbation training has a good theoretic basis and may be an effective method of training coordinated muscle responses, but if not employed with care these exercises may facilitate inappropriate, nonfunctional patterns such as general co-contraction.

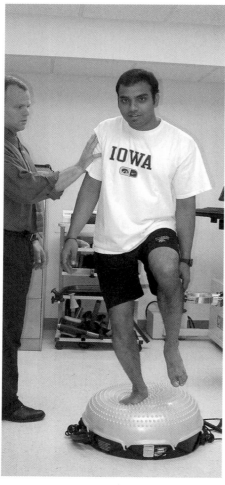

Figure 6-7: Manual perturbation by a rehabilitation specialist as the patient stands in single-leg stance on an air-filled dome.

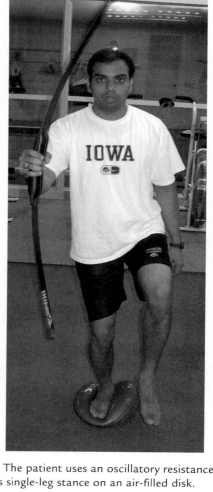

Figure 6-9: The patient uses an oscillatory resistance device as he performs single-leg stance on an air-filled disk.

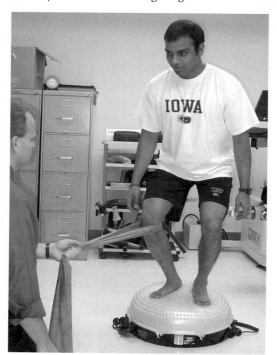

Figure 6-8: The rehabilitation specialist applies an anterior-directed destabilizing load to the patient's tibia while the patient stands in single-leg stance on a dome. The patient is instructed to recruit a specific response rather than employing general co-contraction to stiffen the knee.

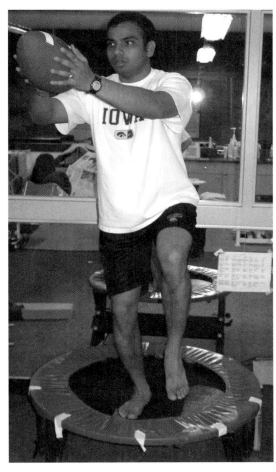

Figure 6-10: Sport-specific training in single-leg stance. The patient catches a football while balancing in single-leg stance on a rebounder with the knee in slight flexion.

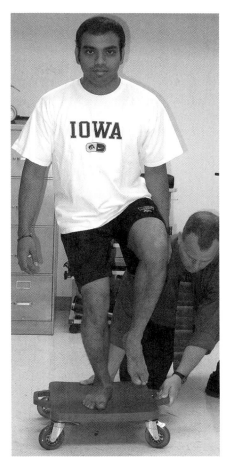

Figure 6-11: Perturbation training using a roller board. The rehabilitation specialist translates or rotates the roller board to perturb the support surface. The patient is instructed to recruit a specific, coordinated response rather than employ generalized co-contraction to stiffen the knee.

Dynamic Control Exercises/Agility Training

The final category of training methods we will discuss includes dynamic exercises and drills directed at progressively taxing the dynamic knee stability system in a functional manner. These are employed in the later phases of postsurgical rehabilitation. These exercises begin with single-plane activities such as jumping rope, stutter steps, shuffling laterally (the defensive posture in basketball), and performing vertical or box jumps. When good control is demonstrated in these activities and the patient appears ready for progression, she or he is advanced to more demanding exercises such as carioca, jumping over hurdles or cones (Figure 6-13), and single-leg hops in the forward or lateral direction with or without obstacles (Figure 6-14). These activities generally begin relatively slow (25% to 50% speed), concentrating on the quality of movement and control in movement, and then progressively increase in speed and complexity. Early in this phase, verbal cueing is used so that directional changes are anticipated, but these cues are later removed so that the directional changes are more random and unanticipated.

Devices such as the Functional Activity System for Testing and Exercise (FASTEX, Cybex Int., Medway, MA) are also a stimulating and challenging method of facilitating agility (Figure 6-15). Once patients are able to perform dynamic drills such as carioca and hopping forward and laterally in an aggressive fashion while maintaining control, they are progressed to tasks that challenge dynamic knee stability to a greater degree, such as figure-of-eight running and shuttle drills. Patient progression in these tasks occurs not only by increasing the intensity and speed of the task, but also by increasing the cutting angles or decreasing the turn radius around a cone. In the final stages of rehabilitation, the emphasis becomes sport-specific training. Advanced agility training should include sport-specific tasks such as running patterns, catching a football, or dribbling a basketball and pivoting or stopping quickly to take a jump shot. These drills are highly informative and assist the sports medicine team in the return-to-sport decision-making process. Many other exercises exist, but those presented in this chapter provide the

Early Phase (Treatments 1–4):

Treatment Goals: Expose the patient to perturbations in all directions
Elicit an appropriate muscular response to applied perturbations (no rigid co-contraction)
Minimize verbal cues

Overview: Perturbations are initially applied slowly and predictably. Verbal cues will be necessary for the onset and direction of the perturbation. Progress to moving in off-plane directions. Then, randomize the direction of the perturbations and decrease verbal cues. As the patient's ability to elicit an appropriate response improves, increase the challenge of the perturbations by performing them with more force, larger magnitude, and increased speed.

Technique	Direction of Board Movement
Rocker Board	Anterior/posterior, medial/lateral
Roller Board/Platform	Initial: Anterior/posterior, medial/lateral Progression: Diagonal, rotation
Roller Board	Initial: Anterior/posterior, medial/lateral Progression: Diagonal, rotation

Middle Phase (Treatments 5–7):

Criteria to Enter Phase: The patient must be able to elicit an appropriate muscular response to perturbations and demonstrate few or no falls during the rocker board and roller board techniques.

Treatment Goals: Add light sport-specific activity during perturbation techniques
Improve accuracy in matching the muscular response to the force, direction, and speed of the applied perturbation

Overview: Initially apply the perturbations as in the Early Phase (slowly, predictably, planes as noted) until the patient elicits an appropriate muscular response while performing the sport-specific activity, then progress according to Early Phase guidelines.

Late Phase (Treatments 8–10):

Criteria to Enter the Phase: While performing light sport-specific activity, the patient must be able to elicit an appropriate muscular response to perturbations and demonstrate few or no falls during the rocker board and roller board techniques.

Goals: Increase the difficulty of the perturbations by using sport-specific stances or performing more difficult sport-specific activity (e.g., on-command drills)
Elicit accurate, selective muscular responses to perturbations in any direction and of any magnitude and speed

Technique	Direction of Board Movement
Rocker Board	Diagonal with respect to the position of the foot
Roller Board/Platform	All directions Stance: Vary stance (e.g., staggered stance)
Roller Board	All directions

Figure 6-12: The University of Delaware perturbation training program. *(Reproduced from Williams GN, Chmielewski T, Rudolph KS, et al: Dynamic knee stability: current theory and implications for clinicians and scientists, J Orthop Sports Phys Ther 31(10):546-566, 2001, with permission of the Orthopaedic and Sports Physical Therapy Sections of the American Physical Therapy Association.)*

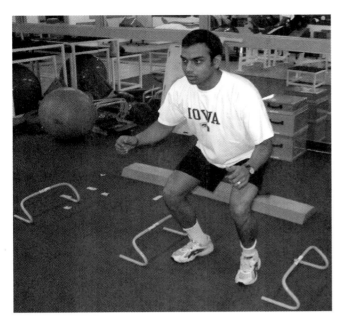

Figure 6-13: The patient jumps over hurdles in the lateral direction to promote dynamic stability in sports tasks.

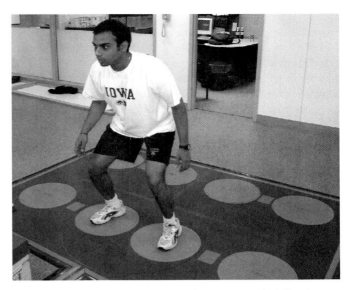

Figure 6-15: Agility training using the FASTEX rehabilitation system. This position provides objective feedback to the patient as the patient moves rapidly from one position to another.

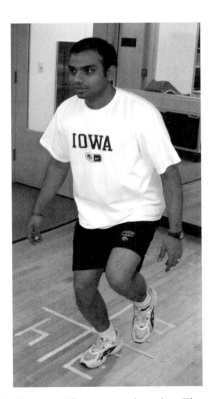

Figure 6-14: Numbered four-square hopping. The patient hops from one box to the next as the rehabilitation specialist calls out numbers. This exercise begins in a controlled and structured fashion and is progressed by increasing the speed and randomness of the patterns.

rehabilitation specialist with a framework for the prescription and progression of neuromuscular training exercises.

Role of Attention

Attention can be defined as the degree of focus or concentration on a specific item or task. The role that attention plays in sensorimotor control, injury, and training is a topic that has been understudied in the past, but is now receiving greater consideration. An important characteristic of attention is that its capacity is limited; in other words, people can only focus on a small number of things at any single point in time. As the amount of information that needs to be processed by the CNS increases, motor performance decreases.[43] Thus dynamic knee stability is at greater risk when the task being performed is complex and there is a lot of different information for the CNS to process. For example, when a football running back is running a play in a stadium filled with 70,000 screaming fans and he sees two players rapidly approaching him from different directions and consequently decides to suddenly decelerate and change direction while holding the ball securely so that it is not fumbled, his dynamic knee stability is in jeopardy not only because of the loads being applied to the knee when performing this high-risk task, but because the complexity and attentional demands associated with the task are significant. It is no surprise that athletes often sustain ACL injuries in situations such as this. Limited attention capacity also has implications for neuromuscular training. In early neuromuscular training, exercises should be simple (e.g., giving cues before perturbations) and there should be few environmental distractions. Increasing the attentional demands of neuromuscular training exercises by removing cues (i.e., making perturbations more random and unanticipated) or having the athlete perform other tasks while performing the training (e.g., counting backward, squatting, catching a ball) is a challenging and practical method of patient progression.

The focus of a patient's attention can also affect the outcomes of neuromuscular training. Evidence suggests that concentrating on external feedback (e.g., a balance system's computer display) rather than internal feedback (e.g., motion at the knee) leads to improved motor skill learning.[103-105] More specifically, external feedback leads to increased automaticity, which equates to reduced attentional costs.[105] These findings have important implications for the way rehabilitation specialists provide feedback to their patients during neuromuscular training. Rather than simply having patients focus on stabilizing their knees, rehabilitation specialists should carefully provide verbal, visual, or auditory feedback (e.g., equipment that provides tones that are associated with task performance). A few examples of visual feedback that may be helpful include computer programs that provide specific visual feedback, videos of patients performing their exercises, and the use of mirrors during training. Researchers have also demonstrated that having patients train in pairs or larger groups may lead to improved motor learning.[103] Thus it may be more effective to have patients train with postsurgical partners (one or more); one patient watches (focuses on) another performing a neuromuscular training task, provides feedback, and then switches roles with the other patient so that she or he now performs the task and receives feedback.

As discussed earlier in this chapter, the exact mechanisms by which neuromuscular training improves sensorimotor control are unknown. It is possible that regular neuromuscular training may lead to a greater awareness (higher level of consciousness) of where the knee is in space. At the same time, these exercises may decrease the attentional demands associated with maintaining dynamic stability, which is likely to reduce response times by decreasing delays associated with information processing.[43] Indeed, it is plausible that neuromuscular training has a greater effect on sensorimotor processing than it has on altering muscle recruitment or joint stiffness. This is not to imply that one effect is more important than another. Neuromuscular training most likely induces important changes in many parameters, which in combination lead to improved dynamic knee stability.

EFFECTS OF SURGERY AND POSTSURGICAL REHABILITATION

In comparison with the number of studies in the injured population, few studies evaluate neuromuscular function or the effects of neuromuscular training after knee surgery. The studies that are available have often used different approaches or measures or are focused on postsurgical neuromuscular function without specifically evaluating the effects of neuromuscular training. Consequently, we are currently unable to draw firm conclusions regarding the effectiveness of neuromuscular training. The scientific bases for many of these exercises are also still largely speculative. With that said, the results of the studies currently available in the literature are very promising.

To date there is only one randomized clinical trial related to the effects of neuromuscular training in the postsurgical sports knee population.[106] Liu-Ambrose and colleagues[106] randomly assigned 10 people to two treatment groups: a strength training group ($n = 5$) and a "proprioceptive" training group ($n = 5$). All subjects had undergone ACL reconstruction with semitendinosus grafts at least 6 months before initiating training, but the mean time since surgery for the strength training group (12.2 months) was nearly twice that of the "proprioceptive" training group (6.7 months). Thus it is no surprise that the quadriceps muscles on the operated side of the strength training group subjects were significantly stronger at pretraining baseline testing. The "proprioceptive" training group performed balance, perturbation, and agility training exercises similar to those described in this chapter at a frequency of three times per week for 12 weeks, whereas the strength training group performed progressive strength training over the same duration. The "proprioceptive" training group demonstrated a significantly greater increase in average isokinetic torque over the study duration. This is also not surprising because the "proprioceptive" training group subjects began the study with significantly weaker quadriceps muscles and were much closer to their surgical dates. It is likely that the differences observed were more a factor of the time since surgery than a treatment effect. The small sample size, the difference in time since surgery between the two groups, and the fact that the training was not initiated until more than 6 months after surgery (range = 6 to 27 months) limit the generalizability of this study.

Williams and co-workers[107] evaluated specificity of muscle action before ACL reconstruction with semitendinosus-gracilis grafts and then again after the subjects had returned to sports participation (approximately 6 months later). The subjects in this study were young athletes who were regular participants in high-risk sports that require quick changes of direction or jumping. This study was designed to assess the neuromuscular status of the subjects shortly after they were cleared to return to sports participation rather than the effect of neuromuscular training. The authors reported that the subjects performed a standard rehabilitation protocol that included neuromuscular training. The study participants exhibited significantly greater specificity of muscle action in the vastus lateralis, lateral gastrocnemius, and biceps femoris muscles at the post–return-to-sports session than they did at the presurgery session. The authors concluded that voluntary muscle control improves following ACL reconstruction with semitendinosus-gracilis grafts, but they stated that it was unclear whether this was the result of the rehabilitation, surgery, or both.[107]

Two randomized controlled trials have evaluated the effect of neuromuscular training in the ACL-deficient population.

Fitzgerald and colleagues[101] compared the outcomes of standard rehabilitation with those of standard rehabilitation plus perturbation of support surfaces. The primary outcome measures used in this study included ratings of patient-based outcomes, functional hop tests, and the incidence of post-training instability events (unsuccessful rehabilitation). Although both groups demonstrated significant improvement at the 6-month follow-up, the group that received perturbation training had a lower rate of unsuccessful rehabilitation.[101] Beard and colleagues[108] performed a double-blind, prospective, randomized controlled trial that compared the results of a strengthening program with a "proprioceptive" training program. Patients in both groups performed 12 weeks of exercises. The primary measures were functional rating scores and the reflex latency of the hamstrings muscle group in response to a destabilizing load. Both groups demonstrated significant improvement, but the "proprioceptive" training group demonstrated significantly greater reductions in hamstrings muscle reflex latencies than those observed in the strengthening group. Although the results of these studies cannot be directly extrapolated to the postsurgical patient population, they suggest that neuromuscular training does alter sensorimotor function.

FUTURE DIRECTIONS

We are in great need of well-designed, systematic lines of research that evaluate the effectiveness of neuromuscular training. These should include prospective, randomized control trials, as well as case-control studies. In addition to evaluating effectiveness, researchers need to clearly identify the effects of neuromuscular training exercises. Dose-response relationships and the optimal exercise sequence, frequency of exercise, and training format are topics that need to be carefully studied. Valid and reliable measures of assessing sensorimotor control are obviously a requisite to much of this research. The relative lack of such measures has been one of the limiting factors in neuromuscular research. Consequently, researchers need to develop or further define these measures before significant progress can be made.

One promising future direction is virtual reality training. One of the problems with contemporary neuromuscular training is that the mode of training and the environment are grossly different than those experienced when competing in an intercollegiate, interscholastic, or professional game. This may limit the degree to which current training improvements translate to the playing field. With virtual reality training, the athlete can be put into a virtual game environment using video game technology and customized treadmills that allow movement in all directions. In theory, this may be a more effective method of training than our current approach.[109] Such training is now becoming feasible, but significant research is needed before widespread application would be practical.

SUMMARY

Dynamic knee stability is the result of a complex integration of articular geometry, soft tissue restraints, and the loads applied by weight bearing and muscle action. Somatosensory mechanoreceptors in the muscles, connective tissues, and skin surrounding the knee joint are constantly sending ensembles of signals related to the conditions at the knee to the CNS. These signals are processed throughout the hierarchy of the CNS. The CNS acts to maintain knee joint homeostasis (stability) by modifying muscle activity and thereby joint stiffness. Although it is common and appropriate to study aspects of the sensorimotor system by isolating one or more of its subcomponents, it should be recognized that dynamic knee stability is built on a multidimensional framework of postural and movement control.

Knee ligament injuries have a profound adverse effect on neuromuscular function, which necessitates neuromuscular retraining. Postsurgical neuromuscular training should be integrated with traditional methods of rehabilitation, including strengthening, building endurance, and functional sport skill training. There are three primary categories of neuromuscular training: (1) detection of movement and joint repositioning exercises, (2) perturbation and postural control exercises, and (3) dynamic exercises targeting movement control and agility. Each of these types of exercises makes unique and important contributions to the restoration of dynamic knee stability. Most postsurgical neuromuscular training exercises are built on the concept of progressively challenging the dynamic stability of the knee. Rehabilitation specialists should seek to promote responses that are specific and functional rather than allow patients to use general cocontraction to stiffen the knee. Although generalized cocontraction may be a successful approach to stabilizing the knee in the clinical setting, it is neither functional nor healthy under typical sports conditions. This chapter presents a number of common training methods used to restore dynamic knee stability after surgery and discusses the typical functional progression of a patient. The process of restoring dynamic knee stability following surgery should be fun, innovative, and as scientifically based as possible. Unfortunately, there are few studies related to the effectiveness of neuromuscular training in the postsurgical patient population. The specific effects of most neuromuscular training exercises, their dose-response relationships, and the appropriate sequencing of exercises are still largely undefined. Although there are not many studies related to neuromuscular training, the results of those currently available are promising and suggest that these exercises are effective at improving stability. The exercises and theories presented in this chapter provide a framework for prescription and progression.

References

1. Allen CR, Wong EK, Livesay GA, et al: Importance of the medial meniscus in the anterior cruciate ligament–deficient knee, *J Orthop Res* 18(1):109-115, 2000.

2. Shoemaker SC, Markolf KL: The role of the meniscus in the anterior-posterior stability of the loaded anterior cruciate–deficient knee. Effects of partial versus total excision, *J Bone Joint Surg Am* 68(1):71-79, 1986.

3. Butler DL, Noyes FR, Grood ES: Ligamentous restraints to anterior-posterior drawer in the human knee. A biomechanical study, *J Bone Joint Surg Am* 62(2):259-270, 1980.

4. Piziali RL, Seering WP, Nagel DA, Schurman DJ: The function of the primary ligaments of the knee in anterior-posterior and medial-lateral motions, *J Biomech* 13(9):777-784, 1980.

5. Seering WP, Piziali RL, Nagel DA, Schurman DJ: The function of the primary ligaments of the knee in varus-valgus and axial rotation, *J Biomech* 13(9):785-794, 1980.

6. Gollehon DL, Torzilli PA, Warren RF: The role of the postero-lateral and cruciate ligaments in the stability of the human knee. A biomechanical study, *J Bone Joint Surg Am* 69(2):233-242, 1987.

7. Grood ES, Noyes FR, Butler DL, Suntay WJ: Ligamentous and capsular restraints preventing straight medial and lateral laxity in intact human cadaver knees, *J Bone Joint Surg Am* 63(8):1257-1269, 1981.

8. Kuo CY, Louie JK, Mote CD Jr: Field measurements in snow skiing injury research, *J Biomech* 16(8):609-624, 1983.

9. DeMorat G, Weinhold P, Blackburn T, et al: Aggressive quadriceps loading can induce noncontact anterior cruciate ligament injury, *Am J Sports Med* 32(2):477-483, 2004.

10. Markolf KL, Bargar WL, Shoemaker SC, Amstutz HC: The role of joint load in knee stability, *J Bone Joint Surg Am* 63(4):570-585, 1981.

11. Torzilli PA, Deng X, Warren RF: The effect of joint-compressive load and quadriceps muscle force on knee motion in the intact and anterior cruciate ligament–sectioned knee, *Am J Sports Med* 22(1):105-112, 1994.

12. Williams GN, Chmielewski T, Rudolph K, et al: Dynamic knee stability: current theory and implications for clinicians and scientists, *J Orthop Sports Phys Ther* 31(10):546-566, 2001.

13. Gandevia SC, Proske U, Stuart DG, editors: *Sensorimotor control of movement and posture,* New York, 2002, Kluwer Academic/Plenum Publishers.

14. Matthews PBC: *Mammalian muscle receptors and their central actions,* Baltimore, 1972, Williams & Wilkins.

15. Grigg P: Nervous system control of joint function. In Finerman G, Noyes F, editors: *Biology and biomechanics of the traumatized synovial joint: the knee as a model,* Rosemont, IL, 1992, American Academy of Orthopaedic Surgeons.

16. Grigg P: Articular neurophysiology. In Zachazewski J, Magee D, Quillen W, editors: *Athletic injuries and rehabilitation,* Philadelphia, 1996, Saunders.

17. Bergenheim M, Johansson H, Pedersen J, et al: Ensemble coding of muscle stretches in afferent populations containing different types of muscle afferents, *Brain Res* 734(1-2):157-166, 1996.

18. Johansson H, Pederson J, Bergenheim M, Djupsjobacka M: Peripheral afferents of the knee: their effects on central mechanisms regulating muscle stiffness, joint stability, and proprioception and coordination. In Lephart S, Fu F, editors: *Proprioception and neuromuscular control in joint stability,* Champaign, IL, 2000, Human Kinetics.

19. Gandevia SC, McCloskey DI, Burke D: Kinaesthetic signals and muscle contraction, *Trends Neurosci* 15(2):62-65, 1992.

20. Matthews PBC: *Mammalian muscle receptors and their central actions,* Baltimore, 1972, Williams & Wilkins.

21. Houk J, Henneman E: Responses of Golgi tendon organs to active contractions of the soleus muscle of the cat, *J Neurophysiol* 30(3):466-481, 1967.

22. Stuart D, Mosher C, Gerlack R, Reinking R: Mechanical arrangement and transducing properties of Golgi tendon organs, *Exp Brain Res* 14:274-292, 1972.

23. Boyd IA, Gladden MH, editors: *The muscle spindle,* New York, 1985, Macmillan.

24. Johansson H, Sjolander P, Sojka P: Receptors in the knee joint ligaments and their role in the biomechanics of the joint, *Crit Rev Biomed Eng* 18(5):341-368, 1991.

25. Johansson H, Sjolander P, Sojka P: A sensory role for the cruciate ligaments, *Clin Orthop* 268:161-178, 1991.

26. Grigg P: Mechanical factors influencing response of joint afferent neurons from cat knee, *J Neurophysiol* 38(6):1473-1484, 1975.

27. Newton RA: Joint receptor contributions to reflexive and kinesthetic responses, *Phys Ther* 62(1):22-29, 1982.

28. Borsa PA, Lephart SM, Irrgang JJ, et al: The effects of joint position and direction of joint motion on proprioceptive sensibility in anterior cruciate ligament–deficient athletes, *Am J Sports Med* 25(3):336-340, 1997.

29. Gandevia SC, Refshauge KM, Collins DM: Proprioception: peripheral inputs and perceptual interactions. In Gandevia SC, Proske U, Stuart DG, editors: *Sensorimotor control of movement and posture,* New York, 2002, Kluwer Academic/Plenum Publishers.

30. Edin B: Cutaneous afferents provide information about knee joint movements in humans, *J Physiol* 531(pt 1):289-297, 2001.

31. McNair PJ, Stanley SN, Strauss GR: Knee bracing: effects of proprioception, *Arch Phys Med Rehabil* 77(3):287-289, 1996.

32. Perlau R, Frank C, Fick G: The effect of elastic bandages on human knee proprioception in the uninjured population, *Am J Sports Med* 23(2):251-255, 1995.

33. Nichols TR, Cope TC, Abelew TA: Rapid spinal mechanisms of motor coordination, *Exerc Sport Sci Rev* 27:255-284, 1999.

34. Nichols TR: A biomechanical perspective on spinal mechanisms of coordinated muscular action: an architecture principle, *Acta Anat* 151(1):1-13, 1994.

35. Ghez C: The control of movement. In Kandel E, Schwartz J, Jessell T, editors: *Principles of neural science,* ed 3, New York, 1991, Elsevier.

36. Evarts EV: Motor cortex reflexes associated with learned movement, *Science* 179(72):501-503, 1973.

37. Lee R, Tatton W: Long loop reflexes in man: clinical applications. In Desmedt J, editor: *Cerebral motor control in man: long loop mechanisms. Prog Clin Neurophys* 4:320-333, Basel, 1978, Karger.

38. Nashner LM: Adapting reflexes controlling the human posture, *Exp Brain Res* 26(1):59-72, 1976.

39. Di Fabio RP, Graf B, Badke MB, et al: Effect of knee joint laxity on long-loop postural reflexes: evidence for a human capsular-hamstring reflex, *Exp Brain Res* 90(1):189-200, 1992.

40. Grabiner MD, Campbell KR, Hawthorne DL, Hawkins DA: Electromyographic study of the anterior cruciate ligament–hamstrings synergy during isometric knee extension, *J Orthop Res* 7(1):152-155, 1989.

41. Grabiner MD, Koh TJ, Miller GF: Further evidence against a direct automatic neuromotor link between the ACL and hamstrings, *Med Sci Sports Exerc* 24(10):1075-1079, 1992.

42. Crago PE, Houk JC, Hasan Z: Regulatory actions of human stretch reflex, *J Neurophysiol* 39(5):925-935, 1976.

43. Schmidt R, Lee T: *Motor control and learning,* ed 3, Champaign, IL, 1999, Human Kinetics.

44. Martin J, Jessell T: Modality coding in the somatic sensory system. In Kandel E, Schwartz J, Jessell T, editors: *Principles of neural science,* ed 3, New York, 1991, Elsevier.

45. Ghez C: Voluntary movement. In Kandel E, Schwartz J, Jessell T, editors: *Principles of neural science,* ed 3, New York, 1991, Elsevier.

46. Hyman R: Stimulus information as a determinant of reaction time, *J Exp Psychol* 45:188-196, 1953.

47. Hick W: On the rate of gain information, *Q J Exp Psychol* 4:11-26, 1952.

48. Lephart S, Reimann B, Fu F: Introduction to the sensorimotor system. In Lephart S, Fu F, editors: *Proprioception and neuromuscular control in joint stability,* Champaign, IL, 2000, Human Kinetics.

49. Sherrington CS: *The integrative action of the nervous system,* New York, 1906, Scribner's.

50. Ashton-Miller JA, Wojtys EM, Huston LJ, Fry-Welch D: Can proprioception really be improved by exercises? *Knee Surg Sports Traumatol Arthrosc* 9(3):128-136, 2001.

51. Winters JM, Woo SLY: *Multiple muscle systems biomechanics and movement organization,* New York, 1990, Springer-Verlag.

52. Zajac FE: Muscle and tendon: properties, models, scaling, and application to biomechanics and motor control, *Crit Rev Biomed Eng* 17(4):359-411, 1989.

53. Sinkjaer T, Toft E, Andreassen S, Hornemann BC: Muscle stiffness in human ankle dorsiflexors: intrinsic and reflex components, *J Neurophysiol* 60(3):1110-1121, 1988.

54. Nichols TR, Lin DC, Huyghues-Despointes CM: The role of musculoskeletal mechanics in motor coordination, *Prog Brain Res* 123:369-378, 1999.

55. Houk J, Rymer W: Neural control of muscle length and tension. In Brooks V, editor: *Handbook of physiology,* vol 2, *Motor control,* Bethesda, MD, 1981, American Physiological Society.

56. Akazawa K, Milner TE, Stein RB: Modulation of reflex EMG and stiffness in response to stretch of human finger muscle, *J Neurophysiol* 49(1):16-27, 1983.

57. Gottlieb GL, Agarwal GC: Response to sudden torques about ankle in man. III. Suppression of stretch-evoked responses during phasic contraction, *J Neurophysiol* 44(2):233-246, 1980.

58. Kearney RE, Stein RB, Parameswaran L: Identification of intrinsic and reflex contributions to human ankle stiffness dynamics, *IEEE Trans Biomed Eng* 44(6):493-504, 1997.

59. Sojka P, Sjolander P, Johansson H, Djupsjobacka M: Influence from stretch-sensitive receptors in the collateral ligaments of the knee joint on the gamma-muscle-spindle systems of flexor and extensor muscles, *Neurosci Res* 11(1):55-62, 1991.

60. Johansson H, Sjolander P, Sojka P: Activity in receptor afferents from the anterior cruciate ligament evokes reflex effects on fusimotor neurones, *Neurosci Res* 8(1):54-59, 1990.

61. Sojka P, Johansson H, Sjolander P, et al: Fusimotor neurones can be reflexly influenced by activity in receptor afferents from the posterior cruciate ligament, *Brain Res* 483(1):177-183, 1989.

62. Wojtys EM, Ashton-Miller JA, Huston LJ: A gender-related difference in the contribution of the knee musculature to sagittal-plane shear stiffness in subjects with similar knee laxity, *J Bone Joint Surg Am* 84A(1):10-16, 2002.

63. Wojtys EM, Huston LJ, Schock HJ, et al: Gender differences in muscular protection of the knee in torsion in size-matched athletes, *J Bone Joint Surg Am* 85A(5):782-789, 2003.

64. Granata KP, Padua DA, Wilson SE: Gender differences in active musculoskeletal stiffness. Part II. Quantification of leg stiffness during functional hopping tasks, *J Electromyogr Kinesiol* 12(2):127-135, 2002.

65. Granata KP, Wilson SE, Padua DA: Gender differences in active musculoskeletal stiffness. Part I. Quantification in controlled measurements of knee joint dynamics, *J Electromyogr Kinesiol* 12(2):119-126, 2002.

66. Arendt E, Dick R: Knee injury patterns among men and women in collegiate basketball and soccer. NCAA data and review of literature, *Am J Sports Med* 23(6):694-701, 1995.

67. Griffin LY, Agel J, Albohm MJ, et al: Noncontact anterior cruciate ligament injuries: risk factors and prevention strategies, *J Am Acad Orthop Surg* 8(3):141-150, 2000.

68. Uhorchak JM, Scoville CR, Williams GN, et al: Risk factors associated with noncontact injury of the anterior cruciate ligament: a prospective four-year evaluation of 859 West Point cadets, *Am J Sports Med* 31(6):831-842, 2003.

69. Nashner LM, Shupert C, Horak F, Black F: Organization of posture controls: an analysis of sensory and mechanical constraints. In Allum J, Hulliger M, editors: *Afferent control of posture and locomotion.* New York, 1989, Elsevier.

70. Shumway-Cook A, Woollacott MH: *Motor control: theory and practical applications,* ed 2, Philadelphia, 2001, Lippincott Williams & Wilkins.

71. Allum J, Honegger F, Pfaltz C: The role of stretch and vestibulospinal reflexes in the generation of human equilibrating reactions. In Allum J, Hulliger M, editors: *Afferent control of posture and locomotion.* New York, 1989, Elsevier.

72. Nashner LM: Fixed patterns of rapid postural responses among leg muscles during stance, *Exp Brain Res* 30(1):13-24, 1977.

73. Horak FB, Nashner LM: Central programming of postural movements: adaptation to altered support-surface configurations, *J Neurophysiol* 55(6):1369-1381, 1986.

74. Adkin AL, Frank JS, Carpenter MG, Peysar GW: Postural control is scaled to level of postural threat, *Gait Posture* 12(2):87-93, 2000.

75. Williams GN, Buchanan TS, Barrance PJ, et al: Quadriceps weakness, atrophy, and activation failure in predicted noncopers after anterior cruciate ligament injury, *Am J Sports Med* 33(3):402–407, 2005.

76. Williams GN, Barrance PJ, Snyder-Mackler L, Buchanan TS: Altered quadriceps control in people with anterior cruciate ligament deficiency, *Med Sci Sports Exerc* 36(7):1089-1097, 2004.

77. Friden T, Roberts D, Zatterstrom R, et al: Proprioceptive defects after an anterior cruciate ligament rupture—the relation to associated anatomical lesions and subjective knee function, *Knee Surg Sports Traumatol Arthrosc* 7(4):226-231, 1999.

78. Good L, Roos H, Gottlieb DJ, et al: Joint position sense is not changed after acute disruption of the anterior cruciate ligament, *Acta Orthop Scand* 70(2):194-198, 1999.

79. Barrack RL, Skinner HB, Buckley SL: Proprioception in the anterior cruciate deficient knee, *Am J Sports Med* 17(1):1-6, 1989.

80. Lephart SM, Pincivero DM, Giraldo JL, Fu FH: The role of proprioception in the management and rehabilitation of athletic injuries, *Am J Sports Med* 25(1):130-137, 1997.

81. Wojtys EM, Huston LJ: Neuromuscular performance in normal and anterior cruciate ligament–deficient lower extremities, *Am J Sports Med* 22(1):89-104, 1994.

82. Beard DJ, Kyberd PJ, O'Connor JJ, et al: Reflex hamstring contraction latency in anterior cruciate ligament deficiency, *J Orthop Res* 12(2):219-228, 1994.

83. Williams GN, Barrance PJ, Snyder-Mackler L, Buchanan TS: Specificity of muscle action after anterior cruciate ligament injury, *J Orthop Res* 21(6):1131-1137, 2003.

84. Howell SM: Anterior tibial translation during a maximum quadriceps contraction: is it clinically significant? *Am J Sports Med* 18(6):573-578, 1990.

85. Beynnon BD, Fleming BC, Johnson RJ, et al: Anterior cruciate ligament strain behavior during rehabilitation exercises in vivo, *Am J Sports Med* 23(1):24-34, 1995.

86. Buchanan TS, Almdale DP, Lewis JL, Rymer WZ: Characteristics of synergic relations during isometric contractions of human elbow muscles, *J Neurophysiol* 56(5):1225-1241, 1986.

87. Dewald JP, Pope PS, Given JD, et al: Abnormal muscle coactivation patterns during isometric torque generation at the elbow and shoulder in hemiparetic subjects, *Brain* 118(pt 2):495-510, 1995.

88. Flanders M, Soechting JF: Arm muscle activation for static forces in three-dimensional space, *J Neurophysiol* 64(6):1818-1837, 1990.

89. Batschelet E: *Circular statistics in biology,* London, 1981, Academic Press.

90. Fisher N: *Statistical analysis of circular data,* Cambridge, 1993, Cambridge University Press.

91. Berchuck M, Andriacchi TP, Bach BR, Reider B: Gait adaptations by patients who have a deficient anterior cruciate ligament, *J Bone Joint Surg Am* 72(6):871-877, 1990.

92. Chmielewski TL, Rudolph KS, Fitzgerald GK, et al: Biomechanical evidence supporting a differential response to acute ACL injury, *Clin Biomech* (Bristol, Avon) 16(7):586-591, 2001.

93. Rudolph KS, Eastlack ME, Axe MJ, Snyder-Mackler L: Movement patterns after anterior cruciate ligament injury: a comparison of patients who compensate well for the injury and those who require operative stabilization, *J Electromyogr Kinesiol* 8(6):349-362, 1998.

94. Rudolph KS, Axe MJ, Buchanan TS, et al: Dynamic stability in the anterior cruciate ligament deficient knee, *Knee Surg Sports Traumatol Arthrosc* 9(2):62-71, 2001.

95. Lass P, Kaalund S, leFevre S, et al: Muscle coordination following rupture of the anterior cruciate ligament. Electromyographic studies of 14 patients, *Acta Orthop Scand* 62(1):9-14, 1991.

96. Limbird TJ, Shiavi R, Frazer M, Borra H: EMG profiles of knee joint musculature during walking: changes induced by anterior cruciate ligament deficiency, *J Orthop Res* 6(5):630-638, 1988.

97. Ciccotti MG, Kerlan RK, Perry J, Pink M: An electromyographic analysis of the knee during functional activities. II. The anterior cruciate ligament–deficient and –reconstructed profiles, *Am J Sports Med* 22(5):651-658, 1994.

98. Swanik CB, Lephart S, Girlado J, et al: Reactive muscle firing of anterior cruciate ligament–injured females during functional activities, *J Athl Train* 34(2):121-129, 1999.

99. Williams GN, Barrance PJ, Snyder-Mackler L, Buchanan TS: Quadriceps femoris muscle morphology and function after ACL injury: a differential response in copers versus non-copers, *J Biomech* 38(4):685–693, 2005.

100. Lewek MD, Chmielewski TL, Risberg MA, Snyder-Mackler L: Dynamic knee stability after anterior cruciate ligament rupture, *Exerc Sport Sci Rev* 31(4):195-200, 2003.

101. Fitzgerald GK, Axe MJ, Snyder-Mackler L: The efficacy of perturbation training in nonoperative anterior cruciate ligament rehabilitation programs for physically active individuals, *Phys Ther* 80(2):128-140, 2000.

102. Chmielewski TL, Rudolph KS, Snyder-Mackler L: Development of dynamic knee stability after acute ACL injury, *J Electromyogr Kinesiol* 12(4):267-274, 2002.

103. McNevin NH, Wulf G, Carlson C: Effects of attentional focus, self-control, and dyad training on motor learning: implications for physical rehabilitation, *Phys Ther* 80(4):373-385, 2000.

104. McNevin NH, Wulf G: Attentional focus on supra-postural tasks affects postural control, *Hum Mov Sci* 21(2):187-202, 2002.

105. Wulf G, McNevin N, Shea CH: The automaticity of complex motor skill learning as a function of attentional focus, *Q J Exp Psychol A* 54(4):1143-1154, 2001.

106. Liu-Ambrose T, Taunton JE, MacIntyre D, et al: The effects of proprioceptive or strength training on the neuromuscular function of the ACL reconstructed knee: a randomized clinical trial, *Scand J Med Sci Sports* 13(2):115-123, 2003.

107. Williams GN, Snyder-Mackler L, Barrance PJ, et al: Neuromuscular function after anterior cruciate ligament with autologous semitendinosus-gracilis graft, *J Electromyogr Kinesiol* 15(2):170–180, 2005.

108. Beard DJ, Dodd CA, Trundle HR, Simpson AH: Proprioception enhancement for anterior cruciate ligament deficiency. A prospective randomised trial of two physiotherapy regimes, *J Bone Joint Surg Br* 76(4):654-659, 1994.

109. Todorov E, Shadmehr R, Bizzi E: Augmented feedback presented in a virtual environment accelerates learning of a difficult motor task, *J Mot Behav* 29(2):147-158, 1997.

CHAPTER 7

Neuromuscular Static and Dynamic Stability of the Shoulder: The Key to Functional Performance

George J. Davies, DPT, MEd, PT, SCS, ATC, LAT, CSCS, FAPTA
Daniel J. R. Krauscher, MPT, CSCS
Kristen F. Brinks, MS, PT, ATC
Jason Jennings, DPT, MSPT, SCS, ATC, CSCS

CHAPTER OUTLINE

NEUROMUSCULAR DYNAMIC STABILITY

of the shoulder is the key to functional performance. All joints in the body are dependent on stability being provided by the osseous, ligamentous/capsular complex (noncontractile tissue); muscular components (contractile unit); and the proprioceptive/kinesthetic system. When these systems work in harmony, the shoulder is one of the more marvelous joints in the body, particularly considering the demands placed on it. The shoulder is expected to effectively place the hand in a position of function for a variety of tasks, including extremely delicate procedures such as performing surgery, powerful activities such as lifting hundreds of pounds overhead in Olympic weightlifting, and sport-specific movements such as throwing a baseball over 90 miles per hour with the shoulder exceeding 7000 degrees per second in angular velocity. However, when there is an injury or dysfunction to any one of the aforementioned components, it disrupts the shoulder complex and creates impairments and functional limitations. Surgical interventions are usually required to correct osseous or ligamentous/capsular problems. Physical therapy interventions can significantly influence the remaining two components of shoulder stability, the muscular and proprioceptive systems, and often are effective in treating patients with shoulder dysfunction. Coupling the components of the muscular and proprioceptive systems together is what is described as *neuromuscular dynamic stability.*

This chapter describes the neuromuscular control system of the shoulder, including various joint receptors and their role in joint stability, along with the motor response pathways; presents techniques to assess and evaluate shoulder neuromuscular control; looks at the effect of injury on neuromuscular control; provides a progressive intervention strategy that can be used to enhance neuromuscular dynamic stability in patients with shoulder pathology; and looks at possible injury prevention techniques.

NEUROMUSCULAR CONTROL SYSTEM OF THE SHOULDER JOINT COMPLEX

The ability to accurately and effectively examine, evaluate, and rehabilitate the shoulder requires a comprehensive understanding of the intricate interplay among the shoulder's articular geometry, static and dynamic restraints, and the neuromuscular system. Because it is beyond the scope of this chapter to cover the anatomy in its entirety, the reader is referred to Jobe,[1] Ernlund and Warner,[2] and Nyland and colleagues[3] for further information.

The shoulder's articular geometry allows considerable range of motion (ROM) afforded to the entire upper extremity, but this comes at the expense of joint stability. The glenohumeral articulation is often analogized to a golf ball resting on a tee, with only 30% of the humeral head in contact with the glenoid fossa throughout the shoulder's ROM.[4] This articular incongruence receives reinforcement from static and dynamic restraints. Static structures include the fibrous glenoid labrum, which nearly doubles the surface area of the glenoid fossa and acts as a "chock block" to prevent translation of the humeral head out of the glenoid fossa. The remaining static restraints consist of the glenohumeral joint capsule and ligament complex. These structures possess the difficult task of being compliant enough to allow sufficient mobility, yet restrictive enough to provide protective stability. This task becomes even more challenging in the presence of extreme positions and torques incurred by the shoulder during functional and recreational activities. Of clinical significance, the capsuloligamentous structures have been shown to become taut and thus provide enhanced glenohumeral restraint primarily at end-ranges of motion,[5,6] leaving increased reliance on the dynamic restraint system for mid-ROM stability.

The rotator cuff (RTC) muscle complex makes up the dynamic restraint system of the glenohumeral joint. Visualization of the fiber orientation of this complex reveals the fibers' medial and inferior arrangement when traversing from their respective insertions along the lateral aspect of the humerus to their origins on the scapula. Consequently, contraction of the RTC creates a concavity compression phenomenon, seating the humeral head into the glenoid for increased stability while simultaneously depressing the humeral head, creating a dynamic caudal glide. The RTC works with the deltoid muscle to form a force couple, which is crucial in maintaining proper arthrokinematics and joint stability during humeral elevation.[2,7]

Of equal importance is the intimate relationship between the RTC tendons and the capsuloligamentous tissues of the glenohumeral joint in which activation of the RTC results in tensioning of the capsuloligamentous structures, further enhancing dynamic stability.[8,9] Working hand-in-hand, stimulation of the neuromuscular system located within the capsuloligamentous tissue can influence the activation of the RTC musculature and similarly enhance dynamic stability. The RTC has been shown to be the primary stabilizer of the glenohumeral joint through mid-ROM and assists the static structures with stability at end-ranges of motion.[6,7] As a result of the articular incongruence in association with the extreme ROM and torques characteristically placed on the shoulder, the synergistic interplay between the static and dynamic stabilizers that is facilitated by the neuromuscular system becomes vital for maintaining dynamic functional stability of the shoulder.

The ultimate goal of this integrative system is to maintain, or restore, joint homeostasis in the presence of a deforming force. To perform this task, the body utilizes reflexive responses known as either feedback or feed-forward control systems. The feedback mechanism relies on sensors, located within the joint's static and dynamic restraints, to monitor specific parameters and report these "data" to the system controller. The system controller compares these data with a predetermined reference "value," and any difference between these two "numbers" results in the production of an error signal.[10] In response, a compensatory reaction is triggered by the controller that is intended to match the reference "value" and therefore reestablish joint homeostasis. This is achieved through numerous reflex pathways that continually adjust muscle activity to produce a desired corrective response.[10-12] The overall function of this system is analogous to the way a thermostat regulates temperature within an environment.

The feed-forward control system also relies on sensors located within the joint's static and dynamic restraints. These sensors work differently in that they function to anticipate and detect potential disturbances that would alter the status of the regulated variable. The systems controller is notified of this potential disturbance, and a preparatory command is instituted in an attempt to counteract this perceived disturbance and maintain joint homeostasis.[10] Past experiences with similar disturbances serve as the basis for the preparatory command instituted by the system. This is analogous to the conditioned reflexes demonstrated by Pavlov's earlier work on dogs.[13] It is unlikely that these control systems work independently of one another, but rather in a complementary fashion, with afferent input being used initially for feed-forward control until a feedback control response can be initiated.

NEUROMUSCULAR CONTROL

The integration of feedback and feed-forward control involves a hierarchic organizational system, spanning from the cellular to the organ level, contributing to the ultimate goal of neuromuscular control for dynamic joint stability. Neuromuscular control, as defined by Myers and Lephart,[14] is an unconscious activation of dynamic restraints occurring in preparation for and in response to joint motion and loading for the purpose of maintaining functional joint stability. The neuromuscular control system consists of a complex interaction between the sensory, motor, and central integration and processing centers of the central nervous system (CNS), collectively termed the *sensorimotor system*.[15] Because of the relative complexity of neuromuscular control, we present this information using a whole-part-whole model, with the objective of providing the reader with an understanding of the function of each "subsystem" in the sensorimotor system, and then how the subsystems are integrated to maintain functional joint stability.

The sensorimotor system is divided into two components: the sensory (afferent) component and the motor response (efferent) component. The sensory component is frequently termed *proprioception,* which includes the perception of position or perception of movement. The motor component is frequently referred to as *neuromuscular control,* which involves coordinated movement patterns and strategies generated by the CNS in response to proprioceptive input.

In its most simplistic description, the sensorimotor system is activated when a sensory receptor becomes stimulated by a perturbation that alters joint homeostasis. In response, sensory (afferent) information regarding this alteration is sent to the CNS for integration. A plan to regain homeostasis is developed and a corrective motor (efferent) response is elicited. This response leads to the production of coordinated muscle activity directed to regain homeostasis and provide functional joint stability. The ability to appreciate sensory stimulation from the periphery and convert this mechanical stimulus into a neural signal that is transmitted to the CNS for processing is referred to as *proprioception.*[11] Proprioception provides the conscious or subconscious appreciation of joint position sense, joint movement sense (kinesthesia), and force of application to the joint.[11-16] The sensory organs of the sensorimotor system responsible for detecting mechanical stimulation are called *mechanoreceptors.* Mechanoreceptors are found within skin, joints, ligaments, tendons, and muscles, and are sensitive to various forms of mechanical deformation.[17,18] These receptors are broadly classified into three groups based on the tissues in which they are found: joint receptors, cutaneous receptors, and muscle receptors.

Joint receptors are further classified into four distinct types based on the stimuli to which they respond, as well as the following characteristics (Table 7-1):

- The joint state in which they are active (static, dynamic, or both)
- The stimulus intensity at which they reach their threshold for activation (low threshold vs. high threshold)
- Whether they remain active with persistent stimuli (slow adapting) or respond quickly and then become quiet (rapid adapting)[10]

At mid-ROM, joint receptors have been identified as being only minimally active, thus providing only a small degree of joint movement sense (kinesthesia) secondary to insufficient tissue tension in the capsuloligamentous tissue to generate adequate stimulus.[5,6] However, at extreme positions of movement, or nearing end-ranges of motion, these structures become subjected to relatively strong tensions, generating maximal receptor response.[3,6] Therefore one could conclude that the primary proprioceptive role of the joint receptor is to signal changes near end-ranges of motion, leading to the creation of a protective motor response to prevent joint injury.

Cutaneous receptors are the neural organs of the sensorimotor system located within the skin. Activation of these receptors occurs through detection of potentially harmful mechanical or thermal stimuli, leading to the initiation of a protective withdrawal reflex. Some evidence suggests that these receptors are stimulated, and therefore may contribute to the detection of joint position and kinesthesia, when the skin becomes stretched.[19] However, Goodwin and colleagues[20] and Zuckerman and colleagues[21] demonstrated that the introduction of an anesthetic to joint and cutaneous afferents failed to disrupt conscious kinesthesia and joint position sense. In response to this, several authors have shown that the sensitivity, and therefore overall contribution of cutaneous receptors to proprioception, can be heightened through the utilization of compression garments, bracing, and taping, thus providing a means of sensory manipulation for stability enhancement.[22-24] The extent to which cutaneous receptors aid in supplying proprioceptive information remains unclear, but it appears to be less substantial than that which is provided by the system's muscle receptors. Further research in this area, especially as it pertains to the upper extremity, is needed.

The muscle receptors of the sensorimotor system consist of the Golgi tendon organs (GTOs) and the muscle spindles, both of which are unique in their location and proprioceptive role. The GTOs are located within the musculotendinous junction and are sensitive to changes in muscle tension from passive tension (stretching) or active muscle contraction. Information concerning muscle tension is provided to higher levels in a continuous manner, such that at rest, low-level steady-state firing occurs, whereas sudden increases in tension result in an increase in the previous level of neural signal transmission.[17] Therefore GTO reflexes are considered to occur under both static and dynamic conditions, providing the CNS with instantaneous information regarding the tension of each muscle.[17] The reflexive activity of the GTO is inhibitory in nature, functioning to prevent muscle tension from reaching damaging levels through a negative feedback mechanism that inhibits further muscle contraction.

Muscle spindles are intrafusal muscle fibers that are located parallel to the muscle fibers within a muscle belly. These neural structures are sensitive to the degree and rate of change in length (stretch) of a muscle and, similar to the GTOs, function under both static and dynamic conditions. When a muscle is rapidly stretched, a dynamic stretch reflex is initiated to modulate muscle length through the production of agonistic muscle contraction. The spindles continue to cause muscle contraction in a static state if the muscle is maintained at an excessive length, signaling potential damage.[17] Theoretically, perturbations with enough magnitude to disrupt joint stability would alter muscle receptor activity and result in reflex activation of the muscles surrounding the joint to increase joint stability and thus prevent injury. There is substantial evidence suggesting that muscle receptors are the greatest contributor to joint position and movement sense throughout mid-ROM (functional ROM).[5,7,20,21] However, the passive structures (labrum or capsule), active structures (RTC), and neural structures (joint, cutaneous, or muscle receptors) do not work in isolation to maintain stability. Instead, a proprioceptive and stability alliance is formed between the static and dynamic structures to detect afferent information that is sent to the

TABLE 7-1*

Mechanical Receptor Classifications

TYPE	RECEPTOR NAME	LOCATION	SENSITIVE OR RESPOND TO	ACTIVATION THRESHOLD	RESPONSE TO PERSISTENT STIMULI
I	Ruffini endings	Capsuloligamentous tissue	Sensitive to joint position sense Respond to tissue stress (loads) Sensitive to limit detectors	Low threshold	Slow adapting
II	Pacinian corpuscles	Capsuloligamentous tissue	Sensitive to movement/ velocity sensors Respond to compression and tensile loading	Low threshold	Fast adapting
III	Golgi tendon organs	Musculotendinous junction of tendons	Sensitive to tension sensors Assist in position sense during volitional muscle activation and passive musculotendinous stretching	High threshold	Slow adapting
IV	Free nerve endings (nociceptors)	Throughout capsular tissue	Sensitive to pain of mechanical or chemical origin	High threshold	Slow adapting

*From Williams GN, Chmielewski T, Rudolph KS, et al: Dynamic knee stability, J Orthop Sports Phys Ther 31:546-566, 2000.

CNS for integration and processing to develop a response for maintaining dynamic neuromuscular control.[3]

Motor Response Pathways

The motor response pathway is the efferent response to the sensory information. This response system is the neuromuscular component of the sensorimotor system. Afferent signals from the peripheral mechanoreceptors are mediated at three levels within the CNS: the spinal cord, the brainstem and cerebellum, and the cerebral cortex.[17] Integration of vast sensory input occurs at each of these higher levels. Integration is the process of summating, gating, and modulating this incoming information to allow for the production of coordinated, fluid motor control response strategies.[12] The higher levels of motor control are arranged in a hierarchic and parallel manner.[25] Hierarchic organization allows lower motor centers to automatically control common motor activities, letting higher centers devote attention to the control of more precise and dexterous motor activities. Their parallel arrangement provides each motor control center the ability to issue independent descending motor commands.[25]

Sensory integration primarily begins at the spinal cord level where it is integrated and processed at a subconscious level. Stimuli received at the spinal cord level result in the production of spinal reflexes. These elementary patterns of motor control provide a direct motor response to peripheral sensory input, with a latency of response ranging from 30 to 50 ms.[26] Sensory information is transmitted via afferent pathways, terminating through bifurcation on anterior motor neurons, interneurons, and ascending tract cells in the dorsal horn of the spinal cord.[11] Anterior motor neurons consist of both alpha and gamma motor neurons. Alpha motor neurons innervate skeletal muscle fibers, with their activation resulting in excitation of associated fibers.[17] Gamma motor neurons innervate the muscle spindles, which provide the CNS with direct control over spindle sensitivity and therefore allow for direct influence of muscle stiffness.[17] Interneurons regulate the innervation of these anterior motor neurons, and the ascending tract cells provide an afferent "copy" to higher levels of control for further integration and processing.[15,17] This bifurcation and interneuronal network provides the spinal cord with its efferent integrative function, such that even the most basic monosynaptic reflex (stretch reflex) is influenced by other sources of afferent input, as well as descending commands from higher control centers.[15]

The brainstem, which connects the brain to the spinal cord, also integrates and processes input at a subconscious level. Information obtained at the brainstem and cerebellar level comes from visual, vestibular, and somatosensory sources. Through integration of incoming sensory input, the brainstem and cerebellum can directly regulate and modulate motor activity, leading to control of postural equilibrium and numerous automatic and stereotypic movements.[25] The latency time for this reflex has been shown to range from 50 to 80 ms.[26] As a result of its central location between the brain and spinal cord, the brainstem also functions as an indirect relay station between these two levels of motor control, with the capability of modifying descending motor commands as necessary. The brainstem and cerebellum do so by comparing the intentions of the cerebral cortex with continuously updated sensory information to determine the best plan of action to produce intended movement.[27] Medial and lateral descending pathways, which are continuous from the brainstem to the spinal cord, are used to elicit finalized motor commands.[25]

The highest level of motor control occurs at the level of the cerebral cortex. The cerebral cortex is made up of a sensory cortex, which registers sensory stimuli from the periphery, and a motor cortex, which provides for voluntary control over complex movement patterns. To implement its motor plan and thus activate a muscular response, the cortex simultaneously stimulates functions of the spinal cord, brainstem, basal ganglia, and cerebellum.[17] The advantage of this complex processing system is its high level of flexibility in the motor response produced. Conversely, the greater number of variables requiring processing associated with such flexibility results in a longer latency of response time, ranging from 80 to 120 ms.[26] The cerebral cortex uses the corticospinal tract to convey its motor plan to the spinal cord, terminating on the interneurons.[17]

In summary, activation of motor neurons can result from direct afferent sensory input (spinal level) or from descending pathways of the higher motor levels (brainstem, cerebellum, or cerebral cortex). Regardless of the source, the skeletal muscle activation produced to create dynamic neuromuscular control occurs through signal convergence from all levels onto the motor neurons.[25] This concept, referred to by Sherrington and reported by Riemann and Lephart,[15] is called the *final common path*.

ASSESSMENT OF PROPRIOCEPTION AND NEUROMUSCULAR CONTROL

Assessment of the sensorimotor system can be performed looking for afferent (proprioceptive) changes or alterations in muscle response patterns (neuromuscular control). Evaluating both or one of the components is important for documenting deficits and identifying the need for neuromuscular training in the rehabilitation program. Proprioception, as previously defined as the sensory (afferent) part of the sensorimotor system, can be assessed by kinesthetic ability, which is the perception of joint motion, and joint position sense, which is the ability to recognize the position of a body part in space.

Proprioception and Joint Position Sense Testing

Determining joint position sense involves measuring the accuracy of joint angle replication. Assessment tools in the laboratory setting include custom-made devices[28-31] and electromagnetic motion analysis systems.[14,31] Although these tools may offer the best controlled environment, they are not readily available in most clinical settings. Tools that are clinically accessible include goniometry (Figure 7-1),[30,32] isokinetics,[6,14,33] and inclinometers.[31,34,35]

Dover and Powers[34] investigated the reliability of joint position sense measurement using an inclinometer. Inclinometers are small, lightweight, affordable, and easily used in a clinical setting.[34,35] Shoulder internal and external ROM measurements were assessed followed by active joint position sense. The results identified the inclinometer as a reliable instrument providing affordable and accurate measurements of ROM and joint position sense.[34]

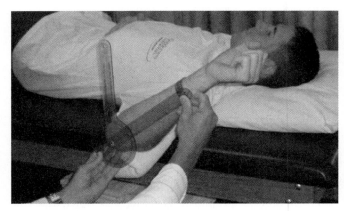

Figure 7-1: Goniometric measurements.

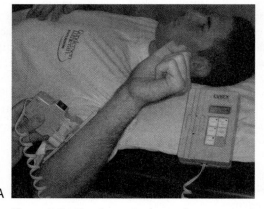

A

Figure 7-2: Gundersen Lutheran Sports Medicine proprioception testing protocol.

SHOULDER PROPRIOCEPTION

DX: _____

DOI/DOS: _____ DOM SIDE: R / L

Procedure: **Active Angular Replication**
1. Patient seated on table with shoulder/arm in neutral position.
2. Patient closes his/her eyes.
3. Patient's arm is **passively** raised to a particular angle as per the protocol.
4. Patient is told to hole and "internalize" the angle while the angle is measured.
5. Patient's arm is **passively** returned to the starting position.
6. Patient is asked to **actively** replicate the angle and hold that position.
7. Patient's arm angle is measured and written as the difference in degrees (**DID**) from the angle the examiner asked to patient to replicate.
8. The procedure is repeated until all 7 measurements are taken or as many measurements allowed based on ROM.
9. Calculate the mean DID for each arm and compare to norms.

Date							
Weeks							
Side							
Flexion < 90 DID							
Flexion > 90 DID							
Abduction < 90 DID							
Abduction > 90 DID							
Extern Rotation < 45 DID							
Extern Rotation > 45 DID							
Internal Rotation DID							
Mean DID							
Initials							

B

Norms	Male	Female
Average	+/− 3	+/− 4
Range	+/− 5	+/− 7

Active or passive angle replication can be performed in shoulder flexion, abduction, external rotation, internal rotation, or a combination of planes of movement.[31,35] Standardized testing protocols are used and include minimizing visual and tactile clues.[6,14,28,32-43] An example of a testing protocol is illustrated in Figure 7-2, **B**.

Normative data are listed in Figure 7-2, **B**, for males and females,[43] while Figure 7-2, **A**, illustrates testing procedure. Multiple angles are used incorporating mid-ROM, where most functional activities occur. Additionally, angles near the end of the ROM, which is closer to a position of possible mechanism of injury, are measured. Absolute end-range of motion is avoided secondary to possible nociceptor firing with pain response or potential apprehension in subjects with a history of instability. Active angular replication was chosen over passive replication because it is functional and most injuries occur during active muscle contraction.

Different methods for calculating target angles have been described in the literature.[6,33-35,43] Using one target angle[33] or using multiple angles both at mid-ROM and near end-ROM has been reported.[33,43] The advantage of using multiple angles is getting a more comprehensive picture of proprioceptive abilities. Another method for calculating target angles using a specific percentage of ROM has also been described.[34,35] This technique ensures that subjects are tested at the same proportional point of their ROM.[6] The disadvantage of this technique is that serial retesting to document progress may lead to a learning response, which has been shown to influence joint position sense acuity.[6]

Proprioception and Kinesthetic Testing

Kinesthesia is assessed by determining the threshold to detection of passive movement (TTDPM).[14] TTDPM quantifies the ability to consciously detect shoulder motion using a custom-made device[21,31,44] or an isokinetic dynamometer.[21] Visual and tactile cues are minimized as in joint angle replication testing.[14,21,43-45] Testing often includes internal and external rotation motions both at mid-ROM and end-ROM.[32,45] The arm is passively moved at a slow velocity from a preset reference angle. Speeds of 5 deg/sec have been shown to produce a more reliable test.[14,45,46] Subjects are instructed to signal or stop the machine as soon as motion is noted (Figure 7-3). The amount of movement occurring before detection is recorded. Although testing at slow speeds has been shown to be more reliable, the results may not be clinically applicable to assess functional movements, because functional movements occur at faster angular velocities and in multiple planes.

NEUROMUSCULAR CONTROL TESTING

Neuromuscular control assessment documents the muscular response to proprioceptive input. This can be accomplished through nerve conduction testing, electromyography, and muscle performance analysis.[32] Clinically applicable techniques in the physical therapy setting include muscle per-

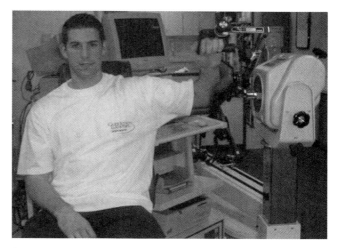

Figure 7-3: Isokinetic dynamometer kinesthetic testing.

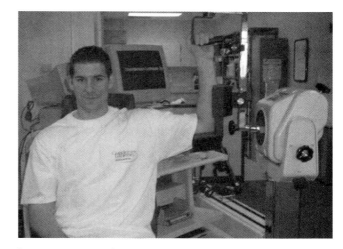

Figure 7-4: Internal rotation/external rotation isokinetic test.

formance on isokinetic testing and functional performance on tests such as the lateral scapular slide test, the closed kinetic chain stability test, and the functional throwing performance index.

Isokinetic Glenohumeral Internal Rotation/External Rotation Testing

Isokinetic testing can be used to quantify torque, work, and power for bilateral comparison, unilateral ratios, and relationship to body weight.[47] The most commonly performed isokinetic power test for the shoulder includes internal rotation/external rotation assessment at the modified neutral position (30/30/30) or at the 90/90 position for overhead athletes (Figure 7-4).

Descriptive normative data (Table 7-2) that are often used for muscular performance analysis include bilateral comparison, unilateral ratios, and relationship to body weight.[47] Typically less than 10% deficit on bilateral comparison and a

TABLE 7-2

Peak Torque/Body Weight Ratios (%) Normative Data for External and Internal Shoulder Rotators

	60 DEG/SEC	180 DEG/SEC	300 DEG/SEC
External rotation (%BW)	10%-15%	5%-10%	5%
Internal rotation (%BW)	15%-20%	10%-20%	10%
Ratio: external rotation/internal rotation	60%-70%	60%-70%	60%-70%

BW, Body weight.

unilateral ratio for external rotation/internal rotation of 66% is targeted for normal subjects.[47] Calculating the patient's peak torque development relative to his or her body weight allows for individualization of the test results.

Isokinetic Scapulothoracic Testing

Scapulothoracic isokinetic testing may also be used as a method to assess neuromuscular control. Scapular protraction and retraction strength is important to prevent scapular winging and to provide proximal stability for proper rotator cuff function and also distal mobility. Normative data are presented in Table 7-3.[43]

Modified Lateral Scapular Slide Testing

The lateral scapular slide test has been described to objectively document scapulothoracic position in varying arm positions.[48] The test evaluates the position of the scapula on the injured side and uninjured side in relationship to a fixed point on the spine. Kibler[48] described three testing positions: arms relaxed at the sides, hands on hips, and 90 degrees of abduction with internal rotation. More than 1 cm of asymmetry is correlated to impingement syndrome in the shoulder.[48] Davies and Dickoff-Hoffman[43] later developed a modified lateral scapular slide test using the three positions described by Kibler, as well as 120 degrees and 150 degrees of abduction. The additional positions were included in testing because symptom provocation most often occurs

in overhead positions. The testing protocol is presented in Figure 7-5.

Gibson and colleagues[49] performed a reliability study and demonstrated that Interclass/Intraclass Correlation Coefficients (ICCs) for the three scapulothoracic positions were .93, .91, and .89, respectively. However, studies on reliability and sensitivity have found the lateral scapular slide test as described by Kibler to have low reliability and poor sensitivity.[50,51] It was found that scapular asymmetry was common in asymptomatic individuals and did not necessarily indicate a dysfunction.[51] Therefore Koslow and colleagues[51] do not recommend the test for determining shoulder dysfunction. Further research may be necessary to determine validity and reliability of the lateral scapular slide test. Furthermore, future studies could investigate positions in the scapular plane rather than the front plane and correlate values to shoulder pathology.

Closed Kinetic Chain Upper Extremity Stability Test

The closed kinetic chain (CKC) upper extremity stability test was designed to objectify dynamic stabilization and determine whether there are deficits in CKC upper extremity performance.[52] The test is easily administered in a clinical setting requiring only athletic tape and a stopwatch. Subjects are positioned in a push-up or modified push-up position with hands on a target line on the floor. Subjects are instructed to move their hands back and forth from the target line to

TABLE 7-3

Peak Torque/Body Weight Ratios (%) Normative Data for Scapulothoracic Protraction and Retraction

	PROTRACTION	RETRACTION	RETRACTION/PROTRACTION RATIO
30 deg/sec	41%	38%	92%
60 deg/sec	31%	33%	105%
120 deg/sec	16%	19%	116%

scapulothoracic lateral slide test

1. The inferior angle of the scapula is at the level of T7.
2. The test is normal if both measurements are within 1 cm bilaterally.
3. The measurements should increase by approximately 0.5 cm with each successive position.

Data:

Date: _____	U (R/L)	I (R/L)	Date: _____	U (R/L)	I (R/L)
Neutral	_____cm	_____cm	Neutral	_____cm	_____cm
Hand on top of iliac crest	_____cm	_____cm	Hand on top of iliac crest	_____cm	_____cm
90 ABD/IR	_____cm	_____cm	90 ABD/IR	_____cm	_____cm
120 ABD	_____cm	_____cm	120 ABD	_____cm	_____cm
150 ABD	_____cm	_____cm	150 ABD	_____cm	_____cm
Date: _____	U (R/L)	I (R/L)	Date: _____	U (R/L)	I (R/L)
Neutral	_____cm	_____cm	Neutral	_____cm	_____cm
Hand on top of iliac crest	_____cm	_____cm	Hand on top of iliac crest	_____cm	_____cm
90 ABD/IR	_____cm	_____cm	90 ABD/IR	_____cm	_____cm
120 ABD	_____cm	_____cm	120 ABD	_____cm	_____cm
150 ABD	_____cm	_____cm	150 ABD	_____cm	_____cm
Date: _____	U (R/L)	I (R/L)	Date: _____	U (R/L)	I (R/L)
Neutral	_____cm	_____cm	Neutral	_____cm	_____cm
Hand on top of iliac crest	_____cm	_____cm	Hand on top of iliac crest	_____cm	_____cm
90 ABD/IR	_____cm	_____cm	90 ABD/IR	_____cm	_____cm
120 ABD	_____cm	_____cm	120 ABD	_____cm	_____cm
150 ABD	_____cm	_____cm	150 ABD	_____cm	_____cm

Figure 7-5: Data form for modified lateral scapula slide test.

another target line 3 feet from the original line. The number of lines touched by both hands in 15 seconds is recorded. Test-retest reliability with ICCs of .922 has been established.[52] Test procedures, data collection, and normative data are presented in Figure 7-6, **C**, while the actual testing procedure is shown in Figure 7-6, **A** and **B**.

Functional Throwing Performance Index

The functional throwing performance index (FTPI) has been described as a clinically oriented test that is easily administered, cost effective, and space efficient.[43] Reliability testing, using ICCs, demonstrated test-retest reliability of .91.[43] Test procedures, data collection, and normative data are presented in Figure 7-7, **B**, while the actual testing procedure is shown in Figure 7-7, **A**.

EFFECT OF INJURY ON THE SENSORIMOTOR SYSTEM

Both the afferent (proprioception) and efferent (neuromuscular control) portions of the sensorimotor system have been shown to be affected by injury.[29,38,53-60]

Shoulder Instability and Proprioception

Several studies have investigated the effect of traumatic dislocations and instability on shoulder proprioception.[38,53-55] Smith and Brunolli[53] reported proprioceptive deficits in patients who sustained anterior shoulder dislocations. They found significant differences in position sense and threshold to detection of motion when comparing involved shoulders with uninvolved shoulders. Lephart and colleagues[28] investigated kinesthetic ability and passive angular replication for external and internal rotators in three study groups: normal shoulders, unstable shoulders, and surgically repaired shoulders. They concluded that subjects with instability demonstrated a decrease in kinesthesia and joint position sense compared with the uninvolved side, whereas normal shoulders and surgically repaired shoulders revealed no significant difference in proprioception. Similarly, Zuckerman and colleagues[55] studied kinesthesia and joint position sense for shoulder flexion, abduction, and external rotation in subjects following traumatic shoulder instability and subsequent surgical correction. Their findings revealed a significant decrease in proprioception when comparing the unstable shoulder

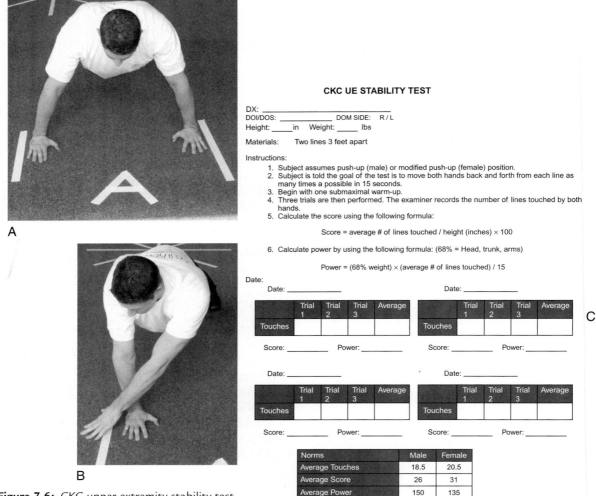

CKC UE STABILITY TEST

DX: _____
DOI/DOS: _____ DOM SIDE: R / L
Height: _____ in   Weight: _____ lbs

Materials: Two lines 3 feet apart

Instructions:
1. Subject assumes push-up (male) or modified push-up (female) position.
2. Subject is told the goal of the test is to move both hands back and forth from each line as many times a possible in 15 seconds.
3. Begin with one submaximal warm-up.
4. Three trials are then performed. The examiner records the number of lines touched by both hands.
5. Calculate the score using the following formula:

Score = average # of lines touched / height (inches) × 100

6. Calculate power by using the following formula: (68% = Head, trunk, arms)

Power = (68% weight) × (average # of lines touched) / 15

Norms	Male	Female
Average Touches	18.5	20.5
Average Score	26	31
Average Power	150	135

Figure 7-6: CKC upper extremity stability test.

with the contralateral shoulder. Warner and colleagues[38] also reported that patients with a history of traumatic instability demonstrated a significantly decreased proprioceptive ability in the involved shoulder following injury.

Subacromial Impingement Syndrome and Proprioception

Subacromial impingement syndrome also has been shown to affect shoulder proprioception. Machner and colleagues[57] analyzed proprioception in 15 patients with a diagnosis of shoulder impingement syndrome with a documented type II acromion on radiographs. Proprioception was assessed by determining the threshold for perception of passive movement. The results revealed a decrease in kinesthetic sense and proprioception in the impingement shoulder compared with the uninvolved shoulder. They suggested that changes in the mechanoreceptors in the subacromial bursa and the coraco-

acromial ligament may have caused the alterations in shoulder proprioception.

Joint Injury and Altered Neuromuscular Response

In addition to changes in proprioception and kinesthesia, joint injury also appears to contribute to alterations in the neuromuscular response.[29] Decreased anterior and middle deltoid activity with shoulder flexion and abduction has been documented in subjects with instability compared with normative controls.[58] Increased supraspinatus and biceps brachii activity along with decreased subscapularis, pectoralis major, and latissimus dorsi activity was reported following fine-wire electromyographic analysis in baseball pitchers with anterior instability.[56] McMahon and colleagues[59] performed comparative electromyographic analysis of shoulder muscles in subjects with glenohumeral instability and normal shoulders.

**FUNCTIONAL THROWING
PERFORMANCE INDEX**

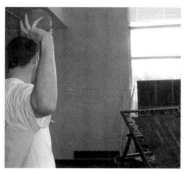

A

Figure 7-7: Functional throwing performance index.

DX: _____

DOI/DOS: _____ DOM SIDE: R / L

Materials:
  Distance: 15 feet from the wall   Height: 4 feet from the floor
  Target size: 1×1 foot square   Ball: 21" diameter rubber playground ball

Instructions:
  1. Normal throwing mechanics are encouraged. Patient should use the "crow-hop" technique when throwing and not standing still at the start line.
  2. The patient performs 4 gradient sub-maximal to maximal warm-up throws.
  3. The patient then performs 5 maximal controlled practice throws, catching the ball of the rebound.
  4. The patient then performs as many throws with control and accuracy in 30 seconds, The examiner records the number of throws and the number of throws that land within the target area.
  5. Three 30 second trials are performed.
  6. Calculate the average for throws in target and total throws.
  7. Functional Throwing Performance Index (FTPI) is then calculated:

FTPI (%) = Throws in target / Total number of throws × 100

Date: _____   Date: _____   B

Throws in target:		Trial 1	Trial 2	Trial 3	Average
	Throws in target				
	Total throws				

FTPI: _____ / _____ × 100 = ____ %

Date: _____

Throws in target:		Trial 1	Trial 2	Trial 3	Average
	Throws in target				
	Total throws				

FTPI: _____ / _____ × 100 = ____ %

Norms	Male	Female
Total Throws	15	13
Target Throws	7	4
FTPI	47%	29%
Range	33-60%	17-41%

The results showed significantly less supraspinatus activity during abduction and flexion, as well as a decrease in serratus anterior firing during abduction, forward flexion, and scaption in shoulders with anterior instability compared with normal shoulders. Additionally, Kim and colleagues[60] completed an analysis of electromyographic activity of the biceps brachii following traumatic unilateral anterior shoulder instability. Biceps brachii muscle activity was significantly greater in the unstable shoulder than in the opposite shoulder in all positions of abduction with near end-range external rotation. Muscle activity was the greatest at 90 degrees and 120 degrees of abduction with external rotation, suggesting that the biceps muscle plays an active compensatory role in the unstable shoulder in positions of vulnerability.[60]

These studies, in addition to the studies mentioned previously, document the deleterious effect injuries can have on the sensorimotor system's ability to properly sense information and then generate appropriate muscular responses.

Connection between Injury and Neuromuscular Control

The connection between joint injury and neuromuscular control has been described by Lephart and Henry.[29] Joint injury leads to tissue deformation, which causes damage to mechanoreceptors and collagen fibers. The damaged mechanoreceptors result in decreased position sense and proprioceptive deficits that can alter motor response and diminish

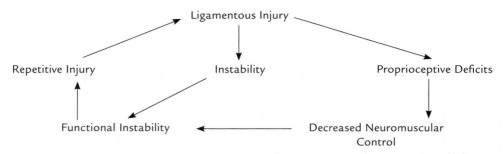

Figure 7-8: Functional stability paradigm depicting the progression of functional instability of the shoulder caused by the interaction between mechanical instability and decreased neuromuscular control. *(Adapted from Lephart SM, Henry TJ: The physiological basis for open and closed kinetic chain rehabilitation for the upper extremity,* J Sport Rehabil *5:71-87, 1996.)*

neuromuscular stabilization. The damaged collagen fibers in the capsule and ligaments result in mechanical instability. This mechanical instability, in conjunction with the decrease in neuromuscular control, results in functional instability of the shoulder and can contribute to a pattern of repetitive injury[29] (Figure 7-8).

SURGICAL MANAGEMENT AND PROPRIOCEPTION

Surgical management for shoulder instability followed by physical therapy has been shown to restore proprioception.[28,37-40,55] Thermal capsulorrhaphy patients tested at least 6 months postoperatively demonstrated normalized kinesthetic and joint position sense.[39,40] Likewise, subjects 6 months postoperative following arthroscopic repair of shoulder instability revealed no significant difference between surgical and contralateral shoulders with active angle replication testing.[37] Kinesthesia testing and passive angle replication testing following open or arthroscopic Bankart repair also demonstrated normalization of proprioception.[38] Zuckerman and colleagues[55] proprioceptively tested 30 patients with unilateral glenohumeral instability at three different phases of recovery: 1 week before surgical correction, 6 months postoperatively, and 12 months postoperatively. These intervals were chosen because a progressive return to full activity usually begins 6 months after surgery and is completed by 1 year.[55] The results revealed significant proprioceptive deficits preoperatively, partial restoration at 6 months, and full restoration at 12 months. These findings further emphasize the importance of continued proprioceptive activities throughout the first year of rehabilitation and recovery.

THEORIES FOR RETURN OF PROPRIOCEPTION FOLLOWING SURGERY

The return of proprioception following surgery may be related to the retensioning of the soft tissue, the rehabilitation program, or both.[37,46,62] Capsular tightness has been suggested as one possible mechanism for shoulder proprio

ception.[46] Retensioning soft tissue may restore proprioception by reestablishing appropriate tension of the joint capsule and ligaments, which contain mechanoreceptors.[37,62] These receptors need to be mechanically deformed or loaded to transmit impulses to the CNS in order to relay information regarding joint position. If tissues are lax, it may be difficult to develop enough tension to activate a neural impulse to the CNS to provoke an appropriate muscular response.[37,62]

The rehabilitation program following surgery may also play a role in the return of proprioception following surgery. It is recommended that most rehabilitation programs incorporate joint position sense activities, dynamic stabilization, and proprioceptive reactive training in order to regain proprioception and dynamic neuromuscular control.* Rhythmic stabilization perturbations, reciprocal isometric contractions for internal and external rotation, rhythmic stabilization with slow reversal holds, axial loading exercises, and plyometric activities are some techniques described to enhance return of proprioceptive function in the shoulder.[29,30,41,43,64,65] Using these techniques postoperatively may be part of the reason that proprioception is restored following surgery. Many of these treatments are described in the following section.

INTERVENTION STRATEGIES

Rehabilitation of the shoulder complex, depending on the particular injury or pathology, goes through a series of many phases with a multitude of recommended interventions (see Chapter 31 on SLAP lesions). The rehabilitation program identifies the specific goals of treatment based on the condition and healing time since the injury. It also outlines a systematic progression through multiple phases incorporating many of the following characteristics: patient education, protecting the area from further injury, decreasing pain, decreasing inflammation, decreasing swelling, increasing ROM, development of motor control of the involved area, improving proprioception/kinesthesia/balance, increasing muscular strength/power/endurance, increasing neuromuscular dynamic stability, and developing functional abilities for return to activity.

---

*References 29, 30, 37, 43, 44, 56, and 63-65.

Coactivation of the dynamic stabilizers (RTC) at the shoulder joint is essential for stability and proper functioning. Dynamically, the glenoid must follow the movement of the humeral head to maintain its instant center of rotation and glenohumeral congruency.[43] Without appropriate neuromuscular control of the scapulothoracic articulation, the RTC will not function around a stable base of support.[43,53] This unstable base of support results in decreased efficiency of the RTC musculature and can impair its ability to provide glenohumeral stability and segmental control of the shoulder. Therefore synergistic control strategies of both the glenohumeral and scapulothoracic joints are essential in providing dynamic stability of the shoulder complex.[43]

The rehabilitation strategies often involve both open kinetic chain (OKC) and closed kinetic chain (CKC) exercises. Previous information in this chapter has shown that injuries to the joint can damage the joint mechanoreceptor system, as well as the surrounding soft tissues. When these structures are injured, the mechanisms responsible for providing neuromuscular static and dynamic stability are disrupted. There is minimal research demonstrating the most effective way to enhance neuromuscular dynamic stability of the shoulder complex. Consequently, this chapter describes various intervention strategies and progressions that can be used to focus on this parameter during the rehabilitation stages.

Traditionally, much of shoulder rehabilitation has incorporated emphasis on OKC exercises and activities. This is appropriate because many functional activities include the use of the upper extremity in the OKC position. Because of specificity of activity, it makes sense to train the shoulder complex based on the functional demands that the patient will be returning to, whether it be activities of daily living (ADLs), vocational requirements, or sports activities. Specificity of rehabilitation in a controlled progressive manner in the clinic in order to prepare for the demands of the functional activities is a mandatory part of the rehabilitation process. OKC exercises have demonstrated their effectiveness in increasing muscular strength, power, and endurance of the shoulder complex.[47]

Over the last decade, there has been an increased awareness in the application of CKC activities for the upper extremity. Previously, CKC activities were primarily reserved for lower extremity rehabilitation programs. Specificity of activities increased our awareness and highlighted the need to incorporate these activities into shoulder rehabilitation programs. Common examples of the upper extremity being used in CKC activities include pushing or pulling objects at work, gymnastics, swimming, blocking in football, and wrestling. Some research has demonstrated that CKC activities for the shoulder complex can enhance dynamic stability and can train the receptors responsible for the static and dynamic stability of the joint.[66] The mechanoreceptors responsible for proprioception and neuromuscular control are maximally stimulated when the joint surfaces are compressed,[30,43,67] which can be accomplished through CKC exercises. If appropriate, the use of CKC exercises during the initial phases in the rehabilitation program can stimulate the mechanoreceptors in the injured joint and thus help restore neuromuscular control.

Closed Kinetic Chain Exercises

Ubinger and colleagues[66] demonstrated that a 4-week upper body CKC training program resulted in improved ability to stabilize the shoulder joint. The results suggest that CKC training can increase the accuracy of joint position sense because of increased stimulation of the mechanoreceptors. Moreover, performing CKC exercises bilaterally is beneficial by increasing stabilization for both extremities. Including the uninjured arm in the CKC exercise program might also cause some carryover to the injured arm throughout the rehabilitation process. There is evidence that training one extremity causes a physiologic overflow to the contralateral untrained extremity.[66,68]

There are many examples of CKC exercises that can be included in the rehabilitation program to enhance the total arm strength concept.[69] Many of these are illustrated as examples of CKC exercises that can be performed during different phases of the rehabilitation program to develop the muscular co-contractions and neuromuscular dynamic stability.

Open Kinetic Chain Exercises

Davies and Dickoff-Hoffman[43] were among the first to describe the clinical applications and use of rhythmic stabilization/perturbation training exercises on a regular basis in the rehabilitation program of various upper extremity injuries. There are numerous OKC exercises, with specific examples and progressions, to be outlined in the different phases of the rehabilitation program.

FUNCTIONAL REHABILITATION

Functional rehabilitation is preparing the patient to return to his or her previous level of function (ADLs, vocational activities, or competitive sports) with no residual functional limitations and prevention of recurrence of injury. Functional rehabilitation restores the proprioception/kinesthesia and resultant neuromuscular dynamic control. Functional rehabilitation is believed to increase the sensitivity of peripheral afferents present in both the capsuloligamentous and musculotendinous structures, facilitate coactivation of the force couples, elicit preparatory and reactive muscle contractions, and increase muscle stiffness.[70] The terminal stages of the rehabilitation program should replicate the demands placed on the shoulder joint during the functional activities.

Sackett and colleagues[71] described evidence-based practice considering the following: (1) patient values; (2) best research evidence available; and (3) clinical experience, education, and expertise. The following rehabilitation program focuses on a whole-part-whole program. Consequently, based on the limited scientific evidence available, review of clinical journals, and empirically based clinical experiences, the following four-stage shoulder neuromuscular dynamic stabilization program is recommended:

- Stage I: proprioception and kinesthesia phase (baseline dynamic stability)
- Stage II: neuromuscular control phase
- Stage III: dynamic neuromuscular stabilization phase
- Stage IV: functional movements and return to activities

Stage I: Proprioception and Kinesthesia Phase (Baseline Dynamic Stability)

Goals

- **Diminish pain and inflammation.**

It is important to decrease pain and inflammation to prevent reflex dissociation, which distorts the normal afferent and efferent pathways.

- **Normalize arthrokinematics and restore range of motion.**

This is critical for the joint mechanoreceptors to receive normal sensory input. If there is ligamentous/capsular hypomobility, the deformation of the mechanoreceptors occurs with an altered pattern and consequently leads to abnormal motor patterns. Using a methodical approach to treating shoulder hypomobility is recommended for restoration of the normal joint arthrokinematics.[72] It is more difficult to treat joint hypermobility, which also alters the input to the joint receptors. Using braces or tape is one method, but there is limited research demonstrating the efficacy of these procedures. Dynamic neuromuscular control is another method to treat hypermobility and is the focus of this chapter. Finally, surgical stabilization procedures may be required to eliminate the functional instability.

- **Restore proprioception and kinesthesia.**

Reestablishing afferent pathways from the mechanoreceptors at the injured joint to the CNS and to facilitate supplementary afferent pathways as a compensatory mechanism for proprioceptive deficits is a goal of the rehabilitation program.[14] Early training of conscious awareness of proprioception is believed to eventually lead to unconscious awareness. Because the risk of injury aggravation with proprioception training is low, both kinesthesia and joint position sense training can be initiated early in rehabilitation.[70]

Proprioception training can be performed by including a variety of different exercises to stimulate the joint receptors. One example is angular joint replications using both active and passive repositioning exercises (Figure 7-9). The passive repositioning exercises primarily target the joint capsule/

ligament mechanoreceptors. The positions in the range of motion should be varied from the mid-ROM to the end-ROM. The end-ROM positions also deform the joint mechanoreceptors and provide stimulation for developing the neural pathways. Moreover, it is also important to have the patient perform active angular replication exercises so the patient has to use volitional muscle contractions. In some cases, active muscle contraction may be contraindicated because of pain and soft tissue healing restraints. If indicated, these exercises are initially performed in the mid-ROM because the musculotendinous unit is the most active in these positions. Commonly, OKC submaximal mid-ROM perturbation training is performed (Figure 7-10). Ultimately, the patient progresses to replicating the specific movement patterns used in the functional activities. Additionally, the joint position training can be performed in both OKC and CKC positions (Figure 7-11). Another example of progressing the difficulty of these exercises is to go from eyes open to eyes closed to eliminate visual input.

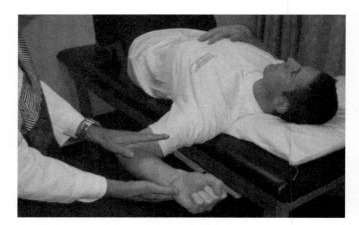

Figure 7-9: OKC angular joint replications.

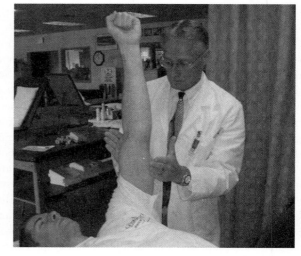

Figure 7-10: OKC submaximal mid-ROM rhythmic stabilization (perturbation).

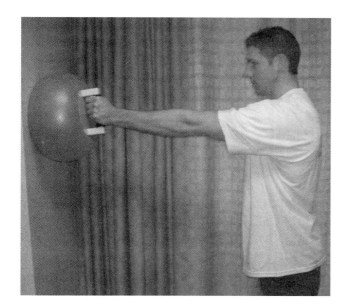

Figure 7-11: CKC wall circles.

Kinesthetic training, TTDPM, can be performed by having the patient indicate when joint motion is sensed. This can be performed using different instrumentation, but from a practical standpoint in a busy clinic, it is commonly performed with manual motions. With eyes closed to eliminate visual clues, the patient is requested to indicate as quickly as possible when he or she perceives movement of the shoulder (Figure 7-12).

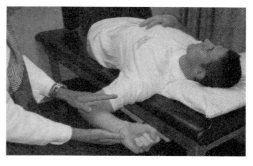

Figure 7-12: OKC manual kinesthetic training for threshold to the detection of passive movement.

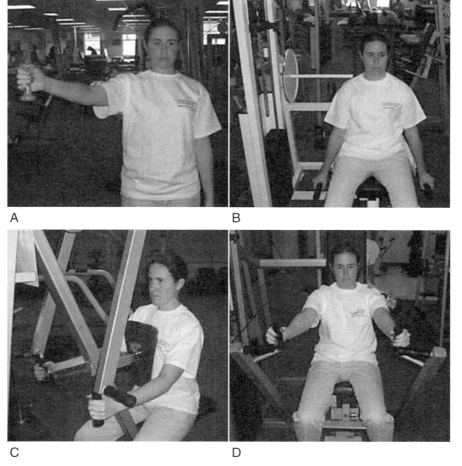

Figure 7-13: Four Moseley scapulothoracic exercises. **A**, Scaption with thumb up (superset) with **B**, press down. **C**, Rowing (neutral grip) (superset) with **D**, bench press (neutral grip).

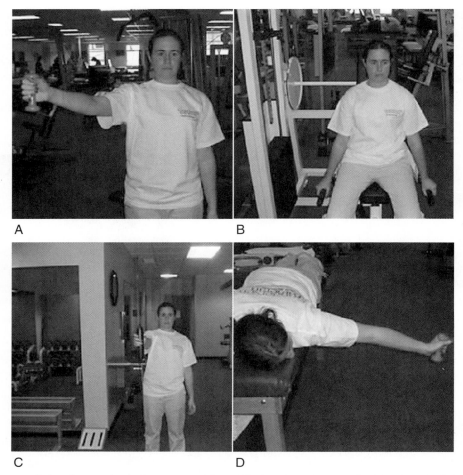

Figure 7-14: Four Townsend glenohumeral exercises. **A,** Scaption with thumb up (superset) with **B,** press-down. **C,** Flexion with thumb up (superset) with **D,** external rotation with horizontal extension.

- **Restore muscle balance of shoulder complex, core, and total kinetic chain.**

For clinical efficiency, the scapulothoracic exercises recommended by Moseley and colleagues[73] (Figure 7-13) and the glenohumeral exercises recommended by Townsend and colleagues[74] (Figure 7-14) can be used. Total arm strength exercises for the biceps and triceps are also included.[69] All of these exercises are performed in a super-set format; agonist muscle exercises are followed by antagonist muscle exercises. Using super-sets is efficient, saves time in the clinic, and helps maintain muscle balance. Based on a recent meta-analysis of the literature,[75] one set of 10 repetitions for untrained patients early in the rehabilitation program is recommended because it is as effective as three sets of 10 repetitions. After 4 to 6 weeks, sets need to be increased. If the patient is a trained subject, three sets of 10 repetitions are recommended to create a muscular training response. Developing normal muscle function for the muscular dynamic stability of the shoulder complex is an important component of the total rehabilitation program.

To focus on the RTC muscles, strengthening exercises are initially performed in the 30/30/30 position (Figure 7-15).

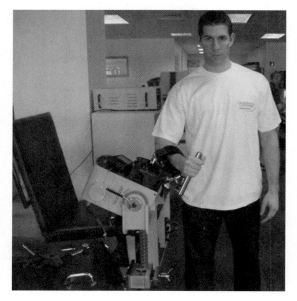

Figure 7-15: 30/30/30 isokinetic exercises.

The first 30 degrees is glenohumeral abduction to prevent the "wringing out effect" of the microcirculation of the supraspinatus tendon. The second 30 degrees is the scaption position. This is the functional arc of motion of the shoulder complex; it protects the anterior shoulder joint and pre-stretches the posterior RTC muscles. The third 30 degrees is a diagonal angle because it places the lower rotator cuff muscle fibers in a direct line of pull to enhance this muscle's ability to develop force and is inherently more comfortable for the patient.[43]

Davies' exercise progression[76] forms the foundation of the exercise program. The exercise progression continuum goes through the following stages:

1. Submaximal-intensity, pain-free, multiple-angle isometrics
2. Maximal-intensity, multiple-angle isometrics
3. Submaximal-intensity, short-arc exercises

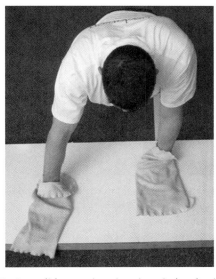

Figure 7-16: Euroglide exercises (tracing circles, horizontal motion, flexion motions).

4. Maximal-intensity, short-arc exercises
5. Full-ROM, submaximal-intensity exercises
6. Full-ROM, maximal-intensity exercises

As the patient progresses through the various stages of the rehabilitation program, the exercises are concurrently progressed to increasing difficulty.

Stage II: Neuromuscular Control Phase

Goals

- **Maintain normalized arthrokinematics and joint range of motion.**
- **Maintain muscle balance of shoulder complex, core, and total kinetic chain.**
- **Maintain proprioception and kinesthesia.**
- **Develop neuromuscular proactive control.**

Besides the obvious muscle contractions providing compressive forces of the glenohumeral joint with resultant osseous stability, the forces likewise tension the capsuloligamentous structures, increasing the neural stability via the joint mechanoreceptors.

It is commonly thought that using CKC exercises creates a co-contraction of the surrounding muscles, creating the force couples commonly seen in shoulder function. Henry and colleagues[77] demonstrated that push-ups and three slide board exercises (tracing circles, horizontal motion, and flexion motion) produced coactivation of the force couples around the shoulder complex (Figure 7-16). Other examples include CKC quadruped position on Swiss ball (Figure 7-17) and CKC tripod position on tilt board (Figure 7-18). Subsequently, CKC exercises are indicated to create the coactivation of muscles for neuromuscular proactive control. Ubinger and colleagues[66] demonstrated that a 4-week CKC training program improved one's ability to remain stable by using the neuromuscular control mechanisms in the joints. The results suggest that CKC training can increase the accuracy of joint position sense because of increased

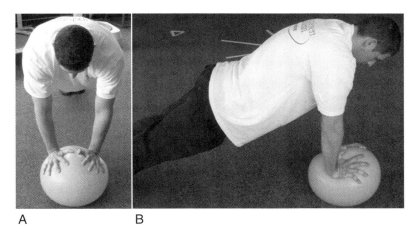

A   B

Figure 7-17: CKC quadruped position using Swiss ball.

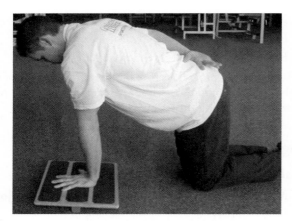

Figure 7-18: CKC tripod position using tilt board.

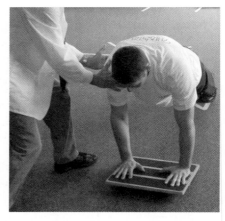

Figure 7-20: CKC tilt board training with superimposed perturbation exercises.

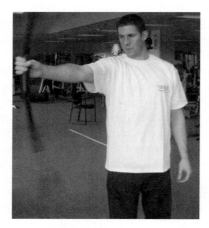

Figure 7-19: Body Blade.

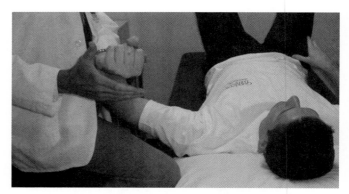

Figure 7-21: Reactive maximal perturbation training in OKC provocative position (90/90).

stimulation of the mechanoreceptors. There is a need for more scientific, prospective, randomized, controlled clinical trial studies to add scientific efficacy to the treatment of neuromuscular deficiency.

- **Restore dynamic functional stability.**

Additional examples to incorporate functional stability exercises include use of the Body Blade (Figure 7-19), as well as CKC tilt board training with perturbations superimposed (Figure 7-20).

Stage III: Dynamic Stabilization Phase

Goals

- **Maintain muscle balance of shoulder complex, core, and total kinetic chain.**
- **Maintain proprioception and kinesthesia.**
- **Develop neuromuscular reactive control.**

One of the goals during this stage of the training program is to get the muscles firing quickly in a "reactive" manner. Consequently, when perturbation training is performed, it is performed in a random pattern so the patient must react to the perturbation (Figures 7-21 and 7-22). This helps develop synergistic co-contraction of the muscles in a reactive pattern to create muscle stiffness and provide dynamic control of the shoulder joint. Furthermore, this synergistic coactivation of the glenohumeral and scapulothoracic force couples provides neuromuscular reactive control of the shoulder complex, which is similar to most functional activities. Additionally, these reactive responses stimulate the unconscious reflexive patterns that are necessary for successful return to activities.

- **Maintain dynamic functional stability.**

Plyometric exercises are important to incorporate into a rehabilitation program because of their functional movement patterns. Many activities in ADLs and sports rely on the

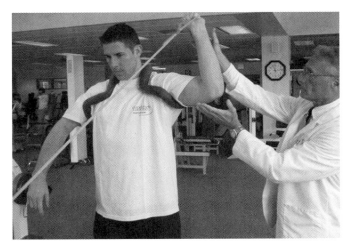

Figure 7-22: Reactive maximal perturbation training progressing to functional 90/90 position/shoulder horn/using surgical tubing (for external rotation strengthening to create a posterior dominant shoulder).

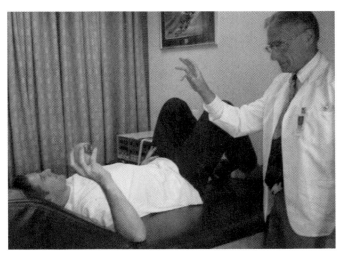

Figure 7-23: Plyometrics.

plyometric (stretch-shorten cycle) to occur. Plyometric exercise incorporates a stretch-shorten cycle in which a prestretch to the series and parallel elastic components and the muscle spindles results in facilitation to the resultant muscle contraction. The stored potential kinetic energy of the prestretch is transferred to help generate a forceful concentric contraction. Plyometrics include three phases: (1) prestretch/preparatory phase, (2) amortization phase, and (3) shortening/concentric power production phase. The key to plyometrics is to keep the amortization phase as short as possible to utilize the stored potential kinetic energy, enhancing the concentric power phase.

Numerous benefits of plyometrics have been described; however, there are limited studies on plyometrics and their application to shoulder rehabilitation.[78-83] The rationale and beneficial reasons for incorporating plyometrics include the following: replicates functional movement patterns such as pitching, reproduces the eccentric-concentric muscular contractions, creates neural adaptations, desensitizes the GTOs, increases muscle spindle gamma bias, increases muscle stiffness, increases muscle power, and enhances performance (Figure 7-23). Fortun and colleagues[79] demonstrated the effectiveness of plyometric training with trained subjects in increasing shoulder external rotation ROM, increasing shoulder power, and improving a functional throwing test.

Schulte-Edelmann and colleagues[83] demonstrated the effectiveness of a novel form of plyometrics ("retro-plyometrics"), which increased the power of the triceps muscles. The triceps contribute to the velocity of the ball when throwing. Additionally, the retro-plyometrics help with conditioning the eccentric deceleration response of the posterior RTC muscles.

- **Improve muscular strength, power, and endurance.**

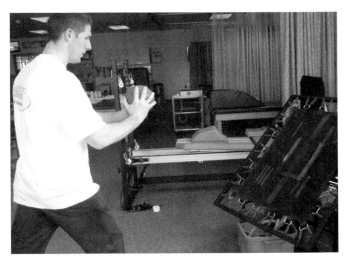

Figure 7-24: Plyoback (rebounder plyometrics).

Stage IV: Functional Movements and Activities

Goals

- **Maintain balance of shoulder complex, core, and total kinetic chain.**

- **Maintain neuromuscular gains and improve performance.**

In the terminal phases of the rehabilitation program, the key is to integrate the exercises back into the functional patterns, such as rebounder plyometrics (Figure 7-24), manual Diagonal 2—Proprioceptive Neuromuscular Facilitation (D2 PNF) exercises (Figure 7-25), and sport-specific activities

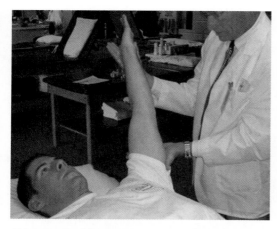

Figure 7-25: Manual Diagonal 2—Proprioceptive Neuromuscular Facilitation exercises.

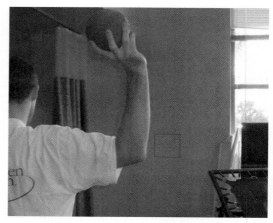

Figure 7-26: Gradual return to activities (e.g., throwing).

(Figure 7-26). Most of the previous components have worked on isolated activation, but now things are integrated back into synergistic function. During this stage, the focus is on specificity of rehabilitation.

CAN SHOULDER INJURIES BE PREVENTED?

A large majority of shoulder injuries occur very rapidly and are traumatic in nature. A load that is greater than the shoulder's static or dynamic restraints will result in injury (i.e., traumatic dislocations). These types of injuries probably are not preventable. However, subtle injuries such as repetitive microtrauma (i.e., impingement) may provide an avenue for prevention.

Fatigue is believed to affect proprioception and neuromuscular control.[14,33,36,41,84] Voight and colleagues[33] examined the effects of muscle fatigue and its relationship with shoulder proprioception. Their data suggest that proprioception acuity was greatest with prefatigue active repositioning. Conversely, the acuity was significantly decreased in the presence of muscle fatigue.[33] This proprioceptive acuity supported the important role of the muscle receptors in the glenohumeral joint.[30,33] Implications of this research are important from a program design standpoint; consequently, the emphasis on endurance training is applied to the shoulder complex.

Knowing that muscle fatigue affects proprioception, some injuries may be preventable by emphasizing muscle endurance exercises in home exercise and rehabilitation programs. Most activities performed during work and daily living involve muscular endurance. A classic example seen regularly in the clinic is shoulder impingement/tendinosus in the overhead worker. Perhaps muscle fatigue leading to decreased proprioceptive feedback was the primary cause of this patient's pathology. If an individual's ability to recognize joint position is altered, especially in a position of vulnerability, he or she may be prone to increased mechanical stress placed on both the static and dynamic structures responsible for joint stability.[14]

Fatigue has also been shown to increase ligamentous laxity that occurs with exercise.[14,85,86] Capsuloligamentous structures increase in tension when the joint approaches the limit of movement in different directions.[6] This increased laxity may desensitize the mechanoreceptors present within the glenohumeral ligaments, leading to altered proprioceptive shoulder function. We have observed clinically that strengthening and proprioceptive training at end-ranges have accelerated our patients in returning to activity. Moreover, the patient's ability to contract the muscles quickly to attempt to stabilize the joint during functional activities is critical to prevent impairments. In an outcome study, Manske and Davies[87] demonstrated the importance of isokinetic testing of the shoulder and looking for muscle power production. Torque acceleration energy (TAE) was measured in a heterogeneous group of patients with shoulder-related problems. After completing a rehabilitation program incorporating many of the aforementioned activities, the patients normalized the TAE deficits compared with the uninvolved side.

Perhaps applying many of these similar principles of exercise may have a greater importance for preventive measures. Can shoulder injuries be prevented? The answer remains complex. Currently, no definitive conclusions can be drawn because the exact mechanism leading to diminished neuromuscular control and the epidemiology of these injuries are yet to be established. Further research in this area is warranted.

SUMMARY

This chapter describes the neuromuscular system and its importance in rehabilitation following shoulder injury or surgery. Although there is limited research on the best method of increasing the neuromuscular dynamic stability of the shoulder complex, it probably requires a multimodal approach in a progressively staged format as described here. As described by Sackett and colleagues,[71] one part of evidence-based practice is clinical experience, education, and expertise when there is no best research available. Empirically based clinical experiences for over 30 years (of the senior author) using the methods and techniques described in this chapter have been successful with thousands of patients with shoulder-related conditions.

Specific assessment techniques are identified, as well as the effects of injury on proprioception and neuromuscular control. A four-stage rehabilitation program is presented, complete with goals and possible treatment interventions. The chapter concludes with a brief discussion of theories for injury prevention.

References

1. Jobe CM: Gross anatomy of the shoulder. In Rockwood CA Jr, Matsen FA III, editors: *The shoulder,* Philadelphia, 1990, Saunders.

2. Ernlund LS, Warner JJP: Gross anatomy of the shoulder: bony geometry, static and dynamic restraints, sensory and motor innervation. In Lephart SM, Fu FH, editors: *Proprioception and neuromuscular control in joint stability,* Champaign, IL, 2000, Human Kinetics.

3. Nyland JA, Caborn DNM, Johnson DL: The human glenohumeral joint: a proprioceptive and stability alliance, *Knee Surg Sports Traumatol Arthrosc* 6:50-61, 1998.

4. Boardman ND, Fu FH: Shoulder biomechanics. In McGinty JB, Caspari RB, Jackson RW, Poehling GG, editors: *Operative arthroscopy,* Philadelphia, 1996, Lippincott-Raven.

5. Bigliani LU, Kelkar R, Flatow EL, et al: Glenohumeral stability: biomechanical properties of passive and active stabilizers, *Clin Orthop* 330:13-30, 1996.

6. Janwantanakul P, Magarey ME, Jones MA, et al: Variation in shoulder position sense at mid and extreme range of motion, *Arch Phys Med Rehabil* 82:840-844, 2000.

7. Lee SB, Kim KJ, O'Driscoll SW, et al: Dynamic glenohumeral stability provided by the rotator cuff muscles in the mid-range and end-range of motion, *J Bone Joint Surg* 82(6):849-857, 2000.

8. Clarke J, Sidles JA, Matsen FA: The relationship of the glenohumeral joint capsule to the rotator cuff, *Clin Orthop* 254:29-34, 1990.

9. Warner JP, Caborn DNM, Berger R, et al: Dynamic capsuloligamentous anatomy of the glenohumeral joint, *J Shoulder Elbow Surg* 2:115-133, 1993.

10. Williams GN, Chmielewski T, Rudolph KS, et al: Dynamic knee stability: current theory and implications for clinicians and scientists, *J Orthop Sports Phys Ther* 31:546-566, 2000.

11. Lephart SM, Reimann BL, Fu FH: Introduction to the sensorimotor system. In Lephart SM, Fu FH, editors: *Proprioception and neuromuscular control in joint stability,* Champaign, IL, 2000, Human Kinetics.

12. Riemann BL, Lephart SM: The sensorimotor system part II: the role of proprioception in motor control and functional joint stability, *J Athl Train* 37(1):80-84, 2002.

13. Pavlov IP: *Conditioned reflexes,* London, 1927, Clarendon Press.

14. Myers JB, Lephart SM: The role of the sensorimotor system in the athletic shoulder, *J Athl Train* 35(3):357-363, 2000.

15. Riemann BL, Lephart SM: The sensorimotor system part I: the physiologic basis of functional joint stability, *J Athl Train* 37(1):71-79, 2002.

16. Myers JB, Lephart SM: Sensorimotor deficits contributing to glenohumeral instability, *Clin Orthop* 400:98-104, 2002.

17. Biedert RM: Contribution of the three levels of nervous system motor control: spinal cord, lower brain, cerebral cortex. In Lephart SM, Fu FH, editors: *Proprioception and neuromuscular control in joint stability,* Champaign, IL, 2000, Human Kinetics.

18. Hogervorst T, Brand R: Current concepts review: mechanoreceptors in joint function, *J Bone Joint Surg* 80(9):1365-1378, 1998.

19. Edin BB, Johansson N: Skin strain patterns provide kinesthetic information to the human central nervous system, *J Physiol* 487:243-251, 1995.

20. Goodwin GM, McCloskey DI, Matthews PBC: The persistence of appreciable kinesthesia after paralyzing joint afferents but preserving muscle afferents, *Brain Res* 37:326-329, 1972.

21. Zuckerman JD, Gallagher MA, Lehman C, et al: Normal shoulder proprioception and the effect of lidocaine injection, *J Shoulder Elbow Surg* 8:11-16, 1999.

22. Chu JC, Kane EF, Arnold BL, et al: The effect of a neoprene shoulder stabilizer on active joint-repositioning in subjects with stable and unstable shoulders, *J Athl Train* 37(2):141-145, 2002.

23. McNair PJ, Stanley SN, Strauss GR: Knee bracing effects on proprioception, *Arch Phys Med Rehabil* 77:287-289, 1996.

24. Perlau R, Frank C, Fick G: The effect of elastic bandages on human knee proprioception in the uninjured population, *Am J Sports Med* 23:251-255, 1995.

25. Ghez C: The control of movement. In Kandel ER, Schwartz JH, Jessell TM, editors: *Principles of neural science,* ed 3, New York, 1991, Elsevier Science.

26. Schmidt R, Lee T: *Motor control and learning: a behavioral emphasis,* ed 3, Champaign, IL, 1999, Human Kinetics.

27. Dye SF: Functional anatomy of the cerebellum. In Lephart SM, Fu FH, editors: *Proprioception and neuromuscular control in joint stability,* Champaign, IL, 2000, Human Kinetics.

28. Lephart SM, Warner JJP, Borsa PA, et al: Proprioception of the shoulder joint in healthy, unstable, and surgically repaired shoulder, *J Shoulder Elbow Surg* 3:371-380, 1994.

29. Lephart SM, Henry TJ: The physiological basis for open and closed kinetic chain rehabilitation for the upper extremity, *J Sport Rehabil* 5:71-87, 1996.

30. Borsa PA, Lephart SM, Kocher MS, et al: Functional assessment and rehabilitation of shoulder proprioception for glenohumeral instability, *J Sport Rehabil* 3:84-108, 1994.

31. Riemann BL, Myers JB, Lephart SM: Sensorimotor system measurement techniques, *J Athl Train* 37(1):85-98, 2002.

32. Bradley JP, Tibone JE: Electromyographical analysis of muscle action about the shoulder, *Clin J Sports Med* 10:789-805, 1991.

33. Voight ML, Hardin JA, Blackburn TA, et al: The effects of muscle fatigue and the relationship of arm dominance to shoulder proprioception, *J Orthop Sports Phys Ther* 23(6):348-352, 1996.

34. Dover G, Powers ME: Reliability of joint position sense and force reproduction measures during internal and external rotation of the shoulder, *J Athl Train* 38(4):304-310, 2003.

35. Dover GC, Kaminski TW, Meister K et al: Assessment of shoulder proprioception in the female softball athlete, *Am J Sports Med* 31(3):431-437, 2003.

36. Carpenter JE, Blasier RB, Pellizzon GG: The effects of muscle fatigue on shoulder joint position sense, *Am J Sports Med* 26(2):262-265, 1998.

37. Aydin T, Yildiz Y, Yamis I, et al: Shoulder proprioception: a comparison between the shoulder joint in healthy and surgically repaired shoulders, *Arch Orthop Trauma Surg* 121:422-425, 2001.

38. Warner JP, Lephart S, Fu F: Role of proprioception in pathoetiology of shoulder instability, *Clin Orthop* 330:35-39, 1996.

39. Lephart SM, Myers JB, Bradley JP, et al: Shoulder proprioception and function following thermal capsulorrhaphy, *Arthroscopy* 18(7):770-778, 2002.

40. Myers JB, Lephart SM, Riemann BL, et al: Evaluation of shoulder proprioception following thermal capsulorrhaphy, *Med Sci Sports Exerc* 32:123, 2000.

41. Davies GJ, Lawson K, Jones B: The acute effects of fatigue on shoulder rotator cuff internal/external rotation kinesthesia, *Phys Ther* 78(5):87, 1993.

42. Davies GJ, Giangarra C: Open anteriocapsulolabral reconstruction in overhead athletes. In DeCarlo M, editor: *Current Topics in Musculoskeletal Medicine: A Case Study Approach.* Thorofare, NJ, 2001, Slack, Inc.

43. Davies GJ, Dickoff-Hoffman S: Neuromuscular testing and rehabilitation of the shoulder complex, *J Orthop Sports Phys Ther* 18(2):449-458, 1993.

44. Safron MR, Borsa PA, Lephart SM, et al: Shoulder proprioception in baseball pitchers, *J Shoulder Elbow Surg* 10(5):438-444, 2001.

45. Allegrucci M, Whitney SL, Lephart SM, et al: Shoulder kinesthesia in healthy unilateral athletes participating in upper extremity sports, *J Orthop Sports Phys Ther* 21(4):220-226, 1995.

46. Blasier RB, Carpenter JE, Huston LJ: Shoulder proprioception effects of joint laxity, joint position, and direction of motion, *Orthop Rev* 23(1):45-50, 1994.

47. Davies GJ, Ellenbecker TS: Application of isokinetics in testing and rehabilitation. In Andrews, Harrelson, Wilk, editors: *Physical rehabilitation of the injured athlete*, ed 2, Philadelphia, 1998, Saunders.

48. Kibler BW: The role of the scapula in athletic shoulder function, *Am J Sports Med* 26(2):325-337, 1998.

49. Gibson MH, Goebel GV, Jordan TM, et al: A reliability study of measurement techniques to determine static scapular positions, *J Orthop Sports Phys Ther* 21:100-106, 1995.

50. Odom CJ, Taylor AB, Hurd CE, et al: Measurement of scapular asymmetry and assessment of shoulder dysfunction using the lateral scapular slide test: a reliability and validity study, *Phys Ther* 81(2):799-809, 2001.

51. Koslow PA, Prosser CA, Suchicki SL, et al: Specificity of the lateral scapular slide test in asymptomatic athletes, *J Orthop Sports Phys Ther* 33(6):331-336, 2003.

52. Goldbeck TG, Davies GJ: Test-retest reliability of the closed kinetic chain upper extremity stability test: a clinical field test, *J Sport Rehabil* 9(1):35-45, 2000.

53. Smith RL, Brunolli J: Shoulder kinesthesia after anterior glenohumeral joint dislocations, *Phys Ther* 69:106-112, 1989.

54. Lephart SM, Kocher MS, Fu FH, et al: Proprioception following ACL reconstruction, *J Sport Rehabil* 1(3):188-196, 1992.

55. Zuckerman JD, Gallagher MA, Cuoma F, et al: The effect of instability and subsequent anterior shoulder repair on proprioceptive ability, *J Shoulder Elbow Surg* 12:105-109, 2003.

56. Glousmann R, Jobe FW, Tibone JE, et al: Dynamic electromyographic analysis of the throwing shoulder with glenohumeral instability, *J Bone Joint Surg* 70A:220-226, 1988.

57. Machner A, Merk H, Becker R, et al: Kinesthetic sense of the shoulder in patients with impingement syndrome, *Acta Orthop Scand* 74(1):85-88, 2003.

58. Kronberg M, Brostrom LA, Nemeth G: Differences in shoulder muscle activity between patients with generalized joint laxity and normal controls, *Clin Orthop* 269:181-192, 1991.

59. McMahon PJ, Jobe FW, Pink MM, et al: Comparative electromyographic analysis of shoulder muscles during planer motions: anterior glenohumeral instability vs normal, *J Shoulder Elbow Surg* 5:118-123, 1996.

60. Kim SH, Ha KI, Kim HS, et al: Electromyographic activity of the biceps brachi muscle in shoulders with anterior instability, *Arthroscopy* 17(8):864-868, 2001.

61. Quincy R, Davies GJ, Kolbeck K, et al: Isokinetic exercise: the effect of training specificity on shoulder torque, *J Athl Train* 35:S-64, 2000.

62. Lephart SM, Pincivero DM, Giraldo JL, et al: The role of proprioception in the management and rehabilitation of athletic injuries, *Am J Sports Med* 25(1):130-137, 1997.

63. Wilk KE, Arrigo CA, Andrews JR: Current concepts: the stabilizing structures of the glenohumeral joint, *J Orthop Sports Phys Ther* 25(1):362-378, 1997.

64. Wilk KE, Meister K, Andrews JR: Current concepts in the rehabilitation of the overhead throwing athlete, *Am J Sports Med* 30(1):136-151, 2002.

65. Dines DM, Levinson M: The conservative management of the unstable shoulder including rehabilitation, *Clin Sports Med* 14(4):797-816, 1995.

66. Ubinger ME, Prentice WE, Guskiewicz KM: Effect of closed kinetic chain training on neuromuscular control in the upper extremity, *J Sport Rehabil* 8:184-194, 1999.

67. Ellenbecker TS, Davies GJ: *Closed kinetic chain exercise: a comprehensive guide to multiple joint exercise*, Champaign, IL, 2001, Human Kinetics.

68. Arai M, Shimizu H, Shimizu ME, et al: Effects of the use of cross-education to the affected side through various resisted exercises of the sound side and settings of the length of the affected muscles, *Hiroshima J Med Soc* 50:65-73, 2001.

69. Davies GJ, Ellenbecker TS: Total arm strength for shoulder and elbow overuse injuries. In Timm K, editor: *Home study course*, LaCrosse, WI, 1993, Orthopaedic Section of American Physical Therapy Association.

70. Swanik CB, Lephart SM, Giannantonio FP, et al: Reestablishing proprioception and neuromuscular control in the ACL-injured athlete, *J Sport Rehabil* 6:182-206, 1997.

71. Sackett DL, Rosenberg WMC, Gray JAM, et al: Evidence based medicine: what it is and what it isn't, *BMJ* 312:71-72, 1996.

72. Davies GJ, Ellenbecker TS: Focused exercise aids shoulder hypomobility, *Biomechanics* 6:77-81, 1999.

73. Moseley JB, Jobe FW, Pink M, et al: EMG analysis of the scapular muscles during a shoulder rehabilitation program, *Am J Sports Med* 20:128-134, 1992.

74. Townsend H, Jobe FW, Pink M, et al: Electromyographic analysis of the glenohumeral muscles during a baseball rehabilitation program, *Am J Sports Med* 19:264-272, 1991.

75. Wolfe BL, Le Mura LM, Cole PJ: Quantitative analysis of single vs multiple-set programs in resistance training, *J Strength Cond Res* 18:35-47, 2004.

76. Davies GJ: *A compendium of isokinetics in clinical usage and rehabilitation techniques*, ed 4, Onalaska, WI, 1992, S&S Publishers.

77. Henry TJ, Lephart SM, Stone D, et al: An electromyographic analysis of dynamic stabilization exercises for the shoulder, *J Athl Train* 33:S14, 1998.

78. Heiderscheit B, Palmer-McLean K, Davies GJ, et al: The effects of isokinetics versus plyometric training of the shoulder internal rotators, *J Orthop Sports Phys Ther* 23:125-133, 1996.

79. Fortun C, Davies GJ, Kernozek TW: The effects of plyometric training on the internal rotators of the shoulder, *Phys Ther* 78:S87, 1998.

80. Davies GJ, Matheson JW: Shoulder plyometrics, *Sports Med Arthrosc Rev* 9:1-18, 2001.

81. Davies GJ, Ellenbecker TS, Briddell D: Upper extremity plyometrics as a key to functional shoulder rehabilitation and performance enhancement, *Biomechanics* 9:18-28, 2002.

82. Swanik KA, Lephart SM, Swanik B, et al: The effects of shoulder plyometric training on proprioception and selected muscle performance characteristics, *J Shoulder Elbow Surg* 11:579-586, 2002.

83. Schulte-Edelmann JA, Davies GJ, Kernozek TW, et al: The effects of plyometric training of the posterior shoulder and elbow, *J Strength Cond Res* 19(1):129-134, 2005.

84. Myers JB, Buskiewicz KM, Schneider RA, et al: Proprioception and neuromuscular control of the shoulder after muscle fatigue, *J Athl Train* 34:362-367, 1999.

85. Skinner HB, Wyatt MP, Stone ML, et al: Exercise-related knee joint laxity, *Am J Sports Med* 14:30-34, 1986.

86. Grana WA, Muse G: The effect of exercise on laxity in the anterior cruciate ligament deficient knee, *Am J Sports Med* 16:586-588, 1988.

87. Manske RC, Davies GJ: Postrehabilitation outcomes of muscle power (torque acceleration energy) in patients with selected shoulder dysfunctions, *J Sport Rehabil* 12:181-198, 2003.

Knee Ligament Injuries

CHAPTER 8

Reconstruction Using Ipsilateral Patellar Tendon Autograft

Robert E. Mangine, MEd, PT, ATC

Stephen J. Minning, MPT

Marsha Eifert-Mangine, EdD(c), PT, ATC

W. Bays Gibson, MPT

Angelo J. Colosimo, MD

CHAPTER OUTLINE

NO STRUCTURE IN SPORTS MEDICINE

literature has received as much attention as the anterior cruciate ligament (ACL). From the first attempt to surgically correct the anatomic integrity of the ligament in 1898 by Mayo Robards to today, the fascination with its function is precedent setting.[1] Rehabilitation protocols for the ACL patient have evolved in the literature, encompassing programs from both a conservative nature as well as more accelerated pathways.[2,3] As Frank[4] states, "It is generally acknowledged that rehabilitation is critical to the success of the treatment of the anterior cruciate ligament." The current trend in rehabilitation is to establish pathways according to evidence-based principles; these attempt to provide us with a defined pathway. However, patient variability leads to failure because outlying patient models go unrecognized; this increases our failure rate secondary to arthrofibrosis versus redevelopment of joint laxity.

The evolution of the ACL in terms of the existing methods for surgical intervention has taken many twists and turns in the last quarter century. Although the initial trial of surgical intervention is over 100 years old, anatomic and mechanical studies since the 1970s have refined the procedure to significantly improve the outcome.[5-7] Simultaneous with the advancement of surgical technique was the scientific rationale of the rehabilitation pathway. Because of the wide variance in surgical procedures, the rehabilitation specialist is required to manipulate protocols to match the given surgery. These concepts fueled the development of a model for protocol design based on evaluation methods; this has produced rehabilitation techniques resulting in sufficient latitude to adjust for patient variance.

In 1990 the senior author of this chapter undertook a process to identify key elements of postsurgical ACL rehabilitation and to strengthen the techniques used by providing a scientific foundation.[2,8,9] The development of a consensus panel composed of rehabilitation specialists explored the various facets of the rehabilitation process and provided evidence. The effort culminated in the published works identified as *evaluation-based rehabilitation*. This chapter both explores and outlines a postsurgical management algorithm based on this format, which heightens the reader's success in this patient population. The therapist must evaluate the following areas: joint mechanics, surgical techniques, soft tissue response, muscle function, articular cartilage function, joint neurology, and psychologic factors.

HISTORICAL EVOLUTION OF POSTSURGICAL REHABILITATION

Just as surgical intervention has evolved, so too has the rehabilitation process. In the 1960s most postsurgical programs were designed with the foundation based on classic healing models, identifying initial healing in a 3- to 4-week period. ACL patients were placed in a cast for a short-term period, after which the patients were pushed to resume normal activity in an 8- to 10-week period. Studies in the 1970s demonstrated that intraarticular graft models did not follow traditional healing models, but required a prolonged period for full maturation; this development became known as the *ligamentization process*.[7,10] Rehabilitation in this era was based on the slow response of the graft to revascularize and form mature collagen. The result of these studies translated into prolonged periods of casting, beginning initially for 12 weeks and then dwindling to 6 weeks. Weight bearing also required an extended period of restriction for upward of 14 weeks. The long-term sequelae of this process resulted in significant complications and led to new models of research to improve rehabilitation outcomes and decrease morbidity to the joint. In the 1980s the trend changed yet again, this time doing away with casting entirely, while incorporating early continuous passive motion. In the 1970s and 1980s a great deal of work was performed that analyzed the effect of motion on the traumatized joint without deleterious side effects.[8,11-15]

The intent of this chapter is to describe a protocol designed to account for the wide variance of ACL graft selection because there is no conventional standard procedure. Attempts to define the ideal graft over the last 20 years have evolved to the current trend, which supplies the surgeon with several options. The three most popular methods involve the patellar tendon, the hamstring, or a variety of allograft tissues[16-18] (Figure 8-1). When working with past patients, the senior author has had the opportunity to rehabilitate patients with the aforementioned grafts, as well as using Gore-Tex, carbon-fiber, and ligament augmentation devices. In most cases, long-term outcome did not demonstrate an improved joint stability or changes in functional outcomes, which has led to the current graft choices.[19-21]

Several recent studies comparing patellar tendon and hamstring grafts show no significant difference in long-term functional outcome and minimal biologic differences.[18,19] However, it is again important to note that the key variable

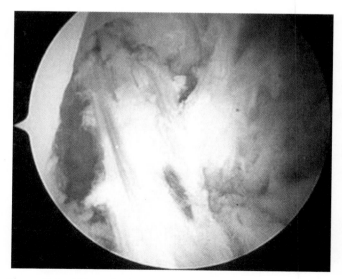

Figure 8-1: ACL graft placement.

is the patient, which requires the clinician to profile the patient's rehabilitative capability, and that time frame–based protocols may enhance the risk of biologic failure while still permitting functional activities.

PATIENT PROFILING

Outcome success is dependent on the understanding that patients have intrinsic and extrinsic variable factors that influence the level of activity to which they return. Intrinsic factors include but are not limited to tissue type, muscle type, potential for excessive scar formation, general medical well-being, osseous alignment, lower extremity mechanics, and compliance with the program. Extrinsic variables include but are not limited to social habits, use of nicotine products, environmental situations, and economic factors. Rehabilitation requires the therapist to address many of these issues, but patient morphologic type is critical.[2,8]

A select group of patients demonstrate hyperelasticity of joint motion, which results in the clinician having to factor in an altered collagen tissue variable in the rehabilitation pathway (Figure 8-2). Postsurgically these patients have the potential to lay down poor collagen tissue that may compromise the biologic graft. Hypoelastic patients demonstrate tight joint arthrokinematics, and postsurgically may have a tendency to develop arthrofibrosis, which must be recognized early on to avoid motion complications. Normal elasticity, as demonstrated in the majority of patients, best fits the traditional postsurgical time frame–based rehabilitation pathways.

PROGRAM OBJECTIVES

The key is to identify the rehabilitation components that the therapist must address in order to restore the ability to perform activities of daily living, and then titrate the exercise program to higher levels of activity until the patient achieves an optimal level of function. The therapist considers a staged approach and must assess the interaction of how one component is influenced by another. The program includes the following components:

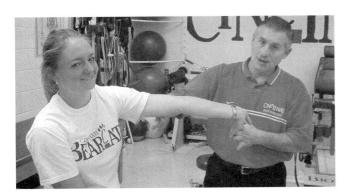

Figure 8-2: Patient demonstrating hyperelasticity with hyperextension at the elbow and wrist.

- Reestablish joint range of motion (ROM) to avoid deleterious motion loss (primary objective)
- Regulate postsurgical pain to avoid influence on ROM and muscle contraction
- Reduce postsurgical hemarthrosis to avoid muscle shutdown and arthrofibrosis
- Advance weight bearing and development of normal gait mechanics without affecting the biologic graft
- Establish early exercise sequences to recondition the muscular system while minimizing risk to the biologic graft
- Retrain the mechanoreceptor system through proprioception program
- Establish subjective and objective data to identify deviations from norm to minimize influence on outcome
- Establish a functional algorithm to verify functional progression
- Maintain progressive functional return to activity and sport

This chapter discusses each of these areas of the rehabilitation process and integrates acceptable exercises or procedures that minimize the risk of biologic failure of the graft.

REESTABLISHING RANGE OF MOTION

The use of continuous passive motion (CPM) after surgical procedures arose from a combination of animal and human studies in the late 1970s and early 1980s.[11-14] The primary focus of these studies was to assess forces applied by early motion on the biologic graft and surrounding tissues. This was a 180-degree shift in postsurgical management. The rationale for the changing philosophy was the negative morbidity of the joint associated with prolonged immobilization. Early studies were undertaken to determine if early use of CPM would provide a positive influence on graft revascularization and collagen regeneration, but findings demonstrated no cause-and-effect relationship. The positive findings identified with these studies included the following:

- Earlier redevelopment of ROM
- Decreased postsurgical pain
- Decreased joint hemarthrosis
- Decreased scar tissue
- Maintaining viability of the articular cartilage in the joint

Currently, we continue to recommend the use of a CPM machine (Figure 8-3) immediately after surgery for 10 to 12 hours per day until the unit is at maximum range. Most patients are able to tolerate gradual increase in motion with discontinuing the unit by 7 to 10 days. On average, the patients adjust their motion 10 to 15 degrees per day. If CPM is not desired, self-ranging exercise can be performed using the contralateral extremity on an hourly basis. Clinically, the

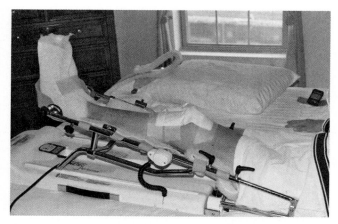

Figure 8-3: Continuous passive motion machine.

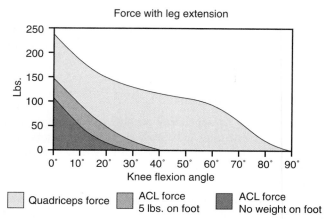

Figure 8-4: Forces applied on ACL during open kinetic chain extension.

use of a Biodex extremity system (Biodex Medical Systems Inc., Shirley, NY) either as a warm-up before the exercise sessions or in the cool-down phase is beneficial.

Active-assistive ROM and active ROM are also permitted by the patient in the early phase to stimulate extensor mechanism training. Although some data suggest that open chain exercise movement may stress the healing tendon, no direct study has identified this as problematic[22,23] (Figure 8-4).

Two key side effects after surgery that delay the redevelopment of motion in the immediate phase are pain and joint hemarthrosis. To maximize pain relief in the initial 24 hours, the patient is provided not only narcotics but also a femoral nerve block for a longer period of pain suppression. The use of a nonsteroidal antiinflammatory drug (NSAID) may be recommended to control the postsurgical hemarthrosis. This intervention may also have a secondary effect on the joint hemarthrosis. With the trend in endoscopic procedure for ACL surgery, there is generally a lesser amount of hemarthrosis. Minimizing joint hemarthrosis has led to the discontinued use of a joint hemovac, which can cause further inhibition to the extensor mechanism.

The second influence on ROM is joint pressure, which is created by the hemarthrosis. This pressure within the joint is applied to the capsular mechanoreceptors, resulting in a heightened pain level, exhibiting a limiting influence.[24-26] Although CPM may aid in the joint effusion reabsorption, as well as NSAIDs, standard cryotherapy is a must. Aggressive use of ice, elevation, and compression is essential in controlling joint swelling.[27,28] Several modalities have been developed that, when applied postsurgically, appear to be beneficial in controlling the swelling. Immediately after surgery we have recommended that the patient use a Game Ready system (CoolSystems Inc., Berkeley, CA) (Figure 8-5) on a continuous basis. The patient can wear some of these devices even while in the CPM machine. Clinically, the utilization of the Game Ready system (see Figure 8-5) has proven to be an added benefit by way of applying a pneumatic

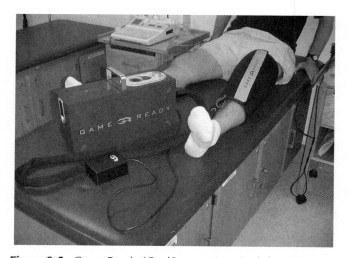

Figure 8-5: Game Ready (CoolSystems Inc., Berkeley, CA) system of vasopneumatic cryotherapy.

cold device. This is applied for the traditional 20 to 30 minutes because it simultaneously generates pressure, allowing a deeper penetration.

Protocols that have evolved in the last 15 years have placed a reduced emphasis on regaining ROM, instead concentrating on accelerating weight bearing and return to function. In these protocols the patients are placed in a long leg immobilizer and permitted full weight bearing. Little mention is made of the need to regain ROM. Although it is eventually regained, two questions arise:

- How long does it take to regain ROM?
- Is the potential for an arthrofibrotic complication increased?

Multiple studies have described motion complication rates ranging from 9% to 74%.[13,28-35] The implementation of an immediate motion program minimizes the risk for this unwarranted side effect. If the patient has not regained full ROM by 3 weeks, the need to initiate a more aggressive program is essential. The senior author has developed an algorithm that was published in 1992 dealing with this patient population.[32] Changes can occur in the periarticular tissues, decreasing ROM. The structures most involved commonly include the infrapatellar fat pad, which can result in a patella infra; the posterior capsule; and the medial and lateral retinaculum of the patellar capsule.[29-32]

The use of manual mobilization techniques may be minimized if an expedited motion program is implemented. Because the primary intervention is motion in this phase, the constant cycling of the joint capsule provides self-stress forces, maintaining capsular elasticity and self-mobilization. In this initial phase the primary concern centers on the patella and its normal superior mechanics. In the 1980s it was not uncommon to have a patient develop a patella infra position with an incident rate of 11% to 15%. A patella infra is a distally translated patella, which leads to an extensor lag. Tambrello and colleagues[33] described abnormal inferior displacement of the patella in a population of patellar tendon–reconstructed patients, resulting in a mechanical block. The conclusion was that early patellar glides and extensor mechanism reeducation were needed. Wojtys and colleagues[34] described altered collagen alignment in patients who developed a patella infra, which was not reversible. The patients in each of these studies also had a high percentage of patellofemoral complaints. Therefore our program emphasizes a clinical and self-directed program of patellar glides for a minimum of six cycles per day. Table 8-1 summarizes the first weeks of the postsurgical phases and flows through the ROM procedures.

WEIGHT BEARING

The second goal in the early rehabilitation period is the titration of the weight-bearing process. Again, there is a range of weight-bearing progression in current protocols, some of which advocate immediate full weight bearing in a locked extension brace, whereas others advocate the use of crutches for up to 4 to 5 weeks. The concept of immediate full weight bearing has prevailed with the thought that it facilitates faster extensor mechanism return. There appear to be no data supporting this claim, and in our experience the patient accommodates for a poor extensor mechanism by ambulating in a leg vault gait pattern.[3,32] Allowing an asymmetric gait pattern secondary to extensor mechanism weakness leads to the potential development of a recurvatum midstance position. This may result in an unwarranted side effect of a prolonged altered gait pattern at midstance caused by poor extensor eccentric control as the knee attempts to go into flexion of 15 to 20 degrees, which is unable to be achieved. Our approach has evolved to allow immediate partial weight bearing in either a protective ROM device or no brace at all. From the initial phase, gait mechanics are retrained without

compensation beginning on day 1. Concurrently, the patient is placed in a gait-training program to emphasize the proper positions and strength.

To progress the weight-bearing program, it is key for the clinician to assess the factors that influence the gait pattern and the biologic graft:

- Motion must progress as weight bearing advances but is not to be compromised at the expense of ROM.
- Extensor strength is able to control 0-degree ROM without extensor lag.
- Joint effusion is resolving as demonstrated by objective measures.
- Joint arthrometer evaluation is not significantly changed on a test-retest basis.
- Pain control has been achieved to avoid sympathetically maintained pain patterns.

Joint laxity evaluation has now become established as a standard measure to objectively assess the biologic graft. The use of joint arthrometry as part of the comprehensive evaluation process provides information that aids and integrates the findings to the rehabilitation pathway.[36] The KT-1000 arthrometry system (MEDmetric Corporation, San Diego, CA) (Figure 8-6) is designed to measure joint translation, in one degree of freedom. This evaluation defines the ligament's ability to restrain forces by an objective analysis. For maximum reliability several factors must be taken into consideration. The patient must be relaxed, without muscle guarding of either the quadriceps or hamstrings. Accurate placement of the arthrometer is critical, as well as maintaining neutral positioning of the tibia. Consistent force must be applied and the test performed for three trials to avoid patient accommodations.

Force application by the clinician is 20 to 30 pounds, and the total anteroposterior translation should be compared

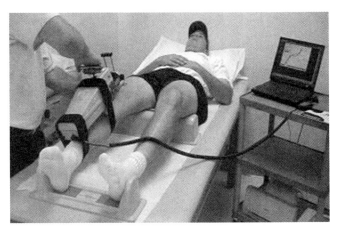

Figure 8-6: KT-1000 arthrometry system (MEDmetric Corporation, San Diego, CA) for testing ligamentous laxity.

TABLE 8-1

Clinical Pathway for Postoperative Management of ACL Reconstruction

WHEN	PHASE 1 MAXIMAL PROTECTION DAY 1 TO WEEK 4	PHASE 2 MODERATE PROTECTION WEEKS 5 TO 10	PHASE 3 MINIMAL PROTECTION WEEKS 11 TO 24	PHASE 4 RETURN TO ACTIVITY 6 MONTHS AND LATER
Patient presentation	· Postoperative day 1–3 · Postoperative hemarthrosis · Postoperative pain · Decreased ROM · Decreased voluntary quadriceps contraction · Dependent ambulation · Postoperative brace (may or may not have)	· Pain controlled · Joint swelling controlled · No increased joint instability · Full or near-full ROM · Fair-plus to good muscle strength (MMT) · Muscular control of joint · Independent ambulation	· No instability · No swelling · No pain · Good to normal strength (MMT) · Unrestricted ADL function	· No instability · Muscle function 70% of noninvolved · No symptoms of instability, pain, or swelling in the previous phase
Key evaluation procedures	· Pain scale · Hemarthrosis—girth · Ligament stability—joint arthrometer (day 7-14) · ROM · Patellar mobility · Muscle control · Functional status	· Pain scale · Effusion—girth · Ligament stability—joint arthrometer · ROM · Patellar mobility · Muscle strength · Functional status	· Ligament stability—joint arthrometer · Muscle strength · Functional status	· Full clinical examination · Ligament stability · Muscle strength · Functional status
Treatment intervention	**Early: Days 1-14** · Protective bracing, ice, compression, elevation (PRICE) · Ambulation training: crutches—WB 25%-50% · PROM/AAROM (range-limiting braces may or may not be used during this phase) · Patellar mobilization, grades I and II	**Early: Weeks 5-6** · Continue isometric exercise, multiple angles · Advance PRE program: quadriceps, hamstrings, gastrocnemius, hips · Advance closed chain strengthening · LE flexibility program · Advance trunk stability · Endurance training: bike, pool, ski machine, etc.	· Continue LE flexibility · Advance PRE strengthening · Advance closed chain exercise · Advance proprioceptive training · Agility drills specific to skill · Advance endurance training · Isokinetic training (if desired)	· Continue as Phase 3, advance as appropriate · Advance agility drills · Advance running drills · Implement drills specific to sport or occupation · Determine the need for protective bracing before return to sport or work

- Muscle setting/isometrics: quadriceps, hamstrings, and adductors, multiple angles (may augment with electrical stimulation)
- SLRs—supine
- Stretching: hamstrings, gastrocnemius/soleus
- Ankle pumps to reduce gravity effects on swelling

Late: Weeks 2-4
- Continue as above
- Progress weight bearing to 75% to full
- Initiate weight-shifting exercises
- SLRs in four planes
- Heel/toe raises
- Initiate open chain knee extensions (range 90°-40°)
- Initiate closed chain squats
- Hamstring PREs
- Trunk/pelvis stability program
- Well-body exercises

- Proprioception training: tilt boards, BAPS board, beam walking, single-leg stance, challenged stance
- Rhythmic stabilization: manual resistance, band kicks, band walking

Late: Weeks 7-10
- Continue as above, advancing strengthening, endurance, and flexibility as indicated
- Advance proprioceptive training to high-speed stepping drills, unstable surface challenge drills, and balance beam
- PNF patterns
- Initiate a walk/jog program at the end of this phase
- Initiate plyometric training: box jumps, jump rope, double-leg/single-leg bounding
- Initiate skill-specific drills at the end of this phase

- Progress running program: full-speed jog, sprints, figure-of-eight, running and cutting

Goals

- Protect healing tissues
- Prevent muscle shutdown
- Decrease joint effusion
- Decrease pain
- ROM 0°-125°
- Muscular control of ROM
- WB 75%—full
- Establish HEP

- Full pain-free ROM
- Good to normal muscular strength (MMT)
- Dynamic control of joint
- Normalize gait pattern
- Normalize ADL function
- Compliance with HEP

- Increase strength
- Increase power
- Increase endurance
- Improve neuromuscular control and dynamic stability

- Increase strength
- Increase power
- Increase endurance
- Regain ability to function at highest desired level
- Develop maintenance program

Adapted from Mangine RE, Kremchek TE: Evaluation based protocol of the anterior cruciate ligament, *J Sport Rehabil* 6:157, 1997. Evaluation based clinical pathway design based on Noyes FR, DeMaio M, Mangine RE: Evaluation-based protocol: a new approach to rehabilitation, *J Orthop* 14(12):1383–1385, 1991.
AAROM, Active-assistive range of motion; *ADL,* activities of daily living; *BAPS,* balance and proprioceptive system; *HEP,* Home Exercise Program; *LE,* lower extremity; *MMT,* manual muscle test; *PNF,* proprioceptive neuromuscular facilitation; *PRE,* progressive resistive exercises; *PROM,* passive range of motion; *ROM,* range of motion; *SLR,* straight leg raise; *WB,* weight bearing.

bilaterally. Differences of 3 mm or less have been reported to be acceptable following reconstruction. Testing every 2 weeks provides the rehabilitation specialist with objective data and allows for the rehabilitation program to be individualized. Generally, if there is a 1.5 mm increase between test dates, the clinician may elect to decrease the intensity of the program until the joint is proven stable.

A postsurgical knee orthosis is fitted at the time of surgery, to allow for early weight bearing with crutch support. The brace is unlocked to allow for normal gait mechanics and avoidance of deviations commonly seen with patients in a locked brace. These deviations include a vaulting gait, circumduction of the involved lower extremity, and avoidance of weight bearing on the limb. The exercises used in the early-phase program are outlined in Table 18-1, and specific gait-training techniques are staged in the pathway.

The second evaluation tool recently developed is the Biodex Gait Trainer system (Biodex Medical Systems Inc., Shirley, NY) allowing for assessment of gait mechanics. Historically, little objective research exists on gait normalization following ACL reconstruction. Timoney and colleagues[37] and DeVita and colleagues[38] demonstrated that, even at a year following ACL surgery, gait biomechanics are not normalized but the tendency toward a true "quad-avoidance" gait is no longer present. The missing factors from these studies, however, are what gait-training protocol was followed in the postsurgical phase and whether an immobilizer was used. There is no research on objective gait mechanics and gait normalization after the use of a specific ACL protocol. The use of the gait trainer has evolved from the senior author's study of the influence of rehabilitation training and the normalization of gait. The system has demonstrated reliability in a controlled study of normal subjects and is both objective and easy to administer in the clinic, as compared with complex gait studies in biomechanics laboratories.[39] Recently, we have demonstrated that normal gait can be achieved in a 12-week time frame with emphasis on gait mechanical training immediately following surgery.[40] The gait training progression used to achieve these results is outlined in Table 8-2.

MUSCLE REEDUCATION

Reestablishing muscle control after joint surgery has many different pathways and has changed dramatically over the last 20 years. This process of reestablishing muscle control is initiated immediately, compared with 30 years ago, when the patient sat in a cast for 6 weeks or longer. The evolution has been brought about by basic science studies allowing a better understanding of the following:

- Joint compression forces
- Exercise forces applied to the ligament
- Improved surgical techniques
- Avoiding joint morbidity effects

Initially, our goal is to simply retard the effects that joint hemarthrosis and surgical pain have on the muscle by causing reflex shutdown. The classic use of isometrics, open chain isotonics such as active range of motion with the weight of the ankle, and straight leg raises can be beneficial but are generally low load and independently may not prevent the disuse muscle atrophy that affects the knee joint.

Over the years, many exercise approaches have been advocated and in some cases are associated with several complications. Although the trend is to accelerate today's patients, patellar tendonitis is common, with a 9% occurrence rate.[32] Of greater concern is the development of patellofemoral arthrosis, which has been reported in a 7% to 51% range in association with ACL reconstructions. Early-phase extensor mechanism exercises may generate large forces across the articular surfaces of the patella. Therefore rehabilitation must account not only for the healing graft, but also for patella protection. Patella degeneration is unpredictable and varies among patients, especially with reference to age range. Shino and colleagues[35] reported that on second-look arthroscopy, 51% of allograft patients demonstrated patellar changes, yet only 17% of the patients reported subjective complaints. Autograft studies describe subjective complaints ranging from 7% to 29%.[8,19,20] Another associated complication leading to patella complaints is infrapatellar contracture syndrome, described as a distal migration of the patella secondary to scarring in the fat pad or a shortening of the patellar tendon, which can occur after surgery.[33] In this scenario the patella is displaced into the trochlear surface, consequently increasing patellar compression and shear load. Maintaining adequate extensor mechanism control in the 0-degree position can prevent these complications. In addition, emphasizing early patellar mobilization immediately following surgery can help prevent infrapatellar contracture later in the rehabilitation process.

To understand the process of neurologically induced muscle shutdown and to develop rational treatment approaches, the therapist must understand the reflex inhibitory mechanism. The key to this process is historical and well defined. Newton[26] identified four neural components to the mechanoreceptor system; these either inhibit or facilitate muscular response to input. Kennedy and colleagues[24] demonstrated the influence of joint pressure on mechanoreceptors as inhibitors resulting in extensor mechanism shutdown; however, this study did not quantify muscle loss percentages. In 1984, the senior author described how a mere 70 ml of injected saline reduced isometric output of the knee by 37% in a normal joint[25] (Figure 8-7). Further theories on pain generated by the type IV mechanoreceptor can also suppress muscle activity. Interpreting this information requires a program that bypasses the mechanoreceptor influence.

In the last 15 years the use of muscle stimulation has gained wider acceptance and is now considered standard of care.[8,40,41] Attempting to achieve two objectives, our program utilizes electrical currents by means of a five-step progression series. To reestablish muscle control of joint motion, this

TABLE 8-2

Gait Training Progression

EXERCISE	PURPOSE	WEEK 1	WEEK 2	WEEK 3	WEEKS 4-6	WEEKS 6-8	WEEKS 8-10	WEEKS 10-12
Quad setting	Facilitates extensor mechanism for heel strike	10-second hold/10 repetitions	10-second hold/30-40 repetitions	10-second hold/50 repetitions	Discontinue use with good control of knee extension			
Closed chain terminal knee extension	Facilitates extensor mechanism for heel strike in closed chain position	25% weight bearing/30 repetitions in controlled fashion	50% weight bearing/40 repetitions with increasingly stronger band resistance	85% weight bearing/40 repetitions with increasingly stronger band resistance	100% weight bearing/50 repetitions with increasingly stronger band resistance	Discontinue use with good control of active extension in closed chain position		
Mini-squats	Aids pelvic control during gait and acceptance of equal weight between limbs		30-40 repetitions in slow, controlled manner	50 repetitions in slow, controlled manner	Discontinue use and transition to eccentric leg press			
Weight shifting	Aids pelvic control during gait and acceptance of equal weight between limbs		30 weight shifts laterally/30 weight shifts forward and back	50 weight shifts laterally/50 weight shifts forward and back	Discontinue use with initiation of single-leg positioning			
Toe/heel rocking	Establishes stance phase of gait		50 rocks forward and back	100 rocks forward and back	Discontinue with good stance phase mechanics			

TABLE 8-2

Gait Training Progression, continued

EXERCISE	PURPOSE	WEEK 1	WEEK 2	WEEK 3	WEEKS 4-6	WEEKS 6-8	WEEKS 8-10	WEEKS 10-12
Cup programming	Reestablishes hip positioning and stresses normal mechanics of foot clearance and heel strike	25% weight bearing/over and back 10 cups 5 times each way	50% weight bearing/over and back 10 cups 5 times each way	85% weight bearing/over and back 10 cups 5 times each way, progressing to one crutch as appropriate	100% weight bearing/over and back 10 cups 5 times each way	Lateral cup stepping/over and back 10 cups 5 times each way	Lateral cup stepping with ball toss/over and back 10 cups 5 times each way	Lateral cup stepping with ball toss and band resistance/over and back 10 cups 5 times each way
Single-leg positioning	Aids ability to control limb at midstance			Hold 5 seconds/10 repetitions with table support as needed	Hold 10 seconds/10 repetitions on floor and progress to unstable surface as indicated	15 seconds/10 repetitions on challenging surface with rebounder	20-30 seconds/4 repetitions with band perturbation and ball toss	20-30 seconds/4 repetitions with sport-specific challenge
Eccentric step-downs	Retrain ability to descend stairs in controlled fashion				6" step-down/30 repetitions	8-10" step-down with band resistance at hip/30-40 repetitions	12-18" step-down with band resistance at hip and outside knee for valgus control/40 repetitions	18-24" step-down with band resistance at hip and outside knee for valgus control and with ball toss challenge/3 sets of 20 repetitions

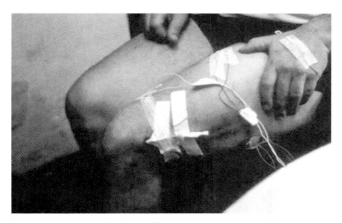

Figure 8-7: Joint effusion influence on neuromuscular performance: 70 ml of saline injected into the joint resulted in 37% reduction in force output of the muscles.

series attempts to reduce the influence of pain as well as the added demands associated with joint pressure on the joint receptors.

- Program 1 (Figure 8-8, *A*):
  - The use of a stimulation unit to modulate pain and influence joint effusion provides effective control of early subjective complaints. Although multiple studies have reported effectiveness, location of electrode placement needs to be optimal.[42,43] Our goal is to control pain in postsurgical patients using transcutaneous electrical nerve stimulation (TENS). In our current protocol, an Empi system (Empi, St. Paul, MN) is preprogrammed to control postsurgical pain and is used 24 hours per day. This program is discontinued when the patient ends the use of narcotic medication.
- Program 2 (Figure 8-8, *B*):
  - Voluntary muscle control of the extensor mechanism is facilitated with the assistance of muscle stimulation applied to the vastus medialis oblique region and the femoral nerve's proximal location. The goal is to augment and produce a stronger contraction of the extensor mechanism. Program 1 of the Empi 300PV is used for this neuromuscular reeducation phase. The patient is instructed to volitionally contract the extensor mechanism musculature during the on cycle of the electrical stimulation. Training occurs at various angles during the 10- to 15-minute session, six to eight times per day. An on/off ratio of 10 seconds on/30 seconds off is programmed on the home unit. The most common angles include 60, 30, 15, and 0 degrees.
- Program 3 (Figure 8-8, *C*):
  - Permitting early weight bearing requires techniques to facilitate the extensor mechanism in a closed chain position. This process is implemented within

5 to 10 days of surgery based on the evaluation of the joint's ability to control this position. The patient is positioned standing, with the feet shoulder-width apart; support from the arms is permitted to maintain a balanced position. The use of stimulation in this position is principally for neurodevelopmental progression of ambulation. The settings are placed at 10 seconds on and 10 seconds off for shorter rest periods. While the electrical stimulation is in process, the patient is instructed to perform a mini-squat. Emphasis is placed on correct performance to decrease trunk lean; to increase weight shifting over the involved extremity; and, most important, to promote a controlled movement pattern.

- Program 4 (Figure 8-8, *D*):
  - This position continues to use the muscle stimulation portion of the 300PV to promote muscular control of the terminal phase of extension. The patient stands with electrode pads placed in the previously described position. The patient actively extends the knee into the fullest extension possible. This technique is implemented if the patient experiences difficulty when holding the terminal-degree ROM. Despite control of contractile potential in the supine position, the patient now has a lever arm weakness, leading to poor extension control. The unit is set at a 10- to 20-second on/off time period, and a 20-cycle program is performed.
- Program 5 (Figure 8-8, *E*):
  - This series is similar to program 3, except the patient performs the exercise in a single-leg balance position. This is an end-stage procedure and is used only after the patient is full weight bearing. Functional and dynamic progression of this exercise includes manual perturbations, plyo-ball toss, and balance on altered surfaces.

It is our experience that by 6 weeks the patient has regained ROM and volitional control of extension during ambulation. At this point the electrical stimulation program is discontinued.

MUSCLE FUNCTION PHASE II

Typically at the 6- to 12-week time period, patients graduate to advanced neuromuscular and functional training.[3,9,44] At this time, exercise intensity is increased to allow for muscle adaptation, a requisite for sport-specific demands. Areas of importance and emphasis during this time period are muscle strength, power, endurance, and control. Aspects of acceleration, deceleration, and reflex response are slowly integrated into the rehabilitation program. The progression of training should increase the duration of the exercise session first, then increase the intensity of the workload, and finally integrate functional training with sport-specific drills.

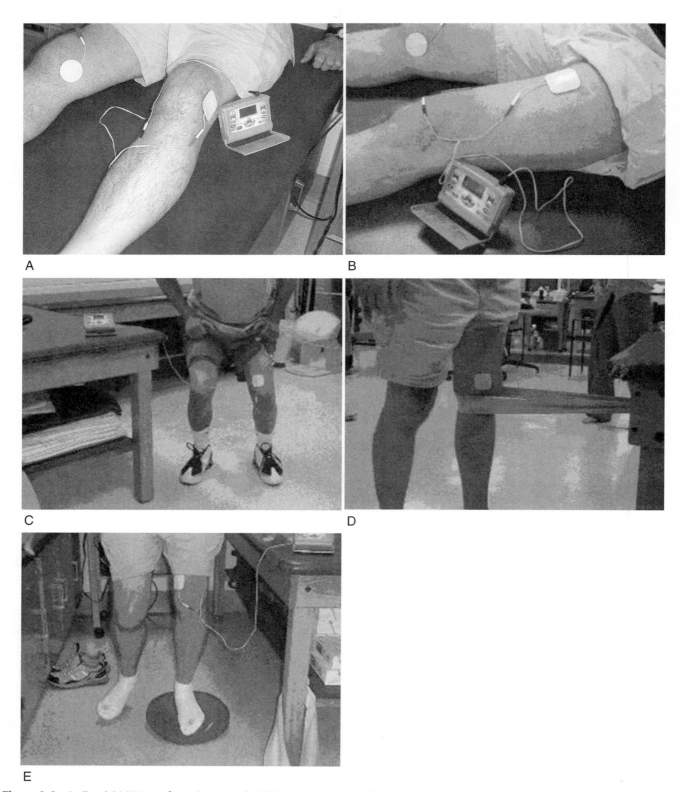

Figure 8-8: A, Empi 300PV set for pain control (TENS setting). **B,** Empi 300PV quad setting neuromuscular reeducation. **C,** Empi 300PV mini-squat reeducation. **D,** Empi 300PV closed chain terminal knee extension. **E,** Empi 300PV single-leg balance neuromuscular reeducation.

During rehabilitation, emphasis should be placed on training the entire kinetic chain, not just the involved lower extremity. Proximal stabilization is of particular importance to the athlete and should be incorporated from the early postoperative phase until return to sport. The hips, pelvis, lumbar spine, and abdominal musculature are areas of primary focus. Straight leg raises are initiated early and progress to higher resistance, providing early-stage training but limited functional carryover. In essence, these exercises are isometric to the vasti group; the long lever arm minimizes the total amount of resistance.

To initiate training for rapid response time of the muscles required to control tibial translation, the transition in this time period involves incorporating high-speed training of the proximal stabilizers of the hip and pelvis. This proximal strategy is part of our core stabilization program (Figure 8-9). Core muscle group training includes bridges using bilateral lower extremities, which progress to bridges with single-limb support and alternate leg extension. Single-leg bridges are held for 10 seconds at a time. Single-leg bridges are a more advanced core-stability exercise and should be performed for both involved and uninvolved extremities. At this point, side-lying bridges should also have been implemented, advancing by abducting the contralateral arm and using weights to increase the balance component. It is important to continuously reinforce proper lumbo-pelvic positioning while avoiding faulty patterns. Abdominal and oblique exercise advancement is paramount during this phase of rehabilitation. Dynamic rotation, plyometric sit-ups, and power training are progressed at this time. All of these exercises can be performed in supine, standing, and sport- and position-specific athletic positions, all of which emphasize total body control and stabilization.

Open kinetic chain knee exercises are continued during this phase. Both isotonic workloads and isokinetic training sessions are helpful. Care must be taken to protect the healing graft and to avoid patellofemoral joint irritation. Isotonic extension work should be limited to 90-30 degrees, and heavy resisted loads should be avoided. Hamstring workload is not limited unless there is posterolateral capsule or meniscal involvement. The senior author has advocated an approach using higher velocity for evaluation and training to protect the patella and graft.[9,44] In closed chain training, 0-degree stops are used to prevent knee hyperextension. Markolf and colleagues[45] reported that this ROM placed the highest forces on the ACL.

Closed kinetic chain training also plays a primary role in ACL rehabilitation. This rationale is based on the performance of functional training and strengthening simulating both sport-specific movements and those associated with activities of daily living. The literature supports this training, based on data from both cadaveric and in vivo models. Both Beynnon and colleagues[17] (performing in vivo measurement) and Wilk and colleagues[46] (by mechanical methods) predicted low strain on the ACL in the closed chain position. They also reported that the quadriceps and hamstrings muscles co-contract to protect the ACL graft against strain.[17,46] Others also have found that the closed chain position allows exercises for early resistance training to the lower extremity before 8 weeks.[47]

Particular emphasis should be placed on single-leg training to enhance neuromuscular control of the knee. Focus on

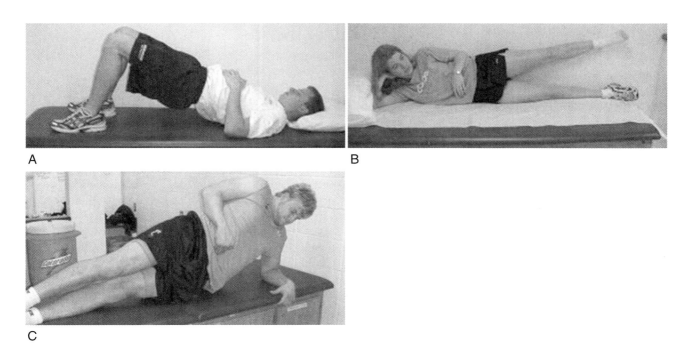

A

B

C

Figure 8-9: Core stabilization program, including **A**, bridges; **B**, rose-wall slides; and **C**, side-lying bridges.

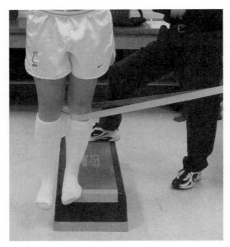

Figure 8-10: Eccentric step-down maneuver for control during stair descent.

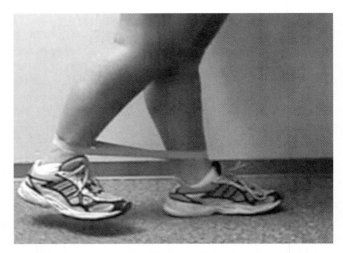

Figure 8-11: Rhythmic stabilization high-speed band kicking.

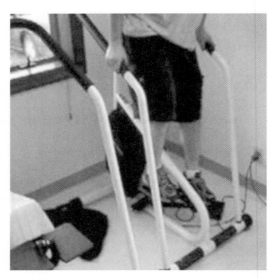

Figure 8-12: Retro aerobic conditioning using a StairMaster (StairMaster, Vancouver, WA).

postural awareness and postural stability in the single-limb supported position is paramount for an athlete to return to competition. Athletes in competition spend a critical amount of time in the single-leg position, executing movements such as running, cutting, pivoting, and jumping, as well as various acceleration and deceleration maneuvers. As part of the rehabilitation continuum to successfully return an athlete to a prior competitive level, training and assessment of proper landing mechanics is performed early in the program. In patients with weak proximal joint segments, valgus (at the knee) and internal rotation (at the hip) increase the strain on the ACL. Landing training begins with the eccentric step-down program (Figure 8-10) and builds to dynamic and responsive stability in the single-leg exercise position.[48]

Training in the single-leg position is progressed from a very controlled environment, focusing on balance in addition to posture and control of the entire kinetic chain. Dynamic stability is gradually introduced by altering the base of support, involving the upper extremities, incorporating sport-specific activities, and implementing rotational components to the program. Kicking exercises (Figure 8-11) with resistive bands at high speeds can be performed at the 5- to 6-week time period as a rhythmic stabilization drill. Lunging exercises are progressed by means of altering surfaces, providing manual perturbations, and, eventually, performing sport-specific tasks. Single-limb training promotes stabilization of the entire lower extremity and should be performed concurrently with the hip/pelvis/trunk stabilization program previously described. The athlete must learn to control the body as it transitions from one point to the next.

Although little information exists in the literature, it is recommended that an athlete should also undergo "retro" training (Figure 8-12). In the early stages of rehabilitation, retro treadmill walking is initiated in a safe and controlled manner. When indicated, retro exercises are progressed gradually. Retro lunges are added to the rehabilitation program along with retro StairMaster (StairMaster, Vancouver, WA) work and resisted retro band work. When the patient begins a jogging program, retro jogging and backpedaling should also be addressed. Progression toward a forward sprint, deceleration, and retro work need to be performed with various tasks and sport drills. Retro training will enable the athlete to safely and efficiently transition from an acceleration phase to a deceleration phase, ultimately leading to change-of-direction ability.

Between weeks 6 and 12, overall strengthening and stabilization of the lower extremity continues; however, speed of performance is also progressively emphasized. Many exercise variations can be implemented early that slowly progress toward higher-speed maneuvers. Elastic bands, lunges, and many stepping and footwork drills can progress toward higher speeds. Over time, repetitions and durations of exercise should increase; this ensures a combination of both submaximal and aerobic training. The critical element at this time period is endurance activity to counterbalance muscle fatigue.

Other chapters in this text discuss in-depth training programs, both as prevention tools and end-stage rehabilitation guides. The clinician at this point is generally transitioning the patient into a performance enhancement program for final activity training. However, before return we recommend a range of evaluation tools.

RETURN TO ACTIVITY

Return to activity in our program, on the average, yields a bell-shaped curve. The range of return is 12 weeks for the hypoelastic patient and up to 12 months for the hyperelastic patient. On average, 6 months serves as our mean time for a safe return to activity, based on biologic healing of the graft. For return to activity, the following objective and subjective evaluations should occur:

1. Subjective rating on the International Knee Documentation Committee (IKDC) scoring system[49] as compared with preinjury status

2. Joint arthrometer score of 3 mm or less (patients above this parameter may be held longer)[50]

3. Objective muscle scoring within 85% of the contralateral extremity[51]

4. Functional hop scores within 85% of the contralateral extremity[52,53]

5. Progressive drill reenactment to simulate activity anticipated on return to sports

6. Confidence by patient to psychologically perform skill-specific activity

Patients are presented with appropriate information on their scores and given the risk/return ratio so they can decide for themselves to which level to return.

SUMMARY

The procedures and techniques that have evolved for the ACL-injured patient have resulted in reconstruction becoming a common surgery with a high percentage of positive outcomes. The postoperative risks that were identified early on, by various studies, have been minimized. As in all surgical procedures, there are certain inherent risks, but the outcomes have been proven beneficial for maintaining long-term knee function.

References

1. Naranja RJ, Corsetti J, Kuhlman JR, Torg JS: The search for the Holy Grail: a century of anterior cruciate ligament reconstruction, *Am J Orthoped* 26(11):742-752, 1997.

2. Noyes FR, DeMaio M, Mangine RE: Evaluation based protocols: a new approach to rehabilitation, *J Orthoped* 14(12):1383-1385, 1991.

3. Shelbourne KD, Nitz P: Accelerated rehabilitation after anterior cruciate ligament reconstruction, *Am J Sports Med* 18:292-299, 1990.

4. Frank CB: The science of reconstruction of the anterior cruciate ligament, current concept review, *J Bone Joint Surg* 79:1556-1567, 1997.

5. Noyes FR: Functional properties of knee ligaments and alteration induced by immobilization, *Clin Orthop* 123:210-242, 1977.

6. Kennedy JC, Weinberg HW, Wilson AS: The anatomy and function of the anterior cruciate ligament, *J Bone Joint Surg* 56:223-235, 1974.

7. Clancy WG, Narechania RG, Rosenberg TF, et al: Anterior and posterior cruciate ligament reconstruction in rhesus monkeys: a histological, microangiographic, and biochemical analysis, *J Bone Joint Surg* 70:1483-1488, 1988.

8. DeMaio M, Noyes FR, Mangine RE: Principles for aggressive rehabilitation after reconstruction of the anterior cruciate ligament, *J Orthop* 15:505-515, 1992.

9. DeMaio M, Mangine RE, Noyes FR, Barber SD: Advanced muscle training after ACL reconstruction: weeks 5 to 52, *Orthopaedics* 15:757-767, 1992.

10. Amiel D, Kleiner JB, Roux RD, et al: The phenomenon of ligamentization: anterior cruciate ligament reconstruction with autogenous patellar tendon, *J Orthop Res* 4:162-172, 1986.

11. Burks R, Daniel D, Losse G: The effect of continuous passive motion on anterior cruciate ligament reconstruction stability, *Am J Sports Med* 12:323-326, 1984.

12. Drez D, Paine RM, Neuschwander DC, Young JC: In-vivo measurement of anterior tibial translation using continuous passive motion, *Am J Sports Med* 19:381-383, 1991.

13. Noyes FR, Mangine RE, Barber SD: Early knee motion after open and arthroscopic anterior cruciate ligament reconstruction, *Am J Sports Med* 15:149-160, 1984.

14. Salter RB: The biologic concept of continuous passive motion on synovial joints, *Clin Orthop* 242:12-25, 1989.

15. Butler D: Personal communication, 2001.

16. Noyes FR, Butler DL, Grood ES: Biomechanical analysis of human ligament grafts used in knee-ligament repairs and reconstruction, *J Bone Joint Surg* 66:344-352, 1984.

17. Beynnon BD, Fleming BC, Johnson RL, et al: Anterior cruciate ligament strain behavior during rehabilitation exercises in vivo, *Am J Sports Med* 23:24-34, 1995.

18. Jansson KA, Linko E, Sandelin J, Harilainen A: A prospective randomized study of patellar versus hamstring tendon autografts for anterior cruciate ligament reconstruction, *Am J Sports Med* 31:12-18, 2003.

19. Beynnon BD, Johnson RJ, Fleming BC, et al: Anterior cruciate ligament replacement: comparison of bone-patellar tendon-bone grafts with two strand hamstring grafts, *J Bone Joint Surg* 84A:1503-1513, 2002.

20. Noyes FR, Barber SD, Mangine RE: Bone-patellar ligament-bone and fascia lata allografts for reconstruction of the anterior cruciate ligament, *J Bone Joint Surg* 71:1125-1132, 1990.

21. Noyes FR, Barber SD: The effect of a ligament augmentation device on allograft reconstructions for chronic ruptures of the anterior cruciate ligament, *J Bone Joint Surg* 74(7):960-968, 1992.

22. Grood ES, Suntay WJ, Noyes FR, Butler DL: Biomechanics of the knee-extension exercise, *J Bone Joint Surg* 66A:725-733, 1984.

23. Yasuda K, Sasaki T: Muscle exercise after anterior cruciate ligament reconstruction: biomechanics of the simultaneous isometric contraction method of the quadriceps and the hamstring, *Clin Orthop* 220:266-274, 1987.

24. Kennedy JC, Alexander IJ, Hayes KL: Nerve supply of the human knee and its functional importance, *Am J Sports Med* 10:329-335, 1982.

25. Mangine RE, Brownstein B: Effects of joint effusion on muscle performance. Abstract in Cybex proceedings manual, education conference, Kansas City, MO, May 1984.

26. Newton RA: Joint receptor contribution to reflexive and kinesthetic responses, *Phys Ther* 2:22-29, 1982.

27. Martin SS, Spindler KP, Tarter JW, et al: Cryotherapy: an effective modality for decreasing intraarticular temperature after knee arthroscopy, *Am J Sports Med* 29:288-291, 2001.

28. Konrath GA, Lock T, Goitz HT: The use of cold therapy after anterior cruciate ligament reconstruction: a prospective, randomized study and literature review, *Am J Sports Med* 24:629-633, 1996.

29. Dodds JA, Keene JS, Graf BK, Lange RH: Results of knee manipulations after anterior cruciate ligament reconstruction, *Am J Sports Med* 19:283-287, 1991.

30. Graf B, Uhr F: Complications of intra-articular anterior cruciate reconstruction, *Clin Sports Med* 7:835, 1988.

31. Harner CD, Fu FH, Irrgang JJ, Paul JJ: Recognition and management of the stiff knee following arthroscopic anterior cruciate ligament reconstruction. Presented at the AAOS meeting, Anaheim, CA, March 1991.

32. Noyes FR, Mangine RE, Barber SD: The early treatment of motion complications following reconstruction of the anterior cruciate ligament, *Clin Orthop* 220:275-283, 1992.

33. Tambrello MT, Personius WJ, Lamb RL, et al: Patella hypomobility as a cause of extensor lag. Presented at Total Care of the Knee: Before and after Injury. Cybex Conference, Overland Park, KS, May 17-19, 1985.

34. Wojtys EM, Noyes FR, Gikas P: Patella baja syndrome. Presented at the annual meeting of the AAOS. New Orleans, LA, February 1986.

35. Shino K, Inouse M, Horibe S, et al: Maturation of allograft tendons transplanted into the knee: an arthroscopic and histological study, *J Bone Joint Surg* 70:103-121, 1988.

36. Barber SD, Noyes FR: The effect of rehabilitation and return to activity on anterior-posterior knee displacement following anterior cruciate ligament reconstruction. Unpublished data, 1991.

37. Timoney JM, Inman WS, Quesada PM, et al: Return of normal gait patterns after anterior cruciate ligament reconstruction, *Am J Sports Med* 21(6):887-889, 1993.

38. DeVita P, Lassiter T Jr, Hortobagyi T, Torry M: Functional knee brace effects during walking in patients with anterior cruciate ligament reconstruction, *Am J Sports Med* 26(6):778-784, 1998.

39. Eifert-Mangine MA, Minning S, Mangine RE: Reliability of the Biodex gait trainer system. Submitted to APTA Combined Section Meeting, New Orleans, LA, 2004.

40. Minning S, Mangine RE, Eifert-Mangine MA, Colosimo AJ: Gait normalization and relationship to KT laxity following anterior cruciate ligament reconstruction. Submitted to APTA Combined Section Meeting, New Orleans, LA, 2004.

41. Snyder-Mackler L, Delitto A, Bailey SL, Stralka SW: Strength of the quadriceps femoris muscle and functional recovery after reconstruction of the anterior cruciate ligament: a prospective, randomized clinical trial of electrical stimulation, *J Bone Joint Surg* 77:1166-1173, 1995.

42. Berlant SR: Method of determining optimal stimulation sites for transcutaneous electrical nerve stimulation, *Phys Ther* 64:924-928, 1984.

43. Gould N, Donnermeyer D, Pope M, Ashikaga T: Transcutaneous muscle stimulation as a method to retard disuse atrophy, *Clin Orthop* 164:215-220, 1982.

44. Mangine RE, Heckmann TP, Eldridge VL: Muscle response to strength training. In Scully RM, Barnes MR, editors: *Physical therapy*, Philadelphia, 1989, JB Lippincott.

45. Markolf KL, Gorek JF, Kabo M, Shapiro MS: Direct measurement of resultant forces in the anterior cruciate ligament, *J Bone Joint Surg* 72:557-562, 1990.

46. Wilk KE, Escamilla RF, Flesig GS, et al: A comparison of tibiofemoral joint forces and electromyographic activity during open and closed kinetic chain exercises, *Am J Sports Med* 24:518-527, 1996.

47. Jenkins WL, Munns SW, Jayaraman G, Werzberger KL: A measurement of anterior tibial displacement in the closed and open kinetic chain, *J Orthop Sports Phys Ther* 25:49-56, 1997.

48. Hewett TE, Paterno MV, Meyer GD: Strategies for enhancing proprioception and neuromuscular control of the knee, *Clin Orthop* 402:76-94, 2002.

49. Irrgang JJ, Anderson AF, Boland AL, et al: Development and validation of the International Knee Documentation Committee subjective knee form, *Am J Sports Med* 29:600-612, 2001.

50. Daniel DM, Malcom LL, Stone ML, et al: Quantification of knee stability and function, *Contemp Orthop* 5:83-91, 1982.

51. Wilk KE, Johnson RD, Levine B: Reliability of the Biodex B-2000, isokinetic dynamometer, *Phys Ther* 68:792, 1988 (abstract).

52. Noyes FR, Barber SD, Mangine RE: Abnormal lower limb symmetry determined by function hop tests after anterior cruciate ligament rupture, *Am J Sports Med* 19:513-518, 1991.

53. Tegner Y, Lysholm J, Lysholm M, Gillquist JA: Performance test to monitor rehabilitation and evaluate anterior cruciate ligament injuries, *Am J Sports Med* 14:156-159, 1986.

CHAPTER 9

Rehabilitation after Anterior Cruciate Ligament Reconstruction with a Contralateral Patellar Tendon Graft: Philosophy, Protocol, and Addressing Problems

K. Donald Shelbourne, MD
Mark S. DeCarlo, PT
Timothy D. Henne, MD

PHILOSOPHY

The use of the contralateral patellar tendon as a preferred graft source in anterior cruciate ligament (ACL) reconstruction has been driven by a recognition that appropriate preoperative and postoperative rehabilitation programs are critical for a successful surgical outcome. Over the course of 20 years' experience with nearly 5000 ACL reconstructions, a steady decrease in complication rates and a corresponding increase in successful outcomes has been caused not by changes in surgical techniques, but by changes in rehabilitation techniques. A well-performed ACL reconstruction and rehabilitation can protect the knee from further injury and allow return to a high level of athleticism. A poorly performed ACL reconstruction or rehabilitation program results in a worse outcome than if the ACL had not been reconstructed at all.[1] Even a well-performed surgery can still result in a poor outcome if rehabilitation is not conducted appropriately. Despite a properly positioned graft, complications such as loss of knee motion, graft site pain, or persistent weakness can still occur. An appropriate rehabilitation process that prevents these complications is the key to successful ACL surgery. Logically, whatever can be done surgically to facilitate postoperative rehabilitation should lead to improved outcomes. The contralateral graft is valuable in this regard because it allows rehabilitation to be a more reliable and effective process.

On first reflection this concept is somewhat counterintuitive. It may seem that the added burden of rehabilitating the previously uninjured knee could only complicate postoperative rehabilitation. However, regardless of whether an ipsilateral or a contralateral graft is chosen, the residual defect is the same.

Targeted rehabilitation that is specific to the graft site still must occur for the best result possible to be achieved. The rehabilitation of the graft site is complicated and slowed by a concomitant ACL reconstruction within the same knee. The rehabilitation of an intraarticular ACL reconstruction and that of a patellar tendon that has had its central portion removed are different and conflicting. In a knee that has undergone only an intraarticular ACL reconstruction, the extensor mechanism has not been injured, and therefore return of strength is expected. In this case the primary goal of rehabilitation is full range of motion because of the risk of arthrofibrosis. Limited range of motion (ROM) makes return to full function of a joint difficult, and pain is more likely. Furthermore, data show that the factor with the greatest negative effect on long-term outcome is a lack of full symmetric hyperextension, with a significant decrease in subjective scores noted in the presence of more than 2 degrees of extension loss compared with the opposite knee (Shelbourne, KD, unpublished data, 2004).

On the other hand, regaining knee motion is not a problem associated with the patellar tendon graft harvest. Because graft harvest is an extraarticular procedure with no injury occurring inside the joint, there should be no risk for arthrofibrosis if appropriate rehabilitation is done. Decreased flexion can be a problem if the patellar tendon is allowed to contract and scar tissue forms that causes the patellar tendon to shorten. The process of graft harvest directly affects the extensor mechanism of the knee and has a significant effect on postoperative strength. The muscle itself is not intrinsically affected, but the postoperative rehabilitation must emphasize strengthening the patellar tendon while returning its native elasticity. Patellar tendon strength is evaluated by tracking quadriceps strength, while tendon elasticity is evaluated objectively by measuring knee flexion ROM.

Rehabilitation after any ACL reconstruction requires exercise for full knee motion to be regained. Rehabilitation after ACL reconstruction with patellar tendon graft harvest also requires healing of the tendon and regaining of quadriceps muscle strength. Regaining motion and strength at the same time is difficult and involves conflicting goals. Separating the goals by taking a graft from the contralateral knee is beneficial. When using an ipsilateral graft, strengthening may come at the expense of knee ROM in the early postoperative period. Conversely, halting strengthening exercises to regain necessary ROM delays the return to function. This conflict has been demonstrated clinically when ipsilateral and contralateral graft populations have been compared at 1 year after surgery.[2]

The contralateral graft offers an additional benefit. A contralateral graft simplifies postoperative rehabilitation by separating the conflicting goals of regaining motion in the ACL-reconstructed knee and strength in the graft-donor knee. Use of a contralateral graft can allow return to function and sport more quickly.[2] However, simply harvesting a contralateral graft itself, in the absence of appropriate rehabilitation, cannot prevent postoperative complications or speed the return to sport. The therapeutic principles of rehabilitation described subsequently still must be applied postoperatively.

Another important concept in ACL rehabilitation is symmetry. An uninjured athlete has two knees in which strength and motion are symmetric. For an injured athlete to return to peak performance, it is important that symmetry be reestablished because he or she will function only at the level of the deficient knee. A patient who has undergone ACL reconstruction with a contralateral graft regains symmetry more quickly and reliably than does a patient who has undergone ACL reconstruction with an ipsilateral graft.[2] When both knees have undergone surgery, a patient will use both knees equally in everyday life, inadvertently accelerating rehabilitation and helping to ensure recovery. The use of a contralateral graft is helpful to the unmotivated patient or the nonathlete as well. Given that both legs are used equally during rehabilitation, the "bad leg" phenomenon is avoided. In contrast, patients who have ACL reconstruction with an ipsilateral graft usually favor the uninjured leg for many months after surgery. In simple activities such as hopping off a table or going up steps, use of the ACL-reconstructed leg is avoided and the benefit of such daily activities is lost. As mentioned, the chance that both legs subsequently will return to a symmetric state is reduced.

SURGICAL PROCEDURE

Intraarticular ACL reconstruction is performed using a miniarthrotomy technique as described by Shelbourne and Rask.[3] An arthroscopy is performed on the ACL-deficient knee to evaluate for and treat meniscus tears and articular cartilage damage. Routine incisions and tibial and femoral bone tunnels are made in the involved knee. After the femoral tunnel is drilled, the tourniquet is inflated on the contralateral extremity. A medial parapatellar incision is made, and a 10 mm autogenous patellar tendon graft with bone plugs on each end is harvested regardless of patellar tendon width. Three sutures are placed in each bone plug. The patellar bone plug is placed into the tibial tunnel, and the tibial bone plug is placed into the femoral tunnel of the involved knee. The graft is secured tightly with the sutures tied over tibial and femoral buttons with the knee in 30 degrees of flexion. To prevent putting too much tension on the graft, the ACL-reconstructed knee is moved through full knee ROM. This movement ensures that the graft placement has not captured the joint.

To eliminate a permanent patellar and tibial defect caused by harvesting the bone plugs, the bone shavings obtained from the notchplasty and drilling of the femoral and tibial tunnels are packed into the defects on the contralateral knee. The patellar tendon defect is loosely closed. To reduce the tendon soreness that often occurs on the night of surgery, the graft knee is moved through full knee ROM after closure of the tendon.

Routine closure is performed on both knees. Light dressings are applied to both knees and are secured into place with antiembolism stockings. A cold-compression device is applied immediately to the ACL-reconstructed knee to prevent a hemarthrosis.

REHABILITATION PROTOCOL

It is essential that rehabilitation for ACL reconstruction, regardless of graft source, begin before surgery itself. An acutely torn ACL results in a knee hemarthrosis and an intraarticular inflammatory state. It has been shown that surgery during this inflammatory state predisposes patients to arthrofibrosis and that waiting until the knee has returned to more normal physiology is vital for preventing this difficult complication.[4] Clinically, a normal physiologic state is reached when the injured knee has full ROM equal to the opposite knee, gait becomes normal, and effusion resolves. This process typically takes up to 4 weeks to achieve when expedited by rehabilitation. During this period, normal ambulation is encouraged and the patient is asked to work on regaining normal extension before flexion. Again, before surgery can be scheduled, patients must demonstrate full

ROM, little or no swelling, and enough functional strength to walk and climb stairs normally.

Achieving these preoperative goals presents a conflict for the physical therapist. It is not possible to attain both motion and strength at the same time without one inhibiting the other. Indeed, it is unadvisable to work on extension and flexion simultaneously for the same reason. Our priorities are initially to emphasize knee extension and a normal gait and stance while waiting to achieve flexion. Strengthening is rarely important preoperatively when using a contralateral patellar tendon graft. The rehabilitation process starts with the initial examination. Virtually all patients with an acute ACL injury will demonstrate loss of knee extension. The reason for this is anatomic. In an uninjured knee the ACL fits perfectly into the roof of the intercondylar notch with the knee in full extension. In a knee with a torn ACL, however, the ACL stump is compressed against the roof of the intercondylar notch as the knee attempts to achieve extension. The compression causes pain, and because of this, the patient avoids extension.

Correcting this phenomenon is the first preoperative goal. With sustained and gentle extension pressure, pathologic tissue can be forced from the intercondylar notch, and full extension can be achieved. In practice, this is accomplished by the series of exercises described subsequently. The frequency of each exercise and the number of repetitions recommended is at the discretion of the physical therapist and should be modified for continued daily progress. The recommended frequencies should serve only as guidelines.

Preoperatively the patient will be seen weekly by a physical therapist. Motion and gait are assessed at each visit. Extension is examined with the patient lying supine. One of the examiner's hands is placed in the area of the suprapatellar pouch while the other hand grasps the plantar midfoot and lifts gently. The distance from the heel to the table is noted and compared bilaterally (Figure 9-1). This maneuver not only allows for an objective measurement of extension but also allows the examiner to get a kinesthetic "feel" for the ease with which the knee goes into extension. The following exercises are used to achieve full hyperextension in the knee.

1. Towel stretches (Figure 9-2): This exercise is considered the cornerstone of extension exercise. While sitting, the patient pushes down on the leg, with the hand just proximal to the patella. A towel is looped around the ball of the foot and held in the opposite hand. The patient then pushes down on the leg while pulling on the towel, bringing the knee into hyperextension and holding for 5 seconds. Then, without letting the heel fall, and using only the quadriceps muscle, the patient contracts the quadriceps and holds the knee in hyperextension for 5 more seconds.

2. Correct stance (Figure 9-3): While standing, the patient's weight is shifted to the involved knee, which is

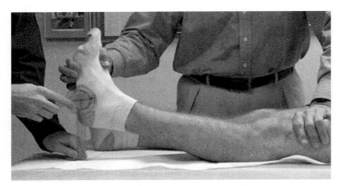

Figure 9-1: Evaluating knee hyperextension. One of the examiner's hands is placed in the area of the suprapatellar pouch while the other hand grasps the plantar midfoot and lifts gently.

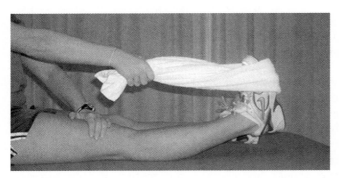

Figure 9-2: Towel stretches. While sitting, the patient pushes down on the leg, with the hand just proximal to the patella. A towel is looped around the ball of the foot and held in the opposite hand. The patient then pushes down on the leg while pulling on the towel, bringing the knee into hyperextension.

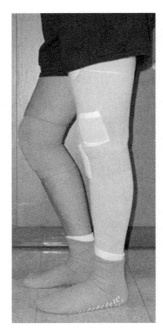

Figure 9-3: Correct stance. While standing, the patient's weight is shifted to the involved knee, which is locked and held into hyperextension by a quadriceps muscle contraction.

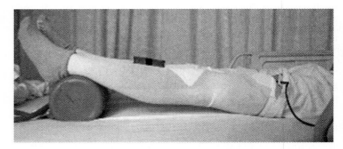

Figure 9-4: Heel props. With the patient lying supine, a bolster is placed under the patient's heel, allowing the knee to fall into hyperextension.

locked and held into hyperextension by a quadriceps muscle contraction.

3. Heel props (Figure 9-4): With the patient lying supine, a bolster is placed under the patient's heel, allowing the knee to fall into hyperextension.

4. Prone hangs (Figure 9-5): With the patient lying prone and the leg support ending just proximal to the knee, a 3 lb weight is placed around the ankle.

5. Gait training: A normal heel-to-toe gait with proper push off is emphasized.

6. Cold compression: The patient is provided a Cryo/Cuff (Aircast, Inc., Summit, NJ) and instructed in appropriate use. The Cryo/Cuff allows for joint space compression and cold therapy and is effective for controlling the volume of effusion.

Once full knee extension and normal gait are achieved, the patient advances to working on achieving full knee flexion, which is typically easier to achieve than extension. It is important to maintain knee extension while working on flexion exercises. If knee extension becomes tight or decreases,

flexion exercises should be curtailed. If knee flexion has normalized, the patient should be able to sit on his or her heels comfortably and symmetrically (Figure 9-6). Recommended knee flexion exercises are as follows.

1. Heel slides (Figure 9-7): The patient begins in a supine position. With the help of a towel looped under the thigh, flexion is initiated by the patient and continued until further flexion is difficult. At this point the patient is assisted in looping the towel around the ankle with both hands, and continued flexion is encouraged. If range of motion allows, the patient may grasp the ankle and pull the leg into further flexion. Terminal flexion is held for 30 seconds.

2. Wall slides (Figure 9-8): The patient lies supine with hips flexed and both legs extended up the wall. With the

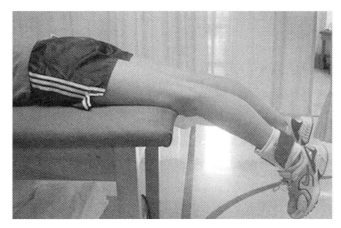

Figure 9-5: Prone hangs. With the patient lying prone and the leg support ending just proximal to the knee, a 3 lb weight is placed around the ankle.

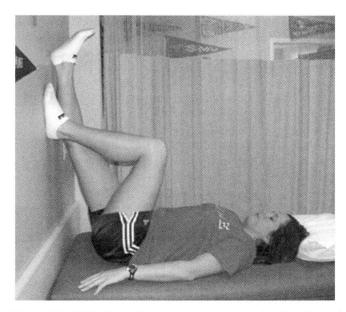

Figure 9-8: Wall slides. The patient lies supine with hips flexed and both legs extended up the wall. With the patient as close to the wall as comfortable, the affected side is allowed to slide down the wall with gravity assistance.

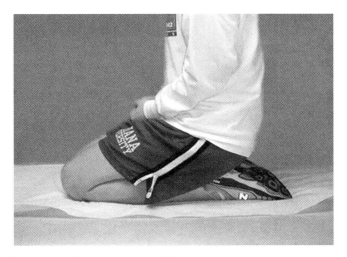

Figure 9-6: Sitting on heels. If flexion has normalized, the patient should be able to sit on his or her heels comfortably and symmetrically.

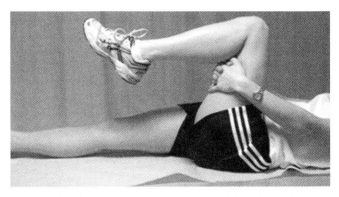

Figure 9-9: Flexion hangs. In a supine position the patient flexes both hips and allows gravity to maximally flex both knees. Next, the foot of the uninjured extremity is placed on top of the foot of the injured extremity, and the weight of the leg is allowed to further flex the involved knee.

patient as close to the wall as comfortable, the affected side is allowed to slide down the wall with gravity assistance. Flexion gains beyond 115 degrees will prove difficult with wall slides.

3. Flexion hangs (Figure 9-9): In a supine position the patient flexes both hips and allows gravity to maximally flex both knees. Next, the foot of the uninjured extremity is placed on top of the foot of the injured extremity, and the weight of the leg is allowed to further flex the injured knee. Multiple repetitions of the above exercises are typically prescribed.

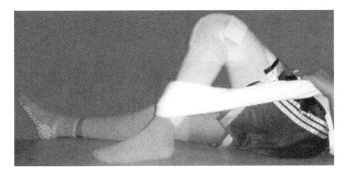

Figure 9-7: Heel slides. The patient lies supine. The patient loops a towel around the ankle with both hands and gently pulls the leg into further flexion.

In practice, time spent doing each exercise is variable according to each patient's need. Exercises during the first week after injury emphasize knee extension, stance, and gait only. During this time, the towel stretch is the exercise of key importance. Patients are generally encouraged to perform exercises three times daily. Typically, a 10 minute heel prop will be followed by 10 to 15 towel stretches. However, there is no maximum number of towel stretches, and the patient is allowed to increase both frequency and repetitions if the knee is tight. The other exercises are added at the discretion of the physical therapist. As surgery draws near, the patient is asked to perform a towel stretch early in the morning to check extension, as this reflects progress more accurately.

In the preoperative phase, it is important not to mistake the rare locked bucket-handle meniscus tear for the normal loss of extension after an ACL tear. In the latter case, passive extension should gradually attain near symmetric hyperextension by the end of the first physical therapy visit. In the event of a locked displaced meniscus tear, the knee will be unable to attain full hyperextension, and extension exercise will cause the patient to have anteromedial or anterolateral pain. If doubt exists as to which is the case, magnetic resonance imaging should be used to confirm the diagnosis. It is important to make this diagnosis early on, as a locked meniscus will prevent extension, and lack of extension can lead to arthrofibrosis if meniscal surgery and ACL reconstruction are attempted concurrently. A safer approach would be to treat meniscal pathology first, then allow the knee to again recover before ACL reconstruction is attempted.[5] In the senior author's experience, less than 1% of acute ACL tears and less than 18% of chronic tears will have this complication.

Another benefit of preoperative rehabilitation is that the patient begins a working relationship with the physical therapist before surgery. Education about postoperative care can be discussed, then reinforced after surgery—a practice that increases both understanding and compliance.

Finally, objective strength is tested. These scores become useful information that give the clinician objective criteria to gauge a patient's progress and response to exercise. These tests include concentric isokinetic testing at 180 degrees/second and 60 degrees/second, leg press test, and single leg hop test. The single leg hop is tested on the uninjured leg only; all other tests are administered bilaterally.

Phase I: Immediate Postoperative Phase

It is common in ACL surgery to perform reconstruction in the outpatient setting. Typically, patients are immobilized, given crutches, and discharged to home. They are then seen in a physician's office a few days to weeks after surgery and eventually referred to a physical therapist to begin rehabilitation. This practice both invites a delay in return to activity and compromises rehabilitation goals. In contrast, we begin postoperative rehabilitation immediately in the operating room. After graft fixation the surgeon checks to ensure that full knee flexion and extension are attainable. Next, the patellar tendon of the graft knee is injected with local anesthetic. Anesthetizing the tendon allows immediate full, relatively painless flexion exercise, permitting the tendon to remain at its full length. Later, quadriceps muscle contraction during weight bearing will similarly draw the patella proximally and stretch the tendon to full length. The combination of these two exercises decreases patellar tendon stiffness and contracture, processes that could otherwise occur after graft harvest and cause graft site pain. Initiating full knee flexion immediately after surgery makes this goal attainable more reliably and earlier in the postoperative course.

Another important technique that allows the patient to participate in phase I rehabilitation is the avoidance of narcotics in the perioperative period. Although occasionally patients will require oral narcotics, parenteral narcotics decrease a patient's ability to physically and cognitively participate in exercise. With the use of a ketorolac infusion, continuous cold-compression therapy, supplemental oral nonnarcotic pain medication, and immediate motion, narcotics can be avoided altogether in most instances. A regimen focused on pain prevention rather than on treating pain after it is already present increases both patient participation and satisfaction.[6] It is interesting to note that patients almost unanimously report that participating in immediate postoperative rehabilitation decreases their subjective pain. Finally, in the operating room, external drains are placed in the region of the fat pad. Along with leg elevation and cold-compression therapy, external drains decrease the incidence and volume of postoperative hemarthrosis, which is the enemy of obtaining full knee motion. Patients are kept in 23-hour outpatient observation primarily to prevent hemarthrosis and allow initiation of immediate rehabilitation. Initiating rehabilitation days after reconstruction fails to exploit the full value of a contralateral graft harvest.

Before the patient leaves the operating room, antiembolism stockings are placed bilaterally, and the ACL-reconstructed knee is placed in a Cryo/Cuff cold-compression device. An elastic sleeve with an incorporated frozen gel package (DuraSoft Patellar Tendon Wrap, dj Orthopedics, Inc., Vista, CA) is placed over the graft harvest site. Suprapatellar compression is not needed on this knee because graft harvest is an extraarticular procedure; there is no risk for an intraarticular effusion. As the patient arrives in the postoperative recovery area, the ACL-reconstructed leg is placed in a continuous passive motion (CPM) machine set at 0 to 30 degrees. Continuous passive motion not only provides gentle motion, but it also, more importantly, elevates the leg. The graft leg is elevated on pillows to the same level. Both knees are then elevated above the level of the heart (Figure 9-10).

Phase I rehabilitation continues immediately on arrival in the outpatient observation unit, where targeted physical therapy begins. The patient and his or her family are given

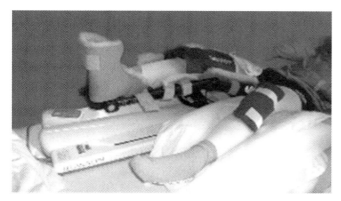

Figure 9-10: Elevation with cold-compression therapy. The ACL-reconstructed knee is placed in a continuous passive motion machine for elevation and a Cryo/Cuff is applied for cold compression. The Cryo/Cuff is unique in that it allows both joint space compression and cold therapy. A DuraSoft knee sleeve is placed on the graft-donor knee.

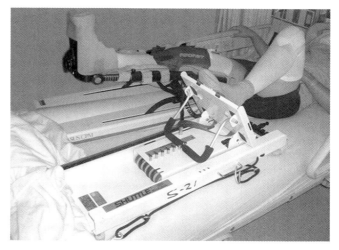

Figure 9-11: The Shuttle. The Shuttle is a lightweight, low-resistance portable leg press machine. Resistance is afforded by the placement of weighted rubber cords, each corresponding to increasing resistance.

an exercise diary outlining activities to perform. Check marks or measurements are placed in boxes next to each exercise as it is completed. This practice aids in compliance by giving the patient a visual reference to specific exercises. To initiate therapeutic exercise, the cold-compression device, CPM, and pillows are removed. The patient then proceeds through the list of exercises as follows:

1. CPM-assisted flexion: Before the CPM machine is removed, maximum flexion is achieved. The maximum flexion allowable by the CPM machine is 125 degrees. This is arrived at slowly and incrementally as tolerated by the patient.

2. Heel slides: From a supine position, heel slides are performed with both legs in turn. A yardstick is positioned next to the leg, with the zero end of the yardstick placed at the heel. With the help of a towel looped under the thigh, flexion of the graft-donor knee is initiated by the patient and continued until further flexion is difficult. At this point the patient is assisted in looping the towel around the ankle with both hands, and continued flexion is encouraged. Terminal flexion is held for 3 minutes. The number of centimeters the heel has traveled is recorded. This number is easy for the patient and physical therapist to discuss over the phone during the subsequent week. Immediately, heel-to-buttock flexion is routine and encouraged in the graft knee. Typical flexion in the ACL-reconstructed knee is approximately 130 degrees immediately postoperatively.

3. Heel props: Both legs are then propped in extension with the heels resting on the cold-compression cooler, allowing the knees to sag into hyperextension. A 3 lb weight is placed just distal to the incision on the ACL-reconstructed knee. This posture is maintained for 10 minutes.

4. Thunks: After 10 minutes with the knee being propped in hyperextension, each knee is bent slightly and gently "thunk" down into hyperextension. This is completed twice for each leg. It can be difficult for the patient to achieve a satisfactory thunk on the ACL-reconstructed leg. Typically, thunks are first performed on the graft leg so that the patient understands how hyperextension feels.

5. Straight leg raises: The patient initiates quadriceps muscle contraction and then lifts each leg in turn several times so that the heel is 2 to 3 feet above the mattress.

6. Towel stretches: Five repetitions are completed on each side in the manner described above.

7. Shuttle exercises: The Shuttle (Contemporary Design, Inc., Glacier, WA) is implemented on the graft leg only as it is meant to strengthen the donor tendon. The Shuttle is a lightweight, low-resistance portable leg press machine (Figure 9-11). Resistance is afforded by the placement of weighted rubber cords, each corresponding to increasing resistance. This weight is applied in both eccentric and concentric contraction. The ACL-reconstructed knee is placed into the CPM machine again, and the Shuttle is placed under the graft-donor leg. Twenty-five repetitions of 7 lb of resistance are then completed.

After these exercises are performed, the cold-compression devices are applied to each leg and changed every waking hour. The CPM is again set at 0 to 30 degrees. The graft-donor leg is placed on pillows, and the patient is confined to bed rest with the use of a portable urinal and bedpan if needed. The patient may ambulate during this time, but does so at the risk of hemarthrosis.

The drains are removed the following morning, and an identical set of exercises is carried out, with a few exceptions. The Shuttle will be used only three times daily, while all other exercises are performed six times daily. The number of centimeters traveled by the heel on the yardstick is recorded in the exercise diary. Patients are advised that knee flexion may decrease from the previous day in the ACL-reconstructed knee, but the flexion obtained initially after surgery should return gradually by 2 to 3 days after surgery. In general, patients are counseled against overemphasizing knee flexion in this period, as extension remains more important. Knee flexion in the graft-donor knee should remain full.

At the end of this session the patient ambulates for the first time. This is accomplished carefully to avoid a fall. First, the patient sits at the edge of the bed. When it is clear that the patient is steady and not dizzy, standing is encouraged. Standing is allowed for a few minutes, with a clinician close by to make sure a vagal episode does not occur. Next, the patient is instructed to shift his or her weight over to the ACL-reconstructed leg and to lock that leg into hyperextension with a quadriceps muscle contraction. The patient then ambulates to the door of the room, taking small steps and focusing on a point high on the wall in the direction in which he or she is ambulating. When the door is reached the patient turns around, again locks the ACL knee into hyperextension, and ambulates back to either the bathroom or the bed. This pattern of ambulation is encouraged whenever the patient rises from bed throughout the first week.

Before release from the hospital, the patient must have full extension of the ACL-reconstructed leg equal to that in the graft-donor leg, flexion of at least 110 degrees on the ACL-reconstructed leg, near full flexion of the graft leg, the ability to lift both legs with quadriceps muscle contraction, the ability to ambulate independently, and an understanding of the home exercise program.

After discharge, patients are called daily for the first week to monitor progress and answer questions that might arise. The exercises listed previously are performed six times daily, with the exception of the Shuttle, which is used three times daily and on the graft-donor leg only. Patients are instructed not to use the Shuttle at the first morning exercise session and to discontinue its use if they become too sore at the graft site or begin to lose knee flexion on daily measurements. Barring these events, they are allowed to add 10 repetitions per session. When 100 repetitions become easy, weight can be added incrementally. With each addition of resistance, the starting point again becomes 25 repetitions and is increased to 100 repetitions before more weight is added. If knee flexion in the graft-donor leg decreases, the patient is advised to similarly decrease Shuttle exercise. In the ACL-reconstructed leg, knee extension is emphasized more than knee flexion during this phase. If the amount of knee extension plateaus or decreases, the amount of exercises to increase knee flexion should be decreased accordingly. Patients are warned that exercises will become more difficult at day two or three after

surgery before gradually improving. If the patient is progressing well and requests additional exercise, the extension towel stretch is permitted more often. During the first week, patients are allowed out of bed only three times daily for bathroom needs.

The first postoperative visit takes place 1 week after surgery. The primary goal at the first visit is full extension of the ACL-reconstructed leg; approximately 110 degrees of knee flexion is a secondary goal and represents the average flexion in this period. No patients should have less than 90 degrees of knee flexion. For the graft-donor leg, full flexion where the heel is brought to the buttocks is expected. These motion goals are carefully documented. Next, quadriceps muscle control is assessed. The patient should be able to ambulate stairs using only the handrail for balance. Furthermore, the patient should be able to strongly contract the quadriceps muscle with the knee in a hyperextended position. If achieving a hyperextended position through a voluntary contraction is not possible, the condition is a result of quadriceps inhibition. Treatment of this problem is discussed later in this chapter.

Phase II: Intermediate Phase

If goals have been satisfactorily achieved, the patient progresses to the intermediate phase of rehabilitation. Specific exercises in this phase are discussed in the following paragraphs. Again, a diary, with spaces to record progress, and detailed instructions are provided to the patient. Rehabilitation remains unique to each leg. The patient continues to work on maintaining full extension of the ACL-reconstructed knee while concentrating on patellar tendon remodeling and regrowth in the graft-donor knee through the use of strengthening exercise and maintenance of flexion. Leg control is emphasized bilaterally with gait and stance training. Techniques reinforced during this phase include the following:

1. Correct stance: In standing, weight is shifted to the involved knee, which is locked into hyperextension.

2. Gait training: A mirror can provide helpful feedback to correct deviations.

3. Heel props: This exercise is performed three times daily for 10 minutes each time.

4. Prone hangs: With the patient prone and leg support ending just proximal to the knee, a 3 lb weight is placed around the ankle. The goal is to perform the exercise three times daily for 10 minutes.

5. Towel stretches: Five repetitions are completed three times daily.

The importance of full symmetric knee hyperextension cannot be overemphasized. If asymmetric hyperextension is noted and not correctable by the end of this follow-up appointment, then more vigorous techniques described in the final part of this chapter are recommended.

Secondly, knee flexion exercises are implemented. The goal for flexion is 120 degrees by the end of week 2. Techniques include the following:

1. Heel slides: This exercise is completed three times daily.

2. Flexion hangs: This exercise typically precedes heel slides, as heel props precede extension exercises.

3. Wall slides: As previously discussed, this exercise can be added at the discretion of the physical therapist.

Additional emphasis is placed on leg control, as evidenced by the ability of the patient to walk smoothly with good quadriceps muscle function. Leg control is achieved with the previously described gait instruction and by continued work with the Shuttle. Strength should also be assessed by the quality of a straight leg raise and eccentric leg curl. However, quantified objective strength is not tested at the initial postoperative visit.

During week 2, use of the CPM machine is discontinued, but cold-compression therapy continues. Shuttle exercises are continued as long as the patient retains heel-to-buttock flexion. If the patient continues to maintain motion and avoid effusion, he or she is allowed to increase upright time by an hour at a time. One week postoperatively, patients usually can attend school or work for half the day. By day 10, if motion remains good and effusion is not an issue, patients are allowed to be up for a full day with brief periods of elevated rest as needed. During this period of increased mobility, a self-contained cold-compression device can be worn underneath clothing.

The second postoperative visit takes place 2 weeks after surgery. ROM, gait, and quadriceps muscle control are again carefully examined. In the ACL-reconstructed knee, 120 degrees of flexion is expected in addition to full extension. Effusion should be well controlled. Excessive effusion is indicative of an overly intense activity level. Full flexion and extension in the graft-donor knee should be maintained. Strength testing, with the exception of single leg hop test, is performed.

The goal of rehabilitation between weeks 2 and 4 is remodeling and regrowth of the donor patellar tendon through high-repetition, low-resistance exercise carried out several times daily. These exercises are essential to avoid graft-site pain. It remains vital to maintain full extension of the ACL-reconstructed knee and to make continued progress in flexion. By the 1-month postoperative visit, patients should be able to comfortably sit on their heels with their feet in maximum dorsiflexion, a position indicative of full knee flexion. However, the main emphasis of the physical therapy visit at 2 weeks is outlining a strengthening program for the donor tendon. Use of the Shuttle is discontinued, and a step box is provided for the patient. The step box is a hinged, foldable device that allows step exercises from heights up to eight inches. The step box is adjustable in 2-inch increments. In addition, patients are guided in leg press exercises and knee extension exercises. Typically, patients are asked to lift

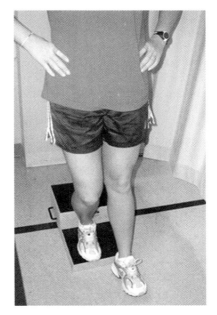

Figure 9-12: The step box. The step box is a hinged, foldable device that allows step exercises from heights up to 8 inches. The patient first stands with hands placed on hips. Balancing on either leg, the patient bends and straightens the involved leg so that the heel of the opposite leg is lowered to touch the floor and then raised off the floor. It is important to keep the pelvis neutral and keep the hip, knee, and toe facing directly anteriorly.

less than half of their body weight, or less weight if this is difficult, for leg press exercises. Knee extension repetitions are carried out initially at 2 to 3 lb.

The use of the step box, however, is the cornerstone of early donor site strengthening and should be the primary focus. It can occasionally be introduced to an advanced patient at the first preoperative visit. The step box is effective and portable and does not require access to a gym. Proper technique is essential (Figure 9-12). Beginning at the lowest setting, the patient first stands in front of the box with hands placed on hips. Balancing on either leg, the heel of the opposite leg is placed on the lowest step and then back to the floor. It is important to keep the pelvis neutral during this step to prevent recruiting of more proximal musculature. In addition, the hip, knee, and toe must face directly anterior with no lateral movement allowed by the moving foot. The foot must progress along a straight line perpendicular to the axis of the body. This is done with both legs in turn and provides more proprioception and balance benefits than strengthening. This initial exercise can be introduced if the patient is doing well at the 1-week visit. Whenever the lowest setting becomes easy, the patient progresses to a higher step. At each subsequent level, exercises are done only with the graft-donor knee.

When progressed the patient stands on the 2-inch step and with similar technique slowly lowers the heel of the ACL-reconstructed leg until it lightly touches the floor. The foot is returned to the platform and the activity is repeated. Progression through the step box heights is achieved under supervision of the physical therapist. The leg press, knee extension, and the step box may be used in conjunction with one another if a patient is doing well and maintains full flexion. At this point a typical step box regimen would include one set of 20 repetitions completed six times daily. Repetitions are added in increments of 10 until 50 repetitions are easy, which is demonstrated by perfect form and minimal tendon soreness after exercise. Soreness should be relieved with cryotherapy, should not interfere with normal gait, and should be absent by the next session. When this occurs, the patient is progressed to the next step height.

During this time, leg press exercises are typically performed twice daily, starting with four sets of 10 repetitions at a comfortable weight. When this weight becomes easy per the previously described criteria, the patient is progressed to four sets of 15 repetitions. From this point, progression occurs in 5 lb to 10 lb increments, and four sets of 10 repetitions are again performed. Leg extensions may be done once or twice daily, again starting at four sets of 10 to 15 repetitions with 2 to 3 lb. In our experience, patients often overdo this particular exercise and develop graft site soreness. If a patient develops soreness with either leg press or leg extension exercises, these exercises may be discontinued. The most important thing is that the patient demonstrates continued improvement without developing unrelenting donor-site pain.

At the 4-week physical therapy appointment, the patient again undergoes strength testing with the exception of the single leg hop. These data will be helpful to assess progress and give objective evidence of initial strength. The patient may receive some satisfaction during this phase by noting that the patellar tendon is becoming palpably thicker than in the immediate postoperative period. Increasing strength scores represent increasing tendon strength. Typically, quadriceps muscle strengthening is limited by tendon soreness rather than muscle soreness. When muscle soreness outweighs tendon soreness, this is a sign that more advanced strengthening is indicated. Generally, this will not occur before 4 weeks postoperatively.

Phase III: Advanced Strengthening

Four weeks after surgery, the patient undergoes full strength testing excluding the single leg hop test. The results are helpful to assess progress over the previous 2 weeks and to develop a plan for further activity. At this point the recovery of preoperative strength is not as important as symmetry between legs. For a patient to be doing well, isokinetic strength in the graft-donor knee should be within 10% of that in the ACL-reconstructed knee and should be notably improved from previous test results.

The ability to return to activities at between 4 and 8 weeks depends on the strength of the graft-donor knee, the presence of full ROM, and the lack of an effusion in the ACL-reconstructed knee. If symmetric quadriceps muscle strength and knee ROM exist, the patient begins bilateral strengthening and conditioning exercises, progressing to exercise on a stair-stepping machine or an elliptical trainer as tolerated. Straight line forward and backward running can be introduced, as can lateral slides, crossovers, shooting baskets, or other sport-specific drills as tolerated. These activities are added only in the continued presence of minimal effusion, full motion, symmetric strength, and continuing improvement in donor tendon soreness. If these criteria are not met, activities are reduced accordingly. No competitive situations are performed at this time.

Phase IV: Return to Competition

There are no strict guidelines as to when a patient may safely return to sports. The principles outlined above continue to be followed at the 2-, 4-, and 6-month visits. Rehabilitation continues to be monitored as the patient returns to the preoperative, fully competitive level of activity. Symmetry, in the form of strength, knee ROM, and effusion, is evaluated at each visit. Typically, between 2 and 4 months patients proceed through a functional progression for their sport. Strength, comfort, and confidence are all factors to consider when allowing the return to a fully competitive level of activity. It is important to counsel the athlete returning from ACL reconstruction that it typically takes 2 months of competition before the athlete will achieve a level of performance similar to the accustomed preinjury level. By 6 months after surgery the majority of athletes report that their knees feel normal enough that the athletes compete without thinking about them and can participate in their sports easily (Table 9-1).

It is interesting to note that we have found the conventional dictum that good leg strength is protective of the ACL-reconstructed knee to be untrue during this phase. Strength may allow an athlete to more effectively return to his or her sport, but in general it is the stronger of the two knees that is at greater risk for subsequent ACL injury (Shelbourne, KD, unpublished data, 2004). This is another reason to focus on symmetry between legs during rehabilitation rather than on strengthening the ACL-reconstructed leg alone.

ADDRESSING PROBLEMS

As previously mentioned, the key to successful ACL surgery is avoiding complications. Extensive experience has shown that these complications are much easier to prevent than to treat. The entire protocol described previously has been created in an effort to avoid these complications while returning an athlete to sport expediently and safely. However, despite the best efforts of the surgeon and physical therapist, whether because of compliance issues, deviation from principles, or physiology, problems do arise and should be dealt with appropriately.

Lack of Knee Motion

No other complication has as much potential to create a poor outcome as lack of motion—hence the obvious emphasis throughout this chapter. Lack of motion is best prevented with a return to physiologic normalcy before ACL reconstruction. A return to full extension can be encouraged with the presented regimen. In the patient for whom attaining full preoperative extension is difficult, it is advisable to discontinue strengthening and flexion exercises. Second, the use of an extension board (O and P Associates, Inc., Indianapolis, IN) or an Elite Seat (Kneebourne Therapeutics, Noblesville, IN) can be advantageous. Both of these devices passively stretch the knee into extension, compressing or forcing aside tissue within the notch. The chief difference is that the extension board is controlled with local Velcro straps and necessitates a second person for correct use (Figure 9-13). The Elite Seat works from proximally controlled pulleys (Figure 9-14). Both are used under the supervision of a physical therapist to aid in attaining full extension.

Similar principles are used postoperatively. If full extension is difficult to achieve or is not achievable at any point, the Elite Seat or extension board should immediately be added as an adjunct activity, and patients should be closely followed to assure quick return to full extension. Similarly, flexion and strengthening exercises are discontinued or decreased until full extension is again achieved. With close follow-up, it is rare that a patient requires additional intervention. However, a persistent asymmetry of extension is an indication for operative intervention.

Lack of knee flexion is typically easier to treat. In the absence of extension loss, aggressive flexion exercise should be instituted immediately if continued improvement is not noted according to the goals described previously. As emphasized, persistent swelling can be the enemy of motion.

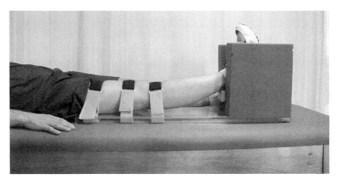

Figure 9-13: Extension board. The heel of the foot is placed in the foam padding that is raised above the board. Velcro straps are secured above and below the knee to push the knee into hyperextension as allowed.

TABLE 9-1

Rehabilitation Phases

PHASE	GOALS	SPECIFIC EXERCISES
Preoperative	Attaining normal physiology and motion	Heel props, towel stretches, prone hangs. Gait and stance training. Heel slides, flexion hangs, wall slides.
Immediate postoperative through first week	ACL knee: Full extension, 115 degrees of flexion; limited effusion	CPM flexion, heel slides, thunks, straight leg raises, heel props, towel stretch, Shuttle.
	Graft knee: Full motion	Cold compression. Early step box.
	Both: Unassisted leg lifts and ambulation with normal gait	
Intermediate phase: weeks 2 to 4	ACL knee: Full extension, 120 degrees of flexion, progressing to full flexion; improving effusion	ACL knee: Heel props, prone hangs, towel stretches, correct stance and walking, heel slides, wall slides, flexion hangs.
	Graft knee: Donor site strengthening	Graft knee: Step box, leg press, knee extension.
		Both: Cold compression.
Advanced strengthening phase: weeks 4 to 8	Full motion and symmetric strength in both knees	Progressing from above to straight-line running, Stairmaster, elliptical trainer, progression to sport-specific exercise. Cold compression as needed.
Return to competition: beyond 2 months	Symmetric, normal knees, full competition	Sport-specific exercise, functional progression, return to competition.

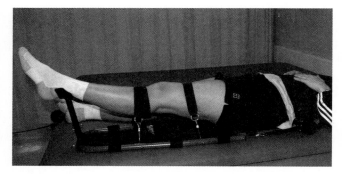

Figure 9-14: The Elite Seat. The heel of the foot is placed in a raised position while the patient lies supine, which allows the hamstring muscles to relax. The patient places the straps across, above, and below the knee. The patient pushes a controlled handle to apply force that will put the knee into hyperextension.

If persistent effusion is problematic, it is recommended that activity level and strengthening be decreased and the use of cold-compression therapy increased until a more normal state is achieved.

Quadriceps Inhibition

Occasionally a patient will have poor quadriceps muscle function postoperatively. The hallmark of this condition is an inability to initiate quadriceps muscle contraction when the knee is brought into hyperextension. Normally, a patient should be able to use the quadriceps muscle to hold the knee in a hyperextended position. The examiner's hand, when placed between the table and the popliteal fossa, should feel increased pressure during this maneuver. The opposite will occur in the presence of quadriceps muscle inhibition. The patient will not be able to hold the affected foot off the examining table using the quadriceps muscle, and the examiner will feel decreased pressure under the popliteal fossa. More important, the lack of contraction will be visible. Clinically this condition manifests itself in a poor gait pattern. Quadriceps inhibition does not represent femoral nerve palsy, as it is often labeled. Helpful exercises to treat this phenomenon include the following:

1. Hyperextension quadriceps muscle contraction: With the patient seated or supine, a hand on the quadriceps may provide enough biofeedback to help initiate quadriceps muscle contraction during hyperextension.

2. Stance and gait training: Standing in front of a mirror in the sagittal plane may assist a patient to understand the correct position of a hyperextended knee in stance.

3. Step box: As previously described, the patient balances on the functional leg in front of the step box and

practices placing the heel of the quadriceps muscle–inhibited leg on the lowest platform, and vice versa.

4. Tubing exercise: The patient is asked to hyperextend the knee against tubing wrapped around the popliteal fossa.

Persistent Weakness

A contralateral graft is useful in preventing persistent weakness. However, patients will occasionally experience persistent weakness of graft-donor leg strength, which may be accompanied by donor-site tendon pain. It is important to keep in mind that this asymmetry cannot be remedied with bilateral exercise. Rather, decreasing bilateral activity and focusing on unilateral exercises such as step downs or leg press exercises is recommended. Donor-site tendon pain should guide the progression through these exercises. Patients will be more comfortable and compete more effectively when symmetry is attained.

Anterior Knee Pain

Much has been written about anterior knee pain with concomitant ACL reconstruction. Anterior knee pain is the best example of a complication best prevented. It is important to keep in mind that anterior knee pain is not a diagnosis, but rather a symptom. Donor-site tendon soreness, loss of motion, and weakness may all cause pain in the front of the knee. Indeed, some donor-site tendon soreness is universal and is useful as a guide to progression through exercise. Early high-repetition and low-resistance exercise, immediate full flexion, and early weight bearing are essential to make this pain temporary. An injured tendon tends to become stiffer and contracted if left alone or immobilized. Over an extended period of time, a stiff contracted tendon can cause pain in the front of the knee because of a poor ability to transmit stress and from its effect on the patellofemoral joint. It has long been recognized in orthopedics that tissues, given physiologic stress while healing, will heal with increased strength and improved collagen orientation.[7] The same principle is applied to the donor patellar tendon. Frequent transmission of physiologic loads and exercises designed to draw the tendon out to its full length can ensure the tendon heals as anatomically normally as possible in terms of strength and elasticity. Early donor-site pain should not be confused with the more malignant long-term entity caused by an unrehabilitated patellar tendon. Loss of motion or weakness should be treated as described previously. Another clinical entity that can contribute to anterior knee pain is a lack of quadriceps muscle flexibility. Even in the face of good knee flexion, the proximal quadriceps muscle can remain tight. This is best examined with the patient's hip in extension and the patient lying prone. In this position the heel should still easily reach the buttock. If this is not the case, appropriate stretching should begin.

SUMMARY

The contralateral patellar tendon graft is the logical result of years of experience rehabilitating patients with ACL reconstructions. It is a tool that allows the physical therapist to successfully target the donor site for early strengthening and flexibility and the reconstructed knee with motion exercises unimpeded by conflicting goals. In this regard, the use of the contralateral patellar tendon graft for ACL reconstruction can contribute to improved outcomes.

References

1. Daniel DM, Stone ML, Dobson BE, et al: Fate of the ACL-injured patient. A prospective outcome study, *Am J Sports Med* 22:632-644, 1994.

2. Shelbourne KD, Urch SE: Primary anterior cruciate ligament using the contralateral autogenous patellar tendon, *Am J Sports Med* 28:651-658, 2000.

3. Shelbourne KD, Rask BP: Anterior cruciate ligament reconstruction using a mini-open technique with autogenous patellar tendon graft, *Tech Orthop* 13:221-228, 1998.

4. Shelbourne KD, Wilckens JH, Mollabashy A, DeCarlo M: Arthrofibrosis in acute anterior cruciate ligament reconstruction. The effect of timing of reconstruction and rehabilitation, *Am J Sports Med* 19:332-336, 1991.

5. Shelbourne KD, Johnson GE: Locked bucket-handle meniscal tears in knees with chronic anterior cruciate ligament deficiency, *Am J Sports Med* 21:779-782, 1993.

6. Shelbourne KD, Liotta FJ, Goodloe SL: Preemptive pain management program for anterior cruciate ligament reconstruction, *Am J Knee Surg* 11:116-119, 1998.

7. Akeson WH: The response of ligaments to stress modulation and overview of the ligament healing response. In Daniel DM, Akeson WH, O'Conner JJ, editors: *Knee Ligaments. Structure, Function, and Repair*, New York, 1990, Raven Press.

CHAPTER 10

Anterior Cruciate Ligament Reconstruction Using the Hamstring–Gracilis Tendon Autograft

Robert C. Manske, DPT, MPT, MEd, SCS, ATC, CSCS
Daniel Prohaska, MD
Ryan Livermore, MD

RECONSTRUCTION OF THE ANTERIOR

cruciate ligament (ACL) is one of the most commonly performed procedures in orthopedic sports medicine. ACL reconstruction has become the procedure chosen by not only the elite athlete but also the "weekend warrior" for maintaining knee stability and function. With loss of the ACL primary restraint, secondary restraints, including menisci, articular surfaces, and other structures around the knee, are generally accepted to be at risk for recurrent episodes of instability. The importance of reconstruction in the athlete and active patient is no longer questioned. However, the ideal method, choice of graft, and choice of fixation remain debated.

Numerous grafts have been used for ACL reconstruction as techniques have been developed and improved. The basic options include allografts, autografts, and synthetic or prosthetic augmentation. Allograft and autograft sources have been successfully used, but at this time synthetic grafts as well as ligament augmentation devices (LADs) are no longer used in the United States because of poor results.[1-4] ACL reconstruction aims to restore stability to the knee. The surgeon chooses which graft will best accomplish this goal. The ideal graft reproduces the anatomy as well as the biomechanics, strength, and stiffness of the native ACL. In addition, it allows rapid and complete biologic incorporation, has strong initial fixation, and causes low or no morbidity from harvest to the patient. Such a graft does not exist at this time. With current techniques, however, excellent knee stability can be achieved with different graft sources.

HISTORY OF HAMSTRING AUTOGRAFTS FOR ANTERIOR CRUCIATE LIGAMENT RECONSTRUCTION

It was in 1939 that Harry B. Macey of Rochester, Minnesota first described a technique using the semitendinosus tendon for ACL reconstruction.[5] Macey left the tendon attachment to the tibia intact before passing the proximal portion through a tibial and femoral tunnel and before suturing this to the medial femoral periosteum. The tendinous portion of the semitendinosus was harvested, stopping short of the musculotendinous junction. Tunnels were made in the tibia and distal femur and the graft was fixed with the knee in full extension. The knee was then immobilized with plaster in full extension for 4 weeks, and normal activity was resumed at 8 weeks.

In 1950 K. Lindemann, a German orthopedic surgeon, described the semitendinosus being detached from the tibia before being rerouted with the muscle belly through the popliteal space.[6] From there the tendon was brought through the femoral notch and into an anterior tibial tunnel. The distal portion was then fixed to the anterior tibia with a wire suture tied to a nail.

Cho in 1975[7] reported five successful outcomes using the Macey technique after an average follow-up of 21 months.

Cho stated that "with this method less anteroposterior instability persists than with other methods."

In 1980 Puddu published a study of 12 cases of ACL tears with "chronic combined anteromedial-anterolateral rotatory instability."[8] These patients underwent ACL reconstruction with the semitendinosus left attached to the tibial insertion with the proximal portion detached, brought through tibial and femoral tunnels, then sutured to the iliotibial band laterally. This was combined with an extraarticular reconstruction and augmented with a posterior oblique ligament and semimembranosus advancement for the medial compartment and biceps advancement for the lateral compartment. Results were promising at 8 months when all subjects in the study had a 1+ anterior drawer sign.

In 1981, noting complications of stiffness and extensor mechanism weakness of the patellar tendon graft method described by Jones, A.B. Lipscomb[9] began using a composite graft of free semitendinosus and gracilis tendons pedicled on the tibia for ACL reconstruction. This was an improvement on Cho's technique, which used only the semitendinosus. In this paper, Lipscomb also described posterior cruciate ligament (PCL) reconstruction with the composite graft.

Gomes and Marczyk[10] reported the use of a looped, double-thickness semitendinosus tendon to reconstruct the ACL in 26 patients. The tensile strength of the looped graft became greater than the tensile strength of the normal ACL. Good results were found in 23 of the patients, and a fair result in three cases. Grafts were fixed in the femoral and tibial tunnels with press-fit bone plugs taken with a trephine at the time of tunnel creation.

As arthroscopically assisted ACL reconstruction became more popular in the late 1980s, M.J. Friedman pioneered the use of the hamstring graft.[11] As graft strength research continued to emerge, multiple strand techniques began to evolve as the norm.

Research then turned to the methods of fixation of the hamstring grafts to both the tibia and the femur. In 1994 Pinczewski[12] described fixation with an "all inside" technique using 8 mm, round-headed interference screws known as *RCI screws*. Later, Rosenberg and Deffner[13,14] described fixation using two femoral tunnels and tying the four-stranded graft over the device termed the *Endo-Button,* which locked itself against the lateral femoral condyle. Howell[15] then described the double-loop gracilis and semitendinosus technique, with which a screw and spiked washers are used for fixation in the proximal tibia. Other methods were devised as well: Paulos used a polyethylene anchor; Barrett described using bone graft; Howell and Wolf developed cross-pinning; Staehelin used biodegradable interference screw fixation; and Johnson used staple fixation. There has been no shortage of ideas for graft fixation, and there is every prospect that even greater progress will be made to enhance the efficacy of this surgical procedure.

ANATOMY AND BIOMECHANICS OF THE ANTERIOR CRUCIATE LIGAMENT

The ACL is a complex ligament that originates on the posterior-medial aspect of the intercondylar notch and inserts on the tibial plateau medial to the insertion of the lateral meniscus.[16,17] In this position the ACL acts as the primary restraint against anterior translation of the tibia on the femur.[18] The ACL consists of two bundles—an anteromedial bundle and a posterolateral bundle. These bundles have dynamic properties that allow the anteromedial bundle to be tight in flexion, while the posterolateral bundle is tight with knee extension.[19] Most ACL surgeries are focused on reconstructing the anteromedial bundle.

One biomechanical property of the graft to consider is the ultimate tensile load. The strongest construct among graft choices offered is the quadruple hamstring tendon graft, followed by quadriceps tendon grafts, bone–patellar tendon–bone (BPTB) grafts, and single strand semitendinosus grafts. The ultimate tensile strength of the ACL has been measured at 1725 to 2195 N.[20-24] The stiffness of the ACL has been determined from cadaver knees and is reported to vary from 242 N/mm[24] to 306 N/mm.[23] The ACL changes approximately 2.5 mm in length when the knee is moved through its normal arc of motion.[17,25] The graft used should have similar characteristics.

WHY HAMSTRINGS?

Many autografts have been used, most commonly the central third of the patellar tendon (ipsilateral and contralateral), quadriceps tendon, fascia lata, and iliotibial band, and the semitendinosus-gracilis or hamstring graft. There has been heated debate over the ideal graft choice for ACL reconstruction. There are proponents for each graft source with innumerable arguments for why a particular graft is better indicated than others in a particular patient or subset of patients based on age, activity level, concomitant injuries, instability, and other factors. Because all grafts have their own individually substantiated merits, it is important to delineate which factors are most debated. Factors that should be considered when comparisons are to be made among graft sources include strength of the graft, fixation methods and strength, donor site morbidity, and ease of early rehabilitation.

BPTB grafts and hamstring grafts have emerged as the most commonly used autografts. The strength of the hamstring semitendinosus-gracilis autograft has been compared with the native ACL and other grafts in multiple studies. Noyes and colleagues first reported the strength of a single-stranded graft in 1984. A single-strand semitendinosus graft provides 70% of the initial strength of the native ACL, whereas gracilis alone provides 49%.[26] This spawned the idea of using multiple strands of the semitendinosus or gracilis for ACL reconstruction. With the number of strands doubled,

the strength can also be doubled, although Hamner and co-workers showed this increase in strength to be additive only if the strands are tensioned in an equal manner.[27] Brahmabhatt and co-workers found the double-stranded semitendinosus to have a higher peak load to failure than both the patellar tendon and quadriceps tendon grafts, with increased strength of 11.5% and 10.3%, respectively.[28] Brown and colleagues showed that the strength of the graft could be greatly increased by increasing the number of graft strands to form bundles, as high as 4108 N with a four-strand technique.[29,30] This is nearly double the strength of the BPTB ultimate tensile load of approximately 2300 N.[31] The diameter of the quadruple semitendinosus-gracilis tendon graft averages 7 to 8 mm, similar to that of the native ACL. The quadruple-bundle hamstring tendon graft also approximates the function of the two-bundle ACL and is thought to be advantageous.[32] This has brought about the idea of braiding and twisting the bundles, although this has not proven to be useful, as it may place collagen fibrils in a suboptimal orientation for loading, resulting in a weaker graft.[33,34]

The advantages of using autograft over allograft include low risk of adverse inflammatory reaction as well as the absence of significant risk of disease transmission. However, allograft use does allow for decreased surgical time, decreased morbidity associated with the donor site, and less pain postoperatively. Common allograft options include Achilles tendon, patellar tendon, and anterior tibialis tendon.

The method of fixation of the graft is another important factor to consider when choosing the autograft. The optimal means of fixation must be strong enough to provide sufficient stiffness to supply knee stability as well as give anatomic fixation to prevent or minimize graft motion within the femoral and tibial tunnels.[35-37] Especially important in rehabilitation, the fixation must also minimize slippage of the graft with cyclic loading and be strong enough to withstand early physical therapy and function until biologic healing and fixation can occur. Graft fixation can be divided into direct and indirect fixation methods. Interference screws, washers, cross-pins, and staples are examples of direct fixation; suture-posts and polyester tape-titanium buttons are indirect fixation devices. Although it has been shown that the biomechanical strength of the quadruple-bundled semitendinosus-gracilis graft is superior to the patellar tendon graft, the strength of fixation of the semitendinosus-gracilis graft is the weakest link in the stability of ACL reconstruction until graft incorporation occurs. This has been one of the biggest concerns when using the hamstring as an acceptable autograft. More specifically, hamstring tendon grafts have been shown to have increased anterior-posterior laxity, slower healing of the tendon graft to the bone tunnel, and graft tunnel motion leading to tunnel widening compared with bone–patellar tendon grafts.[35,36] However, this is now known to be somewhat fixation dependent. Soft tissue graft fixation is technically more difficult for obvious reasons. Decreasing

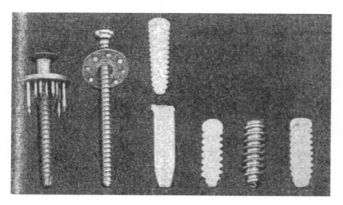

Figure 10-1: Tibial implants. Left to right: WasherLoc, tandem spiked washer, Intrafix, BioScrew, SoftSilk interference screw, and SmartScrew ACL. *(From Kousa P, Jarvinen TLN, Vihavainen M, Kannus P, Jarvinen M: The fixation strength of six hamstring tendon graft fixation devices in anterior cruciate ligament reconstruction. Part II: Tibial site, Am J Sports Med 31(2):182-188, 2003.)*

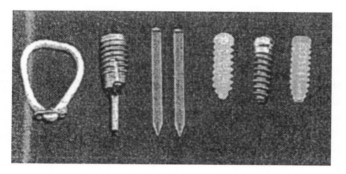

Figure 10-2: Femoral implants. Left to right: Endo-Button CL, Bone Mulch Screw, RigidFix, BioScrew, RCI screw, and SmartScrew ACL. *(From Kousa P, Jarvinen TLN, Vihavainen M, Kannus P, Jarvinen M: The fixation strength of six hamstring tendon graft fixation devices in anterior cruciate ligament reconstruction. Part I: Femoral site, Am J Sports Med 31(2):174-181, 2003.)*

the distance between the site of fixation and the aperture of the bone tunnel may reduce the laxity of the semitendinosus-gracilis graft.[38] Likewise, the stiffness of the graft can be increased with fixation closer to the tunnel aperture. The ultimate tensile loads of fixation devices in hamstring graft ACL reconstruction have been studied closely for both tibial and femoral fixation (Figures 10-1 and 10-2 and Tables 10-1 and 10-2).[39,40] Advances in design and technique have decreased tunnel motion and subsequent tunnel widening and stabilized fixation to allow for early rehabilitation and healing.

Donor site morbidity is another consideration in choosing autograft for ACL reconstruction. The use of the semitendinosus-gracilis graft is advantageous in that there is very little morbidity associated with harvest. Reports of hamstring weakness after harvest and ACL reconstruction have proven not to be clinically significant.[7] In a retrospective study, Lipscomb and co-workers showed no significant loss of overall hamstring strength in 51 ACL reconstructions using semitendinosus and gracilis tendons, alone, or in combination.[41] Other reports concur with this finding.[42-44] It has been reported that the hamstring tendons regenerate in a near-anatomic position and are functional.[45] It is believed that the regrowth occurs in the distal cut end of the muscle belly following the fascial planes to the insertion site. In contrast, BPTB graft has been correlated with a higher incidence of anterior knee pain postoperatively as well as increased risk of patella fracture.

With ACL reconstruction surgery, as with most orthopedic procedures, early and aggressive rehabilitation is essential to a successful outcome. The use of the semitendinosus-gracilis autograft does not preclude this rule. Marder[46] showed in a prospective, randomized study that there was no difference in final knee rating or stability between BPTB grafts and hamstring grafts treated with early and aggressive

TABLE 10-1

Results of Single-Cycle Loading after Cyclic Loading for Each Tibial Fixation Device*

FIXATION	N	YIELD LOAD (N) (MEAN ± SD)	STIFFNESS (N/MM) (MEAN ± SD)
WasherLoc	10	917 ± 234[a]	127 ± 22[b]
Tandem spiked washers	10	675 ± 190[b,c]	108 ± 26[b,d]
Intrafix	10	1309 ± 302	267 ± 36
BioScrew	10	567 ± 156[b,e]	125 ± 23[b,d]
SoftSilk	9	423 ± 75[b,f]	120 ± 18[b,d]
SmartScrew ACL	10	694 ± 173[b]	159 ± 25[b]

[a]Significantly different from Intrafix ($P < 0.01$).
[b]Significantly different from Intrafix ($P < 0.001$).
[c]Significantly different from WasherLoc ($P < 0.05$).
[d]Significantly different from SmartScrew ACL ($P < 0.05$).
[e]Significantly different from WasherLoc ($P < 0.01$).
[f]Significantly different from WasherLoc ($P < 0.001$).
*Data from Kousa P, Jarvinen TLN, Vilahavainen M, et al: The fixation strength of six hamstring tendon graft fixation devices in anterior cruciate tendon reconstruction, *Am J Sports Med* 31:182-188, 2003.

rehabilitation. We believe, however, that early graft protection decreases the likelihood of fixation loss at the bone tunnel–graft healing interface.

Hamstring tendon autograft provides a popular alternative to the BPTB autograft with advantages of cosmesis from harvest and less donor site morbidity. With continued studies demonstrating long-term success rates of hamstring repairs, the patellar tendon may no longer be considered the "gold standard," allowing more and more surgeons to choose this as their graft of choice.

PREFERRED METHOD OF HAMSTRING ANTERIOR CRUCIATE LIGAMENT RECONSTRUCTION

Our preferred method of hamstring ACL reconstruction is as follows. Before surgery the affected proximal thigh is placed in a padded tourniquet with the leg placed in a leg holder. The surgeon sits on a draped rolling stool in front of the patient. This position allows adequate mobility of the surgeon so that careful control of knee flexion and extension can be obtained, which is a critical factor during this surgical procedure.

The semitendinosus graft harvest is performed with the surgeon sitting and the patient's affected extremity in 90 degrees of knee flexion. A 3 to 4 cm longitudinal incision is made over the pes tendons approximately 2 to 3 cm distal to the apex of the tibial tubercle and 2 cm medial to the tibial tuberosity. The sartorius fascia is incised in line with its fibers and retracted. The gracilis and semitendinosus tendons are digitally palpated and are then carefully dissected off their insertion, with caution taken to avoid injury to the underlying superficial medial collateral ligament, although this is medial to their insertion on the tibia. A #2 Ethibond suture is placed

in the distal end before harvest, and the tendon is cut at 20 to 21 cm in length after harvest. While traction is applied to the free end, the deep fascial bands of the medial gastrocnemius fascia are released. This helps prevent premature amputation of the tendon, which can easily occur if these attachments are not removed. The surgeon's finger inserted along the tendons should be able to allow the tendon to slide in a 360-degree arc around the finger to confirm the absence of adhesions. After the gracilis and semitendinosus tendons are isolated and dissected off of the distal tibial attachment (Figure 10-3), a #2 nonabsorbable suture is placed in the distal 20 mm; then they are harvested using a tendon stripper (Figure 10-4). Tendons are then prepared on a back table. The tendons are cut at a length of 20 to 21 cm proximally. All muscle tissue is removed using a flat edge of a metal ruler

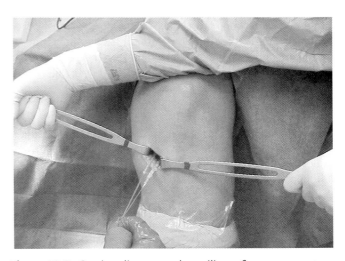

Figure 10-3: Semitendinosus and gracilis graft procurement from tibia.

TABLE 10-2

Results of Single-Cycle Loading after Cyclic Loading for Each Femoral Fixation Device*

FIXATION	N	YIELD LOAD (N) (MEAN ± SD)	STIFFNESS (N/MM) (MEAN ± SD)
EndoButton CL	10	781 ± 252	105 ± 13[a,b,c]
Bone Mulch Screw	10	925 ± 280	189 ± 38
RigidFix	10	768 ± 253	136 ± 13[a]
BioScrew	9	565 ± 137[d]	113 ± 15[a,e]
RCI screw	9	534 ± 129[d,f]	134 ± 23[a]
SmartScrew ACL	10	842 ± 201	162 ± 28

[a]Significantly different from Bone Mulch Screw ($P < 0.001$).
[b]Significantly different from RigidFix ($P < 0.05$).
[c]Significantly different from Smart Screw ACL ($P < 0.001$).
[d]Significantly different from Bone Mulch Screw ($P < 0.05$).
[e]Significantly different from SmartScrew ACL ($P < 0.01$).
[f]Significantly different from SmartScrew ACL ($P < 0.05$).
*Data from Kousa P, Jarvinen TLN, Vilahavainen M, et al: The fixation strength of six hamstring tendon graft fixation devices in anterior cruciate ligament reconstruction, *Am J Sports Med* 31:174-181, 2003.

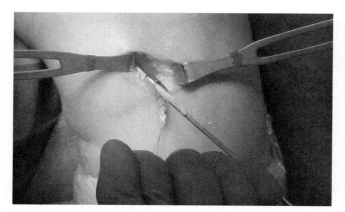

Figure 10-4: Use of tendon stripper during graft harvest.

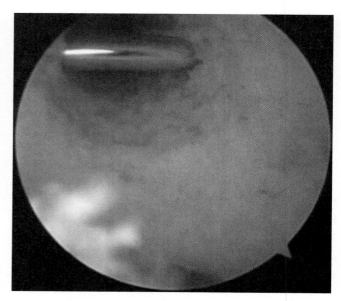

Figure 10-5: Intraarticular view of cross-pin fixation in femoral tunnel.

or other blunt surface. Tendons are doubled over a #5 Ethibond suture to create a four-stranded graft, and sutures are placed in a boxlike fashion through the proximal end of the tendon for 25 mm. The tendons are then sized to the nearest half-millimeter and kept moist with a wet sponge to prevent issue desiccation. The tendons are then kept on the stretcher with 15 to 20 lb of traction until implementation. We generally like to see a graft length of at least 20 to 21 cm after harvest, because a minimum of 15 mm of quadruped graft is needed within each of the femoral and tibial tunnels.

Tibial tunnels are drilled 1 to 2 mm smaller than graft size, then dilated to fit the size of the tendon graft. Correct placement of tunnels is critical for successful outcomes. The tibial tunnel is prepared first using an endoscopic aimer adjusted to the 45-degree position, with the guide tip positioned intraarticularly through the anteromedial portal. This guide tip is positioned so that it will exit the tibia along the central fibers of the tibial ACL stump. The femoral tunnel is prepared second using the femoral guide pin positioned at the 10:30 position for the right knee and 1:30 position for the left knee and advanced up to 2 to 3 cm into the femur while 90 degrees of knee flexion is maintained.

We use bioabsorbable cross-pin fixation at the femoral tunnel (Figure 10-5). This allows for close-to-aperture fixation (8 mm from tunnel opening). This form of fixation also allows the graft to incorporate in a complete 360-degree fashion into the tunnel wall. The system is the Mitek (Ethicon Inc., Sommerville, NJ) Rigid-Fix device and incorporates two cross-pins. In case of revision the pins are easily drilled through or have absorbed, which is an important factor to consider when choosing fixation device.

Tibial fixation is performed with the Mitek (Ethicon Inc., Sommerville, NJ) Intrafix device. This gives 180 degrees of graft incorporation and is believed to give adequate early fixation strength (see Table 10-1). The device is flush on the tibia, reducing the chances for hardware pain. This device is also available in a bioabsorbable material; previously it was offered only in polyethylene. The remaining distal tendon is then amputated flush with the tibial surface. This fixation

allows for rehabilitation to occur early as the graft incorporates into the tunnels.

POSTOPERATIVE REHABILITATION

Rehabilitation after ACL reconstruction has undergone drastic changes in the last two decades. Long gone are the days of extended immobilization, prolonged use of crutches, and delayed quadriceps facilitation.[47-52] A rapid approach to rehabilitation of hamstring autografts similar in many ways to that described by Shelbourne and Nitz[53] is used by our therapists. This rapid rehabilitation approach emphasizes immediate motion, full passive extension, and immediate weight bearing (Box 10-1).[54-60]

Although some centers reserve hamstring reconstruction for the less active older patient who is not returning to demanding sports,[61] we choose to use this form of repair when appropriate for even the most active of patients. Recent evidence supports that the use of the hamstring reconstruction enables a greater return of function than use of the BPTB reconstruction.[62]

Phase I: Immediate Postoperative Phase

Unless there have been any surgical complications, the patient is sent home the day of the surgery. Because of our emphasis on immediate full passive knee extension, all patients are placed in a postoperative knee brace that is locked in full extension and are allowed to bear weight as tolerated using bilateral axillary crutches. Postoperative bandages are covered with a continuous flow cryotherapy device, which circulates cool water around the knee that underwent surgery in an attempt to decrease both postoperative pain and intraarticular effusion. The patient is instructed not to remain sitting

BOX 10-1

Postoperative Rehabilitation Guidelines after Anterior Cruciate Ligament Hamstring Autograft Reconstruction

General Guidelines

Assume 8 weeks for complete graft revascularization

Rarely use CPM

Begin isolated hamstring strengthening 6 weeks after surgery

Undertake supervised physical therapy for 3-9 months

Activities of Daily Living Progression

Bathing or showering without brace acceptable after suture removal

Patient should sleep with brace locked in extension for 1 week

Driving

- 1 week for automatic vehicles with left leg repair
- 4-6 weeks for standard vehicles, or right leg repair

Brace locked in extension for 1 week for ambulation

Crutches and brace for ambulation as needed for 6 weeks

Weightbearing as tolerated immediately after surgery

Phase I: Immediate Postoperative Phase (Immediately after Surgery through 6 Weeks)

Goals

Protect graft fixation (8 weeks)

Minimize effects of immobilization

Control inflammation and swelling

Immediate full knee passive extension

Quadriceps activation

Patient education

Restrictions

Weight bearing as tolerated with axillary crutches as needed for 6 weeks

Hamstring mobilization and stretching in 4 weeks

Brace

0-1 week: Locked in full extension for weightbearing and sleeping

1-6 weeks: Unlocked for ambulation, remove for sleeping

Therapeutic Exercises

Gentle heel slides

Quadriceps setting

Patellar mobilization

Non–weightbearing, gastrocnemius and soleus stretching

SLR in all planes (SLR × 4) with brace locked in full extension until quadriceps prevents extensor lag

Quadriceps isometrics at 60 and 90 degrees

Gluteal setting

Weight shifting

Static balance exercises

Heel raises—bilateral progressing to unilateral

Clinical Milestones

Full knee extension

SLR without extensor lag

No limp or antalgia during gait

Knee flexion of 90 degrees

No signs of active inflammation

No increased effusion or edema

No increased pain

Phase II: Intermediate Phase (6-8 Weeks)

Goals

Restore normal gait

Maintain full knee extension

Progress flexion ROM

Protect graft

Initiate open kinetic chain hamstring exercises

Comments

DC brace and crutches as allowed by physician when the patient has full extension and can perform SLR without extensor lag

Therapeutic Exercise

Wall slides 0-45 degrees, progressing to minisquat

Multihip (four-way hip machine)

Stationary bike (high seat, low tension, promoting ROM)

Closed chain terminal extension with resistive tubing or weight machine

Heel raises

(continued)

with the leg in a dependent position for any length of time, as this will only increase the amount of swelling and or edema in the distal lower leg and foot. When the patient is convalescent for any significant length of time, the lower leg should be elevated with the foot higher than knee (in the supine position), the knee higher than the hip, and the hip higher than the heart. In addition to using the cryotherapy device, the patient is sent home with a prescription for a narcotic medication, as well as a cyclooxygenase (COX)-2 antiinflammatory medication to decrease pain and knee inflammation. The narcotic medication should be taken for severe pain, as instructed by physician and per prescription on bottle label. Formal physical therapy most commonly commences 2 to 3 days after surgery.

Goals of the immediate postoperative phase include (1) protecting the graft fixation while minimizing the effects of immobilization (we assume the full fixation is not complete until around the eighth to twelfth postoperative week)[63]; (2)

controlling inflammation, pain, and swelling; (3) caring for the knee and dressing; (4) achieving and maintaining full knee extension range of motion (ROM); (5) preventing quadriceps shutdown; and (6) educating the patient regarding the surgical procedure and expectations during therapy.

When the patient arrives for therapy, postoperative dressings are removed and the knee is inspected and evaluated to determine the extent of the patient's present impairment. The patient should be instructed to keep incisions dry for the first 7 to 10 days. The patient can shower; however, a waterproof plastic covering must be placed over the incision.

To adequately protect the reconstructed graft the patient will wear the postoperative hinged knee brace locked in full extension for weight bearing during ambulation and while sleeping for the first week. In addition, during the first week the patient can unlock or remove the brace only during gentle ROM exercise sessions. After the first postoperative week, once the quadriceps muscle function is adequate (ability to

---

BOX 10-1, continued

Balance exercises (e.g., single-leg balance, Kinesthetic Awareness Trainer [KAT])

Hamstring curls

Aquatic therapy with emphasis on normalization of gait

Continuing hamstring stretches, progressing to weight-bearing gastrocnemius and soleus exercises

Clinical Milestones

Maximize ROM

Good quadriceps recruitment

Maintenance of full passive knee extension

Advanced Strengthening Phase III (8 Weeks to 6 Months)

Goals

Attain full range of motion

Improve strength, endurance, and proprioception of lower extremity to prepare for full functional activities

Avoid overstressing graft or graft fixation

Protect patellofemoral joint

Therapeutic Exercise

Continue flexibility exercises as appropriate

Stairmaster (begin short steps, avoid knee hyperextension)

NordicTrack knee extension: 90-45 degrees of knee flexion

Advanced closed kinetic chain strengthening (single-leg squats, leg press 0-45 degrees, step-ups beginning at 2 inches and progressing to 8 inches)

Progressive proprioceptive activities (slide board, use of ball, racquet with balance activities, etc.)

Progressive aquatic program to include pool running, swimming (no breaststroke)

Clinical Milestones

Criteria for Advancement

- Full pain-free ROM
- No evidence of patellofemoral joint irritation
- Strength and proprioception approximately 70% of uninvolved leg
- Physician clearance to initiate advanced closed kinetic chain exercises and functional progression

Return to Activity: Phase IV (9 Months +)

Goals

Safe return to athletics

Maintenance program for strength, endurance

Comments

Physician may recommend a functional brace for use during sports for the first 1-2 years after surgery

produce good quadriceps set and perform a straight leg raise [SLR] with no extensor lag), we allow the patient to ambulate with the brace unlocked through a pain-free ROM, and for sleeping. Throughout the first 6 weeks the patient will ambulate weight bearing as tolerated.

Inflammation, pain and swelling are minimized with narcotic pain medication, antiinflammatory medication, and liberal use of electrical stimulation. One of the initial postoperative goals is to decrease swelling and effusion. Several classic studies have demonstrated that knee effusion can cause an inhibition of the quadriceps muscles.[64-66] Moreover, it takes approximately 50 to 60 ml of fluid in the normal knee joint to inhibit the rectus femoris and vastus lateralis, whereas it takes only 20 to 30 ml of fluid to selectively inhibit the vastus medialis oblique.[65] Swelling and joint effusion can be managed in several ways. We commonly recommend continued use of cold therapy and elevation. Electrical stimulation with settings at the level of induced muscle contraction as well as sensory level can be used to decrease edema and joint effusion.[67] Electrical induction of a muscle contraction can be used initially after surgery to duplicate the regular muscle contractions of the knee, helping to stimulate circulation by pumping fluid and blood through venous and lymphatic channels back into the heart.[68] For this type of treatment, pulse duration should be set to approximately 300 to 600 microseconds, and the pulses per second should be in the range of 35 to 50.[67] If swelling and edema are also present distal to the knee after reconstruction, a compressive stocking can be used around the lower extremity to help decrease and minimize distal swelling.

Graft protection during the early phases of rehabilitation is critical. Because the BPTB autograft has been studied in great detail, we can use biomechanical knowledge gained during testing of its tensile strength and healing to guide the hamstring repairs. This autograft source, which was initially an extraarticular structure when placed in the knee, becomes an intraarticular structure. The strength of the graft at initial implantation is of extreme importance. Autografts are thought to be the strongest immediately after implantation. It has been shown that the tensile strength of a 10 mm central third patellar tendon graft has strength of 57% at 3 months, 56% at 6 months, and 87% at 9 months.[69] We also know that autogenic graft sources go through a process of ligamentization. With ligamentization, the graft undergoes a biologic transformation with four distinct phases. Necrosis of the graft occurs within the first 3 weeks after surgery. This graft source consists of a collagen network that has previously had a consistent blood supply. Without this blood supply the tissue becomes "necrotic." This process lasts for the first 2 to 3 weeks, while the native cells diminish. As early as the first week, replacement cells begin to repopulate the graft. Early full ROM is needed because the formation of these new collagen cells is dictated by the stress that is placed on the graft. During this phase of healing the graft is nourished by synovial fluid and bone blood supply to allow collagen cells to repopulate the ligament. Revascularization begins within the

first 6 to 8 weeks and continues until approximately week 16.[55] Inflammatory response should be diminished and under control, and the graft should be nourished by the fat pad and the synovium. Further inflammatory problems after the 8- to 10-week time frame may imply a prolonged inflammatory response, delayed healing process, and potential graft problems. Scranton and colleagues[70] showed that in the sheep model of autogenous ACL tissue repair Sharpey's fibers were prominent and already anchoring to the bone with a fibroproliferative response. Despite this bone anchoring the autograft was still avascular at 6 weeks. At 3 months, there were focal areas of remodeling, and vascular channels were adjacent to necrotic tendon yet tendon was devoid of inflammation that if present would hinder further ligamentization. At 6 months they found that the control ligament and the reconstructed ligament were very similar. In reports of their study they describe human specimens obtained from failed hamstring reconstruction. One subject was noncompliant and playing sports at 6 weeks after surgery when his graft failed. Cross sectioning of this specimen showed abundant intratunnel Sharpey's fibers at 6 weeks. Another hamstring reconstruction specimen was obtained at 9 weeks after surgery, when the patient's ligament failed while the patient was attempting to leap onto a horse that moved. Neovascularization was seen adjacent to the necrotic intraarticular graft. The final phases of cell proliferation and collagen replacement occur throughout the maturation process and may take up to 3 years.[71]

Falconiero and colleagues[72] concluded, through ACL tissue biopsies after autogenous repair, that revascularization and ligamentization occur over a 12-month period after reconstruction, with peak maturity evident at 1 year. They also believe that the vascularity and fiber pattern show significant evidence that maturity may occur earlier, from 6 to 12 months after surgery.

Because we know that the application of physiologic tension and motion has been shown to aid in ligament repair, causing fibroblast and collagen fibrils to align parallel to the direction of force,[73-75] we recommend early joint mobilization and ROM exercises. Therapeutic exercises initially include heel slides with the foot on a wall (Figure 10-6) or doorjamb to increase knee flexion ROM. Standard supine heel slides will require use of the hamstring muscle group, which has been partially removed during this surgical procedure and which may be hindered secondary to pain and discomfort. In addition, sitting on the edge of a treatment table, allowing the knee to flex to 90 degrees, is an acceptable alternative to gain motion. If the knee can be easily flexed to 90 degrees, passive overpressure can be applied with the opposite lower extremity. We prefer that at least 90 degrees of knee flexion be present in the first 5 to 7 days, and up to 120 degrees by 2 to 3 weeks.

Early passive extension is important after any ACL repair so that the intraarticular notch is not allowed to fill in with scar tissue, thereby preventing full knee extension. Passive extension of the knee can be performed by placing a towel

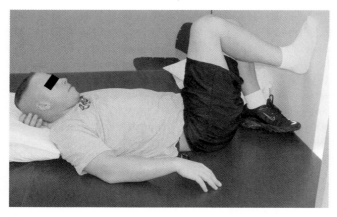

Figure 10-6: Wall slide to increase knee flexion range of motion.

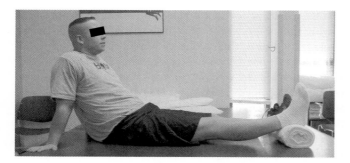

Figure 10-7: Supine static passive knee extension mobilization.

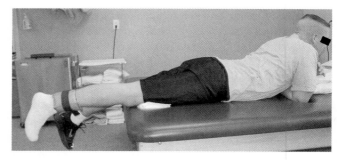

Figure 10-8: Prone hang to increase passive knee extension range of motion.

roll under the patient's foot and ankle (Figure 10-7). This towel roll must be high enough to raise the calf and thigh off the table. Once the leg is in the correct position the patient is asked to sag the knee into full extension for 10 to 15 minutes. Sitting in a chair and supporting the heel on the edge of the stool, table, or another chair by letting the unsupported knee sag into full extension can also be beneficial. We like the patient to perform this maneuver every waking hour for up to 10 minutes during the first postoperative week. Two other methods to help achieve full knee extension are to use the opposite leg and its quadriceps muscle to straighten the knee from the 90-degree position to that of full knee extension, or to use the prone hang (Figure 10-8).

Quadriceps atrophy and weakness can begin immediately after ACL repair[76]; the quadriceps appears to be the major muscle group that undergoes atrophic changes after ACL injury and should therefore be addressed immediately after surgery.[77] Continued weakness of the quadriceps muscle group after surgery can result in poor knee neuromuscular control during functional activities, recurrent knee effusion, and an increased incidence of patellofemoral symptoms throughout the remainder of the rehabilitation process. Quadriceps setting is performed to return motor control to the anterior musculature of the thigh. Quadriceps setting should begin as soon as possible to help retard muscle atrophy and to start recruiting motor fibers to the knee extensor

muscles. These quadriceps contractions should be performed with the knee in its fully extended position and do not necessarily need to be at maximal level. Not only does this exercise help with increasing motor recruitment to the quadriceps, but because of the muscular contraction around the knee, swelling and effusion are often squeezed out of the knee joint. We like to see the patient have the ability to perform a forceful quadriceps contraction by the fourth postoperative day. An SLR exercise should be initiated once full knee extension can be maintained. This exercise is done by first performing a quadriceps contraction with the leg in full extension. Once the leg can achieve full extension an adequate contraction will lock the knee in its terminally extended position, commonly called the "screw home" position. In this position the knee is very stable, and minimal to no stress will be placed on the replaced graft. Once the contraction is held, the entire leg is lifted to about 30 to 45 degrees and held for a count of 6 seconds. If the patient exhibits a quadriceps lag or the inability to achieve full knee extension, he or she should perform the exercise with the brace on and locked at 0 degrees so that excessive stress will not be placed on the graft. The clinician cannot always be assured that because an SLR is performed the quadriceps is firing adequately. Because of hip flexor muscle substitution, quadriceps strength may still be inadequate. We instruct the patient to please remember to remove the leg from the knee brace and perform exercises at leas six to eight times per day to maintain full knee extension. Quadriceps isometrics can also be performed in a safe ROM that does not stress the replaced graft source. These would include isometrics at the angles of 60 degrees and 90 degrees of knee flexion. In these positions the stress on the ACL is very minimal.

If after the third or fourth postoperative day the patient is unable to initiate a strong quadriceps contraction, electrical muscle stimulation units will be used to maintain quadriceps tone (Figure 10-9). A "Russian current," which is a medium-frequency current, is most often used to help facilitate a muscle contraction. This current is a 2000 to 10,000 Hz polyphasic AC waveform generated in 50 burst–per-second envelopes, which makes the intensity of this current much more tolerable for the patient. Various studies have given credence to the use of electrical muscle stimulation as an

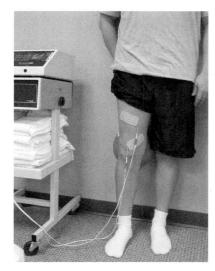

Figure 10-9: "Russian" electrical stimulation in a closed kinetic chain position to increase neuromuscular function.

adjunct during rehabilitation. Wigerstad-Lossing and colleagues[78] looked at quadriceps muscle function after ACL reconstruction in the late 1980s, when casting the knee for up to 6 weeks was common practice. They compared the effects of electrical muscle stimulation combined with a voluntary muscle contraction with those of a program of only voluntary muscle contractions during immobilization after ACL reconstruction. At the end of the 6-week immobilization period the voluntary contraction–only cohort demonstrated a significantly reduced amount of isometric knee extension strength compared with the group that received electrical muscle stimulation superimposed by a volitional contraction of the quadriceps muscle.[78] Moreover, the researchers also found that the experimental group demonstrated a larger quadriceps muscle cross-sectional area than the controls after the immobilization period. Using a single-case experimental design, Delitto and co-workers[79] found that simultaneous stimulation of the quadriceps and hamstrings using a "Russian current" in a patient 6 weeks after ACL reconstruction elicited increases in both knee extension and flexion torque and thigh circumferential measurements. Snyder-Mackler and colleagues[80] placed 10 postoperative ACL patients in one of two groups including a group that received neuromuscular electrical stimulation and volitional exercise and a group that received volitional exercise alone. After 4 weeks of treatment the group that received electrical stimulation with volitional exercise demonstrated a dramatic decrease in strength loss as compared with the group that performed volitional exercise alone. In addition, the researchers also found that the group receiving electrical stimulation and exercise had significant improvements in functional performance of gait including cadence, walking velocity, stance time of involved limb, and flexion-excursion of the knee during stance. They report equivocally that the patients who received neuromuscular electrical stimulation had stronger

quadriceps muscles and more normal gait patterns than those in the volitional only group. In a more recent study, Snyder-Mackler and colleagues[75] randomly assigned 110 patients to several groups, including those who received high-intensity neuromuscular stimulation ($n = 31$), high-level volitional exercise ($n = 34$), low-intensity neuromuscular stimulation ($n = 25$), or combined high- and low-intensity neuromuscular stimulation ($n = 20$). After 4 weeks of treatment, all subjects performed a knee extension isometric contraction in 65 degrees of knee flexion. Quadriceps strength averaged 70% or more of the uninvolved side in the two groups treated with high-intensity neuromuscular stimulation but averaged only 57% and 51% in the groups of high-level volitional exercise and low-intensity neuromuscular stimulation, respectively. Most recently Rebal and co-workers[81] evaluated the effects of a sample of 10 "sportsmen" randomly assigned to neuromuscular electrical stimulation with either 80 Hz intensity or 20 Hz intensity. All patients received electrical stimulation of the quadriceps 5 days per week for 12 weeks. Isokinetic testing after 12 weeks revealed that quadriceps peak torque, at 180 degrees/second and 240 degrees/second, was significantly greater in the 20 Hz group.

Depending on the size of the patient we will commonly place one or two pairs of electrodes on the patient's anterior thigh to deliver the intended current. It is best to ensure that at least one of the pads is over the motor point on the vastus medialis oblique, because it is the muscle most affected by swelling or pain that is causing a quadriceps shutdown. The intensity of current should be high enough that the clinician can observe an actual motor contraction from the patient's quadriceps muscles. The electrical stimulation should be performed with a volitional maximal quadriceps contraction by the patient. Quadriceps contractions can be performed while in a supine position, but in many instances they are done in the standing position in an attempt to gain greater muscle recruitment and cocontraction from other, surrounding muscles.

Recent evidence has revealed that the gastrocnemius and to a larger extent the soleus muscles may play a dynamic role in stabilizing the knee by reducing anterior tibial translation.[82] Seated or limited weight-bearing gastrocnemius and soleus muscle exercises are usually tolerated well. Full body weight can be unloaded by the use of a leg press machine, total gym, or any other form of resistance that does not require full body weight, progressing to full body weight resistive exercises for the gastrocnemius and soleus group.

Because portions of the hamstring muscles are used for this surgical procedure, excessive stress to these muscles may be contraindicated early. Early aggressive exercises after graft harvest may irritate the remaining portion of the semitendinosus or cause a tendinopathy of the semimembranosus. For this reason, resistance exercises for the hamstrings are delayed for up to 6 weeks after harvest. Gentle hamstring stretches can be begun at approximately 4 weeks. Because the hamstrings can be accidentally stretched by leaning forward to pick things up from the ground, putting on pants, or tying

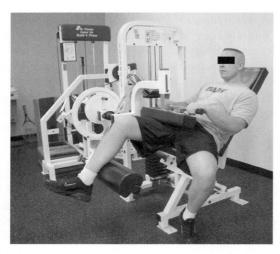

Figure 10-10: Progressive resistive single-leg seated hamstring machine curl.

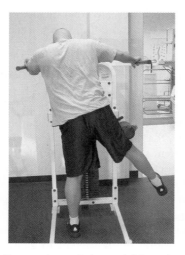

Figure 10-11: Progressive resistive multihip unit to increase total leg strength.

shoes, the patient should be advised to bend the knee during any of these maneuvers, which will place the muscles on slight slack. After about 6 weeks the hamstrings can be exercised again, beginning with gentle multiple angle isometrics and progressing to supine heel slides. After about 9 weeks, more aggressive resistance exercises such as hamstring curls (Figure 10-10) or straight leg dead lifts can be initiated as the patient comfortably tolerates these exercises. Regardless of this delay in applying resistance exercises to the hamstrings, their strength normally returns after hamstring harvest.[41-43]

The four-way multihip unit is an excellent choice to increase core hip strength (Figure 10-11). To continue to facilitate improvement in ROM, a stationary bike can be ridden with the seat high with very little tension for more of an emphasis on ROM than on strength. Riding the stationary bike has been shown to place very little stress on the

reconstructed graft; therefore we generally recommend little limitation on how much it is used. Full or partial weight-bearing heel raises are excellent exercises for total leg strength.

Phase II: Intermediate Phase

Phase II of the quadruple hamstring rehabilitation protocol begins at approximately 6 weeks after surgery and extends to approximately 8 weeks after surgery. Allowing the patient to leave phase I requires that the patient be able to obtain a good quadriceps contraction during an SLR with minimal to no quadriceps lag. In addition, knee flexion ROM should be at minimum 90 degrees. The patient should have full knee extension by this time frame. Any sign of active inflammation at this point should be of great concern and requires that the patient maintain in the phase I portion of the protocol. By week 6 the patients should have a close-to-normal gait pattern. Full extension of the knee is imperative now for progression of functional activities. The graft should still be protected at 6 to 8 weeks. Open kinetic chain hamstring exercises can be used with caution and a gradual progression of loading.

Weight-bearing status has been as tolerated from day 1; therefore the patient should be off crutches at 6 weeks. If the patient can ambulate with a normal gait cycle and achieve full active knee extension without an extension lag, the brace may be discontinued with the physician's approval.

Limited ROM wall slides can be begun (0 to 45 degrees), with gentle progression to partial squats, commonly known as *minisquats*. Partial squats are performed with the feet directly under the shoulders with a very slight externally rotated position. To begin, the patient may want to use a handhold for support as he or she slowly lowers the buttocks backward and downward. Because many patients have trouble with the basic squatting technique, we commonly describe the squatting technique as similar to sitting on the toilet. In this manner the patients usually understand to also flex at the hip rather than only flexing at the knees, which would take the knee farther anteriorly than appropriate, substantially increasing patellofemoral joint stress. Squatting is a very useful exercise to facilitate cocontraction between both the quadriceps and hamstring muscle groups, allowing an increase in knee joint stability.

Balance and proprioceptive exercises are emphasized to a greater extent when full weight bearing is tolerated. Examples of balance training include the use of the single-leg stance, single-leg stance with contralateral lower extremity movement, balance boards, or other balance training devices such as the Dyna Disc (Exertools, Inc., Vavato, CA) (Figure 10-12).

During this phase of rehabilitation, the hamstrings have had a sufficient amount of time to begin the healing process and strengthening is no longer contraindicated. The patient may begin with simple gravity-resisted hamstring curls and progressing to cuff weights or machine weights as tolerated.

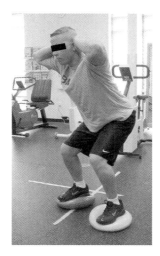

Figure 10-12: Balance exercise using Dyna Disk.

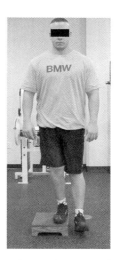

Figure 10-13: Unilateral step-down exercise for lower extremity neuromuscular control.

During rehabilitation after cruciate repair patients commonly ask when they may drive a vehicle. In most cases those who have had surgery on the left knee and have an automatic transmission may drive when they can comfortably get into and out of their vehicle. Patients who have had surgery on the left knee and have a standard transmission should not drive until they have good muscular control of the leg, which most often occurs around the fourth postoperative week. Patients who have had surgery on the right knee can usually be expected to drive safely in 4 to 6 weeks.

Phase III: Advanced Strengthening

Our phase III protocol begins at approximately 8 weeks and extends through 6 months. Goals during this time are (1) to achieve full functional knee ROM, (2) to improve strength, endurance, and proprioception of the lower extremity to prepare for functional activities, (3) to avoid overstressing the graft fixation, and (4) to protect the patellofemoral joint.

During this time ROM and flexibility exercises will be continued if and as appropriate. Higher-level exercises can be begun, including StairMaster (Nautilus Group, Inc., Vancouver, WA) with short steps and being sure to avoid knee hyperextension. NordicTrack (Icon Health and Fitness, Logan, UT) can be performed as tolerated. We also place more emphasis on advanced closed kinetic chain exercises including single-leg squats, leg presses from 0 to 45 degrees of knee flexion, and step ups progressing from 2 inches initially up to 8 inches (Figure 10-13).

Proprioception exercises at this time frame are advanced as well and include use of slide boards and balance board and perturbation exercises.

Unilateral closed kinetic chain exercises are stressed during this time. Rudrud and colleagues[83] have demonstrated asymmetric weight bearing for at least 6 to 12 months after surgical repair of the ACL. Patients often subconsciously unload the surgically injured extremity at the expense of

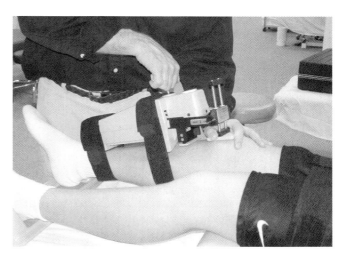

Figure 10-14: KT1000 knee ligament arthrometer testing device.

muscular recruitment and firing patterns. Single-leg closed kinetic chain exercises require the patient to rely solely on the postsurgical extremity. The weight the patient has been using while performing bilateral leg presses can in most cases be reduced by 50% and used by the single postsurgical leg. This forces the single surgical leg to work in isolation, performing neuromuscular recruitment exercises to facilitating strength gains.

At approximately 12 weeks after surgery we perform a ligament arthrometer test with the KT1000 (Medmetric Corp., San Diego, CA) to determine ligament stability (Figure 10-14). If ligament stability is within 3 mm bilaterally, open kinetic chain (OKC) isokinetic tests to determine quadriceps and hamstring strength are performed at all functional speeds using a velocity spectrum protocol. If ligament stability is greater than 3 mm with bilateral comparison, the physician is consulted to determine appropriate interventions before testing is continued. Isokinetic strength testing is performed at 60, 180, and 300 degrees/second. If ligament stability and muscle strength are within normal ranges the patient is allowed to begin light jogging activities. Jogging is initiated in a linear fashion with no running on hills, curves, or uneven surfaces. Occasionally a trampoline can be used when beginning to run, allowing a gradual increase in tolerance to loading and landing on the involved extremity. Because returning to running is not taken lightly, we use a graduated return-to-running protocol that allows the patient to slowly, safely, and painlessly increase the running mileage. This return-to-running program (Table 10-3) is performed every other day or as the directions allow. The patient is instructed to never run into pain and also to use cold therapy liberally after runs to prophylactically combat any swelling, inflammation, or delayed-onset muscle soreness that may result from increasing running endurance.

Immediate jumping and hopping on the involved extremity unilaterally are not recommending. Gentle "miniplyometrics" are begun at the 3-month period if clinically acceptable. If no actual jumping has yet been performed, these can be performed initially on a Total Gym (EFI Sports Medicine, San Diego, CA); the patient is actually unloaded during the first several jumps (Figure 10-15). These plyometrics will transition to "miniplyos" or very small jumps bilaterally in single classic straight planes such as forward/backward and right/left, progressing to diagonal patterns. Next we slowly add rotational jumping movements, all begun gently with emphasis on soft bent-knee landings. Jumping should start with about 10 to 15 jumps only, with a gradual systematic increase in jumping quantity as tolerated. Once the patient demonstrates adequate stability with the double leg jumps, we incorporate single-leg hops. Again these hops begin in straight patterns and progress to diagonals as tolerated. Often it is very helpful when beginning these "miniplyos" to use an unloading device, such as those described previously, with which the patient is not required to load the joint with full bodyweight. A gradual progression of stress loading to the joint and ligament is always preferred to provide a more

accommodating environment for the patient. During these advanced higher-level activities the patient should be closely monitored for pain and swelling, and ROM and flexibility should be assessed, to ensure that the patient is not being progressed too fast. Careful assessment of landing techniques should begin immediately so as not to allow faulty motor patterns to develop early. The clinician should pay careful attention to the presence of the landing patterns that place the athlete in the at-risk position of hip and knee internal rotation and genu valgus with foot pronation. Furthermore, a bent-knee landing should always be advised so that the patient does not use a knee position that might perpetuate knee hyperextension.

Phase IV: Return to Activity Phase

Phase IV begins at approximately 6 months and extends to 9 months after surgery. Criteria for advancement to phase IV include freedom from pain; full ROM; no evidence of patellofemoral irritation; and strength of quadriceps and hamstrings at approximately 70% of those of the uninvolved leg; and proprioception at 70% of that of the uninvolved leg.

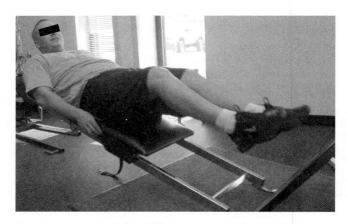

Figure 10-15: Unweighted bilateral plyometric jumping.

TABLE 10-3

Return to Running Protocol

SUN.	MON.	TUES.	WED.	THURS.	FRI.	SAT.
5.0 min	0	5.0 min	0	7.5 min	0	7.5 min
0	10.0 min	0	10.0 min	0	12.5 min	0
12.5 min	0	15.0 min	0	15.0 min	0	17.5 min
0	17.5 min	0	20.0 min	0	20.0 min	0
10.0 min	20.0 min	0	10.0 min	20.0 min	0	15.0 min
20.0 min	0	15.0 min	20.0 min	0	15.0 min	25.0 min
0	15.0 min	25.0 min	0	20.0 min	25.0 min	0
20 min	25 min	0	20.0 min	30.0 min	0	0

At 6 months we use an algorithm-based functional testing progression very similar to that described by Davies and Zilmer.[84,85] Using this approach the clinician is able to systematically and objectively evaluate return to activity both qualitatively and quantitatively to progress a patient from one level of performance to the next.[84-86] We initially perform basic tests and measurements such as measuring knee joint circumference and knee active and passive ROM. After these initial tests we determine knee ligament stability, balance and proprioception, and muscle strength and follow with functional tests.

At this time a second ligament arthrometer test and isokinetic strength test are performed. Again we would like to see less than 3 mm of laxity of the graft during a side-by-side comparison. Isokinetic strength of the quadriceps and hamstrings should be 90% or above as compared with the uninvolved extremity to allow full return of activity and release to competitive sports activities. The functional testing sequence we use begins with the lower extremity functional reach test (LEFRT), which assesses dynamic neuromuscular stability. During this testing procedure the patient stands on the uninvolved leg first, then on the involved extremity. The patient is then asked to reach with the involved extremity as far as possible in multiple directions including anterior, anterior medial 45 degrees, medial, posterior medial 45 degrees, posterior, posterior lateral, lateral, anterolateral. Manske and Anderson have shown the LEFRT to be a very reliable testing method.[87] Three attempts are given to each extremity and then averaged to obtain a score. We like the involved extremity to reach at least 90% of the uninvolved in each direction.

Despite the fact that numerous studies have found correlations between scores on an isokinetic strength test and jump performance assessment,[88-93] we do not feel confident with only information gained by strength tests alone. Therefore we use a spectrum of functional testing procedures to back up our other objective data when determining ability to return to play.

The next set of functional tests we perform includes the bilateral and unilateral vertical jump tests. These tests were originally described by Sargent[94] and Seminick.[95] The vertical jump test has been found to be very reliable by numerous authors,[88,95-97] whereas the single-leg vertical jump has been found reliable by Bandy and co-workers[98] and Manske and colleagues.[88] Because using tape or chalk methods can generate substantial measurement error, we use the Vertec jump apparatus (Sports Imports, Inc., Columbus, OH). After a standing baseline reach flatfooted, the patient is asked to jump as high as possible off of both feet initially, followed by unilateral vertical jumping. Using the Vertec the patient jumps as high as possible and displaces a movable plastic vane in $\frac{1}{2}$-inch increments. Countermovements with upper extremities are allowed with this test, because reaching is part of the measurement. We are currently in the process of determining standards for various patient populations.

Next in the progression of tests is the jump test, which is defined as a double leg jump. The patient is asked to place the hands on the hips[99] or behind the back. The patient is allowed up to four gradient warm-up jumps to become accustomed to the testing procedure (25%, 50%, 75%, and 100% effort). The patient is then instructed to explode horizontally as far as possible; again, it is stressed that the patient should land with a bent knee to decrease risk of further injury. The patient must be able to "stick" the landing without a loss of balance requiring use of the upper extremities or taking an extra step. Distance is measured from the takeoff stripe to the posterior portion of the more posterior heel. In addition to the distance measurement, the quality of the jump is assessed as part of the performance. Next is the single-leg hop test. Like the other tests used in the algorithm, the single-leg hop test has been proven very reliable by numerous authors.[88,98,100-102] The patient is asked to first hop off of the uninvolved lower extremity. The patient is asked to hold his or her hand on the hips to avoid gaining momentum with the upper extremities. The patient is then asked to hop as far horizontally as possible, making sure to land with a bent knee on the same leg. The distance from the starting mark to the heel of the landing leg is measured. The patient has to "stick" the landing with both jumps and hops, without relying on the upper extremity for assistance. A failed jump would include taking a short hop after landing, falling forward and using the upper extremity to catch oneself, or having to use the contralateral lower extremity to catch oneself during the single-leg hop for distance.

Although some clinicians may believe that performing numerous functional tests after an isokinetic test may decrease reliability of those tests, it been clearly shown that the tests described are very reliable after up to 6 sets of isokinetic testing.[87]

If and when the patient passes all of his or her isokinetic and functional tests, the patient is allowed full return to sports activity. This in most instances does not occur before 6 months after surgery.

SUMMARY

There are many accepted graft choices for ACL reconstruction. We believe that the hamstring graft provides excellent stability with limited patient morbidity for harvest compared with other potential grafts sources. Critical to the success of any reconstructive procedure is surgical technique and postoperative rehabilitation designed for specific graft sources. The rehabilitation for the patient with a hamstring ACL reconstruction requires a series of transitional phases with increasing applied and functional stresses to the knee. This gradual, systematic progression provides a healthy stimulus for the maturing graft that is safe enough to not cause damage. We have found the hamstring construct to be an excellent choice for successful ACL reconstruction.

References

1. Denti M, Bigoni M, Dodaro G, et al: Long-term results of the Leeds-Keio anterior cruciate ligament reconstruction, *Knee Surg Sports Traumatol Arthrosc* 3:75-77, 1995.

2. Jadarvinen M, Jozsa L, Johnson RJ, et al: Effect of anterior cruciate ligament reconstruction with patellar tendon or prosthetic ligament on the morphology of the other ligaments of the knee joint. An experimental study in dogs, *Clin Orthop* 311:176-182, 1995.

3. Klein W, Jensen KU: Synovitis and artificial ligaments, *Arthroscopy* 8:116-124, 1992.

4. Savarese A, Lunghi E, Budpassi P, et al: Remarks on the complications following reconstruction using synthetic ligaments, *Ital J Orthop Traumatol* 19:79-86, 1993.

5. Macey HB: A new operative procedure for repair of ruptured cruciate ligament of the knee joint, *Surg Gynecol Obstet* 69:108-109, 1939.

6. Lindemann K: Plastic surgery in substitution of the cruciate ligaments of the knee-joint by means of pedunculated tendon transplants, *Z Orthop Ihre Grenzgeb* 79(2):316-334, 1950.

7. Cho KO: Reconstruction of the anterior cruciate ligament by semitendinosus tenodesis, *J Bone Joint Surg Am,* 57A:608-612, 1975.

8. Puddu G: Method for reconstruction of the anterior cruciate ligament using the semitendinosus tendon, *Am J Sports Med* 8:402-404, 1980.

9. Lipscomb AB, Johnston RK, Snyder RB: The technique of cruciate ligament reconstruction, *Am J Sports Med* 29:77, 1981.

10. Gomes JLE, Marczyk LRS: Anterior cruciate ligament reconstruction with a loop or double thickness of semitendinosus tendon, *Am J Sports Med* 12:199, 1984.

11. Friedman MJ: Arthroscopic semitendinosus reconstruction for anterior cruciate deficiency, *Tech Orthop* 2:74, 1988.

12. Pinczewski L: Clinical results: Pinczewski endoscopic hamstring technique utilizing the DonJoy RCI fixation screw. Australian Orthopaedic Meeting, Adelaide, Australia, 1994.

13. Rosenberg TD, Deffner KT: ACL reconstruction: semitendinosus is the graft of choice, *Orthopedics* 20:396, 1997.

14. Rosenberg TD: *Technique for endoscopic method of ACL reconstruction. Technical bulletin,* Mansfield, MA, 1993, Acufex Microsurgical.

15. Howell SM: Brace-free rehabilitation with early return to activity for knees reconstructed with double looped semitendinosus and gracilis graft, *Arthroscopy* 6:594, 1999.

16. Furman W, Marshall D, Girgis F: The anterior cruciate ligament: a functional analysis based on postmortem studies, *J Bone Joint Surg* 58A:179-185, 1976.

17. Girgis F, Marshall J, Monajem A: The cruciate ligaments of the knee joint, *Clin Orthop* 106:216-231, 1975.

18. Butler D, Noyes F, Grood E: Ligamentous restraint to anterior-posterior drawer in the human knee: a biomechanical study, *J Bone Joint Surg* 62A:256-270, 1980.

19. Hefzy M, Grood E: Sensitivity of insertion locations on length patterns of anterior cruciate ligament fibers, *J Biomech Eng* 108:73-82, 1986.

20. Noyes F, Butler D, Grood E, et al: Biomechanical analysis of human ligament grafts used in knee-ligament repairs and reconstructions, *J Bone Joint Surg* 66A:344-352, 1984.

21. Noyes F, Butler D, Paulos L, Grood E: Intra-articular cruciate reconstruction: perspectives on graft strength, vascularization, and immediate motion after replacement, *Clin Orthop* 172:71-77, 1983.

22. Noyes F, Grood E: The strength of the anterior cruciate ligament in humans and rhesus monkeys, *J Bone Joint Surg* 58A:1074-1082, 1976.

23. Rowden N, Sher D, Rogers G, Schindhelm K: Anterior cruciate ligament graft fixation: initial comparison of patellar tendon and semitendinosus autografts in young fresh cadavers, *Am J Sports Med* 25:472-478, 1997.

24. Woo S, Hollis M, Adams D, et al: Tensile properties of the human femur-anterior cruciate ligament-tibia complex, *Am J Sports Med* 19:217-225, 1991.

25. Arms SW, Pope MH, Johnson RJ, et al: The biomechanics of anterior cruciate ligament rehabilitation and reconstruction, *Am J Sports Med* 12:8-18, 1984.

26. Noyes FR, Vutler DL, Grood ES, et al: Biomechanical analysis of human ligament grafts used in knee ligament repairs and reconstructions, *J Bone Joint Surg Am* 66:334, 1984.

27. Hamner DL, Brown CH, Steiner ME: Hamstring tendon grafts for reconstruction of the anterior cruciate ligament: biomechanical evaluation of the use of multiple strands and tensioning techniques. *J Bone Joint Surg Am* 81:549-557, 1999.

28. Brahmabhatt V, Smolinski R, McGlowan J, et al: Double-stranded hamstring tendons for anterior cruciate ligament reconstruction, *Am J Knee Surg* 12:141-145, 1999.

29. Brown CH: Biomechanics of the semitendinosus and gracilis tendon grafts. American Orthopaedic Society for Sports Medicine (AOSSM),Toronto, Canada, 1995.

30. Brown CH, Steiner ME, Carson EW: The use of hamstring tendons for anterior cruciate reconstruction: technique and results, *Clin Sports Med* 12:723, 1996.

31. Schatzmann L, Brunner P, Staubli HU: Effect of cyclic preconditioning on the tensile properties of human quadriceps tendons and patellar ligaments, *Knee Surg Sports Traumatol Arthrosc* 6:S56-S61, 1998.

32. Woo SL-Y, Fox RJ, Sakane M, et al: Force and force distribution in the anterior cruciate ligament and its clinical implications, *Sportorthopaedie-Sporttraumatologie* 13:37-48, 1997.

33. Millett PJ, Miller BS, Close M, et al: Effects of braiding on tensile properties of four-strand human hamstring tendon grafts, *Am J Sports Med* 31:714-717, 2003.

34. Kim DH, Wilson DR, Hecker AT, et al: Twisting and braiding reduces the tensile strength and stiffness of human hamstring tendon grafts used for anterior cruciate reconstruction, *Am J Sports Med* 31:861-867, 2003.

35. Fu FH, Bennett CH, Ma CB, et al: Current trends in anterior cruciate ligament reconstruction. Part I: Biology and biomechanics of reconstruction, *Am J Sports Med* 27:821-830, 1999.

36. Fu FH, Bennett CH, Ma CB, et al: Current trends in anterior cruciate ligament reconstruction. Part II: Operative procedures and clinical correlations, *Am J Sports Med* 28:124-130, 2000.

37. Brand JC Jr, Weiler A, Caborn DNM, et al: Current concepts. Graft fixation in cruciate ligament reconstruction, *Am J Sports Med* 28:761-774, 2000.

38. Isibashi Y, Kim KS, Rudy T: Robotic evaluation of the effect of the tibial fixation level on the ACL reconstructed knee. 41st Meeting of the Orthopedic Research Society, Orlando, FL, 1995.

39. Kousa P, Jarvinen TLN, Vihavainen M, et al: The fixation strength of six hamstring tendon graft fixation devices in anterior cruciate ligament reconstruction. Part I: Femoral Site, *Am J Sports Med* 31:174-181, 2003.

40. Kousa P, Jarvinen TLN, Vihavainen M, et al: The fixation strength of six hamstring tendon graft fixation devices in anterior

cruciate ligament reconstruction. Part II: Tibial Site, *Am J Sports Med* 31:182-188, 2003.

41. Lipscomb AB, Johnston RK, Snyder RB: Evaluation of hamstring strength following use of semitendinosus and gracilis tendons to reconstruct the anterior cruciate ligament, *Am J Sports Med* 10:340, 1982.

42. Carter TR, Edinger S: Isokinetic evaluation of anterior cruciate ligament reconstruction: Hamstring versus patellar tendon, *Arthroscopy* 15:169-172, 1999.

43. Simonian PT, Harrison SD, Cooley VJ, et al: Assessment of morbidity of semitendinosus and gracilis tendon gravest for ACL reconstruction, *Am J Knee Surg* 10:54-59, 1997.

44. Yasuda K, Tsujino J, Ohkoshi Y, et al: Graft site morbidity with autogenous semitendinosus and gracilis tendons, *Am J Sports Med* 23:706-714, 1995.

45. Cross MJ, Roger G, Kujawa, P: Regeneration of the semitendinosus and gracilis tendon following their transection for repair of the anterior cruciate ligament, *Am J Sports Med* 20:221-223, 1992.

46. Marder RA: Prospective evaluation of arthroscopically assisted anterior cruciate ligament reconstruction: Patellar tendon versus semitendinosus and gracilis tendons, *Am J Sports Med* 19:478, 1991.

47. Blackburn TA: Rehabilitation of anterior cruciate ligament injuries, *Orthop Clin North Am* 16:240-269, 1985.

48. Brewster CE, Moyens DR, Jobe FR: Rehabilitation for anterior cruciate reconstruction, *J Orthop Sports Phys Ther* 5:121-126, 1983.

49. Henning CE, Lynch MA, Glick KR: An in-vivo strain gauge study of the anterior cruciate ligament, *Am J Sports Med* 12:22-26, 1985.

50. Johnson RJ, Ericksson E, Haggmark T: Five to ten year follow-up evaluation after reconstruction of the anterior cruciate ligament, *Clin Orthop* 183:122-140, 1984.

51. Yasuda K, Sakaki T: Muscle exercises after anterior cruciate ligament reconstruction. Biomechanics of the simultaneous isometric contraction method of the quadriceps and hamstrings, *Clin Orthop* 22:266-274, 1987.

52. Yasuda K, Sasaki T: Exercises after anterior cruciate ligament reconstruction. The force exerted on the tibia by the separate isometric contraction of the quadriceps and hamstrings, *Clin Orthop* 22:275-286, 1987.

53. Shelbourne KD, Nitz APA: Accelerated rehabilitation after anterior cruciate ligament reconstruction, *Am J Sports Med* 18:292-299, 1990.

54. Mangine RE, Noyes FR: Rehabilitation of the allograft reconstruction, *J Orthop Sports Phys Ther* 15:294-302, 1992.

55. Wilk KE, Andrews JR: Current concepts in the treatment of anterior cruciate ligament disruptions, *J Orthop Sports Phys Ther* 15:279-293, 1992.

56. Shelbourne KD, Wilckens JH, Mollabashy A, et al: Arthrofibrosis in acute anterior cruciate ligament reconstruction. The effect of timing of reconstruction and rehabilitation, *Am J Sports Med* 19:332-336, 1991.

57. Sach RA, Reznik A, Daniel DM, et al: Complication of knee ligament surgery. In Daniel DM, Akeson WH, O'Connor W, editors: *Knee ligaments; structure, function, injury and repair,* New York, 1990, Raven Press.

58. Wilk KE, Arrigo C, Andrews JR, et al: Rehabilitation after anterior cruciate ligament reconstruction in the female athlete, *J Athl Train* 34:177-193, 1999.

59. Lephart SM, Kocher MS, Fu FH, et al: Proprioception following ACL reconstruction, *J Sports Rehabil* 1:188-196, 1992.

60. Lephart SM, Pincivero DM, Giraldo JL, et al: The role of proprioception in the management and rehabilitation of athletic injuries, *Am J Sports Med* 25:130-137, 1997.

61. Wilk KE, Reinold MM, Hooks TR: Recent advances in the rehabilitation of isolated and combined anterior cruciate ligament injuries, *Orthop Clin North Am* 34:107-137, 2003.

62. Rudroff T: Functional capability is enhanced with semitendinosus than patellar tendon ACL repair, *Med Sci Sports Exerc* 35(9):1486-1492, 2003.

63. West RV, Harner CD: Graft selection in anterior cruciate ligament reconstruction, *J Am Acad Orthop Surg* 13(3):197-207, 2005.

64. deAndrade JR, Grant C, Dixon A: Joint distention and reflex muscle inhibition in the knee, *J Bone Joint Surg* 47A:312-322, 1965.

65. Spencer JD, Hayes KC, Alexander, IJ: Knee joint effusion and quadriceps reflex inhibition in man, *Arch Phys Med Rehab* 65:279-283, 1981.

66. Stokes M, Young A: Investigations of quadriceps inhibition: Implications for clinical practice, *Physiotherapy* 70:425-428, 1984.

67. Prentice WE: *Therapeutic modalities for physical therapists,* ed 2, New York, 2002, McGraw-Hill.

68. Cook H, Morales M, La Rosa E, et al: Effects of electrical stimulation on lymphatic flow and limb volume in the rat, *Phys Ther* 74:1040-1046, 1994.

69. Clancy W, Nelson D, Reider B: Anterior cruciate ligament reconstruction using one third of the patellar ligament augmented by extra-articular tendon transfers, *J Bone Joint Surg* 62A:352, 1982.

70. Scranton PE, Lanzer WL, Ferguson MS, et al: Mechanisms of anterior cruciate ligament neovascularization and ligamentization, *Arthroscopy* 14:702-716, 1998.

71. Rougraff B, Shelbourne KD, Gerth PK, Warner J: Arthroscopic and histologic analysis of human patella tendon allografts used for anterior cruciate ligament reconstruction, *Am J Sports Med* 21:277-284, 1993.

72. Falconiero RP, DiStefano VJ, Cook TM: Revascularization and ligamentization of autogenous anterior cruciate ligament grafts in humans, *Arthroscopy* 14:197-205, 1998.

73. Woo SLY, Gomez MA, Sites TJ, et al: The biomechanical and morphological changes in the medial collateral ligament of the rabbit after immobilization and remobilization, *J Bone Joint Surg* 69A:1200-1211, 1987.

74. Kielty CM, Shuttleworth CA: Synthesis and assembly of fibrillin by fibroblasts and smooth muscle cells, *J Cell Sci,* 106:167-173, 1993.

75. Snyder-Mackler L, DeLitto A, Bailey SL, Stralka SW: Strength of the quadriceps femoris muscle and functional recovery after reconstruction of the anterior cruciate ligament, *J Bone Joint Surg* 77A:1166-1172, 1995.

76. Sachs R, Daniel DM, Stone ML, Garfein RF: Patellofemoral problems after anterior cruciate ligament reconstruction, *Am J Sports Med* 17:760-765, 1989.

77. Gerber C, Hoppeler H, Claassen H, et al: The lower extremity musculature in chronic symptomatic instability of the anterior cruciate ligament, *J Bone Joint Surg* 67A:1034-1043, 1985.

78. Wigerstad-Lossing I, Grimby G, Jonsson T, et al: Effects of electrical muscle stimulation combined with voluntary contractions after knee ligament surgery, *Med Sci Sports Exerc* 20:93-98, 1988.

79. Delitto A, McKowen JM, McCarthy JA, et al: Electrically elicited co-contraction of thigh musculature after anterior cruciate

ligament surgery. A description and single-case experiment, *Phys Ther* 68:45-50, 1988.

80. Snyder-Mackler L, Ladin Z, Schepsis AA, Young JC: Electrical stimulation of the thigh muscles after reconstruction of the anterior cruciate ligament. Effects of electrically elicited contraction of the quadriceps femoris and hamstring muscles on gait and on strength of the thigh muscles, *J Bone Joint Surg* 73A:1025-1036, 1991.

81. Rebal H, Barra V, Laborde A, et al: Effects of two electrical stimulation frequencies in thigh muscle after knee surgery, *Int J Sports Med* 23:604-609; 2002.

82. Sherbondy PS, Queale WS, McFarland EG, et al: Soleus and gastrocnemius muscle loading decreases anterior tibial translation in anterior cruciate ligament intact and deficient knees, *J Knee Surg* 16:152-158, 2003.

83. Rudrud JA, Kollwelter KA, Davies GJ, et al: Closed kinetic chain weight bearing response following knee surgery, *Phys Ther* 30:A-48, 2000 (abstract).

84. Davies GJ, Zilmer DA: Functional progression of a patient through a rehabilitation program, *Orthop Phys Ther Clin North Am* 9:103-118, 2000.

85. Davies GJ, Zilmer DA: Functional progression of exercise during rehabilitation. In Ellenbecker TS, editor: *Knee Ligament Rehabilitation*, Philadelphia, 2000, Churchill Livingstone.

86. Manske RC, Davies GJ: A nonsurgical approach to examination and treatment of the patellofemoral joint. Part 1: Examination of the patellofemoral joint, *Crit Rev Phys Rehabil Med* 15:141-166, 2003.

87. Manske RC, Anderson J: Test retest reliability of the lower extremity functional reach test, *J Orthop Sports Phys Ther* 34(1): A52-53, 2004 (abstract).

88. Manske RC, Smith B, Wyatt F: Test-retest reliability of lower extremity functional tests after a closed kinetic chain isokinetic testing bout, *J Sports Rehabil* 12:119-132, 2003.

89. Malliou P, Ispirlidis I, Beneka A, et al: Vertical jump and knee extensors isokinetic performance in professional soccer layers related to the phase of the training period, *Isokin Exerc Sci* 11:165-169, 2003.

90. Blackburn JR, Morrissey M: The relationship between open and closed kinetic chain strength of the lower limb and jumping performance, *J Orthop Sports Phys Ther* 27:430-435, 1998.

91. Destaso J, Kaminski TW, Perrin DH: Relationship between drop vertical jump heights and isokinetic measures utilizing the stretch-shortening cycle, *Isokin Exerc Sci* 6:175-179, 1997.

92. Genuario SE, Dolgener FA: The relationship of isokinetic torque at two speeds to the vertical jump, *Res Q Exerc Sport* 51:593-598, 1980.

93. Pincivero DM, Lephart SM, Karunakara RG: Relation between open and closed kinematic chain assessment of knee strength and functional performance, *Clin J Sport Med* 7:11-16, 1997.

94. Sargent DA: The physical tests of a man, *Am Phys Ed Rev* 26:188-194, 1921.

95. Seminick D: The vertical jump, *J Strength Cond Res* 12:68-69, 1990.

96. Considine WJ, Sullivan WJ: Relationship of selected tests of leg strength and leg power on college men, *Res Q* 44:404-416, 1973.

97. Glencross DJ: The nature of the vertical jump test and the standing broad jump, *Res Q* 37:353-359, 1966.

98. Bandy WD, Rusche KR, Tekulve FY: Reliability and limb symmetry for five unilateral functional tests of the lower extremities, *Isokin Exerc Sci* 4:108-111, 1994.

99. Manske RC, Smith BS, Rogers ME, Wyatt F: Closed kinetic chain (linear) isokinetic testing: Relationships to functional testing, *Isokin Exerc Sci* 11:171-179, 2003.

100. Bolga LA, Keskula DR: Reliability of lower extremity functional performance tests, *J Orthop Sports Phys Ther* 3:138-142, 1997.

101. Booher LD, Hench KM, Worrell TW, Stikeleather J: Reliability of three single-leg hop tests, *J Sports Rehabil* 2:138-142, 1993.

102. Greenberger HB, Paterno MV: The test-retest reliability of a one-legged hop for distance in healthy young adults, *J Orthop Sports Phys Ther* 15:51, 1992 (abstract).

CHAPTER 11

Anterior Cruciate Ligament Reconstruction with Allograft

John H. Fernandez, PT, ATC, OCS, CSCS
Naomi N. Shields, MD

CHAPTER OUTLINE

GRAFT SELECTION FOR ANTERIOR CRU-CIATE ligament (ACL) reconstruction is based on numerous factors including patient choice, surgeon preference, surgeon and patient philosophy, surgeon experience, graft or tissue availability, patient expectations, patient activity levels, and patient desires. ACL injuries are common. Each year, 95,000 ACL injuries are seen by U.S. physicians and approximately 50,000 ACL reconstructions are performed.[1] This chapter discusses both surgical and rehabilitation considerations for performing an allograft (i.e., tissue from another human being) ACL reconstruction.

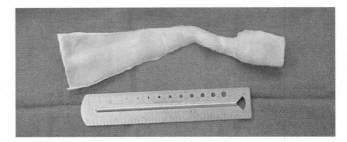

Figure 11-1: Achilles tendon allograft as received from the tissue bank. Not the calcaneal portion on the right.

ALLOGRAFT DEFINITIONS

Allograft by definition is tissue taken from another person, usually deceased. Approximately 1,000,000 allografts obtained from tissue banks were distributed in 2002 and used for orthopedic surgical procedures (ACL, meniscus transplant, spine surgery, etc.).[2] Recommended tissues banks are accredited by the American Association of Tissue Banks (AATB) (http://www.aatb.org), which sets standards for allograft harvesting (retrieval), processing, storage, and distribution. Initial standards for allograft harvesting were devised in 1984 and have been updated six times, most recently in 1996. The AATB sets the minimal standards for tissue bank accreditation, including record keeping, quality control, donor selection criteria, patient history, and safety.

ALLOGRAFT

Allograft anatomic choices useful for ACL reconstruction include the Achilles tendon; patella bone-tendon-bone; quadriceps tendon bone; anterior or posterior tibial tendon bone; tensor fascia lata; and hamstring tendon. Grafts are harvested and then processed as either fresh frozen (stored at −70°C); freeze dried; or irradiated with low-dose radiation. The most commonly used allografts currently are fresh frozen bone-patella-tendon-bone (BPTB) or Achilles tendon (Figure 11-1). Allograft alternatives include autograft (tissue taken from the host); synthetic tissue; or xenograft (grafts from another species). Allografts are extensively tested before being released for use. Tests for both viral and bacterial contamination are performed. Allografts are harvested, processed, and sterilized and ideally would be rendered incapable of transmitting viral or bacterial infection. Sterilization options include chemical sterilants, antimicrobial solutions, radiation, deep freezing (at −70° to −80°C), or freeze drying. Gamma irradiation typically consists of 1 to 2 megarads. All these methods, however, affect the material properties of allograft tissue.[3] Ethylene oxide (EtO) has been used to "sterilize" tissue during processing. However, seven of 109 patients receiving a freeze-dried, EtO-sterilized BPTB allograft developed a persistent intraarticular reaction characterized by persistent synovial effusion with collagenous particulates and cellular inflammatory response.[4] Gas chromatography demonstrated detectable levels of ethylene chlorohydrin, a toxic reaction product of EtO. Use of freeze-dried, EtO-sterilized allograft is not recommended for reconstruction of the ACL.[4]

The most common harvesting and processing tissue technique is fresh freezing to −70°C in liquid nitrogen. The effect of cryopreservation on ligament strength and relative performance of both autograft and allograft ACL transplants up to 18 months was studied in a dog model by Nikolaou and coworkers.[5] The cryopreservation process and duration of storage were found to have no effect on the biomechanical or structural properties of the ligament. The mechanical integrity of the allografts was similar to that of the autografts, with both achieving nearly 90% of control ligament strength by 36 weeks. Revascularization approached normal by 24 weeks in both allograft and autograft.[5] The most common method of tissue processing is aseptic. This restricts contamination of allograft tissue but cannot be considered sterile and carries the risk of bacterial infection.[6]

Allograft use raises concerns regarding bacterial infections. Group A *Streptococcus pyogenes* infection was reported in September 2003.[2,6] Bacterial *Clostridium* was reported in 13 of 26 reported cases of infections associated with musculoskeletal tissue allografts reported to the Centers for Disease Control and Prevention (CDC).[2,6] One tissue-processing facility processed 14 of 26 grafts. Viral transmission, especially of human immunodeficiency virus (HIV), hepatitis, and human T-lymphotropic virus, remains a concern. The majority of reported cases occurred before the implementation of guidelines for donor screening and before availability of currently validated serologic tests.[1] In April 2003 the CDC reported hepatitis C virus (HCV) transmission in a patella tendon allograft. Additional disease transmission was found in 8 of 40 organ and tissue graft recipients from the same donor with more sensitive HCV RNA assay. There are no reports of HCV transmission in recipients of irradiated bone.[3] Screening of donor allograft tissue is extremely effective for active viral infections, but there is a "window period" during which the donor may be infectious but have negative test results, with no detectable antibodies to the virus. Present screening and testing protocols put risk of implanting tissue from an HIV-infected donor at <1:1,000,000.[7] Risk of hepatitis B virus (HBV) or HCV infection is higher because of the greater prevalence of these viruses in the general population.

Tissue rejection of allografts in ACL reconstructions is low, as grafts are washed and cleansed of blood and marrow elements. Tendon is primarily collagen, which has a low antigenicity. Failure to incorporate or an inflammatory response to the graft may be seen. This is usually evidenced by delayed graft incorporation and/or tunnel widening. With delayed graft incorporation or tunnel widening, graft remodeling and maturation may be prolonged by as much as 50%. Once graft remodeling is complete, allograft ACLs are histologically similar to native ACLs, although strength may be decreased. Cost and availability are issues that must be considered with allografts. Cost does vary widely within a region.

ANTERIOR CRUCIATE LIGAMENT ALLOGRAFT

Outcomes for allograft ACL reconstructions in the literature are varied. Siebold and co-workers reviewed 183 fresh frozen patellar vs. 42 Achilles tendon allografts with a mean follow-up of 37.7 months. Using an International Knee Documentation Committee (IKDC) score, they found normal or near-normal results in 75.3% of the patella tendon group vs. 76.2% of the Achilles tendon group. Laxity failures were found in 4.4% of the patella tendon and 2.5% of the Achilles tendon group. Reruptures of the ACL graft occurred in 10.4% of the patella tendon and 4.8% of the Achilles tendon group.[8] Siebold also reviewed 325 fresh-frozen allografts (BPTB and Achilles tendon) in primary and revision ACL reconstructions with a mean follow-up of 38 months. This group reported an overall subjective rating using the Cincinnati knee score of 82 points. The IKDC score was normal or nearly normal in 75.6% primary and 67% revision ACL reconstructions. Total failure rate (rerupture and laxity failures) was reported as 13.7% in the primary and 15% in the revision ACL reconstructions. No specific complications were noted with the use of allograft tissue.[9] Gorschewsy and colleagues reviewed 132 BPTB allografts (Tutoplast) vs. 136 autograft BPTB ACL reconstructions. The BPTB Tutoplast allografts had a 2.6% rerupture rate within 11.75 months. The autograft BPTB ACL reconstructions had a 4.8% rerupture rate within 17 months. Histologic appraisal indicated delayed incorporation and extended reconstruction in the BPTB allograft. Further analysis of the BPTB allograft group indicated that especially in patients who were young and very active in sports there was increased elongation of the implant and a higher rerupture rate.[10] Noyes evaluated 70 allograft patients at 4- and 7-year follow-up and found no significant deterioration of allograft ACLs.[11] Shelton and colleagues evaluated 30 autografts vs. 30 allograft reconstructions with 24 months of follow-up. There were 15 acute and 15 chronic ACL injuries in the allograft group and 24 acute and six chronic in the autograft group. There was a trend for 20% of allografts to have a glide on pivot shift at 24 months

vs. 7% of autografts. No difference in patellofemoral crepitus or thigh circumference was noted.[12] Chang and co-workers retrospectively reviewed BPTB allograft ACL reconstructions vs. autografts. Both were augmented with an iliotibial band tenodesis. Good to excellent Lysholm II scores were obtained in 91% of allograft and 97% of autograft ACL reconstructions. Patients returned to their preinjury activity level in 65% of allograft and 73% of autograft ACL reconstructions. No significant difference was found in KT1000 testing. A traumatic graft rupture at 12, 19, and 43 months occurred in three of 46 allograft and zero of 33 autograft ACL reconstructions.[13] In 1993 Shino and colleagues reported on 92 patients who had undergone fresh frozen allogenic (tibialis anterior or posterior, Achilles, or peroneus) tendon (47) and autograft BPTB (45) ACL reconstructions. They found the ACL-reconstructed knees to have greater anterior laxity or less quadriceps torque than the contralateral normal knees. Knees treated with allografts showed better results then those treated with autografts for static anterior stability and in recovery of quadriceps muscle strength.[14] The results in the literature both supporting and criticizing allograft use for ACL reconstructions have led to much debate.

Current indications for allograft ACL reconstructions are divided into primary ACL reconstructions, revision ACL reconstructions,[15,16] and multiligamentous reconstructions. Primary ACL reconstructions are believed by some to be controversial.[17] Suggested indications include age older than 45 years,[16] skeletal immaturity,[18] previous patella tendon pathology, decreased donor site morbidity, patients who must kneel as part of their daily occupation or sports activity, the presence of a contraindication to autogenous graft harvest, and patient and/or surgeon preference.

An examination under anesthesia of both injured and uninjured knee is performed including range of motion (ROM) and ligamentous instability of the ACL, posterior cruciate ligament (PCL), medial collateral ligament (MCL), and lateral collateral ligament (LCL). Diagnostic arthroscopy is used to evaluate the entire knee for associated intraarticular pathology (Figure 11-2) and to verify the ACL tear (Figure 11-3). Associated pathology is treated as appropriate. Meniscal lesions may be repaired or resected as appropriate. Chondroplasty, abrasionplasty, or cartilage transplant is performed for chondral lesions. In some patients with varus malalignment, a high tibial osteotomy may be performed in conjunction with the ACL reconstruction. The intracondylar notch is then débrided, and the graft tunnels are prepared (Figure 11-4). Success of an ACL reconstruction is improved by accurate tunnel placement and secure anchoring of the ACL graft, allowing early functional motion. The graft must not impinge on the femoral notch roof or the PCL. Once intraarticular preparation is complete, a longitudinal incision 2 to 4 cm in length is made over the proximal medial tibia medial to the tibial tubercle. The pes anserine is incised longitudinally. The tibial tunnel is then drilled to the graft size (usually 10 to 11 mm). Through the tibial tunnel, the

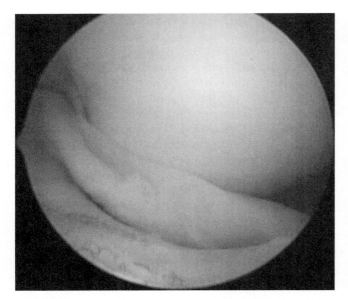

Figure 11-2: Intraoperative view of a bucket handle medial meniscal tear.

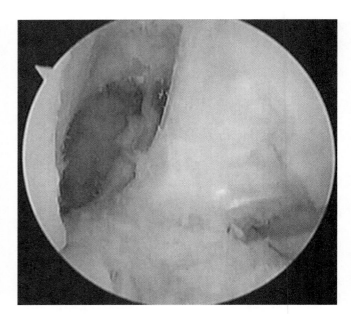

Figure 11-4: Intraoperative view of tunnel placement and the completed notch preparation for the graft.

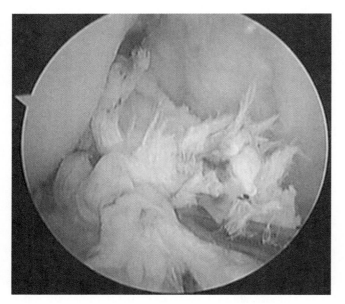

Figure 11-3: Intraoperative view of a torn anterior cruciate ligament. Note the complete disruption of the proximal portion of the anterior cruciate ligament.

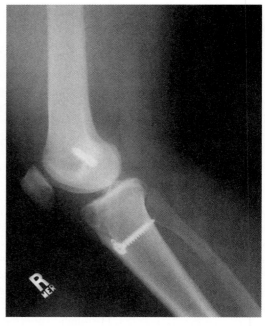

Figure 11-5: Lateral radiograph demonstrating the fixation used for the anterior cruciate ligament allograft.

femoral guide is passed and the femoral tunnel drilled. Bony debris from the tunnel drillings should be removed. The graft is then passed into the knee using a passing pin through the tibial tunnel into the femoral tunnel and out the anterior lateral thigh. The knee should be flexed to 90 degrees for drilling of the femoral tunnel, passage of the graft, and anchoring of the graft in the femoral tunnel using a metal or bioabsorbable interference screw. The knee is flexed approxi-

mately 45 degrees, the graft put under tension, and the graft anchored in the tibial tunnel using interference screws (metal or bioabsorbable) and/or transtibial screw and washer (Figures 11-5 and 11-6). A bone plug may be shaped from extra allograft bone and placed superior to the tendon portion of the graft within the tibial tunnel to augment fit and decrease risk of synovial fluid leakage. The pes anserine is repaired. Failure to obtain a good repair may lead to hamstring symp-

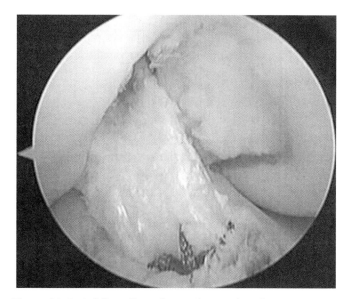

Figure 11-6: Achilles allograft anterior cruciate ligament.

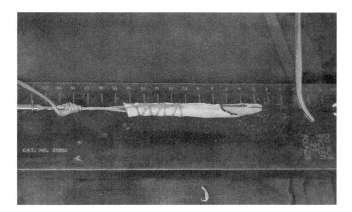

Figure 11-7: The prepared Achilles allograft. Note the calcaneal portion on the right.

toms and anterior medial pain during rehabilitation. Appropriate subcutaneous and skin sutures are placed, along with dressings. Intraarticular bupivacaine (Marcaine) may be injected for postoperative pain control, and a polar pack placed if available. A hinged knee immobilizer locked at 0 degrees flexion and extension is placed on the knee postoperatively.

Preparation of the fresh frozen allograft during the surgical procedure begins with obtaining the graft (Figure 11-7). Documentation in the patient record of the graft type, donor number, company graft was procured from, and site of implantation is important for tracking purposes in case of tissue recalls or infectious complications. The graft is usually thawed in warm antibiotic containing saline. It is important to not bend the graft during thawing, because this will break some graft fibers and result in graft weakening Once the graft is thawed it is sized and shaped. For an Achilles tendon

allograft, the bone from the calcaneal portion of the graft is shaped into a bullet or conical shape equal to the planned tunnel size (usually 10 to 11 mm) and a length of 20 to 25 mm. The tendon length is usually approximately 70 mm. Pull-out sutures for passing of the bone plug end into the femoral tunnel are placed through one or two small drill holes using #2 PDS or other equivalent absorbable sutures. Nonabsorbable sutures (#5 Mersilene or #2 FiberWire) are placed using a Krackow grasping stitch in the 25 mm of the distal portion of the tendon. The completed graft is placed on a tension board under 10 to 20 lb and kept moist until needed.

MEDICAL POSTOPERATIVE MANAGEMENT

Postoperative management includes pain control accomplished with a combination of narcotics and antiinflammatory medications, femoral blocks, and cold therapy. Motion is limited for the first 2 days in the hinged knee immobilizer brace locked at 0 degrees of knee extension. The brace is opened per the ACL allograft rehabilitation protocol beginning on day 3 by the physical therapist. Progressive protected weight bearing is continued until full weight bearing is tolerated, usually approximately 7 to 10 days after surgery. Patients return to the surgeon's office at 1 week for suture removal, 4 weeks for examination and fitting of a functional ACL brace, 12 weeks for recheck with strength test results, 6 months, and 1 year. They are released to full sports participation at approximately 6 months *if* they have full motion, good stability, good strength, and no pain. If a patient does not meet these criteria at 6 months, return to sports is delayed. Patients are encouraged to continue wearing the functional knee brace for running, jumping, and pivoting activities until 12 to 24 months after surgery to allow for maximum graft maturity and return of proprioception.

REHABILITATION AFTER ANTERIOR CRUCIATE LIGAMENT ALLOGRAFT

Preoperative Rehabilitation Considerations and Management

Preoperatively, after acute ACL rupture the major thrust of rehabilitation should be to do the following:

1. Obtain full knee ROM (minimum 0 to 90 degrees).
2. Minimize joint effusion.
3. Maintain quadriceps strength.
4. Minimize any further damage to the knee joint.
5. Prepare patient for the rehabilitative process.

As early as 24 to 48 hours postinjury, passive ROM (PROM) exercises may be started. These may include heel slides and seated pendulums. Assisted motion on a stationary bike may also be used to gradually increase ROM. (See the postoperative exercise section for a description of these exercises.) ROM can be restored to approximately 0 to 110 degrees in approximately 2 weeks postinjury.

Quadriceps activation and joint ROM are both decreased when a joint effusion is present. Therefore minimizing joint effusion before ACL reconstruction should be addressed. Joint effusion can typically be minimized in 1 to 2 weeks by the use of ice, compression, elevation, and electrical stimulation.[19,20]

Exercises have the dual effect of minimizing swelling and maintaining muscle strength. A preoperative home program of straight leg raises in all directions, ankle pumps, and seated knee extension (90 to 40 degrees) can be initiated to help maintain quadriceps function and hip strength.

Gait training instruction with assistive devices should ideally be done preoperatively in order to minimize the risk of fall postoperatively. Weight-bearing status preoperatively will vary depending on the physician and suspected collateral damage (articular cartilage, meniscal, or chondral bone damage), which may have occurred at the time of the ACL rupture.

In addition to these goals, it is of utmost importance to have the patient not only aware of the entire rehabilitation process, but also prepared for a protracted rehabilitation. Although the goals during the preoperative phase seem simple, having the patient both physically and psychologically prepared for surgery can minimize postoperative complications.

Postoperative Rehabilitation Management

Elements of the postoperative rehabilitation of the ACL allograft patient are essentially the same as that of the patient who has undergone an ACL autograft procedure. However, because of the inherent differences between the allograft and the autograft, some aspects of the rehabilitation process are emphasized and others are delayed (Box 11-1).

Restoration of Motion after Surgery

Paramount after any joint surgery is to restore motion. During the early phases of rehabilitation after BPTB midpatellar

---

BOX 11-1
Rehabilitation Guidelines after ACL Allograft

Phase 1: Preoperative Phase

Goals

Minimize joint effusion

Restore quadriceps control

Improve ROM (at least 90 degrees of flexion)

Independent ambulation with crutches

Independent with home exercise program

Restrictions

Protective weight bearing

Minimize prolonged weight-bearing activities

Treatment

Quadriceps setting

Heel slides

Straight leg raises in all directions

Stationary biking for ROM

Protection, rest, ice, compression, and elevation (PRICE)

Clinical Milestones

+1 effusion

Good quadriceps set

No pain at rest

PROM 0-90 degrees at a minimum

Phase 2: Immediate Postoperative Phase (Weeks 1-2)

Goals

Wound healing

Minimized risk of deep venous thrombobosis (DVT)

Quadriceps activation

Improved PROM

Weight bearing with assistive device

Improve patellar femoral joint mobility

Restrictions

Weight bearing as tolerated (WBAT) with crutches; brace opened slowly according to patient's pain-free PROM tolerance, not to exceed 120 degrees by the end of week 2

Treatment

Pain management

Ice, compression, elevation

Patella mobilization

BOX 11-1

Rehabilitation Guidelines after ACL Allograft—cont'd

Scar mobilization

PROM manually

Heel slides

Quadriceps setting

Hamstring isometrics

Stationary biking for PROM

Gait training with crutches increasing weight at tolerated

Electrical stimulation (for both edema and muscle reeducation)

Clinical Milestones

Reduction in effusion by half a grade to one grade by the end of 2 weeks

Full knee hyperextension

110 degrees of knee flexion

Good patellar mobility

Ability to perform straight leg raises without gross quad lag

Weight bearing at least 75% without gross compensation

Phase 3: Intermediate Postoperative Phase (Weeks 2-4)

Goals

Full weight bearing (FWB) with brace with or without one crutch, with good gait pattern

Decreased effusion

Minimized adhesions

Improvement in muscular control

Closed kinetic chain exercises begun

Minimized pain

Improvement in gait pattern

Restrictions

No forced flexion past 125 degrees

Treatment

Pain management

Electrical stimulation

Scar mobilization

Control of effusion

Minisquats (wall squats)

Calf raises (bilateral)

Hip strengthening

Hamstring isotonic exercises

Gait activities (forward and backward walking)

Stationary biking

Open chain 90-40 degrees active range of motion (AROM)

Unilateral standing activities for balance

Cryotherapy after exercise

Clinical Milestones

FWB

Minimal gait compensation

125 degrees of knee flexion

Full knee hyperextension

One third effusion

Uncorrected unilateral stance for 20 seconds

Normal patella mobility

Straight leg raise without lag

Phase 4: Early Strengthening Phase (Weeks 4-6)

Goals

FWB without assistive devices and without compensation

No effusion

Improved eccentric quadriceps control

Ability to ascend stairs without compensation

Absence of overstretching of the graft

Restrictions

No forced flexion beyond 125 degrees

Treatment

Stationary bike (warm-up and cardiovascular training)

Scar massage

Minisquats progressing to body-weight squats (BWS)

Step-ups forward and to the side

Half lunges

Hamstring, isotonic exercise

Balance activities (trampoline ball toss)

Open chain 90-40 degrees AROM

Calf raises (bilateral to single leg)

Cryotherapy after treatment

(continued)

BOX 11-1
Rehabilitation Guidelines after ACL Allograft—cont'd

Clinical Milestones

FWB without compensation

No effusion

Improved eccentric control (4-inch step-down with good control)

Ascent and descent of stairs without use of assistive devices or guard rail

Absence of overstretching of the graft

Uncorrected unilateral stance (on trampoline) held for 30 seconds

Phase 5: Intermediate Strengthening Phase (Weeks 6-8)
Goals

Independent activities of daily living without pain or compensation

No effusion

Increased quadriceps and hamstring strength

Good hip stability with closed chain activity

Restrictions

No forced flexion past 125 degrees

Treatment

Stationary biking (warm-up and cardiovascular training)

Body-weight squats

Step-ups forward, side, and eccentric

Lunges

Hamstring, isotonic exercise

Balance activities (Airex [Alusuisse Composites, St. Louis, MO], progressing to ball toss)

Open chain 90-40 degrees AROM

Calf raises (single leg to bilateral with weight)

Dot drills

Cryotherapy after exercise

Clinical Milestones

No effusion

Good eccentric control of the quadriceps (6-inch step)

Ascent and descent of stairs without compensation

Absence of overstretching of the graft

Unilateral stance for 30 seconds on Airex

Phase 6: Advanced Strengthening Phase (Weeks 8-12)

At this point exercises are changed to circuit training. This allows for increased flexibility in the volume of the program as well as increased cardiovascular exertion. The intensity may be increased by decreasing the rest periods between sets or by weighting the patient.

Goals

Improved power, strength, and endurance

No effusion

Normal balance and proprioception

Restrictions

No forced flexion beyond 125 degrees

Treatment

Progressive circuit training; when the patient is able to complete one circuit, he or she progresses to the next.

- Circuit 1
  Start with two sets, and progress to four sets
  Stationary bike for warm-up
  Step-ups (6 inches)
  Body-weight squats
  Lunges
  Calf raises (single leg)
- Circuit 2
  Start with two sets, and progress to four sets
  Stationary bike for warm-up
  Step-ups (12 inches)
  Body-weight squats (at one per second unweighted)
  Lunges (with weight)
  Calf raises (single leg with weight)
  Monster walks
- Circuit 3
  Start with two sets, and progress to four sets
  Stationary bike for warm-up
  High step-ups (18-20 inches)
  Body-weight squats (weighted or jump squats)
  Lunges (with weight)
  Calf raises (single leg with weight)
  Monster walks

tendon ACL reconstruction, obtaining full ROM can sometimes be quite difficult. Pain and stiffness in the infrapatellar region can make passive flexion and active knee extension painful. In contrast, motion after an allograft reconstruction is gained more easily. Because there has been no trauma to the extensor mechanism, the incidence and risk of infrapatellar contracture or anterior knee pain with passive motion or with active knee extension are markedly reduced. Because ACL allograft ROM gains are easier, the therapist needs to be careful not to permit motion too soon, as this may result in graft stretching. For this reason, deep knee flexion is not emphasized during the first 8 weeks. As with other ACL rehabilitation protocols, patella femoral mobility also needs to be restored. Again, the time needed to restore full patella femoral mobility is less with the allograft than with the BPTB autograft surgery secondary to less anterior knee insult.

Full knee extension should be achieved within the first 2 weeks after surgery.[21-23] The use of low-load prolonged stretch is started in the immediate postoperative phase. This may start by simply having the patient's leg lie flat on the plinth. The use of prone hangs is another common method of using low-load prolonged stretching in order to achieve full extension. Investigators have studied the effects of different stretching techniques—high load, short duration vs. low load, long duration—in the permanent elongation of collagenous tissue and have found low-load, long-duration stretching more effective.[24,25]

Low-load high-repetition exercises are also employed early in the rehabilitation phase.[26] With this type of exercise, tensile loads remain small, minimizing the risk of injury. The use of a stationary bike to assist with gaining range is typically started on the second postoperative session. The patient is instructed to begin using half-revolutions, keeping knee movement in a pain-free range. As the patient gains confidence, he or she is instructed to slowly increase the arc or amount of motion. Once full revolutions can be made at a given seat height, the amount of knee flexion can be increased by lowering the seat height.

Joint mobilization techniques are employed for reducing capsular restrictions.[27] Tibial femoral joint mobilization techniques are typically started with the knee in its resting position of approximately 20 degrees of knee flexion; however the amount of knee flexion during mobilization may be modified according to the patient's available ROM. For example, if the patient has only mild capsular restrictions at the end range of flexion, the knee may be placed at 90 degrees of flexion before application of mobilization techniques.

Continuous PROM may be used after ACL reconstruction. As stated earlier, with the ACL allograft ROM gains are made more easily than with ACL autograft, negating the need for PROM machines. However, based on Salter's original work on continuous passive motion (CPM), when there is articular cartilage damage the use of CPM is advocated for the ACL allograft patient.[28]

BOX 11-1

Rehabilitation Guidelines after ACL Allograft—cont'd

At each treatment session, after whichever circuit the patient is performing, the patient also continues with the following:

Hamstring isotonics

Balance activities

Static stretching

Agility activities (dot drills and agility ladder)

Cryotherapy

Clinical Milestones

No effusion

Improved confidence in knee

Hamstring strength equal to uninvolved side

Quadriceps strength 70% of uninvolved side

Full pain-free hyperextension

130 degrees of flexion

No compensation with squat

Ability to jog straight line without compensation

Balance equal to uninvolved side

Phase 7

Typically, after achieving the described milestones the patient is transitioned to an independent home-exercise program. Patients are expected to continue with their circuit training and start a progressive running program. This is continued until 6-12 months after surgery. Patients who will be returning to cutting sports are encouraged to enroll in an ACL injury–prevention program before returning to sports.

Our clinic employs the Sportsmetrics (Cincinnati Sports Medicine Research and Education Foundation, Cincinnati, OH) program, and we have found that patients respond better to the program after completing a progressive running program. This progressive running program and Sportsmetrics program usually occurs at least 6 months after undergoing ACL reconstruction.

Ambulation after Surgery

Depending on the procedure used, complications in surgery, or concurrent surgeries, such as abrasion arthroplasty or meniscal repair, weight bearing after surgery may range from weight bearing as tolerated to non–weight bearing. When to wean the patient from assistive devices should be based both on the surgical procedure and the patient's ability to ambulate without gross gait compensation. Far too often, in a patient's zeal to walk without crutches a poor gait pattern is reinforced, resulting in an excessive limp, a flexed-knee gait pattern, increased knee pain, and joint effusion. The patient whose surgeon allows weight bearing as tolerated should be kept on assistive devices until the ability to walk with a near-normal gait pattern is proven. Patients who can ambulate with minimal compensation but continue to have pain or swelling should resume using assistive devices.

The surgeon should relate the weight-bearing restrictions after ACL surgery. Weight-bearing status is dependent on a multitude of factors. For example, weight bearing after a meniscal repair along with ACL reconstruction can vary from full weight bearing immediately with a knee brace locked at 0 degrees to non–weight bearing for 6 weeks.[29-32] With an ACL allograft without meniscal repair or any other weight bearing–contraindicated procedure, the patient may begin ambulating using toe-touch weight bearing on postoperative day 1. Weight bearing is increased according to the patient's response to treatment. As the patient regains quadriceps motor control, weight bearing is progressed. Typically, by postoperative weeks 3 to 4, the patient is ambulating with full weight bearing without assistive devices.

Modalities after Surgery

Cryotherapy is effective in reducing pain and swelling and is used routinely postoperatively.[33] Commercial cryotherapy units now available have made the use of cryotherapy much simpler. With such systems, cold can be applied continually, without the risk of contaminating the surgical site and without the need to change ice bags frequently. The use of such devices is now common after ACL surgery.

Electrical stimulation for control of pain and edema after ACL reconstruction is used routinely in rehabilitation. If rehabilitation is to begin in the first 24 hours after surgery, electrical stimulation parameters should be different from electrical stimulation later in the rehabilitation course. In the first 24 to 48 hours a high-frequency setting—approximately 80 to 150 Hz with a submotor response—is used so as to not dislodge the platelet plug, which would result in increased swelling.[34] After 24 to 48 hours, a fibrin clot has replaced the platelet plug and the wound site is far more stable. At this time the parameters of electrical stimulation should be changed to a lower frequency with a motor response in order take advantage of the muscle pump.[34,35] Electrical stimulation is also used postoperatively for muscle reeducation of quadriceps muscles. Snyder-Mackler and colleagues reported that improved quadriceps strength was achieved using high-frequency electrical stimulation in conjunction with an aggressive rehabilitation program.[36]

Biofeedback is another modality that may be used during the muscle reeducation phase of rehabilitation. Biofeedback devices give the patient audio and visual feedback describing muscle activity. Depending on the desired goal, biofeedback may be used to encourage muscle contraction or to quiet increased muscle activity, such as to enhance muscle contraction of the quadriceps to restore terminal extension, or may be used in conjunction with low-load prolonged stretching to reducing hamstring spasm.

Rehabilitation Exercises

Both open kinetic and closed kinetic chain exercises are employed during the rehabilitation course. Whenever possible exercises for the ACL allograft patient are started before surgery. During the preoperative phase of the rehabilitation, a patient is instructed on quadriceps-setting exercises and ankle pumps to be started postoperatively. The submaximal isometric contractions of the quadriceps aid the postoperative patient in two ways. First, the exercises help restore quadriceps control and decrease the frequency of quadriceps shutdown. Second, the isometric exercises take advantage of the muscle pump reducing effusion within the joint.[37,38] Ankle pumps aid in venous return and may decrease the risk for deep vein thrombophlebitis.

Quadriceps-setting exercises are continued until the patient has regained quadriceps control. Straight-leg raises are also started early in the rehabilitation phase, typically at the second postoperative visit. It should be noted that the patient must have enough quadriceps control to perform straight-leg raises without greater than a 5- to 10-degree quadriceps lag before initiating this exercise. Hamstring submaximal isometrics are also started in the first week postoperatively. Because the hamstrings provide a posterior shear to the joint, reducing strain on the ACL, there is no risk of stretching the ACL. However, the rehabilitation specialist must be aware of the surgical technique that was employed. For example, in some cases when making the tibial tunnel the surgeon may lift part of the pes anserine. The patient may have increased anterior medial knee pain consistent with a pes anserine bursitis if hamstring exercises are started too early when the surgeon's technique involved lifting the pes anserine.

Hip strengthening. Hip strengthening exercises are started as early as the preoperative phase. The simplest consist of straight-leg raises in supine, prone and side lying. As the patient progresses weights are added proximal to the knee in order to minimize the forces being transmitted through the knee. Commercial equipment such as the multihip or pulleys may be used with the weights or the resistance proximal to the knee (Figures 11-8 to 11-11).

Step-ups. The step-up is used to assist in regaining both concentric and eccentric quadriceps control. Traditionally

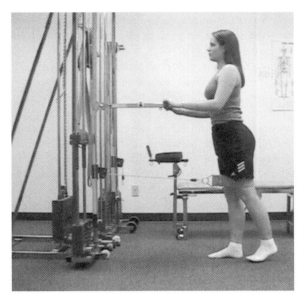

Figure 11-8: Resisted hip extension. Note that the resistance is maintained above the knee.

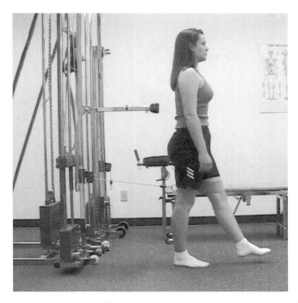

Figure 11-10: Resisted hip flexion. Note that the resistance is maintained above the knee.

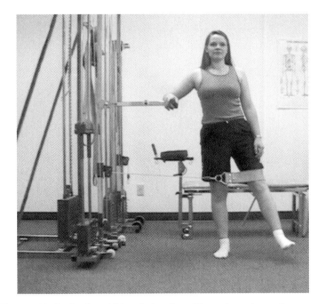

Figure 11-9: Resisted hip abduction. Note that the resistance is maintained above the knee. During the exercise the patient needs to maintain erect posture without leaning to the side.

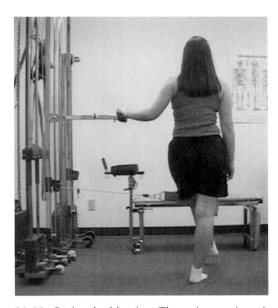

Figure 11-11: Resisted adduction. The resistance is maintained above the knee. During this exercise with this type of equipment, pure adduction is not possible, so slight flexion is added to allow the involved limb to cross the unaffected limb.

step-ups were started only after the patient was able to bear full weight. However, there are now commercially available devices that make it possible to start step-ups before the patient has good quadriceps control. With such devices the patient's weight is unloaded with the assistance of an overhead "lat-pull" pulley system (Figure 11-12). As the patient's quadriceps control improves, the weight is decreased, resulting in an increased load through the knee.

Forward step-ups. With this exercise the patient lifts himself or herself onto a step with the affected limb (Figure 11-13). Once both feet are on the step, the patient can then step to the rear with the affected or unaffected limb. If the unaffected limb remains on the step, there is minimal to no eccentric load placed on the affected limb. However, if the affected limb remains on the step, there will be a greater eccentric load. This exercise can be varied to produce greater

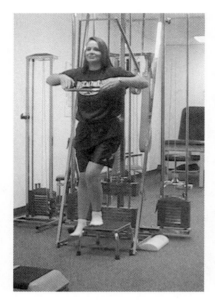

Figure 11-12: Deloaded step-down. With this type of equipment the patient is allowed to step down with only a portion of the body weight. This allows the patient to perform closed-chain exercises even when the quadriceps cannot lift body weight.

eccentric control by placing the affected limb on the step and lowering the unaffected limb to the front, thereby performing a forward step-down.

Side step-ups. If a greater effort of both concentric and eccentric force is desired, side step-ups can be used. This exercise begins with the affected limb placed on the step and the unaffected limb on the floor. The patient is instructed to concentrically lift himself or herself by straightening the affected leg. Once the patient has completed this first maneuver, instructions are to eccentrically lower the unaffected limb to the floor by flexing the affected knee (Figure 11-14). Exercise intensity can be varied by changing the speed of each phase. Intensity can also be increased by not allowing the unaffected foot to bear weight before the next concentric phase is begun.

Wall squats. Once the patient demonstrates good eccentric and concentric control when performing step-ups, the patient may progress to wall squats (Figure 11-15). This exercise is used as a precursor to a traditional squat. The patient is placed with the back against a wall with a ball in the small of the back. The patient is asked to move the feet away from the wall so that during hip and knee flexion, the tibia remains perpendicular to the floor. The intensity of this exercise may be increased by increasing the amount of hip and knee flexion during the eccentric lowering phase of the exercise. Feedback to the patient is required during this exercise to minimize compensation.

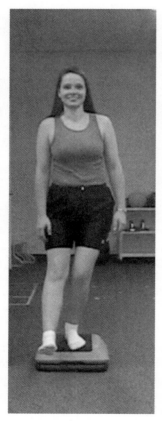

Figure 11-13: Forward step-down. As the patient's unaffected limb is lowered to the ground, the affected limb performs a controlled eccentric contraction.

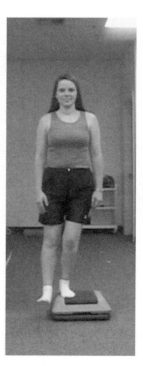

Figure 11-14: Side step-up. The patient stands with the affected limb on the step and the unaffected limb on the ground. The patient then extends the affected knee, thereby lifting the affected limb off the floor. Note the patient should flex and extend the knee, not drop the hip. The hips should remain parallel.

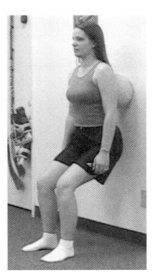

Figure 11-15: Wall squat. When the wall squat is performed, the tibia remains perpendicular to the ground.

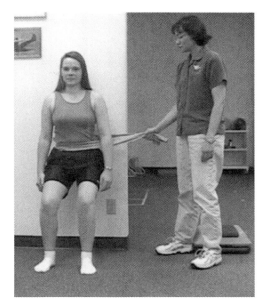

Figure 11-16: Assisted wall squats. When a patient is unable to maintain equal weight on both legs, weight bearing may be increased on the affected side by bringing the patient back to a neutral position.

When viewed from the front, the patient may compensate by shifting weight onto the unaffected limb. The patient should be instructed to eccentrically flex the knees without shifting weight. A mirror may be used to give visual feedback to the patient. Additionally, the use of an assistant to shift the patient back to a neutral position may be helpful (Figure 11-16).

Squats. The squat has been used for years in the areas of strength training and rehabilitation. After ACL surgery this exercise in various forms can be used throughout rehabilitation.[38,39] Squatting may be performed with or without an external load or support. The amount of knee and trunk flexion and cadence can be varied. The execution of the squat has been described in several ways. In one of these the tibia is kept perpendicular to the floor with no ankle movement until the knee is flexed to 90 degrees (Figure 11-17).[38] If this method is used, the arms must be raised to 90 degrees of flexion to serve as a counterbalance. Another method is to lower the body toward the floor until the thigh is parallel to the floor while keeping the trunk erect (Figure 11-18).[39]

As noted previously, another method is to place a ball between the patient's back and a wall, then have the patient step away from the wall so that when the trunk is lowered the patient's knees do not move in front of the patient's feet. The squat is also described in terms of the amount of knee flexion (quarter squat, parallel squat, or full squat). Although the increased tibial femoral compression produced when using the squat is desirable to decrease the amount of sheer forces through the tibial femoral joint, the same compressive forces may provoke pain in patients with articular cartilage damage. With greater knee flexion angles the compressive force of the tibial femoral joint increases.[39,40] By modifying the squat so that the patient is flexing the knee only from 0 to 50 degrees, patellar femoral forces and tibial femoral compressive forces are minimized.[40]

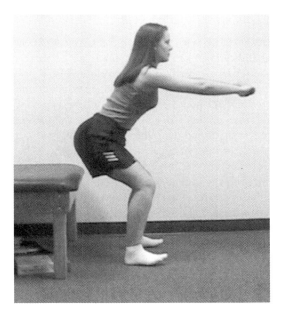

Figure 11-17: Squat method 1. In this exercise the arms are brought parallel to the floor in forward flexion. This allows the patient to maintain the tibia perpendicular to the floor without loosing balance.

The progression of squats used in ACL allograft rehabilitation is as follows:

1. Quarter wall squat with a ball
2. Wall squat parallel with ball
3. Squat with arms flexed and no ankle movement

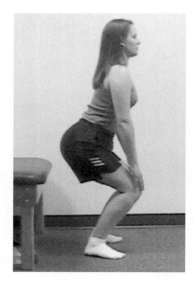

Figure 11-18: Squat method 2. In this exercise the arms are no longer parallel to the ground. The weight is shifted slightly forward as compared with method 1; however, in this method the patient's arms are now free, allowing for the use of external weights.

4. Squat, maintaining erect trunk and without external load

5. Squat with an external load

External loads with the squat are used in the last phase of the rehabilitation. The external load can be in the form of dumbbell, barbell, medicine ball, weighted vest, or any other weighted materials. If space is a concern, medicine balls or weighted collars may be preferred. These types of weights not only take up less space but also allow the patient to "bail out" of the squat and drop the weight if necessary, minimizing the risk of injury to the patient and others. As with other forms of exercise, the intensity of the squat can be increased by increasing the cadence of the exercise. Morrissey and colleagues studied the effects of cadence of the squat on vertical and long jumps, maximal squat lift, and isokinetic strength testing at both slow and fast speeds.[41] The cadences used were one repetition per second or one repetition every 2 seconds. It was shown that those exercising with a faster cadence demonstrated greater strength improvements on both slow and fast isokinetic testing.[41]

Proprioception. Foot placement during weight-bearing activities is so instinctive that it is rarely given thought during the course of a normal day. However, the integrated systems of muscle spindle, joint mechanoreceptors, reflexes, and vestibular function, which normally work seamlessly, may be severely impaired after joint insult. It has been suggested that the nervous system simultaneously processes feedback from the joint, cutaneous receptors, and muscle receptors rather than dealing with each signal separately.[42-44] This instantaneous recognition from several sources allows the body to maintain near-normal response times after an injury even though one of the systems may be slowed.

In the orthopedic and sports community, finding a way to enhance the proprioceptive system has been gaining interest in the past 10 years. There are now many commercially available devices for proprioceptive training, but the basic tenets are still applicable. In order to have adequate balance one needs input from the middle ear, visual cues, and the complex proprioceptive system. It is the least demanding to start balance training with a situation in which all systems are giving input, such as unilateral stance on a firm stationary surface with the eyes open. To make any balancing maneuver more difficult, one can simply challenge any of the proprioceptive systems or decrease the available cues. For example, standing on a trampoline with eyes open is more challenging than standing on a firm surface with eyes open. A second way of increasing the level of difficulty is to have the patient move in the cardinal planes then progress to diagonal patterns. Once the patient has mastered static forms of training, such as balance board or Airex pad (Alusuisse Composites, St. Louis, MO), perturbation training can be started. The progression of proprioception-balance training after ACL allograft is as follows:

1. Unilateral stance, eyes open
2. Unilateral stance, eyes closed
3. Unilateral stance on trampoline, eyes open
4. Unilateral stance on trampoline, eyes closed
5. Unilateral stance, Airex pad, eyes open
6. Unilateral stance, Airex pad, eyes closed
7. Unilateral stance, trampoline, ball toss
8. Unilateral stance, Airex pad, ball toss
9. Agility ladder
10. Agility ladder, ball toss
11. Sport-specific perturbation training

Calf raises. Calf raises are started once full weight bearing is allowed. Calf raises are used to increase the strength of both the gastrocnemius and the soleus. This exercise can be used with or without external weights. The exercise is started with the patient standing on the floor with knees extended. The patient is instructed to lift the heels up as high as possible, then slowly lower (Figure 11-19). Once the patient demonstrates good control with bilateral calf raises, single-leg raises are started with knees extended. Because a higher level of knee control is needed to perform bent-knee calf raises, this exercise is started after the patient has gained good eccentric knee control. As the patient gains control and strength, the addition of a 2-inch by 4-inch piece of wood or a half roll of foam may be used to increase the excursion of motion during both straight- and bent-knee calf raises.

Lunges. The lunge maneuver may be used as both a stretching and a strengthening move. The forward lunge can be broken down into the beginning phase, forward movement phase, backward movement phase, and end position.[45]

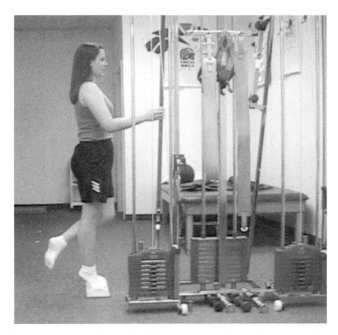

Figure 11-19: Unilateral calf raises. Note the patient using her arm for balance. Although the patient may need assistance for balance, the therapist needs to ensure the patient is not using the arm to help lift his or her body weight.

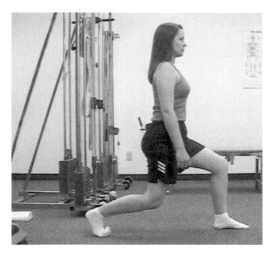

Figure 11-20: Forward lunge. The patient maintains an erect trunk while the forward limb is kept perpendicular to the ground.

- *Beginning phase:* Patient stands erect with the feet approximately shoulder width apart. While the lunge is performed, there are many positions in which a weight can be held, including on the chest, at the shoulders, or behind the neck. If weights are to be used, a spotter is beneficial to ensure that the patient's hips are under the external load before the next phase is begun.

- *Forward movement phase:* This phase begins with the patient taking an exaggerated step directly forward. The lead leg should be placed squarely on the floor with the toes pointing forward. The lead knee is slowly flexed while the trailing knee is lowered to the floor. The weight is maintained over the hips, and the torso remains perpendicular to the floor. To accomplish this the patient "sits back" on the trailing leg. This phase ends when the trailing knee is 1 to 2 inches off the floor and the lead tibia is perpendicular to the floor.

- *Backward movement phase:* This phase begins immediately after the conclusion of the forward movement phase. The patient forcefully pushes off the lead leg while simultaneously extending the trailing knee. The weight is maintained over the hips. This phase ends when the feet return to the starting position.

- *End position:* When the patient's lead leg returns to the starting position, there is a pause until the patient leads with the other leg. At this time the weight is shifted to the new trailing leg. Again, the weight needs to remain over the hips and the trunk should remain erect (Figure 11-20).

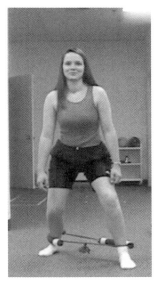

Figure 11-21: Monster walks. Note that tension is maintained in the resistive band throughout the exercise.

Monster walks. Monster walks are a form of resisted walking. Resistive bands are placed around the ankles, and the patient is instructed to achieve a good athletic stance (slight hip and knee flexion with feet at least shoulder width apart). The patient then walks forward while maintaining the wide base of support (Figure 11-21). Changing the stiffness of the band, distance walked, or walking speed can vary the intensity of the exercise. This exercise can be performed walking forward or backward.

High step-ups. Although this form of step-up is performed in the same manner as the forward or side step-up, it is mentioned separately because of its place in the rehabilitation progression. A high step is classified as a step of a height at which the knee and hip need to be flexed to 90 degrees in order for the foot to be placed on the platform (Figure 11-22). The high step-up is performed slowly both concentrically and eccentrically. In order to properly perform this exercise the patient must have good knee, hip, and core strength. For this reason the high step-up is introduced in the later strengthening phase of rehabilitation.

Hamstring strengthening. Restoring hamstring strength after ACL reconstruction is essential if the hamstrings are to be dynamic stabilizers. However, as mentioned earlier, if the surgical technique used has invaded the pes anserine, hamstring strengthening is delayed until postoperative week 5 in order to allow soft tissue healing. Postoperative hamstring strengthening is started with submaximal isometrics. As the patient's motor response improves, standing submaximal isotonic hamstring curls are started. Weights are added as the patient's strength improves. Later other equipment with greater resistance may be employed. In our clinic pulley exercises with the patient in the prone position are used. Hamstring strength should be fully restored before the patient is permitted to run.

Agility activities. Being able to move quickly and precisely is a necessary component if one is to return to sports. As stated earlier in the proprioception section, integrating the vestibular system, mechanoreceptors, and motor control is complex. After ACL reconstruction, basic everyday tasks such as walking can be difficult. To help regain proprioception and limb control, the speed of exercises may be changed throughout the rehabilitation program. For example, as soon as the patient can ambulate without assistive devices, the speed of gait is altered in the clinic to enhance body awareness. Dot drills are started as soon as the patient is released

to full weight bearing without assistive devices. In the early phase of this exercise it is accuracy, not speed, that is emphasized.

Dot drills allow the patient to receive visual feedback as to foot placement (Figure 11-23). Dot drills employ a variety of foot patterns and speeds. In later phases of rehabilitation and in sport-specific drills, jumping or single leg techniques are used. However, during early phases of the ACL rehabilitation, the goal is to increase proprioception while minimizing the joint reaction forces, so speed is started at walking pace and a stepping motion is used. For this drill, five marks or dots are placed on the floor. As seen in the diagram, the first two dots *(1 and 2)* are placed approximately 20 inches apart. A center dot *(3)* is placed 10 to 15 inches above the first two. Then two more dots *(4 and 5)* are placed 10 to 15 inches above the center dot. The patient starts by placing the left foot on dot 1 and the right foot on dot 2. Then the patient steps forward with the left foot to the center number 3 dot. The patient then places the right foot on the top right dot number 5. Then the patient places the left foot in the top left dot number 4 and the right foot in the center dot number 3. The patient continues by placing the left foot on the bottom left dot number 1 and the right foot on the bottom right dot number 2. Speed is increased as the patient's balance and body awareness allow. The order in which the first foot strikes the center dot is also changed during the drill.

Agility ladder drills are the next agility exercise used. In such drills a variety of foot sequences are used in conjunction with a cloth ladder placed on the floor. This exercise requires the patient to move in a variety of planes. Proper foot placement is emphasized throughout the exercise. As the patient progresses, the speed of the foot drills is increased. The patient is instructed to perform the assigned drill as fast as possible while maintaining proper foot placement and good balance (Figure 11-24). The therapist watches for any signs of loss of balance, difficulty with maintaining the sequence and drill rhythm, or performance of the drill at a speed that

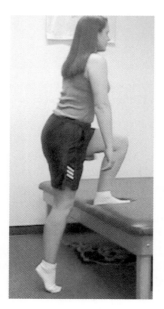

Figure 11-22: High step-ups. Note starting position, with the hip and knee in approximately 90 degrees of flexion.

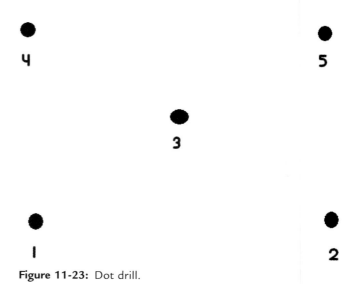

Figure 11-23: Dot drill.

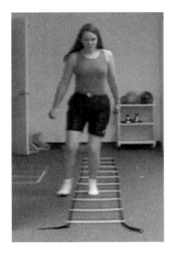

Figure 11-24: Agility ladder. With this exercise the patient performs the drill as fast as possible while maintaining balance and form.

is not challenging. The optimal drill is one performed at the patient's maximal speed with maintenance of balance throughout the drill, and with proper foot placements and sequence. Later in the progression the therapist can have the patient perform the drills while a ball is tossed between therapist and patient. The patterns used can be varied according to the patient's ability and specific sport.

RETURN TO ACTIVITY

When the patient has met all of the following rehabilitation milestones, he or she is started on a straight-line running program:

1. Improved confidence in knee
2. Hamstring strength equal to uninvolved side
3. Quadriceps strength 70% of uninvolved side
4. Full pain-free knee hyperextension
5. 130 degrees of knee flexion
6. No compensation with squat
7. Ability to jog in a straight line without compensation
8. Balance equal to uninvolved side

The patient is instructed on a progressive running program starting with a half-mile jog three times per week, increasing the distance and speed only after having run at one speed and distance for at least 2 weeks without signs of knee pain or swelling. The running program is continued, and low-demand cutting activities are started for the next 2 months. The time for this phase is quite varied and dependent on the individual. Strength and joint stability guide the rehabilitation progression from 3 month postoperatively until the patient is released to full sporting activity. Isokinetic strength testing using concentric-concentric contraction at 60 and 120 degrees/second is performed at 3, 6, and 12 months postop-

eratively. Goals for the 3-month test are hamstring strength equal to the unaffected side and affected quadriceps at 70% of unaffected side. At the 6-month test quadriceps strength should be 80% or higher, and at 12 months within 10% of the uninvolved side. Full release to sports after ACL surgery is usually accomplished by 6 to 12 months after surgery.

SUMMARY

Although the role of the primary ACL allograft reconstruction remains controversial, suggested indications for the use of allograft include the complex injured knee, ACL revision, patients older than 45 years of age, and skeletally immature patients. The major complication of disease transmission is quite low. The postoperative course is fairly straightforward. As can be seen in Box 11-1, the rehabilitation progression is divided into seven phases including a preoperative phase. The postoperative phase begins on postoperative day 2 and continues for 3 months, transitioning from a protective and healing emphasis to a motion and proprioceptive period, a strength period, and a running phase. The overall progression mirrors that of the ACL reconstruction with autograft. The major difference one encounters when rehabilitating the patient with an allograft is that ROM and motor function return more quickly. This rapid return allows the patient to increase activity at an advanced rate. Although this decreases the incidence of joint contracture, the rehabilitation professional needs to be aware that the graft may overstretch secondary to the time needed for complete graft incorporation.

References

1. American Academy of Orthopaedic Surgeons (AAOS): *ACL Reconstruction,* AAOS Bulletin, Feb 2004.
2. Centers for Disease Control and Prevention (CDC): Invasive *Streptococcus pyogenes* after allograft implantation—Colorado, 2003. *MMWR Morb Mortal Wkly Rep* 52:1173-1176, 2003.
3. Vangsness, CT: *Overview of allograft soft tissue processing,* AAOS Bulletin, Feb 2004.
4. Jackson, DW, Windler, GE, Simon TM: Intraarticular reaction associated with the use of freeze-dried, ethylene oxide–sterilized bone-patella-tendon-bone allografts in the reconstruction of the anterior cruciate ligament, *Am J Sports Med* 18(1):1-10, 1990.
5. Nikolaou PK, Seaber AV, Glisson RR, et al: Anterior cruciate ligament allograft transplantation. Long-term function, histology, revascularization, and operative technique, *Am J Sports Med* 14: 348-360, 1986.
6. Centers for Disease Control and Prevention (CDC). CDC update: allograft-associated bacterial infections—United States, 2002, *MMWR Morb Mortal Wkly Rep* 51:207-210, 2002.
7. Mellonig JT, Prewett AB, Moyer MP: HIV inactivation in a bone allograft, *J Periodontol* 63:979-983, 1992.
8. Siebold R, Buelow JU, Bos L, Ellerman A.: Primary ACL reconstruction with fresh-frozen patellar versus Achilles tendon allografts, *Arch Orthop Trauma Surg* 123:180-185, 2003.
9. Siebold R, Buelow JU, Boes L, Ellermann A: Primary- and revision-reconstruction of the anterior cruciate ligament with

allografts: a retrospective study including 325 patients, *Zentralbl Chir* 127:850-854, 2002.

10. Gorschewsy O, Browa A, Vogel U, Stauffer E: Clinico-histologic comparison of allogenic and autologous bone tendon-bone using one-third of the patellar tendon in reconstruction of the anterior cruciate ligament, *Unfallchirurg* 105:703-714, 2002.

11. Noyes FR, Barber-Westin SD: Reconstruction of the anterior cruciate ligament with human allograft: comparison of early and later results, *J Bone Joint Surg* 78A:524-537, 1996.

12. Shelton WR, Papendick L, Dukes AD: Autograft versus allograft anterior cruciate ligament reconstruction, *Arthroscopy* 13: 446-449, 1997.

13. Chang SK, Egami DK, Shaieb MD, et al: Anterior cruciate ligament reconstruction: allograft versus autograft, *Arthroscopy* 19: 453-462, 2003.

14. Shino K, Nakata K, Horibe S, et al: Quantitative evaluation after arthroscopic anterior cruciate ligament reconstruction: allograft versus autograft, *Am J Sports Med* 21:609-616, 1993.

15. Lawhorn KW, Howell SM: Scientific justification and technique for anterior cruciate ligament reconstruction using autogenous and allogeneic soft-tissue grafts, *Orthop Clin North Am* 34:19-30, 2003.

16. Stickland SM, MacGillivray JD, Warren RF: Anterior cruciate ligament reconstructions with allograft tendons, *Orthop Clin North Am* 34:41-47, 2003.

17. Miller SL, Gladstone JN: Graft selection in anterior cruciate ligament reconstruction, *Orthop Clin North Am* 33:675-683, 2002.

18. Fuch R, Wheatley W, Uribe JW, et al: Intra-articular anterior cruciate ligament reconstruction using patellar tendon allograft in the skeletally immature patient, *Arthroscopy* 18:824-828, 2002.

19. Bettany JA, Fish DR, Mendel FC: Influence of high voltage pulsed direct current in edema formation following impact injury, *Phys Ther* 70:219-224, 1990.

20. Hopkins JT, Ingersoll CD, Edwards J, et al: Cryotherapy and transcutaneous electric neuromuscular stimulation decrease arthrogenic muscle inhibition of the vastus medialis after knee joint effusion, *J Athl Train* 37:25-31, 2001.

21. Noyes FR, Berrios-Torres S, Barber-Westin SD, et al: Prevention of permanent arthrofibrosis after anterior cruciate ligament reconstruction alone or combined with associated procedures: a prospective study in 443 knees, *Knee Surg Sports Traumatol Arthrosc* 8: 196-206, 2000.

22. Wilk KE, Arrigo C, Andrews JR, et al: Rehabilitation after anterior cruciate ligament reconstruction in the female athlete, *J Athl Train* 34:177-193, 1999.

23. Shelbourne KD, Nitz P: Accelerated rehabilitation after anterior cruciate ligament reconstruction, *Am J Sports Med* 18:292-299, 1990.

24. Warren CG, Lehman JF, Koblanski NJ: Elongation of rat tail tendon: effects of load and temperature, *Arch Phys Med Rehabil* 52:465, 1971.

25. Warren CG, Lehman JF, Koblanski NJ: Heat and stretch technique: an evaluation using rat tail tendon, *Arch Phys Med Rehabil* 57:122, 1976.

26. Faugli HP, editor: *Medical exercise therapy*, Abildsø N-Oslo, Lærergruppen for Medisinsk Treningsterapi AS, 1996.

27. Dutton M: *Orthopaedic examination, evaluation, and intervention*, New York, McGraw-Hill, 2004.

28. Salter RB: *Textbook of disorders and injuries of the musculoskeletal system*, Baltimore, Williams and Wilkins, 1983.

29. DeLee JC, Drez Jr D, editors: *Orthopaedic sports medicine: principles and practice*, vol 2, Philadelphia, 1994, Saunders.

30. Brotzman SB, editor: *Clinical orthopaedic rehabilitation*, St. Louis, 1996, Mosby.

31. Fritz JM, Irrgang JJ, Harner CD: Rehabilitation following allograft meniscal transplantation: a review of the literature and case study, *J Sports Phys Ther* 24:98-106, 1996.

32. Gray JC: Neural and vascular anatomy of the menisci of the human knee, *J Sports Phys Ther* 29:23-30, 1999.

33. Lessard LA, Scudds RA, Amendola A, et al: The efficacy of cryotherapy following arthroscopic knee surgery, *J Sports Phys Ther* 26:14-22, 1997.

34. Prentice WE: *Therapeutic modalities for physical therapists*, ed 2, New York, 2002, McGraw-Hill.

35. Nelson RM, Currier DP, editors: *Clinical electrotherapy*, ed 2, East Norwalk, 1991, Appleton & Lange.

36. Snyder-Mackler L, Delitto A, Stralka SW, et al: Use of electrical stimulation to enhance recovery of quadriceps femoris muscle force production in patients following anterior cruciate ligament reconstruction, *Phys Ther* 74:901-907, 1994.

37. Fitzgerald GK: Open versus closed kinetic chain exercise: issues in rehabilitation after anterior cruciate ligament reconstructive surgery, *Phys Ther* 77:1747-1754, 1997.

38. Yack HJ, Collins CE, Whieldon TJ: Comparison of closed and open kinetic chain exercise in the anterior cruciate ligament–deficient knee, *Am J Sports Med* 21:49-54, 1993.

39. Hattin HC, Pierrynowski MR, Ball KA: Effect of load, cadence, and fatigue on tibiofemoral joint force during a half squat, *Med Sci Sports Exerc* 21:613-618, 1989.

40. Escamilla RF, Fleisig GS, Zheng N, et al: Biomechanics of the knee during closed kinetic chain and open kinetic chain exercises, *Med Sci Sports Exerc* 30:556-569, 1998.

41. Morrissey MC, Harman EA, Frykman PN, et al: Early phase differential effects of slow and fast barbell squat training, *Am J Sports Med* 36:221-230, 1998.

42. Williams GN, Chmielewski T, Rudolph KS, et al: Dynamic knee stability: current theory and implications for clinicians and scientists, *J Orthop Sports Phys Ther* 10:546-566, 2001.

43. Fridén T, Roberts D, Ageberg E, et al: Review of knee proprioception and the relation to extremity function after an anterior cruciate ligament rupture, *J Orthop Sports Phys Ther* 10:567-576, 2001.

44. Tyler TF, McHugh MP: Neuromuscular rehabilitation of a female Olympic ice hockey player following anterior cruciate ligament reconstruction, *J Orthop Sports Phys Ther* 10:577-587, 2001.

45. Baechle TR, editor: *Essentials of strength training and conditioning*, Champaign, 1994, National Strength and Conditioning Association.

CHAPTER 12

Complications in Anterior Cruciate Ligament Reconstruction

Robert C. Manske, DPT, MPT, MEd, MPT, SCS, ATC, CSCS
Charles E. Giangarra, MD
Kimberly A. Turman, MD
Bryan C. Heiderscheit, PhD, PT

ANTERIOR CRUCIATE LIGAMENT (ACL)

reconstruction has become an increasingly common procedure encountered in orthopedic surgery and sports medicine. It is estimated that approximately 100,000 ACL reconstructions were performed in 1997, with an incidence of 1 in 3000 persons in the general population.[1] As athletics continues to become more competitive and the general population strives to become more active and physically fit, the incidence of ACL injuries will undoubtedly continue to increase. Therefore improvements in both surgical and rehabilitative aspects of care need to occur to minimize the complications that develop all too frequently.

The technical aspects of ACL surgery have evolved since the early 1900s, with the first attempts at ACL reconstruction performed by Hey Groves in 1917 using a strip of fascia lata.[2] Surgical technique and graft options have continued to evolve since that time, as indicated by long-term success rates of good to excellent currently being achieved in 75% to 90% of primary cases. In comparison, equivalent results are achieved in only 50% to 70% of ACL revisions.[1] It is therefore vital to obtain success with the primary surgical procedure and initial rehabilitation period, thereby avoiding the need for revision.

As with any surgical procedure, complications may arise both intraoperatively and in the postoperative period. Surgical pitfalls may be grouped into several distinct categories including graft harvest, notch preparation, tunnel placement, and graft tensioning and fixation. Intraoperative technical errors are reported as the cause of failure in 77% to 95% of revision ACL cases,[3] with close attention to surgical detail being imperative to prevent these potential technical errors. During the postoperative rehabilitation period, frequent complications involve the loss of knee motion, donor-site morbidity, and anterior knee pain, with the occasional development of complex regional pain syndrome (CRPS), infection, and deep vein thrombosis (DVT) also creating difficulties. Alternative options must also exist within the clinician's arsenal in the event of intraoperative or rehabilitation complications. Familiarity with these options will allow successful outcomes in spite of such complications.

PREOPERATIVE CONSIDERATIONS

Graft Selection

Before surgical technique and pitfalls can be considered, one must first address the issue of graft selection. Various grafts have been used over the course of time, and selection should be individualized to optimize the outcome for each patient. The bone-patella-tendon-bone (BPTB) construct is currently considered the gold standard. Use of the hamstrings (semitendinosus and gracilis) as a quadruple loop autograft is also increasing in popularity. Each of these two grafts is most commonly taken from the ipsilateral extremity but may also be harvested from the contralateral side. The third option commonly used in current practice is allograft. Each

of these graft options has unique characteristics and indications and will be briefly discussed. A final graft option is the quadriceps tendon. This graft is less commonly employed and therefore will not be discussed further; however, its availability should not be forgotten.

BPTB autografts consist of the central third patellar tendon with a bone plug on both ends—the distal pole of the patella and the tibial tubercle. Advantages of this graft include its inherent strength and the benefit of bone-to-bone healing. The initial strength of BPTB grafts is comparable to the native ACL.[4] Healing of the bone plugs within the femoral and tibial tunnels results in quicker biologic incorporation in comparison to soft tissue healing to bone. This biologic incorporation determines the ultimate fixation strength of ACL reconstructions and has important implications for the rehabilitation period. Potential disadvantages of BPTB grafts include anterior knee pain and quadriceps weakness. Less commonly reported disadvantages include patellar tendon rupture, patellar fracture, patellar tendonitis, and paresthesia secondary to interruption of the infrapatellar branch of the saphenous nerve during graft harvest. These complications are discussed in greater detail later in this chapter.

Hamstring autografts, as noted, typically use the semitendinosus and gracilis tendons (STG). When the tendons are looped on themselves to form a quadruple loop construct, the strength and stiffness are greater than those of the native ACL,[5] and strength is greater than that of BPTB constructs.[6] This graft is being used more and more commonly, as it has the benefit of decreased donor site morbidity and preservation of the extensor mechanism. Donor site discomfort rarely persists beyond 3 months. An area of numbness from the medial calf to the medial malleolus may persist secondary to interruption of the saphenous nerve during dissection for graft harvest. Hamstring weakness is minimal, with function returning to normal with proper rehabilitation.[7] Hamstring grafts do, however, require the healing of soft tissue within bone tunnels. There has been a reported 18% decrease in the percentage of patients returning to preinjury level of activity with this graft as compared with BPTB.[5,8]

Allografts may also be used in certain circumstances and have the advantage of no donor site morbidity and decreased surgical time. The premiere drawback, however, is the possibility of disease transmission. Other potential disadvantages include slower incorporation, cost, availability, and potential for immune reactions and infection. Allograft options include fascia lata, tibialis anterior, BPTB, and Achilles grafts.

Based on these many considerations, each graft has created its own niche for use. For the high-demand athlete or younger individual, the BPTB graft is often used. Historically, the STG graft has been more commonly used for the lower demand or older athlete, but recently, due to improved soft tissue fixation, this graft has been used for increasingly active patient populations. This graft is also better for patients with preexisting patellofemoral pain or pathology (patella alta or baja, previous surgery or trauma to the extensor mechanism) and for the skeletally immature patient. Allografts are typically used in older individuals, in those who fully understand the risks and benefits, and for multiligament knee injuries.

OVERVIEW OF SURGICAL PROCEDURE

The surgical technique of ACL reconstruction can be broken down into several basic steps. The first step involves graft harvest and preparation. This is followed by diagnostic arthroscopy. During this part of the procedure any additionally identified intraarticular pathology should be addressed and may include chondroplasty as well as meniscal repair versus partial meniscectomy. Next, the intercondylar notch is carefully explored and the femoral and tibial stumps of the ACL debrided. Care must be used to protect the posterior cruciate ligament (PCL). A notchplasty is also performed at this point to aid in visualization and later acts to protect the graft against impingement. Tunnel placement is then determined, and the tibial and femoral tunnels are sequentially drilled. The prepared graft is then passed within the tunnels and its position verified. Finally, the graft is tensioned and fixed. Each of these steps may be complicated by potential pitfalls and technical errors.

Graft Harvest

Patellar Tendon

Patellar tendon autografts are harvested through a longitudinal incision just medial of midline from the inferior pole of the patella to the tibial tubercle. The central third (approximately 10 mm) of the tendon is incised, and 2 to 2.5 cm bone plugs are created on either end. The patellar defect is later bone grafted.

Potential complications are numerous. As noted, the goal is to obtain a 10 mm graft. If the patellar tendon is too narrow (<25 mm), the residual tendon is significantly weakened and there is increased risk of tendon rupture. Most tendon ruptures occur distally and must be repaired. Inadequate bone plug size and bone plug fracture are also possible and result in the need for alternate fixation or augmentation of fixation. Whereas patellar fractures are more commonly encountered in the postoperative period, they may occur intraoperatively as well during proximal bone plug harvest. Bone grafting the patella defect decreases the incidence of later fractures. If fracture does occur, open reduction and internal fixation are performed.

Hamstring

Hamstring autografts are typically harvested through a longitudinal incision located 2 cm medial to the tibial tubercle and 2 cm distal to the medial joint line. The semitendinosus and gracilis tendons are then exposed and isolated. The distal insertions may be detached before or after proximal harvest.

The primary and perhaps most dreaded complication is premature transection of the tendons secondary to fascial bands that divert the tendon stripper and lead to a truncated graft. To prevent this error, careful dissection and isolation of the tendons is imperative before harvesting. To maximize length obtained, the distal aspect should be detached at the tendons' periosteal insertions. A good harvest should yield approximately 25 to 30 cm of tendon. If the graft remains of inadequate length (<18 cm) or width, alternate graft options must be considered. Lastly, care must also be taken to protect the medial collateral ligament (MCL) during hamstring graft exposure and harvest. The MCL lies deep to the semitendinosus and gracilis tendons.

The potential for saphenous nerve damage exists with either graft harvest. The saphenous nerve passes superficial to the gracilis at the posteromedial joint line. As mentioned previously, damage may result in paresthesias as well as CRPS. Placing the extremity in the figure-of-four position during dissection decreases risk of damage. The infrapatellar branch of the saphenous nerve is often disrupted with BPTB autograft harvest and also results in a local area of paresthesia.

One final complication of either graft is graft contamination (e.g., dropped graft). In case of this unfortunate situation, an alternate graft must be available for use. Sterilization procedures have been shown to be ineffective, with positive culture results in up to 30% of grafts after sterilization attempts.[3,9]

Notch Preparation and Tunnel Placement

Proper tunnel placement is crucial in recreating the biomechanics and function of the native ACL. Nonanatomic tunnels are reported as a major reason for failure in ACL reconstructions, accounting for up to 70% to 80% of failures.[3] Improper placement leads to instability, difficulties with range of motion, and early graft failure secondary to impingement or abnormal tension. Femoral tunnel placement is considered more important biomechanically as the femoral tunnel is closer to the center of axis of knee motion. One of the primary causes of improper tunnel placement is inadequate visualization. Notchplasty is therefore vital in most cases to improve visualization and help ensure appropriate tunnel placement.

Notchplasty

Not only does notchplasty improve visualization, but it also helps protect the graft from impingement. The notch should be examined with the knee in flexion to evaluate the posterior wall and in extension to evaluate the roof and assess for possible impingement. The lateral wall can also lead to graft abrasion with knee motion and should therefore be contoured.

One of the most common places for improper femoral tunnel placement involves the so-called "resident's ridge," located anterior to the femoral attachment of the ACL at the midportion of the roof of the lateral femoral condyle. Failure to address this area leads to anterior placement of the tunnel. Care must also be taken, however, to avoid removing excessive bone from the femoral attachment site such that abnormal knee kinematics result. Attention is therefore concentrated on the anterior and superior surfaces.

Notchplasty must be performed in a controlled manner to avoid damage to other structures around the knee. The primary concern is damage to the PCL caused by careless use of the shaver. Other structures to be mindful of include the transverse meniscal ligament, ligament of Humphrey, and articular cartilage.

Tibial Tunnel

The tibial tunnel is ideally placed at the posteromedial insertion of the ACL stump. After debridement of the ACL stump, the footprint of the native ACL is identified anteromedial to the tibial spine (Figure 12-1, *A1*). Finding landmarks for tibial tunnel placement also includes identifying the intersection of the posterior border of the anterior horn of the lateral meniscus and the ACL stump, approximately 7 mm anterior to the PCL. If the tibial tunnel is placed too far anterior, it results in graft impingement in extension and increased graft tension in flexion (see Figure 12-1, *A2* and *B2*, and Figure 12-2, *B*). Placing the tunnel posterior results in impingement on the PCL, increased graft tension in

extension, and laxity in flexion (see Figure 12-2, *A*). Excessive medial or lateral placement is also problematic and leads to graft abrasion or impingement. Proper placement of the tibial tunnel is also important because it dictates to a large degree femoral tunnel placement.

Femoral Tunnel

The femoral tunnel is ideally placed within 1 to 2 mm of the posterior intercondylar wall at the 10:30 to 11 o'clock position for the right knee and 1 o'clock to 1:30 position for the left knee. The most common error in femoral tunnel placement is placing the tunnel too far anterior, often as a result of inadequate notchplasty and debridement of resident's ridge (Figure 12-3, *A*). In this position there is an increased intraarticular distance between the two tunnels with flexion that results in loss of flexion or stretching and failure of the graft with flexion. In extension, there is impingement of the graft against the roof of the notch and the graft may be lax. If the tunnel is too far posterior, the graft will be lax in flexion and taut in extension with resultant loss of terminal extension (see Figure 12-3, *B*). With posterior placement there is also the risk of posterior wall blowout. For interference screw fixation to function properly, there must be 1 to 2 mm of posterior wall present. Breaching the posterior wall during drilling of the femoral tunnel requires use of alternate fixation. Finally, a femoral tunnel placed at the 12 o'clock position results in a vertical graft and persistent rotational

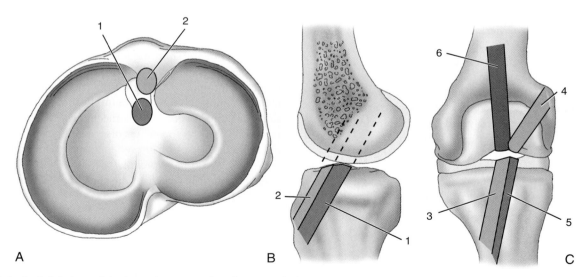

Figure 12-1: A, Axial view of the knee demonstrating the normal "footprint" of the tibial insertion of the anterior cruciate ligament and the optimal position of the tibial tunnel (1). Anterior tunnel placement (2) leads to anterior impingement on the roof of the intercondylar notch. **B,** Lateral view demonstrates ideal tibial tunnel placement (1) in the second quartile of the tibia as measured from anterior to posterior, with the graft lying posterior to the roof of the femoral notch *(arrow)*. Anterior tunnel placement (2) leads to impingement on the roof of the intercondylar notch. **C,** Anteroposterior view of the left knee demonstrates the ideal placement of the tibial tunnel (3) and the femoral tunnel (4). Lateral tunnel placement (5) can lead to impingement on the lateral condyle. Vertical femoral tunnel placement (6) leads to poor rotational control and recurrent instability. *(From Petsche TS, Hutchinson MR: Loss of extension after reconstruction of the anterior cruciate ligament, J Am Acad Orthop Surg 7:119-127, 1999.)*

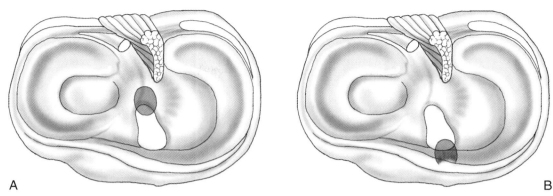

Figure 12-2: Improper tibial tunnel placement. **A,** Posterior tibial tunnel placement resulting in impingement on the PCL, with increased graft tension in knee extension or laxity in knee flexion. **B,** Anterior tibial tunnel placement resulting in graft impingement in full extension, excessive graft tension in flexion, or anterior tibial tunnel breakout. *(From Cain EL, Gillogly SD, Andrews JR: Management of intraoperative complications associated with autogenous patellar tendon graft anterior cruciate ligament reconstruction, AAOS Instructional Course Lectures, 52:359-367, 2003.)*

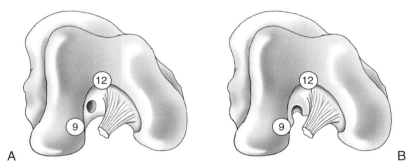

Figure 12-3: Improper femoral tunnel position. **A,** Anterior femoral tunnel placement. **B,** Posterior femoral tunnel placement and posterior wall blowout. The numbers 9 and 12 denote the 9 o'clock and 12 o'clock positions. *(From Cain EL, Gillogly SD, Andrews JR: Management of intraoperative complications associated with autogenous patellar tendon graft anterior cruciate ligament reconstruction, AAOS Instructional Course Lectures 52:359-367, 2003.)*

instability. Although anterior-posterior stability is achieved, rotational instability leads to a persistent pivot shift on examination.

Techniques for avoiding these pitfalls include performing an adequate notchplasty to improve visualization, using femoral guides, avoiding resident's ridge, and checking the back wall during femoral drilling to avoid blowout. The two-incision technique is a good salvage procedure for improper femoral tunnel placement, and a rear entry guide should always be available. Some surgeons may also prefer to use the two-incision technique on a routine basis. Advantages of this technique include consistent femoral tunnel placement; elimination of the potential for posterior wall blowout, graft-tunnel mismatch, and screw divergence; and the fact that the angle of the graft is purportedly more anatomic.[10]

Graft Tensioning and Fixation

Once proper tunnel placement is achieved and the graft is prepared, the graft is passed within the tunnels and subsequently tensioned and securely fixed. Studies have shown that the weakest link in the early postoperative period (6 to 8 weeks) is the fixation sites and not the graft itself.[11] With the trend towards early range of motion and weight bearing in postoperative rehabilitation, there are increased demands on initial fixation of the graft. The ultimate goal is biologic incorporation of the graft to the host, which has been shown to occur at 6 to 12 weeks postoperatively.[1] Once biologic incorporation has occurred, the graft itself becomes the weaker link. Graft tensioning and fixation are therefore of utmost importance in the early rehabilitation period.

Graft Tensioning

Proper tensioning of the graft is an important step in the ultimate success of ACL reconstructions. Undertensioning of the graft results in continued instability. Overtensioning leads to decreased range of motion and potential for articular degeneration secondary to altered joint mechanics. After femoral fixation, the graft should be cycled multiple times through full range of motion to optimize tension and strength within the graft. The tibial side is then fixed with the knee in 10 to 30 degrees of flexion. After fixation is completed, the knee is reexamined. If persistent laxity is noted within the graft, tibial fixation may be revised with the knee in increased flexion. If the graft is overtensioned with decreased range of motion, tibial fixation may be revised with the knee in full extension. If poor motion and an overconstrained graft persist despite these measures, improper tunnel placement should be considered.

Graft Fixation

Multiple fixation options are available for ACL reconstructions and include interference screws, Endo-Buttons, staples, cross-pins, washers, and suture posts. It is generally accepted that the tibial side of fixation is weaker than femoral fixation.[11] Interference screws are considered the gold standard for fixation in BPTB grafts. Typically, 7 and 9 mm screws are used for femoral and tibial fixation, respectively. This form of fixation is believed to be the strongest option available and is therefore used whenever possible. A number of potential pitfalls exist with the use of interference screws and include suture or guidewire failure, eccentric graft placement or malrotation, divergent screw placement, excessive or inadequate screw advancement, and graft injury. Screw divergence of 15 degrees or more leads to failure with loose fixation or graft laceration.[1] The ultimate strength of interference screw fixation is based on bone quality, gap distance between the screw and bone, and screw divergence. Poor fixation may be remedied with use of larger screw fixation, stacking screws, or alternate means of fixation such as Endo-Button on the femoral side and supplementing with post and washer on the tibial side. Posterior wall blowout also requires alternate femoral fixation as discussed previously.

Another commonly encountered difficulty with BPTB graft fixation is graft-tunnel mismatch. The incidence of graft-tunnel mismatch is reported to be as high as 26%.[12] If the graft is too short, the femoral side is fixed normally with an interference screw and an alternate method of fixation is used for the tibial side—for example, stacking of screws or suture posts. If the graft is too long, the femoral side is once again fixed in the traditional fashion. The tibial bone plug, however, protrudes from the tibial tunnel and therefore poses a dilemma for tibial fixation. Multiple options are available and include changing the angle and starting point of the tibial tunnel to lengthen the tunnel, insetting the femoral bone plug up to 5 to 10 mm within the femoral tunnel, flipping the bone plug on itself to effectively shorten the graft, or making a trough along the tibia and fixing the graft with a staple. An additional solution that has been recently studied is graft rotation.[12] The amount of graft shortening is proportional to the degree of graft rotation, with 540° degrees leading to an approximate 10% or 5 mm of shortening.

More variability exists in hamstring graft fixation. Initial fixation is paramount, as biologic incorporation of the graft is believed to be slower secondary to the need for soft tissue healing within bone. Some believe this may necessitate less aggressive rehabilitation in the early postoperative period. As with BPTB grafts, tibial fixation is considered the weaker side. Options for femoral fixation include Endo-Button and cross-pin techniques with interference screw fixation less reliable as compared to BPTB fixation. Tibial fixation may be achieved via multiple methods, based on surgeon preference. Use of a compaction dilator may prevent problems with bone quality or tunnel expansion. It is important to apply equal tension to all four limbs of the hamstring graft during fixation to maximize graft strength. Poor femoral or tibial fixation may be augmented as BPTB grafts are, with the use of larger screws, stacking screws, tying over post with screw, and staples.

After surgery a host of complications can occur in the postoperative period. These rehabilitation dilemmas can include loss of motion because of arthrofibrosis, cyclops lesions, and infrapatellar contracture syndrome. Other postoperative pitfalls include anterior knee pain, CRPS, knee infection, DVT, and problems related to workers' compensation.

POSTOPERATIVE COMPLICATIONS

Loss of Motion

Motion loss after ACL reconstruction has been cited as one of the most common complications observed.[13] Loss of knee motion after surgery is truly a multifactorial problem that can change normal knee biomechanics and lead to stiffness and abnormal joint contact pressures, leading to overuse or early degenerative arthritis. Common postoperative causes can include arthrofibrosis, cyclops lesion, and infrapatellar contracture syndrome.

Terminology

In current literature, motion loss is described in many different ways (Box 12-1). Furthermore, motion loss terminology abounds in the scientific literature related to postoperative complications. *Arthrofibrosis* generally refers to motion loss that is symptomatic and resistant to rehabilitation. This

---

BOX 12-1

Terms Used to Describe Motion Loss

Arthrofibrosis

Flexion contracture

Loss of extension

Extension contracture

Loss of extension

Cyclops lesion

Infrapatellar contracture syndrome

common term can be used for both loss of flexion or extension range of motion. Some use the term *arthrofibrosis* to mean merely loss of knee extension and report it to be the most common postoperative complication of ACL reconstruction, occurring in as many as 4% to 59% of cases.[14,15] Others use the term to describe a specific form of motion loss resulting from scar tissue and fibrous adhesions that can form throughout the joint.[14] Used in this sense, arthrofibrosis would describe a globally restricted joint in which very little motion can occur. An ankylosed joint is a very restricted joint in which minimal movement occurs. True ankylosis means a fusion of a given joint. At the knee this can occur as a result of severe arthritis, or fibrous overgrowth. A final term commonly used to describe loss of motion at the knee is *flexion contracture*. Most use this term to denote an inability to attain full knee extension because of either soft tissue or capsular tightness. Millett and colleagues[16] report that this term is often used to denote loss of knee extension for various reasons and should be used only to denote that extension is lost because of soft tissue restrictions.

Shelbourne and co-workers[17] have devised a classification for motion loss, otherwise known as *arthrofibrosis* (Table 12-1). Regardless of the name or terminology used, loss of motion can be debilitating to the postoperative ACL patient.

As little as 5 to 10 degrees' loss of extension results in abnormal gait, quadriceps weakness, and patellofemoral pain. This loss of extension and its consequences may be more debilitating to the patient than the preoperative instability. Loss of flexion is less common and better tolerated. It was previously thought that time from injury until time of reconstruction was the critical factor in predicting postoperative loss of motion, with 3 weeks the typically cited duration. More recently it has been shown that time is not as crucial as certain other criteria, including ability to use a range of motion of 0 to 120 degrees, quadriceps control with performance of straight leg raise, and resolution of edema.[18] If these criteria are met, regardless of the time period, the incidence of arthrofibrosis is diminished. If sufficient time

TABLE 12-1

Classification Scheme for Arthrofibrosis Developed by Shelbourne and Colleagues

TYPE	FLEXION (DEGREES)	EXTENSION (DEGREES)
I	Normal	<10
II	Normal	>10
III	>25	>10
IV	>30	>10 with patella infera

Data from Shelbourne KD, Patel DV, Martin DJ: Classification and management of arthrofibrosis of the knee after anterior cruciate ligament reconstruction, Am J Sports Med *24: 857-862, 1996.*

is not allowed for attainment of these goals preoperatively, postoperative results are poorer.

Arthrofibrosis

It is thought that surgical trauma during ACL reconstructive surgery initiates the clotting cascade, which is followed by migration of inflammatory cells, then fibroblasts, to the injured tissue.[19] An abnormal expression of platelet-derived growth factor, fibroblast growth factor, insulin-like growth factor 1, and transforming growth factor beta may accentuate the degree of fibrous tissue formation, resulting in excessive periarticular scarring. This overzealous scarring response occurs in the anterior compartment and frequently in the posteromedial and posterolateral capsule as well.[16] Recent evidence has demonstrated a possible link between human leukocyte antigen and primary arthrofibrosis.[20]

Cyclops Lesion

A fibroproliferative scar nodule in the femoral notch located adjacent to the tibial attachment of the cruciate graft can mechanically block extension.[21] This nodule is typically attached to the graft as well as the soft tissue overlying the proximal tibia.[16] Patients who develop this form of entrapment usually develop clinical symptoms of a painful mechanical block to knee extension, crepitus, and physical sensation of grinding with knee extension. Marzo and colleagues[22] performed histologic studies of these nodules and found that they contained disorganized, dense fibroconnective tissue that underwent modulation to fibrocartilage. Other authors have thought that these nodules are most likely the result of debris from the tibial tunnel, remnants of the ACL stump, or a result of broken fibers of the ACL graft.[23-25]

Prevention may be divided into three phases. Preoperatively, prevention consists of allowing time for resolution of edema and the return of quadriceps function and adequate range of motion. Intraoperatively, anatomic placement of the graft and tensioning of the graft with the knee in full extension are important considerations. Postoperative rehabilitation should then focus on early motion, with emphasis on full extension and avoidance of immobilization in flexion. Promoting full extension engages the ACL graft in the notch and occupies this space, thereby preventing the formation of the anterior scar tissue or cyclops lesion. Full knee extension after surgery can be facilitated with judicious use of prone hangs (Figure 12-4). Adequate pain control is also necessary to produce these results. Treatment of arthrofibrosis consists of further physical therapy, which may include serial casting or the use of a dynamic splint and potentially arthroscopic debridement.

Infrapatellar Contracture Syndrome

The infrapatellar contracture syndrome (IPCS) was first described by Paulos and co-workers as "an infrequently

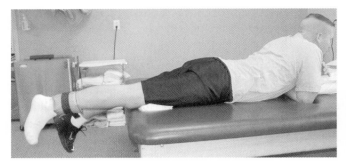

Figure 12-4: Prone hang to increase knee extension.

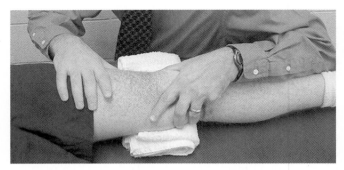

Figure 12-5: Performance of superior patellofemoral glide joint mobilization.

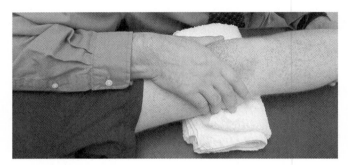

Figure 12-6: Performance of inferior patellofemoral glide joint mobilization.

recognized cause of posttraumatic knee morbidity."[26] In addition to causing limitation of knee extension and flexion because of fibrosclerotic changes of the infrapatellar fat pad, IPCS also causes pain and knee stiffness. Paulos and colleagues[26] revealed that tissue that underwent biopsy during surgery demonstrated a dense, fibrosclerotic reaction with disorganized collagen. The patella was firmly adherent to a fibrotic fat pad, with the fat pad occupying the entire anterior space, extending from the intercondylar notch and the medial and lateral joint lines forward to the patellar tendon. Prolonged patellar entrapment caused destructive changes of the articular surfaces of the tibia, femur, and patella. Paulos and colleagues[26] have described three different stages of IPCS that can be distinguished. Stage I is the prodromal stage, which is considered a normal stage of healing. This stage usually occurs approximately 2 to 8 weeks after surgery; however, some patients can progress to stage II of IPCS during this time. Patients in the prodromal stage of IPCS will progress through therapy, as one would expect, being hindered by abnormal pain and swelling and the inability to achieve full knee extension. Patellar glide tests demonstrate decreased patellar mobility, as does patellar tilt. The active stage (stage II) usually begins from 6 to 20 weeks after surgery and has the hallmark signs of dramatically decreased patellar mobility (global), while fat pad induration and patellar tendon rigidity are present.[26] Quadriceps atrophy is apparent, and on active contraction of the quadriceps the patella does not move superiorly. Stage III is the residual stage and may occur at any time from 8 months to years after the onset of IPCS. Stage III reveals significant patellofemoral arthrosis, demonstrated by patellofemoral crepitation, and decreased joint space seen on radiographs.[26] After enough time, many signs indicative of IPCS may no longer be present; however, residual patella infera and patellofemoral arthrosis may remain.[26] In stage III both flexion and extension range of motion may be substantially restricted.[26]

Treatment

Treatment of IPCS appears to be dependent on the stage of the disorder.[27] During stage I, therapy should focus on regaining motion, with emphasis on full knee extension, regaining strength, and diminishing swelling. Aggressive patellar superior and inferior joint mobilizations are essential for patellar mobility to be regained (Figures 12-5 and 12-6). When therapy does not help to resolve the situation, arthroscopic lysis and gentle manipulation may be warranted. Debridement of the suprapatellar pouch, medial and lateral gutters, and anterior fat pad should be performed.[28] When stage II is entered, open debridement is necessary through a midline approach allowing release of the suprapatellar pouch, along with lateral and medial retinacular release as needed. When this condition has extended to stage III, a patella infera will usually be present, and soft tissue releases will be inadequate to correct the permanent shortening of the patellar tendon.[28] Patients in this stage have frequently undergone multiple corrective surgeries with inconsistent improvement in symptoms. Continuation of physical therapy may be indicated; however, restoration to preinjury status is unlikely.

Anterior Knee Pain

Ranging from mild, intermittent irritation to activity-limiting pain, anterior knee pain is considered one of the major problems after ACL surgery. Its incidence has been reported to be as high as 55% after surgery,[29] with most authors reporting an incidence ranging from 15% to 25%.[30-33] A variety of reasons related to donor site morbidity have been suggested as contributing to this high incidence, including:

tendon-bone defects after patellar tendon autograft, loss of range of motion, and anterior knee sensitivity.

Tendon-Bone Defects

After the harvesting of the central third of the patellar tendon and the adjacent tibial and patellar bone plugs, defects remain at the donor site. These defects have been implicated in the occurrence of patellar tendon ruptures and fracture of the patella and lateral femoral condyle, leading many to use alternative graft sources (e.g., hamstring tendons) for the ACL reconstruction.

Although the gap in the patellar tendon significantly reduces within 6 months of surgery, a thinning of the central tendon is still apparent at 6 years.[34] Furthermore, the healing tendon is frequently observed to shorten an average of 10% relative to the contralateral side, potentially creating a patella baja or infera.[35-37] This shortening has been demonstrated to occur after ACL reconstruction regardless of whether the tendon defect is left open or is closed with multiple absorbable sutures at the time of surgery.[38] It is interesting to note that the shortened patellar tendon after ACL reconstruction has not been demonstrated to correlate to the incidence of anterior knee pain.[35,37] This is likely related to the maintenance of normal patellofemoral alignment, as Muellner and colleagues[39] demonstrated that a shortening of the patellar tendon of up to 20% does not significantly influence the alignment of the patellofemoral joint.

With donor site morbidity seemingly related to the remaining patellar tendon and bone defects, some advocate the closure of the defects at the time of reconstruction. Filling the patellar defect has been demonstrated to restore axial strain during flexion of cadaver knee joints to normal presurgical values.[40] Although it improves knee joint mechanics, closure of the defects does not appear to improve surgical outcomes. At 2-year follow-ups after ACL reconstruction, closure of the patellar tendon defect and bone grafting of the patellar defect did not reduce donor site morbidity or improve the functional results.[41] Moreover, the prevalence of anterior knee pain was not different between subjects with an open or closed defect. This may be largely a result of the similarity in patellofemoral contact regardless of whether the patellar defect is filled.[40]

When compared with the use of the patellar tendon graft during ACL reconstruction, the use of a hamstring tendon graft is generally thought to reduce the risk of development of anterior knee pain postoperatively. Through use of the hamstring tendon graft, disruption of the extensor mechanism is avoided, and surgical trauma to the tissues adjacent to the patellofemoral joint is minimized. Therefore postoperative complications involving these structures, such as anterior knee pain, are likely diminished. However, recent literature has revealed conflicting results as to the validity of this theory.

Long-term incidence of anterior knee pain between patients receiving a patellar tendon autograft compared with those receiving a hamstring autograft is largely equivalent.[30, 31, 42, 43] This does not suggest that anterior knee pain did not occur, but rather that the incidence appeared unrelated to the type of graft used. Marder and co-workers[30] found 17 of the examined 72 patients to have experienced postoperative anterior knee pain; however, the presence of knee pain was not specific to the type of autograft used during the reconstruction. Although knee function scores and general symptoms were reported to be similar between groups, Corry and colleagues[44] did identify a decreased incidence of anterior knee pain with kneeling at 2 years postsurgery among persons receiving a hamstring tendon autograft (6%) relative to those receiving a patellar tendon autograft (31%). In contrast, Spicer and colleagues[45] reported the incidence of anterior knee pain with kneeling after a hamstring tendon autograft procedure to be 12%. During early postoperative healing, Eriksson and co-workers[46] reported a greater incidence of anterior knee pain among persons receiving an infrapatellar tendon graft than among those having a hamstring tendon graft. It is interesting to note that the subjective evaluation of knee function (Lysholm score and Tegner activity level score) did not differ between the two groups, suggesting that the reported anterior knee pain had minimal impact on activity. Feller and colleagues[47] also observed a greater incidence of anterior knee pain among patellar tendon autograft recipients compared with those receiving hamstring tendon autografts. However, the functional outcomes were similar between groups, leading the authors to conclude the clinical impact of the knee pain to be insignificant.

When all literature is taken into consideration, the occurrence of anterior knee pain does not appear to be specific to the type of autograft used during the reconstruction. Although early postoperative anterior knee pain and pain with kneeling have been reported by some investigators, the impact of these symptoms on activity and sport are minimal.

Loss of Range of Motion

As described earlier in this chapter, loss of motion can have profound effects on the success of the ACL reconstruction. Most notably, the development of anterior knee pain has been repeatedly linked to the loss of full extension.[33,48-51] Kartus and colleagues[49] observed an extension deficit (>5 degrees) in 13% of ACL patients (81 of 604 patients) during 2- to 5-year follow-up, with one third of these patients requiring surgical correction. It has been suggested that the occurrence of anterior knee pain after ACL reconstruction can be prevented by restoring knee extension comparable to that in the contralateral limb, including obtaining full hyperextension if present.[52] Therefore obtaining and maintaining full extension early in the rehabilitative process can reduce the risk of developing anterior knee pain.

In addition to the loss of extension, knee flexion loss has also been implicated with the development of anterior knee pain. Some investigators argue that knee flexion loss is only of concern if total flexion is less than 110 degrees,[48] whereas others state that even subtle losses in flexion significantly increase the likelihood of anterior knee pain.[32,49] This lack of agreement regarding a minimum knee flexion angle requirement is likely related to the diverse activities of the patients. Unlike the nearly universal agreement that full knee extension is a requirement after ACL reconstruction, it is unlikely that a knee flexion threshold that would apply to all individuals can be identified, because fewer tasks involve knee flexion beyond 110 degrees. It is likely that the majority of ACL-reconstructed patients perform tasks daily that would press the knee extension deficit (e.g., walking, stair climbing), whereas a knee flexion deficit is likely to affect fewer people throughout the day. This lack of agreement on a knee flexion threshold does not suggest that the loss of knee flexion is less important. For those individuals who frequently perform tasks requiring full motion, a subtle loss of either extension or flexion would increase the risk for anterior knee pain.

Anterior Knee Sensitivity

After ACL reconstruction, regions of decreased or altered sensation along the incision are common. In addition, surgical injury to the saphenous nerve or its infrapatellar branches has been identified as a cause of sensation loss across the anterior knee region.[50] This loss of sensation has been correlated to difficulty in kneeling or knee-walking.[49] Given the anatomic distribution of the infrapatellar nerve(s), it seems likely that the risk of injury is greater when the patellar tendon autograft is used, because of the 7 to 8 cm central vertical incision required during the harvesting. This has led many to suggest alternate incisions including a lateral parapatellar incision,[53] two horizontal incisions,[54] and two 25 mm vertical incisions.[55] However, anterior knee sensation loss along the distribution of the infrapatellar nerve(s) has also been identified after the use of hamstring tendon autografts.[45] Kartus and colleagues[50] suggest that although both patellar tendon and hamstring tendon autografts are associated with comparable sensation loss, the difficulties with kneeling and knee-walking is reduced with the hamstring tendon autograft. Despite the greater difficulty with kneeling or knee-walking secondary to anterior knee sensation loss reported with patellar tendon autografts, functional outcome scores do not appear to be affected.[44,46]

Gender Differences

Considering the disparity in ACL tears between males and females, a gender difference in response to surgery and rehabilitation may exist. Based on an average follow-up of 5 years using the Cincinnati scale and the ACL Quality-of-Life scale and the Tegner activity rating scale, no gender differences in outcome were revealed among a group of 151 ACL reconstruction patients (74 males and 77 females) who received patellar tendon autografts.[56] In addition, no differences were identified with respect to complaints of anterior

knee pain. This is in contrast to the twofold increase in incidence of anterior knee pain in females reported by Aglietti and colleagues[32] after ACL reconstruction and the increased severity of knee pain in females after ACL reconstruction observed by Asano and co-workers.[51]

Complex Regional Pain Syndrome

A less frequent but potentially severe complication of anterior cruciate reconstruction is CRPS (also termed *reflex sympathetic dystrophy*). Among a sample of 60 patients with CRPS, 66% developed CRPS after knee surgery, with 60% of the surgeries being arthroscopic.[57] Characterized by burning pain and hypersensitivity, CRPS is often accompanied by tissue swelling and temperature changes. Although the severity and duration of symptoms can vary among patients, the reported pain is typically disproportionate to physical findings and progressively worsens. This pain reduces the patient's use of the knee, with eventual joint stiffness and atrophy of accompanying muscle and bone. Incidents of patellar tendon contracture secondary to CRPS have also been observed.[58] In addition to the presence of the noted physical examination findings, test results used to diagnose CRPS may include findings from a bone scan and lumbar sympathetic blockade.[57,59] However, it should be noted that no diagnostic test specific to CRPS is available.[60]

Although the cause of CRPS remains unknown, successful response to treatment has been correlated to the presence or absence of a persistent anatomic lesion (e.g. articular cartilage loss, meniscal tear, intraarticular adhesions, flexion contracture). Individuals without an anatomic lesion are four times more likely to respond favorably to treatment.[57] Among patients who do have an anatomic lesion, surgical correction of the lesion after a sympathetic blockade consistently resulted in favorable outcomes.[57] Nonsurgical treatment of CRPS may include serial lumbar sympathetic blockade and physical therapy interventions specific for pain relief and functional restoration.

Knee Infection

Despite attempts to achieve a completely aseptic surgical technique, knee sepsis can and occasionally does occur. Knee arthroscopic surgery is a common cause of a knee bacterial infection.[61-65] Once in the joint cavity, bacteria rapidly multiply in the warm liquid culture of the joint cavity and synovial fluid. With continued progression, inflammatory exudates called *panni* can erode the articular cartilage, joint capsule, and subchondral bone.[66] Most studies have reported a cumulative incidence of septic arthritis between 0.1% and 0.9%.[61,62,67-71] With an average infection rate of 0.2%, Matava and colleages[72] could not find any correlation between rate and graft choice, reconstruction method, or duration of prophylactic antibiotic use.

In a majority of cases, the physical therapist may be the first contact with the patient after infection; therefore it is critical to know the classic signs and symptoms of infection. In addition, diagnosis is often delayed, as many of the presenting features are similar to typical postoperative symptoms. Symptoms of knee infection include progressive knee pain with fast onset, knee effusion, erythema, incisional drainage, and localized warmth, which may or may not be accompanied by chills and fever.[67] Although common, these classic signs of infection may not always be present.[65] Patients may acutely show signs of mild local pain and effusion, which can easily be interpreted as signs of ordinary postoperative status, overuse inflammation, or the initial stages of the common cold.[65] The symptoms of infection are most common within 3 weeks of ACL reconstriction.[67] In most cases a fever with an acute exacerbation of inflammation should be an indication to the clinician to suspect the presence of sepsis in a joint and must be managed as a medical emergency.[73,74] In addition, patients who undergo ACL reconstruction should be given strict instruction to contact the surgeon if any sign of infection appears after surgery.[65]

Diagnosis of sepsis in a knee joint can be made by analysis of joint aspirate, which is liberally recommended if infection is suspected.[65] Recommended laboratory analysis includes a combination of C-reactive protein level and erythrocyte sedimentation rate,[65] which are elevated with an active infection. A high index of suspicion is necessary, because if left untreated this condition may result in articular cartilage damage and arthrofibrosis. Increased incidence has been associated with the use of drains postoperatively. The recommended treatment for a very slight infection may consist of taking oral culture-specific antibiotics or intravenous antibiotics. As the condition worsens, arthroscopic irrigation and debridement of the joint may be required; removal of graft and hardware are reserved for resistant infections.[13] Prevention with preoperative antibiotics is standard. Use of postoperative antibiotics is more controversial.

Deep Vein Thrombophlebitis

As with postoperative infection, the physical therapist is usually the first to notice symptoms of a DVT. Also known as *thrombophlebitis, venous thromboembolism,* or *phlebothrombosis,* a DVT occurs when a thrombus completely or partially occludes a vein. The human venous system uses a series of one-way valves to prevent backflow of blood. In the healthy human, muscular contractions "pump" blood through the venous system. After orthopedic knee surgery, blood may pool in the veins and form into a clot.

Although DVT is an uncommon complication of ACL reconstruction, its importance lies in its possible progression. Although it is often clinically silent and therefore difficult to diagnose through clinical examination alone, if not identified it can progress to a pulmonary embolism, which is potentially life threatening. It is reported that nearly 50% of people who develop a DVT are without symptoms initially.[75] Approximately 5% to 20% of calf DVTs progress to pulmonary

embolism, as compared with nearly 50% of DVTs with more proximal involvement.

A patient with a DVT may initially complain of or manifest symptoms including chronic swelling or edema, paresthesia, engorged veins, pain, tenderness, cramping, redness and discoloration, and warmth in the affected calf or thigh. Temperature in the affected extremity should be palpated with the posterior surface of the hand for best results. Examination may reveal nonspecific findings of calf tenderness, warmth, erythema, and/or swelling. In some instances a clinician can easily mistake a DVT for a grade I strain of the gastrocnemius or soleus muscle complex or a ruptured Baker cyst.[75] One of the more common tests used to diagnose DVT is Homans' sign. To perform this test the clinician passively dorsiflexes the foot of the involved leg with the patient's knee extended. Significant pain in the calf indicates a positive sign. In addition, the patient may have pain on palpation of the gastrocnemius or soleus muscle. To complicate matters, Goodman reports that the diagnosis of DVT by Homans' sign is unreliable because similar results occur with a variety of musculoskeletal conditions.[75] Diagnosis is typically confirmed with duplex ultrasound. The incidence of DVT after arthroscopic surgery has been reported as ranging from 2% to 18% overall.[76]

Diagnosis of DVT can be made with several well-known testing procedures. Venography is considered the gold standard for diagnosing DVT. This form of testing is invasive in that a radiopaque contrast medium is injected into a vein in the dorsum of the foot. The major drawback to this form of testing is that it is very painful to the patient; therefore repeat testing is generally not tolerated well. Impedance plethysmography uses electrodes on the lower legs to measure maximum venous capacity while the cuff is inflated. After this measurement maximal venous outflow can be measured on release of the cuff. This form of testing is most efficient for proximal vein thrombi that produce a critical obstruction, but it is not very sensitive for distal calf vein thrombi. Doppler ultrasonography has recently become the most accepted method for determination of DVT. This form of testing is noninvasive and does not cause discomfort and therefore is a favorite of patients. Ultrasound submits sound waves directed toward the veins; these sound waves are reflected at varying frequencies according to the rate of movement of blood through the veins.

Once DVT is diagnosed, initial treatment involves preventing the clot from becoming a pulmonary embolus, preventing another clot from forming and becoming dislodged, and attempting to lessen the extent of damage to the involved vein. Several forms of treatment are currently used. Immediate anticoagulation with heparin is the first defense in treatment of the patient with a DVT. This can be accomplished in two ways: with unfractionated heparin or with low-molecular-weight heparin. Conservative treatment for DVT can include physical therapy to provide gentle mobilization once the physician believes that the chance for dislodging an embolus is minimal. Moist heat to the affected area can increase circulation to the area that may be devoid of adequate blood flow. Compressive dressings can be applied as a conservative measure to decrease the risk for developing a DVT. A gradual increase in pressure applied with the dressing is used, with the highest pressure at the ankle and with progressively decreasing pressure as the dressing is applied proximally. Intermittent compression pumps are also used to decrease venous stasis that can lead to DVT. In each of these situations it is imperative that the physician and physical therapist work together to identify and institute appropriate treatment promptly to ensure overall successful outcomes.

WORKERS' COMPENSATION

A survey of 397 members of the American Academy of Orthopaedic Surgeons revealed that 40% of the surgeons considered Workers' Compensation to be a negative factor influencing their decision to perform ACL reconstruction.[77] The surgeons reluctance to perform surgery is likely reflective of their perception that a Workers' Compensation patient is less motivated to return to preinjury status and may experience and/or describe greater complications during the necessary rehabilitation. This perception was supported by Barrett and colleagues,[78] who reported that Workers' Compensation patients' self-rating scores were three times worse than non–Workers' Compensation patients undergoing identical surgeries and rehabilitation. These poor self-rating scores were in stark contrast to the objective physical examination findings. In addition, the non–Workers' Compensation patients obtained a 6.02 postoperative Tegner score, with the Workers' Compensation patients scoring 3.05 with a preoperative score of 4.75. It should be noted that these striking difference were not supported by a similar study that found no significant difference in subjective rating between these two patient groups.[79]

SUMMARY

Complications during and after ACL reconstruction can be greatly minimized or prevented with adequate preoperative and postoperative planning. Although careful attention to detail and adequate preoperative preparation may prevent many of the intraoperative problems, well-thought-out postoperative rehabilitation with a keen eye toward slight variances in the patient's condition will avert potential problems after surgical reconstruction.

References

1. Bealle D, Johnson DL: Technical pitfalls of anterior cruciate ligament surgery, *Clin Sports Med* 18:831-845, 1999.
2. Colombet P, Allard M, Bousquet V, et al: Anterior cruciate ligament reconstruction using four-strand semitendinosus and gracilis tendon grafts and metal interference screw fixation, *Arthroscopy* 18:232-237, 2002.
3. Cain EL, Gillogly SD, Andrews JR: Management of intraoperative complications associated with autogenous patellar tendon graft

4. Noyes FR, Butler DL, Grood ES, et al: Biomechanical analysis of human ligament grafts used in knee-ligament repairs and reconstructions, *J Bone Joint Surg Am* 66A:344-352, 1984.
5. Miller SL, Gladstone JN: Graft selection in anterior cruciate ligament reconstruction, *Orthop Clin North Am* 33:675-683, 2002.
6. Chen L, Cooley V, Rosenberg T: ACL reconstruction with hamstring tendon, *Orthop Clin North Am* 34:9-18, 2003.
7. Solman CG, Pagnani MJ. Hamstring tendon harvesting. Reviewing anatomic relationships and avoiding pitfalls, *Orthop Clin North Am* 34:1-8, 2003.
8. Gladstone JN, Andrews JR: Endoscopic anterior ligament reconstruction with patella tendon autograft, *Orthop Clin North Am* 33:701-715, 2003.
9. Sekiya JK, Ong BC, Bradley JP: Complications in anterior ligament surgery, *Orthop Clin North Am* 34:99-105, 2003.
10. Gill TJ, Steadman R: Anterior cruciate ligament reconstruction. The two incision technique, *Orthop Clin North Am* 33:727-735, 2002.
11. Martin SD, Martin TL, Brown CH: Anterior cruciate ligament graft fixation, *Orthop Clin North Am* 33:685-696, 2002.
12. Verma N, Noerdlinger MA, Hallab N, et al: Effects of graft rotation on initial biomechanical failure characteristics of bone-patellar tendon-bone constructs, *Am J Sports Med* 31:708-713, 2003.
13. D'Amato MJ, Bach B: Anterior cruciate ligament reconstruction in the adult. In DeLee JC, Drez D, Miller MD, editors: *DeLee and Drez's orthopedic sports medicine*, ed 2, Philadelphia, 2003, Saunders.
14. DeHaven KE, Cosgarea AJ, Sebastianelli WJ: Arthrofibrosis of the knee following ligament surgery, *Instr Course Lect* 52:369-381, 2003.
15. Petsche TS, Hutchinson MR: Loss of extension after reconstruction of the anterior cruciate ligament, *J Am Acad Orthop Surg* 7:119-127, 1999.
16. Millett PJ, Wickiewicz TL, Warren RF: Motion loss after ligament injuries to the knee. Part I: Causes, *Am J Sports Med* 29:664-675, 2001.
17. Shelbourne KD, Patel DV, Martini DJ: Classification and management of arthrofibrosis of the knee after anterior cruciate ligament reconstruction, *Am J Sports Med* 24:857-862, 1996.
18. Sterett WI, Hutton KS, Briggs KK, Steadman JR: Decreased range of motion following acute versus chronic anterior cruciate ligament reconstruction, *Orthopedics* 26:151-154, 2003.
19. Eakin CL:. Knee arthrofibrosis: Prevention and management of a potentially devastating condition, *Phys Sportsmed* 29:31-42, 2001.
20. Skutek M, Elsner HA, Slateva K, et al: Screening for arthrofibrosis after anterior cruciate ligament reconstruction: analysis of association with human leukocyte antigen, *Arthroscopy* 20:469-473, 2004.
21. Heiderscheit BC: Optimizing treatment of joint contracture following reconstruction. In Ellenbecker T, editor: *Knee ligament rehabilitation*, Philadelphia, 2000, Churchill Livingston.
22. Marzo JM, Bowen MK, Warren RF, et al: Intraarticular fibrous nodule as a cause of loss of extension following anterior cruciate ligament reconstruction, *Arthroscopy* 8:10-18, 1992.
23. Aglietti P, Buzi R, DeFelice R, et al: Results of surgical treatments of arthrofibrosis after ACL reconstruction, *Knee Surg Sports Traumatol Arthosc* 3:83-88, 1995.
24. Bach BR, Jones GT, Sweet FA, et al: Arthroscopy-assisted anterior cruciate ligament reconstruction using patellar tendon substitution. Two-to four-year follow-up results, *Am J Sports Med* 22:758-767, 1994.

25. Bents RT, Jones RC, May DA, et al: Intercondylar notch encroachment following anterior cruciate ligament reconstruction. A prospective study, *Am J Knee Surg* 11:81-88, 1996.

26. Paulos LE, Rosenberg TD, Drawbert J, et al: Infrapatellar contracture syndrome. An unrecognized case of knee stiffness with patella entrapment and patella infera, *Am J Sports Med* 15:331-341, 1978.

27. Veltri DM: Surgical treatment of infrapatellar contracture syndrome, *Tech Orthop* 12:192-199, 1997.

28. Theut PC, Fulkerson JP: Anterior knee pain and patellar subluxation in the adult. In DeLee JC, Drez D, Miller MD, editors: *DeLee and Drez's orthopaedic sports medicine principles and practice,* vol II, Philadelphia, 2003, Saunders.

29. Arendt EA, Hunter RE, Schneider WT: Vascularized patella tendon anterior cruciate ligament reconstruction, *Clin Orthop* 244:222-232, 1989.

30. Marder RA, Raskind JR, Carroll M: Prospective evaluation of arthroscopically assisted anterior cruciate ligament reconstruction. Patellar tendon versus semitendinosus and gracilis tendons, *Am J Sports Med* 19:478-484, 1991.

31. Karlson JA, Steiner ME, Brown CH, Johnston J: Anterior cruciate ligament reconstruction using gracilis and semitendinosus tendons. Comparison of through-the-condyle and over-the-top graft placements, *Am J Sports Med* 22:659-666, 1994.

32. Aglietti P, Buzzi R, D'Andria S, Zaccherotti G: Patellofemoral problems after intraarticular anterior cruciate ligament reconstruction, *Clin Orthop* 288:195-204, 1993.

33. Sachs RA, Daniel DM, Stone ML, Garfien RF: Patellofemoral problems after anterior cruciate ligament reconstruction, *Am J Sports Med* 17:760-765, 1989.

34. Svensson M, Kartus J, Ejerhed L, et al: Does the patellar tendon normalize after harvesting its central third? A prospective long-term MRI study, *Am J Sports Med* 32:34-38, 2004.

35. Muellner T, Kaltenbrunner W, Nikolic A, et al: Shortening of the patellar tendon after anterior cruciate ligament reconstruction, *Arthroscopy* 14:592-596, 1998.

36. Breitfuss H, Fröhlich R, Povacz P, et al: The tendon defect after anterior cruciate ligament reconstruction using the midthird patellar tendon—a problem for the patellofemoral joint? *Knee Surg Sports Traumatol Arthrosc* 3:194-198, 1996.

37. Tria AJ, Alicea JA, Cody RP: Patella baja in anterior cruciate ligament reconstruction of the knee, *Clin Orthop* 299:229-234, 1994.

38. Krosser BI, Bonamo JJ, Sherman OH: Patellar tendon length after anterior cruciate ligament reconstruction. A prospective study, *Am J Knee Surg* 9:158-160, 1996.

39. Muellner T, Menth-Chiari WA, Funovics M, et al: Shortening of the patellar tendon length does not influence the patellofemoral alignment in a cadaveric model, *Arch Orthop Trauma Surg* 123:451-454, 2003.

40. Sharkey NA, Donahue SW, Smith TS, et al: Patellar strain and patellofemoral contact after bone-patellar tendon-bone harvest for anterior cruciate ligament reconstruction, *Arch Phys Med Rehabil* 78:256-263, 1997.

41. Brandsson S, Faxén E, Eriksson BI, et al: Closing patellar tendon defects after anterior cruciate ligament reconstruction: absence of any benefit, *Knee Surg Sports Traumatol Arthrosc* 6:82-87, 1998.

42. Aglietti P, Buzzi R, Zaccherotti G, De Biase P: Patellar tendon versus doubled semitendinosus and gracilis tendons for anterior cruciate ligament reconstruction, *Am J Sports Med* 22:211-217, 1994.

43. Otero AL, Hutcheson LA: A comparison of the doubled semitendinosus/gracilis and central third of the patellar tendon autografts in arthroscopic anterior cruciate ligament reconstruction, *Arthroscopy* 9:143-148, 1993.

44. Corry IS, Webb JM, Clingeleffer AJ, Pinczewski LA: Arthroscopic reconstruction of the anterior cruciate ligament. A comparison of patellar tendon autograft and four-strand hamstring tendon autograft, *Am J Sports Med* 27:444-454, 1999.

45. Spicer DDM, Blagg SE, Unwin AJ, Allum RL: Anterior knee symptoms after four-strand hamstring tendon anterior cruciate ligament reconstruction, *Knee Surg Sports Traumatol Arthrosc* 8:286-289, 2000.

46. Eriksson K, Anderberg P, Hamberg P, et al: There are difference in early morbidity after ACL reconstruction when comparing patellar tendon and semitendinosus tendon graft. A prospective randomized study of 107 patients, *Scand J Med Sci Sports* 11:170-177, 2001.

47. Feller JA, Webster KE, Gavin B: Early post-operative morbidity following anterior cruciate ligament reconstruction: patellar tendon versus hamstring graft, *Knee Surg Sports Traumatol Arthrosc* 9:260-266, 2001.

48. Irrgang JJ, Harner CD: Loss of motion following knee ligament reconstruction, *Sports Med* 19:150-159, 1995.

49. Kartus J, Magnusson L, Stener S, et al: Complications following arthroscopic anterior cruciate ligament reconstruction. A 2-5-year follow-up of 604 patients with special emphasis on anterior knee pain, *Knee Surg Sports Traumatol Arthrosc* 7:2-8, 1999.

50. Kartus J, Movin T, Karlsson J: Donor-site morbidity and anterior knee problems after anterior cruciate ligament reconstruction using autografts, *Arthroscopy* 17:971-980, 2001.

51. Asano H, Muneta T, Shinomiya K: Evaluation of clinical factors affecting knee pain after anterior cruciate ligament reconstruction, *J Knee Surg* 15:23-28, 2002.

52. Shelbourne KD, Trumper RV: Preventing anterior knee pain after anterior cruciate ligament reconstruction, *Am J Sports Med* 25:41-47, 1997.

53. Berg P, Mjöberg B: A lateral skin incision reduces peripatellar dysaesthesia after knee surgery, *J Bone Joint Surg Br* 73:374-376, 1991.

54. Mishra AK, Fanton GS, Dillingham MF, Carver TJ: Patellar tendon graft harvesting using horizontal incisions for anterior cruciate ligament reconstruction, *Arthroscopy* 11:749-752, 1995.

55. Kartus J, Ejerhed L, Eriksson BI, Karlsson J: The localization of the infrapatellar nerves in the anterior knee region with special emphasis on central third patellar tendon harvest: a dissection study on cadaver and amputated specimens, *Arthroscopy* 15:577-586, 1999.

56. Ott SM, Ireland ML, Ballantyne BT, et al: Comparison of outcomes between males and females after anterior cruciate ligament reconstruction, *Knee Surg Sports Traumatol Arthrosc* 11:75-80, 2003.

57. O'Brien SJ, Ngeow J, Gibney MA, et al: Reflex sympathetic dystrophy of the knee: causes, diagnosis, and treatment, *Am J Sports Med* 23:655-659, 1995.

58. Soubrier M, Dubost JJ, Urosevic Z, et al: Contracture of the patellar tendon: an infrequently recognized complication of reflex sympathetic dystrophy of the knee, *Rev Rhum (Engl Ed)* 62:399-400, 1995.

59. Bach BR, Wojtys EM, Lindenfeld TN: Reflex sympathetic dystrophy, patella infera contracture syndrome, and loss of motion following anterior cruciate ligament surgery, *Instr Course Lect* 46:251-260, 1997.

60. Vacariu G: Complex regional pain syndrome, *Disabil Rehabil* 24:435-442, 2002.

61. Armstrong RJ, Bolding F, Joseph R: Septic arthritis following arthroscopy: clinical syndromes and analysis of risk factors, *Arthroscopy* 8:213-223, 1992.

62. D'Angelo GL, Ogilvie-Harris DJ: Septic arthritis following arthroscopy, with cost/benefit analysis of antibiotic prophylaxis, *Arthroscopy* 4:10-14, 1988.

63. DeLee JC: Complications of arthroscopy and arthroscopic surgery: results of a national survey, *Arthroscopy* 1:214-220, 1985.

64. Kieser C: A review of the complications of arthroscopic knee surgery, *Arthroscopy* 8:79-83, 1992.

65. Schollin-Borg M, Michaelsson K, Rahme H: Presentation, outcome, and cause of septic arthritis after anterior cruciate ligament reconstruction: a case control study, *Arthroscopy* 19:941-947, 2003.

66. Boissonnault WG, Goodman CC: Introduction to pathology of the musculoskeletal system. In: Goodman CC, Boissonnault WG, Fuller KS: *Pathology. Implications for the physical therapist,* ed 2, Philadelphia, 2003, Saunders.

67. McAllister D, Parker R, Cooper A, et al: Septic arthritis in postoperative anterior cruciate ligament reconstruction, *Am J Sports Med* 27:562-570, 1999.

68. Viola R, Marzano N, Vianello R: An unusual epidemic of *Staphylococcus*-negative infections involving anterior cruciate ligament reconstruction with salvage of the graft and function, *Arthroscopy* 16:173-177, 2000.

69. Austin KS, Sherman OH: Complications of arthroscopic meniscal repair, *Am J Sports Med* 21:864-868, 1993.

70. Williams RJ, Laurencin CT, Warren RF, et al: Septic arthritis after arthroscopic anterior cruciate ligament reconstruction. Diagnosis and management, *Am J Sports Med* 25:261-267, 1997.

71. Armstrong RW, Bolding F: Septic arthritis after arthroscopy: the contributing roles of intraarticular steroids and environmental factors, *Am J Infect Control* 22:16-18, 1994.

72. Matava MJ, Evans TA, Wright RW, Shively RA: Septic arthritis of the knee following anterior cruciate ligament reconstruction: results of a survey of sports medicine fellowship directors, *Arthroscopy* 14:717-725, 1998.

73. Erkan D, Yazici Y, Paget SA: Fever and arthritis. Narrowing the diagnosis, *J Musculoskelet Med* 17:676-687, 2000.

74. Ignacia EM: Pediatric septic arthritis, *Trauma* 5:67-81, 2001.

75. Goodman CC: The cardiovascular system. In Goodman CC, Boissonnault WG, Fuller KS, editors: *Pathology. Implications for the physical therapist,* ed 2, Philadelphia, 2003, Saunders.

76. Jaureguito JW, Greenwald AE, Wilcox JF, et al: The incidence of deep venous thrombosis after arthroscopic knee surgery, *Am J Sports Med* 27:707-710, 1999.

77. Marx RG, Jones EC, Angel M, et al: Beliefs and attitudes of members of the American Academy of Orthopaedic Surgeons regarding the treatment of anterior cruciate ligament injury, *Arthroscopy* 19:762-770, 2003.

78. Barrett GR, Rook RT, Nash CR, Coggin MRH. The effect of Workers' Compensation on clinical outcomes of arthroscopic-assisted autogenous patellar tendon anterior cruciate ligament reconstruction in an acute population, *Arthroscopy* 17:132-137, 2001.

79. Noyes FR, Barber-Westin SD: A comparison of results of arthroscopically assisted anterior cruciate ligament reconstruction between workers' compensation and noncompensation patients, *Arthroscopy* 13:474-484, 1987.

CHAPTER 13

Strain Gauge Studies: A Historical Review with Implications for Postoperative Anterior Cruciate Ligament Rehabilitation

Karl Glick, PT
Kelly Ashton, PT

CHAPTER OUTLINE

SINCE 1938 SURGEONS HAVE BEEN striving to perfect the cure for knee ligament injuries. Their road has been long, but to their credit they have persisted with great tenacity. Blackburn[1] stated in 1985 that rehabilitation programs for the knee, especially for injured anterior cruciate ligaments (ACLs), have "acquired a new outlook with the development of greater diagnostic skill and the complexity of new surgical techniques." It was a statement that could not have been truer in 1985 or in 2004. Modifications, improvements, and the collection of objective critical data have aided this trek to progress us to where we find ourselves today. One might wonder where we will go next.

The purpose of this chapter is to discuss, with some analysis, the significance that the collection of scientific evidence has had in the role of defining rehabilitation of knee ligament injuries, specifically ACL reconstruction. We will look back introspectively at early rehabilitation ideas, how they developed, and how they influence what we do today.

Many creative thinkers have carried the banner of anterior cruciate reconstruction forward to the twenty-first century. Eriksson[2] acknowledged that internationally the approach to knee ligament injuries was very diverse. One common thread at the time, however, was that all repairs or reconstructions of ligaments were casted.[2-6] The most frequently chosen position was with the knee in 30 to 45 degrees of flexion.[4] Ellison[3] speculated that full extension too soon would almost certainly compromise the integrity of the ACL. Eriksson[2] discussed his concerns with atrophy of the quadriceps muscle and introduced the idea of a moveable cast brace. This cast brace functioned at 20 to 60 degrees of knee flexion. He noted that athletes had better motion and less muscle atrophy of the quadriceps than those placed in a traditional cylinder cast.

Almost all orthopedic surgeons in the 1970s and early 1980s immobilized ACL repairs or reconstructions in a cylinder cast postoperatively for 6 to 8 weeks. In his quest to reduce atrophy and stimulate type II fast-twitch muscle fibers, Eriksson had postoperative patients hopping on the involved leg while still in the cast brace.[7]

With Clancy's[5] contribution of the free patellar tendon graft in the early 1980s, the advancement of both the surgical procedure and rehabilitation of the ACL began to take shape. With this new published technique for ACL reconstruction came numerous published postoperative protocols.[6,8-10]

EARLY ANTERIOR CRUCIATE LIGAMENT REHABILITATION PROTOCOLS

Jones[8] described a four-phase program designed to progress the patient from injury to return to sport activity. The protocol used a progressive strength and motion program, being very mindful of slow return to full knee extension. Hamstring strength was emphasized early and "traditional quadriceps exercises are downplayed and modified because of their anterior pull on the tibia." Phase I ended approximately 6 weeks after cast removal, and motion expected was from 15 to 90 degrees of knee flexion. In phase II, as described by McCleod and Blackburn,[9] cycling along with general strengthening of hamstrings begins. Still motion was limited in extension to −10 degrees, but full flexion was achieved. Phase III began at approximately 6 months after injury or surgery. Strength development with isokinetic exercise began at that time. Running was initiated in phase IV, somewhere between 9 and 12 months. Stressed throughout the program was an ever vigilant monitoring of full knee extension.

Paulos and colleagues[10] described a five-phase program with maximum protection through 12 weeks, moderate protection through 24 weeks, and minimum protection through 48 weeks. Return to running activity was achieved at 60 weeks. They described a very detailed plan with regard to range-of-motion and strength, along with progressive loading of the ACL graft. This was really the first detailed published protocol and was quickly adopted by most programs. In the same publication they described using a buckle transducer to measure stress through a cadaveric ACL. This gave the first confirmation of knowledge that had previously been reported by biomechanical studies. Quadriceps activities routinely performed postoperatively could in fact rupture the reconstruction in the early phases. That information along with the results of the authors' earlier canine studies formed the scientific evidence on which the protocol was based. No longer was there speculation about what would work best; now scientific evidence was being used to design rehabilitation programs. Dr. Frank Noyes,[11] who coauthored the Paulos work, had previously published work on ligament healing and failure after reconstruction in rhesus monkeys. This study gave the first direct insight into what happens to the tensile strength of a ligament while it is immobilized. The dramatic loss of strength in the immobilized ligament helped fuel concerns that although failure of the bony fixation needed to be guarded against, too much protection may have a deleterious effect on the graft itself. In a later study Noyes and co-workers[12] cited Woolf's Law and suggested that loading may be very important to the postoperatively healing anterior cruciate reconstruction. Noyes indicated that his group had, for the period of a year, not used traditional cast immobilization but instead used removable splinting. This allowed for earlier mobilization postoperatively. The study also introduced the idea that 0 degrees of knee extension may be healthy and not harmful for the graft. There was caution, however, that graft placement and fixation were critical. "The point made here is that immediate motion under very prescribed protective conditions is beneficial for the joint." During the same period that Noyes and colleagues[12] advocated early mobility and 0 degrees of extension to purposely load the anterior cruciate graft, Brewster and colleagues[6] described a 52-week program, stressing again protected extension through 18 weeks, followed by the use of a 0-degree stop brace during physical activity until 1 year after surgery.

STRAIN GAUGE STUDIES

After the strong investigative effort by Noyes and Paulos a litany of work involving the ACL and strain gauges began to emerge (Figure 13-1). In 1984 Arms and colleagues[13] used a tiny Hall transducer that could be directly implanted on the ligament itself in such a way as to facilitate better motion and duplication of rehabilitation activities. Using the Hall effect strain transducer (HEST) in cadaveric knees and comparing both intact and reconstructed anterior cruciate knees, they determined that a simulated isometric quadriceps contraction from 0 to 45 degrees of flexion increased strain, whereas a simulated contraction at 60 degrees or higher decreased the strain through the ACL. Strain during passive movements of the knee was also measured; it was determined that the flexion angles associated with the least strain were from full extension to 35 degrees of knee flexion and the strain continued to increase with further flexion to 120 degrees, with a maximum strain of 1.25% of normal at 120 degrees. The researchers concluded that the reconstructed ACL should be positioned so as to duplicate the important anteromedial fibers and that careful attention should be directed toward proper tensioning of the graft.

Henning and colleagues[14] described a strain gauge study using two live patients with grade II ACL sprains (Figure 13-2). This in vivo study measured ACL loads during ligament integrity testing techniques and compared them with activities commonly performed during rehabilitation after reconstruction. This study was the first to look at ligamentous strain in vivo, allowing ACL strain to be determined during various functional activities. Each activity was compared against an 80 lb Lachman test, which strained the anteromedial fibers of the ACL more than the anterior drawer or the pivot shift tests. The activity proving to strain the ACL the most was downhill running, which placed 125% of

the strain that the Lachman test placed on the ACL. Normal walking on the floor produced 36% of the elongation that the Lachman test produced. Quadriceps isometric contraction from 0 to 22 degrees flexion produced greater elongation than testing at 45 degrees flexion. It was determined that strain generated within the ACL during quadriceps contraction in these ranges has the potential to damage recently reconstructed ligaments. Activities producing small amounts of strain were walking at 2.25 mph on the treadmill, stationary cycling, and isometric hamstring contractions. Based on data from this study the authors were able to determine a recommended order of physical activity after ACL reconstruction: crutch walking, cycling, walking, slow running, and faster running (Figure 13-3).

In 1986 Renstrom and co-workers[15] measured ACL strain in cadaveric knees during simulated hamstring, quadriceps, and hamstring-quadriceps co-contraction activities. Again, strain was measured using the HEST. This was the first study to look directly at the effect of hamstring activity on the strain of a reconstructed ACL. As in previous cadaveric studies, it was determined that strain was least during passive movement from extension to approximately 35 degrees of flexion. Strain increased from 105 to 120 degrees of passive flexion. With the passive motion findings used as a reference, it was determined that isometric quadriceps activity significantly increased ACL strain from 0 to 45 degrees of flexion. Isotonic quadriceps activity resulted in strain patterns similar to those during isometric contraction, with greatest strain values in full extension. Alternately, hamstring activity in all ranges demonstrated strain values lower than those found during passive motion. During a hamstring and quadriceps co-contraction it was determined that ACL strain was highest at angles closer to extension (primarily from 0 to 30 degrees

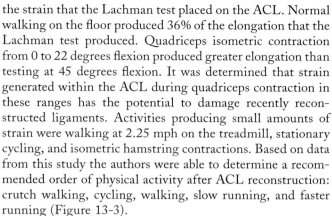

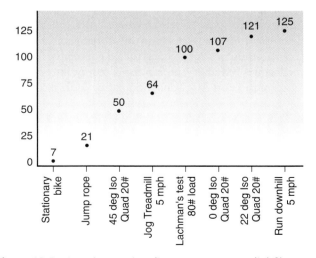

Figure 13-3: Anterior cruciate ligament anteromedial fiber elongation relative to 80 lb Lachman test. *(Adapted from Henning C, Lynch M, et al: An in vivo strain gauge study of elongation of the anterior cruciate ligament, Am J Sports Med 13:22-26, 1985.)*

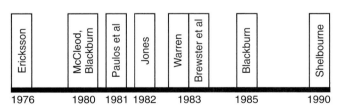

Figure 13-1: Published ACL rehabilitation protocol timeline.

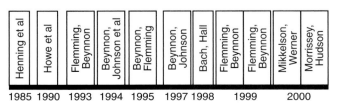

Figure 13-2: In vivo strain gauge studies timeline.

of flexion) and lowest at flexion angles beyond 60 degrees. These data suggest that hamstring function cannot mask the strain placed on the ACL by quadriceps activity between full extension and 30 degrees of flexion.

Similarly, Howe and colleagues[16] described strain measurement in vivo in five persons with normal ACLs under local anesthesia. Using a HEST within the anteromedial band (AMB) of the ACL, strain was determined during anterior-posterior tibial shear testing at 30 degrees and at 90 degrees (Lachman and drawer tests) as well as during isometric quadriceps contractions at 30 degrees and 90 degrees. During Lachman and drawer testing using an anterior shear force of 150N placed on the tibia, it was determined that Lachman testing, at 30 degrees flexion, placed significantly greater strain on the AMB than drawer testing at 90 degrees. The shear testing results allowed the authors to quantitatively conclude that Lachman testing is the preferred method of assessing ACL integrity. In relation to quadriceps rehabilitation activity, no strain was detected in the AMB during isometric quadriceps contractions at 90 degrees of knee flexion. Conversely, at 30 degrees of flexion strain was increased significantly during an isometric quadriceps contraction creating 27 Nm of torque, leading the authors to recommend using this activity with caution during rehabilitation after an ACL injury or reconstruction.

In 1994 Fleming and co-workers[17] compiled data and performed further statistical analysis, drawing the same conclusions as the previously described work. The purpose of this analysis was to determine whether tibial translation could be used as a predictor of AMB strain. Correlational data showed that when the knee is flexed at 30 degrees as in a Lachman test, the amount of tibial translation may be used as a reliable predictor of strain. On the other hand, data suggested that tibial translation may not be used as a reliable indicator of strain in the AMB when the knee is flexed to 90 degrees, as during the drawer test when shear forces of 150 N are placed on the tibia.

Further strain research was able to use data collected over previous years to compare strain measurements in normal ACLs with strain in newly reconstructed ligaments. Beynnon and colleagues[18] studied the effects of 20 cycles of passive flexion-extension on ACL elongation after ACL reconstruction. No significant difference was determined in elongation patterns during varied ranges of passive flexion in the newly reconstructed ACLs versus normal ACL patterns derived from previously obtained data. Other results from this study indicate that passive motion immediately after fixation of the graft may increase the length of the graft, although further study is needed to determine whether this will help or hinder restoration of normal knee kinematics.

Beynnon and colleagues continued their study of in vivo ACL strain behavior with further experimentation during exercises specific to ACL rehabilitation.[19] At the time, there was little agreement existing within the literature as to which rehabilitation activities were best after ACL reconstructions. Emphasis within the rehabilitation program used was restoration of knee mobility and enhancement of lower extremity strength while placing a minimal amount of strain on the graft. During anterior-posterior shear loading with the thigh fixed to the table, the ACL became strained during anterior shear loading at 25 degrees of knee flexion with a force of up to 200 N. The ligament remained slack during posterior loading. Next, the study evaluated ACL shear during active ranges of flexion and extension of the knee (5 to 90 degrees) with and without resistance. It was determined that maximum strain was produced when the knee approached full extension. Results were augmented with the use of resistance primarily at 10 and 20 degrees of flexion. Adding resistance also created increased strain during the flexion phase of active motion, possibly secondary to internal tibial rotation during flexion. Transition from unstrained to strained ACL during both flexion and extension phases occurred at slightly greater ranges of flexion with weights than without weights. Next tested were isometric quadriceps and hamstrings contractions at 15, 30, 60, and 90 degrees. Strains during quadriceps isometric contractions were significantly greater at 15 and 30 degrees than at the greater ranges. No significant changes in strain levels were detected during hamstrings activity. Finally, strain was studied during a simultaneous hamstring and quadriceps contraction at each range. Again, strain was highest at 15 and 30 degrees of flexion. This study is useful for applying results to activities actually performed during rehabilitation.

Research through the years brought on additional clinically adapted studies looking at the effect of bracing on the strain of the ACL.[20] Research has shown that bracing significantly reduces strain with loading in both weight-bearing and non–weight-bearing situations. Strain of the ACL has been studied with subjects placed in varied positions mimicking common mechanisms of ACL injury with and without a brace such as one that the surgeon might prescribe after ACL reconstruction. Significant strain values were found in the ACL of an unbraced knee with simple standing, a posture thought to be safe because of straight compressive forces through the joint. With an anterior-directed load of 140 N placed on the unbraced tibia, subjects demonstrated no difference in ACL strain between either a seated or a standing position. On the other hand, braced knees demonstrated significantly lower ACL strain as compared with unbraced knees within the varied positions, with variable loads placed on the tibia. In addition, the placement of the strap tension within the brace, whether high or low in magnitude, demonstrated no significant difference in strain values under the different conditions.

Strain gauge studies were able to be further refined in the late 1990s by looking at the differences in strain within the AMB versus the posterior lateral band (PLB) of the ACL under various loads.[21] Previous strain gauge studies focused primarily on the AMB alone. Passive range-of-motion activity beyond 90 degrees of knee flexion continued to increase strain on the AMB, whereas PLB strain remained nonexistent. During quadriceps loading activities both bundles increased in strain from 0 to 60 degrees of knee flexion. Further load testing comparisons revealed similar results. Statistical analyses were unable to find significant differences between the AMB and PLB, although the authors caution that when there were differences in strain, the PLB strain was usually higher than that of the AMB. Bach and Hull[21] concluded that an injury model should be based on the PLB, as this will fail at a lower strain than the AMB.

Further study became more clinically relevant by taking the subjects through functional and sport-specific activity.[22] Fleming and colleagues studied the strain produced on the ACL during stationary bicycling. Subjects rode the stationary bike at varied power levels, which simulated downhill, level, and uphill riding conditions at 60 and 90 revolutions per minute (rpm). Highest strain levels were found when the knee was flexed to 38 degrees, where strain occurred at the latter portion of the pedal stroke. Peak values did not differ significantly at the different power levels or at the varied pedaling speeds. ACL strain and the knee flexion angle did vary inversely, with strain values at their highest as the knee was extended. Based on these data, the authors concluded that stationary bicycling is an appropriate rehabilitation exercise with which subjects' lower extremity musculature and endurance may be challenged while avoiding any undue strain on the new ACL graft.

In a separate study, Fleming and colleagues[23] went on to look at ACL strain during stair climbing. The StairMaster (Nautilus Health and Fitness Group, Vancouver, WA) simulated closed-chain activity commonly used in rehabilitation. Strain of the AMB of the ACL was measured while subjects performed varied cadences on the StairMaster. As in the previous study of subjects on the stationary bike, strain values tended to increase as the knee extended. No significant differences were found in strain values at the faster versus slower cadence levels. The authors determined a ranking of varied rehabilitation activities according to the peak strain placed on the ACL. According to the ranking, highest strain levels occurred during isometric quadriceps contraction at 15 degrees, followed by squatting with a sport cord and active flexion-extension of the knee with a 45 N weight boot. Lowest strain values were found during hamstring activity, various quadriceps-hamstring co-contraction activities, and isometric quadriceps contraction with the knee flexed to 60 and 90 degrees. Stair-climbing and stationary bicycling were ranked in the middle of the comparison.

With the turn of the century much of the research regarding strain of the ACL turned to open kinetic chain (OKC) versus closed kinetic chain (CKC) activities.[24,25] Mikkelsen and colleagues[24] compared ACL strain between two groups performing quadriceps strengthening in CKC and OKC activities after ACL reconstruction with a bone-patella-tendon-bone autograft. Group 1 performed only CKC quadriceps exercises, whereas group 2 performed the same CKC exercises until 6 weeks after surgery, when they began OKC activities for the quadriceps. Laxity was measured with the KT-1000 arthrometer (Medmetric Corp., San Diego, CA)

preoperatively and 6 months postoperatively for comparison. For the first 6 weeks after surgery, both groups performed traditional postoperative activities with quadriceps exercises in a CKC only. After week 6, group 2 began isokinetic concentric and eccentric quadriceps exercises, which were continued through the course of rehabilitation for 6 months. Results after rehabilitation determined that group 2 demonstrated a laxity of 1.2 mm, whereas group 1 demonstrated a laxity of 1.7 mm. The results were not significantly different between the two groups. A higher proportion of the group 2 subjects did return to sports at the same level as before the injury, however. Authors concluded that a combination of OKC and CKC exercises should be included postoperatively in order to gain adequate quadriceps muscle torque and to allow earlier return to sports at the same level. Further research was suggested to verify long-term results.

Similarly Morrissey and colleagues[25] compared ACL laxity in two groups who performed OKC and CKC exercises postoperatively. The OKC group performed knee and hip extensor exercises without fixing the tibia in the kinetic chain using varied levels of resistance. The CKC group performed knee and hip extension activities with a fixed distal lower extremity using a leg press machine. After a 4-week regimen, subjects were retested for ACL laxity. Results indicated that the two groups did not differ significantly in laxity. Because of lack of experimental control, the authors concluded that until there is evidence that OKC training is preferable to CKC training after ACL reconstruction, CKC should be used.

LATEST REHABILITATION PROTOCOLS

In 1990 Shelbourne and co-workers[26] published the first in a series of accelerated rehabilitation protocols. Oddly enough, with all the scientific data presented at the time, the original push toward early activity was a result of a prospective look at compliant versus noncompliant patients. It was noted that the noncompliant patients had earlier mobility and appeared to do better than the conservative compliant patients. Mindful of that and with well-documented databases, the genesis of accelerated rehabilitation occurred.

The protocol matured through the late 1980s, and although most had lengthened the time for return to play to 9 to 12 months, Shelbourne kept his in the 4- to 6-month range, if all criteria were met. The accelerated protocol was visited again in 1997 by Shelbourne.[27] By this time Beynnon and colleagues[18-20] had given the orthopedic community a plethora of in vivo strain gauge studies. These, along with more current histologic studies,[28-30] supported the theory of both Shelbourne and Noyes that loads could be applied sooner to postoperative ACL reconstructions. Early, safe activities that gradually stress the graft actually stimulate healing. Now supported by scientific evidence, protocols can be written to simultaneously protect and strengthen postoperative ACL reconstructions.

SUMMARY

It should be stressed that frequent assessments for instability, edema and pain not typical during rehabilitation are all warnings that care must be taken not to force the patient into expected parameters. As Noyes noted, protocols are guidelines, not cookbooks. Therapists must be ever vigilant, especially for changes in stability of ACL reconstructions during the entire postoperative phase. Too much early emphasis on strength, especially of the quadriceps, can overload a graft and have deleterious effects on the outcome.

Even with an accelerated rehabilitation program, the mean-average return to sport competition is 6.2 months. Ironically, that is the same time frame used nearly 27 years ago by early advocates of ACL reconstruction. Improvements in surgical techniques, especially graft placement and evidence-based rehabilitation, have played important roles in decreasing the failure rate of reconstructions and returning a more complete athlete to competition.

References

1. Blackburn, TA Jr: Rehabilitation of anterior cruciate ligament injuries, *Orthop Clin North Am* 16:241-269, 1985.
2. Eriksson E: Sports injuries of the knee ligaments: their diagnosis, treatment, rehabilitation and prevention, *Med Sci Sports* 8:133-144, 1976.
3. Ellison AE: Distal iliotibial-band transfer for anterolateral rotatory instability of the knee, *J Bone Joint Surg* 16A:330-337, 1979.
4. Warren RF: Primary repair of the anterior cruciate ligament, *Clin Orthop* 172:65-70, 1983.
5. Clancy WG Jr, Nelson DA, Reider B, et al: Anterior cruciate ligament reconstruction using one-third of the patellar tendon, augmented by extra-articular tendon transfers, *J Bone Joint Surg* 64A:352-359, 1982.
6. Brewster CE, Radovich Moynes D, Jobe FW: Rehabilitation for anterior cruciate reconstruction, *J Orthop Sports Phys Ther* 5:121-126, 1983.
7. Eriksson E: Intra-articular anterior cruciate ligament reconstruction technique: patellar tendon. AOSSM Annual Meeting, Atlanta, GA, 1980.
8. Jones AL: Rehabilitation for anterior instability of the knee: preliminary report, *J Orthop Sports Phys Ther* 3,121-128, 1982.
9. McCleod WD, Blackburn TA Jr: Biomechanics of knee rehabilitation with cycling, *Am J Sports Med* 8:175-179, 1980.
10. Paulos L, Noyes FR, Grood E, et al: Knee rehabilitation after anterior cruciate ligament reconstruction and repair, *Am J Sports Med* 9:140-149, 1981.
11. Noyes FR, Torvik PJ, Hyde WS et al: Biomechanics of ligament failure II: An analysis of immobilization, exercise and reconditioning effect in primates, *J Bone Joint Surg* 56A:1406-1418, 1974.
12. Noyes FR, Butler DL, Paulos LE, et al: Intra-articular cruciate reconstruction I: perspectives on graft strength, vascularization and immediate motion after replacement, *Clin Orthop* 172:71-77, 1983.
13. Arms S, Pope M, Johnson RJ, et al: The biomechanics of anterior cruciate ligament rehabilitation and reconstruction, *Am J Sports Med* 12:8-18, 1984.
14. Henning C, Lynch M, Glick K: An in vivo strain gauge study of elongation of the anterior cruciate ligament, *Am J Sports Med* 13:22-26, 1985.
15. Renstrom P, Arms S, Stanwyck T, et al: Strain within the anterior cruciate ligament during hamstring and quadriceps activity, *Am J Sports Med* 14:83-87, 1986.
16. Howe J, Wertheimer C, Johnson R, et al: Arthroscopic strain gauge measurement of the normal anterior cruciate ligament, *Arthroscopy* 6:198-204, 1990.
17. Fleming B, Beynnon B, Nichols C, et al: An in vivo comparison of anterior tibial translation and strain in the anteromedial band of the anterior cruciate ligament, *J Biomech* 26:51-58 1993.
18. Beynnon B, Johnson R, Fleming B, et al: The measurement of elongation of anterior cruciate ligament grafts in vivo, *J Bone Joint Surg* 76A:520-531, 1994.
19. Beynnon B, Fleming B, Johnson R, et al: Anterior cruciate ligament strain behavior during rehabilitation exercises in vivo, *Am J Sports Med* 23:24-34, 1995.
20. Beynnon B, Johnson R, Fleming B, et al: The effect of functional knee bracing on the anterior cruciate ligament in the weightbearing and nonweightbearing knee, *Am J Sports Med* 25:353-359, 1997.
21. Bach J, Hull M: Strain homogeneity in the anterior cruciate ligament under application of external and muscular loads, *J Biomech Eng* 120:497-503, 1998.
22. Fleming B, Beynnon B, Renstrom P, et al: The strain behavior of the anterior cruciate ligament during bicycling: an in vivo study, *Am J Sports Med* 26:109-118, 1998.
23. Fleming B, Beynnon B, Renstrom P, et al: The strain behavior of the anterior cruciate ligament during stair climbing: an in vivo study, *Arthroscopy* 15:185-191, 1999.
24. Mikkelsen C, Werner S, Eriksson E, et al: Closed kinetic chain alone compared to combined open and closed kinetic chain exercises for quadriceps strengthening after anterior cruciate ligament reconstruction with respect to return to sports: a prospective matched follow-up study. *Knee Surg Sports Traumatol Arthrosc* 8:337-342, 2000.
25. Morrissey M, Hudson Z, Drechsler W, et al: Effects of open versus closed kinetic chain training on knee laxity in the early period after anterior cruciate ligament reconstruction, *Knee Surg Sports Traumatol Arthrosc* 8:343-348, 2000.
26. Shelbourne KD, Nitz P: Accelerated rehabilitation after anterior cruciate ligament reconstruction, *Am J Sports Med* 18:292-299, 1990.
27. Shelbourne KD, Gray T: Anterior cruciate ligament reconstruction with autogenous patellar tendon graft followed by accelerated rehabilitation. A two- to nine-year follow-up, *Am J Sports Med* 25:786-795, 1997.
28. Rougraff B, Shelbourne KD, Gerth PK, et al: Arthroscopic and histologic analysis of human patellar tendon autografts used for anterior cruciate ligament reconstruction, *Am J Sports Med* 21:277-284, 1993.
29. Kleiner JB, Amiel D, Harwood FL, et al: Early histologic, metabolic, and vascular assessment of anterior cruciate ligament autografts, *J Orthop Res* 7:235-242, 1989.
30. Hannafin JA, Arnoczky SP, Hoonjan A, et al: Effect of stress deprivation and cyclic tensile loading on the material and morphologic properties of canine flexor digitorum profundus tendon: an in vitro study, *J Orthop Res* 13:907-914, 1995.

CHAPTER 14

Rehabilitation after Posterior Cruciate Ligament Reconstruction

James J. Irrgang, PhD, PT, ATC
Robin West, MD
Amit Sahasrabudhe, MD
Christopher D. Harner, MD

CHAPTER OUTLINE

HISTORY OF POSTERIOR CRUCIATE REPAIR TECHNIQUE

Surgical treatment of the posterior cruciate ligament (PCL) has varied and progressed dramatically since it was first described by Hey Groves in 1917.[1] Hey Groves reconstructed the PCL by using the semitendinosus tendon through femoral and tibial drill holes. Later he modified the procedure by adding the gracilis tendon.[2] In 1980 Trickey described using the semitendinous and gracilis tendons as free grafts passed through drill holes in the femur and tibia.[3] Methods of reconstructing the PCL have ranged from using other structures around the knee such as a slip of iliotibial band or the lateral meniscus to using the proximally detached medial head of the gastrocnemius as a dynamic transfer. Unfortunately, all of these methods either have lacked good postoperative data or have had disappointing clinical results.

Since the early 1980s the results of several series describing primary repair for PCL injuries have been published. All the reports concluded that direct suture repair of the PCL does not restore its function.[4] Use of the patellar tendon became popular in the late 1980s when Augustine described a technique of PCL reconstruction using a distally detached portion of the patellar tendon placed through a tibial bone tunnel intraarticularly.[5] Clancy then reported the use of free bone-patella-tendon-bone autograft for anterior cruciate ligament (ACL) and PCL reconstruction in rhesus monkeys, followed by successful use of these autografts in humans.[6,7]

Other types of grafts have since been reported, including a long flap of quadriceps and a prosthetic ligament. All have had less than optimal results. Most recently, Achilles tendon allograft has been described for PCL reconstruction.[8,9] This technique has had good clinical outcomes and has a number of advantages, including decreased surgical and tourniquet time, injury-free graft-site harvesting, easier passage of a soft tissue end, increased size of graft material, and ample graft length. Disadvantages include the potential for disease transmission and the requirement for soft tissue fixation at one end.

SURGICAL INDICATIONS AND CONTRAINDICATIONS

The indications for PCL reconstruction remain controversial. This is partly because of the lack of knowledge about the true natural history of the PCL-deficient knee. Nonoperative management is advocated by many physicians because functional instability is usually not a symptom after isolated PCL injury, and most patients are able to lead active lives despite the injury. However, degenerative arthritis of the patella and medial femoral condyle has been reported as a late sequela of PCL tears.[10]

In order to grade PCL injuries a classification system based on posterior tibial translation on the femur was developed. The test is performed at 90 degrees of knee flexion because posterior tibial translation is greatest at 70 to 90

degrees of flexion in the PCL-deficient knee. Also, the posterior capsule is lax at 90 degrees, and therefore posterior tibial translation better reflects the status of the PCL than at 30 degrees, where the posterior capsule is tighter.

Grade I PCL injuries demonstrate a palpable but diminished tibial step-off. The tibial plateau remains anterior to the femoral condyles, such that the amount of posterior displacement is less than 5 mm. This is indicative of a partial PCL disruption. Grade II PCL injuries have no palpable tibial step-off. The tibial plateau is flush with the femoral condyles. The amount of posterior displacement is between 5 and 10 mm. This occurs with either a complete PCL disruption or a significant PCL injury. With grade III PCL injuries the tibial plateaus are posterior to the femoral condyles. The amount of posterior displacement is more than 10 mm. This is usually indicative of a complete PCL disruption with concomitant major ligamentous injury.

In general, a nonoperative approach is taken with grade I injuries. Disability from these injuries is typically not extensive, and results from conservative management have been reported in the literature to be quite good. On the other hand, patients with combined ligamentous injuries (grade III) become functionally unstable after injury and require surgical intervention. Surgical reconstruction will improve a grade III injury to a grade II or sometimes even a grade I injury.[4]

Grade II injuries represent a "gray zone."[1] Treatment for affected patients is individualized based on age, activity, associated injury, symptoms, objective laxity, and injury acuteness. For example, someone with a concomitant medial meniscal tear would likely be treated operatively because of the high risk of developing medial compartment arthritis. Acute grade III PCL tears, with an associated posterolateral (PL) corner injury to the knee, are usually treated surgically within 3 weeks of the injury.

Contraindications to PCL reconstruction include neurovascular injury that has not yet been addressed (e.g., injury to the popliteal artery), complex regional pain syndrome, open wounds, infection, and advanced degenerative arthritis.

SURGICAL TECHNIQUE

A few factors must be reviewed before any PCL reconstruction is undertaken. First, the anatomy, specifically the insertion sites of the PCL, must be known. Second, the appropriate graft must be selected. Finally, before the procedure is begun, a systematic examination must be performed with the patient under anesthesia to confirm the pattern of instability. Both knees should be examined to allow for side-to-side comparison.

After standard preparation and draping, arthroscopy is performed. Standard anteromedial (AM) and anterolateral portals are used for the initial diagnostic arthroscopy; PCL disruption is confirmed. While this is being done, an assistant may prepare the Achilles tendon allograft on a side table (Figure 14-1).

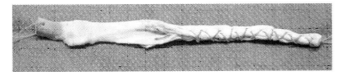

Figure 14-1: Prepared Achilles allograft.

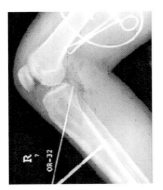

Figure 14-2: Intraoperative x-ray film confirming correct tibial tunnel placement.

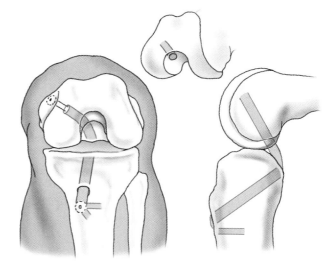

Figure 14-3: Line drawing of the tibial and femoral tunnels during posterior cruciate ligament reconstruction.

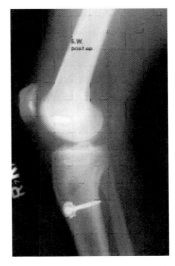

Figure 14-4: Postoperative posterior cruciate ligament reconstruction radiograph, demonstrating the hardware fixation.

An arthroscope, basket punch, and mechanized shaver are used to debride the PCL stump. Commonly, only the PL bundle is disrupted. The AM bundle of the PCL is often intact. During the reconstruction, the AM bundle is preserved and the remainder of the disrupted PCL is debrided. The arthroscopic PCL drill guide for the tibial insertion is set to approximately 55 degrees and is introduced through the AM portal, with the tip seated in the distal and lateral aspect of the tibial footprint. A guidewire is then advanced from the AM tibial cortex to the tibial footprint. After confirmation of accurate guidewire placement by fluoroscopy (Figure 14-2), a cannulated reamer is used to create the tibial tunnel. The diameter of the tunnel should accommodate the size of the graft.

The PCL femoral tunnel is placed several millimeters off the articular cartilage of the medial femoral condyle. The tunnel is placed at approximately the 10:30 position in a left knee and the 1:30 position in a right knee. As for the tibial tunnel preparation, a guidewire is advanced through the femoral footprint. After confirmation of accurate guidewire placement, a femoral tunnel is reamed to the same diameter as the tibial tunnel.

The Achilles tendon allograft is then passed from the tibial tunnel through the femoral tunnel using an 18-gauge wire and a Beath (passing) pin. The bone block on the Achilles allograft is placed into the femoral tunnel. A cannulated interference screw or a post and washer are used to secure the graft into the femoral tunnel. Distal fixation is then accomplished by using a bioabsorbable screw and a metal screw with a spiked soft tissue washer. Double fixation is used on the tibial side because of the poor bone density of the proximal tibia. The knee is placed in 70 to 90 degrees of flexion, and an anteriorly directed force is applied to the tibia to recreate the normal AM tibial step-off of approximately 1 cm. While manual tension is maintained on the graft, the tibial fixation is secured into place (Figures 14-3 and 14-4).

The reconstruction is then checked by performing a posterior drawer test, followed by arthroscopic assessment of the graft. Finally, a layered closure is performed and a sterile dressing is applied. The knee is then placed in a long-leg hinged brace, locked in full extension.

BIOLOGIC AND BIOMECHANICAL CONSIDERATIONS FOR REHABILITATION AFTER POSTERIOR CRUCIATE LIGAMENT RECONSTRUCTION

Before we provide the details for rehabilitation after PCL reconstruction, it is necessary to briefly discuss the biologic and biomechanical factors that affect rehabilitation. Much of our understanding of graft healing and maturation is based on animal models, and relatively little is known about this process in humans. After reconstruction in animals the graft undergoes avascular necrosis, revascularization, invasion and proliferation of fibroblasts, collagen formation, and remodeling of the graft.[6] During this time mechanical strength of the graft gradually increases.[6] In rhesus monkeys, Clancy and colleagues[6] found that tensile strength of the PCL graft was 31% of the native PCL 8 weeks after implantation, 51% at 3 months, 68% at 6 months, 93% at 9 months, and 47% at 12 months. In interpreting these data, it must be remembered that only one specimen was tested at each time point. A similar process has been described for healing of the ACL graft in humans; however, the time frame was slightly longer.[12] By 18 months after implantation the graft progressed to a thick ligamentous structure that was enveloped by a thin synovial membrane that appeared similar to the native ACL. In the animal model, allografts demonstrate slower biologic incorporation and healing than autografts.[13] Six months after ACL graft implantation in goats, strength of the autograft was 62% and strength of the allograft was 27% of the native ACL.

Another factor to consider after PCL reconstruction is healing of the graft in the bone tunnels. When the PCL is reconstructed using Achilles tendon allograft, the bone block is fixed in the femoral tunnel and soft tissue is fixed in the tibial tunnel. Rodeo and co-workers[14] investigated tendon-to-bone healing in a dog model and found that by 12 weeks failure occurred by pull-out of the graft from the clamp as opposed to pull out of the graft from the tunnel that occurred before 12 weeks. Tomita and colleagues[15] in a dog model found soft tissue healing within bone tunnels via Sharpey's fibers at 12 weeks, whereas bone plugs healed within the tunnels by 3 weeks. Therefore it appears that healing of soft tissues within bone tunnels takes longer than healing of bone plugs. As a result, the method of initial fixation is of greater concern when soft tissue is placed in the bone tunnels. An area of healing of soft tissue to bone should be protected from excessive stress for 12 weeks.

Despite the research that has been done, relatively little is known concerning the process of healing and maturation of the graft after reconstruction of the PCL in humans. Given this, we believe it is prudent to protect the graft from potentially stressful activities for 6 months.

Anatomically the PCL consists of the AM and PL bundles. Tension within the PCL is dependent on the angle of knee extension-flexion. With the knee in extension, there

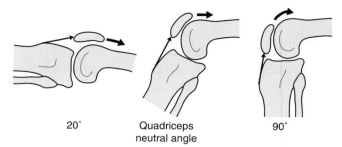

20°   Quadriceps neutral angle   90°

Figure 14-5: Quadriceps neutral position is the angle of knee flexion at which the patellar tendon is perpendicular to the tibial plateaus and contraction of the quadriceps produces no anterior or tibial translation. At angles less than the quadriceps neutral angle, contraction of the quadriceps causes anterior translation of the tibia, and at angles greater than the quadriceps neutral angle, contraction of the quadriceps causes posterior translation of the tibia. (*From Daniel DM, Stone ML, Barnett P, Sachs R: Use of the quadriceps active test to diagnose posterior cruciate-ligament disruption and measure posterior laxity of the knee,* J Bone Joint Surg 70-A: 386-391, 1988.)

is increased tension within the PL bundle that decreases as the knee is passively flexed. Conversely, tension on the AM bundle increases as the knee is passively flexed.

When planning an exercise program after PCL reconstruction, it is important to understand the effects of muscle forces on stress and strain of the PCL. During open chain exercises, in which the lower leg and foot are free to move, contraction of the quadriceps is synergistic to the PCL and contraction of the hamstrings is antagonistic to the PCL. During open chain knee extension, the quadriceps neutral angle is that angle of knee flexion at which contraction of the quadriceps does not create anterior or posterior translation of the tibia.[16] The quadriceps neutral angle occurs at 60 to 75 degrees of knee flexion. At this position of knee flexion the patellar tendon is perpendicular to the tibial plateau, and contraction of the quadriceps produces only compression of the tibiofemoral joint.[16] At knee flexion angles less than the quadriceps neutral angle (i.e., toward knee extension) the quadriceps causes anterior translation of the tibia, which is synergistic to the PCL. At knee flexion angles greater than the quadriceps neutral angle (i.e., greater knee flexion) the quadriceps causes posterior translation of the tibia, which is antagonistic to the PCL (Figure 14-5). Therefore after PCL reconstruction we restrict open chain knee extension exercises from 60 degrees of flexion to full extension are restricted.

Open chain knee flexion is produced by unopposed contraction of the hamstrings. Unopposed contraction of the hamstrings causes posterior translation of the tibia, which is least with the knee in full extension and increases as the knee flexes. This posterior translation is antagonistic to the healing PCL graft. Therefore after PCL reconstruction we do not advocate the use of open chain knee flexion exercises to increase strength of the hamstrings. Alternate methods to strengthen the hamstrings include hip extension with the knee extended and closed chain exercises.

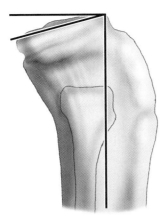

Figure 14-6: Tibial slope is measured as the angle formed by a line perpendicular to the mid diaphysis and a line parallel to the tibial plateaus. (*From Griffin JR, et al: Effects of increasing tibial slope on the biomechanics of the knee,* Am J Sports Med *32:376-382, 2004.*)

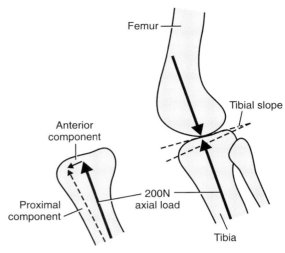

Figure 14-7: Analysis of the effects of tibial slope. An axial load can be resolved into a compressive load that is perpendicular to the tibial plateaus and an anteriorly directed load that is parallel to the tibial plateaus. (*From Griffin JR, et al: Effects of increasing tibial slope on the biomechanics of the knee,* Am J Sports Med *32:376-382, 2004.*)

Closed chain exercises are those in which the distal aspect of the extremity is fixed, such as weight-bearing exercises. During closed chain exercises for the lower extremity, each joint moves in a predictable manner, and movement is controlled by co-contraction of muscles. With regard to the quadriceps and hamstrings, the quadriceps contracts to counter the flexion moment at the knee and the hamstrings contract to counter the flexion moment at the hip. Closed chain exercises are thought to decrease tibial translation, thereby decreasing load on the cruciate ligaments, because of co-contraction of the quadriceps and hamstrings as well as because of the compressive forces acting on the tibiofemoral joint.

Another factor that needs to be considered in terms of closed chain exercises after PCL reconstruction is the effect of tibial slope. The tibial plateaus slope posteriorly. Tibial slope is defined as the angle formed by a line that is perpendicular to the mid diaphysis of the tibia and a line defining the posterior inclination of the tibial plateaus (Figure 14-6). Application of an axial force applied to the tibiofemoral joint can be resolved into a vector component that is perpendicular to the tibial plateaus and an anteriorly directed component parallel to the tibial plateaus (Figure 14-7). Therefore during weight bearing an axial load applied to the tibiofemoral joint causes a tendency for the tibia to shift anteriorly, which is synergistic to the PCL.[17] This implies that closed chain exercises can be initiated in the early postoperative period without undue stress on the healing PCL graft.

Development of tension within the muscle is the stimulus needed for increasing strength. Progressive overload of the muscle creates increasing levels of tension within the muscle, which stimulates muscle fiber hypertrophy. Therefore resisted exercises designed to enhance strength should maximally activate the muscle. Muscle activation during resisted exercise is dependent on a number of factors including whether movement occurs with the distal extremity fixed or free to move.

The success of rehabilitation after PCL reconstruction is dependent on strength of the quadriceps, which acts as a synergist to the PCL. During closed chain exercises, activation of the quadriceps is minimal with the knee in extension and increases as the angle of knee flexion increases. In a study to determine the effects of hip rotation during an Olympic squat, Ninos and co-workers[18] found electromyographic activity of the quadriceps reached 20% to 25% of a maximal voluntary isometric contraction at approximately 60 degrees of knee flexion during squatting against body weight with 25% body weight added to the shoulders. Therefore unless heavy loads or deep angles of knee flexion are used, which are contraindicated during rehabilitation after PCL reconstruction, closed chain exercises produce a relatively inefficient stimulus for quadriceps strengthening.

An alternative to closed chain exercises to strengthen the quadriceps is open chain knee extension exercises, during which the lower leg is free to move against resistance. Open chain knee extension from 90 degrees of flexion to full extension requires progressively increasing quadriceps force.[19] From 90 to 60 degrees of flexion an increasing level of quadriceps force is required to extend the knee. From 60 to 30 degrees of knee extension, the amount of quadriceps force to extend the knee remains relatively constant because of the biomechanical advantage provided by the patella. A marked increase in quadriceps force is required to produce the final 20 to 30 degrees of knee extension.[19] The amount of quadriceps force required to extend the knee increases with the application of resistance. Therefore open chain knee extension exercises produce an efficient stimulus for strengthening the quadriceps.

A final consideration for exercises to strengthen the quadriceps is the biomechanical effect of open and closed chain exercises on the patellofemoral joint. Starting with the knee in full extension, the inferior pole of the patella makes initial contact with the trochlear grove of the patella at approximately 20 degrees of knee flexion. The area of patellofemoral contact migrates superiorly on the patella as the knee continues to flex, so that by 90 degrees of flexion the entire posterior surface of the patella, except for the odd medial facet, has articulated with the trochlear grove. As knee flexion continues, the patella drops down into the intercondylar notch of the femur.[20] From 20 to 90 degrees of flexion the area of patellofemoral contact increases, which acts to distribute patellofemoral joint reaction forces over a larger area.[20] The patellofemoral joint reaction force is a force that tends to compress the patellofemoral joint; it is a function of the angle of knee flexion and amount of quadriceps force. The patellofemoral joint reaction force increases with an increasing angle of knee flexion and increasing levels of quadriceps force.[20] Quadriceps force increases as a function of the external flexion moment arm of the tibiofemoral joint.

During open chain knee extension exercises, in which the knee extends against gravity from 90 degrees of flexion to full extension, there is an increasing external knee flexion moment arm, which requires greater quadriceps force to progressively extend the knee. As quadriceps force increases, there is an increase in patellofemoral joint reaction force that peaks at approximately 35 degrees of knee flexion; this increasing patellofemoral joint reaction force is distributed over a smaller contact surface area, resulting in increased patellofemoral contact stress (i.e., force per unit of area).[20]

During closed chain exercises, as the individual performs squats from 0 to 90 degrees of flexion, the external knee flexion moment arm increases, requiring increased quadriceps force. The increasing angle of knee flexion and quadriceps force results progressively in increased patellofemoral joint reaction forces. These patellofemoral joint reaction forces are distributed over a larger contact, which helps to minimize the increase in patellofemoral contact stress.[20]

Given these biomechanical considerations, we use a combination of open and closed chain exercises to strengthen the quadriceps after PCL reconstruction. Unless the individual has patellofemoral symptoms, which often accompany longstanding PCL deficiency, we perform open chain knee extension exercises in the range of 60 degrees of flexion to full extension and closed chain exercises from 0 to 90 degrees of flexion. If the individual has patellofemoral symptoms, we restrict open chain knee extension exercises to 20 to 0 degrees of knee flexion.

REHABILITATION AFTER POSTERIOR CRUCIATE LIGAMENT RECONSTRUCTION

Rehabilitation after PCL reconstruction focuses on resolving impairments and lessening functional limitations and disability. Impairments associated with PCL reconstruction include pain, swelling, loss of motion, decreased muscle performance (strength, endurance) and decreased neuromuscular control. Our rehabilitation efforts are primarily directed at resolving these resulting impairments. Modifications that we make in the postoperative guidelines for concomitant surgical procedures, such as reconstruction of the PL corner, will be discussed at the end of this section (Table 14-1).

Postoperative Bracing

In the immediate postoperative period the patient is immobilized in a postoperative knee brace locked in extension for 4 weeks. After 4 weeks the brace is unlocked for ambulation, and the brace is discontinued after 6 weeks.

Weight-Bearing Considerations

Immediately after surgery patients bear weight as tolerated with crutches, with the postoperative brace locked in full extension. Four weeks after surgery the patient may begin walking weight bearing as tolerated with the brace unlocked. Crutches may be discontinued 6 weeks after surgery, provided the patient has full passive and active knee extension, 100 degrees of flexion, no extensor lag, minimal swelling, and ability to walk without a flexed-knee gait pattern.

Range of Motion

Immediately after surgery, passive and active extension exercises are permitted as tolerated by the patient. Full knee extension symmetric to the noninvolved side should be achieved within 1 week. If full extension is not achieved within 3 weeks, we begin to use passive stretching techniques, such as prone hangs (Figure 14-8) to restore passive knee extension. If the patient has not achieved at least 0 degrees of knee extension by 3 weeks after surgery, communication with the physician is warranted.

Range-of-motion exercises for knee flexion may be started 1 week after surgery. These include passive knee flexion exercises, as well as standing partial squats with the patient's body weight evenly distributed on each extremity. To perform passive knee flexion, the patient is taught to apply an anteriorly directed force to the proximal tibia, lifting the lower leg to passively flex the knee (Figure 14-9). Supporting the tibia during passive knee flexion is necessary to prevent posterior sagging of the tibia, which is antagonistic to the graft. To avoid stretching the graft, the range of passive knee flexion is restricted to 90 degrees for the first 4 weeks after surgery. After 4 weeks the patient may gradually flex the knee beyond 90 degrees. Passive stretching exercises, in which the knee is flexed beyond the available range of motion, may be initiated after 6 weeks. Active contraction of the hamstrings to flex the knee should be avoided for the first 6 weeks. Full knee flexion symmetric to the uninvolved side is expected within 8 to 10 weeks. Patellar mobilization, particularly inferior glide of the patella, may be used as necessary to restore flexion. We believe that use of a continuous passive motion

TABLE 14-1

Summary of Postoperative Rehabilitation Guidelines after PCL Reconstruction

	0 TO 6 WEEKS	6 WEEKS TO 6 MONTHS	6 TO 12 MONTHS
Postoperative bracing considerations	Brace locked in full extension for 4 weeks; may be unlocked several times daily for ROM exercises up to 90 degrees		
	After 4 weeks, brace unlocked up to 100 degrees for ambulation		
	Discontinued after 6 weeks		
Weight-bearing considerations	Weight bearing as tolerated with crutches with brace locked in extension for 4 weeks		
	After 4 weeks brace may be unlocked for ambulation Discontinue use of crutches 6 weeks after surgery, provided milestones have been achieved (see text)		
ROM	Passive and active extension exercises; full extension symmetric to noninvolved knee expected within 1 week	Begin passive stretching exercises beyond available ROM at 6 weeks	
	Begin passive flexion exercises 1 week after surgery; limit to 90 degrees for 4 weeks	Expect full flexion symmetric to noninvolved side within 8 to 10 weeks after surgery	
	After 4 weeks passive flexion may be gradually progressed beyond 90 degrees		
	Include patellar mobilization as necessary to improve flexion		
	Avoid active contraction of hamstrings		
Muscle performance	Begin quadriceps sets and SLR immediately after surgery	Progress resistance with open chain knee extension from 60 degrees to full extension	Progress resisted open and closed chain exercises as tolerated
	Use high-intensity electrical stimulation and biofeedback as necessary to improve quadriceps activation Initiate limited arc open chain knee extension from 60 degrees to full extension as ROM improves	Progress closed chain exercises as tolerated; may include wall-slides, unilateral step-ups, leg presses, and squats	
	No open chain knee flexion exercises	Begin open chain hip extension with knee extended to enhance hamstring strength	
	Begin partial squats with weight evenly distributed on both legs 1 week after surgery		

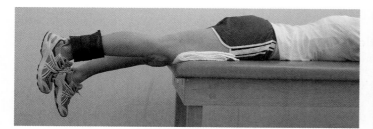

Figure 14-8: Prone knee hangs to restore full passive knee extension.

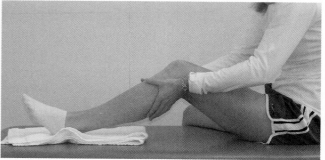

Figure 14-9: Passive knee flexion is performed by lifting the proximal tibia to prevent posterior sagging of the tibia.

TABLE 14-1

Summary of Postoperative Rehabilitation Guidelines after PCL Reconstruction—cont'd

	0 TO 6 WEEKS	6 WEEKS TO 6 MONTHS	6 TO 12 MONTHS
Neuromuscular control	Begin weight-shifting exercises to involved leg Progress to standing unilateral balance on stable surface as tolerated	Progress unilateral standing balance activities to unstable surface, such as foam mat or balance board Add perturbations to support surface once able to balance on balance board Incorporate sport-specific activities during balance activities as tolerated	
Functional progression for return to sport		Resume normal walking provided milestones have been reached (see text) Begin low-impact aerobic activities, such as walking, step machines, or cycling when patient can walk without symptoms or gait deviations	Begin running, provided quadriceps strength is at least 75% that of noninvolved side Begin agility drills at half-effort once patient can run 1 to 2 miles without symptoms and quadriceps strength is at least 80% of that of noninvolved side Progress agility drills to full effort as tolerated Add sport-specific tasks as tolerated Begin gradual return to sports once patient can tolerate full effort agility and sport-specific drill and quadriceps strength is at least 85% that of the noninvolved side

ROM, Range of motion; *SLR,* straight leg raises.

machine after PCL reconstruction is contraindicated because most machines do not adequately prevent posterior sagging of the tibia during flexion.

Muscle Performance

Isometric quadriceps exercises in full extension (e.g., quadriceps sets and straight leg raises) should be initiated immediately after surgery. High-intensity electrical stimulation and biofeedback are indicated if the patient has a knee extensor lag. If the knee extensor lag is a result of limited superior glide of the patella, patellar mobilization should be used. As range of motion of the knee improves, limited arc open chain quadriceps exercises from 60 degrees of flexion to full extension are permitted. If the patient has patellofemoral symptoms, it may be necessary to limit the amount of exercise in which extension from 20 degrees of flexion to full extension. Open chain hamstring exercises should be avoided. Closed chain exercises in the form of bilateral partial squats can be performed beginning 1 week after surgery. After 6 weeks, closed chain exercises can be progressed to increase quadriceps loading. These may include wall-slides, unilateral step-ups, leg presses, and squats. Resistance during closed chain exercises must be sufficient to stimulate quadriceps strength development. Open chain hip extension with the knee extended may be initiated after 6 weeks to enhance strength of the hamstrings.

Neuromuscular Control

Once sufficient strength of the lower extremity musculature has been established it is necessary to incorporate activities to develop neuromuscular control to enhance dynamic stability of the knee. This requires learning how to recruit muscles with the proper force, timing, and sequence to prevent abnormal joint motion. A variety of activities can be used to develop neuromuscular control, including balance activities on stable and unstable surfaces, perturbation training, and a variety of agility drills such as acceleration, deceleration, sprinting, jumping, cutting, pivoting, and twisting. These activities are generally progressed from slow to fast speed, from low to high force, and from controlled to uncontrolled activities. Initially the performance of these activities requires conscious effort; however, through practice and repetition, control of abnormal joint motion should become automatic and occur subconsciously.

A number of factors should be considered when planning interventions that are designed to promote compensatory lower extremity neuromuscular responses after PCL reconstruction. Because individuals will encounter a variety of potentially destabilizing forces on the knee during many functional activities, it would seem logical that they are provided with experiences in dealing with these forces during rehabilitation. Therefore treatment techniques should be designed that would allow for application of potentially destabilizing loads to the knee in a controlled manner.

Another factor to consider is that destabilizing loads encountered during functional activities usually occur very rapidly and without warning to the individual, making voluntary neuromuscular responses inadequate for protecting the knee. Therefore treatment techniques should be designed that would promote quick, automatic, protective neuromuscular responses to potentially destabilizing loads. This may be encouraged by applying potentially destabilizing loads to the knee in a quick, random, manner during treatment. Finally, it is important to ensure that treatment techniques designed to enhance the development of protective neuromuscular responses to destabilizing loads provide carryover of learned responses to functional activities. Therefore these techniques may be more successful if they are practiced in the context of functional and sport-specific tasks.

A number of treatment options are available that have the potential for promoting protective neuromuscular responses in the lower extremity to maintain knee stability during physical activity. Balance and agility training techniques, such as shuttle runs, cut and spin drills, cariocas, lateral sliding, and uniaxial and multiaxial balance boards, can be used to provide the individual with experience in dealing with potentially destabilizing loads on the knee during rehabilitation. Wojtys and colleagues[21] reported that subjects who underwent 6 weeks of agility training exhibited improved reaction times in the quadriceps, hamstrings, and gastrocnemius muscles to anterior tibial translational perturbations. It appears that agility training techniques may be useful to enhance protective neuromuscular responses to potentially destabilizing loads on the knee.

Another treatment option for improving neuromuscular control after PCL reconstruction involves perturbing support surfaces, such as roller boards and tilt boards (Figure 14-10). For these techniques the patient stands on the support surface on the involved limb, and potentially destabilizing loads are applied to the knee by the therapist through multidirectional perturbations of the roller board or tilt board. The therapist is able to apply the load in a random manner without warning to the patient in an attempt to encourage quick, automatic responses to the destabilizing loads. These techniques can also be modified so that patients can experience the perturbations during performance of activity-related tasks, which may enhance carryover of learned protective responses to functional performance situations. Ihara and Nakayama[22] and Beard and colleagues[23] have shown that hamstring reaction time and functional ability were improved after training with these techniques. Recently, Fitzgerald and co-workers[24] reported that subjects who were ACL deficient demonstrated a greater likelihood of success of returning to preinjury level sport activities if they received perturbation training than those subjects who did not receive this type of training as part of the rehabilitation program. No studies to date have examined the effectiveness of these treatments in patients after PCL reconstruction; however, it seems logical that these types of training techniques may be useful for rehabilitation of patients after PCL reconstruction.

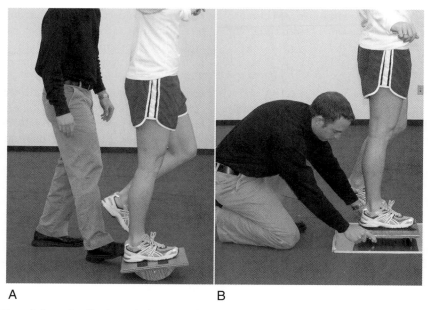

Figure 14-10: A and **B,** Use of tilt and roller boards for perturbation training to enhance neuromuscular control.

The neuromuscular training program after PCL reconstruction begins as soon as the patient can bear full weight on the reconstructed extremity. We begin with standing unilateral balance on a stable support surface. As indicated by the absence of symptoms and the ability to perform the task, we progress the balance activities to unilateral balance on unstable surfaces, such as a foam mat or balance board. When the patient is able to balance on the balance board, we begin to add perturbations to the support surface and also introduce perturbation activities on a roller board. Initially the perturbations are done systematically, but over time we progress to random perturbations to allow the patient to develop quick, automatic responses to the potentially destabilizing loads. To enhance carryover of learned protective responses to functional performance situations we incorporate sport-specific activities such as catching and throwing or dribbling a ball. The incorporation of agility and sports-specific tasks to enhance neuromuscular control are described in the following discussion of the patient's functional program.

Functional Progression for Return to Sport

Once the patient is able to walk normally without symptoms or gait deviations we incorporate a variety of low-impact aerobic activities such as walking, step-machines, or cycling. Typically these activities are initiated 6 to 8 weeks after surgery. Running is initiated once the patient has at least 75% quadriceps strength compared with the uninvolved side. This typically occurs 6 months after surgery. Running is initiated on a treadmill or level running surface. Generally the running program is progressed 10% to 20% per week as indicated by the absence of signs and symptoms (e.g., pain, swelling, instability) or deviations in running form. Agility drills are initiated once the patient has at least 80% quadriceps strength

compared with the uninvolved side and is able to run 1 to 2 miles without symptoms. Agility drills include line drills that incorporate forward and backward running with change in direction, lateral slides, shuttle runs, cut and spin drills, cariocas (i.e., braiding). These activities are begun at half-effort and are progressed to full effort as tolerated. The agility drills are progressed to sport-specific tasks that include reacting to a training partner. Agility drills are typically introduced 7 to 9 months after surgery. The athlete is allowed a gradual return to sport once he or she is tolerating full effort agility and sport-specific drills without signs or symptoms and has at least 85% to 90% quadriceps strength compared with the uninvolved leg. Return to sport begins with a gradual resumption of practice, then return to limited competition and eventual return to full participation. After PCL reconstruction, return to sport typically occurs 9 to 12 months after surgery. Throughout the functional progression for return to sport, the patient should be monitored closely to ensure the absence of symptoms and use of appropriate movement patterns.

Modification of the Rehabilitation Program when PCL Reconstruction Is Combined with Other Procedures

In the multiple ligament–injured knee, PCL reconstruction is often combined with other ligament procedures, most notably ACL reconstruction or reconstruction of the PL corner. Rehabilitation after combined anterior and posterior reconstruction generally follows the guidelines established for rehabilitation after PCL reconstruction described earlier. To avoid undue stress on the grafts after combined PCL and ACL reconstruction, open chain knee extension exercises should be restricted to the range of 75 to 60 degrees of

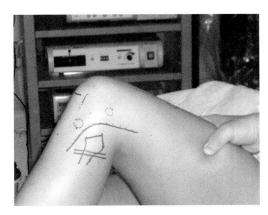

Figure 14-11: Curvilinear lateral incision for repair or reconstruction of the lateral collateral ligament and/or posterolateral corner.

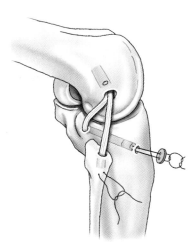

Figure 14-13: Split patellar or Achilles tendon for reconstruction of the popliteus and popliteofibular ligament.

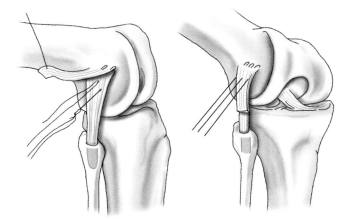

Figure 14-12: Use of allograft to reconstruct the lateral collateral ligament.

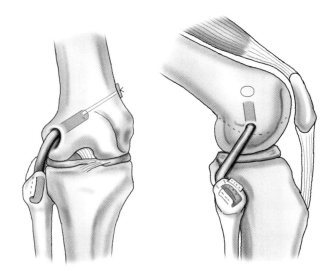

Figure 14-14: The reconstruction of the popliteofibular ligament with advancement of the popliteus muscle (not shown).

flexion. Open kinetic chain knee flexion exercises should be avoided, since unopposed contraction of the hamstrings produces posterior translation of the tibia. Closed kinetic chain exercises should be used to improve quadriceps and hamstring strength. Hamstring strength can be developed by performing open kinetic chain hip extension with the knee in terminal extension.

The PL corner consists of the capsule, arcuate ligament, and popliteus tendon. Injury to the PL corner results in increased PL rotatory laxity. There may be associated varus laxity if the lateral collateral ligament (LCL) is involved. Surgery to reconstruct the PL corner is performed through a curvilinear lateral incision (Figure 14-11). For acute injuries to the LCL and the PL corner, a primary repair of the structures can usually be performed. When the LCL is torn through its midsubstance or in the case of the chronically LCL-deficient knee, reconstruction using a patellar tendon or Achilles tendon allograft is performed (Figure 14-12). For a chronic PL corner injury a reconstruction of the popliteus and popliteofibular ligament is performed using anterior tibialis allograft or hamstring autograft (Figures 14-13 and 14-14).

When PCL reconstruction is combined with reconstruction of the PL corner and/or LCL, patients are placed in a postoperative brace for 6 weeks to minimize varus stress on the knee. During this period limited arc passive range-of-motion exercises at 0 to 90 degrees of flexion can be performed as described earlier for isolated PCL reconstruction. During this time excessive hyperextension of the knee should be avoided. During the first postoperative week isometric quadriceps sets and straight leg raises may be initiated. A touchdown weight-bearing gait is used for the first 4 to 6 weeks after surgery to minimize stress on the PL reconstruction. We have found that early full weight bearing, particularly in the knee, that demonstrates a varus thrust leads to increased varus laxity. After 4 to 6 weeks the patient is progressed to weight bearing as tolerated. The use of assistive devices can be discontinued once the patient has full knee extension without a quadriceps lag and is able to demonstrate a normal gait pattern. This typically occurs 8 weeks after surgery.

The rehabilitation brace is discontinued 6 weeks postoperatively. At this time, emphasis is placed on regaining full motion of the knee, taking care to avoid excessive hyperextension. Muscle strength and endurance are developed using open and closed kinetic chain exercises. Open kinetic chain knee extension exercises from 60 degrees of flexion to full extension may be performed through the arc of motion as tolerated by the patellofemoral joint. Open kinetic chain knee flexion exercises place undue stress on both the PCL and PL corner and should be avoided. Closed kinetic chain exercises may be performed to increase quadriceps and hamstring strength. Hip abduction with resistance applied to the distal aspect of the leg should be avoided. Balance and proprioceptive activities are initiated once the patient is fully weight bearing to regain neuromuscular control of the knee. Low-impact aerobic exercises such as walking, swimming, and cycling may be initiated 8 to 12 weeks after surgery. Running may be initiated 6 months after surgery provided the individual has at least 80% quadriceps strength compared with the contralateral leg. Return to sports activities may begin 9 to 12 months after surgery.

SUMMARY

Rehabilitation after PCL reconstruction requires an understanding of the surgical procedure as well as of the biologic and biomechanical factors that affect rehabilitation. Rehabilitation after PCL reconstruction should focus on resolving impairments and lessening functional limitations and disability. Impairments associated with PCL reconstruction include pain, swelling, loss of motion, decreased muscle performance, and decreased neuromuscular control. Rehabilitation should be directed at resolving these impairments. Guidelines for postoperative bracing, weight bearing, range of motion, muscle performance, neuromuscular control, and functional progression for return to sport have been provided. Guidelines for modifying rehabilitation after PCL reconstruction when concomitant ACL reconstruction or repair or reconstruction of the PL corner is performed have also been provided.

References

1. Hey Groves EW: Operation for the repair of the crucial ligaments, *Lancet* 2: 674-675, 1917.
2. Hey Groves EW: The crucial ligaments of the knee joint. Their function, rupture, and operative treatment of the same, *Br J Surg* 17:505-515, 1919.
3. Trickey EL: Injuries to the posterior cruciate ligament. Diagnosis and treatment of early injuries and reconstruction of late instability, *Clin Orthop* 147:76-81, 1980.
4. Andrews J, Soffer S: Posterior cruciate reconstruction with bone-patellar tendon-bone autografts. In Scott WN, editor: *The knee,* Baltimore, 1994, Williams & Wilkins.
5. Augustine RW: The unstable knee, *Am J Surg* 92:380, 1956.
6. Clancy WG, Narechania RG, Rosenberg TD, et al: Anterior and posterior cruciate ligament reconstruction in rhesus monkeys. A histological microangiographic and biochemical analysis, *J Bone Joint Surg Am* 63:1270-1284, 1981.
7. Clancy WG Jr, Nelson DA, Reider B, Narechania RG: Anterior cruciate ligament reconstruction using one third of the patellar ligament augmented by extra-articular tendon transfers, *J Bone Joint Surg Am* 64:352-359, 1982.
8. Schulte KR, Harner CD: Management of isolated posterior cruciate ligament injuries, *Op Tech Orthop* 5: 270, 1995.
9. Swenson TM, Harner CD, Fu FH: Arthroscopic posterior cruciate ligament reconstruction with allograft, *Sports Med Arthrosc Rev* 2:120-128, 1994.
10. Parolie JM, Bergfeld JA: Long-term results of nonoperative treatment of isolated posterior cruciate ligament injuries in the athlete, *Am J Sports Med* 14:35-38, 1986.
11. Arnoczky SP, Tarvin GB, Marshall JL: Anterior cruciate ligament replacement using patellar tendon. An evaluation of graft revascularization in the dog, *J Bone Joint Surg Am* 64:217-224, 1982.
12. Yasuda K, Tomiyama Y, Ohkoshi Y, Kaneda K: Arthroscopic observations of autogeneic quadriceps and patellar tendon grafts after anterior cruciate ligament reconstruction of the knee, *Clin Orthop* 246:217-224, 1989.
13. Jackson DW, Grood ES, Goldstein JD, et al: A comparison of patellar tendon autograft and allograft used for anterior cruciate ligament reconstruction in the goat model, *Am J Sports Med* 21:176-185, 1993.
14. Rodeo SA, Arnoczky SP, Torzilli PA, et al: Tendon-healing in a bone tunnel. A biomechanical and histological study in the dog, *J Bone Joint Surg Am* 75:1795-1803, 1993.
15. Tomita F, Yasuda K, Mikami S, et al: Comparisons of intraosseous graft healing between the doubled flexor tendon graft and the bone-patellar tendon-bone graft in the anterior cruciate ligament reconstruction, *Athroscopy* 17:461-476, 2001.
16. Daniel DM, Stone ML, Barnett P, Sachs R: Use of the quadriceps active test to diagnose posterior cruciate-ligament disruption and measure posterior laxity of the knee, *J Bone Joint Surg* 70-A:386-391, 1988.
17. Giffin JR, Vogrin TM, Zantop T, et al: Effects of increasing tibial slope on the biomechanics of the knee, *Am J Sports Med* 32:376-382, 2004.
18. Ninos JC, Irrgang JJ, Burdett R, Weiss JR: Electromyographic analysis of the squat performed in self-selected lower extremity neutral rotation and 30° of lower extremity turn-out from the self-selected neutral position, *J Orthop Sports Phys Ther* 25:307-315, 1997.
19. Grood ES, Suntay WJ, Noyes FR, Butler DI: Biomechanics of the knee-extension exercise, *J Bone Joint Surg* 66A:725-733, 1984.
20. Hungerford DS, Barry M: Biomechanics of the patellofemoral joint, *Clin Orthop* 144:9-15, 1979.
21. Wojtys EM, Huston LJ, Taylor P, Bastian SD: Neuromuscular adaptations in isokinetic, isotonic, and agility training programs, *Am J Sports Med* 24:187-192, 1996.
22. Ihara H, Nakayama A: Dynamic joint control training for knee ligament injuries, *Am J Sports Med* 14:309-315, 1986.
23. Beard DJ, Dodd CAF, Trundle HR, Simpson AHRW: Proprioception enhancement for anterior cruciate ligament deficiency, *J Bone Joint Surg Br* 76:654-659, 1994.
24. Fitzgerald GK, Axe MJ, Snyder-Mackler L: The efficacy of perturbation training in non-operative anterior cruciate ligament rehabilitation programs for physically active, *Phys Ther* 80:128-140, 2000.

CHAPTER 15

Treatment of Collateral Ligament Injuries of the Knee

Gary Sutton, PT, MS, SCS, OCS, ATC, CSCS
Julious P. Smith III, MD

THE KNEE JOINT IS FREQUENTLY IN-JURED during participation in athletics. Of all the injuries sustained at the knee, injury to the ligamentous structures accounts for 25% to 40% of the total.[1] These ligamentous structures that offer the primary static stability to the knee are collectively referred to as the *cruciate* and *collateral ligaments.* The cruciate ligaments, the anterior cruciate and posterior cruciate, are well recognized for their contribution to knee function in gait, as well as in athletic endeavors. Conversely, the collateral ligaments present somewhat of a paradox.

The medial, or tibial, collateral ligament is the most frequently sprained ligament of the knee.[2] Although frequency of injury is high, current management of isolated medial collateral ligament (MCL) tears rarely favors surgical repair. The lateral, or fibular, collateral ligament (LCL) is rarely injured,[1,3] but the stability afforded by this ligament and adjacent soft tissues to the posterior and lateral sides of the knee is significant. Persistent posterolateral rotatory instability is recognized as one of the causes of poor outcomes following surgical reconstruction of the anterior cruciate ligament (ACL)–deficient knee or the posterior cruciate ligament (PCL)–deficient knee.[2]

Controversy exists regarding the most accurate methods of assessing posterolateral instability of the knee. In addition, clinical parameters used to determine the necessity for surgical repair of torn collateral ligaments when observed in conjunction with ACL or PCL deficiency in the traumatized knee remain vague.

This chapter discusses anatomy, biomechanics, mechanisms of injury, and clinical examination techniques of the medial and lateral compartments of the knee. A review of current operative approaches to the medial and lateral compartments is presented. Consideration is given to the operative and nonoperative rehabilitation of the collateral ligaments of the knee and development of a functional exercise progression emphasizing multiple-plane stability.

FUNCTIONAL ANATOMY OF THE COLLATERAL LIGAMENTS

The medial aspect of the knee is supported by a broad, flat connective tissue band that runs from the medial epicondyle of the femur to a point of insertion two to three finger widths below the medial joint line on the tibia. This tibial collateral ligament, or MCL, has been described as a thickening of the medial capsule of the knee and is divided into superficial and deep layers. The deep layer of the MCL attaches intimately with the medial meniscus, forming a superior meniscofemoral ligament and an inferior meniscotibial ligament. Slocum and colleagues[4] considered the deep fibers of the MCL to be the middle third of the medial joint capsule (Figure 15-1).

The superficial portion of the MCL lies further from the instant center of the knee and becomes the first ligament loaded in withstanding valgus stresses applied to the knee. Warren and colleagues[5] described the anterior 5 mm of the MCL as tightening when the knee flexes and relaxing when

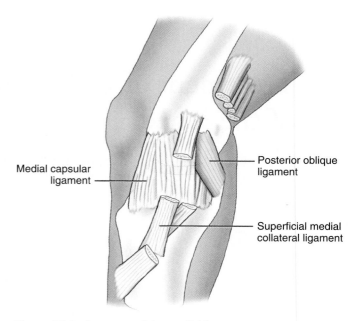

Figure 15-1: Anatomy of the medial knee.

Medial capsular ligament

Posterior oblique ligament

Superficial medial collateral ligament

the knee extends, suggesting varying degrees of stability afforded by the superficial MCL at varying angles of sagittal plane motion. Grood and colleagues[6] reported on tissue-sectioning studies that demonstrated that the superficial MCL primarily functions to provide 78% of the valgus restraint when the knee is flexed to 25 degrees. The ACL and PCL account for 13% of the total stability at 25 degrees of flexion, and the deep anterior, middle, and posterior capsular ligaments provide just over 7% of the valgus restraint. When the knee is positioned in full extension, the superficial MCL contributes 57% of the valgus restraint; the deep capsular ligaments afford 25%, particularly the posterior third of the medial capsule; and the cruciate ligaments provide 15% of the stability.

A second function of the medial capsular ligaments is to prevent external rotation of the tibia on the femur.[5] Sectioning studies have demonstrated only minimal increase in tibial external rotation when the deep fibers of the MCL were cut. Conversely, sectioning of the superficial portion of the MCL results in tibial external rotation of approximately 6 degrees with the knee held in extension and external rotation of 18 degrees with the knee flexed to 90 degrees.

A third function of the MCL recognizes this structure as a secondary restraint against anterior tibial translation, particularly in the absence of an intact ACL.[7] Cutting the superficial and deep fibers of the MCL and the anterior and posterior thirds of the medial capsule did not increase anterior tibial translation in an ACL-intact knee. Sectioning of the ACL first, followed by the superficial MCL, allowed significant increases in anterior tibial translation.

The lateral aspect of the knee is likewise supported by superficial and deeper-positioned ligamentous structures, although the deep structures are subject to anatomic varia-

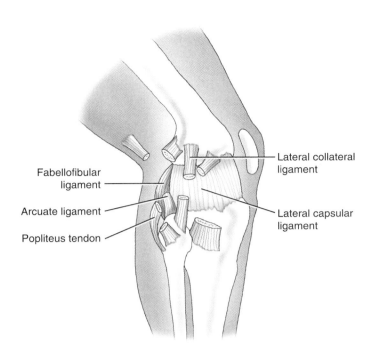

Figure 15-2: Anatomy of the lateral knee.

Labels: Fabellofibular ligament, Arcuate ligament, Popliteus tendon, Lateral collateral ligament, Lateral capsular ligament

tion and primary stabilizing function is more difficult to define (Figure 15-2).

The LCL runs from the lateral femoral condyle to the fibular head and provides primary restraint against varus forces at 5 and 25 degrees of knee flexion, much the same as the superficial MCL.[6] Seebacher and colleagues[8] describe the deeper ligamentous structures supporting the lateral capsule as being the fabellofibular ligament and the arcuate ligament. The fabellofibular ligament originates from the head of the fibula, inserts into the fabella (the sesamoid bone sometimes found in the lateral head of the gastrocnemius muscle), and inserts into the posterior capsule. The arcuate ligament likewise originates from the fibular head and merges into the posterior capsule. When the fabella is present, the fabellofibular ligament is considered the primary stabilizer of the posterolateral corner of the knee. When the fabella is absent, the arcuate ligament provides the primary posterolateral support.[8]

MECHANISMS OF INJURY OF THE COLLATERAL LIGAMENTS

The frequently injured MCL is damaged as a result of a valgus or combined valgus and external rotation force that exceeds the tensile strength of the ligament.[9] This mechanism of injury is commonly seen in collision sports such as football and hockey in which blows are sustained on the lateral aspect of the knee, but the forces are translated to the medial ligamentous restraints. The MCL can also be damaged by a fall laterally over a fixed foot that frequently results in a combined injury to the MCL and ACL.

Age of the injured subject will affect the site of MCL failures.[9] In animal studies, Tipton and colleagues[10] and Woo and colleagues[11] reported that in the skeletally immature the bone-MCL-bone complex failed at the tibial attachment because of attachment site proximity to the open tibial growth plate. Once the epiphysis was closed, midsubstance tears of the MCL were more common. Conversely, subjects older than 50 years of age demonstrate a higher incidence of bony avulsion fractures than do their younger counterparts in similar loading of the bone-ligament-bone complex.[12]

Isolated injuries of the LCL are the least common injury to the knee and account for only 2% of all knee injuries that result in pathologic motion.[3] The force that injures the LCL is direct varus, generally with the foot planted and knee positioned in extension. Injuries to the LCL seldom occur in sports as a result of a direct medial-to-lateral blow, but instead are the result of high-energy activities that cause sudden imbalance in stance. Such an imbalance may result from stepping in a hole such that the center of gravity is quickly shifted toward the midline, away from the stance leg, applying an immediate load to the lateral aspect of the knee.[13]

Straight varus forces directed on the knee tend to generate LCL tears with or without avulsion from the fibular head in 75% of cases, from the femoral attachment in 20%, and from midsubstance tears in 5%.[14] Straight-plane varus injuries of the knee may generate injury to the peroneal nerve as a result of tethering as it courses around the fibular head, often with poor prognosis for complete recovery. The varus mechanism of injury is often associated with injuries to other ligaments of the knee. A large varus force directed through the knee sequentially damages the LCL, then the posterolateral capsule, and then the PCL.

For several reasons, each of these structures when injured presents a challenge to initial clinical examination. First, the mechanism of injury is less obvious than other mechanisms at the knee. Second, the degree of knee effusion for injuries to the posterolateral capsule and posterior cruciate ligament is most often negligible, and the LCL, being extraarticular, does not generate knee effusion. Third, clinical tests for these conditions are subtle and varied, particularly for injuries of the posterolateral capsule.

CLINICAL EXAMINATION OF THE COLLATERAL LIGAMENTS

For every individual with a complaint of knee pain, a thorough history of the cause and progression of the pain should be ascertained to ensure an accurate diagnosis. Determination of the mechanism of injury is the key to solving the puzzle of pain. Athletes are typically adept in recollection of body position, forces applied, resultant motions, noises emulating from the joint in question, initial site of pain, and any observed deformity. Further answers to questions concerning the time of injury; the onset of joint effusion; symptoms of locking, buckling, or giving way; current aggravating activities; progression and current level of pain; and history of previous injury should provide the examiner with the information needed to establish a hypothesis for the cause of the knee pain.

Physical examination of the knee must be represented by a standard battery of manual techniques used to gain an appreciation of the individual's current localization of pain, active and passive ranges of motion, strengths of muscles supporting the joint, functional activity level available (including gait pattern), degree of joint effusion present, and level of ligamentous stability present at the joint. Each of these manual techniques should be performed in rote sequence while observing deviations from expected normative measures. Because each standard battery of manual techniques for the most part takes on the personality of the examiner based on that examiner's skill and experience, further discussion of these techniques is beyond the scope of this chapter.

However, further review of tests used to determine ligamentous stability of the knee is necessary in defining injury of the collateral ligaments. Whereas the standard tests to observe point tenderness, range of motion (ROM), strength, gait, and effusion are routinely performed on all individuals with knee pain, special tests used to define knee stability are selected in an effort to confirm the examiner's hypothesis of injury based on findings from the patient's history.

A patient history is described by a football offensive lineman attempting to maintain a block on a defender when he perceived a teammate being pushed onto the lateral aspect of his right knee. A "pop" was felt, with immediate right medial knee pain. Swelling was immediate along the medial knee, spread throughout the knee in subsequent hours. Active and passive range of motion (PROM) of the knee was limited to lacking 30 degrees from full extension to 60 degrees of flexion at 4 days postinjury, limited by complaints of pain at the ends of the patient's available range. Strength of the

patient's quadriceps muscles was 4/5 within the available ROM, but limited by complaints of medial knee pain on attempts to straighten into extension beyond 30 degrees. His hamstring strength was 3-/5, limited by complaints of medial knee pain throughout his ROM. He ambulated in an antalgic gait on right lower extremity midstance, with weight bearing on the ball of his right foot secondary to complaints of pain in attempts to walk with greater foot contact.

Based on his history and on the hypothesis of injury to the MCL, the valgus stress test should be performed at full extension and at 30 degrees of flexion. This test is recognized to assess the integrity of the MCL and medial capsule in one plane.[14] The test begins with the patient lying supine with the thigh supported on the treatment table and leg supported by the examiner off the treatment table. The examiner's hand is positioned over the lateral joint line and the examiner's opposite hand supports the patient's medial ankle, holding the extremity in slight external rotation. The knee is first tested in full extension by applying a lateral-to-medial force through the examiner's proximal hand while stabilizing the ankle (Figure 15-3). Next, the knee is flexed 30 degrees by lowering the patient's ankle below the level of the table. Again, a lateral-to-medial force, or valgus force, is directed through the knee while stabilizing the patient's ankle.

Severity of MCL and LCL tears is determined by extent of the tear as visualized by the degree of laxity observed when the ligament is specifically stressed. A grade I sprain is conceptualized as microscopic tearing of the ligament substance, but no appreciable change in length of the ligament can be observed. Changes in ligament length are measured against the amount of laxity observed in performing the same ligament stress test on the noninvolved extremity. Further determination of the degree of ligament laxity is based on the experience and skill of the examiner in assessing "normal"

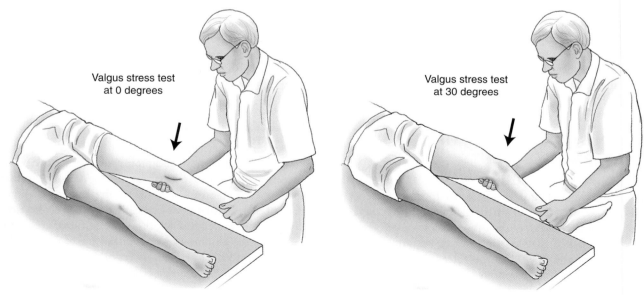

Figure 15-3: Valgus stress test performed at 0 degrees and at 30 degrees.

ligament stability recognized in previously examined knees. A grade II sprain also represents a partial tear, but results in partial loss of ligament function in that a slight increase in joint opening is observed while maintaining a definite end point when stressed. In valgus testing of the MCL in 30 degrees of flexion, a 3 to 5 mm opening of the medial joint line may be noted, but the knee demonstrates less than 2 mm difference compared with the noninvolved knee when the valgus is stressed in full extension. A grade III sprain is categorized as a complete tear of the ligament causing loss of function demonstrating greater than 5 mm opening of the medial joint line in 30 degrees of flexion, as well as greater than 3 mm of medial opening in full knee extension for MCL tears.[14]

An additional special test to identify medial capsular instability of the knee was described by Slocum and colleagues.[15] The test represents a modification to the anterior drawer test. The anterior drawer test,[14] used to determine single-plane instability in a posterior-to-anterior direction, is demonstrated by positioning the patient supine on an examination table with the ipsilateral hip flexed to 45 degrees and the knee flexed to 90 degrees. The examiner sits on the patient's forefoot to stabilize the leg while grasping the posterior aspect of the proximal tibia. With bilateral index fingers palpating the hamstring muscle insertions to ensure relaxation and bilateral thumbs positioned over the anterior joint lines to appreciate anterior tibial translation, the examiner applies an anteriorly directed force. The amount of perceived anterior translation and the firmness of the end point of the motion are compared with those of the contralateral knee and with recollections of previous tests performed by the examiner.

Slocum's modification of the anterior drawer test for medial laxity involves positioning the patient's foot and leg in approximately 15 degrees of external rotation, sitting on the forefoot to stabilize the leg, and applying a similar anteriorly directed force (Figure 15-4). A positive test for "anteromedial rotatory instability" is observed when a greater amount of anterior translation occurs in the medial compartment, generating a relative increase in tibial external rotation, or the amount of anterior tibial translation is the same as or greater than when the force is applied with the tibia in neutral or internal rotation. Rotatory instabilities as classified by Hughston and colleagues[16] maintain that ligamentous instability may occur in a straight plane or follow a rotatory path if the integrity of the PCL is maintained. If the PCL is intact, the medial and lateral knee compartments may sublux anteriorly in simple or combined instabilities medially or laterally (or both) with the intact PCL acting as a pivot point. The instability is named for the direction of tibial translation followed by the name of the compartment that subluxes. Thus anteromedial, anterolateral, posteromedial, and posterolateral rotatory instabilities must be recognized in the evaluation of collateral ligaments of the knee.

As with the case history of the patient who has injured his or her MCL, individuals suspected to have injured their LCL

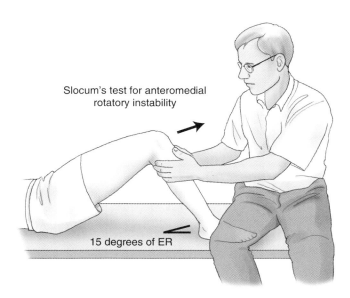

Slocum's test for anteromedial rotatory instability

15 degrees of ER

Figure 15-4: Slocum's test for anteromedial rotatory instability.

and lateral capsular ligaments have common mechanisms in their case histories. A recreational runner describes hearing a pop in his left knee when he inadvertently stepped in a hole while running at dawn. He complains of left lateral knee pain without swelling and describes a "shifting sensation" when attempting to walk on uneven ground. Active range of motion (AROM) of the left knee is within normal limits, as is manual muscle testing except for hamstring strength graded 4/5 with complaints of pain on resisted testing. Ambulation is accomplished without assistive device and may demonstrate a slight lateral shift, or varus thrust through the left lower extremity in midstance position. Complaints of left lateral knee pain may develop after maintained stance or with ambulation. Such a scenario prompts the examiner to perform special tests to determine the integrity of the lateral ligamentous structures.

Palpation of the LCL is easily accomplished by positioning the patient supine and placing the ankle of the involved extremity across the opposite knee, which has been flexed to a 90-degree angle, creating a "figure of 4." With the knee maintained in a relaxed posture, the LCL can be palpated as a firm, taut band in its normal state, or pathologically as being soft, mushy, or indistinguishable. The examiner should palpate the noninvolved LCL for comparison.

Based on the previous case history, the varus stress test should be performed with the knee maintained in full extension, and then with the knee flexed to 30 degrees. With the patient positioned supine, the examiner stabilizes the ankle while applying a medial-to-lateral force to the knee of the extremity in question with the knee maintained in full extension (Figure 15-5). This test position, maintained in full extension, enables the clinician to examine the stability afforded by the LCL, posterolateral capsule, arcuate-popliteus complex, iliotibial band, biceps femoris tendon, ACL, PCL, and lateral head of the gastrocnemius muscle.[14] The

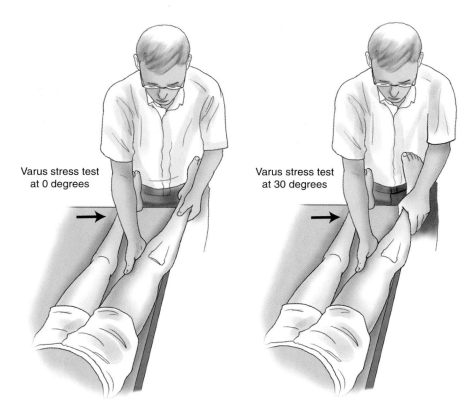

Figure 15-5: Varus stress test performed at 0 degrees and at 30 degrees.

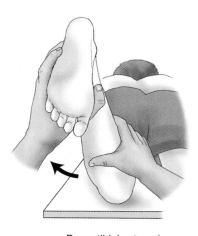

Prone tibial external
rotation test at 30 degrees

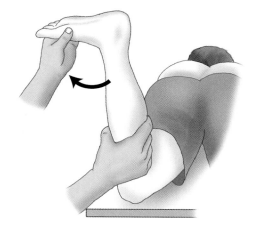

Prone tibial external
rotation test at 90 degrees

Figure 15-6: Prone external rotation test.

test movement is repeated with the knee flexed to 30 degrees (see Figure 15-5). Slight flexion serves to relax the previously mentioned secondary constraints, allowing primary testing of the LCL. As with testing the MCL, the degree of laxity of the lateral structures is determined by measurement of lateral joint line opening and firmness of the end points palpated in single-plane, varus stress testing.

Veltri and Warren[17] describe the prone external rotation test in assessment of lateral capsular laxity (Figure 15-6).

With the patient lying prone, the examiner attempts to externally rotate the leg with the knee positioned at 30 degrees of flexion and again at 90 degrees of flexion. The medial border of the foot, held in neutral alignment, is used as the reference point for external rotation, and the tibial plateaus are palpated to determine their relationship to the femoral condyles. The "normal" knee is compared with measurements of the "involved" knee, and differences of 10 degrees are considered to be evidence of pathology. If laxity is apparent at the 30-

degree test position, injury to the posterolateral capsule is indicated. If laxity is apparent at 90 degrees of flexion, injury to both the PCL and the posterolateral capsule is expected.

Additional tests used to discern lateral ligamentous laxity of the knee are numerous. Several tests attempt to determine lateral compartment instability in light of injury to the ACL and PCL. The pivot shift test, Losee test, Hughston jerk test, posterolateral drawer test, reverse pivot shift test, and external rotation recurvatum test have been described by Irrgang,[14] as well as the Slocum test,[15] and are beyond the scope of detailed description in this chapter.

TREATMENT OF COLLATERAL LIGAMENT INJURIES OF THE KNEE

As previously described, the surgical treatment of MCL injuries has changed greatly over the last 65 years. Whereas all medial ligament injuries were previously treated with surgical repair,[18-22] the indications for operative treatment of an acute, isolated MCL injury are now very limited. The movement away from operative care was not a condemnation of the results of those treated surgically; results on these patients were actually quite good.[20-24] The change was instead due to a realization that those treated nonoperatively could attain the same excellent results seen with operative treatment.[25-27] Basic science studies have since shown that the similarities between the two different treatments extend to histologic and biomechanical levels,[2,28,29] with most studies showing no difference in tensile strength or microscopic variation between MCL injuries that were repaired and those treated conservatively. As a result of these findings, nearly all isolated acute MCL injuries are presently treated nonoperatively. Operative treatment still has its indications, however, especially in combined ligament injuries and chronic MCL tears. These indications are reviewed in the following section. Because of the differences in treatment algorithms, acute and chronic injuries are discussed separately.

As nonoperative treatment has become more accepted in acute injuries, much of the focus of research has turned to the factors that influence outcomes. Some papers have focused on how the grade of the injury (I, II, or III) affects results.[25,27,30-33] Others have focused on the success in the treatment of isolated MCL injuries compared with that of combined ligament knee injuries.[27,30,34] Both of these factors remain important in the decision of how to approach MCL injuries.

Since first described in detail by Fetto and Marshall,[25] isolated grade I and grade II injuries of the MCL have been almost universally treated nonoperatively.[27,28,30-33] The results of studies have shown such excellent healing that there has been little push to investigate other options. Much of the work has instead focused on the best method of rehabilitating these injuries, which has evolved from cast immobilization to early intervention encouraging ROM.[2,29,35] Much of the success in recovery of grade I to II injuries is related to the fact that the ACL is often intact and acts as a secondary stabilizer against valgus stress at the knee, giving the MCL a chance to heal in a normal position. There are very few cases in which acute grade II injuries of the MCL should be treated operatively, and no real indications for operative treatment of grade I injuries. Grade II injuries are sometimes repaired if the injury is severe and mimics a grade III injury. Most other indications for repairing a grade II lesion involve injuries to other knee structures. These combination injuries include concomitant damage to the meniscus, ACL, PCL, LCL, or posteromedial corner of the knee. These combined injuries are discussed in a later section.

Treatment of isolated grade III MCL injuries is one of the few aspects of the treatment of medial knee injuries that remains controversial. While many papers have shown good results at biomechanical, histologic, and clinical levels by treating grade III lesions conservatively,[19,25,26,28-30,36] there remain those who endorse operative treatment of these complete ligament ruptures. The present opinion of the majority of orthopedic surgeons supports conservative management of these injuries with bracing and rehabilitation after determination that the lesion is definitely isolated. Grade III lesions involve a significant force and often disrupt other structures in addition to the MCL, so good diagnostic evaluation is critical. Although magnetic resonance imaging (MRI) has made this much easier, the physical examination is still the most important evaluation tool. Evaluation of the posteromedial corner of the knee is critical to ensure that the posterior capsule is intact. Failure to recognize injury of the posterior capsule will result in persistent symptomatic instability if not repaired. Complete tear of the MCL in conjunction with injury to any of the other knee ligaments or the meniscus also requires operative intervention.

Grade II and III injuries to the MCL that also involve other major knee structures often require operative treatment, although the MCL is not always the structure that is repaired. The structures that are most commonly injured along with the MCL are the ACL, the medial meniscus, the posteromedial capsule, and the PCL. Combined tears of the MCL and ACL usually require at minimum ACL reconstruction, but the need to openly repair the MCL has been debated. Many surgeons are now recommending reconstruction of the ACL, reexamination of valgus stability, and allowing the MCL to heal conservatively if stability is adequate.[37-40] Although early studies yielded poor results with this technique,[25,41] more recent data show that nonoperative treatment of the MCL leads to less postoperative stiffness with equal outcomes.[39] If the ACL is not reconstructed in an ACL/MCL injury, open repair of the MCL is necessary to avoid persistent medial instability, because the ACL cannot provide the secondary support needed to allow the MCL to heal. The same is true when an incomplete tear of the ACL occurs in conjunction with an MCL tear and the ACL is damaged enough that medial stability is compromised.

Treatment of combined MCL/meniscal injuries is somewhat variable. Some recommend open repair of the meniscus with concomitant open MCL and capsular repair. Others recommend inside-out suture repair of the meniscus with capsular repair, if necessary, but no MCL repair. Both techniques have seen good results and are reasonable if no other injury is present. As mentioned, posteromedial corner injuries, which involve injury to the posteromedial capsule, the posterior oblique ligament, and often the medial meniscus, require open repair of all of the structures to their anatomic position. Failure to do this will result in chronic instability.

Treatment algorithms for PCL/MCL injuries are also variable. Whereas some advocate repair of the PCL and MCL, others recommend repair of either the PCL or MCL and rehabilitation of the other.[42,43] Complicating the decision is the fact that the posteromedial corner is also often involved and must be repaired. Staged treatment with repair of the medial structures followed by delayed reconstruction of the PCL is an option in this situation. Staging the operation can decrease the amount of postoperative arthrofibrosis,[43] but it requires a second operation. Obviously the decision is patient dependent.

Chronic cases of medial instability are rarely limited to the collateral ligament alone. Most cases are the result of a fairly significant injury that involves the posterior oblique ligament or posteromedial corner of the knee (or both). Although these injuries can be difficult to treat, most can be managed conservatively with a combination of therapy and bracing. Unless there is an obvious bony deformity or gait disturbance caused by instability, rehabilitation should be the first-line treatment for these problems. There are some instances in which conservative measures fail, mostly in those athletes who place higher demands on their knees. In those circumstances, surgical intervention with repair of the affected structures is undertaken.

OPERATIVE TREATMENT OF THE MEDIAL KNEE

Unlike the reconstruction seen with cruciate ligament injury, most surgical intervention involving the MCL involves repair of the affected structures. Very rarely do autografts or allografts play a role in the procedure, because the affected structures can usually be identified and restored. Thorough knowledge of the anatomy and the ability to re-create that anatomy are the essential factors in successful repair of the medial side.

Most surgical repairs of the medial side of the knee are preceded by arthroscopic evaluation to determine intraarticular damage in the knee. Once the joint has been thoroughly inspected, the scope is removed and a medial incision is made along the midline curving distally parallel to the patella tendon and just medial to it. The underlying retinaculum is incised in line with the skin incision and reflected to expose the underlying ligament and capsule. The damaged structures are then identified and dissected out. The MCL is examined first and the site of its injury is identified. The posterior oblique ligament and capsule are then carefully

identified, and their injury is evaluated. With careful planning, the surgical repair is begun.

First, the MCL is repaired. Avulsions of the bony MCL attachments can be repaired either with suture anchors or with a screw and washer. Midsubstance tears are repaired with end-to-end opposition and then reinforced with capsular tissue. After the MCL has been re-created, necessary meniscal repair is performed. The capsule is then reattached to the bone, taking care to advance the capsule anteriorly as necessary to tighten any area that might have been stretched. At the same time, the posterior oblique ligament is advanced anteriorly and superiorly to again tighten the posteromedial corner. Reattachment of all of the structures can be done using either drill holes through the tibia/femur or suture anchors at the insertion sites. Special care should be taken to ensure that the ligament is attached to the proper position on the bone and that the ligament is not in any way shortened. Shortening the ligament alters the flexion-extension characteristics of the knee and can change the kinematics of the knee. The fascia and skin are then closed and the patient is placed in a double upright brace to prevent varus and valgus stress to the repair. If the posteromedial corner of the knee is involved, the last 10 to 30 degrees of extension is often blocked to protect the repair for the first 2 to 3 postoperative weeks.

NONOPERATIVE TREATMENT OF MEDIAL COLLATERAL LIGAMENT INJURY

Historically, treatment approaches for ligamentous injuries of the knee have focused on restoring normal anatomy by primary repair of the injured tissues. Isolated tears of the MCL were similarly treated by surgical reapproximation of the tissue ends by arthrotomy of the knee.[20] More recent clinical studies suggest excellent outcomes from a nonoperative approach in the treatment of grade I and II injuries[44] and complete isolated tears of the MCL.[45] These nonoperative rehabilitation strategies focused on immediate ROM, early weight bearing in ambulation, and progressive strength training. Immediate motion and progressive exercise are theorized to provide a stimulus to the medial ligamentous structures to facilitate earlier and enhanced healing of these injured tissues. Unfortunately, healing rates and mechanical properties of the injured MCL are altered and often delayed when combined with complete ACL tears.[9] As previously stated, controversy exists regarding the need for surgical repair of both torn ligaments, as well as the timing of the repair, in combined MCL/ACL injuries.[46]

Wilk and colleagues[9] outline "optimal conditions for MCL healing" as (1) maintenance of the torn fibers in close continuity, (2) an intact and stable ACL along with stability afforded by other ligamentous structures, (3) immediate controlled motion and controlled progressive loading of the healing ligament, and (4) protection of the MCL against deleterious stresses that would cause further injury, including valgus and external rotation.

These "optimal conditions" can be promoted in a phased rehabilitation program. The concept of rehabilitation "phases" dictates progression through the program based on therapist interpretation of ligament healing and the need for ligament protection. As a result, progression through the phases is based on accomplishing the "criteria for progression" as opposed to a timeline based on lapsed time from injury or surgery. Phase I, a period for maximal protection of the injured MCL, emphasizes protected active motion of the injured knee in a pain-free arc of motion. Other objectives in phase I include prevention of quadriceps atrophy and reduction of pain and joint effusion. Phase II, a period of moderate ligament protection, can be entered as signs of acute injury diminish, including stabilization of joint effusion, degree of instability, and tenderness to palpation. Tolerance to having the injured knee moved as demonstrated by PROM of 10 to 100 degrees is also required. Goals of phase II include full pain-free AROM, restoration of normal quadriceps and hamstring muscle strengths, and independent ambulation. Phase III, a period of minimal ligament protection, requires a knee that demonstrates full AROM and PROM, as well as absent effusion, tenderness, and instability. Goals of phase III involve restoration of strength and power. Phase IV describes criteria for return to competition. In addition to full ROM, absence of effusion, instability, and palpation tenderness are necessary. Functional parameters such as muscle strength at 85% or better compared with the noninvolved extremity, acceptable quadriceps muscle strength–to–body weight ratios, and proprioceptive abilities comparable with the noninvolved extremity are measured. Once these criteria are achieved, allowing for return to competition, phase IV emphasizes a program to maintain current levels of strength, flexibility, and proprioception, allowing the athlete to enter sport-specific training cycles based on proximity to his or her competitive season. Such a non-operative rehabilitation program for the isolated grade I or II MCL sprain has been detailed by Wilk and colleagues[9] (Box 15-1).

TREATMENT OF THE LATERAL SIDE OF THE KNEE

Restoration of patient function remains the standard of care in treating patients with posterolateral instability of the knee. Determination of an operative or a nonoperative approach is required in the treatment of posterolateral instability, but current strategies stand in contrast to the conservative approaches used in the care of grade III MCL injuries. Kannus[47] performed an 8-year follow-up on 11 patients diagnosed with grade II lateral ligament sprains and 12 patients with grade III lateral ligament sprains. Outcomes for patients with grade II injuries demonstrated an 82% return to preinjury activities with the injured knee supported by quadriceps and hamstring muscle strength comparable to the nonin-

volved extremity, negligible thigh atrophy, and no radiographic evidence of posttraumatic osteoarthritis despite maintained lateral ligament laxity observed in varus stress testing at 30 degrees of flexion. In contrast, 8-year follow-up of the patients with grade III injuries revealed decreased physical activity as a result of the injury in 75% of the cases. Strength was assessed to be deficient by 23% in the quadriceps and 14% in the hamstring muscles measured isokinetically, and thigh circumference was reduced an average of 1.5 cm. Ligament laxity was maintained and believed to have developed additional straight-plane instabilities anteriorly and posteriorly. More significant was the finding that 50% of the sample had developed posttraumatic osteoarthritis. Although retrospective and descriptive in nature, this report questions the efficacy of nonoperative treatment of grade III LCL tears.

OPERATIVE TREATMENT OF THE LATERAL KNEE

Operative treatment of injury to the lateral side of the knee is highly patient dependent, much like treatment of the medial knee. Decisions are made based on which lateral structures are injured and the severity of those injuries. Isolated injuries to the LCL are much less common than the MCL,[48,49] so management usually requires treatment of the posterolateral structures as well as the LCL. Again, knowledge of the anatomy and the ability to re-create that anatomy are the keys to successful treatment.

The LCL is quite strong, and injuries to that structure often involve significant force, causing injury to other structures at the same time. When isolated injuries do occur, treatment is largely based on the grade of the injury. All grade I and most grade II isolated injuries can be treated conservatively using bracing and rehabilitation. Severe grade II and all grade III isolated injuries do poorly with conservative care and require operative treatment.[47] Persistent instability will result if severe LCL injuries are not repaired. Decisions on treatment of grade II lesions are based on the degree of laxity, the medical state of the patient, and the desired activity level of the patient. Because most grade II and III LCL injuries involve the injury of other structures around the lateral knee, this decision is not often required. Operative procedures in acute lateral ligament injury usually involve simple repair of the torn ligament, although use of a graft can be necessary in more severe circumstances.

As previously described, the posterolateral corner of the knee involves multiple structures, which can be injured in various combinations and levels of severity. The main stabilizing structures (the LCL, the arcuate ligament complex, the popliteus muscle, and the posterior knee capsule) are the most commonly injured, and each must be carefully evaluated when a varus-extension knee injury is encountered. Although there can certainly be minor damage to these structures, most symptomatic injuries tend to be more severe. Unlike the MCL, however, there is not an efficient grading

BOX 15-1

Treatment Protocol for Nonoperative Grade I or II MCL Sprains

This program can be accelerated for grade I MCL sprains or can be extended depending on the severity of the injury. The following schedule serves as a guideline to help in the expediency of returning an athlete to his or her preinjury state.

Please note that if there is any increase in pain or swelling or loss of range of motion, these serve as signs that the progression of the patient may be too rapid.

I. MAXIMAL PROTECTION PHASE
   Goals:　Early protected ROM
   　　　　Prevent quadriceps atrophy
   　　　　Decrease effusion/pain

   A. Time of Injury: Day 1
      • Ice, compression, elevation
      • Hinged knee brace, nonpainful ROM; if needed
      • Crutches, weight bearing as tolerated
      • Passive ROM/active-assistive ROM to maintain mobility
      • Electrical muscle stimulation to quads (8 hours a day)
      • Isometric quadriceps exercises: quadriceps sets, straight-leg raises (flexion)

   B. Day 2
      • Continue above exercises
      • Quadriceps sets
      • Straight-leg raises (flexion, abduction)
      • Hamstring isometric sets
      • Well-leg exercises
      • Whirlpool for ROM (cold for first 3-4 days, then warm)
      • High-voltage galvanic stimulation to control swelling

   C. Days 3-7
      • Continue above exercises
      • Crutches, weight bearing as tolerated
      • ROM as tolerated
      • Eccentric quadriceps work
      • Bicycle for ROM stimulus
      • Resisted knee extension with electrical muscle stimulation
      • Initiate hip adduction and extension
      • Initiate mini-squats
      • Initiate leg-press isotonics
      • Brace worn at night, brace during day as needed

II. MODERATE PROTECTION PHASE
   Criteria for Progression:
   1. No increase in instability
   2. No increase in swelling
   3. Minimal tenderness
   4. Passive ROM 10-100 degrees
   Goals:　Full painless ROM
   　　　　Restore strength
   　　　　Ambulation without crutches

   A. Week 2
      • Continue strengthening program with progressive resistive exercise (PRE)
      • Continue electric muscle stimulation to quads during isotonic strengthening
      • Continue ROM exercise
      • Emphasize closed kinetic chain exercises; lunges, squats, lateral lunges, wall squats, lateral step-ups
      • Bicycle for endurance
      • Water exercises, running in water forward and backward
      • Full ROM exercises
      • Flexibility exercises, hamstrings, quadriceps, iliotibial band, etc.
      • Proprioception training (balance drills)
      • StairMaster endurance work

   B. Days 11-14
      • Continue all exercises in week 2
      • PREs emphasis on quadriceps, medial hamstrings, hip abduction
      • Initiate isokinetics, submaximal → maximal fast contractile velocities
      • Begin running program if full painless extension and flexion are present

III. MINIMAL PROTECTION PHASE
   Criteria for Progression:
   1. No instability
   2. No swelling or tenderness
   3. Full painless ROM
   Goals: Increase strength and power

   A. Week 3
      • Continue strengthening program

(continued)

system that has proven helpful with clinical decision making for this condition. Careful physical examination is still essential in evaluating these injuries because any significant laxity is usually treated operatively.

Posterolateral rotatory instability is the term used to describe combined injury to the LCL, popliteus, and arcuate ligament complex. Damage to these structures can be of varying severity.[48,50] If the injury involves more extension than varus stress, the arcuate complex can be more involved. More varus stress will impart greater damage to the LCL. Although MRI can be helpful, physical examination is the most important tool used to differentiate these injuries and determine the appropriate treatment. Acute mild injury can be treated with bracing and rehabilitation, using the brace to block excessive extension and protect against varus stress. Moderate or severe injury to any of these structures should almost always be treated operatively to prevent persistent instability.

Because of the myriad structures involved in the lateral knee, combined injury is the most common injury pattern. Rarely are these injuries isolated to the LCL or even the posterolateral corner. More commonly, the injury will involve many of these structures and include the ACL or PCL (or both), as well as the lateral meniscus. With more severe injuries, especially those involving a strong varus stress, other structures in this region are often injured, including the iliotibial tract, the lateral hamstring, and the peroneal nerve. With these more traumatic, multiple-structure injuries, surgery is almost always required to provide any chance of the knee regaining normal function. These are complex surgeries that have to be carefully planned to address all of the injuries, especially when multiple ligaments are involved. Different opinions exist as to whether these injuries should be treated all at once or staged with cruciate repair occurring at a later time to avoid postoperative arthrofibrosis. Although most surgeons prefer to repair all at the same time, staged reconstruction is also performed, and each case must be evaluated independently. Again, a thorough knowledge of the anatomy is essential in these procedures because restoration of the normal anatomy is the ultimate goal.

MANAGEMENT OF LATERAL LIGAMENT INJURIES OF THE KNEE

As with all knee reconstructions, surgical treatment is always preceded by careful examination of the knee under anesthesia to fully evaluate the integrity of the various structures. The procedure often begins with a diagnostic arthroscopy to carefully inspect the intraarticular structures. If the cruciate ligaments are injured, preparation for their reconstruction, including removal of the remnants and drilling of the bone

---

BOX 15-1, continued

- Wall squats
- Vertical squats
- Lunges
- Lateral lunges
- Step-ups
- Leg press
- Knee extension
- Hip abduction and adduction
- Hamstring curls
- Emphasis:
  - Functional exercise drills
  - Fast speed isokinetics
  - Eccentric quadriceps
  - Isotonic hip adduction, medial hamstrings
- Isokinetic test
- Proprioception training
- Endurance exercise
- Stationary bike 30-40 minutes

- NordicTrac, swimming, etc.
- Initiate agility program, sport-specific activities

IV. MAINTENANCE PROGRAM
Criteria for return to competition:
1. Full ROM
2. No instability
3. Muscle strength 85% of contralateral side
4. Proprioception ability satisfactory
5. No tenderness over MCL
6. No effusion
7. Quadriceps strength; torque/body weight ratios
8. Lateral knee brace (if necessary)
Maintenance Program
Continue isotonic strengthening exercises
Continue flexibility exercises
Continue proprioceptive activities

Developed by Kevin E. Wilk, PT; revised 1/98; from Wilk KE et al. In Ellenbecker TS: *Knee ligament rehabilitation*, Philadelphia, 2000, Churchill Livingstone.
ROM, range of motion.

tunnels, is often done at this time if the integrity of the joint capsule is intact. The joint integrity is usually restored by 5 to 7 days after the injury, allowing arthroscopy without leakage of fluid into the surrounding tissue. After arthroscopy is completed, the knee is flexed to 90 degrees and a lateral incision is made along the midline of the lateral distal femur, curving distally at the knee to end at Gerdy's tubercle. A deep incision is then made through the iliotibial tract at the junction of the posterior one third and anterior two thirds. In severe injuries, the iliotibial tract may be ruptured, making dissection and visibility easier. The peroneal nerve should then be located behind the biceps femoris and protected. If the nerve is injured, the ends of the peroneal nerve should be tagged and then reapproximated at the end of the case.

The posterolateral corner of the knee and the upper portion of the LCL are now visible and can be evaluated. The anatomy should be thoroughly inspected, especially in areas where hematoma is evident. If the capsule is not detached enough to see directly into the joint, a vertical capsulotomy can be made directly anterior or posterior to the popliteus tendon. The intraarticular structures, including the popliteus and the meniscus, are then carefully inspected and palpated, as is the LCL. A second deep incision is then made between the posterior aspect of the iliotibial tract and the anterior portion of the biceps femoris to allow inspection of the fibular insertion of the LCL, as well as the insertion of the biceps. After all of these structures have been exposed, the damage is surveyed and the repair is planned.

The order of lateral repair usually requires attention to the meniscus first, followed by the popliteus, and then the joint capsule. The arcuate ligament is evaluated, and, if injured, it should be repaired back onto the femur or tibia to the original attachment site. The final step is to repair the LCL. If the ligament is torn off of the femur, a screw and washer or suture anchors are often used to repair the LCL. If the avulsion is off of the fibula, the injury can be repaired with sutures through drill holes or anchors. Midsubstance tears in the LCL (or the popliteus or arcuate ligament) are repaired using Bunnell or Kessler sutures. If the cruciate ligaments are involved, all grafts should be passed and secured before the lateral structures are repaired. Exact anatomic repair should be attempted if at all possible.

There are two important factors when considering surgical treatment of chronic lateral knee ligament injuries. First, chronic injuries are usually more complex than acute ones. Rarely are these injuries restricted to one structure, or even to the lateral side of the knee. These are symptomatic instabilities that have usually worsened over time and are multifactorial in nature. Most involve one or both cruciate ligaments, and they sometimes involve articular cartilage injury or bony deficiency. Careful evaluation of the entire lateral knee must be done to delineate all deficient structures and address all of the problems.

Second, it is common during surgical treatment to find structures that are damaged or irreparable. This is different from repair of acute injuries, during which most injured lateral structures can be repaired primarily. Because of this destruction of the normal anatomy, reconstruction and graft use are common with chronic lateral knee injuries. It is also common to see multiple procedures performed at the same setting to correct the various deficiencies.

The procedures done to correct chronic lateral knee instability can be divided into surgical techniques that restore the anatomy and those that attempt to restore stability despite altered anatomy. "Anatomy-restoring procedures" are in some ways similar to acute repair. The goal of these procedures is to restore function by returning damaged structures to their preinjury state. This type of procedure is possible only when the structures themselves have not been damaged beyond the point of functional repair. There can be no bony deficiency, and the tissues must not be irreversibly stretched or attenuated. If the situation is favorable for this type of procedure, repair proceeds exactly as if one were doing an acute repair. The procedure begins with careful examination under anesthesia, followed by arthroscopy to identify and address all intraarticular pathology, including cruciate ligament injury. A midlateral incision is then made, and the iliotibial tract is incised to expose the lateral knee. All structures are carefully identified and evaluated. Special attention must be given to the posterolateral structures, especially the popliteus and arcuate ligament. If these are irreparable, they must be reconstructed with grafts. Structures are repaired from deepest to most superficial, starting with the meniscus, the popliteus, and the capsule.

In chronic injury, the damaged structures often attempt to heal in a nonanatomic position. This situation requires "function-restoring procedures," including advancement of the tissues, especially the posterior capsule and the arcuate ligament, to remove the laxity and stabilize the posterolateral corner. The LCL is also evaluated and, when possible, repaired. If it is too severely damaged, it also must be reconstructed with a graft. Although the many different procedures that have been described as treatments for this problem cannot all be discussed here, most of them are founded on the aforementioned concepts.

In situations with severe injury to the lateral knee, the structures cannot always be preserved. Severe stretch of the lateral structures often renders them irreparable and can even lead to a lateral thrust while walking. These situations require the restoration of stability by nonanatomic means. Many procedures have been described to do this, including redirection of the biceps femoris tendon, creation of a ligamentous sling in the posterolateral corner, and other artificially created constraints of the lateral side designed to provide a nonanatomic posterolateral stability. Each of these situations is obviously different, and each instability must be evaluated carefully.

Surgery, unlike in acute repairs, is more often performed to restore function than to re-create anatomy, so each reconstruction can be tailored to the specifics of the instability. The posterolateral sling, for example, can be used in situations where the entire posterolateral corner is stretched and incompetent, but it does not address any insufficiency of the LCL. Redirection of the biceps tendon with tenodesis to the femur can address LCL laxity but does little to address the posterolateral corner laxity. In situations of lateral thrust, a valgus proximal tibial osteotomy is sometimes required in addition to soft tissue reconstruction to protect the posterolateral corner. Although none of these treatments is anatomically correct, all can provide stability in cases of severe chronic damage.

TREATMENT OF LATERAL LIGAMENT INJURIES OF THE KNEE

Little has been written regarding rehabilitation for posterolateral instability of the knee.[13,46,51,52] Because of the infrequent occurrence of injury to the lateral ligamentous structures, few clinical trials have been reported in the enormous amount of literature written about knee injuries. As a result, the posterolateral aspect of the knee remains the least understood region of the knee, but when injured can lead to severe disability because of pain, instability, and articular cartilage degeneration.[51]

Acute nonoperative management of isolated grade III LCL injuries follows a pattern similar to MCL injuries where initial goals include pain control and reduction of swelling.[14] Early AROM is performed in a pain-free range, and isometrics for the quadriceps and hamstring muscles are initiated in a submaximal- to maximal-intensity range as tolerated to prevent muscle atrophy. Patients with grade III LCL injury demonstrating laxity in varus stress testing with a soft end point are placed in a hinged knee brace with ROM preset from full extension to 90 degrees of flexion for 4 to 6 weeks. Patients with grade I and II LCL sprains with minimal laxity and solid end point on varus stress testing may not require a brace.

Weight-bearing status for patients with LCL injury is determined by resolution of symptoms; good quadriceps eccentric muscle control; recognition of joint stability, particularly a firm end point on varus testing; and limited appearance of gait deviations, primarily a varus thrust, observed in the midstance phase of weight bearing on the affected limb. Crutches can be discontinued when the patient achieves full passive knee extension and can control his or her body weight while performing a single-leg mini-squat through approximately 30 degrees of knee flexion on the involved extremity.

Although crutches are discontinued when these criteria are achieved, additional strategies to minimize the long-term effects of the varus thrust should be considered for the patient with a grade III LCL sprain. Functional bracing that provides "good medial and lateral support" has been recommended for athletes returning to contact sports to prevent reinjury.[14] Bracing designed to unload the arthritic medial compartment of the knee in an osteoarthritic patient by creating a slight valgus moment has been recommended to control the varus thrust in grade III LCL injuries.[51] Gait

retraining has been suggested in which the patient is coached to maintain slight knee flexion throughout the stance phase of gait, limiting the thrusting motions at the knee.[53] Strategies to train hip musculature necessary to control varus movements of the knee have been cited and are discussed in greater detail later in this chapter.[54] Use of orthotics with a lateral heel wedge has been described to minimize tensile forces on lateral knee structures and control varus thrust in the stance phase of gait.[51] Taping to support fibular head position has been discussed as a method of providing proprioceptive feedback to support a patient with a grade II LCL sprain.[55]

Postoperative management of grade III injuries of the LCL place the greatest restrictions on patient activity through immediate protected ROM of the surgical knee and maximum protection against undue loads in gait that would cause the repair to stretch or fail.[52] Hyperextension and varus loading of the surgical knee in gait are forces to be avoided.

Following operative repair of the LCL, patients are placed in a knee immobilizer or long leg postoperative brace locked at 0 degrees for the first 4[52] to 6 weeks,[14] particularly if the surgical repair also involved reconstruction of the PCL.[54] Ambulation begins in a non–weight-bearing gait progressing to partial weight bearing at week 4 with slow progression to full weight bearing by week 8.[52] Limited ROM exercises are performed in a 0- to 90-degree range immediately after surgery, but flexion greater than 90 degrees is deferred until the fifth postoperative week in an effort to limit varus tensioning and posterior shear forces that might overload the repair. Patients are also taught to place a hand on the lateral aspect of the knee to create a "10-pound valgus load" to protect the lateral repair when attempting knee flexion beyond 90 degrees.[52]

Isometric contractions of the quadriceps and hamstring muscle groups are initiated during the first postoperative week. Further strengthening exercises continue with quadriceps active knee extensions through a 90- to 0-degree ROM around 5 weeks after surgery and hamstring knee flexion to 90 degrees beginning around 9 weeks after surgery.[52]

Because of the propensity for lateral repairs to loosen with weight-bearing activities, running programs are restricted until at least the ninth postoperative month. Plyometric and further sport-specific training are restricted until the twelfth postoperative month after the athlete has accomplished appropriate indices on stress radiographs, KT-2000 tests, and strength and functional testing. Examples of these performances for the athlete anticipating return to moderately heavy running, cutting, or twisting activities include the following[52]:

- Stress radiographs and KT-2000 tests demonstrating less than 5 mm of lateral joint line opening when tested at 70 degrees of knee flexion

- Less than or equal to 20% deficit on Biodex isometric testing of the involved quadriceps and hamstring muscles versus the noninvolved knee

BOX 15-2

Protocol for Operative Treatment of Grade III LCL Sprains
Cincinnati Sportsmedicine and Orthopaedic Center Rehabilitation Protocol for Lateral, Posterolateral Ligament Reconstruction

	Postoperative Weeks			Postoperative Months	
	1 to 4	5 to 8	9 to 12	4 to 6	7 to 12
Brace					
Bledsoe 0 degrees locked	X				
Custom medial unloader		X	X	X	X
Range-of-motion goals (degrees)					
0-90	X				
0-110		X			
0-120		X			
1-130			X		
Weight bearing					
None	X				
Toe-touch to one-quarter to one-half body weight	X				
Full body weight		X			
Patella mobilization	X	X			
Modalities					
Electrical muscle stimulation (EMS)	X	X			
Pain/edema management (cryotherapy)	X	X	X	X	X
Stretching					
Hamstring, gastroc-soleus, iliotibial band, quadriceps	X	X	X	X	X
Strengthening					
Quadriceps isometrics, straight-leg raises	X	X	X		
Active knee extension	X	X	X		
Closed-chain (gait retraining, toe raises, wall sits, mini-squats)	X	X	X	X	
Knee flexion hamstring curls (90 degrees)			X	X	X
Knee extension quads (90-0 degrees)		X	X	X	X
Hip abduction-adduction, multi-hip			X	X	X
Leg press (50-0 degrees)			X	X	X
Balance/proprioceptive training					
Weight-shifting, mini-trampoline, BAPS, KAT, plyometrics		X	X	X	X
Conditioning					
Upper body ergometer (UBE)	X	X			
Bicycling (stationary)			X	X	X
Aquatic program			X	X	X
Swimming (kicking)			X	X	X
Walking				X	X
Stair-climbing machine			X	X	X
Ski machine				X	X
Running: straight					X
Cutting: lateral carioca, figure-of-eights					X
Full sports					X

BAPS, Biomechanical Ankle Platform System; *KAT*, Kinesthetic Awareness Trainer.

- Scores of greater than or equal to 85% symmetry on functional testing such as hopping for distance comparing involved versus noninvolved knees

Further explanation of postoperative protocols for repair of grade III LCL injuries can be found in Box 15-2.

CONSIDERATIONS FOR REESTABLISHMENT OF KNEE STABILITY

Traditional rehabilitation programs created for athletes following knee ligament injury had focused on the restoration of muscle strength, power, endurance, and flexibility as parameters necessary for prevention of recurrence of injury. Currently, more attention has been placed on the prevention of injury in sports through improved functional joint stability offered by enhanced neuromuscular control mechanisms.[56]

Neuromuscular control refers to the integration of sensory input balanced with appropriate motor output mediated by the central nervous system. Sensory input is derived from visual, vestibular, and somatosensory sources. Somatosensory sources include both tactile and proprioceptive senses transmitted from peripheral sensory receptors located in skin, muscles, and connective tissues supporting joints. Detailed description of these sensory receptors is beyond the scope of this chapter; briefly, these receptors function to convey information regarding joint position and movement to the central nervous system. This information from the peripheral receptors is processed by the central nervous system at three levels. First, information is relayed at the spinal level where spinal reflexes transmit responses, quickly serving to provide a dynamic muscle balance about the joint in question. Second, information is transmitted to the cerebellum where processing of incoming messages serves to mediate posture and balance. Third, information is sent to the higher cortical centers where volitional responses are created based on the input from the peripheral receptors.[56]

More specific to the knee, Hewett and colleagues[57] summarize the findings of other authors in stating that the ACL has sensory and proprioceptive functions, in addition to its role as a static stabilizer of the knee. Proprioceptive receptors located in fibers of intact ACLs in humans, when stretched, generate changes in cerebral activity following stimulation.[58] Further, muscle responses around the knee are coincident to forced anterior tibial translation such that hamstring activation increased and quadriceps inhibition occurred when the ACL was loaded.[57] Thus a motor response affording increased stability to the knee has been observed in response to a proprioceptive stimulus, which verifies the presence of a protective sensorimotor loop.

Unfortunately, this protective sensorimotor loop appears to be disrupted with injury to the ACL.[59-61] Patients with ACL-deficient knees have demonstrated proprioceptive deficits in ability to reposition their knees to pretest positions once moved either passively or actively. Decreased sensitivity to detect onset of passive motion has been reported.[59] Also, deficits in motor performance initiated by the sensorimotor

loop have been described as decreased muscle response time and recruitment following forced anterior tibial translation in ACL-deficient knees.[62] Further research is needed to define the influences of collateral ligament laxity on sensorimotor loop deficits contributing to knee instability, particularly in the frontal and transverse planes, attributed to collateral ligament function in static postures.

Proprioceptive function in ACL-deficient knees has been reported to improve following ligament reconstruction,[60,63,64] but it also has been reported to improve in individuals without reconstruction through training.[61,65]

Training programs to improve proprioception of the knee have incorporated non–weight-bearing postures to regain the ability to sense small changes in joint position, as well as maintenance of balance in weight-bearing positions. Weight-bearing activities emphasize maintenance of static balance. Weight-bearing activities can also challenge the athlete to maintain balance in response to planned movement patterns and to test patient reaction to external forces attempting to disrupt stability. Use of unstable balance platforms, treadmills, slide boards, steps, grids, partially deflated balls, foam rollers, rubber tubing, patterned trunk movements, and plyometric drills has been described in the development of proprioceptive training programs.[56,66-68] Exercise progression moves from double-leg stance to single-leg stance, stable surfaces to unstable surfaces, slow speeds to fast speeds, eyes open to eyes closed, general tasks to sport-specific tasks, nonimpact to impact, and planned perturbations to unexpected perturbations of balance. These training programs are constructed to "integrate peripheral somatosensory, visual, and vestibular afferent input and improve motor control through spinal reflex, brainstem, and cognitive programming."[56]

Early aggressive initiation of neuromuscular conditioning has been advocated in an attempt to overcome deficits associated with joint injury before progressing to high-level strengthening exercises,[69] particularly with female athletes.[57] According to Paterno and colleagues,[70] females frequently possess three neuromuscular imbalances, making them more prone to noncontact mechanisms of knee injury. First, females demonstrate "ligament dominance" in control of the knee as opposed to muscular control of medial-lateral knee motion, resulting in high valgus knee torques and high ground reaction forces on landing from jumps. Second, females frequently exhibit quadriceps muscle dominance over hamstring muscles to stabilize the knee during sport-related movements. Third, females frequently exhibit "dominant leg dominance," alluding to disparity of muscular strength and recruitment in the nondominant leg, predisposing that knee to injury. Therefore neuromuscular conditioning programs must address these imbalances by promoting stability in the coronal, sagittal, and transverse planes of motion,[70] while training muscular control of the trunk and both lower extremities.

Although phased protocols have previously been described detailing progression of ROM, weight-bearing status,

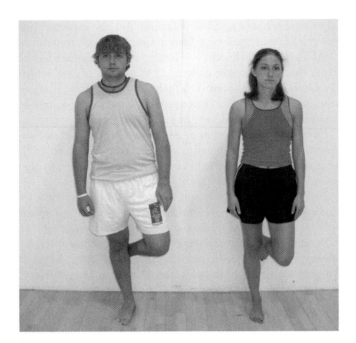

Figure 15-7: Single-leg stance.

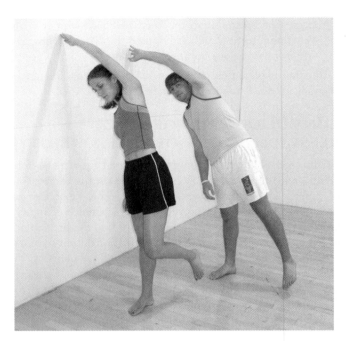

Figure 15-9: Frontal plane motion in erect trunk posture.

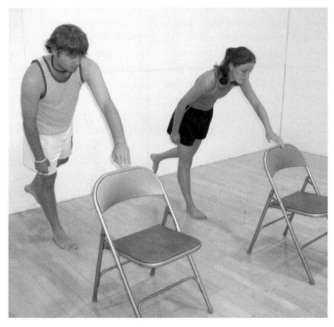

Figure 15-8: Sagittal plane motion in erect trunk posture.

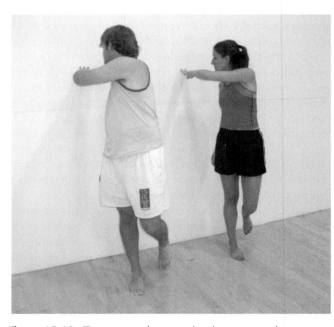

Figure 15-10: Transverse plane motion in erect trunk posture.

strength, endurance, and flexibility training for the collateral ligament–injured athlete, discussion of neuromuscular conditioning for this athlete warrants greater attention. Particular attention focuses on activities early in the rehabilitation process that progress the athlete from ability to achieve double-leg stance on the involved extremity to tolerance of multiplanar posturing of the trunk and extremities in single-leg stance while seeking to maintain the center of gravity within the base of support, the essence of balance.[71]

Initial phases of neuromuscular conditioning involve double-leg stance, relative neutral trunk posture, and movement of upper extremities in three planes of motion. Progression occurs by moving to single-leg stance on the involved lower extremity and performing upper extremity patterns with one or two hands, depending on extremity or trunk strategies requiring emphasis (Figures 15-7 to 15-10).

Figures 15-11 through 15-13 illustrate a hip strategy performed with relative trunk extension requiring quad-

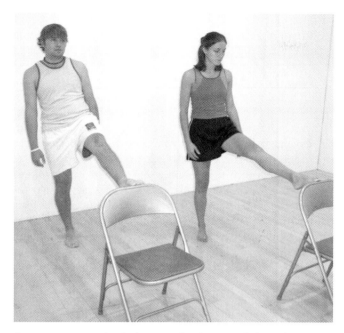

Figure 15-11: Sagittal plane motion in extended trunk posture.

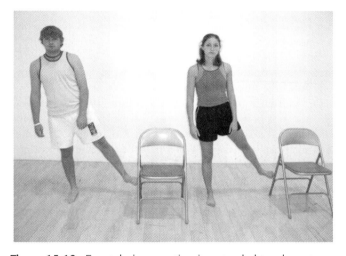

Figure 15-12: Frontal plane motion in extended trunk posture.

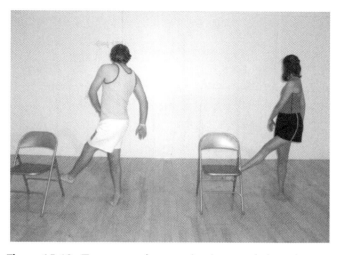

Figure 15-13: Transverse plane motion in extended trunk posture.

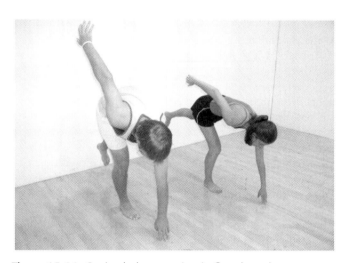

Figure 15-14: Sagittal plane motion in flexed trunk posture.

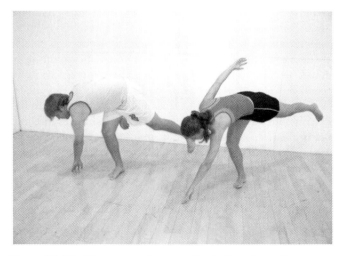

Figure 15-15: Transverse plane motion in flexed trunk posture.

riceps control. Movements are initially conducted in slow, coordinated reciprocal patterns incorporating vestibular and visual cues as the athlete is required to process commands such as "touch your right big toe on the top of the backrest on the chair." Objects such as chairs, tables, or stickers attached to doorways can serve as "targets," and the balance tasks can be performed in a doorway or in proximity to a wall if the task is particularly challenging. Combining balance postures with commands to contact various targets is used to integrate responses at the spinal, brainstem, and cortical levels.

Figures 15-14 through 15-16 are used to encourage hamstring control through upper extremity patterns performed in single-leg stance in trunk flexion. Commands instructing

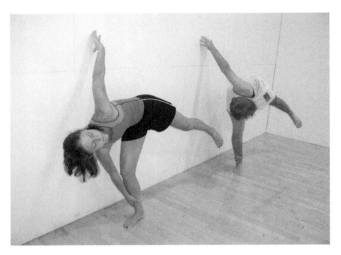

Figure 15-16: Frontal plane motion in flexed trunk posture.

the athlete to touch targets with his or her fingers are given to allow the athlete to explore movement in the sagittal, frontal, and transverse planes while attempting to stabilize on the supporting involved extremity in trunk flexion.

As the athlete masters static balance in the previously described poses, dynamic control is promoted by seeking more rapid reciprocal and alternating upper extremity movements through the described cardinal planes, as well as diagonal patterns,[72] with varied trunk postures while maintaining balance over the involved knee. Such exercise protocols have been reported to be more effective than isolated stretching and strengthening in returning athletes to competition and preventing recurrence in athletes suffering from acute hamstring strains.[73] Additional interventions employed to challenge the athlete involve changing the surfaces on which to balance, removing visual cues, and perturbing the athlete in predicted and unpredictable manners.

Each task previously described asks the athlete to balance his or her center of gravity over the base of support. As formidable as these tasks have appeared in the previous exercises, sports participation demands even more from the injured athlete. Even the basic activity of running straight ahead demands more than balance. This activity requires momentary loss of balance by moving the center of gravity off the base of support, followed by immediate regaining of balance at foot-strike, only to repeat the sequence in rapid succession. For neuromuscular conditioning to be complete, the sensorimotor loop must transmit information pertaining not only to maintenance of balance, but also how to lose and regain balance. A balance retraining strategy that demonstrates progressions from static balance to dynamic balance to cyclic loss and recovery of balance may prove helpful.

BALANCE TRAINING PROGRESSIONS

For the athlete who has sustained a collateral ligament injury of the knee, a loss of sensory input from the damaged tissue

has been described. Efforts of sports specialists to integrate sensorimotor responses in retraining the neuromuscular support system of the knee may benefit from examination of progressions used to generate appropriate motor responses in the neurologic patient populations. The phases of mobility, stability, controlled mobility, and skill are considered by the rehabilitation specialist in retraining the patient after cerebrovascular accident.[74] *Mobility* pertains to facilitating movement of the patient into a posture or position the patient has not attained on his or her own. *Stability* refers to the patient's ability to maintain the previously unexplored posture. *Controlled mobility* describes the ability to hold the new posture while performing purposeful movements from that posture. *Skill* pertains to the ability to accomplish coordinated movements in and out of the posture with minimal effort.

Theories of mobility, stability, controlled mobility, and skill can be used as a framework in conceptualizing neuromuscular training programs for the purpose of balance retraining. *Balance* has previously been defined as the ability to maintain the center of gravity over the base of support.[71] In athletics the definition of *static balance* could be expanded to a more dynamic ability to momentarily lose balance to initiate quick movement and then regain the center of gravity over the base of support with equal speed so as to generate movement in an alternative direction.

Box 15-3 illustrates balance training progressions in phases of maintaining and regaining balance, categorizing activities based on the strategies of mobility, stability, controlled mobility, and skill. The first column illustrates *mobility* as movement into static balance postures with progressions requiring increasing stability. Column two, *stability*, describes dynamic balance tasks in which balance must be maintained over the involved extremity in light of trunk and extremity movements in planned and reactive progressions. Columns three and four list activities requiring displacement of the center of gravity outside the base of support, providing opportunities to learn the skill of regaining lost balance. Column three, *controlled mobility*, outlines tasks requiring vertical displacement of the center of gravity in jumping and, of greater importance, in controlled landings. Column four, *skill*, lists more athletic tasks performed in multiple responses that more closely simulate movement patterns performed during sport activities.

Balance training progressions should not be viewed as a continuum through which each athlete should progress in sequence. The arrangement of tasks may not be consistent with the skills of the individual athlete. Also, the thought that all athletes should be capable of demonstrating all drills in the skill column may be inconsistent with the demands of the sport in question. Instead, balance training progressions offer a framework that recognizes that in sports balance needs to be regained, as well as maintained, and trained within phases of mobility, stability, controlled mobility, and skill.

SUMMARY

The collateral ligaments of the knee present a paradox in etiology of injury and strategies for treatment. The MCL is a frequently injured structure from athletic mechanisms of injury, yet current strategies seldom recommend surgical repair. The LCL is rarely injured, but if injured and unrecognized can contribute to the failure of reconstructive procedures performed on other ligaments, notably the ACL.

Phased rehabilitation is the foundation for recovery in both operative and nonoperative care of injury to the collateral ligaments. Neuromuscular reeducation initiated early in the rehabilitation process attempts to counter the loss of proprioceptive input sustained in the damaged tissues. Weight-bearing exercises are used to relearn neuromuscular control, maintaining the center of gravity over the involved knee. Higher-level tasks train the athlete to "lose balance" to initiate movement, only to quickly regain balance in prepara-

---

BOX 15-3

Balance Training Progressions

Maintain Center of Gravity over Base of Support		Lose and Regain Center of Gravity over Base of Support	
Mobility: Static Balance	Stability: Dynamic Balance	Controlled Mobility: Regain Balance from Vertical Displacement	Skill: Regain Balance from Horizontal Displacement
Weight shift to momentary hold on involved lower extremity	Single-leg stance/reciprocal movements of opposite leg: single plane and multiplane	Single-leg stance/mini-squats: slow to fast speed	Single-leg/single-response hop in three planes: "hopscotch"
Weight shift from three planes to momentary hold on involved extremity	Single-leg stance/reciprocal movements of upper extremities: single plane and multiplane, unilateral and bilateral upper extremity patterns	Single-leg/hop-in-place emphasizing controlled landings	Single-leg/multiple hops in three planes emphasizing controlled landings
Maintained single-leg stance: timed responses with eyes open	Single-leg stance/movement of trunk and three extremities in sport-specific patterns: kicking and throwing motions	Single-leg/hop-in-place emphasizing slow to fast speed	Single-leg/multiple hops for height and distance: hopping up/down stairs
Single-leg stance: timed responses with eyes closed	Single-leg stance/movement of trunk and three extremities in reactive patterns: catch a ball	Single-leg/jumps for height: double-leg landing to single-leg progression	Single-leg/standing long jump; lateral jump; 90-, 180-, and 360-degree jumps
Single-leg stance: decreased base of support—on toes, heel, lateral foot	Single-leg stance/movements of trunk and three extremities in reactive patterns on unstable surfaces: trampoline, balance board	Single-leg/jumps from a height with immediate vertical jump: double-leg landing to single-leg progression	Single-leg/sport-specific skills: rebound to outlet pass, catch and throw, trap and kick with opposite leg
Single-leg stance: perturbations of balance while performing the above static tasks	Single-leg stance/movements of trunk and three extremities in reaction to perturbations of balance while attempting to stabilize in the above movements	Single-leg/perturbations of balance while performing the above vertical displacements	Single-leg/perturbations of balance while performing the above skills

tion for the next movement. Balance training progressions should seek to train mobility, stability, controlled mobility, and skill based on the needs of the athlete as those needs coincide with the demands of the sport.

References

1. Dehaven KE, Litner DM: Athletic injuries: comparison by age, sport and gender, *Am J Sports Med* 14:218-224, 1986.

2. Woo SLY, Inoue M, McGuik-Burleson E, et al: Treatment of the medial collateral ligament injury: structure and function of the canine knee in response to differing treatment regimens, *Am J Sports Med* 15:22-29, 1987.

3. Miyasaka KC, Daniel DM, Stone ML, Hirschman P: The incidence of knee injuries in the general population, *Am J Knee Surg* 4:3-8, 1991.

4. Slocum DB, Larson RL, James SI: Late reconstruction of ligamentous injuries of the medial compartment of the knee, *Clin Orthop* 100:23-55, 1974.

5. Warren LF, Marshall JL, Girgis F: The prime static stabilizer of the medial side of the knee, *J Bone Joint Surg* 56A:665-670, 1974.

6. Grood ES, Noyes FR, Butler DL, et al: Ligamentous and capsular restraints preventing straight medial and lateral laxity in intact human cadaver knees, *J Bone Joint Surg* 63A:1257-1269, 1981.

7. Sullivan DJ, Levy IM, Shesikier S, et al: Medial restraints to anterior-posterior motion of the knee, *J Bone Joint Surg* 6A:930-939, 1984.

8. Seebacher JR, Inglis AE, Marshall JL, et al: The structure of the posterolateral aspect of the knee, *J Bone Joint Surg* 64A:536, 1982.

9. Wilk KE, Clancy WG, Andrews JR, Fox GM: Assessment and treatment of medial capsular injuries. In Ellenbecker TS: *Knee ligament rehabilitation*, Philadelphia, 2000, Churchill Livingstone.

10. Tipton CM, Mathies RD, Martin RK: Influence of age and sex on strength of bone-ligament junctions in knee joints of rats, *J Bone Joint Surg* 60A:230-234, 1978.

11. Woo SLY, Orlando CA, Gomez MA, et al: Tensile properties of the medial collateral ligament as a function of age, *J Orthop Res* 4:133-136, 1986.

12. Noyes FR, Grood ES: The strength of the anterior cruciate ligament in humans and rhesus monkeys: age-related and species-related changes, *J Bone Joint Surg* 58A:1074, 1976.

13. DeLee JC, Riley MB, Rockwood CA: Acute straight lateral instability of the knee, *Am J Sports Med* 11:404-411, 1983.

14. Irrgang JJ, Safran MR, Fu FH: The knee: ligamentous and meniscal injuries. In Zachazewski JE, Magee DJ, Quillen WS: *Athletic injuries and rehabilitation*, Philadelphia, 1996, Saunders.

15. Slocum DB, James SL, Larson RL, Singer KM: Clinical test for anterolateral rotatory instability of the knee, *Clin Orthop* 118:63-69, 1976.

16. Hughston J, Andrews J, Cross M, Moschi A: Classification of knee ligament instabilities. Part I. The medial compartment and cruciate ligaments, *J Bone Joint Surg* 58A:2, 1976.

17. Veltri DM, Warren RF: Anatomy, biomechanics, and physical findings in posterolateral knee instability, *Clin Sports Med* 13(3):599-614, 1994.

18. Oster A, Okhum K, Hulgaard J: Operative treatment of rupture in the medial collateral ligament, *Acta Orthop Scand* 42(5):439, 1971.

19. Palmer I: On the injuries to the ligaments of the knee joint: a clinical study, *Acta Chir Scand Suppl* 53, 1938.

20. O'Donoghue DH: Surgical treatment of fresh injuries to the major ligaments of the knee, *J Bone Joint Surg* 32A:721-737, 1950.

21. O'Donoghue DH: An analysis of end results of surgical treatment of major injuries of the ligaments of the knee, *J Bone Joint Surg* 37A:1-12, 1955.

22. Godshall RW, Hansen CA: The classification, treatment, and follow-up evaluation of medial collateral ligament injuries of the knee, *J Bone Joint Surg* 56A:1316, 1974.

23. England RL: Repair of the ligaments about the knee, *Orthop Clin North Am* 7:195-205, 1976.

24. Hughston JC, Eilers AF: The role of the posterior oblique ligament in repairs of the acute medial (collateral) ligament tears of the knee, *J Bone Joint Surg* 55A:923-940, 1973.

25. Fetto JF, Marshall JL: Medial collateral ligament injuries of the knee: a rationale for treatment, *Clin Orthop* 132:206-218, 1978.

26. Sanberg R, Balkfors B, Nilsson B, Westlin N: Operative versus non-operative treatment of recent injuries to the ligaments of the knee, *J Bone Joint Surg* 69A:1120-1126, 1987.

27. Indelicato PA: Non-operative treatment of complete tears of the medial collateral ligament of the knee, *J Bone Joint Surg* 65A:323-329, 1983.

28. Weiss JA, Woo SLY, Ohland KJ, et al: Evaluation of a new injury model to study medial collateral ligament healing: primary repair versus nonoperative treatment, *J Orthop Res* 9:516-528, 1991.

29. Hart DP, Dahners LE: Healing of the medial collateral ligament in rats, *J Bone Joint Surg* 69A:1194-1199, 1987.

30. Mok DW, Good C: Non-operative management of acute grade III medial collateral ligament injury of the knee: a prospective study, *Injury* 20(5):277-280, 1989.

31. Elsasser JC, Reynolds FC, Omohundro JR: The non-operative treatment of collateral ligament injuries of the knee in professional football players, *J Bone Joint Surg* 56A:1185-1190, 1974.

32. Hastings DE: The non-operative management of collateral ligament injuries of the knee joint, *Clin Orthop* 147:22-28, 1980.

33. Jokl P, Kaplan N, Stovell P: Non-operative treatment of severe injuries to the medial collateral and anterior cruciate ligaments of the knee, *J Bone Joint Surg* 66A:741-744, 1984.

34. Holden DL, Eggert AW, Butler JE: The nonoperative treatment of grade I and II medial collateral ligament injuries to the knee, *Am J Sports Med* 11(5):340-344, 1983.

35. Reider B, Sathy MR, Talkington J, et al: Treatment of isolated medial collateral ligament injuries in athletes with early functional rehab. A five year follow-up study, *Am J Sports Med* 22(4):470-477, 1994.

36. Jones RE, Henley MB, Francis P: Nonoperative management of isolated grade III collateral ligament injury in high school football players, *Clin Orthop* 213:137-140, 1986.

37. Campbell JD: The evolution and current treatment trends with anterior cruciate, posterior cruciate, and medial collateral ligament injuries, *Am J Knee Surg* 11(2):128-135, 1998.

38. Harner CD, Irrgang JJ, Paul J, et al: Loss of motion following anterior cruciate ligament reconstruction, *Am J Sports Med* 20:507-515, 1992.

39. Shelbourne KD, Baele JR: Treatment of combined anterior cruciate ligament and medial collateral ligament injuries, *Am J Knee Surg* 1:56-58, 1988.

40. Shelbourne KD, Porter DA: Anterior cruciate ligament–medial collateral ligament injury: nonoperative management of medial collateral ligament tears with anterior cruciate ligament reconstruction—a preliminary report, *Am J Sports Med* 20:283-286, 1992.

41. Fetto JF, Marshall JL: The natural history and diagnosis of anterior cruciate ligament insufficiency, *Clin Orthop* 147:29-38, 1980.

42. Spindler KP, Walker RN: General approach to ligament surgery. In Fu FH, Harner CD, Kelly KG: *Knee surgery,* Baltimore, 1994, Williams & Wilkins.

43. Miller MD, Harner CD, Koshiwaguchi S: Acute posterior cruciate ligament injuries. In Fu FH, Harner CD, Kelly KG: *Knee surgery,* Baltimore, 1994, Williams & Wilkins.

44. Derscheid GL, Garrick JG: Medial collateral ligament injuries in football: nonoperative management of grade I and grade II sprains, *Am J Sports Med* 9:365-368, 1981.

45. Indelicato PA, Hermansdorfer J, Huegel M: Nonoperative management of complete tears of the medial collateral ligament of the knee in intercollegiate football players, *Clin Orthop* 256:174-177, 1990.

46. Shelborne KD, Patel DV: Management of combined injuries of the anterior cruciate and medial collateral ligaments, *J Bone Joint Surg* 77A:800-806, 1995.

47. Kannus P: Nonoperative treatment of grade II and III sprains of the lateral ligament compartment of the knee, *Am J Sports Med* 17:83-88, 1989.

48. Grana WA, Janssen T: Lateral ligament injury of the knee, *Orthopedics* 10:1039-1044, 1987.

49. Rettig A: Medial and lateral ligament injuries. In Scott W, editor: *Ligament and extensor mechanism injuries of the knee: diagnosis and treatment,* St Louis, 1991, Mosby.

50. Hughston JC, Andrews JR, Cross MJ: Classification of knee ligament instability. II. The lateral compartment, *J Bone Joint Surg* 58A:173-179, 1976.

51. Wilk K: JOSPT commentary. In DeLeo AT, Woodzell WW, Snyder-Mackler L: Resident's case problem: diagnosis and treatment of posterolateral instability in a patient with lateral collateral ligament sprain, *J Orthop Sports Phys Ther* 33(4):185-195, 2003.

52. Noyes FR, Heckmann TP, Barber-Westin SD: Posterior cruciate ligament and posterolateral reconstruction. In Ellenbecker TS: *Knee ligament rehabilitation,* New York, 2000, Churchill Livingstone.

53. Noyes FR, Dunworth LA, Andriacchi TP, et al: Knee hyperextension gait abnormalities in unstable knees. Recognition and preoperative gait retraining, *Am J Sports Med* 24:35, 1996.

54. Wilk K: Rehabilitation of nonoperative and operative injuries to the posterior cruciate ligament and posterolateral knee structures, *Clin Sports Med* 13(3):649-677, 1994.

55. DeLeo AT, Woodzell WW, Snyder-Mackler L: Resident's case problem: diagnosis and treatment of posterolateral instability in a patient with lateral collateral ligament sprain, *J Orthop Sports Phys Ther* 33(4):185-195, 2003.

56. Griffin LYE: Neuromuscular training and injury prevention in sports, *Clin Orthop* 409:53-60, 2003.

57. Hewett TE, Paterno MV, Myer GD: Strategies for enhancing proprioception and neuromuscular control of the knee, *Clin Orthop* 402:76-94, 2002.

58. Pittman MI, Nainzadeh N, Menche D, et al: The interoperative evaluation of the neurosensory function of the anterior cruciate ligament in humans using somatosensory evoked potentials, *Arthroscopy* 8:442-447, 1992.

59. Barrack RL, Skinner HB, Buckley SL: Proprioception in the anterior cruciate deficient knee, *Am J Sports Med* 17:1-6, 1989.

60. Barrett DS: Proprioception and function after anterior cruciate reconstruction, *J Bone Joint Surg* 73B:833-837, 1991.

61. Beard DJ, Dodd CAF, Trundle HR, Simpson AHRW: Proprioception enhancement for anterior cruciate ligament deficiency: a prospective randomized trial of two physiotherapy regimes, *J Bone Joint Surg* 76B:654-659, 1994.

62. Wojtys EM, Huston LJ: Neuromuscular performance in normal and anterior cruciate ligament–deficient lower extremities, *Am J Sports Med* 22:89-104, 1994.

63. Co FH, Skinner HB, Cannon WD: Effect of reconstruction of the anterior cruciate ligament on proprioception of the knee and the heel strike transient, *J Orthop Res* 11:696-704, 1993.

64. Harrison EL, Duenkel N, Dunlop R, Russell G: Evaluation of single-leg standing following anterior cruciate ligament surgery and rehabilitation, *Phys Ther* 74:245-252, 1994.

65. Fitzgerald GK, Axe MJ, Snyder-Mackler L: The efficacy of perturbation training in nonoperative anterior cruciate ligament rehabilitation programs for physically active individuals, *Phys Ther* 80:128-140, 2000.

66. Voight M, Blackburn T: Proprioception and balance training and testing following injury. In Ellenbecker TS: *Knee ligament rehabilitation,* Philadelphia, 2000, Churchill Livingstone.

67. Brody LT: Balance impairment. In Hall CM, Brody LT: *Therapeutic exercise: moving toward function,* Philadelphia, 1999, Lippincott Williams & Wilkins.

68. Lefever-Button S: Closed kinetic chain training. In Hall CM, Brody LT: *Therapeutic exercise: moving toward function,* Philadelphia, 1999, Lippincott Williams & Wilkins.

69. Johnston RB, Howard ME, Cawley PW, Losee GM: Effect of lower extremity muscular fatigue on motor control performance, *Med Sci Sports Exerc* 30(12):1703-1707, 1998.

70. Paterno MV, Myer GD, Ford KR, Hewett TE: Neuromuscular training improves single-limb stability in young female athletes, *J Orthop Sports Phys Ther* 34(6):305-316, 2004.

71. Crutchfield CA, Shumway-Cook A, Horak FB: Balance and coordination training. In Scully RM, Barnes MR, editors: *Physical therapy,* Philadelphia, 1989, JB Lippincott.

72. Knott M, Voss D: *Proprioceptive neuromuscular facilitation, patterns and techniques,* ed 2, Philadelphia, 1968, Harper & Row.

73. Sherry MA, Best TM: A comparison of two rehabilitation programs in the treatment of acute hamstring strains, *J Orthop Sports Phys Ther* 34(3):116-125, 2004.

74. Minor MAD: Therapeutic exercise class notes. Northwestern University Physical Therapy, 1978.

CHAPTER 16

The Multiple Ligament–Injured Knee: Evaluation, Treatment, and Rehabilitation

Richard L. Romeyn, MD
George J. Davies, DPT, MEd, PT, SCS, ATC, LAT, CSCS, FAPTA
Jason Jennings, DPT, SCS, ATC, MTC, CSCS

MULTIPLE LIGAMENTOUS KNEE INJURY

is a potentially devastating trauma resulting from a range of mechanisms, from high-velocity motor vehicle trauma to recreational athletics. Historically, the diagnosis was confined only to those cases in which knee dislocation was obvious at the scene of an accident or when confirmed radiographically in a hospital emergency center. As such, the incidence of these knee injuries was considered to be rare. It is now realized that polyligamentous disruption and its associated neurologic and vascular complications can occur without frank dislocation, and that dislocations, when they do occur, may spontaneously reduce before the patient is able to seek treatment. Conversely, it is possible for a knee dislocation to occur without complete disruption of both cruciate ligaments. Thus a better and more encompassing term for the injury complex is probably *multiple ligamentous knee injury* (MLKI), rather than *knee dislocation*. Because its incidence is much greater than once supposed, most orthopedic surgeons, emergency department physicians, and physical therapists will be called on to treat this injury more than once in the course of their careers.

The severity of traumatic knee dislocation has been recognized for centuries. In 1824 Sir Astley Cooper stated that "there are scarcely any accidents to which the body is liable, which more imperiously demand immediate amputation than these."[1] Because neurovascular injuries were so frequently associated with knee dislocation, any outcome other than amputation was considered a success, even if the result was severe loss of motion or significant residual laxity. The first reported description of surgical intervention was by Thomas Annandale in 1881.[2] However, until recently, the treatment of traumatic knee dislocation generally consisted of closed reduction and cast or brace immobilization.[3-7] Although the consensus of current opinion is that operative repair/reconstruction is the preferred mode of treatment in most instances, even today there is no uniform agreed-on approach to these injuries.[8-27] Studies addressing treatment protocols are compromised by being retrospective and by having small sample size, multiple treatment and rehabilitation protocols, and definitions of success that often fail to assess a patient's ability to return to high-demand activities such as athletics.

This chapter presents an overview of current opinion regarding the assessment, surgical treatment, and rehabilitation of multiple ligamentous knee trauma, along with the insights gained from our personal experience with these complex injuries.

ANATOMY

Knowledge of the anatomy and biomechanics of the knee is necessary to accurately assess and appropriately treat multiple ligamentous knee trauma. The tibiofemoral joint is the largest joint in the human body, and its stability is primarily a function of soft tissue integrity. Static elements include the two menisci, the two cruciate ligaments, and the respective collateral ligament complexes. The quadriceps, hamstrings, popliteus, and gastrocnemius muscles are the primary dynamic stabilizers that cross and act on the knee joint.

The medial and lateral menisci are C-shaped, fibrocartilaginous structures. A thick peripheral margin tapers centrally to a thin rim, giving each meniscus a triangular shape in cross section, which enhances joint congruity. The menisci also function to absorb shock and dissipate loads across the articular surfaces of the tibiofemoral joint and to diminish friction by dispersing synovial fluid.[28] Their role as secondary stabilizers becomes particularly important with loss of normal ligamentous integrity. The medial meniscus, in particular, has been shown to act as a secondary stabilizer to resist anterior translation of the tibia when the integrity of the anterior cruciate ligament is compromised.[29,30]

Ligaments function as passive restraints that circumscribe joint motion. They serve a significant proprioceptive function, containing neurosensory triggers to initiate muscle actions that, under normal circumstances, help prevent abnormal torsional stresses on the joint.[31-33]

The cruciate ligaments are named for their tibial attachments. The anterior cruciate ligament (ACL) courses obliquely from the lateral femoral condyle to the tibia. It is composed of two functional bundles: the anteromedial bundle, which is tightest in flexion, and the posterolateral bundle, which becomes taut with extension.[31-34] The ACL primarily functions to control anterior translation of the tibia relative to the femur, accounting for 86% of the total resistance to anterior translation.[35] An intact ACL also limits varus and valgus laxity if the integrity of the fibular collateral ligament (FCL) or medial collateral ligament (MCL) is compromised, and it limits both internal and external rotation when the knee is in full extension.[36]

The posterior cruciate ligament (PCL) has a femoral point of attachment high in the intracondylar notch, giving it a nearly vertical course to its insertion in a sulcus below the articular surface of the posterior tibia. The PCL provides 95% of the total static resistance to posterior tibial displacement and, like the ACL, serves also as a secondary restraint to external and varus-valgus rotation.[35] As in the ACL, the PCL has been considered to have two functional components: an anterolateral bundle that is taut in flexion and a posteromedial portion that is tight in extension.[37]

The anatomy of the medial knee can be thought of as a multilayered sleeve of tissue extending from the anterior midline to the posterior midline and including both static and dynamic stabilizers that act synergistically. Based on cadaver dissection, Warren and Marshall[38] described three specific tissue layers and proposed that the medial ligaments represented condensations of these tissue planes, not discrete structures (Figure 16-1).

The superficial MCL, originating from the medial femoral condyle and inserting on the tibia 8 to 10 cm distal to the joint line, is composed of two groups of fibers. A thick, heavy group of vertically orientated parallel fibers forms an anterior band, and an oblique group of fibers courses posteriorly to merge with the capsule at the posteromedial corner. The oblique portion has been referred to as the *posterior oblique*

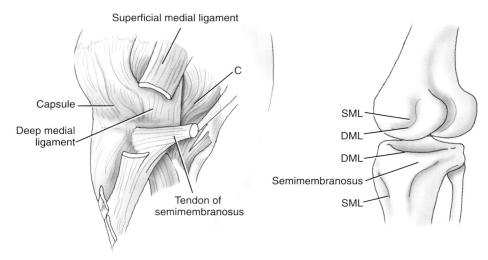

Figure 16-1: Oblique view of posteromedial aspect of the knee. With layer I, the mid-portion of the superficial medial ligament and the medial half of the semimembranosus sheath, removed, the structures composing the posteromedial corner can be seen. The figure on the right is included for orientation and shows the sites of attachment of the superficial medial *(SML)* and deep medial *(DML)* ligaments and the insertions of the semimembranosus tendon. *C* indicates the oblique popliteal ligament. *(From Warren LF, Marshall JL: The supporting structures and layers on the medial side of the knee,* J Bone Joint Surg *61A:59, 1979.)*

ligament (POL). Because the vertically orientated fibers lie within the axis of knee flexion, they show no change in tension during the functional arc of motion. The oblique fibers become lax with knee flexion. The middle capsular ligament (deep MCL) is a short, robust structure spanning the joint deep to the superficial MCL. Its fibers are intimately attached to the periphery of the medial meniscus. It is fused with the superficial MCL proximally, but discrete distally.

The superficial MCL has been shown to provide 78% of the restraining force to valgus stress at 25 degrees of flexion, with the capsule contributing only about 8%.[39] Even at 5 degrees of flexion the superficial MCL continues to be predominant (57%), although the role of the capsule increases (15%).[39] Stability to valgus stress at full extension seems to be provided primarily by the cruciate ligaments in conjunction with the POL and posterior capsule.[40,41]

The semimembranous muscle functions as an active stabilizer of the medial knee.[42,43] Its robust tendon inserts into bone at the posteromedial corner of the tibia just distal to the joint line, but additional insertions reinforce the posterior and posteromedial capsular ligaments. It is primarily a knee flexor, but it can produce some internal rotation of the tibia when the knee is in flexion. The vastus medialis portion of the quadriceps complex and the pes anserinus group (semi-tendinosus, gracilis, and sartorius) also provide some dynamic stability to the medial knee.

The anatomy of the lateral side of the knee is more complex and subject to more individual variation than the medial side. The iliotibial band (ITB) runs between the supracondylar tubercle of the femur and Gerdy's tubercle on the proximal tibia. The ITB is an important stabilizer of the lateral knee. During knee flexion the ITB becomes tight and moves posteriorly, exerting an external rotation and posteriorly directed force on the lateral tibia.[44] With extension the ITB moves anteriorly and in this position functions as an important sec-

ondary restraint to varus stress and posterolateral rotation.[45] The cordlike FCL originates on the lateral femoral epicondyle and inserts on the lateral aspect of the fibular head. Because its course is posterior to the axis of motion, it is tightest in extension and progressively relaxed in flexion. However, the FCL is the primary static restraint to varus stress at all flexion angles.[37,46,47] Secondarily, it resists external rotation and posterior translation.[40,42] Isolated injury is uncommon.[48]

Considerable variation in individual anatomy and confusing terminology have historically made study of the posterolateral corner (PLC) difficult, but its vital role in joint stability and the consequences of its injury have recently received considerable attention.[37,49-59] The PLC is composed of the arcuate complex, popliteus tendon, and popliteofibular ligament (Figure 16-2). Taken as a whole, the primary function of the posterolateral corner is to resist external rotation of the knee, but it also supports the PCL in resisting posterior translation.[37,46,47,60,61]

Perhaps the most important element of the PLC is the popliteus tendon and its attachments. The popliteus muscle originates from the posterior surface of the tibia and courses proximally and laterally, becoming tendinous at the posterolateral corner of the knee and inserting into the femur on the lateral femoral condyle, just anterior and distal to the attachment point of the FCL. The popliteus also has a robust attachment to the posterior fibular head via the popliteofibular ligament (PFL), which joins its tendon just proximal to the musculotendinous junction, and to the deep lateral capsule. The popliteus muscle "unlocks" the knee during flexion by internally rotating the tibia. Its tendon functions in many ways as a ligament in conjunction with the PFL, resisting varus rotation, posterior tibial translation, and posterolateral tibial rotation.[49,55,56,58,59,62] Loss of popliteal and PFL integrity places considerable additional stresses on both cruciate ligaments.[52,54]

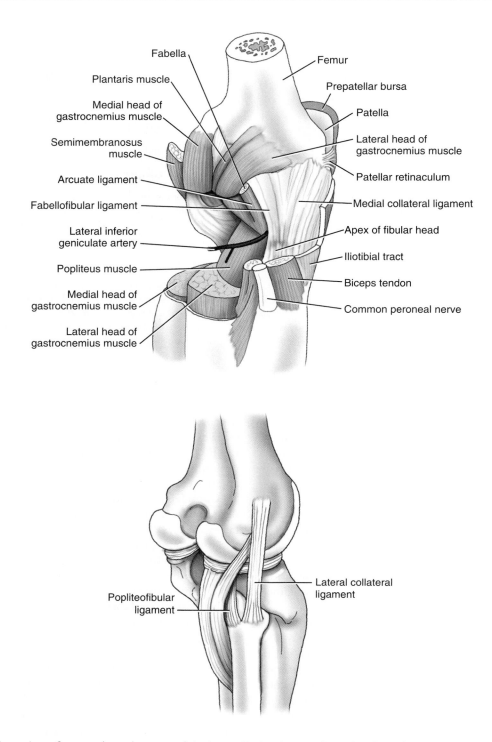

Figure 16-2: Oblique view of posterolateral aspect of the knee. (© *American Academy of Orthopaedic Surgeons. Reprinted from Chen FS, Rokito AS, Pitman MI: Acute and chronic posterolateral rotatory instability of the knee, J Am Acad Orthop Surg 8[2]:97-110, 2000; and Veltri DM, Warren RF: Posterolateral instability of the knee, J Bone Joint Surg 76A:460-472, 1994.)*

The biceps femoris is also an important dynamic stabilizer of the lateral knee. It courses posterior to the ITB, inserting primarily into the fibular head, but also sending strong attachments to the ITB, Gerdy's tubercle, the FCL, and the posterolateral capsule. With the ITB, the biceps is a strong dynamic external rotator of the tibia and a secondary lateral stabilizer.[57] Injury to the biceps femoris is frequently associated with ligamentous disruption of the posterolateral corner.[63]

Dynamic knee extension results from the action of the quadriceps muscle complex acting through the patella and its retinaculum as they insert into the anterior tibia via the infrapatellar tendon. The quadriceps is composed of four muscles that share a common tendinous insertion into the patella. The rectus femoris is the only one that also crosses the hip joint, originating from the ilium and forming the central anterior portion of the quadriceps complex. The vastus lateralis, which originates from the lateral femur, is the largest of the four and has distal attachments to both the lateral patella and the ITB. The vastus medialis originates opposite the vastus lateralis and inserts into both the common tendon and directly into the patella. Its distal fibers, which originate from the tendon of the adductor magnus and have an almost transverse course laterally to insert into the patella, are termed the *vastus medialis obliquus (VMO)*. The obliquus has an important role in dynamic patellar tracking,[64,65] and it is frequently injured during the acute lateral patellar displacement associated with significant medial-sided knee injury. The vastus intermedius arises from the femoral shaft deep to the rectus femoris and blends distally with the vastus medialis.

The two heads of the gastrocnemius originate from the respective femoral condyles. Their muscle bellies converge to form the inferior boundary of the popliteal fossa just distal to the knee joint.

The major neurovascular structures associated with the knee lie posterior to the joint in the popliteal fossa. The popliteal artery and vein are separated from the posterior capsule by a layer of fat. The artery is tethered proximally at the adductor hiatus and distally as it passes through the soleus arch, where it bifurcates into the anterior and posterior tibial arteries. Although the popliteal vein runs in close association with the artery, it is more mobile and thus less prone to injury. The four genicular arteries originate within the popliteal fossa and provide collateral circulation around the joint, as well as supplying the cruciate ligaments. However, this collateral circulation is inadequate to provide viable distal perfusion if popliteal arterial flow is obstructed.[66,67]

The sciatic nerve divides into the peroneal and tibial nerves within the popliteal fossa. The peroneal nerve is especially vulnerable as it courses in close proximity around the neck of the fibula. When mechanisms of injury involve varus angulation or posterolateral displacement of the tibia, the fibula acts as a fulcrum across which the nerve may be attenuated, resulting in varying degrees of injury.

ASSOCIATED INJURIES (VASCULAR AND NEUROLOGIC)

Multiple ligamentous knee injuries are associated with a significant incidence of injury to other organ systems, particularly in cases of high-energy trauma. Ten percent of patients have associated life-threatening chest, abdominal, or head injuries.[68] Additional musculoskeletal trauma, such as ipsilateral or contralateral hip, femur, or tibia fractures, also occurs. Among the most frequent associated injuries are those to the vascular and neurologic structures of the involved knee.

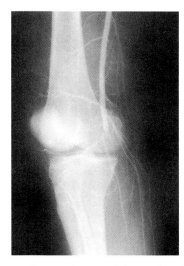

Figure 16-3: Complete occlusion of the popliteal artery occurring after an anterior dislocation of the knee in a 21-year-old motorcycle rider.

The popliteal artery is always at risk in association with MLKI because of anatomic constraints. It is tethered just proximal to the knee as it exits Hunter's canal and just distally at the soleus arch. Displacement of the tibia posteriorly is typically associated with transection of the artery, whereas anterior dislocations tend to cause stretch injury.[67,69] The incidence has been reported as being between 8% and 64%[21,67,70] (Figure 16-3). The incidence of vascular injury does not seem to vary significantly with direction of tibial displacement.[67,71] In general, higher-energy injuries are associated with a greater risk of vascular injury.[21] However, it is important to emphasize that there is no statistical difference in the incidence with respect to whether the patient's knee is dislocated or reduced at the time of initial evaluation.[68,72] Thus patients who manifest the significant laxity reflective of MLKI on initial examination should be transported immediately to a medical center equipped to provide definitive vascular evaluation and care, whether there is a clear history of knee dislocation or not.

Injury to the popliteal artery predictably results in distal vascular insufficiency. This fact was first established after World War II, when DeBacke and Simeone[66] reviewed 2471 popliteal artery injuries from that conflict and found that ligation was associated with a 72.5% amputation rate.

Although collateral circulation about the knee is inadequate for long-term perfusion, it may initially be sufficient to provide normal pulses and thus a false sense of security.[13,66,70] It is vitally important to recognize and treat popliteal artery injury acutely. Successful outcomes after arterial injury are extremely time dependent.[67,73,74] Green and Allen[67] found that when popliteal artery repair was completed within 8 hours of injury, the amputation rate was 11%, but increased dramatically if delayed beyond that time. Even at 6 hours after injury, 66% of patients developed myonecrosis resulting in at least some degree of clinically relevant muscle fibrosis.[67,74]

The orthopedic literature has traditionally recommended that arteriography be performed to access vascular injury in all cases of MLKI.[16,69,75-79] However, several authors have more recently questioned its universal necessity.[80-84] Treiman and colleagues[84] reviewed 115 patients with unilateral knee dislocations who underwent arteriography. They found that of the 86 patients (75%) who had normal arterial pulses, 77 (90%) had a normal arteriogram, 5 (6%) had arterial spasm, and 4 (5%) had an intimal tear. In this review, the finding of a normal pedal pulse was 100% accurate in predicting the need for vascular surgery because those with spasm and intimal tears were managed nonoperatively. Of those 29 patients who had abnormal pulses, 23 (79%) had popliteal artery injuries that required vascular repair.[84] In another study, Dennis and co-workers[80] evaluated 38 knee dislocations and also found that physical examination was 100% accurate in diagnosing those who would require vascular repair. These authors, and others, also point out that arteriography is expensive and is frequently associated with significant time delay before definitive treatment can be initiated; that complications such as pseudoaneurysm, arteriovenous fistula, and contrast reactions can occur in 1% to 2% of patients; and that arteriography has a false-positive rate of 5%.[85]

As an alternative to arteriography, Doppler evaluation of arterial flow with a calculation of ankle-brachial indices (ABIs) has been recommended.[80,82,86,87] The ABI is calculated by dividing the Doppler arterial pressure distal to injury by the Doppler arterial pressure in an uninvolved arm. Johansen and colleagues[81] and Lynch and Johansen[83] have shown that if an ABI of less than 0.90 is considered abnormal, major arterial injury can be predicted with excellent sensitivity and specificity.

The bottom line is that the specific approach chosen will depend on the particular dynamics of the medical center where treatment is being rendered and the comfort level of the orthopedic and vascular surgeons supervising the care. However, basic guidelines always apply. A warm but pulseless foot should never be merely "observed."[67,88] An absent pulse should never be attributed merely to arterial "spasm."[67] Capillary refill is a poor indicator of vascular integrity, because significantly less blood flow is necessary to sustain cutaneous circulation than to meet the metabolic demands of skeletal muscle.[84] If the popliteal artery is transected, loss of circulation will almost always be immediate and obvious. However, in cases of crushing or moderate stretching, the artery may remain grossly intact and disruption of the intimal layer can promote the formation of a thrombus that may lead to progressive arterial occlusion, although clinical studies have demonstrated that this risk is low.[79,89,90] Thus if the orthopedic surgeon decides that the patient does not need to undergo arteriography, hourly serial vascular examination for 72 hours is mandatory. Patients who are good candidates to avoid arteriography are those with isolated low-energy knee injuries who are fully alert and have normal symmetric pulses. Those patients with associated trauma such as a head injury, those who require intubation, or those who will be undergoing a lengthy surgical procedure for treatment of associated

injury should be strongly considered for arteriography even if the initial vascular examination is completely normal. Patients demonstrating any asymmetry of distal pulses or an abnormal neurologic examination should always undergo arteriography as well. Those with frank signs of ischemia should have the radiographic assessment in the operating room as part of the preparation for vascular repair. Even in the absence of any direct signs of ischemia, it can never be considered wrong to obtain an arteriogram.

When repair of a popliteal artery disruption is necessary, an interposed reversed saphenous vein graft is most frequently used.[91,92] The surgical exposure necessary for the vascular surgery may occasionally lend itself to the primary treatment of certain portions of ligamentous pathology, such as fixation of an avulsed PCL from the tibia. An external fixator spanning the reduced knee joint is the best means of providing immobilization after vascular repair. Four compartment fasciotomies of the calf are strongly advisable as a proactive measure against the edema that invariably occurs.[91-93] Provided that normal perfusion and venous return have been reestablished, it is generally safe to perform the definitive ligamentous repair/reconstruction for MLKI within 10 to 14 days.[15]

Popliteal vein disruption may occur in association with arterial injury. Isolated venous injury may also occasionally occur, but the incidence has not been defined. Ligation has been shown to result in prolonged edema and a high incidence of chronic venous stasis. If injury to the popliteal vein is recognized, surgical repair is warranted.[93,94]

Neurologic injury has been reported as accompanying 16% to 40% of MLKIs.* Peroneal nerve palsy is most common, particularly in association with posterior knee dislocation or with varus instability secondary to disruption of significant portions of the lateral structures. The prognosis of peroneal nerve injuries is poor, because the typical traction mechanism of injury generally causes axonotmesis (axon disruption with intact endoneurium) over an extensive segment of the nerve, so that primary repair is not possible.[95-98] Even partial recovery of function does not exceed 50%.[14,95,97] The results of cable grafting have not proven to be reliable.[99] Several authors have reported occasional improvement in neural function after peroneal nerve decompression at 3 to 5 months after injury.[24,100,101] We have not found this to be helpful enough to justify the morbidity of the procedure and generally advise patients that tendon transfers are the best option for improving function if spontaneous neurologic recovery has not occurred within 6 months.

The sensory deficits on the dorsum and lateral aspects of the foot, which occur with peroneal nerve dysfunction, do not present a significant functional deficit, but the footdrop and resulting gait impairment can represent a significant disability.[102] Contracture of the Achilles tendon will occur rapidly and must be prevented. In all cases of peroneal nerve dysfunction, an ankle-foot orthosis must be applied immediately and supplemented with passive range of motion (PROM) exercises to maintain full range of motion (ROM)

---

*References 3, 6, 12, 13, 19, 21, 23, 24, and 71.

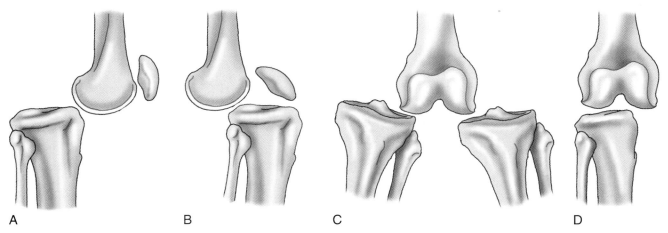

Figure 16-4: Classification of knee joint dislocations. **A,** Anterior; **B,** posterior; **C,** lateral or medial; **D,** rotary. *(From Klimkiewicz JJ, Petrie RS, Harner CD: The dislocated knee. In Insall JN, Scott WN, editors: Surgery of the knee, ed 3, vol 1, Philadelphia, 2001, Churchill Livingstone.)*

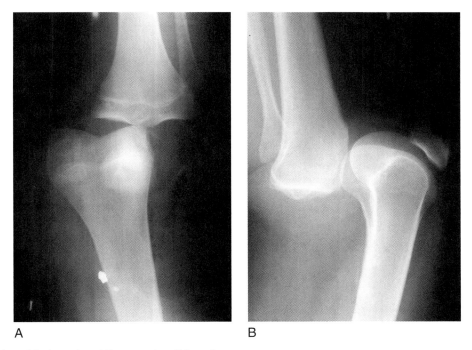

Figure 16-5: Examples of **A,** lateral and **B,** posterior dislocations.

of the ankle and great toe. Electromyography (EMG) testing should be obtained at 3 weeks postinjury to assess whether the nerve lesion is a neuropraxia (demyelination of the nerve without axonal damage), in which case recovery is commonly observed within 1 to 4 months, or a more severe lesion.[100,103] Absent clinical return of nerve function, follow-up testing at 3 to 4 months postinjury may be warranted to investigate any potential for recovery before decisions regarding surgical intervention are made.[100,104] Paresthesias in a stocking distribution should suggest the possibility of compartment syndrome rather than just simple neuropraxia of the peroneal nerve.

Tibial nerve trauma occurring in association with MLKI carries an even worse prognosis than peroneal nerve injury.

Tibial nerve injuries are generally associated with high-energy trauma and popliteal artery disruption.[100] Chronic tibial nerve palsy results in poor function, is refractory to tendon transfer, and generally necessitates below-knee amputation.

CLASSIFICATION AND MECHANISM OF INJURY

Historically, knee dislocations have been classified as one of five types according to the direction of tibial displacement relative to the femur: anterior, posterior, medial, lateral, and rotatory (Figures 16-4 and 16-5). This scheme is well established in the medical literature and may be useful if the

MLKI patient's knee is dislocated, but it is obviously not applicable to those situations in which a dislocation or subluxation has previously spontaneously reduced. Also, the position classification system only suggests, but does not actually define, the pattern of ligamentous injury.

Anterior dislocations predominate in most published series of knee dislocations.[67,71,105] The typical mechanism of injury is hyperextension. Biomechanical studies performed by Kennedy[71] demonstrated that with hyperextension the posterior capsule failed initially, followed by the ACL and then potentially the PCL. The popliteal artery was torn if hyperextension reached approximately 50 degrees.[71] The pattern and magnitude of collateral ligament involvement vary. Less force is required to produce an anterior dislocation than to produce posterior or collateral displacements, and an anterior dislocation may be produced by such a seemingly innocuous mechanism as missing a step while descending stairs or lunging to beat a throw to first base during a softball game.

Posterior dislocation requires considerable force and is most often associated with high-energy vehicular trauma.[20] The most common mechanism of injury is that of a direct, posteriorly directed force striking the anterior tibia just below the knee, as exemplified when the upper shin hits the dashboard during a deceleration motor vehicle accident. As a posterior dislocation occurs, the PCL, as the primary stabilizer to posterior translation, is always disrupted, but injury to the ACL is not inevitable.

Medial or lateral dislocations are encountered less frequently than anterior or posterior dislocations. The mechanism of injury is most often a high-energy direct blow to the side of the knee, such as occurs in a vehicle-pedestrian collision. Fracture-dislocations are more frequent than purely ligamentous injury.[12,68,106] Disruption of both collateral ligaments and one of the cruciate ligaments typically occurs.

Multiple ligamentous knee injuries can also be classified according to the specific structures injured and the extent of the disruption (total vs. partial). Many combinations of cruciate and collateral ligament injury are potentially possible. Eastlack and colleagues[107] and Schenck[108] have developed and advocated such an anatomically based system (Table 16-1 and Figure 16-6). This approach allows the description of pathology to be objective, consistent, and reproducible, which is crucial for clinical research and outcome studies; however, it requires an exacting physical examination. Recognized patterns of injury include the following: (1) knee dislocated

TABLE 16-1

Anatomic Classification System

TYPE	DESCRIPTION
KDI	Dislocation with single cruciate + single collateral ligament
KDII	Both cruciate ligaments torn, collateral ligaments intact
KDIIIM	ACL + PCL + MCL
L	ACL + PCL + LCL/PLC
KDIV	Both cruciate ligaments + both collateral ligaments torn
KDV	Fracture-dislocation

The letters C and N can be added to denote arterial and neurologic injury, respectively.[107]

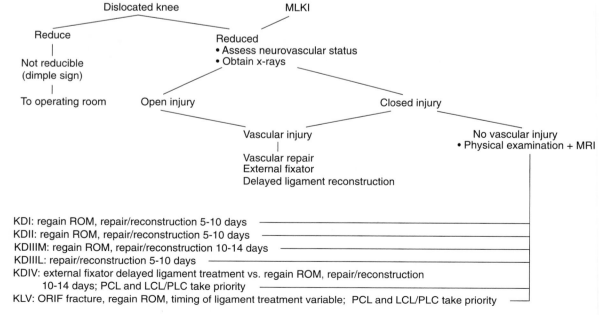

Figure 16-6: Treatment algorithm for multiple-ligamentous knee injury.

BOX 16-1
Gundersen Lutheran Sports Medicine Rehabilitation Protocol for MLKI

Phase I (Weeks 1-6)

Long Leg Postoperative Brace/Splint

Locked at 0 degrees weeks 0-2 for ADLs and gait

0-90 degrees (controlled supervised motion of the knee) (protect PCL with counterforce motion) weeks 2-6

Weight Bearing

Weeks 0-2 NWB with brace locked at 0 degrees

Weeks 2-4 toe-touch WB with brace locked at 0 degrees

Weeks 5-6, with brace unlocked 0-90 degrees (if LE control) (PWB week 5—50%-75%, PWB week 6—75%-100%)

If applicable begin aquatic therapy at week 4

Range-of-Motion Goals

	Extension	Flexion
ACL/PCL/medial	Full physiologic extension of 0 degrees (weeks 1-3)	0-90 degrees
ACL/PCL/lateral	No greater than 10 degrees recurvatum (week 3-6)	0-90 degrees

Proprioception/Kinesthesia

NWB → PWB activities

Proactive training (eyes open)

Single-plane → multiplane board

Perturbation training: submaximal

Strengthening

Quadriceps sets, single-leg raise (with brace → without brace)

Electrical stimulation as needed

Biofeedback as needed

Weeks 4-6 (with brace)

- CKC leg press (0-60 degrees)
- CKC knee extension (0-60 degrees)
- Wall squats (0-60 degrees)—two legs
- Total leg strengthening (LE kinetic chain)
  - Avoid adduction exercise—medial side injury
  - Avoid abduction exercise—lateral side injury

Exercise

Core stability exercises (as tolerated but protect surgical repair)

Upper extremity exercises (as tolerated but protect surgical repair)

Return to Sedentary Work

2-4 weeks (leg must be elevated at work, continuous ankle pumps to prevent DVT)

Phase II (Weeks 6-12)

Long Leg Postoperative Brace/Splint

Unlocked to allow full range of motion

Discharge brace at week 7 (no quadriceps lag with straight leg raise, good LE control, and no antalgic gait)

Functional knee brace 7-8 weeks (atrophy pads as needed)

Weight Bearing

Full WB (must have at least neutral extension, no quadriceps lag with straight leg raise, good LE control, and no antalgic gait)

Discharge crutches week 8 (no quadriceps lag with straight leg raise, good LE control, and no antalgic gait)

Range-of-Motion Goals

Gradual increase of knee flexion

Full range of motion at weeks 8-12

Proprioception/Kinesthesia

FWB

Double-leg exercises → single-leg exercises

Single-plane tilt board → multiplane tilt board

Eyes open → eyes closed

Perturbation training (proactive training), submaximal

Strengthening

3 sets × 10 reps at approximately 50%-75% maximum

FWB CKC exercises, 0-60 degrees

Weeks 8-12: OKC quadriceps exercises from 75-60 degrees

(continued)

DVT, Deep vein thrombosis; *FWB,* full weight bearing; *LE,* lower extremity; *NWB,* non–weight bearing; *PWB,* partial weight bearing; *WB,* weight bearing; *ADLs,* activities of daily living.

with a single cruciate and collateral ligament disrupted (KDI), the most frequent pattern being ACL plus PLC injury;[76,109] (2) both cruciate ligaments disrupted, collateral ligaments grossly intact (KDII)—a rare injury in which there is magnetic resonance imaging (MRI) evidence of injury to one or both collateral ligament complexes, but without increased clinical laxity; (3) both cruciate and one collateral ligament complex disrupted (KDIII), the most frequently encountered pattern of MLKI and further subdivided into M or L to distinguish medial or lateral collateral involvement; (4) both cruciate and both collateral ligaments disrupted (KDIV), occurring secondary to high-energy trauma and resulting in profound loss of joint integrity; and (5) fracture-dislocation of the knee (KDV); MLKI in association with intraarticular fractures of the tibial plateau or femoral condyles, a separate entity described by Moore[110] and Schenck and colleagues.[111] Clinical studies using this system demonstrate that, in general, the higher the number, the greater the magnitude of injury, the rate of complications, and the length of recovery and the poorer the outcome as measured on objective standardized scales.[106,112] Injuries involving MCL rupture are associated with the highest rate of extensor mechanism injury.[113] The incidence of medial-sided injury is higher than lateral collateral complex disruption.[18,25]

Dislocations must also be classified as either compound (open) or closed. Compound injury is not uncommon, with a reported incidence of between 19% and 35%.[4,23,106] An open knee dislocation, in general, carries a worse prognosis, secondary to more severe injury to the soft tissue envelope and the more complicated nature of the treatment protocol, which generally must involve multiple, staged surgical procedures.

BOX 16-1

Gundersen Lutheran Sports Medicine Rehabilitation Protocol for MLKI—cont'd

Exercise

Core stability exercises (as tolerated but protect surgical repair)

Upper extremity exercises (as tolerated but protect surgical repair)

Low-Impact Aerobics

Weeks 8-12: cycling, elliptical, NordicTrack, etc.

Return to Work

Return to low-demand work activities

Phase III (Weeks 12-24)
Proprioception/Kinesthesia

Continue phase II exercises; progress to more advanced exercises

Perturbation training exercises

- Submaximal → maximal
- Slow → fast
- Known (proactive) → unknown (reactive) patterns

Strengthening

3 sets × 10 reps at approximately 75%-100% maximum

Weeks 12-18:

- 30-90 degrees for OKC knee extension exercises (approximately week 12 depending on joint stability, surgical repairs, comorbidities, and physician approval)

Weeks 18-24:

- 0-90 degrees for OKC knee extension exercises (depending on joint stability, surgical repairs, comorbidities, and physician approval)
- 0-90 degrees for OKC knee flexion exercises (depending on joint stability, surgical repairs, comorbidities, and physician approval)

Return to Work

Return to moderate-demand work activities

Phase IV (Week 24 and Beyond)
Functional and Sport-Specific Activities

Straight-ahead running, approximately 6-7 months

Agility, approximately 7-8 months

Functional knee brace for strenuous manual labor or sports participation

Strenuous manual labor, approximately 9-12 months

Return to full sports activity, approximately 9-12 months (patient must meet criteria identified in phase IV for functional testing algorithm)

EVALUATION AND INITIAL TREATMENT

The pronounced deformity of a knee dislocation is usually obvious on initial examination; however, spontaneous reduction of dislocations and subluxations does occur. Several authors have reported the incidence as being between 20% and 50%.[25,68,72,73,107] Thus the appearance of the knee at the time that the patient seeks treatment is not necessarily reflective of the degree of structural injury. Abrasions, contusions, gross crepitus, or bogginess about the joint should suggest substantial knee trauma, but a multiple ligament–injured knee may occasionally look misleadingly benign. Rupture of the posterior capsule and gross disruption of collateral ligaments allow blood and synovial fluid to be dispersed into the periarticular soft tissue, and effusion is thus an inconsistent sign. A high index of suspicion must prevent such a knee from escaping detection in a patient with polytrauma; a patient who is intubated, who is sedated, or who cannot give a history; or a patient in whom more obvious injury may be present and deflect attention. That same attention to detail will prevent the underdiagnosis of MLKI in low-velocity trauma. There is a tendency among medical practitioners to doubt that so significant an injury could occur from recreational athletic participation, but we have seen a number of dislocated and bicruciate ligament–injured knees from such seemingly benign activities as running the bases in softball, playing backyard volleyball, and dunking a basketball on the playground.

The importance of immediate recognition of MLKI lies not in the treatment of its instability, but as a prompt to the recognition of associated occult vascular injury, which may have limb-threatening consequences. Thus a through examination for ligamentous instability is mandatory in all patients who give a history, or have evidence, of knee trauma. Knees that fall into recurvatum beyond 15 degrees compared with the contralateral side, or are grossly unstable with soft "floppy" endpoints when collateral stresses are applied at neutral extension, likely have disruption of at least one cruciate ligament, an entire collateral ligament complex, and a portion of the posterior capsule. Until proven otherwise, such knees must be presumed to be multiple ligamentous deficient and referred promptly to an orthopedic surgeon experienced in the diagnosis and treatment of that condition (see Table 16-1).

Some controversy exists as to whether a dislocated knee should be reduced before or after radiographs have been obtained. In the controlled setting of a hospital emergency center, and when the limb shows no evidence of neurovascular compromise, radiographs should be obtained initially to document the direction of displacement and rule out associated fractures. However, they are not absolutely mandatory and should never delay reduction of a knee dislocation if there are findings of a neurovascular nature. On an athletic field, we believe that a dislocation should be reduced as soon as recognized if competent personnel are in attendance. The limb is then splinted and the athlete immediately transported

to an appropriate medical center for definitive care. Physicians in community hospital emergency departments should also strongly consider reduction of a dislocation before transportation of the patient to a larger medical center. It goes without saying that it is essential that anyone reducing a dislocation, and then referring the patient elsewhere for definitive care, should provide accurate documentation accompanying the patient as to the direction of tibial displacement and initial neurovascular status of the limb. In general, prompt reduction decreases the likelihood of neurologic injury secondary to prolonged stretching, helps reestablish circulation, and minimizes soft tissue edema.

Reduction of a knee dislocation can usually be accomplished with simple longitudinal traction delivered through the tibia while an assistant provides countertraction by stabilizing the femur. As the tibia is disengaged from the femur, it is lifted or gently pushed into an anatomic relationship. Hyperextension is to be avoided, particularly when reducing anterior dislocations. Simple longitudinal traction is not likely to cause additional injury, even if performed before radiographs are obtained. When performed promptly at the scene of injury, no anesthesia is generally necessary to effect prompt reduction of a dislocation. Otherwise, intramuscular analgesia or intravenous sedation is generally sufficient, and general anesthesia is rarely necessary.

Occasionally, closed reduction is prevented by the interposition of soft tissue. This occurs most often in posterolateral dislocations and is due to the infolding of the medial collateral ligament and capsule. An indentation on the skin over the medial knee serves as an indicator of these extremely rare "complex" dislocations.[95,96]

After reduction, high-quality anteroposterior and lateral radiographs must be obtained to confirm an anatomic reduction and to reassess the knee for periarticular fractures. Fractures about the knee and ipsilateral limb are common. *Fracture-dislocation of the knee* refers to the combination of MLKI plus an intraarticular fracture of the femoral condyles or tibial plateau.[110,111] This entity is distinct from the purely ligamentous injury discussed in this chapter. Avulsion fractures, such as those from the fibular head, cruciate attachments, or anterolateral capsule (Segond's fracture), frequently accompany knee dislocations and multiligamentous injury.[11,24,107] They should be considered within the context of a ligamentous injury because they do not change basic treatment and prognosis, as do joint-destabilizing intraarticular fractures associated with fracture-dislocations of the knee.

Particularly in high-energy trauma, a significant rate of associated remote musculoskeletal trauma coexists with MLKI and should be suspected and ruled out. High-energy dislocations are also associated with injuries to other body systems. Management of high-energy knee dislocation is initially the same as that for any polytrauma patient. The examiner ensures an adequate airway, respiration, and cardiac output. A primary survey documents the neurovascular status of all four extremities. A trauma series of radiographs always includes lateral cervical spine, chest, and anterior/posterior pelvis films.

If associated unstable fractures have been ruled out on postreduction radiographs, a ligament examination is performed immediately after closed reduction. In cases of coexisting unstable fractures, vascular injury, or open injuries requiring emergent care, this examination is performed with the patient under anesthesia. It is important that all elements of potential pathologic laxity be defined. No knee is too painful or too swollen for a gentle and specific knee examination. If the patient is in too much pain for a thorough examination, brief conscious sedation will allow the assessment. We have found the following approach to be helpful.

We begin by visually inspecting the knee. Abrasions provide clues to the mechanism of injury and resultant pathology in instances when the injury occurred secondary to direct violence. Bogginess and ecchymosis suggest areas where capsular or collateral complexes have been disrupted (Figure 16-7).

The stability examination begins with evaluation of the contralateral knee, if it is uninjured. In this way, the baseline laxity of the patient's injured knee can be inferred. An individual with significant generalized physiologic laxity may otherwise demonstrate translation during testing, which may seem pathologic. The stability examination of the injured knee begins with Lachman's test for ACL integrity. It is performed in the standard position of 30 degrees of knee flexion. In a knee with multiplanar instability, it is particularly important to control rotation during the test to avoid false-positive results. The Lachman's test is positive or negative based solely on the quality of the end point to anterior translation,[114] but the extent of excursion may be influenced by associated pathology in a MLKI. Significant additional excursion may result when the PCL is incompetent, which reflects the reduction of the posterior drop-back of the tibia.

The most accurate clinical test to assess PCL integrity is the posterior drawer test.[115-120] With the knee flexed to 90 degrees and with the tibia maintained in neutral rotation, a posteriorly directed force is applied to the proximal tibia. The extent of posterior translation is evaluated by noting the change in the distance of the step-off between the medial tibial plateau and the medial femoral condyle. Normally, the plateau is positioned approximately 10 mm anterior to the condyle. Complete tears of the PCL demonstrate a greater than 10 mm translation, so that the plateau assumes a position posterior to the condyle[117] (Figure 16-8). Partial tears demonstrate less displacement. Bilateral comparison is important. Rubinstein and colleagues[119] found that the posterior drawer test, when performed in conjunction with palpation of the anterior tibial step-off, was 96% accurate, 90% sensitive, and 99% specific, and had an 81% interobserver agreement of grade in diagnosing PCL insufficiency. The posterior sag sign (Godfrey's test) is also helpful. With the patient lying supine, the examiner grasps the heels of both feet and supports them while the knees are flexed to 90 degrees. Under normal circumstances the tibial tubercle is slightly prominent on the anterior tibia. With even partial PCL insufficiency the profile of the tibia becomes flat, and with complete disruption it becomes concave.[120] If PCL integrity is compromised, it is important to remember to correct the posterior sag to neutral when examining for collateral ligament integrity.

The medial collateral structures are examined initially at 30 degrees of flexion and then at neutral extension. The superficial MCL is the primary restraint to valgus force at 30 degrees of flexion, and laxity with the knee in that position, which decreases as the knee is further extended, reflects isolated disruption of that structure. Because inadvertent external rotation of the tibia as load is applied may cause the examiner to overestimate medial laxity on clinical examination, valgus stress testing should be performed with the foot already maximally externally rotated. Subtle increases in laxity are meaningful. During laboratory testing, Grood and colleagues[39] measured only 5 mm of medial opening during the application of valgus stress after the superficial MCL was completely sectioned. Laxity at neutral extension reflects disruption of the posteromedial corner, as well as the superficial MCL. Medial injury of this magnitude rarely occurs without

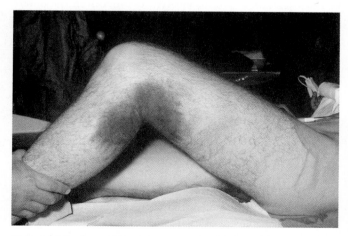

Figure 16-7: Extensive ecchymosis is evident and suggestive of the disruption of the lateral collateral ligament complex and posterolateral corner that occurred in association with an anteromedial (KDIIIL) dislocation of the knee in a college football player.

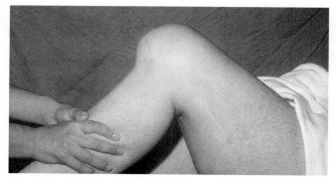

Figure 16-8: Grade III posterior drawer test.

associated disruption of at least one cruciate ligament. Lack of integrity of the medial hinge in the multiple ligament–injured knee will render the pivot shift and reverse pivot shift tests invalid. It is frequently difficult to separate vastus medialis tenderness from MCL pain during clinical examination. Because valgus injuries are associated with a high incidence of damage to the extensor mechanism with resultant acute patellar instability, a high index of suspicion is warranted. A 9% to 21% incidence of damage was reported in one study.[113]

Examination for integrity of the FCL and the PLC is the most difficult part of the examination and is of crucial importance. Because MRI scans often have a lower sensitivity in this portion of the knee, they cannot be relied on to replace a careful physical examination. Failure to recognize and properly treat disruption of the anatomically complex PLC is a significant cause of failure in reconstructive knee surgery. Occult PLC injuries can occur in association with either PCL or ACL disruption.[52,121-124]

The external rotation recurvatum test (ERRT), posterolateral drawer test (PLDT), and assessment of external tibial rotation (dial test) have demonstrated efficacy in assessing the integrity of the PLC.[122,125-127] However, no one test is completely sensitive or specific. The ERRT is performed with the patient supine (Figure 16-9). The great toe of each foot is grasped and the patient's knees are allowed to fall toward full passive extension as the feet are lifted off the examination table. The test is considered positive when the affected knee assumes a posture of varus angulation, hyperextension, and external rotation of the tibia.[122] Several authors have considered this to be the most specific test for PLC insufficiency.[63,128] It is generally not particularly uncomfortable for the patient and so can be performed even in the acutely injured knee. It must be carefully performed in cases of acute multiple ligament disruption, however, because disruption of the posterior capsule may allow dangerously excessive hyperextension and the knee may sublux or redislocate. The PLDT is performed by applying a posteriorly directed force to the tibia with the knee flexed 80 degrees while the foot is externally rotated 15 degrees. It is positive when the lateral tibial plateau moves posteriorly while the medial half of the knee maintains its resting position[122] (Figure 16-10). If PCL integrity is compromised, it is important to differentiate the amount of posterior displacement that occurs when the foot is maintained in neutral rotation versus that when it is externally rotated. Additional displacement or a softer end point with 15 degrees of external rotation reflects PLC injury in addition to PCL disruption. The dial test for external tibial rotation is most accurately assessed with the patient prone or sitting with the knees hanging at 90 degrees of flexion over the edge of the examination table. This is not generally possible in the acute setting, so the test is performed supine (Figure 16-11). While an assistant maintains both knees at 30 and then at 90 degrees of flexion, the examiner grasps the forefeet and provides a symmetric external rotation force.[126] The amount of external rotation of the feet relative to the axis of the femur is assessed. Because the

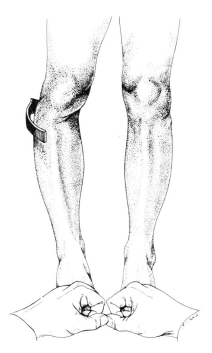

Figure 16-9: External rotation recurvatum test. *(From Hughston JC, Norwood LA Jr: The posterolateral drawer test and external rotational recurvatum test for posterolateral rotatory instability of the knee, Clin Orthop 147:82-87, 1980.)*

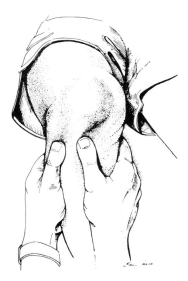

Figure 16-10: Posterolateral drawer test. *(From Hughston JC, Norwood LA Jr: The posterolateral drawer test and external rotational recurvatum test for posterolateral rotatory instability of the knee, Clin Orthop 147:82-87, 1980.)*

normal range of external rotation varies widely within the population, bilateral comparison is mandatory. If structural injury to the PLC exists, there will be an increase in external rotation of at least 10 to 15 degrees at 30 degrees of flexion, because the PLC is the primary stabilizer preventing external rotation. As the knee is flexed to 90 degrees, a reduction in this increased rotation, though remaining greater than the

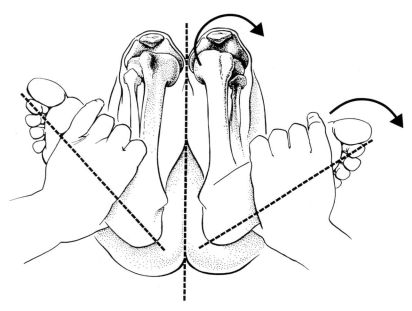

Figure 16-11: Tibial external rotation test (supine). Excessive tibial rotation, as well as posterior translation of the lateral tibial plateau, is noted in cases of posterolateral rotational instability. *(From Loomer RL: A test for knee posterolateral rotary instability, Clin Orthop 264:235-238, 1991.)*

contralateral side, reflects PCL integrity, because the PCL is the secondary stabilizer resisting external rotation and gains mechanical advantage as the knee is flexed. An increase in the amount of external rotation at 90 degrees compared with 30 degrees indicates combined PLC and PCL disruption.[37,129] In all cases, palpation of the tibial plateau should be done for confirmation that the appreciated external rotation is due to the lateral tibial plateau moving posteriorly, as it will in PLC disruption, versus the medial plateau moving anteriorly, as will occur in posteromedial corner disruption causing anteromedial rotatory instability. The reversed pivot shift test may also be used to assess the PLC, provided that prior examination has established that the MCL complex is structurally intact. An intact medial hinge is necessary for the test. It is performed by bringing the flexed knee toward full extension, with a valgus load applied and with the tibia externally rotated. It is positive when the posteriorly subluxed tibia abruptly reduces as the knee passes through the arc of 20 to 30 degrees.[125] This reduction is theorized to occur secondary to the tension of the ITB, and thus the reverse pivot shift may be diminished or eliminated if its integrity is compromised.[130] Because as many as 35% of uninjured subjects have been found to exhibit a positive reverse pivot shift, comparison with the contralateral knee is necessary.[50,125]

Injury to the FCL rarely occurs in isolation, so a knee that manifests increased varus laxity on examination must prompt the assessment of PLC integrity.[48,63,130] In contradistinction, although posterolateral instability frequently manifests some degree of increased varus laxity, particularly if the injury to the posterolateral corner occurred because of a varus mechanism, varus laxity is not essential to the diagnosis of posterolateral instability.[128,129]

After examination, the knee should be immobilized at 20 degrees of flexion in a hinged brace. This position relaxes tension on the neurovascular structures and minimizes the likelihood that anterior subluxation will occur secondary to disruption of the posterior capsule. Circumferential wraps or casting should be avoided. As soon as comfort allows, limited ROM and quadriceps setting exercises are initiated; ROM of 0 to 30 degrees is usually tolerated. The arc of motion is gradually increased, depending on maintenance of reduction, until definitive surgery is performed. An external fixator may be used to immobilize the joint and maintain reduction in cases where profound instability makes maintenance of concentric reduction impossible, or when open wounds, skin compromise, or vascular compromise necessarily delays definitive ligament surgery.

An MRI scan should be obtained within a few days of injury. In the multiple ligament–injured knee, MRI is an extremely helpful adjunct to physical examination in defining the extent of soft tissue trauma. The extent and pattern of collateral ligament injury, the type of cruciate ligament injury (avulsion vs. midsubstance rupture), meniscal pathology, and potential occult injury to the extensor mechanism are generally well delineated (Figure 16-12). The PLC is generally not adequately demonstrated during routine studies, so additional thin section imaging sequences, orientated in the coronal oblique plane and including the entire fibular head, are helpful.[53,131,132] Overall, MRI scanning is extremely useful for decision making and preoperative planning. If there is periarticular osseous injury, a computed tomography (CT) scan may also be helpful.

Approximately 2% to 30% of knee dislocations in most published series are open injuries.[13,23,106] Basic principles of

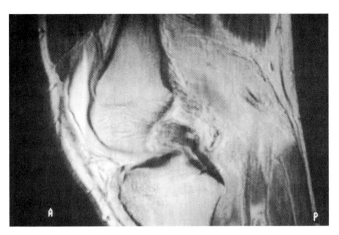

Figure 16-12: Avulsion of the PCL from the femur is well demonstrated on this MRI scan obtained after an anterior knee dislocation (KDIIIM) sustained during cross-country skiing.

wound and compound joint injury management apply.[106,133] Repairs and reconstructions are generally not performed at the time of the initial joint debridement and lavage. Arthroscopically directed irrigation may have occasional utility, but additional incisions beyond the initial wound should not be made unless absolutely necessary.

DEFINITIVE TREATMENT

The current standard of definitive care for most knee dislocations is surgical repair or reconstruction (or both) of the disrupted ligamentous and capsular structures. However, although a majority of authors have concluded that operative management is the treatment of choice for multiligamentous injury, little agreement exists with respect to the optimal timing of surgery and the specifics of ligamentous reconstruction.[*]

Historically, knee dislocations were usually managed with prolonged immobilization. The tradeoff for stability was significant knee stiffness. Early reports suggested that reasonable outcomes could be obtained with nonoperative management and that those results were comparable to surgical intervention.[3,6,13,14,71] However, during those years, the typical surgical treatment involved the reapproximation of cruciate ligaments with suture, rather than reconstruction with grafts, and other techniques that are of historical interest only. As the technique and success rate of single cruciate ligament reconstruction evolved, so too did its application to MLKI, and more recent authors have consistently reported superior results with an approach combining reconstruction of cruciate ligament insufficiency with repair of collateral ligament disruption.[8,15,18,20,26,27] We agree strongly with Montgomery[15] that, although nonoperative management is appropriate in selected instances, in a young and active patient

"there is little likelihood of obtaining excellent or near excellent results unless surgery is performed."

In each case, however, the decision for surgical versus nonoperative treatment must be individualized. A short period of immobilization, followed by ROM bracing, usually restores a physiologic ROM within a few weeks, though there is often severe residual laxity that causes significant functional instability. Therefore to be justified, surgical intervention must offer improved stability without compromising a physiologic ROM, and success is dependent on not only that portion of treatment which occurs in the operating room, but also that which is related to patient enthusiasm and compliance afterward. For success, both the ability of the surgeon to manage a complex and demanding procedure and the full cooperation of the patient during a lengthy convalescence are mandatory. Elements such as patient age and fitness, associated injuries, preinjury level of function, and availability of appropriate physical therapy must be considered. For example, multiple ligamentous injuries sustained during athletic participation typically occur in well-conditioned individuals who are already familiar with physical training and rehabilitation and are motivated to return to a level of function for which knee stability is crucial. In contrast, the risk/benefit ratio for multiple trauma patients is higher. The high-energy dislocations of motor vehicle injury are more likely to involve individuals with multisystem injury and those unaccustomed to regular physical exercise, who are unable or unmotivated to participate in the lengthy and arduous rehabilitation necessary to maximize their recovery.[3,68,134] Rather than improving their prognosis, well-intentioned surgical stabilization may instead increase the likelihood for permanent disabling stiffness. An old adage in orthopedic surgery is that "the enemy of good is better."

Four guiding principles apply to the surgical treatment of MLKI: (1) never jeopardize the life of the patient or the viability of the limb to improve the chance of obtaining a stable knee; (2) residual laxity is easier to treat than arthrofibrosis; (3) when in doubt regarding either patient compliance or tissue quality, delay surgery; and (4) the goal of surgery, regardless of pathology, is the restoration of all instability patterns with methods of fixation such that ROM can be allowed early in the postoperative course.

When early definitive surgery is not advisable, application of an external fixator or a hinged cast brace "burns no bridges." The spanning external fixator is often the best choice for those patients. This technique provides good stability of the knee joint, is readily adjustable, and allows excellent access to open wounds and assessment of neurovascular status. The fixation pins must be placed far enough away from the joint and in such a manner that the pin tracks will not compromise incision placement in future knee surgery. If a nonoperative approach is elected as the definitive treatment, the external fixator is maintained in place for 6 weeks before ROM exercises are begun. Anteroposterior and lateral radiographs should be obtained every 1 to 2 weeks during the 6 weeks of immobilization to confirm that reduction has not been lost.

*References 9, 11, 12, 17, 18, 21, 25, and 26.

Slight subluxation can occur; chronic subluxation is difficult to treat and is generally associated with poorer functional outcomes.

Although a detailed description of surgical technique is beyond the scope of this chapter, some specific points that bear on postoperative recovery and rehabilitation merit emphasis. Almost all knee dislocations involve complete disruption of the anterior and posterior cruciate ligaments (anatomic types KDII to KDIV).[108] The pattern of collateral ligament injury is variable. Knee dislocations are associated with a significant incidence of avulsion injury of both ligament and tendinous insertions. Frassica and colleagues[11] and Sisto and Warren[24] noted PCL avulsion of 77% and 88% and ACL avulsion of 46% and 63%, respectively, associated with MLKI. Our experience has demonstrated a lesser but still significant incidence (Figure 16-13). This is in contrast to the typical presentation of isolated ACL ruptures, where intrasubstance disruption is the rule.[108] Schenck and colleagues[135] have suggested that, at least in PCL disruption, avulsion is associated with higher strain rate (velocity) injury than is interstitial failure. Avulsion fractures are often large enough to be securely reapproximated with screws. Soft tissue avulsions are repaired to their anatomic site of origin with pull-out sutures.[136]

There is general agreement that injuries including the combination of PCL and PLC disruption are at particularly high risk of persistent functional instability, and that the results of early repair/reconstruction are superior to delayed approaches.[8,22,26,27,120] Surgical intervention within 2 weeks of injury is thus highly desirable. Early surgery also seems most appropriate when injury includes ligament avulsions, periarticular fractures, extensor mechanism disruption, or large displaced meniscus tears. For other injury patterns there is far less uniformity of opinion. Shelbourne and Carr[22] recommend initial nonoperative treatment for ACL/PCL/MCL (KDIIIM) injuries when the PCL laxity is grade II or less and PCL reconstruction alone if PCL laxity is grade III. Their approach is predicated on the belief that the PCL and MCL have "intrinsic" abilities to heal, that residual laxity is

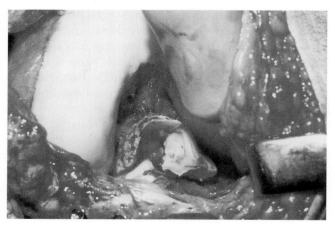

Figure 16-13: Exposure of the intercondylar notch demonstrates avulsion of the PCL from the femur and ACL from the tibia.

preferable to stiffness, and that ACL reconstruction can be performed electively if necessary as a secondary procedure once ROM is reestablished. Fanelli and colleagues[137] have recommended that most ACL/PCL/MCL injuries be treated by initial brace immobilization followed by simultaneous arthroscopic bicruciate ligament reconstruction in 4 to 6 weeks after the MCL has healed. Any residual MCL laxity is treated with reconstructive techniques. Others recommend simultaneous bicruciate and collateral ligament reconstruction/repair performed within 5 to 14 days of injury unless extenuating circumstances exist.[8,24,26,138,139] By this time, postinjury edema and the acute posttraumatic inflammatory response will have largely subsided and the joint's ROM will have been at least partially restored. However, anatomic definition of the collateral ligaments and capsule remains possible. The senior author has consistently followed this approach. Although PCL-only reconstruction may reduce the risk of permanent knee stiffness, bicruciate ligament reconstruction allows the most accurate centering of the tibia on the femur and minimizes stress on repaired collateral ligaments. We do not believe that delayed reconstruction of significant structural injury to the posterior medial or posterior lateral corners can consistently match the quality of the end result obtainable with acute surgical treatment. Although manipulation under anesthesia to obtain physiologic flexion may often be necessary if surgery is undertaken early, we agree with Cole and Harner[8] that more extensive arthrofibrosis has seldom been a problem. However, this approach assumes exacting surgical technique, tissue fixation that will tolerate aggressive rehabilitation, and appropriate patient compliance.

If a delay in operative intervention beyond 3 weeks is necessary, primary repair becomes more difficult as the definition of the collateral and capsular structures is progressively lost in abundant scar formation, and soft tissue contracture makes restoration of normal anatomic relationships difficult to achieve with precision. In that instance, it is usually best to continue to treat the patient nonoperatively for several months and defer overall reconstruction until a full ROM has been reestablished.

Several graft options are available for bicruciate reconstruction. Ipsilateral autografts (patellar tendon for the PCL and semitendinosus/gracilis for the ACL) can be used, but their harvest increases the morbidity of an already severely traumatized knee. Collateral autografts can be used, especially if the patient will not allow the use of allograft tissue, but their use does, at least theoretically, compromise a perfect knee and their harvesting requires additional operative time. The success rates obtained using allograft tissue in the reconstruction of isolated ACL and PCL injuries has been documented to approach that of autografts, and their use in the multiple ligament–injured knee has decided advantages.[17,20,26,140-142] Donor site morbidity is eliminated, and a second surgeon or assistant can prepare the grafts while the primary surgeon prepares the knee, thus saving significant operative time. Sterilely harvested, nonirradiated, fresh frozen allografts are recommended.[20,26,138] One whole patellar tendon may be split to yield the two separate bone-tendon-bone grafts needed for reconstruction of both cruciate ligaments; alternatively, one hemi–bone-tendon-bone graft provides an excellent graft for the ACL while an Achilles tendon allograft is used for the PCL. The only drawbacks to allograft use are potential disease transmission, limited availability, and cost.[143,144]

COMPLICATIONS OF MULTILIGAMENTOUS INJURIES

Possible complications of MLKIs include wound problems, loss of motion, residual laxity, and chronic pain. The incidence of complications may be minimized by careful preoperative planning, exacting surgical technique, and thorough postoperative rehabilitation.

The incidence of wound infections in open knee reconstruction has been documented to range from 0.3% to 12.5%.[3,68,145,146] High-energy injuries and MLKIs are particularly susceptible to wound complications, such as marginal necrosis and superficial infection, because of the exceptional soft tissue stress that invariably accompanies this level of trauma. Significant injury to the skin may occur even without the creation of an open wound, especially on the lateral side of the knee, where the skin and subcutaneous tissue may be sheared off the underlying fascia as the knee is dislocated. When this has occurred, the blood flow to the skin is tenuous and an incision in this area can be prone to wound breakdown. Open procedures are ideally delayed until soft tissues have recovered and posttraumatic edema and inflammation have waned. The reduction of tissue swelling is enhanced by knee joint motion, cryotherapy systems, and the active contraction of the muscles of the thigh and calf. The careful placement of incisions to provide adequate skin bridges, gentle handling of tissue, meticulous hemostasis, and judicious use of tourniquets are important intraoperative variables under the surgeon's control. If excessive swelling is encountered during wound closure, delayed closure or skin grafting should be considered. It is routine to administer a broad-spectrum antibiotic before and for 24 hours after surgery.[147] Any wound complications or any evidence of superficial infection should be managed aggressively to prevent progression. This may include the debridement of necrotic wound edges, drainage of hematomas, and temporary immobilization of the knee to remove tension on the vulnerable area of skin. Two series reviewing the treatment of deep infection after ligament reconstruction have been published.[148,149] Repeated arthroscopic irrigation and a 4- to 6-week course of intravenous antibiotics will often allow intraarticular grafts to be salvaged. Adequate outcomes can occur after deep infection but are generally inferior to those for patients without infection.[148]

Loss of motion is the most frequent and long-term complication affecting knees undergoing multiple ligament reconstruction.[150-153] The etiology is often multifactorial and may occur secondary to extraarticular scarring, intraarticular adhesion formation, improper graft tension, improper graft placement, or an inadequate notchplasty.

To reproduce normal knee kinematics, ACL and PCL grafts must be positioned so that they are as nearly isometric as possible. An isometric graft remains under consistent tension through the knee's entire arc of motion. Because the femoral attachment of the ACL lies so close to the knee's axis of rotation, small changes in the position of the femoral tunnel from that which is anatomic will result in substantial variations in graft tension during motion. A femoral tunnel that is placed too anterior will result in a graft that becomes lax in extension and tight in flexion, and a posteriorly positioned tunnel will cause the converse.[154] Depending on the flexion angle at which it was tensioned, the nonisometric graft will thus either limit motion or undergo progressive plastic deformation. A graft that reproduces the PCL's anterolateral bundle has been shown to provide the most stable reconstruction of that structure's complex geometry.[9,155-158] However, such a graft is inherently slightly nonisometric and will progressively tighten in flexion.[9,157,158] Thus terminal flexion is often lost after PCL reconstruction. The position of the knee at which cruciate grafts are tensioned and fixed has a significant effect on knee mechanics.[159] During bicruciate ligament reconstruction, the knee should be flexed to 90 degrees and tension applied simultaneously at the distal ends of both ACL and PCL grafts. This concomitant tension will center the tibia on the femur and reproduce the normal anatomic tibial step-off. The PCL graft is then fixed to the tibia with the knee maintained at 90 degrees of flexion and in neutral rotation. The ACL graft is tensioned with the knee flexed approximately 20 degrees. Final repair or reconstruction of the collateral ligaments is performed after both cruciate ligaments have been fully secured. Tensioning and fixing the PCL graft at a shallow flexion angle or after the ACL graft has been secured may result in the knee being nonisometrically constrained, resulting in a greater loss of flexion than normally expected or graft attenuation and failure.[155,159]

The uninjured ACL fits into the apex of the intracondylar notch at terminal knee extension with exact tolerance. Grafts are usually larger than the native ACL, have a different configuration, and have been shown to hypertrophy during the healing and remodeling process.[160,161] Thus surgical enlargement of the notch (notchplasty) is generally necessary to minimize the likelihood that graft impingement will cause extension block. Anterior malpositioning of the tibial tunnel during ACL reconstruction is also well known to increase the likelihood of graft impingement.[162]

The tendency toward scar formation is increased in severe knee trauma, being proportional to the magnitude of the injury and the subsequent inflammatory response. However, scar formation can be minimized by proper attention to antiinflammatory measures during the immediate postinjury period, allowing ROM preoperatively, careful surgical technique, and limiting the period of immobilization afterward. Because loss of terminal extension is particularly devastating as a result of its negative effect on the normal gait pattern, and because flexion is easier to obtain than extension if stiffness does occur, knees should be immobilized in extension after surgery. Soft tissue scarring is also minimized by the use of allografts for ligament reconstruction. Their use avoids the superimposition of graft donor site morbidity on an already vulnerable knee. When treating collateral ligament injury, plication procedures are best avoided, because they create nonisometric tethers to physiologic motion. When augmentation grafts are used, they should precisely reproduce anatomic structures. MCL injuries are notorious for causing ROM problems, which has led some to recommend that operative intervention be delayed until MCL healing is complete.[9,153] However, this concern is most applicable only to proximal and middle MCL injuries, which behave somewhat differently than distal tears. The latter are less prone to ROM problems, but frequently heal with residual valgus laxity.[163] Preoperative MRI scanning will clarify the location of pathology and allow appropriate planning.

Infrapatellar contracture syndrome (IPCS) represents the end result of extraarticular inflammation. The condition, first described by Paulos and colleagues,[164] represents an exaggerated fibrous hyperplasia of the periarticular soft tissues about the knee of uncertain etiology. If its course proceeds uninterrupted, IPCS results in significant and refractory stiffness. In its early stages it may be difficult to differentiate from complex regional pain syndrome (CRPS), as discussed in subsequent paragraphs. The two conditions may, in fact, be interrelated. IPCS is initially marked by diffuse warmth and tenderness about the knee, a persistent low-grade effusion, loss of motion (both flexion and extension), and the failure of muscle fitness deficits to resolve.[165-167] Prevention is the key to successful treatment. Encouraging an early ROM after surgery minimizes its occurrence. If IPCS is suspected in its early stages, immediate and vigorous antiinflammatory measures and gentle efforts toward improving ROM and patellar mobility, while avoiding aggressive physical therapy, will often be successful in restoring a normal progression of recovery.[164,165]

Adhesions occur within the synovial cavity more frequently than does extraarticular scarring after MLKI.[9,152,166,168] Persistent hemarthrosis is associated with the development of suprapatellar pouch adhesions that limit knee flexion, intracondylar notch scarring that limits knee extension, and negative effects on quadriceps function, because the pain of capsular distention and afferent signals from the knee lead to muscle inhibition, particularly in the vastus medialis.[32] For these reasons we recommend aspiration of all sizable postoperative hemarthroses at the time of the first postoperative visit. Early ROM is also extremely effective in minimizing intraarticular adhesions. The old adage that "a rolling stone gathers no moss" is particularly applicable.

Despite all appropriate efforts, ROM problems do occur in association with the treatment of MLKI. Cole and Harner[8] have reported a 10% to 20% incidence of arthrofibrosis in their series of patients who underwent multiple ligament reconstructions using fresh frozen allografts. Manipulation under anesthesia performed as necessary 6 to 8 weeks post-

operatively is generally successful in reestablishing physiologic flexion. In cases of refractory arthrofibrosis, particularly those cases involving extension deficits, arthroscopic lysis of adhesions, debridement of the infrapatellar fat pad, and lateral retinacular release may be necessary if improvement has not occurred within 10 to 12 weeks.[8,168]

Residual laxity after ligament reconstruction may result from missed diagnosis, failure of graft incorporation, failure of graft fixation, or technical errors in placing or tensioning grafts. The most common complication is recurrent posterior laxity after PCL reconstruction.[150] This may occur secondary to the failure to diagnose and properly treat concomitant posterolateral or posteromedial structural injury, a PCL graft of inadequate mechanical strength, technical errors during reconstruction, and ill-advised rehabilitation factors such as allowing weight bearing on a flexed knee or open chain hamstring exercise.[150,155,169] Preoperative MRI assessment and a comprehensive examination of knee stability under anesthesia should eliminate the possibility of missed collateral laxity. Injury to the PLC is well understood to require surgical repair/reconstruction rather than immobilization for successful healing. Less well understood is that the grade III MCL injuries associated with a dislocated knee do not heal predictably with simple immobilization as they generally do when occurring in isolation.[147] Graft incorporation requires that the tissue used retain its biomechanical properties as it remodels and undergoes the process of ligamentization, not that it merely heals to the host bone.[160,170] Impingement and the excessive tension and stress shielding that result from nonisometric graft placement are negative influences on this process.[160] Anterior placement of the tibial tunnel during ACL reconstruction has been shown to result in notch impingement at terminal extension that may cause graft failure secondary to repetitive blunt trauma or abrasion.[152,171] Recent attention has focused on the "killer" turn at the posterior tibia, which a PCL graft traverses as it courses from the tibial tunnel into the posterior intracondylar notch. This acute angle may result in graft attenuation or abrasion. Modifications of technique have been suggested by several authors.[172-174]

Complex regional pain syndrome is the currently preferred term for what has been known for years as reflex sympathetic dystrophy (RSD).[175] The International Association for the Study of Pain has defined the condition as a "departure from the orderly and predictable response of an extremity to some form of internal or external trauma."[176] It is not possible to predict patients at risk prospectively, and early recognition can be difficult because it shares many of the clinical symptoms associated with periarticular inflammation. The diagnosis of CRPS is suggested if postinjury pain exceeds the normal range for duration or severity of symptoms. Classically, affected patients exhibit hypersensitivity to stimuli, skin color changes, and subcutaneous edema.[176] Recovery is delayed, muscle atrophy continues, and joint stiffness develops. It has been suggested that injury to the infrapatellar branch of the saphenous nerve can serve as a trigger.[177] The diagnosis is purely clinical. There are no laboratory tests that are helpful. It was once thought that a patient's response to a sympathetic block was the best method for diagnosing this condition. More recent experience indicates that only a minority of those affected with CRPS will respond to a block, although those who do so will often benefit greatly.[178] There is no cure for CRPS, but current treatment recommendations suggest that a combined approach of medication, stress management training, and physical therapy will most effectively provide symptomatic relief and improved function.

Pain after multiple ligament reconstruction can also result from other etiologies. Anterior knee pain may occur, resulting from the posterior tibial sag of an incompetent PCL and secondary to the resultant increase in patellofemoral compression force. These symptoms are best prevented by a sound PCL reconstruction. Anterior knee pain may also occur in association with the failure to regain terminal extension.[179,180] Postinjury synovitis, which may persist secondary to occult chondral trauma, or localized irritation secondary to prominent ligament fixation devices may also cause discomfort. Osteonecrosis of the medial femoral condyle has been reported as a complication of PCL reconstruction, possibly secondary to excessive soft tissue dissection or placement of the femoral tunnel too close to the articular surface, which may injure the single nutrient vessel providing the intraosseous blood supply.[181,182] Care must also be taken to ensure that adequate osseous bone bridges of at least 1 cm are retained between the multiple tunnels drilled through the tibia during the course of multiple ligament reconstructions. Those affected with osteonecrosis manifest pain and tenderness at the site of pathology.

REHABILITATION

The rehabilitation of complex knee injuries has evolved significantly in the past two decades, reflecting advances in the treatment of single ligament repair and reconstruction. Current surgical approaches to MLKI, emphasizing the anatomic restoration of injured tissue, present the therapy team with an unmatched opportunity for optimal functional rehabilitation. However, no two instances of MLKI are exactly alike. Multiple variables affect rehabilitation and recovery, such as specific tissues injured and degree of disruption, specific technique of repair or reconstruction, physiology and psychology of the individual patient, and associated injuries about the knee or elsewhere in the body. The rehabilitation program must be "customized" to the individual patient, and ongoing communication between the surgeon and the rehabilitation team is mandatory.

Detailed rehabilitation protocols for MLKI have seldom been published.[183] There is a lack of research data on the forces imposed on healing tissue during the rehabilitation of these injuries and a lack of prospective, randomized, controlled clinical studies. The exact strategies employed in the rehabilitation of single ligament injury may not be directly applicable to the situation of MLKI, and occasionally may, as in the case of protecting both the reconstructed ACL and PCL concurrently, seem to be diametrically opposed. This creates significant challenges for the clinician. Except in major trauma centers, most therapists may not encounter these patients more than once or twice in a career and thus have little opportunity to learn from experience.

After MLKI, the progression of rehabilitation should occur in a logical sequence (see Box 16-1). Once the patient's impairments and functional limitations have been identified, specific algorithm-based protocols can be implemented for treatment. Issues to be addressed during recovery include the following:

1. Protection of ligament grafts and repaired tissues
2. Interventions to decrease pain, reflex inhibition, effusion, and edema
3. Measures to maximize ROM; initiate, facilitate, and enhance neuromuscular control; improve proprioception; and enhance dynamic stability of the knee through exercises and functional activities

The purpose of this section is to provide clinical pathways and rehabilitation procedures based on the current literature and our personal practical experiences. Many studies regarding the specific advantages/disadvantages and indications/contraindications for the use of open and closed kinetic chain exercise, the reduction of stress on the patellofemoral articulation, and the minimization of stress on cruciate and collateral ligament reconstruction have been published and will be summarized in the next several sections of this chapter.

Scientific Basis and Biomechanics of Knee Rehabilitation for Multiple Ligamentous Knee Injury

An understanding of the biomechanics of knee rehabilitation must be integrated in the examination, evaluation, and rehabilitation program interventions. Rehabilitation of MLKI should include exercises and functional activities to facilitate neuromuscular dynamic stability of the knee. The focus of the therapeutic interventions should be to provide dynamic stability through synergistic support of the injured ligaments.

Open Kinetic Chain Exercises versus Closed Kinetic Chain Exercises

Rehabilitation exercises for the knee can occur in either an open kinetic chain (OKC) or a closed kinetic chain (CKC) pattern. OKC exercises have the distal end of the extremity free in space, are typically non–weight bearing, and involve isolated joint exercises. The classic examples of exercises characterized by OKC in knee rehabilitation are exercises performed on the knee extension machine. CKC exercises are those in which the distal segment is in contact with a surface and meets resistance. Typical examples would be squat exercises, leg presses, and step-ups. OKC and CKC exercises produce different stresses on intraarticular knee ligaments. Appreciating these differences is critical when designing a rehabilitation program for the patient with MLKI.

Open Kinetic Chain Exercises and Ligamentous Stresses

Typically it has been thought that performing OKC exercises would cause significant anterior tibial translation and consequently be detrimental to an ACL injury. Several studies demonstrate that OKC knee extension creates anterior tibial translation and increased strain on the ACL.[184-191] Beynnon and colleagues[192] used a dynamic variable resistance transducer, which was surgically placed on the ACL to monitor in vivo stresses on the ACL. Several exercises were then performed that are commonly used in knee rehabilitation. ACL strain ranged from 0% to 4.4% depending on where the OKC exercise was performed in the ROM and the amount of resistance to the knee extension motion. Strain on the ACL with active knee extension was 2.8%. When a 45 Newton (N) weight was added to the distal end of the kinetic chain, it added an additional 1% strain to the ACL, up to 3.8%. With dynamic exercises, the peak strain occurred at 10 degrees of knee flexion.

When multiple-angle isometric exercises were performed at different positions, they created different stresses on the ACL. The angles of 15, 30, 60, and 90 degrees of knee flexion produce average peak strains of 4.4%, 2.7%, 0%, and 0%, respectively. When co-contraction exercises of both the quadriceps and hamstrings were performed at 15 degrees of knee flexion, they decreased the strain on the ACL by 1.6% to an average peak strain of 2.8%. This demonstrates the synergistic effects the OKC hamstrings contractions have on the ACL. When co-contraction exercises of both the quadriceps and hamstrings were performed at 30, 60, and 90 degrees of knee flexion, no strain was produced on the ACL. Based on this information, it is appropriate to use OKC following ACL reconstructive surgeries from 90 to 60 degrees of knee flexion in the ROM. Furthermore, using co-contraction exercises (particularly for MLKI) empirically may be protective to all of the healing structures by stabilizing the knee joint.[193-195] What are unknown are the specific strain rates that become detrimental to the ACL versus physiologic loading conditions and where the cut-off point should be to protect the healing ligament. As an example, if less than 3% strain on the ACL were within physiological loading limits of the ligaments, the ROM exercises could be performed between 90 and 30 degrees of knee flexion because the average peak strain on the ACL is only 2.7%. This is important because the knee functions more commonly with activities of daily living (ADLs) and sports in both OKC and CKC activities at 30 degrees of ROM compared with 60 to 90 degrees. Aune and colleagues[196] indicated that their research was actually protective to the ACL during a quadriceps contraction.

The quadriceps contractions are synergistic to the PCL because it decreases the strain and increases anterior tibial translation. Consequently, OKC knee extension exercises for rehabilitation of a patient with a PCL injury should be performed between 90 degrees and terminal extension (0 degrees) of the knee.

OKC knee flexion exercises, using the hamstrings, causes a posterior translation of the tibia creating more stress on the PCL. Several studies have demonstrated that the posterior translation increases as the knee flexion angle increases.[185,188,197] Because of the increased stresses on the PCL with isolated hamstring flexion exercises, OKC flexion exercises should be avoided with a PCL injury or PCL reconstruction early in the rehabilitation program. Moreover, because of the posterior shear forces created, it demonstrates that OKC hamstring exercises are synergistic with the ACL and as a result may be performed safely following ACL injuries and reconstructions.

Closed Kinetic Chain Exercises and Ligamentous Stresses

A widely held principle regarding CKC exercises is that because of the position, compressive forces, and co-contraction, less strain occurs to the ACL.[193-195,198,199] However, research by Beynnon and colleagues[191,192] demonstrated that CKC exercises create significant strain on the ACL. Various exercises were compared, including (1) OKC knee flexion to extension from 100 to 0 degrees; (2) CKC squats from 0 to 100 degrees; and (3) CKC squats from 0 to 100 degrees with sport-cord resistance with the load sensor. The average strain values produced by the exercises were (1) OKC of 3.5%; (2) CKC of 3.6%; and (3) CKC with resistance of 4%. Consequently, the original hypotheses that OKC exercises were more stressful to the ACL and perhaps even detrimental were not supported by this research. In all the exercises, the maximum ACL strain occurred near terminal extension and decreased progressively with increasing knee flexion. There were no significant differences in maximum strain values among exercises at 10, 20, and 90 degrees. As a result, the findings of this study are a departure from the previous clinical studies and accepted theory considering ligamentous rehabilitation. The authors speculated that it may not be valid to designate CKC or OKC exercises as "safe" or "unsafe" for rehabilitation of the injured ACL or healing graft.

Another interesting interpretation of research comparing OKC and CKC exercises is in a study by Bynum and colleagues.[200] This was one of the first prospective randomized studies comparing OKC versus CKC exercises. This study reached the following conclusions about the CKC training group:

- Lower mean KT-1000 arthrometer side-to-side differences (20 lb: $p = .057$, not significant; manual maximum: $p = .018$, significant)
- Less patellofemoral pain ($p = .48$, not significant)

- Generally more satisfied with the end result ($p = .36$, not significant)
- Returned to ADLs sooner than expected ($p = .007$, significant)
- Returned to sports activities sooner than expected ($p = .118$, not significant)

Bynum and colleagues[200] stated, "As a result of this study, we now use the CKC protocol exclusively after ACL reconstruction." Surprisingly, these researchers deduced several conclusions that were *not* statistically significant and probably not clinically significant either. Yet they base their entire protocol exclusively on these findings.

Snyder-Mackler and colleagues[201] stated the following:

Rehabilitation after reconstruction of the ACL continues to be guided more by myth and fad than by science. Intensive CKC exercises have virtually replaced OKC exercise of the quadriceps after a reconstruction. . . . The present study confirms the finding that strength of the quadriceps has a substantial impact on functional recovery and suggests that CKC exercise alone does *NOT* provide an adequate stimulus to the quadriceps femoris to permit more normal function of the knee in stance phase in most patients in the early period after reconstruction of the ACL . . . We believe that the judicious application of OKC exercises for the quadriceps femoris muscle (with the knee in a position that does not stress the graft, i.e., 90 to 30 degrees) improves the strength of this muscle and functional outcome after reconstruction of the ACL.

CKC exercises and their relation to PCL shear stress have been investigated. Dahlkuits and colleagues[202] demonstrated an increase in posterior shear up to three times body weight during squatting exercises.

Functional Exercises

CKC exercises are often described as being more functional, particularly in the lower extremities. The obvious reason is that the CKC position closely simulates the movement patterns during activities such as walking, jogging, running, and other recreational activities.

Interestingly, when we analyze most lower extremity functional activities, we find that they consist of continuous reciprocal OKC and CKC exercises. An example is the progression of walking to sprinting. During walking, approximately 65% of the gait cycle is weight bearing (CKC) and 35% is non–weight bearing (OKC). When the patient starts to run, the time spent in CKC and OKC positions essentially reverses. When the patient starts to sprint, the CKC segment decreases to approximately 10% of the running cycle whereas 90% is OKC. So paradoxically, when one becomes more active, the actual time spent in a CKC position decreases. Consequently, this reinforces the importance of understanding and testing and rehabilitation of the patient (due to specificity) with *both* CKC and OKC exercises. Admittedly, many injuries of the lower extremity occur in the CKC position such as ankle sprains and ACL injuries; however, there is no research that demonstrates that performing only CKC exercises will prevent many of those injuries.

Biomechanical Summary

Based on the current research and information presented, it behooves clinicians to incorporate *both* CKC and OKC exercises into the rehabilitation of patients with MLKI. All studies have researched CKC and OKC forces in isolated injuries; therefore we will take this information and apply it to MLKI. The following is a list of recommended "safe" guidelines regarding isolated ACL and PCL initial OKC and CKC exercises. However, because of the complexity of MLKI these guidelines will need to be customized based on concomitant injured structures, surgical procedures, and the patient's response to rehabilitation.

- OKC knee extension
  - 90 to 30 degrees for ACL rehabilitation
  - 90 to 0 degrees for PCL rehabilitation
- OKC knee flexion
  - Full ROM for ACL rehabilitation
  - Contraindicated for PCL rehabilitation in the early phases
- CKC exercises
  - 0 to 60 degrees for ACL and PCL rehabilitation

Because no formal research has been conducted on patients with MLKI, these restrictions will be combined to form the basis of our rehabilitation. Obviously these restrictions may be lifted, as soft tissue healing allows, later during the rehabilitation process.

REHABILITATION PHASES

Phase I (1 to 6 Weeks)

- Protect healing tissue
- Facilitate soft tissue healing
- Decrease pain and effusion
- Restore full physiologic range of motion
- Initiate neuromuscular control to prevent reflex inhibition
- Enhance neuromuscular proactive control and stability
- Improve proprioception and kinesthesia

Protect Healing Tissue

The early phase (phase I) of the postoperative course is constant irrespective of the specifics of the pattern of MLKI and the surgical technique employed to treat it. The priority is to protect the reconstructed and repaired tissues while at the same time implementing strategies to regain ROM, reduce pain and edema, and initiate and facilitate muscle function.

Although these activities have been subdivided into categories for purposes of discussion, they all occur concurrently and are mutually reinforcing. A great deal of insight may be gained from assessing the patient's normal anatomy, especially the opposite knee, before embarking on the rehabilitation of MLKI. Those who demonstrate significant multijoint laxity as a body build characteristic will need greater than usual protection. Those patients with significant preexisting inflexibility, less than average general physical fitness, or scars suggesting a tendency toward keloid formation may need to be more aggressively managed to reduce the risk of ROM deficits and adhesion formation. Insights gained from the degree of pain, swelling, and patient coping skills experienced during the interval between injury and surgery are often applicable to the postsurgical recovery.

During the early postoperative period after multiple ligament reconstruction, the healing and maturation of grafts and of directly sutured tissues must be considered. During the phase I period of rehabilitation, we use a long leg brace. For the first 4 to 6 weeks patients are instructed to maintain the leg brace locked in extension. However, we encourage controlled, non–weight-bearing early flexion, generally beginning approximately 1 week after surgery, but with a proximal pad or counterforce support on the proximal tibia to minimize the effects of gravity and to prevent posterior tibial sag. Arms and colleagues[203] have demonstrated increased strain on the PCL as the knee flexes, with maximum strain recorded at 100 degrees. Therefore we do not allow knee flexion past 90 degrees during the first 6 weeks of the rehabilitation program. Stannard and colleagues[204] demonstrated that the Compass Knee Hinge (CKH) (Smith and Nephew Orthopedic, Memphis, TN) allowed aggressive initial physical therapy without placing repaired or reconstructed ligaments under high stresses that can result in failure. Their study, however, used a staged procedure in which the PCL was initially reconstructed, the CKH was used, and then 8 weeks later an ACL reconstruction was performed. Its applicability to other procedures is untested.

To adequately protect repaired and reconstructed tissues, the patient must be strictly non–weight bearing for the first 4 weeks. Depending on demonstrated patient compliance, the specific pathology of the MLKI, and the characteristics of the surgical technique, we often allow a limited degree of gradually progressive partial weight bearing during the last 2 weeks as pain decreases, ROM increases, and neuromuscular control of the lower extremity improves. Resumption of weight bearing should take into consideration the patient's natural limb alignment. For example, a delay of several weeks would be advisable in a knee with an ACL, PCL, PLC combination injury in a limb with significant genu varum alignment.

The fixation of repaired and reconstructed tissues is an important consideration during early rehabilitation because it generally represents the "weak link" in the system. Bone-to-bone graft fixation may be initially even stronger than the strength of the soft tissue portion of the graft. However, soft tissue–to–bone fixation, even with contemporary "bioscrews" and staples, may be subject to creep and has been shown to take at least 12 weeks before incorporation begins. Suture fixation of soft tissue to bone is even more tenuous and requires even greater protection during the first 6 postoperative weeks.[205] Soft tissue–to–soft tissue repairs with sutures are generally able to withstand considerable stress after 6 weeks. It is crucial that the therapist be aware of the surgical technique employed after MLKI surgeries and that the therapist discuss the specifics with the surgeon.

Facilitate Soft Tissue Healing

There is a predictable progression of soft tissue healing response after severe trauma and surgical intervention. The initial phase of acute inflammation is followed within a week by phases that include collagen fibroplasia, maturation, and then remodeling. During the acute inflammatory phase, various physical therapy modalities are effective in decreasing the severity of pain and effusion, thus facilitating a healing response. Soft tissue healing is a long process, with the latter three stages each taking weeks at a time. During soft tissue healing, it is important that the appropriate stresses be imposed on injured tissues to promote physiologic healing responses, minimize negative changes, and facilitate the proliferation and alignment of collagen fibers. During this vulnerable time, interventions that are overly aggressive can potentially disrupt and stretch the healing structures, or promote a repetition of the inflammatory phase, leading to enhanced scar formation. It is also important to keep in mind that the physiology of soft tissue healing varies widely from one patient to another. Ideally, the graduated stresses of a well-designed rehabilitation program will permit the mutable tissues to adapt and accommodate to the functional demands that occur through the rehabilitation program.

Decrease Pain and Effusion

Both pain and the presence of an effusion are associated with decreased quadriceps muscle function and protective hamstring spasm. Spencer and colleagues[206] have demonstrated that as little as 20 to 30 ml of fluid in the knee joint can retard the muscle contraction of the VMO. We recommend aspiration of any residual postoperative effusion of greater than minimal volume. Various physical therapy modalities such as interferential electrical stimulation, cryotherapy, and compression are effective in decreasing postsurgical effusion, edema, inflammation, and pain. Patients are often provided with a home cryocuff compression unit that is used three times per day for a total of 60 minutes to assist with pain management and reduction of effusion. Edema can also be reduced when vigorous ankle pumps are performed hourly to mechanically transfer interstitial fluid via the venous and lymphatic systems. Furthermore, the ankle pumps also decrease the risk of a DVT (blood clot) by reducing venous stasis. We do not routinely prescribe nonsteroidal antiinflammatory medications, but we use them for 7 to 10 rehabilitation days in those selected patients whose knees manifest a greater than usual inflammatory response that is compromising the progression of recovery.

Restore Full Physiologic Range of Motion

Full physiologic ROM is necessary for normal function of the knee. Prolonged immobilization is associated with many detrimental effects to the joint and surrounding structures, including the development of intraarticular and periarticular adhesions, arthrofibrosis with loss of joint motion, degradation of hyaline cartilage, and decreased bone mass. The surrounding muscles are also negatively affected, with interfiber adhesions, atrophy, and decreased oxidative function. Loss of extension leads to gait abnormalities and subsequently to an increase in patellofemoral joint reaction forces, which often causes pain and progressive deterioration of articular cartilage. Loss of flexion impairs the patient's function, as it interferes with stair climbing, kneeling, and arising from a chair. The goal is the steady and gradual return of motion by setting goals and meeting them weekly. We have found that those patients who make slow but continuous gains in ROM have less laxity and better long-term outcomes.

Obtaining extension must take precedence during the initial phases of rehabilitation. The longer one waits to obtain it, the more difficult it becomes to accomplish. Our goal is to gain at least neutral extension by the end of the second week. This will be most difficult when injury patterns involve MCL pathology. The repaired or reconstructed PCL comes under increasing stress as the knee goes into hyperextension. PCL/PLC combination injuries are especially vulnerable, as the lateral structures also come under increasing tension with terminal extension secondary to the "screw-home" mechanism. In cases in which the patient demonstrates significant physiologic recurvatum on the contralateral knee (evidence of physiologic multijoint laxity), when the PLC has been repaired, or when the posterior capsule has been generally disrupted (as reported by the operating surgeon), we recommend that no more than neutral extension be allowed for the first 3 weeks and no more than 10 degrees of recurvatum be allowed until after 6 weeks. Otherwise, the risk of stretching out the reconstructed/repaired tissue is too great. The return of extension can be accurately assessed by heel height measurements as described by Sachs and colleagues[207] (Figure 16-14). One centimeter in heel height is equal to approximately 1 degree. Reliability of this method has been confirmed.[208]

When the knee is maintained chiefly in extension for 6 weeks, flexibility deficits of posterior muscle groups tend to occur. Hamstring and gastrocnemius flexibility stretching exercises are performed daily for 30 seconds for at least three sets.[209-211] Patellar mobilizations are begun immediately postoperatively. Physiologic patellar glide is necessary for both flexion and extension to occur. Terminal extension can be

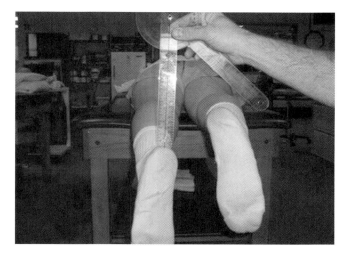

Figure 16-14: Prone measurement of heel-height difference.

prevented by swelling or scarring in the infrapatellar fat pad, secondary to either the trauma of the initial dislocation or that of a surgical incision. Flexion can be limited by intraarticular scarring in the parapatellar gutters and suprapatellar pouch, or within the retinaculum itself. Although obtaining immediate flexion is relatively less crucial than achieving adequate extension, it should not be ignored. The goal must be to have 90 degrees of flexion by the end of phase I.

Additional treatment interventions often need to be performed to regain the motion. For patients with hypomobilities, the total end-range time (TERT) stretching formula is used. The TERT formula is used to create plastic deformation of the noncontractile tissue.[212,213] This formula is based on stretching intensity, duration, and frequency. The intensity is the maximal stretch intensity the patient can tolerate based on comfort. The research indicates that 20 minutes is probably the optimum duration of the stretch.[212] However, we have found that a 10-minute duration is ideal for patient tolerance and from a clinical efficiency perspective. The optimal frequency is three times per day. The first and second TERTs can usually be performed by the passive warm-up at the start of the treatment program and by stretching again at the completion of the treatment. The patient needs to complete the third TERT as part of his or her home exercise program (HEP). This formula can be used on any joint or ROM in the body with noncontractile tissue limitations. The following list is an example of how this concept can be efficiently applied in the clinic setting:

- *Active warm-up:* Exercises that can be used include bicycle, elliptical, and treadmill. In the early stages of rehabilitation, short-arc motions, active-assistive range of motion (AAROM) exercises, and so on should be used for the warm-up phase.

- *Heat in a stretched position:* First TERT (Figure 16-15).

- *Mobilizations/ROM:* Hypomobility of patellofemoral cephalic glide interferes with the normal function of the extensor mechanism. Loss of passive motion or a

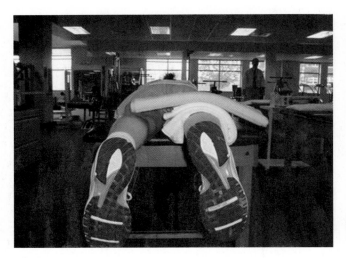

Figure 16-15: Heating in a stretched position—first TERT.

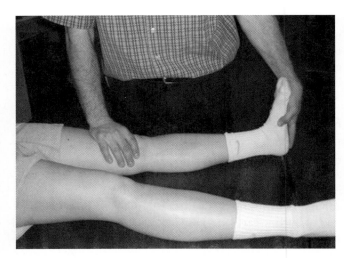

Figure 16-16: Physiologic joint mobilizations.

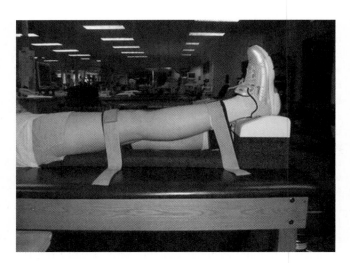

Figure 16-17: Knee extension HEP—third TERT.

quadriceps lag may result. Patellofemoral cephalic glide mobilizations are important to facilitate extension of the knee. Technique is important when performing the cephalic glide; the web space of the hand needs to be positioned at the inferior pole of the patella above the infrapatellar fat pad. If the hand is not carefully positioned to avoid compressing the fat pad against the inferior pole of the patella, it may iatrogenically create inflammation of the fat pad, which may create a block to terminal extension. Overly aggressive manipulation of the patella will aggravate pain and swelling and is always counterproductive. Patellofemoral caudal glides are used to increase flexion of the knee and patellofemoral joint. In contradistinction to single cruciate ligament reconstruction surgeries, mobilization of the tibiofemoral articulation is only occasionally necessary for patients who have had MLKI surgeries.

- Physiologic mobilizations (Figure 16-16).
- Accessory mobilizations:
  - *Static stretching or proprioceptive neuromuscular facilitation (PNF) contract-relax:* Often, the musculotendinous unit adaptively shortens, which also leads to flexibility deficits. Furthermore, because many of the muscles around the knee are biarticular, it often leads to compensatory changes proximally around the hip or distally around the foot and ankle area. Based on research findings published during the 1990s, the static portion of the stretches should be held for 30 seconds for younger patients.[209-211] However, if the patient is older than 65, the stretched position should be maintained for 60 seconds.[214] Moreover, PNF techniques such as contract-relax can be included as part of the treatment program.
  - *Therapeutic exercises:* This is the key to regaining ROM of any joint. After passive range of motion (PROM) is increased, it is useless until the patient

gains dynamic control of the new ROM. The best example of this is the patient who has full PROM of knee extension, but still has a quadriceps lag. This is the typical patient who has a neuromuscular activation and strength problem. Developing the dynamic stabilization is critical to have functional dynamic control to use the newly gained PROM of terminal knee extension.

- *Total leg strengthening (TLS):* Dynamic stabilization exercises for the entire lower extremity are performed, including gastrocnemius/soleus complex, hip muscles, and core stability exercises.[215,216]
- *Ice in a stretched position:* The second TERT is applied at the completion of the physical therapy treatment session.[217]
- *Home exercise program (HEP):* The patient performs a third TERT (Figure 16-17).

Initiate Neuromuscular Control to Prevent Reflex Inhibition

Quadriceps weakness and atrophy in the initial stages post-operatively is unavoidable, but must be promptly addressed if the patient is to satisfactorily progress. Isometric quadriceps sets are initiated immediately postoperatively as soon as pain will allow, with a progression to straight leg raising without the controlled position brace (CPB). In most cases, we supplement quad sets with electrical stimulation to augment strength,[218] as described in the following paragraph. Additionally, the use of biofeedback with quad sets and straight leg raises facilitates internalization of the muscle activity. Patients use the "rule of tens" with a 2-second gradient increase, holding the contraction for 6 seconds[219] (which is the optimum duration for an isometric contraction),[220] then perform a 2-second gradient decrease of the muscle contraction. The patient performs 10 repetitions, 10 sets, 10 times per day. Moreover, research demonstrates that there is a 20-degree physiologic overflow from the angle of application of the isometric contractions.[221] This provides the scientific basis of how to design the rehabilitation program, as well as saving time because of efficiency.

Enhance Neuromuscular Proactive Control and Stability

Several methods can be used during phase I that are safe for the patient and can effectively enhance neuromuscular control. A frequently used technique is electrical stimulation to the extensor mechanism. This helps "fire" the muscles, which the patient volitionally contracts concurrent with the stimulation.[218] This can initially be started in a non–weight-bearing position and then progress to a weight-bearing position. When it is appropriate (approximately 4 to 6 weeks), the electrical stimulation can be applied while the patient is performing short-arc CKC exercises. In the CKC position, the joint compression and the muscle co-contractions help stabilize the joint and the electrical stimulation superimposed on the active contraction may enhance the muscles' functioning. A functional exercise that can be applied at this time is the CKC exercise, during which the hamstrings extend the hip while simultaneously extending the knee (Figure 16-18).

The Davies[219] exercise progression forms the foundation of the exercise program. The exercise progression continuum goes through the following stages:

- Submaximal-intensity pain-free multiple-angle isometrics
- Maximal-intensity multiple-angle isometrics
- Submaximal-intensity short-arc exercises
- Maximal-intensity short-arc exercises
- Full-ROM submaximal-intensity exercises
- Full-ROM maximal-intensity exercises

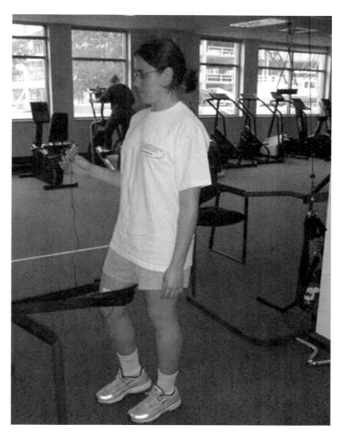

Figure 16-18: Closed kinetic chain knee extension with biofeedback.

During phase I, the emphasis is on the first three stages of this exercise progression. Total leg strengthening can also be performed,[215,216] but using the entire lower extremity and long lever arms may put stresses on the healing ligaments. As an example, if the patient has a lateral side injury, we would not put resistance at the lateral ankle and have the patient perform abduction exercises. By crossing multiple joints in this case, it would put additional contraindicated varus stresses on the knee joint in the early phases of the healing process. One-legged cycling can also be included at this time to create a contralateral overflow response to assist the injured leg.

Improve Proprioception and Kinesthesia

Knee proprioception and kinesthesia are negatively affected by injury.[222] *Proprioception* is defined as the conscious and unconscious recognition of position sense. *Kinesthesia* is the sensation of joint motion or acceleration. Joint position neuromuscular control is where the efferent motor response to afferent (sensory) information occurs. Mechanoreceptors within the cruciate ligaments are destroyed during the ligament failure of MLKI and do not regrow into the grafts when the ACL and PCL are reconstructed. Receptors within the collateral ligaments and capsule are also always damaged to varying degrees.

Specific exercises that are safe for the healing structures early in the rehabilitation program may facilitate the remaining intact mechanoreceptors to compensate for those that are absent. The sooner the patient can improve joint proprioception, the better carryover she or he should have through the progression of the rehabilitation program. Facilitating proprioception during the initial stages of rehabilitation would be expected to minimize the subsequent risk of reinjury, normalize gait, and facilitate the progression to running, agility activities, and return to functional activities. Various exercises that can be used at this time include angular joint replication training, end-ROM reproduction training, and perturbation training.[223] The perturbation training (submaximal) should be performed in a non–weight-bearing position during the initial phases by having the patient sit in a chair, place his or her foot on a single-dimensional tilt board, and then perturb the tilt board. Use of a tilt board is a low-intensity exercise with minimal motion that prevents unduly stressing the healing tissue. Initially, the patient begins with the eyes open so the patient can see the perturbation coming, which constitutes *proactive* training. The majority of the training at this time is performed in a proactive mode. The patient progresses to partial weight bearing using a tilt board during this phase. In the next phase, progression increases to perturbations with the eyes closed so that the training becomes a *reactive* response.

Phase II (6 to 12 Weeks)

- Guarded protection
- Restore full physiologic ROM (normalize arthrokinematics)
- Improve proprioception and kinesthesia
- Increase muscular strength, power, and endurance

Guarded Protection

In phase II, continued protection of repaired and reconstructed tissue is necessary, though to a diminishing extent. Progressive guarded stresses are imposed as the rehabilitation program continues. The patient may generally be allowed full weight bearing in a postsurgical brace at the beginning of the sixth week. We have usually found that crutches remain necessary for balance for several weeks thereafter, except in the exceptional cases where adequate lower extremity function has already returned. Patients must have at least active neutral extension to assume full weight bearing. Walking on a flexed knee merely perpetuates the knee flexion contracture position and can ultimately cause irritation of the extensor mechanism. A normal gait pattern is necessary to dispense with crutches.

We discontinue the long leg postoperative brace when the patient begins to ambulate without crutches at approximately week 8. A functional brace is then employed and is worn for all ADLs until approximately week 12. We recommend that those patients who plan to return to athletic activity or manual labor use the brace for those specific activities until 18 months have passed since the reconstructive surgery. At the present time, there are no published studies that assess the efficacy of functional braces after MLKI. Studies after isolated ACL reconstruction have been inconclusive in demonstrating the objective value of postoperative bracing.[224,225] Nevertheless, we believe that it is important to provide the patient with external support because muscle function and proprioception are so deficient during the early stages of recovery from these devastating injuries.

Restore Full Physiologic Range of Motion (Normalize Arthrokinematics)

Neutral extension should have been obtained by the end of phase I. During phase II the goal is to obtain, and maintain, physiologic recurvatum equivalent to that of the contralateral knee. Flexion should gradually increase until ideally it is symmetric to the uninvolved side by weeks 8 to 12. However, we have found it difficult to consistently obtain full flexion. Flexion of 125 degrees is generally adequate for all ADLs and even high-demand athletics. Occasionally, gains in flexion will be accompanied by some loss of terminal extension. This must not be allowed to occur. Extension always takes precedence, because flexion is easier to obtain later if necessary by manipulation under anesthesia and the arthroscopic release of adhesions. If neutral extension and flexion to 125 degrees have not been obtained by week 12, and gains in ROM have plateaued, we consider surgical intervention. However, we do not proceed with an invasive treatment if improvement continues, no matter how slowly. Once flexion exceeds 90 degrees, gradual improvement is possible and may slowly continue for up to 6 months after injury. In the face of ROM problems, frequent rehabilitation sessions are preferable to aggressive rehabilitation. The key is to maximize the relaxation of the connective tissue, so that creep leads to permanent elongation. The knee cannot be bullied into submission. Overly aggressive manipulation merely engenders a greater inflammatory response and is counterproductive. Application of the TERT formula as described in phase I (for knee flexion or extension) may be continued if needed.

Improve Proprioception and Kinesthesia

Once adequate strength and endurance of the lower extremity musculature have been reestablished, it is necessary to incorporate exercises to further improve proprioception. The patient must learn how to recruit muscles in sequence and, with the proper force, how to minimize abnormal joint motion. Initially, the performance of the exercises will require the patient's conscious attention; however, after adequate repetition, control of abnormal joint motion will become automatic. Neuromuscular stability training requires the patient to learn proper muscle recruitment patterns, appropriate forces, and temporal components. This prevents the creation of abnormal compensatory motor patterns. Progression with the angular joint replications and end-ROM

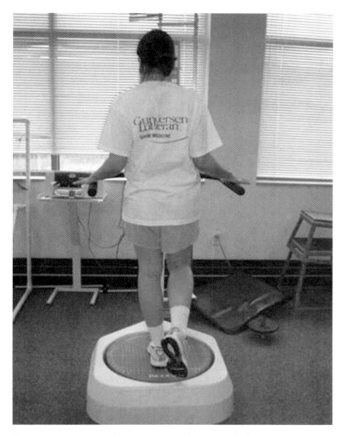

Figure 16-19: Proprioceptive exercises—single leg.

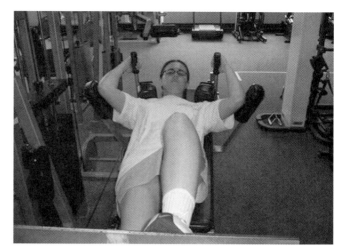

Figure 16-20: CKC exercise—leg press.

reproductions continues. The proprioceptive/kinesthesia progressions are in a systematic sequence:[226-228]

- Partial weight bearing progresses to full weight bearing
- Double-leg exercises progress to single-leg exercises (Figure 16-19)
- Single-plane tilt board progresses to multiple-plane tilt board
- Eyes open progresses to eyes closed
- Perturbation training (proactive), submaximal

Increase Muscular Strength, Power, and Endurance

An important part of the rehabilitation program for the patient with an MLKI is dynamic stability, which helps protect the knee joint and compensates for any residual impairments. Core stability training can also be included for a comprehensive rehabilitation program.

As previously described, the Davies[219] exercise progression forms the foundation of the exercise program. In phase II, the emphasis to enhance neuromuscular dynamic stability is on stages 3 to 6 of the exercise progression continuum. Neitzel and colleagues[229] discovered that following knee surgery, patients have a tendency to unload their surgical extremity. It was demonstrated that patients continued to unload the surgical limb for at least 6 months and then normalized their weight bearing by 1 year. Consequently, we encourage patients to begin single-leg exercises earlier in the rehabilitation program to facilitate the improved weight bearing and increased proprioception.

The initial CKC exercises are used to improve muscular strength and endurance in a functional weight-bearing position.[199] Various CKC exercises include wall slides, short-arc squats, multiple direction step-ups, leg press (Figure 16-20), and variations of squats and lunges. The various exercises are progressed in ROM, repetitions, sets, and resistance. If there are no contraindications, OKC exercises are initially performed in the mid-ROM protecting the healing structures at the respective ends of the ROM. If there are patellofemoral problems, OKC exercises may be contraindicated and avoided.[179,180] If there are significant chondrosis problems from the original injury, modifications are considered as to where in the ROM exercises may be performed. If the patient has a significant bone contusion, aggressive weight bearing and high-impact loading activities are minimized. With these considerations forming the basis of the rehabilitation, communication between the physician and therapist is crucial.

The quantity of therapeutic exercise required for strength gains can be based on recent research by Wolfe and colleagues.[230] A meta-analysis of the literature revealed the following: With untrained subjects, using one set of 10 reps is as effective in strength gains as is three sets of 10 reps in the early stages. As the subjects progress in the program, sets need to increase. However, if the patient is a trained individual, three sets of 10 repetitions are necessary to produce strength gains.

Phase III (12 to 24 Weeks)

- Improve proprioception and kinesthesia
- Increase muscular strength, power, and endurance
- Enhance neuromuscular reactive stability

Improve Proprioception and Kinesthesia

Various proprioceptive/kinesthesia exercises as described previously are continued and progressed to the terminal stages of the exercises. More aggressive progressions include the following:

- Perturbation training exercises
- Submaximal progressing to maximal
- Slow progressing to fast
- Known (proactive) patterns progressing to unknown (reactive) patterns

At approximately week 24, low-intensity agility drills may be initiated. Exercises such as controlled acceleration and deceleration, slide board, and jumping rope form the foundation of these exercises[199] (Figures 16-21 and 16-22).

Increase Muscular Strength, Power, and Endurance

In the later phases of rehabilitation, the resistive exercises for both CKC and OKC exercises use the principles of progression and overload.[231-233] Based on the previous biomechanical discussion, OKC limitations are as follows:

- Weeks 12 to 18:
  - From 30 to 90 degrees for knee extension exercises (approximately week 12; depending on joint stability, surgical repairs, comorbidities, and physician approval).
  - Knee flexion exercises are contraindicated at this time secondary to the stress placed on the PCL.
- Weeks 18 to 24:
  - From 0 to 90 degrees for knee extension exercises (approximately week 18; depending on joint stability, surgical repairs, comorbidities, and physician approval).
  - From 0 to 90 degrees for knee flexion exercises (approximately week 18; depending on joint stability, surgical repairs, comorbidities, and physician approval).

Emphasis on higher resistance and lower repetitions primarily increases muscular strength. Resistive exercises should include both concentric and eccentric exercises. More emphasis can now be placed on eccentric exercises because of the increased force-generating capabilities. Both concentric and eccentric exercises need to be included in the rehabilitation because most functional activities use both modes of muscle actions. To improve muscular power, the patient exercises at faster speeds with maximum-effort activities. This can be done with faster-speed isokinetic training and functional training activities using more dynamic exercises, such as low-intensity plyometric exercises.

Enhance Neuromuscular Reactive Stability

The neuromuscular reactive stability is important to provide dynamic stability of the knee. The neuromuscular stability training requires that the patient learn proper muscle recruitment patterns, appropriate forces, and temporal components. Development of normal functional patterns is one of the goals of the training program at this point. During this phase, the primary motor learning responses redevelop and activities progress from a conscious to an unconscious level where the responses occur automatically.

Research studies have demonstrated that patients who compensate well after an ACL injury usually do so because of compensatory lower extremity patterns that provide dynamic stability to the knee.[234-237] Patients with MLKI may need to rely on neuromuscular reactive compensatory patterns to perform functional activities. Research demonstrates that the primary muscles involved in the compensatory patterns (quadriceps, hamstrings, and gastrocnemius muscles) are important in helping the patient return to various activities.[234-237] Therefore a patient with MLKI may also need to rely on some of these compensatory patterns to create the

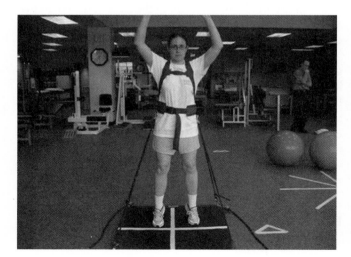

Figure 16-21: Plyometric jumps.

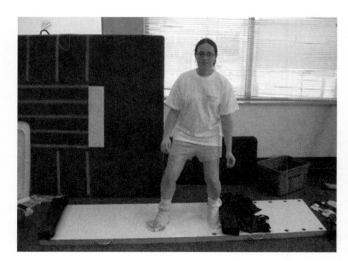

Figure 16-22: Lateral slides.

dynamic stability for the knee. However, because of the complexity of MLKI, there are differences in the way patients are going to compensate to provide dynamic knee stability. Consequently, the rehabilitation program needs to be customized to the patient.

Many functional activities create destabilizing forces across the knee. Most of these activities occur very quickly in true functional situations. Often the activities occur more quickly than volitional muscular responses can react to them. Consequently, treatment strategies need to simulate some of these forces in a controlled clinical environment with progressively increasing forces. That is why this part of the rehabilitation training program is referred to as neuromuscular reactive training. Examples include advanced perturbation (reactive) training, plyometrics, advanced agility drills, and ergonomic/sport-specific simulation.[199]

Phase IV (Greater Than 24 Weeks)

- Functional specificity and return to activities

Functional Specificity and Return to Activities

A functional testing algorithm (FTA), which is a progressive step-by-step process, is used to evaluate and progress a patient through the rehabilitation program. The details and specific criteria are described by Davies and Zillmer.[238] The FTA progresses through a series of stages, with each one becoming progressively more difficult. The patient must pass through each stage in a systematic process in order to progress to higher levels of functional activities. If the patient fails a test of the FTA, the rehabilitation program is then focused on that area until the deficit is adequately addressed. The stages of the FTA include the following:[238]

- Time for soft tissue healing
- Physician approval for testing (typically approximately 9 to 12 months); if all testing is within normal limits, appropriate for progressive return to activity
- Visual analog scale: rest—ideally 0/10
- ADLs—ideally 0/10
- Higher levels of activity—less than 3/10
- Anthropometric measurements—bilateral comparison—within 10%
- AROM/PROM goniometric measurements—bilateral comparison—within 10%
- Balance testing, single leg—bilateral comparison—within 10%

- CKC isokinetic testing (if applicable)—bilateral comparison—within 10% (if isokinetic testing is not applicable, may use handheld dynamometer comparisons of selective muscles within 10%)
- Peak torque/body weight (PT/BW)—within normative data for age, gender, sport, and so on[239]
- OKC isokinetic testing (if applicable)—bilateral comparison—within 10% (if isokinetic testing is not applicable, may use handheld dynamometer comparisons of selective muscles within 10%)
- Unilateral ratios—within normative data based on speed of testing; PT/BW—within normative data for age, gender, sport, and so on[240,241]
- Functional jump test (two legs): within normative data for age, gender, sport, and so on
- Functional hop test (one leg)—bilateral comparison—within 10%
- Lower extremity functional test (LEFT)[242]—within normative data for age, gender, sport, and so on
- Ergonomic or sport-specific testing—within normative data for age, gender, work, sport, and so on

The FTA provides a progressive and efficient method to use test results along with clinical judgment to progress and discharge a patient safely back into activity. Based on test results and our empirical observations, we allow patients to return to jogging at approximately 6 to 7 months. Many patients are ready to return to athletics or strenuous manual labor at 12 months, based on their feedback and responses to functional training. An outline of the complete rehabilitation progression guidelines for a patient who has undergone MLKI can be seen in Box 16-1.

SUMMARY

Because of the complexity of the injury, there are no randomized, controlled trial studies regarding the optimum surgical and rehabilitation guidelines. Because of the uniqueness of the injuries, the surgery and rehabilitation programs have to be customized to meet the specific needs of the patient. Guidelines regarding mechanisms of injuries, classification of injuries, surgical procedures, and limited evidence-based literature on rehabilitation, as well as our empirically based experience with more than 30 patients, are provided. Table 16-2 outlines descriptive information regarding MLKI patients we have seen for surgical treatment and rehabilitation.

TABLE 16-2

Descriptive Information Regarding MLKI Patients We Have Treated

PATIENT	AGE (YR)	GENDER	METHOD OF INJURY	TYPE	LIGAMENTS	VASCULAR	NEUROLOGIC	FRACTURE	REDUCTION
1	29	F	Vehicle accident	Anterior	ACL, PCL, LCL (KDIIIL)	Popliteal artery disruption	N	N	Spontaneous
2	36	F	Vehicle accident with ejection	Posterior	ACL, PCL, MCL, LCL (KDIV)	N	N	N	Emergency department (ED)
3	23	M	Motorcycle accident	Lateral	ACL, PCL, MCL (KDIIIM)	N	N	Avulsion, PCL	Spontaneous
4	21	M	Vehicle accident with ejection	Medial	ACL, PCL, MCL, LCL (KDIV)	N	N	Avulsion, LCL	Spontaneous
5	23	M	Struck by car	Posterior	ACL, PCL, LCL (KDIIIL)	N	N	Avulsion, ACL	Spontaneous
6	59	M	Tractor overturned on leg	Lateral	ACL, PCL, MCL (KDIIIM)	Y, decreased Doppler	N	Tibia and fibula	Spontaneous
7	26	M	Motorcycle accident	Posterior	ACL, PCL, MCL, LCL (KDIV)	Absent PT pulse and DP pulse	N	N	Spontaneous
8	47	F	Vehicle accident	Posterior	ACL, PCL, LCL (KDIIIL)	Absent PT pulse and DP pulse	N	N	Spontaneous
9	33	M	Carrying his girlfriend piggyback	Posterior	ACL, PCL, LCL (KDIIIL)	PT decreased, DP absent	N	N	Spontaneous

	Age	Sex	Mechanism	Direction	Ligaments				Presentation
10	63	M	Fell off ladder	Lateral	ACL, PCL, MCL (KDIIIM)	N	N	Avulsion, MCL, tibial plateau fracture	Spontaneous
11	38	M	Jumping over object	Anterior	ACL, PCL, LCL (KDIIIL)	Popliteal vein thrombosis	N	Avulsion of popliteus tendon	Spontaneous
12	14	M	Macro-trauma; collision with player	Posterior	ACL, PCL, LCL (KDIIIL)	Popliteal artery and vein disruption	N	Avulsion fracture, tibial spine	Spontaneous
13	65	M	Cross-country skiing	Posterior-lateral	ACL, PCL, MCL (KDIIIM)	N	N	Avulsion, quadriceps muscle and adductor longus	ED
14	59	F	Tripped and fell	Posterior	ACL, PCL, MCL (KDIIIM)	N	N	N	ED
15	22	M	Farm accident	Anterior-lateral	ACL, PCL, MCL (KDIIIM)	N	Deep vein thrombosis, popliteal vessels	N	Spontaneous
16	34	M	Playing basketball	Anterior	ACL, PCL, LCL (KDIIIL)	N	N	N	Spontaneous
17	54	M	Vehicle accident with ejection	Posterior	ACL, PCL, MCL (KDIIIM)	N	N	N	ED
18	38	M	Playing softball	Posterior-lateral	ACL, PCL, LCL (KDIIIL)	N	N	N	Spontaneous

(continued)

TABLE 16-2

Descriptive Information Regarding MLKI Patients We Have Treated—cont'd

PATIENT	AGE (YR)	GENDER	METHOD OF INJURY	TYPE	LIGAMENTS	VASCULAR	NEUROLOGIC	FRACTURE	REDUCTION
19	50	M	Fell from height	Lateral	ACL, PCL, MCL (KDIIIM)	N	N	N	ED
20	39	M	Farm accident	Anterior	ACL, PCL, LCL (KDIIIL)	N	N	N	ED
21	39	M	Motorcycle accident	Posterior	ACL, PCL, LCL (KDIIIL)	N	N	N	Spontaneous
22	32	M	Motorcycle accident	Lateral	ACL, PCL, LCL (KDIIIL)	N	N	Cortical fracture MFC	ED
23	20	M	Collided with another player—baseball	Posterior-lateral	ACL, PCL, MCL (KDIIIM)	N	N	N	
24	35	M	Running hurdles	Posterior	ACL, PCL, LCL (KDIIIL)	N	Peroneal nerve	N	ED
25	21	M	Basketball	Posterior	ACL, PCL, LCL (KDIIIL)	N	Peroneal nerve	N	ED
26	19	M	Football	Posterior	ACL, PCL, MCL (KDIIIM)	N	N	N	On field by physician
27	32	M	Football	Unknown	ACL, PCL, MCL (KDIIIM)	N	N	N	Spontaneous

28	18	M	Soccer	ACL, PCL, MCL (KDIIIM)	Medial	N	N	N	N	On field
29	22	M	Skiing	ACL, PCL, MCL (KDIIIM)	Posterior	N	N	N	Avulsion, PCL	ED
30	36	F	Softball	ACL, PCL, MCL (KDIIIM)	Posterior	N	N	N	N	Spontaneous
31	34	F	Softball	ACL, PCL, LCL (KDIIIL)	Unknown	N	Peroneal nerve	N	N	Spontaneous
32	48	M	Vehicle accident	ACL, PCL, LCL (KDIIIL)	Unknown	N	N	N	N	Spontaneous
33	39	M	Snowmobile accident	ACL, PCL, MCL (KDIIIM)	Unknown	N	N	N	N	Spontaneous
34	29	F	Work trauma	ACL, PCL, MCL (KDIIIM)	Medial	N	N	N	N	Spontaneous

There were no compound injuries in our series, all were closed.
DP, Dorsalis pedis; *MFC*, medial femoral condyle; *PT*, posterior tibial.

References

1. Cooper A: *A treatise on dislocations and on fractures of the joints*, Boston, 1824, Lilly, Wait, Carter & Hendee, p 198.

2. Annandale T: On 3 cases of dislocation of the knee-joint, *Lancet* ii:903, 1881.

3. Almekinders LC, Logan TC: Results following treatment of traumatic dislocations of the knee joint, *Clin Orthop* 284:203-207, 1992.

4. Myles JW: Seven cases of traumatic dislocation of the knee, *Proc R Soc Med* 60:279-281, 1967.

5. Reckling FW, Peltier LF: Acute knee dislocations and their complications, *J Trauma* 9:181-191, 1969.

6. Taylor AR, Arden GP, Rainey HA: Traumatic dislocation of the knee: a report of forty-three cases with special reference to conservative treatment, *J Bone Joint Surg Br* 54:96-102, 1972.

7. Thomsen PB, Rud B, Jensen UH: Stability and motion after traumatic dislocation of the knee, *Acta Orthop Scand* 55:278-283, 1984.

8. Cole BJ, Harner CD: The multiple ligament–injured knee, *Clin Sports Med* 18:241-262, 1999.

9. Fanelli GC, Giannotti BF, Edson CJ: Arthroscopically assisted combined anterior and posterior cruciate ligament reconstruction, *Arthroscopy* 12:5-14, 1996.

10. Fanelli GC, Giannotti BF, Edson CJ: Arthroscopically assisted combined posterior cruciate ligament/posterolateral complex reconstruction, *Arthroscopy* 12:521-530, 1996.

11. Frassica FJ, Sim FH, Staeheli JW, et al: Dislocation of the knee, *Clin Orthop* 263:200-205, 1991.

12. Malizos KN, Xenakis T, Xanthis A, et al: Knee dislocations and their management; a report of 16 cases, *Acta Orthop Scand* 68(suppl 275):80-83, 1997.

13. Meyers MH, Harvey JP Jr: Traumatic dislocation of the knee joint. A study of eighteen cases, *J Bone Joint Surg Am* 53:16-29, 1971.

14. Meyers MH, Moore TM, Harvey JP Jr: Traumatic dislocation of the knee joint, *J Bone Joint Surg Am* 57:430-433, 1975.

15. Montgomery JB: Dislocation of the knee, *Orthop Clin North Am* 18:149-156, 1987.

16. Montgomery IJ, Savoie FH, White JL, et al: Orthopedic management of knee dislocations: comparison of surgical reconstruction and immobilization, *Am J Knee Surg* 8:97-103, 1995.

17. Noyes FR, Barber-Westin SD: Reconstruction of the anterior and posterior cruciate ligaments after knee dislocation: use of early protected postoperative motion to decrease arthrofibrosis, *Am J Sports Med* 25:769-778, 1997.

18. Prohaska DJ, Harner CD: Surgical treatment of acute and chronic anterior and posterior cruciate ligament medial side injuries of the knee, *Sports Med Arthrosc Rev* 9:193-198, 2001.

19. Roman PD, Hopson CN, Zenni EJ Jr: Traumatic dislocation of the knee: a report of 30 cases and literature review, *Orthop Rev* 16:917-924, 1987.

20. Shapiro MS, Freedman EL: Allograft reconstruction of the anterior and posterior cruciate ligaments after traumatic knee dislocation, *Am J Sports Med* 23:580-587, 1995.

21. Shelbourne KD, Porter DA, Clingman JA, et al: Low-velocity knee dislocation, *Orthop Rev* 20:995-1004, 1991.

22. Shelbourne KD, Carr DR: Combined anterior and posterior cruciate and medial collateral ligament injury: nonsurgical and delayed surgical treatment, *AAOS Instructional Course Lectures* 52:413-418, 2003.

23. Shields L, Mital M, Cave EF: Complete dislocation of the knee: experience at the Massachusetts General Hospital, *J Trauma* 9:192-215, 1969.

24. Sisto DJ, Warren RF: Complete knee dislocation. A follow-up study of operative treatment, *Clin Orthop* 198:94-101, 1985.

25. Walker DN, Hadison R, Schenck RC: A baker's dozen of knee dislocations, *Am J Knee Surg* 7:117-124, 1994.

26. Wascher DC, Becker JR, Dexter JG, et al: Reconstruction of the anterior and posterior cruciate ligaments after knee dislocation: results using fresh-frozen nonirradiated allografts, *Am J Sports Med* 27:189-196, 1999.

27. Wascher DC, Schenck RC Jr: Surgical treatment of acute and chronic anterior cruciate ligament/posterior cruciate ligament/lateral sided injuries of the knee, *Sports Med Arthrosc Rev* 9:199-207, 2001.

28. Mow VC, Ratcliffe A, Chern KY, et al: Structure and function relationships of the menisci of the knee. In Mow VC, Arnoczky SP, Jackson DW, editors: *Knee meniscus: basic and clinical foundations*, New York, 1992, Raven Press.

29. Levy IM, Torzilli PA, Warren RF: The effect of medial menisectomy on anterior-posterior motion of the knee, *J Bone Joint Surg Am* 68:71-79, 1986.

30. Shoemaker SC, Markolf KL: The role of the meniscus in the anterior-posterior stability of the loaded anterior cruciate-deficient knee, *J Bone Joint Surg Am* 68:71-79, 1986.

31. Barrack RL, Skinner HB, Buckley SL: Proprioception in the anterior cruciate ligament deficient knee, *Am J Sports Med* 17:1-6, 1989.

32. Kennedy JC, Alexander IJ, Hayes KC: Nerve supply of the human knee and its functional importance, *Am J Sports Med* 10:329-335, 1982.

33. Schutte MJ, Dabezies EJ, Zimny ML, et al: Neural anatomy of the human anterior cruciate ligament, *J Bone Joint Surg Am* 69:243-247, 1987.

34. Smith BA, Livesay GA, Woo SL: Biology and biomechanics of the anterior cruciate ligament, *Clin Sports Med* 12:637-670, 1993.

35. Butler DL, Noyes FR, Grood ES: Ligamentous restraints to anterior-posterior drawer in the human knee. A biomechanical study, *J Bone Joint Surg Am* 62:259-270, 1980.

36. Chhabra A, Elliott CC, Miller MD: Normal anatomy and biomechanics of the knee, *Sports Med Arthrosc Rev* 9:166-177, 2001.

37. Gollehon DL, Torzilli PA, Warren RF: The role of posterolateral and cruciate ligaments in the stability of the human knee: a biomechanical study, *J Bone Joint Surg Am* 69:233-242, 1987.

38. Warren LF, Marshall JL: The supporting structures and layers on the medial side of the knee: an anatomic analysis, *J Bone Joint Surg Am* 61:56-62, 1979.

39. Grood ES, Noyes FR, Butler DL, et al: Ligamentous and capsular restraints preventing straight medial and lateral laxity in intact human cadaver knees, *J Bone Joint Surg Am* 63:1257-1269, 1981.

40. Hughston JC, Andrews JR, Cross MJ, et al: Classification of knee ligament instabilities: part I. The medial compartment and cruciate ligaments, *J Bone Joint Surg Am* 58:159-172, 1976.

41. Warren LF, Marshall JL, Girgis F: The prime static stabilizer of the medial side of the knee, *J Bone Joint Surg Am* 56:665-674, 1974.

42. Hughston JC, Eilers AF: The role of the posterior oblique ligament in repairs of acute medial (collateral) ligament tears of the knee, *J Bone Joint Surg Am* 55:923-940, 1973.

43. Muller W: *The knee: form, function, and ligament reconstruction,* Berlin, 1983, Springer-Verlag.

44. Kaplan E: The iliotibial tract: clinical and morphologic significance, *J Bone Joint Surg Am* 40:817-832, 1958.

45. LaPrade RF, Wentorf F: Diagnosis and treatment of posterolateral knee injuries, *Clin Orthop* 402:110-121, 2002.

46. Grood ES, Stowers SF, Noyes FR: Limits of movement in the human knee: effect of sectioning the posterior cruciate ligament and posterolateral structures, *J Bone Joint Surg Am* 70:88-97, 1988.

47. Nielsen S, Rasmussen O, Ovesen J, et al: Rotatory instability of cadaver knees after transection of collateral ligaments and capsule, *Arch Orthop Trauma Surg* 103:165-169, 1984.

48. DeLee JC, Riley MB, Rockwood CA Jr: Acute straight lateral instability of the knee, *Am J Sports Med* 11:404-411, 1983.

49. Chen FS, Rokito AS, Pitman MI: Acute and chronic posterolateral rotatory instability of the knee, *J Am Acad Orthop Surg* 8:97-110, 2000.

50. Cooper DE: Tests for posterolateral instability of the knee in normal subjects: results of examination under anesthesia, *J Bone Joint Surg Am* 73:30-36, 1991.

51. Covey DC: Injuries of the posterolateral corner of the knee, *J Bone Joint Surg Am* 83:106-118, 2001.

52. LaPrade RF, Resig S, Wentorf F, et al: The effects of grade III posterolateral knee complex injuries on anterior cruciate ligament graft force: a biomechanical analysis, *Am J Sports Med* 27:469-475, 1999.

53. LaPrade RF, Gilbert TJ, Bollom TS, et al: The magnetic resonance imaging appearance of individual structures of the posterolateral knee: a prospective study of normal knees and knees with surgically verified grade III injuries, *Am J Sports Med* 28:191-199, 2000.

54. LaPrade RF, Muench C, Wentorf F, et al: The effect of injury to the posterolateral structures of the knee on force in a posterior cruciate ligament graft: a biomechanical study, *Am J Sports Med* 30:233-238, 2002.

55. Maynard MJ, Deng X, Wickiewicz TL: The popliteofibular ligament. Rediscovery of a key element in posterolateral stability, *Am J Sports Med* 24:311-316, 1996.

56. Shahane SA, Ibbotson C, Strachan R: The popliteofibular ligament: an anatomic study of the posterolateral corner of the knee, *J Bone Joint Surg Br* 81:636-642, 1999.

57. Terry GC, LaPrade RF: The biceps femoris muscle complex at the knee. Its anatomy and injury patterns associated with acute anterolateral-anteromedial rotatory instability, *Am J Sports Med* 24:2-8, 1996.

58. Veltri DM, Deng XH, Torzelli PA, et al: The role of the popliteofibular ligament in stability of the human knee: a biomechanical study, *Am J Sports Med* 24:19-27, 1996.

59. Watanabe Y, Moriya H, Takahashi K, et al: Functional anatomy of the posterolateral structures of the knee, *Arthroscopy* 9:57-62, 1993.

60. Harner CD, Vogrin TM, Horer J: Biomechanical analysis of a posterior cruciate ligament reconstruction: deficiency of the posterolateral structures as a cause of graft failure, *Am J Sports Med* 28:32-39, 2000.

61. Noyes FR, Stowers SF, Grood ES: Posterior subluxations of the medial and lateral tibiofemoral compartments: an in vitro ligament sectioning study in cadaveric knees, *Am J Sports Med* 21:407-414, 1993.

62. Staubli HU, Birrer S: The popliteus tendon and its fascicles at the popliteal hiatus: gross anatomy and functional arthroscopic evaluation with and without anterior cruciate ligament deficiency, *Arthroscopy* 6:209-220, 1990.

63. DeLee JC, Riley MB, Rockwood CA: Acute posterolateral rotatory instability of the knee, *Am J Sports Med* 11:199-207, 1983.

64. Koskinen SK, Kujala UM: Patellofemoral relationship and distal insertion of the vastus medialis muscle: a magnetic resonance imaging study in nonsymptomatic subjects and in patients with patellar dislocation, *Arthroscopy* 8:465-468, 1992.

65. Wheatley M, Jahnke W: Electromyographic study of the superficial thigh and hip muscles in normal individuals, *Arch Phys Med Rehabil* 32:508-515, 1951.

66. DeBacke ME, Simeone FA: Battle injuries of the arteries in WWII: an analysis of 2,471 cases, *Ann Surg* 123:534-579, 1946.

67. Green NE, Allen BL: Vascular injuries associated with dislocation of the knee, *J Bone Joint Surg Am* 59:236-239, 1977.

68. Wascher DC, Dvirnak PC, DeCoster TA: Knee dislocation: initial assessment and implications for treatment, *J Orthop Trauma* 11:525-529, 1997.

69. O'Donnell JF Jr, Brewster DC, Darling RC, et al: Arterial injuries associated with fractures and/or dislocations of the knee, *J Trauma* 17:775-784, 1997.

70. Hoover NW: Injuries of the popliteal artery associated with fractures and dislocations, *Surg Clin North Am* 41:1099-1116, 1961.

71. Kennedy JC: Complete dislocation of the knee joint, *J Bone Joint Surg Am* 45:889-904, 1963.

72. Varnell RM, Coldwell DM, Sangeorzan BJ, et al: Arterial injury complicating knee dislocation, *Am J Surg* 55:699-704, 1989.

73. Good L, Johnson RJ: The dislocated knee, *J Am Acad Orthop Surg* 3:284-292, 1995.

74. Miller HH, Welch CS: Quantitative studies of the time factor in arterial injuries, *Ann Surg* 130:428-438, 1949.

75. Alberty RE, Goodfried G, Boyden AM: Popliteal artery injury with fracture dislocation of the knee, *Am J Surg* 142:36-40, 1981.

76. Bratt HD, Newman AP: Complete dislocation of the knee without disruption of both cruciate ligaments, *J Trauma* 34:383-389, 1993.

77. Cone JB: Vascular injury associated with fracture/dislocations of the lower extremity, *Clin Orthop* 243:30-35, 1989.

78. Kremchek TE, Welling RE, Kremchek EJ: Traumatic dislocation of the knee, *Orthop Rev* 18:1051-1057, 1989.

79. Welling RE, Kakkasseril J, Cranley JJ: Complete dislocations of the knee with popliteal vascular injury, *J Trauma* 21:450-453, 1981.

80. Dennis JW, Jagger C, Butcher JL, et al: Reassessing the role of arteriograms in the management of posterior knee dislocations, *J Trauma* 35:692-697, 1993.

81. Johansen K, Lynch K, Paun M, et al: Non-invasive vascular tests reliably exclude occult arterial trauma in injured extremities, *J Trauma* 31:515-522, 1991.

82. Kendall RW, Taylor DC, Salvian AJ, et al: The role of arteriography in assessing vascular injuries associated with dislocation of the knee, *J Trauma* 35:875-878, 1993.

83. Lynch K, Johansen K: Can Doppler pressure measurement replace "exclusion" arteriography in the diagnosis of occult extremity arterial trauma? *Ann Surg* 214:737-741, 1991.

84. Treiman GS, Yellin AE, Weaver FA, et al: Examination of the patient with a knee dislocation: the case for selective arteriography, *Arch Surg* 127:1056-1063, 1992.

85. Snyder WH III, Watkins WL, Whiddon LL, et al: Civilian popliteal artery trauma: an eleven year experience with 83 injuries, *Surgery* 85:101-108, 1979.

86. Abou-Sayed H, Berger DL: Blunt lower-extremity trauma and popliteal artery injuries, *Arch Surg* 137:585-589, 2002.

87. Miranda FE, Dennis JW, Veldenz HC, et al: Confirmation of the safety and accuracy of physical examination in the evaluation of knee dislocation for injury of the popliteal artery: a prospective study, *J Trauma* 52:247-252, 2002.

88. Merrill KD: Knee dislocations with vascular injuries, *Orthop Clin North Am* 25:707-713, 1994.

89. Sawchuk AP, Eldrup-Jorgensen J, Tober C, et al: The natural history of intimal flaps in a canine model, *Arch Surg* 125:1614-1616, 1990.

90. Stain SC, Yellin AE, Weaver FA, et al: Selective management of non-occlusive arterial injuries, *Arch Surg* 124:1136-1141, 1989.

91. Armstrong PJ, Franklin DP: Management of arterial and venous injuries in the dislocated knee, *Sports Med Arthrosc Rev* 9:219-226, 2001.

92. Hafez HM, Woolgar J, Robbs JV: Lower extremity arterial injury: results of 550 cases and review of risk factors associated with limb loss, *J Vasc Surg* 33:1212-1219, 2001.

93. Wagner WH, Calkins ER, Weaver FA, et al: Blunt popliteal artery trauma: 100 consecutive injuries, *J Vasc Surg* 7:736-743, 1988.

94. Rich NM, Hobson RW, Collins GJ, et al: The effect of acute popliteal venous interruption, *Ann Surg* 183:365-368, 1976.

95. Hill JA, Rana NA: Complications of posterolateral dislocation of the knee: case report and literature review, *Clin Orthop* 154:212-215, 1981.

96. Quinlan AG, Sharrard WJW: Posterolateral dislocation of the knee with capsular interposition, *J Bone Joint Surg Br* 40:660-663, 1958.

97. Tomaino MM, Day C, Papageorgiou C: Peroneal nerve palsy following knee dislocation: pathoanatomy and implications for treatment, *Knee Surg Sports Traumatol Arthrosc* 8:163-165, 2000.

98. White J: The results of traction injuries to the common peroneal nerve, *J Bone Joint Surg Br* 50:346-350, 1968.

99. Sedel L, Nizard RS: Nerve grafting for traction injuries of the common peroneal nerve: a report of 17 cases, *J Bone Joint Surg Br* 75:772-774, 1993.

100. Monahan TJ: Treatment of nerve injuries in the multiple-ligament-injured knee, *Op Tech Sports Med* 11:208-217, 2003.

101. Mont MA, Dellon AL, Chen F, et al: The operative treatment of peroneal nerve palsy, *J Bone Joint Surg Am* 78:863-869, 1996.

102. Bateman JE: *Trauma to nerves in limbs*, Philadelphia, 1962, Saunders, p 299.

103. Terranova WA, McLaughlin RE, Morgan RF: An algorithm for the management of ligamentous injuries, *Orthopaedics* 9:1135-1140, 1986.

104. Goitz RJ, Tomaino MM: Management of peroneal nerve injuries associated with knee dislocations, *Am J Orthop* 32:14-16, 2003.

105. Brautigan B, Johnson DL: The epidemiology of knee dislocations, *Clin Sports Med* 19:387-397, 2000.

106. Wright DG, Covey DC, Born CI, et al: Open dislocation of the knee, *J Orthop Trauma* 9:135-140, 1995.

107. Eastlack RK, Schenck RC, Guarducci C: The dislocated knee: classification, treatment, and outcome, *US Army Med Dept J* 11/12:1-9, 1997.

108. Schenck RC Jr: Classification of knee dislocations, *Op Tech Sports Med* 11:193-198, 2003.

109. Cooper DE, Speer KP, Wickiewicz TL, et al: Complete knee dislocation without posterior cruciate ligament disruption: a report of four cases and review of the literature, *Clin Orthop* 284:228-233, 1992.

110. Moore TM: Fracture-dislocation of the knee, *Clin Orthop* 156:128-140, 1981.

111. Schenck RC, McGanit PIJ, Hedman JD: Femoral-sided fracture-dislocation of the knee, *J Orthop Trauma* 6:416-421, 1997.

112. Walker D, Rogers W, Schenck RC: Immediate vascular and ligamentous repair in a closed knee dislocation: a case report, *J Trauma* 35:898-900, 1994.

113. Hunter SC, Marascalco R, Hughston JC: Disruption of the vastus medialis obliquus with medial knee ligament injuries, *Am J Sports Med* 11:427-431, 1983.

114. Torg JS, Conrad W, Kalen V: Clinical diagnosis of anterior cruciate ligament instability in the athlete, *Am J Sports Med* 4:84-93, 1976.

115. Bergfeld JA, McAllister DR, Parker RD, et al: The effects of tibial rotation on posterior translation in knees in which the posterior cruciate ligament has been cut, *J Bone Joint Surg Am* 83:1339-1343, 2001.

116. Covey DC, Sapega AA: Injuries of the posterior cruciate ligament, *J Bone Joint Surg Am* 75:1376-1386, 1993.

117. Harner CD, Hoher J: Evaluation and treatment of posterior cruciate ligament injuries, *Am J Sports Med* 26:471-482, 1998.

118. Markolf KL, Slauterbeck JR, Armstrong KL, et al: A biomechanical study of replacement of the posterior cruciate ligament with a graft: part I. Isometry, pre-tension of the graft, and anterior-posterior laxity, *J Bone Joint Surg Am* 79:375-380, 1997.

119. Rubinstein RA Jr, Shelbourne KD, McCarroll JR, et al: The accuracy of the clinical examination in the setting of the posterior cruciate ligament injuries, *Am J Sports Med* 22:550-557, 1994.

120. Veltri DM, Warren RF: Posterolateral instability of the knee, *J Bone Joint Surg Am* 76:460-472, 1994.

121. Clancy WG Jr, Sutherland TB: Combined posterior cruciate ligament injuries, *Clin Sports Med* 13:629-647, 1994.

122. Hughston JC, Norwood LA Jr: The posterolateral drawer test and external rotational recurvatum test for posterolateral rotatory instability of the knee, *Clin Orthop* 147:82-87, 1980.

123. Hughston JC, Jacobson KE: Chronic posterolateral rotary instability of the knee, *J Bone Joint Surg Am* 67:351-359, 1985.

124. O'Brien SJ, Warren RF, Pavlov H, et al: Reconstruction of the chronically insufficient anterior cruciate ligament with the central third of the patellar ligament, *J Bone Joint Surg Am* 73:278-286, 1991.

125. Jakob RP, Hassler H, Staeubli HU: Observations on rotatory instability of the lateral compartment of the knee: experimental studies on the functional anatomy and the pathomechanism of the true and the reversed pivot shift sign, *Acta Orthop Scand* 191(suppl):1-32, 1981.

126. Loomer RL: A test for knee posterolateral rotary instability, *Clin Orthop* 264:235-238, 1991.

127. Veltri DM, Warren RF: Anatomy, biomechanics, and physical findings in posterolateral knee instability, *Clin Sports Med* 13:599-614, 1994.

128. LaPrade RF, Terry GC: Injuries to the posterolateral aspect of the knee: association of anatomic injury patterns with clinical instability, *Am J Sports Med* 25:433-438, 1997.

129. Nielsen S, Ovesen J, Rasmussen O: The posterior cruciate ligament and rotatory knee instability: an experimental study, *Arch Orthop Trauma Surg* 104:53-56, 1985.

130. LaPrade RF, Konowalchuk B, Wentorf FA: Posterolateral corner injuries. In Schenck RC Jr, editor: *Multiple ligamentous injuries of the knee,* Rosemont, IL, 2002, American Academy of Orthopaedic Surgeons.

131. Yu JS, Goodwin D, Salonen D, et al: Complete dislocation of the knee: spectrum of associated soft-tissue injuries depicted by MR imaging, *Am J Rad* 164:135-139, 1995.

132. Yu JS, Salonen DC, Hodler J, et al: Posterolateral aspect of the knee: improved MR imaging with a coronal oblique technique, *Radiology* 198:199-204, 1996.

133. Olson SA, Finkemeier CG, Moehring HD: Open fractures. In Bucholz RW, Heckman JD, editors: *Fractures in adults,* vol I, Philadelphia, 2001, Lippincott Williams & Wilkins.

134. DeCoster TA: High-energy dislocations. In Schenck RS Jr: *Multiple ligamentous injuries of the knee,* Rosemont, IL, 2002, American Academy of Orthopaedic Surgeons.

135. Schenck RC, Kovach IS, Agarwal A, et al: Cruciate injury patterns in knee hyperextension: a cadaveric model, *Arthroscopy* 15:489-495, 1999.

136. Krakow KA, Thomas SC, Jones LC: A new stitch for ligament-tendon fixation: brief note, *J Bone Joint Surg Am* 68:764-768, 1986.

137. Fanelli GC, Feldman DD, Edson CJ, et al: The multiple ligament–injured knee. In DeLee JC, Drez D Jr, Miler MD, editors: *Orthopaedic sports medicine: principles and practice,* ed 2, vol 2, Philadelphia, 2003, Saunders.

138. Weiss NG, Kaplan, LD, Graf BK: Graft selection in surgical reconstruction of the multiple-ligament-injured knee, *Op Tech Sports Med* 11:218-225, 2003.

139. Sims WF, Simonian PT, Wickiewicz TL: The dislocated knee. In Callaghan JJ, Rosenberg AG, Rubash HE, editors: *The adult knee,* vol 1, Philadelphia, 2003, Lippincott Williams & Wilkins.

140. Harner CD, Olson E, Irrgang JJ, et al: Allograft versus autograft anterior cruciate ligament reconstruction: 3-5 year outcome, *Clin Orthop* 324:134-144, 1996.

141. Indelicato PA, Linton RC, Huegel M: The results of fresh-frozen patellar tendon allografts for chronic anterior cruciate ligament deficiency of the knee, *Am J Sports Med* 20:118-121, 1992.

142. Noyes FR, Barber-Westin SD: Reconstruction of the anterior cruciate ligament with human allograft: comparison of early and later results, *J Bone Joint Surg Am* 78:524-537, 1996.

143. Buck BE, Malinin TI, Brown MD: Bone transplantation and human immunodeficiency virus: an estimate of risk of acquired immunodeficiency syndrome (AIDS), *Clin Orthop* 240:129-136, 1989.

144. Centers for Disease Control and Prevention: Update: allograft-associated bacterial infections, United States, 2002, *JAMA* 287:1642-1644, 2002.

145. Graf B, Uhr F: Complications of intra-articular anterior cruciate reconstruction, *Clin Sports Med* 7:835-842, 1988.

146. Hughston J: Complications of anterior cruciate ligament surgery, *Orthop Clin North Am* 16:237-245, 1985.

147. Hegyes MS, Richardson MW, Miller MD: Knee dislocation: complications of nonoperative and operative management, *Clin Sports Med* 19:519-543, 2000.

148. McAllister DR, Parker RD, Cooper AE, et al: Outcomes of postoperative septic arthritis after ACL reconstruction, *Am J Sports Med* 27:562-570, 1999.

149. Williams RJ III, Laurencin CT, Warren RF, et al: Septic arthritis after arthroscopic anterior cruciate ligament reconstruction. Diagnosis and management, *Am J Sports Med* 25:261-267, 1997.

150. Fanelli GC: Complications of multiple ligamentous injuries. In Schenck RC Jr, editor: *Multiple ligamentous injuries of the knee in the athlete,* Rosemont, IL, 2002, American Academy of Orthopaedic Surgeons.

151. Fu FH, Irrgang JJ, Sawhney R, et al: Loss of knee motion following anterior cruciate ligament reconstruction, *Am J Sports Med* 18:557-562, 1990.

152. Harner CD, Irrgang JJ, Paul J, et al: Loss of motion after anterior cruciate ligament reconstruction, *Am J Sports Med* 20:499-506, 1992.

153. Shelbourne KD, Klootwyk TE, Carr DR: Low velocity knee dislocation associated with sports injury, *Op Tech Sports Med* 11:226-234, 2003.

154. Hefzy MS, Grood ES, Noyes FR: Factors affecting the region of most isometric femoral attachments. Part II. The anterior cruciate ligament, *Am J Sports Med* 17:208-216, 1989.

155. Burns WC II, Draganich LF, Pyevich M, et al: The effect of femoral tunnel position and graft tensioning technique on posterior laxity of the knee, *Am J Sports Med* 23:424-430, 1995.

156. Galloway MT, Grood ES, Mehalik JN, et al: Posterior cruciate ligament reconstruction. An in vitro study of femoral and tibial graft placement, *Am J Sports Med* 24:437-445, 1996.

157. Harner CD, Hoher J: Current concepts: evaluation and treatment of posterior cruciate ligament injuries, *Am J Sports Med* 26:471-482, 1998.

158. Markoff KL, O'Neill G, Jackson SR, et al: Reconstruction of knees with combined cruciate deficiencies: a biomechanical study, *J Bone Joint Surg Am* 85:1768-1774, 2003.

159. Harner CD, Janaushek MA, Ma B, et al: The effects of knee flexion angle and tibial position during graft fixation on the biomechanics of a PCL reconstructed knee, *Am J Sports Med* 28:460-465, 2000.

160. Michaelson JE, Bergfeld JA: Complications of knee ligament surgery. In Callaghan JJ, Rosenberg AG, Rubash HE, editors: *The adult knee,* vol 1, Philadelphia, 2003, Lippincott Williams & Wilkins.

161. Steadman JR, Seemann MD, Hutton KS: Revision ligament reconstruction of failed prosthetic anterior cruciate ligaments, *Instr Course Lect* 44:417-429, 1995.

162. Engebretsen L, Lewis JL: Graft selection and biomechanical considerations in ACL reconstruction (isometry, stress, preload), *Sports Med Arthrosc Rev* 4:336-341, 1996.

163. Robbins AS, Newman AP, Burks RT: Postoperative return of motion in anterior cruciate ligament and medial collateral ligament injuries: the effect of medial collateral ligament rupture location, *Am J Sports Med* 21:20-25, 1993.

164. Paulos LE, Rosenberg TD, Drawbert J, et al: Infrapatellar contracture syndrome: an unrecognized cause of knee stiffness with patella entrapment and patellar infera, *Am J Sports Med* 15:331-341, 1987.

165. Noyes FR, Wojtys EM, Marshall MT: The early diagnosis and treatment of developmental patella infera syndrome, *Clin Orthop* 265:241-252, 1991.

166. Shelbourne KD, Wilckens JH, Mollabashy A, et al: Arthrofibrosis in acute anterior cruciate ligament reconstruction: the effective timing of reconstruction and rehabilitation, *Am J Sports Med* 19:332-336, 1991.

167. Thomas P, Rud B, Jensen U: Stability and motion after traumatic dislocation of the knee, *Acta Orthop Scand* 55:278-283, 1984.

168. Sprague NF, O'Conner RL, Fox JM: Arthroscopic treatment of postoperative knee arthrofibrosis, *Clin Orthop* 166:165-172, 1982.

169. Ogata K, McCarthy JA: Measurements of length and tension patterns during reconstruction of the posterior cruciate ligament, *Am J Sports Med* 20:351-355, 1992.

170. Falconiero RP, DiStefano VJ, Cook TM: Revascularization and ligamentization of autogenous anterior cruciate ligament grafts in humans, *Arthroscopy* 14:197-205, 1998.

171. Brown CH Jr, Carson EW: Revision anterior cruciate ligament surgery, *Clin Sports Med* 18:109-171, 1999.

172. Berg EE: Posterior cruciate ligament tibial inlay reconstruction, *Arthroscopy* 8:95-99, 1995.

173. Bergfeld JA, McAllister DR, Parker RD, et al: A biomechanical comparison of posterior cruciate ligament reconstruction techniques, *Am J Sports Med* 29:129-136, 2001.

174. Miller MD: Posterior cruciate reconstruction: tibial inlay technique, *Sports Med Arthrosc Rev* 7:266-272, 1999.

175. Galer BS: Complex regional pain syndromes, types I (reflex sympathetic dystrophy) and II (causalgia). In Insall JN, Scott WN, editors: *Surgery of the knee,* ed 3, vol 2, New York, 2001, Churchill Livingstone.

176. International Association for the Study of Pain: IASP Pain Terminology. In Merskey H, Bodguk N, editors: *Classification of chronic pain: descriptions of chronic pain syndromes and definitions of terms,* ed 2, Seattle, 1994, IASP Press.

177. Poehling GG, Pollock FE Jr, Kolman LA: Reflex sympathetic dystrophy of the knee after sensory nerve injury, *Arthroscopy* 4:31-35, 1988.

178. Stanton-Hicks M, Baron R, Boas R: Consensus report—complex regional syndromes: guidelines for therapy, *Clin Rev Pain* 14:155, 1997.

179. Sachs RA, Daniel DM, Stone ML, et al: Patellofemoral problems after anterior cruciate ligament reconstruction, *Am J Sports Med* 17:760-765, 1989.

180. Shelbourne KD, Trumper RV: Preventing anterior knee pain after anterior cruciate reconstruction, *Am J Sports Med* 25:41-47, 1997.

181. Athanasian EA, Wickiewicz TL, Warren RF: Osteonecrosis of the femoral condyle after arthroscopic reconstruction of a cruciate ligament: report of two cases, *J Bone Joint Surg Am* 77:1418-1422, 1995.

182. Reddy AS, Frederick RW: Evaluation of the intraosseous and extraosseous blood supply of the distal femoral condyles, *Am J Sports Med* 26:415-419, 1998.

183. Irrgang JJ, Fitzgerald GK: Rehabilitation of the multiple-ligament-injured knee, *Clin Sports Med* 19:545-571, 2000.

184. Beynnon BD, Johnson RJ, Fleming BC, et al: The measurement of elongation of anterior cruciate ligament grafts in vivo, *J Bone Joint Surg* 76A:520-531, 1994.

185. Lutz GE, Palmitier RA, An KN, et al: Comparison of tibiofemoral joint forces during open and closed kinetic chain exercises, *J Bone Joint Surg* 75(5):732-739, 1993.

186. Fleming BC, Beynnon BD, Renstrom PA, et al: The strain behavior of the anterior cruciate ligament during stair climbing: an in-vivo study, *Arthroscopy* 15:185-191, 1999.

187. Henning CE, Lynch MA, Glick KR: An in-vivo strain gauge study of elongation of the anterior cruciate ligament, *Am J Sports Med* 13:22-26, 1985.

188. Lutz GS, Palmitier RA, An KN, et al: Comparison of tibiofemoral joint forces during open and closed kinetic chain exercises, *J Bone Joint Surg* 75A:732-739, 1993.

189. Yack HJ, Collins CE, Whieldon TJ: Comparisons of closed and open kinetic chain exercises in the anterior cruciate ligament–deficient knee, *Am J Sports Med* 21:49-54, 1993.

190. Renstrom PS, Arms SW, Stanwych TS, et al: Strain within the anterior cruciate ligament during hamstring and quadriceps activity, *Am J Sports Med* 14:83-87, 1986.

191. Beynnon BD, Fleming BC, Johnson RJ, et al: Anterior cruciate ligament strain behavior during rehabilitation exercises in vivo, *Am J Sports Med* 23:24-34, 1995.

192. Beynnon BD, Johnson RJ, Fleming BC, et al: The strain behavior of the anterior cruciate ligament during squatting and active flexion-extension: a comparison of open and closed kinetic chain exercise, *Am J Sports Med* 25:823-829, 1997.

193. Draganich LF, Jaeger RJ, Knalj AR: Co-activation of the hamstrings and quadriceps during extension of the knee, *J Bone Joint Surg* 71A:1075-1081, 1989.

194. Isear JA, Erickson JC, Worrell TW: EMG analysis of lower extremity muscle recruitment patterns during an unloaded squat, *Med Sci Sports Exerc* 29:532-539, 1997.

195. More RC, Karras BT, Neiman R, et al: Hamstrings—an anterior cruciate ligament protagonist: an in vitro study, *Am J Sports Med* 21:231-237, 1993.

196. Aune AK, Cawley PW, Ekeland A: Quadriceps muscle contraction protects the anterior cruciate ligament during anterior tibial translation, *Am J Sports Med* 25:187-195, 1997.

197. Grood ES, Stowers SF, Noyes FR: Limits of movement in the human knee: effect of sectioning the posterior cruciate ligament and posterolateral structures, *J Bone Joint Surg* 70A:88-97, 1988.

198. Hsieh HH, Walker PS: Stabilizing mechanisms of the loaded and unloaded knee joint, *J Bone Joint Surg* 58A:87-93, 1976.

199. Ellenbecker TS, Davies GJ: *Closed kinetic chain exercise: a comprehensive guide to multiple joint exercises,* Champaign, IL, 2001, Human Kinetics.

200. Bynum EB, Barrack RL, Alexander AH: Open versus closed kinetic chain exercises after anterior cruciate ligament reconstruction: a prospective randomized study, *Am J Sports Med* 23:401-406, 1995.

201. Snyder-Mackler L, Delitto A, Bailey SL, et al: Strength of the quadriceps femoris muscle and functional recovery after reconstruction of the anterior cruciate ligament, *J Bone Joint Surg* 77A:1166-1173, 1995.

202. Dahlkuits NJ, Mago P, Seedholm BB: Forces during squatting and rising from a deep squat, *Engineering Med* 11:69-76, 1982.

203. Arms SW, Pope MH, Johnson RJ, et al: The biomechanics of the anterior cruciate ligament rehabilitation and reconstruction, *Am J Sports Med* 12:8, 1984.

204. Stannard JP, Sheils TM, McGwin G, et al: Use of hinged external knee fixator after surgery for knee dislocation, *Arthroscopy* 19(6):626-631, 2003.

205. Rodeo SA, Arnoczky SP, Torzilli PA, et al: Tendon-healing in a bone tunnel: a biomechanical and histological study in the dog, *J Bone Joint Surg* 75A:1795-1803, 1993.

206. Spencer JD, Hayes KC, Alexander JJ: Knee joint effusion and quadriceps inhibition in man, *Arch Phys Med Rehabil* 65:171-177, 1984.

207. Sachs RA, Daniel DM, Stone ML, et al: Patellofemoral problems after anterior ligament reconstruction, *Am J Sports Med* 17:760-765, 1989.

208. Schlegel TF, Boublik M, Hawkins RJ, et al: Reliability of heel-height measurement for documenting knee extension deficits, *Am J Sports Med* 30:479-482, 2002.

209. Bandy WD, Irion JM: The effect of time on static stretching on the flexibility of the hamstring muscles, *Phys Ther* 74:845-850, 1994.

210. Bandy WD, Irion JM, Briggler M: The effect of time and frequency of static stretch on flexibility of the hamstring muscles, *Phys Ther* 77:1090-1096, 1997.

211. Bandy WD, Irion JM, Briggler M: The effect of static stretch and dynamic range of motion on the flexibility of the hamstring muscles, *J Orthop Sports Phys Ther* 27:295-300, 1998.

212. McClure PW, Blackburn LG, Dusold C: The use of splints in the treatment of joint stiffness: biological rationale and algorithm for making clinical decisions, *Phys Ther* 74:1101-1107, 1994.

213. Davies GJ, Ellenbecker TS: Focused exercise aids shoulder hypomobility, *Biomechanics,* Nov 1999, pp 77-81.

214. Feland JB, Myrer JW, Schulthies SS, et al: The effect of duration of stretching on the hamstring muscle group for increased range of motion in people aged 65 years and older, *Phys Ther* 81:1110-1117, 2001.

215. Nicholas JA, Strizak AM, Veras G: A study of thigh muscle weakness in different pathological states of the lower extremity, *Am J Sports Med* 4:241-248, 1976.

216. Gleim GW, Nicholas JA, Webb JN: Isokinetic evaluation following leg injuries, *Phys Sports Med* 6:74-82, 1978.

217. Sapega AA, Quedenfeld TC: Biophysical factors in range of motion exercises, *Phys Sports Med* 9:57-65, 1981.

218. Snyder-Mackler L, Ladin Z, Schepsis AA, Young JC: Electrical stimulation of the thigh muscles after reconstruction of the anterior cruciate ligament: effects of electrically elicited contraction of the quadriceps femoris and hamstring muscles on gait and on strength of the thigh muscles, *J Bone Joint Surg* 73A:1025-1036, 1991.

219. Davies GJ: *A compendium of isokinetics in clinical usage,* ed 4, Onalaska, WI, 1992, S&S Publishers.

220. Astrand P, Rodahl K: *Textbook of work physiology,* New York, 1977, McGraw-Hill.

221. Halback JW, Davies GJ, Gould JA, et al: Effect of limited range of motion on non-exercised range of motion strength, *Phys Ther* 65:732-733, 1985 (abstract).

222. Rowinski MJ: Afferent neurobiology of the joint. In Gould JA, Davies GJ, editors: *Orthopaedic and sports physical therapy,* St Louis, 1985, Mosby.

223. Fitzgerald GK, Axe MJ, Snyder-Mackler L: The efficacy of perturbation training in non-operative anterior cruciate ligament rehabilitation programs for physically active individuals, *Phys Ther* 80:128-140, 2000.

224. Smith J, Malanga GA, Yu B, et al: Effects of functional knee bracing on muscle-firing patterns about the chronic anterior cruciate ligament–deficient knee, *Arch Phys Med Rehabil* 84:1680-1686, 2003.

225. Decoster LC, Vailas JC: Functional anterior cruciate ligament bracing: a survey of current brace prescription patterns, *Orthopedics* 26:701-706, 2003.

226. Ohkoshi Y, Yasuda K, Kaneda K, et al: Biomechanical analysis of rehabilitation in the standing position, *Am J Sports Med* 19:605-611, 1991.

227. Palmitier RA, An KN, Scott SG, et al: Kinetic chain exercises in knee rehabilitation, *Sports Med* 11:402-413, 1991.

228. Davies GJ, Heiderscheidt BC, Schulte R, et al: The scientific and clinical rationale for the integrated approach to open and closed kinetic chain rehabilitation, *Orthop Phys Ther Clin North Am* 9:247-267, 2000.

229. Neitzel JA, Kernozek TW, Davies GJ: Loading response following anterior cruciate ligament reconstruction during parallel squat exercise, *Clin Biomech* 17:551-554, 2002.

230. Wolfe GL, LeMura LM, Cole PJ: Quantitative analysis of single vs. multiple-set programs in resistance training, *J Strength Cond Res* 18:35-47, 2004.

231. Rivera JE: Open versus closed kinetic chain rehabilitation of the lower extremity: a functional and biomechanical analysis, *J Sport Rehabil* 3:154-167, 1994.

232. Escamilla RF, Flesig GS, Zheng N, et al: Biomechanics of the knee during closed kinetic chain and open kinetic chain exercises, *Med Sci Sports Exerc* 30:556-569, 1998.

233. Wilk KE, Escamilla RF, Flesig GS, et al: A comparison of tibiofemoral joint forces and EMG activity during open and closed kinetic chain exercises, *Am J Sports Med* 24:518-527, 1996.

234. Ciccotti MG, Kerlan RK, Perry J, et al: An EMG analysis of the knee during functional activities: part II, *Am J Sports Med* 22:651-658, 1994.

235. Gauffin H, Tropp H: Altered movement and muscular-activation patterns during the one-legged jump in patients with an old anterior cruciate ligament rupture, *Am J Sports Med* 20:182, 1992.

236. Kauland S, Sinkjaer R, Arendt-Nielson L, et al: Altered timing of hamstring muscle action in anterior cruciate deficient patients, *Am J Sports Med* 18:245, 1990.

237. Solomonow M, Baratta R, Zhou BH, et al: The synergistic action of the anterior cruciate ligament and thigh muscles in maintaining joint stability, *Am J Sports Med* 15:207, 1987.

238. Davies GJ, Zillmer DA: Functional progression of exercise during rehabilitation. In Ellenbecker TS, editor: *Knee ligament rehabilitation,* ed 2, Philadelphia, 2000, Churchill Livingstone.

239. Davies GJ, Heiderscheit BC: Reliability of the Lido Linea closed kinetic chain isokinetic dynamometer, *J Orthop Sports Phys Ther* 25:133-136, 1997.

240. Davies GJ, Heiderscheidt BC, Clark M: Open kinetic chain assessment and rehabilitation, *Athl Training Sports Health Care Perspect* 1:347-370, 1995.

241. Wilk KE, Andrews JR: The effects of pad placement and angular velocity on tibial placement during isokinetic exercises, *J Orthop Sports Phys Ther* 17:23-30, 1993.

242. Tabor M, Davies GJ, Negrete R, et al: A multi-center study of the test-retest reliability of the lower extremity functional test, *J Sport Rehabil* 11:190-201, 2002.

CHAPTER 17

Preventing Injury to the Anterior Cruciate Ligament

Timothy E. Hewett, PhD
Kim M. Yearout, PT, BS
Robert C. Manske, DPT, MPT, MEd, SCS, ATC, CSCS

CHAPTER OUTLINE

Epidemiology: Incidence and Prevalence
Anatomy Overview
    Anterior Cruciate Ligament
    Posterior Cruciate Ligament
Mechanism of Injury
Intrinsic Factors
    Q-angle
    Notch Size
    Joint Laxity
    Hormonal Factors
Extrinsic Factors
    Muscular Strength and Activation
      Patterns
    Muscular Activation and
      Recruitment Patterns
    Postural Considerations
    Landing and Jumping Characteristics
Programs Designed for the Prevention of
  ACL Injury
Dynamic Neuromuscular Analysis Training
    Rationale
    Dynamic Neuromuscular Analysis
      Training Protocol
Summary

EPIDEMIOLOGY: INCIDENCE AND PREVALENCE

One of the most devastating and disabling injuries to the knee joint is rupture of the anterior cruciate ligament (ACL). The ACL is disrupted more than any other ligament in the knee.[1] In the general population, it is estimated that 1 in 3000 people endure an ACL injury per year in the United States. Griffin and colleagues[2] estimate that 80,000 ACL tears occur annually in the United States; 70% of these injuries are the result of sports participation, with the majority of the injuries occurring in pivoting sports. Age ranged from 15 to 45 years; however, the most prevalent age-group for ACL surgery was in the third decade. Griffin and colleagues point out the economic burden on our health care system, with approximately 50,000 ACL surgeries being performed per year resulting in an estimated $850,000 in medical expense, not to overshadow the emotional and physical burden imposed on the individual who sustained the devastating injury. Whether the ACL is reconstructed or treated conservatively, all are at greater risk for arthritis. Myklebust and colleagues[3] hypothesized that an effective ACL reconstruction increases the risk of future osteoarthritis by enabling the athlete to return to competitive, weight-bearing activities. In concurrence, von Porat and colleagues[4] reported that the prevalence of osteoarthritis among soccer players 14 years after injury was alarming. In their study of 219 male soccer players with ACL injury in 1986, 205 (94%) were available for follow-up at 14 years. Of the original 219 patients, 154 (75%) answered mailed questionnaires and 122 of the athletes consented to weight-bearing radiographs. Despite ACL surgical reconstruction, osteoarthritis was found in 78% of the injured knees, and more advanced changes, comparable with Kellgren-Lawrence grade 2 or higher, were seen in 41% of a group of 122 participants who consented to the radiographs. *Radiographic osteoarthritis* was defined as joint space narrowing grade 1 combined with osteophytes, or joint space narrowing grade 2 or more. Of the 205 participants who were available for follow-up, the majority claimed some type of knee symptomatology affecting their quality of life. These now middle-aged men attempt to earn a living, raise a family, and perform normal activities of daily living on knees that are older than their chronologic age. The indirect costs to this population and society as a whole are still unknown, but must be enormous. This creates even more of an impetus to prevent catastrophic knee injuries that are not the result of direct trauma. Our profession continues to search for ways to prevent catastrophic ACL tears. These injuries interrupt athletic participation, most likely requiring surgical reconstruction, and may affect an athlete's collegiate scholarship and educational opportunities. Adding perplexity and misery to the ACL injury epidemic are separate but similar studies indicating that 70% to 80% of ACL injuries are noncontact (the majority of ACL injuries are self-inflicted). McNair and colleagues[5] reported that 70% of the 23 ACL tears in their study incurred injuries at foot-strike during noncontact situations. Boden and Garrett[6] reported that 71% of recorded injuries were classified as noncontact.

What causes these injuries? What factors, intrinsic and extrinsic, contribute to the high incidence of ACL disruption, especially in the female athlete? Arendt and Dick[7] indicate that female athletes are 2 to 8 times more likely to suffer an ACL injury than their male counterparts. Pearl[8] reported that female basketball players suffer ACL tears 7.8 times more than their male counterparts. If the majority of ACL disruptions are self-inflicted, how can we, as health care professionals, introduce and train preventive measures for all athletes? Numerous published articles reveal the popularity of diagnosing and treating the ACL injury, but only 3% of the publications focus on ACL injury prevention.[9] Clearly, it is a topic long overdue for intense scrutiny, investigation, research, and action in order to reverse the increasing incidence of ACL-injured knees. It becomes our ethical obligation and passion to develop, teach, and train preventive programs.

ANATOMY OVERVIEW

The cruciate ligaments located within the capsule of the knee joint are the primary static stabilizers of the knee joint. They are named according to the attachment site on the tibia. The anterior cruciate attaches to the tibia anteriorly, and the posterior cruciate attaches to the tibia posteriorly. They are contained within the medial and lateral femoral condyles.

Anterior Cruciate Ligament

The anterior cruciate arises from the anterior portion of the intercondylar area of the tibia, just posterior to the attachment of the medial meniscus. It then travels superiorly, posteriorly, and laterally to attach to the posterior portion of the medial side of the lateral femoral condyle (Figure 17-1). The ACL contains two distinct bundles that consist of individual fascicles to add integrity to the ligament. The anteromedial bundle is more taut in flexion and lax in extension; the posterolateral bundle is more taut in extension and more lax in flexion. However, because of the unique design of the ACL, consisting of an interconnection of fibers throughout the two bands, some portion of the anterior cruciate remains taut throughout knee range of motion. The primary function of the ACL is to prevent the tibia from translating anteriorly on the femur. Both of the cruciates help control excessive rotatory motion of the knee joint as well. Of the two cruciate ligaments, the ACL is more commonly injured.

Posterior Cruciate Ligament

The stronger of the two cruciate ligaments, the posterior cruciate ligament (PCL), arises from the posterior part of the intercondylar area of the tibia and passes superiorly and anteriorly on the medial portion of the ACL to insert into the

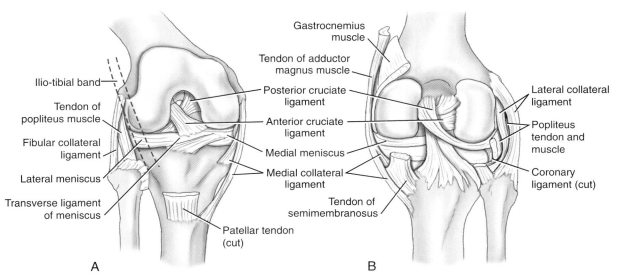

Figure 17-1: Anterior cruciate ligament (ACL) and posterior cruciate ligament (PCL). **A,** Anterior view. Patellar tendon is sectioned and the patella reflected upward. Knee flexed. Note that the cruciate ligament rises in front of the anterior tibial spine, not from it. Note also that the medial meniscus is firmly attached to the medial collateral ligament. **B,** Posterior view, knee extended. Note that the posterior ligament has been removed. The two layers of the medial collateral ligament are shown diagrammatically, as is the tibial portion of the lateral collateral ligament. The PCL rises behind the tibia, not on its upper surface. Observe the femoral attachment of the ACL at the back of the notch. *(From Magee DJ:* Orthopedic physical assessment, *Philadelphia, 1987, WB Saunders.)*

anterior part of the lateral surface of the medial condyle of the femur. The PCL is also composed of two bundles of fascicles. The anterolateral bundle is taut in flexion, and the posteromedial bundle is taut in extension. The primary functions of the PCL are to prevent the tibia from moving posteriorly on the femur, prevent hyperextension, and control rotatory stability. The posterior cruciate defines the knee's central axis of motion.

MECHANISM OF INJURY

To gain a better perspective of ACL injury patterns, several investigators performed interviews and watched countless videotapes of actual ACL injuries. Boden and Garrett[6] interviewed 65 males with 71 ACL injuries and 25 females with 28 ACL injuries (mean age at the time of injury, 26 years; range, 14 to 48 years) using a standardized questionnaire to determine what common characteristics might be found. Contact was involved in only 29% of the injuries. A breakdown of injuries by sport revealed the following: basketball 25%, football 21%, and soccer 21%.

Myklebust and colleagues[3] studied female handball players and found that 51% of the injuries occurred in a noncontact situation. Of those noncontact injuries, 80% were injured during a plant-and-cut maneuver or landing after a jump shot. Yu and colleagues[10] reported that recreational sports accounted for 41% of the injuries, varsity sports accounted for 34%, and intramural sports accounted for 23%. Similar

to previously reported information, 35% of patients reported deceleration to be a causative factor, 31% were landing from a jump, 13% reported accelerating, and 4% were falling backward. Henning's data, presented by Griffis to the American Orthopaedic Society for Sports Medicine (AOSSM), revealed similar statistics[11] (Table 17-1). Sudden change of direction, sudden deceleration, plant-and-cut maneuver, and vertical deceleration are common themes in the noncontact ACL injury. Teitz,[12] after reviewing 54 videotapes of ACL injuries from basketball and soccer participants, noted that 100% of the male basketball players injured the ACL landing from a jump (vertical deceleration), whereas approximately half of the women were injured landing from a jump and the other half were injured when they stopped suddenly while running down court.

After discussion of mechanism of injury in noncontact ACL injuries, a brief look at intrinsic and extrinsic factors that may predispose an athlete to ACL injury is warranted.

INTRINSIC FACTORS
Q angle

Quadriceps femoris angle (Q angle) is defined as the acute angle between the line connecting the anterior superior iliac spine and the midpoint of the patella, and the line connecting the tibial tubercle with the same reference point on the patella. Q-angle theory is implicated as a possible causative factor in ACL injury, especially in the female population. Increased Q-angle lends itself to an increased valgus moment at the knee and may put the athlete at risk. With excessive, uncontrolled femoral internal rotation, a chain reaction may occur with excessive tibial external rotation and increased pronation putting the athlete at high risk for an "overpronation moment" in the lower extremity; this places the ACL in a dangerous situation for rupture. Add to that situation diminished neuromuscular control or unfamiliar neuromuscular demand (i.e., the athlete's proprioceptive system has never been trained to fire in that excessive excursion or range of motion) and the athlete may not be able to recover, resulting in ACL rupture. Consistently, women have greater Q angles than men. The average Q angle, measured with the knee straight, is 13 degrees for males and 18 degrees for females.[13]

Q angles greater than 15 degrees in men and greater than 20 degrees in women are considered to be clinically abnormal (Figure 17-2). Shambaugh and colleagues[14] studied 45 athletes participating in recreational basketball and correlated ACL injury with the average Q angle. Those athletes who sustained knee injury displayed a significantly larger Q angle compared with those athletes who did not suffer a knee injury (14 degrees vs. 10 degrees). Increased Q angle may predispose athletes (especially female athletes) to excessive tibial torsion and excessive foot pronation, which may lead to ACL rupture. More studies must be conducted in order to directly implicate this chain reaction. If increased Q angle is found to be a contributory factor in ACL rupture, it will be critical to condition our athletes to dynamically enhance appropriate muscle groups in order to neuromuscularly control the overpronation moment in the lower extremity.

Notch Size

Huston and colleagues' excellent overview[15] of intercondylar notch studies and the correlation between notch size and

shape with unilateral and bilateral ACL tears questions this particular anatomic location as a potential risk factor in ACL rupture. Reviewed studies included the following:

1. Norwood and Cross[16] illustrated impingement of the ACL on the anterior intercondylar notch with the knee in full extension, and Shelbourne and colleagues[17] concluded that in men and women who sustained ACL tears, the notch width is narrower than a control group.

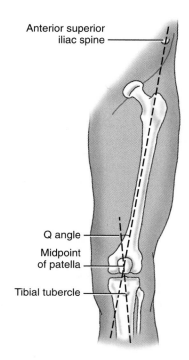

Figure 17-2: Quadriceps angle (Q angle). *(From Magee DJ: Orthopedic physical assessment, Philadelphia, 1987, WB Saunders.)*

TABLE 17-1

Henning's AOSSM[11] Data

SPORT; NUMBER OF SUBJECTS	NOT HIT	HIT	PAC	SKL	OSS
Women's basketball; 84	74 (88%)	10 (12%)	23 (27%)	18 (21%)	19 (23%)
Men's basketball; 96	78 (81%)	18 (19%)	21 (22%)	34 (35%)	12 (13%)
Recreational football; 34	28 (82%)	6 (18%)	20 (59%)	4 (12%)	3 (1%)
Full-contact football; 120	49 (41%)	69 (58%)	31 (26%)	4 (3%)	3 (3%)
Soccer; 61	51 (84%)	10 (16%)	23 (38%)	11 (18%)	5 (8 %)
Volleyball; 28	28 (100%)	0	0	17 (61%)	6 (2%)
Softball; 60	53 (87%)	7 (13%)	10 (18%)	1 (2%)	18 (34%)
Baseball; 4	4 (100%)	0	3 (75%)	0	0

Some interviewed subjects could not identify the exact injury-producing mechanism or situation. They were put into an unknown category. *OSS,* One-step stop; *PAC,* plant-and-cut maneuver, *SKL,* straight-knee landing.

2. Houseworth and colleagues[18] reported a significant difference in the ratio of the posterior arch area to the total area of the distal femur between patients with an ACL injury and control subjects who did not have an ACL injury. They concluded that a narrowed posterior notch might predispose the athlete to an ACL tear.

3. Similar findings by Lund-Hanssen and colleagues[19] illustrate that the noninvolved (healthy) knee of subjects who injured their ACL was remarkably more narrow than the intercondylar notch of the control subjects. Females with a 17 mm or less anterior notch width at the level of the popliteal groove were six times more susceptible to ACL injury compared with players with wider notch widths.

A prospective cohort study by Uhorchak and colleagues[9] revealed that a small femoral notch width, especially in females, predisposes the ACL to rupture. In addition to the notch width, this study looked at other anatomic factors that predisposed West Point cadets to ACL injury and found that the following risk factors were highly predictive of ACL injury in females: small femoral notch width, generalized joint laxity, higher than normal body mass index, and KT-2000 arthrometer values that were 1 standard deviation or more above the mean.

In contrast, numerous studies indicate that there is not a correlation between notch size and ACL disruption.[20,21] Of the numerous studies to date, there is no direct correlation to increase risk for unilateral ACL tear because of a more narrow notch width; however, it is notable that patients with bilateral ACL injuries have a more narrow intercondylar notch width than patients with unilateral ACL injuries.[22] It is our bias that this anatomic risk factor may not be the most paramount factor in preventing ACL injury. Rarely is an athlete going to submit to arthroscopic surgery on the recommendation that a notchplasty may prevent ACL injury. Therefore performance of a prophylactic notchplasty is uncommon. However, in the athlete who is already undergoing an ACL reconstruction, it is common to perform a notchplasty. As medical professionals, our training teaches us to start with the most noninvasive approach; therefore continual investigation of other potential culprits for the ACL injury enigma remains of utmost importance.

Joint Laxity

Laxity is an inherited, genetically predetermined condition of passive joint movement. Females tend to have more inherent laxity than males,[23] but does this lead to an increased incident of ACL tears in the female population? Several studies analyzed the relationship between hypermobility of the joint and increased incidence of ACL injury. Nicholas[24] reported that football players who were categorized as being more loose jointed suffered more ACL injuries than their tight-jointed comrades. However, others such as Grana and Moretz[25] and Godshall[26] disputed these claims. Hypotheti-

cally, there could be a case supporting hypermobility or hypomobility: Hypermobility is viewed as occurring when the joint allows more motion than normal; therefore the ligament does not get pulled taut as quickly, giving the musculoskeletal system an opportunity to proprioceptively react to the increased joint excursion. On the other hand, if the joint is hypomobile the integrity of the joint stability is greater, putting the ligament at less risk for disruption. Unfortunately, to date there is no conclusive evidence to scientifically support either increased or decreased joint laxity with predisposition to ACL injury. This inconclusive evidence reinforces the need for the neuromuscular prevention programs, such as the ones developed by the late Dr. Charles E. Henning and presented by Griffis and colleagues,[11] Caraffa and colleagues,[27] Hewett and colleagues,[28] and Mandelbaum and colleagues.[29] The one thing we do know is that athletes can highly train the neuromuscular system to improve functional joint stability and kinetic awareness.

Hormonal Factors

Statistics prove that females suffer two to eight times more ACL injuries than their male counterparts, so logically the female hormones come under great scrutiny for being a contributing culprit. Hormonal fluctuation throughout the menstrual cycle, in particular estrogen surges, can influence many systems throughout the body, such as the central nervous system[30] and the neuromuscular system,[31] significantly enough to produce changes in skill performance, laxity, and injury rate.[32] In 1996 estrogen and progesterone receptor sites were found in the human ACL.[33] Female sex hormones influence the composition and mechanical properties of the ACL. Liu and colleagues[33] illustrated this linkage of ACL injury with hormonal fluctuations in the menstrual cycle. Wojtys and colleagues[32] and Myklebust and colleagues[3] contradicted the time during the cycle that was most susceptible for the ACL injury. Wojtys and colleagues[32] included women with regular menstrual cycles not taking oral contraceptives, whereas Myklebust and colleagues[3] included 50% of women taking oral contraceptives. Studies such as these are commendable for engaging possible concepts linking ACL injuries and the female athlete. The authors respectfully ask a practical question with regard to preventing ACL injury based on hormonal factors. Can you imagine telling head coach Pat Summit of the University of Tennessee that her top player is in the ovulatory stage of her menstrual cycle and will not be able to participate in the NCAA National Championship game? We think not. Should we administer contraceptives to all female athletes? We think not. Nonetheless, the hormonal influence still requires investigation and may glean insight to assist with preventing ACL injury. Once again the practicality of prevention in noncontact ACL injuries leads back to the work of Henning,[11] Caraffa and colleagues,[27] Hewett and colleagues,[28] and Mandelbaum and colleagues.[29] Eradication of this epidemic requires identification of the mechanism of injury (improper technique); identification of the common injury-producing play situations per sport; and education of coaches, players, trainers, and parents on safe neuromuscular patterns to prevent ACL overload.

EXTRINSIC FACTORS

Muscular Strength and Activation Patterns

Not surprisingly, muscle strength in males is much greater than that in their female counterparts. Males are stronger than females because of differences in muscle mass and possible structural differences in elastic tissue. Quadriceps strength and hamstring strength are significantly less in females. Even when body weight is normalized per sex, females demonstrate significantly less strength in the quadriceps and hamstring muscle groups.[34] Overall, strength and endurance may be controllable, significant variables in ACL injury prevention. Lack of quadriceps and hamstring muscle strength places the female athlete at risk because the muscles surrounding the knee protect the joint from deleterious distress. Watching a team practice "defensive slides" for about 60 seconds allows observation as to how fatigue in the quadriceps changes postural and biomechanical stance. What does the athlete do when fatigue sets into the quadriceps? The athlete alters lower extremity alignment from a knee-flexed position to a near-extended or fully extended knee position, in order to rest the quadriceps, thus placing the ACL at greater risk for injury. Combine the fully extended knee position with a horizontal or vertical deceleration movement and you now have a disastrous combination for the ACL.

Does adequate quadriceps and hamstring strength prevent ACL noncontact injury? How many patients have been rehabilitated following ACL reconstruction (male or female), and on achieving adequate healing requirements (including soft tissue healing constraints, appropriate range of motion, quadriceps and hamstring strength goals, and passing of functional goals) were released to return to play, only to return to your office with an ACL rupture on the contralateral side? The patient had demonstrated good quadriceps and hamstring muscle strength or would not have been allowed to return to play. National statistics indicate that 4% to 5% of unilateral ACL tears become bilateral within 2.4 years of the initial ACL insult. However, many other factors may contribute to the ACL bilateral group, including unrecognized, ingrained favoring patterns; proprioceptive inhibition; decreased stance time caused by lack of proprioceptive confidence; and inadequate stabilization. Another observation with the "strength" risk factor is that the males who rupture the ACL through noncontact maneuvers usually are high-performance athletes ("blue chip" players) who have exceptional quadriceps and hamstring strength. So why do they injure? More studies must be conducted. Perhaps it is not just a matter of strength but, more important, a matter of *strength balance*. In particular, it may be a matter of a healthy balance between the quadriceps and hamstring muscle groups and appropriate and timely coactivation patterns.

Baratta and colleagues[35] investigated coactivation patterns in young male and female subjects. The subjects were categorized into a nonathletic group, a recreational athletic group, and a highly competitive athletic group. Electromyographic data were compiled during an isokinetic strength evaluation that produced maximal muscle contractions. The findings were as follows: High-performance athletes with hypertrophied quadriceps had strong inhibitory effects on the coactivation of the hamstrings compared with a group of healthy subjects who were not involved in athletics. Athletes who consistently strengthened their hamstrings, however, had a coactivation pattern similar to the pattern of the nonathletic subjects. This suggests that a hamstring training program aimed at balancing the quadriceps strength with good hamstring strength may benefit the high-performance athlete in reducing the risk of ACL disruption in a noncontact situation.

Muscular Activation and Recruitment Patterns

Muscle activation and recruitment patterns are essential components in the investigation of how to prevent the noncontact ACL rupture. The study by Huston and Wojtys[36] on elite male and female athletes' muscle recruitment patterns is highly insightful to the female ACL injury. Elite female athletes exhibit quadriceps-dominant muscle patterns; that is, they respond to anterior tibial translation with a primary quadriceps muscle contraction. The elite male athletes and the male and female control subjects, on the other hand, all respond to anterior tibial translation by initially contracting the hamstring muscle group. This may be a contributing factor to the increased incidence of ACL injuries in the female athlete.

Postural Considerations

Static postural analysis of the female athlete with inadequate neuromuscular control illustrates an anteriorly tilted pelvis.[37] Loudon and colleagues[38] have linked this posture to increased incidence of ACL injury. This position can decrease the effectiveness of the gluteus medius and external rotators to maintain a neutral lower extremity alignment position. Decreased hip muscle activation directly affects quadriceps and hamstring activation. Monoarticular muscles (the glutei) facilitate the biarticular muscles; therefore decreased hip muscle activation reduces the maximal possible quadriceps/hamstring activation.[39] Are the elite female athletes' quadriceps dominant because females have a tendency to have weak hip extensors, inefficient external rotators, and less hamstring and gluteus medius activation during stance phase? If hip extensors are weak, the female athlete must pull in the iliopsoas for trunk control, resulting in greater hip extension and therefore greater knee extension. Landing and jumping biomechanics are altered based on the postural influence.

Landing and Jumping Characteristics

Vertical deceleration produces a high percentage of ACL injuries. Landing from a jump, depending on the height, can exert between 3 and 14 times a person's body weight. This amount of force can shred the ACL. Henning described proper landing from a jump as soft and on the toes, with the knees flexed on contact and continuing to flex throughout the landing so that load can be absorbed over a greater amount of time. Peak forces in a short time frame are what potentially tear the ACL. Stacoff and colleagues[40] proposed the same concept, reporting that knee angle on touchdown is extremely important in determining the maximum load absorbed by the ACL. The less knee flexion on impact, the greater the impact forces imparted to the knee and associated ligaments. Hewett and colleagues[41] reported a 22% decrease in landing peak forces for female subjects following a 6-week injury prevention training program for volleyball players. Such studies give hope for reducing the tragedy of noncontact ACL injuries. Hewett and colleagues[28] reported a decreased incidence of serious knee injury rates following the training program.

The work of hundreds of scientists, clinicians, and researchers directs our path to eliminate the noncontact ACL injury through proper neuromuscular reeducation and education training programs. It appears that our medical society is on the verge of attaining a dream of the late Dr. Charles Henning (as well as many of our associates and colleagues), which was someday to put himself out of the business of reconstructing ACL-deficient knees and spend his valuable time educating athletes, coaches, and parents on how to prevent this tragic athletic injury. As clinicians, as educators, as researchers, our greatest influence lies in our ability to minimize extrinsic risk factors that predispose athletes to ACL disruption.

PROGRAMS DESIGNED FOR THE PREVENTION OF ACL INJURY

Although we must concede that a total extinction of ACL injuries is not foreseeable in the immediate future, preventive strategies for reducing the incidence of ACL rupture appear to be a worthwhile goal. Prevention of ACL injuries is imperative for reducing the incidence of acute injury, and also for the prevention of secondary knee disorders that can severely impair independence and adversely affect quality of life of the competitive and recreational athlete alike.

One of the first ACL injury prevention programs to be implemented was designed by Charles Henning in the 1980s. Henning's preventive program was based on what he termed the *quad–cruciate interaction*. It was his belief that a significant strain is placed on the ACL while the knee is in a weight-bearing position of extension. Approximately 86% of the total resistive force caused by forward movement of the tibia on the femur is thought to be restrained by the ACL. With a forceful quadriceps contraction, while the knee is

positioned near full extension, a significant strain may be placed on the ACL, with a possible disastrous end result of ligament rupture. While the knee is flexed greater than 60 degrees or more, the anterior translation of the tibia on the femur is much less, significantly reducing stress to the ACL. As he proposed years ago, the quad–cruciate interaction can be minimized by the knee and hip flexion angle.

Following a 10-year study of ACL-injured female basketball players, Henning and colleagues discovered that the most common mechanisms of injury were as follows: (1) planting and cutting (29%), for example, cutting to maneuver away from an opposing player or when driving to the goal; (2) a straight-knee landing (28%), for example, landing from a rebound with knee fully extended; and (3) a one-step stop (26%), for example, stopping quickly to turn in the other direction to elude an opposing player. Despite the fact that Henning and colleagues' study was never published in peer-reviewed literature, we believe that because of its landmark status, its inclusion is essential.

The preventive program that they describe was developed in an attempt to remedy compromising motor patterns believed to cause ACL rupture. Individuals were taught to practice a rounded accelerated turn off of a bent knee rather than the plant and cut, and landing on a bent knee was substituted for landing with the knee in a fully extended position. These components are of critical importance to their program because it has been shown that the highest amount of anterior tibial translation occurs within 10 to 30 degrees of full extension.[42-45] It has also been reported by some that video analysis of actual knee injuries reveals that the majority of injuries occur with the knee close to full extension.[6] In addition, a three-step stop was used rather than the pathologic one-step stop with the knee in hyperextension. Unpublished data from their center revealed an 89% decrease in ACL injury of Division I female collegiate basketball players following inclusion of their preventive training program.

Caraffa and colleagues[27] revealed dramatic results after instituting a proprioceptive training program to 600 soccer players in 40 semiprofessional or amateur teams. Twenty of the teams agreed to receive a special proprioceptive training program in addition to the standard training program, and the other 20 teams were asked to continue their normal training program. The study group was instructed in a proprioceptive training program that consisted of five phases. Phase I consisted of balance training, in which the athletes were instructed to stand on a single leg for up to 2.5 minutes four times per day. In phase II, athletes were asked to train on a rectangular balance board unilaterally four times per day for up to 2.5 minutes on each leg. In phase III, the athletes were progressed to a round board with the same time frames and repetitions as used in phase II. During phase IV, the athletes trained on a combined round and rectangular board, and in phase V they performed the same training on a Biomechanical Ankle Platform System (BAPS) board (Camp Jackson, MI). During the competitive soccer season the athletes were asked to continue their regimen three times per week at minimum.

The results were outstanding. ACL injuries were tracked for all teams over the following 3 years. A total of 10 verified ACL injuries occurred in the study group, whereas 70 such injuries occurred in the control group. The study group had an incidence of 0.15 injuries per team/season, whereas the control group had an incidence of 1.15 injuries per team/season. This study has clearly demonstrated that some form of proprioceptive training can substantially decrease the incidence of ACL injury in an athletic population.

Hewett and colleagues[28] prospectively evaluated the effectiveness of preventive neuromuscular training on the incidence of knee injury in female athletes. Their study followed two separate groups of female athletes and one group of male athletes; one group consisted of 366 female athletes who participated in their neuromuscular training program while the second group of 463 female athletes were not trained in the program. In addition, a group of 434 untrained male athletes participated in the study. Hewett and colleagues' program was presented to the training groups by certified athletic trainers and physical therapists. The program consisted of a 6-week preseason training program, which incorporated various aspects including flexibility, plyometrics, and weight training in an attempt to increase muscle strength and decrease landing forces.[28] These training sessions typically lasted from 60 to 90 minutes per day, 3 days a week, on alternating days. This training program consisted of three distinct phases: (1) the technique phase, (2) the fundamentals phase, and (3) the performance phase (Table 17-2).

The technique phase is the first phase in which athletes were trained. During this phase, athletes were instructed in proper jump technique through the use of physical drills and demonstration of proper technique. In this initial phase, all the jumping techniques were done in a double-leg fashion. The second phase was the fundamentals phase, in which the main emphasis was on building a base of strength, power, and agility through various lower extremity exercises. During this phase, several single-leg hopping exercises were incorporated into the progression. The final phase was the performance phase, in which focus was placed on achieving maximal vertical jump height. This phase incorporated more strenuous exercises such as bounding and single-leg hopping for maximal distance. Following each session of jump training, a weight training program was performed consisting of various exercises for the trunk and both upper and lower extremities.

All 1263 athletes were monitored throughout their respective seasons, and results were impressive. It was found that the untrained female group demonstrated a significantly higher incidence of injury than either the trained females or the untrained males. There was, however, no significant difference in injury rates between the trained females and the untrained males. When comparing total number of athlete-exposures, the incidence of all knee injuries in the untrained group was 0.43; however, the incidence was significantly lower in the trained female group at 0.12. Surprisingly, the incidence in untrained males was even lower than in the trained females at 0.09. Stated in simpler terms, the untrained female group demonstrated an injury rate 3.6 times higher than the trained female group and 4.8 times higher than the male control group. The trained female group showed an injury incidence of only 1.3 times higher than the male control group.

Hewett and colleagues[28] acknowledge several limitations to their study. Although their study was prospective in nature, it was not randomized or double-blinded. In addition, equal numbers of sports participants were not observed, and subjects were also not randomly placed into trained and untrained groups. However, the sheer number of subjects involved should allow making generalizations to the athletic female population regarding the outcomes of their study. Although it appears hard to ascertain whether the decrease in serious knee injury in the trained female group was due to improvements in technique or from improved strength, most would agree that preventive neuromuscular training is beneficial for the female athlete.

Recently Mandelbaum and associates[29] followed 14- to 18-year-old female soccer players in an attempt to determine the effectiveness of implementing a neuromuscular and proprioceptive sport-specific (soccer) training program to reduce the incidence of ACL injuries. The Prevent Injury, Enhance Performance ACL Prevention Program (PEP program) addresses both biomechanical risk factors and increasing kinesthetic awareness and includes various stretching, strengthening, proprioceptive, and sport-specific drills. Each participating team was mailed a training video, which emphasized proper landing technique with emphasis on "soft landing" and landing with a bent knee, similar to the bent-knee landing drills developed by Henning.

In the first year following inception of the PEP program, only four ACL tears were reported in the intervention group with an incidence rate of 0.2 per 1000 athletes. The control group incurred a total of 32 ACL tears for an incidence rate of 1.7 ACL injuries per 1000 athletes. In the second year four ACL tears were reported in the study group for an incidence of 0.47 injuries per 1000, and the control group incurred 35, equating to 1.8 per 1000.

Myklebust and colleagues[3] have proven it is possible to prophylactically prevent anterior cruciate injuries through specific neuromuscular training drills. Their study examined the effect that a neuromuscular training regimen had on preventing ACL injuries in female team handball players. They followed female team handball players for three seasons (one control season followed by two intervention seasons). They had subjects perform a five-phase program consisting of three different balance exercises, which focused on neuromuscular control and planting and landing skills. (See Box 17-1 for an outline of exercises used in this study.) During the control season, the ACL injury incidence was 0.14 per 1000 playing hours, compared with 0.13 the first intervention season and 0.09 the second season.

Therefore strong evidence suggests that any number of neuromuscular training programs can help significantly lower the risk for ACL injury. The exact reasons for this decreased risk may be multifactorial and include development of neuromuscular control via strengthening exercises, plyometrics, and proprioceptive drills, which enhance the functional biomechanical deficits that are demonstrated by many at-risk athletes. No prospective studies have been performed comparing the various neuromuscular training programs to determine superiority. A summary of the various neuromuscular control programs is listed in Table 17-3.

TABLE 17-2

Hewett and colleagues[28,48] Jump Training Program

	DURATION OR REPETITIONS BY WEEK	
EXERCISE	WEEK 1	WEEK 2
Phase I: Technique		
1. Wall jumps	20 sec	25 sec
2. Tuck jumps*	20 sec	25 sec
3. Broad jumps, stick (hold) landing	5 reps	10 reps
4. Squat jumps*	10 sec	15 sec
5. Double-leg cone jumps*	2 × 30 sec	2 × 30 sec (side/side and back/front)
6. 180-degree jumps	20 sec	25 sec
7. Bounding in place	20 sec	25 sec
Phase II: Fundamentals	WEEK 3	WEEK 4
1. Wall jumps	30 sec	30 sec
2. Tuck jumps*	30 sec	30 sec
3. Jump, jump, jump, vertical jump	5 reps	5 reps
4. Squat jumps*	20 sec	20 sec
5. Bounding for distance	1 run	2 runs
6. Double-leg cone jumps*	2 × 30 sec	2 × 30 sec (side/side and back/front)
7. Scissors jump	30 sec	30 sec
8. Hip, hop, stick landing*	5 reps/leg	5 reps/leg
Phase III: Performance	WEEK 5	WEEK 6
1. Wall jumps	30 sec	30 sec
2. Step, jump up, down, vertical	5 reps	10 reps
3. Mattress jumps	2 × 30 sec	2 × 30 sec
4. Single-leg jumps, distance*	5 reps/leg	5 reps/leg
5. Squat jumps*	25 sec	25 sec
6. Jump into bounding*	3 runs	4 runs
7. Hop, hop, stick landing	5 reps/leg	5 reps/leg

From Hewett TE, Stroupe AL, Nance TA, et al: Plyometric training in female athletes. Decreased impact forces and increased hamstring torques, *Am J Sports Med* 24(6):765-773, 1996.
Note: Each jump exercise is followed by mandatory 30-second rest period.
Stretching (15-20 min), skipping (2 laps), side shuffle (2 laps) before beginning jumping exercises.
Posttraining: cool-down walk (2 min), stretching (5 min).
*Jumps performed on mats.

BOX 17-1

Myklebust and Colleagues[3] Anterior Cruciate Ligament Injury Prevention Program

Floor Exercises

Week 1: Running and planting, partner running backward and giving feedback on the quality of the movement; change position after 20 sec.

Week 2: Jumping exercise—right leg—right leg over to left leg—left leg and finishing with a two-foot landing with flexion in both hips and knees.

Week 3: Running and planting (as in week 1), now doing a full plant-and-cut movement with the ball, focusing on knee position.

Week 4: Two players together; two-leg jump forward and backward, 180-degree turn and the same movement backward; partner tries to push the player out of control but still focusing on landing technique.

Week 5: Expanding the movement from week 3 to a full plant and cut, then a jump shot with double-leg landing.

Mat Exercises

Week 1: Two players standing on one leg on the mat throwing to each other.

Week 2: Jump shot from a box (30-40 cm high) with a two-foot landing with flexion in hips and knees.

Week 3: Step-down exercise from box with one-leg landing with flexion in hip and knee.

Week 4: Two players both standing on balance mats trying to push partner out of balance, first on two legs, then on one leg.

Week 5: The players jump on a mat catching the ball, then take a 180-degree turn on the mat.

Wobble Board Exercises

Week 1: Two players standing two legged on the board throwing to each other.

Week 2: Squats on two legs, then on one leg.

Week 3: Two players throwing to each other, one foot on the board.

Week 4: One foot on the board, bounding the ball with their eyes shut.

Week 5: Two players, both standing on balance boards trying to push partner out of balance, first on two legs, then on one leg.

From Myklebust G, Engebretsen IH, Braekken A, et al: Prevention of anterior cruciate ligament injuries in female team handball players: a prospective intervention study over three seasons, *Clin J Sports Med* 13(2):71-78, 2003.

TABLE 17-3

Summary of Current Anterior Cruciate Ligament Injury Prevention Studies

STUDY	METHODS	PARTICIPANTS	INTERVENTION	OUTCOMES
Griffis ND, Vequist SW, Yearout KM[11]	Retrospective; tracked for 10 years	Female Division I collegiate level basketball players	ACL preventive program	87% decrease in ACL injuries following program
Caraffa et al[27]	Prospective controlled clinical trial; followed 3 years	600 male semiprofessional and amateur soccer players	20 teams participated in proprioceptive program; 20 teams normal program	Research group incidence, 0.15 injuries/team-season; control incidence, 1.15 continued
Hewett et al[28]	Prospective controlled clinical trial; followed 1 season	1263 subjects; 366 trained female subjects; 463 female control; 434 male control	6 week preseason neuromuscular training program	Research group incidence, 0.12 injuries/athlete exposure; untrained females, 0.49; untrained males, 0.09
Mandelbaum et al[29]	Prospective controlled clinical trial; followed 2 years	Female soccer players; numbers of subjects and controls varied each year	PEP neuromuscular training program	First year research group, 0.2/1000; untrained females, 1.7/1000
Myklebust et al[3]	Prospective controlled clinical trial: 1 year control; followed by 2 years' intervention	2647 female team handball players	Control season Balance exercises with focus on neuromuscular control, planting, and landing skills	Control season, 0.14/1000; first season, 0.13/1000; second season, 0.09/1000

DYNAMIC NEUROMUSCULAR ANALYSIS TRAINING

Rationale

Dynamic neuromuscular analysis (DNA) training is a synthesis of the most important findings derived from existing research studies and prevention techniques described earlier in this chapter. DNA training can be broken down into three basic philosophies and four components. DNA training is defined as that which incorporates dynamic sport-specific movement skills, neuromuscular patterning based on the identification of underlying neuromuscular imbalances and biomechanical analysis by the instructor, and feedback to the athlete both during and following training.

Dynamic neuromuscular analysis training should address the neuromuscular imbalances present in the population to be trained. Special attention should be given to the female athlete, because she may display one or more dynamic neuromuscular imbalances. Dynamic movements that are a challenge to the proprioceptive system are a required component of this type of training. The exercises selected must challenge the dynamic joint restraints (muscle-tendon units) that maintain limb and joint position in response to changing loads. Dynamic sport-specific training should provide the athlete with an effective means for facilitating the desired adaptations to the proprioceptive function of the knee joint. The dynamic component progresses the female athlete to high-risk, sport-specific maneuvers that can be performed in a safe and controlled manner. A properly trained athlete is prepared to handle the high joint forces generated during athletic competition in order to reduce the risk of injury and prepare the athlete to achieve peak levels of performance.

The neuromuscular component of DNA training is a balance between challenging the proprioceptive abilities of the athlete and exposing the athlete to movement patterns that generate greater dynamic knee control. This type of proprioceptive stress may aid the development of spinal reflexes that more quickly and effectively stabilize the joint than the voluntary muscular movements, which require an afferent-efferent pathway along with cerebral input. The voluntary muscle response is too slow to manage the ground reaction forces from the high-risk maneuvers encountered during competitive play. As the neuromuscular system develops and adapts to neuromuscular training, reflexive multijoint neuromuscular engrams may be created that employ joint stabilization patterns which control acceleration and deceleration forces on the knee. The enhanced neuromuscular control gained through DNA training can protect the athlete from the ground reaction forces that will be encountered in competitive play when jumping, landing, and cutting.

The analysis component of DNA training involves exercises that provide the instructor with the tools to analyze imperfections in technique.

Progression from double-leg to single-leg power maneuvers is a requirement for correcting dominant leg imbalances. In addition, the incorporation of multiplanar movements that equally recruit both lower extremities for optimal performance is necessary. More complex movement patterns require greater synchronization and coordination in side-to-side performance, which leads to greater balance in side-to-side muscle recruitment and equalization of leg-to-leg coordination and power.

Hewett and colleagues[28] demonstrated that female athletes who underwent a neuromuscular training program demonstrated greater dynamic knee stability than females who had not undergone training. The hypothesis was that female athletes who underwent a neuromuscular training program would demonstrate greater dynamic and passive knee stability than nontrained athletes. They also conducted an epidemiology study with the purpose to prospectively evaluate the effect of neuromuscular training on serious knee injury rates in female athletes.[28]

Preseason screening questionnaires were administered to high school soccer and volleyball athletes. A group of the female athletes underwent a 6-week preseason neuromuscular training program proven to decrease landing forces and increase hamstrings power.[5] Certified athletic trainers submitted weekly team and individual injury reports during the 3-month sports season. The incidence of serious knee injury was 0.43 in untrained females, 0.12 in trained females, and 0.09 in males (injuries per 1000 exposures). Chi-square analysis indicated a significant effect of training on group injury rates ($p = 0.02$). Untrained females had a significantly higher incidence of serious knee injury than trained females ($p = 0.05$) and males ($p = 0.03$). Trained females were not different than untrained males ($p = 0.86$). Training resulted in even greater differences in noncontact ACL injuries between the female groups ($p = 0.01$). These results indicate that neuromuscular training decreases injury risk in female athletes. High landing forces and imbalances in hamstrings and quadriceps strength and recruitment patterns may predispose the female athlete to knee injury. The results also demonstrate the higher incidence of serious knee injury in a female high school athletic population relative to a male population. The mechanism of decreased injury in trained athletes may be increased dynamic stability of the knee joint following training.

This is the first prospective study to report the effects of neuromuscular training on knee injury in the high-risk female sports population. Nontrained female athletes are at higher risk of knee ligament injuries. The study is ongoing, yet these results suggest that preventive measures such as neuromuscular training should be taken with the female athlete in order to decrease the incidence of serious knee injury in this high-risk population.

The training focus should be on perfecting the technique of each training exercise, especially early in the training cycle. If the athlete is allowed to perform the exercise maneuvers improperly, the training will reinforce improper techniques. The trainer should give continuous and immediate feedback to the athlete both during and after each exercise bout.

The trainer should be skilled in recognizing the desired technique for a given exercise, and should learn to encourage the athlete to maintain perfect technique for as long as possible. If the athlete fatigues to a point that she can no longer perform the exercise perfectly and displays a sharp decline in proficiency, the athlete should be instructed to stop training for that exercise session. The duration of each completed exercise should be noted, and the goal of the next training session must be to continue to improve technique and to increase volume (number of repetitions). The goal of increasing the quantity of exercises while maintaining the quality of exercises is critical in achieving good results.

The recent data from several different groups such as Henning and colleagues,[11] Myklebust and colleagues,[3] Caraffa and colleagues,[27] Hewett and colleagues,[28] and Mandelbaum and colleagues[29] strongly suggest that preventive measures such as DNA training should be taken with female athletes in order to decrease the incidence of ACL injury in this high-risk population. Although the benefit of injury prevention training is evident among a wide variety of athletes, it would appear that those demonstrating poor dynamic knee stability might benefit to a greater extent from DNA training. The next logical step in injury prevention is to develop methods to further identify athletes who might be at greater risk of injury. The goal of this approach is to calculate injury risk associated with an athlete playing a particular sport. Recent advances in technology and epidemiology have brought injury screening and prediction of injury risk closer to reality, especially for noncontact ACL injuries. For example, kinematic (motion) and kinetic (force) measurement systems are available to measure complex sports movements with highly repeatable precision.

The examination of high-force sports movements that simulate high-risk athletic maneuvers in a controlled laboratory can lead to significant advances in the field of injury risk prediction. Prospective examination of large numbers of athletes, using protocols that incorporate repeatable measurements coupled with systematic tracking of ACL injuries, should allow the accurate prediction of injury risk in the athletic population. With this type of predictive information, athletes can be better identified in order to complete an injury prevention program and help reduce the risk of injury.

The neuromuscular imbalances observed in female athletes give us a framework for identifying individuals at increased risk of ACL injury. Evaluation of an athlete's pre-injury assessment may demonstrate characteristics that may put her into an identifiable injury risk profile. An athlete may display scores that put her at risk in one, two, or all three of the aforementioned dynamic neuromuscular imbalances. First, ligament dominance can be tested using a box drop combined with a maximum effort vertical leap. The parameter of valgus moment (torque) at the knee can be measured, if a laboratory kinetic measurement system is available. Values

greater than 100 mm of total knee displacement at landing or 40 Newton-meters on the involved leg, respectively, may prove indicative of ligament dominance.[46] Simultaneous measures of ground reaction force at landing from the box drop (in multiples of body weight) may also give indications of ligament dominance. We have previously noted the correlation of peak landing force with valgus moments.[41] The peak landing force and the valgus moment values displayed by an athlete following a volleyball block above the mean plus 1 standard deviation values reported in our 1996 study may be predictive of ligament dominance.[41] Peak forces greater than five times body weight and valgus moments greater than 6% of body weight times height may be predictive of higher injury risk. A valgus knee displacement measurement greater than 100 mm would put the athlete in the lower percentiles of all athletes in respect to their ability to control total knee displacement when landing from a jump.

Athletes can also be screened for indicators of quadriceps dominance using relatively common measurement techniques, such as isokinetic dynamometry or perhaps even simple leg curl and leg extension machines. If the athlete exhibits a high level of quadriceps strength, a low level of hamstring strength, or a low hamstring to quadriceps ratio in one or both limbs, quadriceps dominance is likely present. Hamstring to quadriceps peak torque ratios of less than 55% may be indicative of increased injury risk. More sophisticated measurements of this imbalance can be attained through kinetic analysis of knee flexor-extensor torques during high-force sports movements. Extensor to flexor ratios greater than 2:1 may indicate that DNA training is required.

Dominant leg imbalance can also be assessed using a dynamometer or a leg curl and leg extension machine. A difference in strength or power of 20% or more between limbs is indicative of a neuromuscular imbalance that may underlie significant injury risk. Another test representative of bilateral imbalances between limbs is a measure of the athlete's ability to perform a single-leg balanced stance on an unbalanced platform that can objectively quantitate postural sway (i.e., a stabilometer). An athlete who is significantly more unstable on one side using dynamic stabilometry measures may also be at greater risk of ACL injury.

Although imbalances observed in any one of these measures alone may not pinpoint an athlete with a high-risk profile, a risk profile that incorporates measures from two or three dynamic neuromuscular imbalances might identify the athlete as high risk. Identification of these imbalances will assist the clinician and researcher to intervene with athletes in need of DNA training.

Dynamic Neuromuscular Analysis Training Protocol

The neuromuscular training program outlined in the following paragraphs uses the DNA training principles and is a synthesis of findings derived from published research studies and prevention techniques.[2,22,28,47-52] The four components of the dynamic neuromuscular training protocol are (1) plyometrics and movement training, (2) core strengthening, (3) balance training, and (4) resistance training. Each component of the training focuses on constant biomechanical analysis by the instructor with feedback given to the athlete both during and following training. The training protocol stresses technique perfection for each exercise. The trainers should be able to recognize the desired techniques for a given exercise and should encourage the athletes to maintain proper technique throughout each exercise. When the athlete fatigues to a point that she cannot perform the exercise with near-perfect technique, the exercise should be stopped. The duration and repetitions completed should be recorded by the athlete. The goal of the next training session should be to continue to improve technique, while increasing duration, volume, or intensity of the exercise (i.e., the training sessions must be progressive in nature). The progressive nature of the neuromuscular training is extremely important for achieving successful outcomes from the training. The neuromuscular training should stress performance of athletic maneuvers in a powerful, efficient, and safe manner.

The training protocol should be conducted 3 days per week. Each training session should last approximately 60 to 90 minutes. Before each training session an active warm-up should include jogging, backward running, lateral shuffling, and carioca. Each day of the week, training should include a 20-minute plyometric station, a 20- to 30-minute strength station, and a 20- to 30-minute core strengthening and balance station. At the end of each training session the athletes may perform self-selected stretching exercises for 15 minutes. The training period should be a minimum of 6 weeks in duration.

The plyometrics and dynamic movement training component should progressively emphasize double-leg and then single-leg movements.[41] The majority of the initial exercises should involve both legs to safely introduce the athletes to the training movements. Early training emphasis should be on sound athletic positioning to create dynamic control of the athlete's center of gravity.[3] Soft, athletic landings that stress deep knee flexion are used with verbal feedback to make the athlete aware of biomechanically unsound and undesirable positions. Progressively, a greater number of single-leg movements are introduced, while the focus on correct technique is maintained (Figure 17-3). For example, the single-leg crossover hop-and-hold exercise is used to teach single-leg landings (Figure 17-4). Later training sessions use explosive double- and single-leg movements that focus on maximal effort in multiple planes of movement (Table 17-4). The volume of the initial plyometric bouts should be low because of extensive technique training that is required due to the athlete's decreased ability to perform the exercise with proper technique for the given durations. Volume should be increased as technique improves to the midpoint of training, after which a progressive decrease in volume is followed for the final sessions to allow for increased training intensity.[41]

An important component of the final progressions of the plyometric and movement training is unanticipated cutting movements (Figure 17-5). Single-faceted sagittal plane training and conditioning protocols that do not incorporate cutting maneuvers will not provide similarly challenging levels of external varus/valgus or rotational loads to those seen during

TABLE 17-4

Example of Plyometrics and Movement Training Component from One Session

EXERCISE	SETS	TIME/REPETITIONS
Wall jumps (ankle bounces)	1	15 sec
Squat jumps (frog jumps)	1	10 sec
Tuck jump (with abdominal crunch)	1	10 sec
Barrier jumps (front to back) speed	1	15 sec
Barrier jumps (side to side) speed	1	15 sec
Crossover hop, hop, hop-stick (right-left)	1	6 reps
180-degree jumps (speed)	1	15 sec
Broad jump, jump, jump, vertical	1	6 reps
Jump into bounding	1	6 reps
Forward barrier hops with staggered box	1	6 reps
Lateral barrier hops with staggered box	1	6 reps
Box depth-180 degrees-box depth-max vertical	1	8 reps
180-degree jumps stick landing—unstable surface	1	15 reps

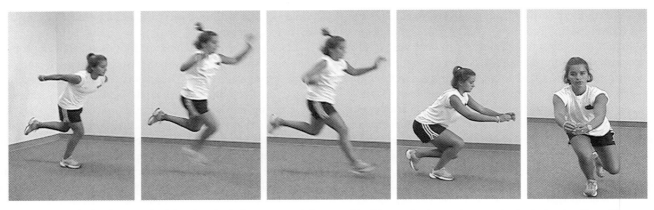

Figure 17-3: Single-leg hop and stick. The single-leg crossover hop-and-hold exercise is used to teach single-leg landings. The athlete focuses on technique with deep knee flexion and holding the position for approximately 3 to 5 seconds.

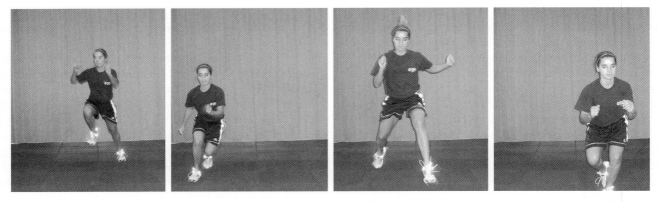

Figure 17-4: Crossover hop. In this exercise the athlete starts on a single limb and jumps at a diagonal across the body, lands on the opposite limb with the foot pointing straight ahead, and immediately redirects the jump in the opposite diagonal direction. Train this jump with care to protect your athlete from injury.

sport-specific cutting maneuvers.[53] Training that incorporates safe levels of varus/valgus stress may induce more "muscle dominant" neuromuscular adaptations.[54] Such adaptations can better prepare an athlete for more multidirectional sport activities, which can improve the athlete's performance and reduce risk of lower extremity injury.[28,41,55] Female athletes perform cutting techniques with increased valgus angles.[56] Knee valgus loads can double when performing unanticipated cutting maneuvers similar to those used in sport.[57] The end point of the training should be designed to reduce ACL loading via valgus torque reduction that may be gained through training the athlete to use movement techniques that produce low abduction knee joint torques.[54] Additionally, by improving reaction times to provide more time to voluntarily precontract the lower extremity musculature and make appropriate kinematic adjustments, ACL loads may be reduced during athletic maneuvers.[57,58]

Before teaching unanticipated cutting, female athletes should be taught to attain proper athletic position (Figure 17-6). The athletic position is a functionally stable position with the knees comfortably flexed, shoulders back, eyes up, feet approximately shoulder width apart, and the body mass

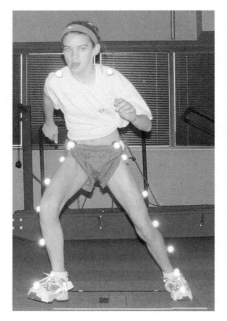

Figure 17-5: Unanticipated cutting maneuver. Unanticipated cutting is an advanced exercise that demonstrates single-limb stance support. One of the final progressions of plyometric and movement training is unanticipated cutting movements.

balanced over the balls of the feet. The knees should be over the balls of the feet and the chest should be over the knees.[41] This athlete-ready position is the starting and finishing position for the majority of the training exercises. This is also goal position before initiating a directional cut. Adding the directional cues to the unanticipated part of training can be done with the trainer pointing out a direction using partner mimic or ball retrieval drills. The goal of this component of the training is to teach the female athlete to employ safe cutting techniques in unanticipated sport situations that might generate adaptations in technique that will more readily transfer onto the field of play.

The resistance training component of a protocol should progress from high-volume, low-intensity to low-volume, high-intensity training. The initial training intensity may be set at approximately 60% of the athlete's predicted 1 repetition maximum. Exercise order can then also be progressed from multijoint exercises to alternating upper and lower body exercises (Table 17-5). Trainers should prescribe the weight to be employed before each training session, and athletes should record the number of repetitions achieved after each completed set. The weight is increased before each training session if the required number of repetitions is achieved. If technique is not near perfect, weight is lowered until proper technique is restored. The assisted Russian hamstring curl can be an important exercise included in training to focus on correction of quadriceps dominance or the low hamstring strength levels common to female athletes.[41,59] Figure 17-7 shows the trainer-assisted performance of this technique. The goal of the resistance training component of the protocol is to strengthen all major muscle groups through the com-plete range of motion and to provide complementary muscular strength and power to the plyometric component of the protocol.

The core strengthening and balance training components of the protocol (Table 17-6) should follow an organized exercise selection specifically directed at strengthening the core stabilizing muscles. This component focuses on an appropriate balance between developing the proprioceptive abilities of the athlete and exposing the athlete to inadequate joint control. The training progressions should take the athlete through a combination of low-risk to higher-risk maneuvers in a controlled situation. The intensity of the exercises should be modified by changing the arm position, opening and closing eyes, changing support stance, increasing or decreasing surface stability with balance training devices (Figure 17-8), increasing or decreasing speed, adding unanticipated movements or perturbations, and adding sport-specific skills. The goal of the functional balance training and core strengthening should be to bring the athlete to a level of core stability and coordination that allows her to properly reduce force, maintain balance and posture, and subsequently regenerate force in the desired direction.

SUMMARY

Multiple factors may underlie the gender difference in ACL injury rates. These include anatomic, hormonal, and neuromuscular factors. Perhaps serendipitously, the neuromuscular factors, which are the most modifiable, may also be the most important. Recent evidence demonstrates that neuromuscular training can bring female ACL injury rates down to near-male levels. This strongly suggests that neuromuscular control plays a major role in the mechanism underlying the difference in males and females. Females demonstrate

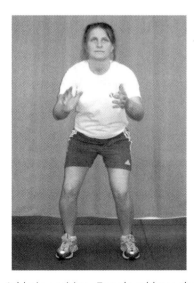

Figure 17-6: Athletic position. Female athletes should be taught to attain proper athletic position. The athletic position is a functionally stable position with the knees comfortably flexed, shoulders back, eyes up, feet approximately shoulder width apart, and the body mass balanced over the balls of the feet.

TABLE 17-5

Example of Resistance Training Component from One Session

EXERCISE	SETS	REPETITIONS
Dumbbell hang snatch	2	8
Squat	2	8
Bench press	2	8
Leg curl	2	8
Shoulder press	2	8
Lat pulldown	2	8
Assisted Russian hamstring curls*	2	15
Back fly	2	12
Bicep circuit	1	12
Ankle: plantar-dorsi	1	12

*The assisted Russian hamstring curl is depicted in Figure 17-7.

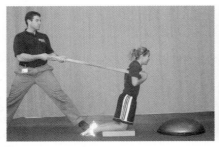
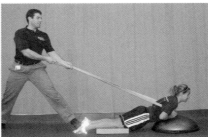
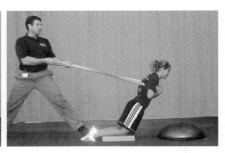

Figure 17-7: Assisted Russian hamstring curl. In this exercise the trainer anchors the athlete by standing on the athlete's feet and provides lift assistance with a strap that is attached around the chest. The Russian hamstring curl can be an important exercise included in training to focus on correction of quadriceps dominance or the low hamstring strength levels common to female athletes. Figure shows the trainer-assisted performance of this technique. Athlete performs full eccentric and concentric movement with the assistance of the trainer.

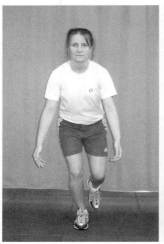
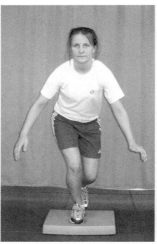
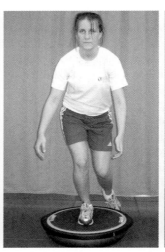
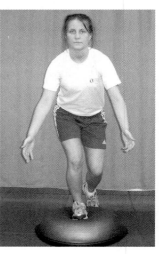

Figure 17-8: Support variations. Increasing or decreasing surface stability with balance training device. A pictorial display of different support stances on unstable surfaces that are used in core strengthening and balance training.

TABLE 17-6

Example of Core Strengthening and Balance Training Component from One Session

EXERCISE	SETS	TIME/REPETITIONS
Broad jump—stick landing	1	4 reps
Crossover hop-stick	1	12 reps
Single-leg X hop	1	5 reps
Box drop medicine ball catch	1	8 reps
180-degree jumps, stick landing—medicine ball catch	1	6 reps
BOSU double-leg perturbations	2	20 sec
BOSU both knees deep hold—medicine ball catch	2	20 reps
BOSU double-leg pick	1	10 reps
BOSU single-leg deep hold	2	20 sec
BOSU crunches	1	55 sec
Double crunch	2	25 reps
BOSU V—sit—toe touches	1	15 reps
BOSU swivel crunch (feet up)	2	30 reps
BOSU superman (right-left)	1	20 reps

dynamic neuromuscular imbalances that can be readily observed in the laboratory. These imbalances include ligament dominance, quadriceps dominance, and dominant leg dominance. Multicomponent DNA training can be used to specifically address and correct these neuromuscular imbalances in female athletes. Correction of neuromuscular imbalances is important for both optimal biomechanics of athletic movements and reduction of ACL injury incidence. Further study on the effects of neuromuscular retraining on ACL injury incidence and on biomechanical performance is important for the advancement of injury prevention initiatives and women's athletics.

References

1. Johnson R: Prevention of cruciate ligament injuries. In Feagin JJ, editor: *The crucial ligaments: diagnosis and treatment of ligamentous injuries about knee,* New York, 1988, Churchill Livingstone.

2. Griffin LY, Angel MJ, Albohm EA, et al: Noncontact anterior cruciate ligament injuries: risk factors and prevention strategies, *J Am Acad Orthop Surg* 8(3):141-150, 2000.

3. Myklebust G, Engebretsen IH, Braekken A, et al: Prevention of anterior cruciate ligament injuries in female team handball players: a prospective intervention study over three seasons, *Clin J Sports Med* 13(2):71-78, 2003.

4. von Porat A, Roos EM, Roos H: High prevalence of osteoarthritis 14 years after an anterior cruciate ligament tear in male soccer players: a study of radiographic and patient relevant outcomes, *Ann Rheum Dis* 63(3):269-273, 2004.

5. McNair PJ, Marshall RN, Matheson JA: Important features associated with acute anterior cruciate ligament injury, *N Z Med J* 103(901):537-539, 1990.

6. Boden BP, Garrett WE: Mechanisms of injuries to the anterior cruciate ligament, *Med Sci Sports Exerc* 28(5S):156, 1996 (abstract).

7. Arendt E, Dick R: Knee injury patterns among men and women in collegiate basketball and soccer. NCAA data and review of literature, *Am J Sports Med* 23(6):694-701, 1995.

8. Pearl AJ: American Orthopaedic Society for Sports Medicine: The athletic female. In *The athletic female,* Champaign, IL, 1993, Human Kinetics.

9. Uhorchak JM, Scoville CR, Williams GN, et al: Risk factors associated with noncontact injury of the anterior cruciate ligament: a prospective four-year evaluation of 859 West Point cadets, *Am J Sports Med* 31(6):831-842, 2003.

10. Yu B, Kirkendall DT, Taft TN, et al: Lower extremity motor control–related and other risk factors for noncontact anterior cruciate ligament injuries, *Instr Course Lect* 51:315-324, 2002.

11. Griffis ND, Vequist SW, Yearout KM: Injury prevention of the anterior cruciate ligament. In *AOSSM 15th annual meeting,* Traverse City, MI, 1989, American Orthopaedic Society for Sports Medicine.

12. Teitz CC: Unpublished data, 1999.

13. Magee DJ: *Orthopedic physical assessment,* Philadelphia, 1987, WB Saunders.

14. Shambaugh JP, Klein A, Herbert JH: Structural measures as predictors of injury in basketball players, *Med Sci Sports Exerc* 23(5):522-527, 1991.

15. Huston LJ, Greenfield ML, Wojtys EM: Anterior cruciate ligament injuries in the female athlete. Potential risk factors, *Clin Orthop* 372:50-63, 2000.

16. Norwood LA Jr, Cross MJ: The intercondylar shelf and the anterior cruciate ligament, *Am J Sports Med* 5(4):171-176, 1977.

17. Shelbourne K, Davis T, Klootwyk T: The relationship between intercondylar notch width of the femur and the incidence of anterior cruciate ligament tears, *Am J Sports Med* 26:402-408, 1998.

18. Houseworth SW, Mauro VJ, Mellon BA, et al: The intercondylar notch in acute tears of the anterior cruciate ligament: a computer graphics study, *Am J Sports Med* 15(3):221-224, 1987.

19. Lund-Hanssen H, Gannon J, Engebretsen L, et al: Intercondylar notch width and the risk for anterior cruciate ligament rupture. A case-control study in 46 female handball players, *Acta Orthop Scand* 65(5):529-532, 1994.

20. Schickendantz MS, Weiker GG: The predictive value of radiographs in the evaluation of unilateral and bilateral anterior cruciate ligament injuries, *Am J Sports Med* 21(1):110-113, 1993.

21. Teitz CC, Lind BK, Sacks BM: Symmetry of the femoral notch width index, *Am J Sports Med* 25(5):687-690, 1997.

22. Souryal TO, Moore HA, Evans JP: Bilaterality in anterior cruciate ligament injuries: associated intercondylar notch stenosis, *Am J Sports Med* 16(5):449-454, 1988.

23. Rozzi S, Lephart SM, Gear WS, et al: Knee joint laxity characteristics of male and female soccer and basketball players, *Am J Sports Med* 27(3):312-319, 1999.

24. Nicholas JA: Injuries to knee ligaments. Relationship to looseness and tightness in football players, *JAMA* 212(13):2236-2239, 1970.

25. Grana WA, Moretz JA: Ligamentous laxity in secondary school athletes, *JAMA* 240(18):1975-1976, 1978.

26. Godshall RW: The predictability of athletic injuries: an eight-year study, *J Sports Med* 3(1):50-54, 1975.

27. Caraffa A, Cerulli G, Projetti M, et al: Prevention of anterior cruciate ligament injuries in soccer. A prospective controlled study of proprioceptive training, *Knee Surg Sports Traumatol Arthrosc* 4(1):19-21, 1996.

28. Hewett TE, Lindenfeld TA, Riccobene JV, et al: The effect of neuromuscular training on the incidence of knee injury in female athletes. A prospective study, *Am J Sports Med* 27(6):699-706, 1999.

29. Mandelbaum BR, Silvers HJ, Watanabe DS, et al: Effectiveness of a neuromuscular and proprioceptive training program in preventing the incidence of ACL injuries in female athletes: a two-year follow-up, *Am J Sports Med* 33(7):1003-1010.

30. Frankovich RJ, Lebrun CM: Menstrual cycle, contraception, and performance, *Clin Sports Med* 19(2):251-271, 2000.

31. Sarwar R, Beltran NB, Rutherford OM: Changes in muscle strength, relaxation rate and fatigability during the human menstrual cycle, *J Physiol* 493(1):267-272, 1996.

32. Wojtys EM, Huston LJ, Lindenfeld TN, et al: Association between the menstrual cycle and anterior cruciate ligament injuries in female athletes, *Am J Sports Med* 26(5):614-619, 1998.

33. Liu SH, Al-Shaikh RA, Panossian V, et al: Primary immunolocalization of estrogen and progesterone target cells in the human anterior cruciate ligament, *J Orthop Res* 14(4):526-533, 1996.

34. Griffin JW, Tooms RE, VanderZwaag R, et al: Eccentric muscle performance of elbow and knee muscle groups in untrained men and women, *Med Sci Sports Exerc* 25(8):936-944, 1993.

35. Baratta R, Solomonow M, Zhou BH, et al: Muscular coactivation. The role of the antagonist musculature in maintaining knee stability, *Am J Sports Med* 16(2):113-122, 1988.

36. Huston LJ, Wojtys EM: Neuromuscular performance characteristics in elite female athletes, *Am J Sports Med* 24(4):427-436, 1996.

37. Ireland ML, Gaudette M, Crook S: ACL injuries in the female athlete, *J Sports Rehabil* 6:97-110, 1997.

38. Loudon JK, Jenkins W, Loudon KL: The relationship between static posture and ACL injury in female athletes, *J Orthop Sports Phys Ther* 24(2):91-97, 1996.

39. van Ingen Schenau GJ, Bobbert MF, Rozendal RH: The unique action of the biarticular muscles in explosive movements, *Int J Sports Med* 5:301-305, 1984.

40. Stacoff A, Kaelin X, Stuessi E: Impact in landing after a volleyball block. In de Groot G et al, editors: *Biomechanics XI,* Amsterdam, 1988, Free University Press.

41. Hewett TE, Stroupe AL, Nance TA, et al: Plyometric training in female athletes. Decreased impact forces and increased hamstring torques, *Am J Sports Med* 24(6):765-773, 1996.

42. Draganich LF, Vahey JW: An in vitro study of anterior cruciate ligament strain induced by quadriceps and hamstrings forces, *J Orthop Res* 8(1):57-63, 1990.

43. Hirokawa S, Solomonow M, Lu Y, et al: Anterior-posterior and rotational displacement of the tibia elicited by quadriceps contraction, *Am J Sports Med* 20(3):299-306, 1992.

44. Renstrom P, Arms SW, Stanwyck TS, et al: Strain within the anterior cruciate ligament during hamstring and quadriceps activity, *Am J Sports Med* 14(1):83-87, 1986.

45. Wilk KE, Escamilla RF, Fleisig GS, et al: A comparison of tibiofemoral joint forces and electromyographic activity during open and closed kinetic chain exercises, *Am J Sports Med* 24(4):518-527, 1996.

46. Hewett TE, Myer GD, Noyes FR: Identification of athletes with increased valgus knee displacement during landing: effects of gender and training. 26th Annual Meeting of the American Orthopaedic Society for Sports Medicine, 2000.

47. Lehnhard RA, Lehnhard HR, Young R, et al: Monitoring injuries on a college soccer team: the effect of strength training, *J Strength Cond Res* 10(2):115-119, 1996.

48. Heidt RS Jr, Sweeterman LM, Carlonas RL, et al: Avoidance of soccer injuries with preseason conditioning, *Am J Sports Med* 28(5):659-662, 2000.

49. Hejna WF, Rosenberg A, Buturusis D, et al: The prevention of sports injuries in high school students through strength training, *Natl Strength Coaches Assoc J* 4(1):28-31, 1982.

50. Kraemer WJ: A series of studies—the physiological basis for strength training in American football: fact over philosophy, *J Strength Cond Res* 11(3):131-142, 1997.

51. Kraemer WJ, Duncan ND, Volek JS: Resistance training and elite athletes: adaptations and program considerations, *J Orthop Sports Phys Ther* 28(2):110-119, 1998.

52. Kraemer WJ, Hakkinen K, Triplett-McBride NT, et al: Physiological changes with periodized resistance training in women tennis players, *Med Sci Sports Exerc* 35(1):157-168, 2003.

53. Lloyd DG, Buchanan TS: Strategies of muscular support of varus and valgus isometric loads at the human knee, *J Biomech* 34(10):1257-1267, 2001.

54. Lloyd DG: Rationale for training programs to reduce anterior cruciate ligament injuries in Australian football, *J Orthop Sports Phys Ther* 31(11):645-654, 661 (discussion), 2001.

55. Cahill BR, Griffith EH: Effect of preseason conditioning on the incidence and severity of high school football knee injuries, *Am J Sports Med* 6(4):180-184, 1978.

56. Malinzak RA, Colby SM, Kirkendall DT, et al: A comparison of knee joint motion patterns between men and women in selected athletic tasks, *Clin Biomech* 16(5):438-445, 2001.

57. Besier TF, Lloyd DG, Ackland TR, et al: Anticipatory effects on knee joint loading during running and cutting maneuvers, *Med Sci Sports Exerc* 33(7):1176-1181, 2001.

58. Neptune RR, Wright IC, van den Bogert AJ: Muscle coordination and function during cutting movements, *Med Sci Sports Exerc* 31(2):294-302, 1999.

59. Huston LJ, Wojtys EM: Neuromuscular performance characteristics in elite female athletes, *Am J Sports Med* 24(4):427-436, 1996.

CHAPTER 18

Meniscal Surgery Rehabilitation

Timothy F. Tyler, MS, PT, ATC
Stephen J. Nicholas, MD
Aruna M. Seneviratne, MD

CHAPTER OUTLINE

THE MENISCI ARE A PAIR OF FIBROCAR-

tilaginous semilunar-shaped discs that play a vital role in the normal functioning of the human knee. They serve an important function in load transmission, shock absorption, joint lubrication, and proprioception and also act as secondary restraints to anterior translation of the tibia. Given these important functions, meniscal surgery has evolved over the years from complete meniscectomy to partial meniscectomy to the modern era, in which meniscal repair and even meniscal allograft transplantations are being performed. This chapter covers the basics of the mechanisms of injury, clinical evaluation, treatment, modalities, and rehabilitation after meniscal surgery.

MENISCAL ANATOMY

Gross Anatomy

The menisci are semilunar-shaped discs of fibrocartilage, situated between the tibia and femur, in the medial and lateral compartments of the knee. They are attached to the tibia by the coronary ligaments and by direct insertion of the anterior and posterior horns into the bone. The horn insertion of the menisci into the tibia is adapted to transmit sheer and tensile loads from the menisci to the tibia.[1] The menisci also attach to the joint capsule. The medial meniscus attaches to the deep layer of the medial collateral ligament, and the lateral meniscus attaches loosely to the lateral capsule. The posterior horn of the lateral meniscus is attached to the medial femoral condyle via the meniscal femoral ligaments.[2] The capsule attachments of the medial meniscus are more secure than those of the lateral meniscus.[3]

Microscopic Anatomy

The meniscus contains fibrochondrocytes and fibroblasts. Fibrochondrocytes are predominantly concentrated in the deeper portion of the menisci and synthesize and maintain the extracellular matrix. Fibroblasts are located on the meniscal surface and produce important matrix proteins (collagen and proteoglycan) that facilitate load transmission across the knee joint. Interactions between collagen and glycosaminoglycan allow the meniscus to behave as a fiber-reinforced solid material, providing resistance to forces of tension, compression, and shearing.[4-6]

The principal meniscal collagen is Type I, although Types II, III, V, and VI are also present. Most of the collagen fibers are oriented circumferentially and provide resistance to "hoop stresses," which are generated during weight bearing. Radially oriented fibers on the meniscal surface help to hold the circumferential fibers together and provide resistance to shear stresses.[5,7]

Meniscal glycosaminoglycans are negatively charged molecules that trap water and provide resistance to compressive loading. Other noncollagenous glycoproteins (such as elastin, fibronectin, and thrombospondin) play an important role by

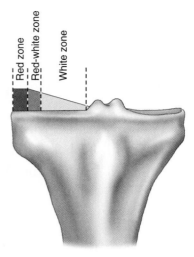

Figure 18-1: Various zones of the meniscus: red zone (peripheral 2 mm), excellent propensity to heal; red-white zone (peripheral 2 to 5 mm), good to excellent propensity to heal; white zone (>5 mm from periphery), poor healing potential. *(From Miller MD, Warner JJP, Harner CD: Meniscal repair. In Fu FH, Harner CD, Vince KG, editors: Knee surgery, Baltimore, 1994, Williams & Wilkins.)*

binding the matrix proteins together. In contrast to articular cartilage, the amount of proteoglycan is very small.[8]

The blood supply to the meniscus originates from the superior and inferior medial and lateral genicular arteries.[9] A perimeniscal capillary plexus is located in the capsular and synovial attachments of the menisci and penetrates 10% to 30% of the width of the medial meniscus and 10% to 25% of the lateral meniscus (Figure 18-1). In addition, a vascular synovial fringe extends 1 to 3 mm over the femoral and tibial surfaces peripherally. This synovial fringe does not contribute vessels to the meniscal substance but does help with healing.

Meniscal vascular anatomy can be described in terms of zones that provide important information about healing and help to determine management. The "red-red" zone is the peripheral third of the meniscus. This zone is highly vascular. A tear in this region has blood supply from both sides of the tear and does have a high potential for healing. The "red-white" zone is located in the meniscal midportion, or the central third. A tear in this region has blood supply from the outside or the peripheral aspect of the tear, but the inner aspect is avascular. The "white-white" zone is located on the inner or central aspect of the meniscus. A tear in this region is avascular on both sides of the tear and does not trigger a healing response. The site of the tear can easily be described by the surgeon using the grid created by Cooper and colleagues[10] illustrated in Figure 18-2. This information may be useful for a physical therapist trying to direct modalities at the healing meniscus or to gain knowledge of the tear site. In addition, it has been documented that the menisci are innervated, with most nerve fibers associated with blood

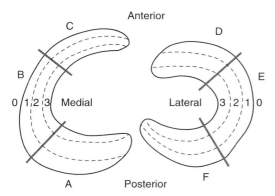

Figure 18-2: The meniscus is divided into different zones for classification of tears. *(From van Trommel MF, Simonian PT, Potter HG, Wickiewicz TL: Different regional healing rates with the outside-in technique for meniscal repair, Am J Sports Med 26:446-452, 1998.)*

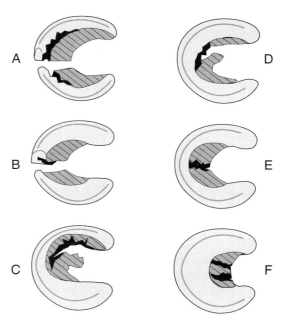

Figure 18-3: Common meniscal tear patterns, with recommended areas of excision shown by dotted lines. **A,** Bucket handle. **B,** Horizontal cleavage tear. **C,** Degenerative flap tear. **D,** Flap tear. **E,** Radial tear. **F,** Double radial tear of a discoid meniscus. *(From Scott WN, editor: Arthroscopy of the knee: diagnosis and treatment, Philadelphia, 1990, Saunders.)*

vessels. Nerve fibers and sensory receptors were found mainly in the peripheral, vascular zone, representing the outer one third of the meniscus, and the innervated area was wider in the anterior and posterior horns. Pacinian and Ruffini corpuscles as well as free nerve endings were identified in these areas. Larger fibers coursed circumferentially in the peripheral zone, with smaller branches of nerve fibers running radially into the meniscus. Research indicates that some of the pain in cases of meniscal tears could originate in the meniscus itself, especially with peripheral tears that may be accompanied by bleeding.[11]

Meniscal Function

The menisci serve several important functions. They facilitate load transmission across the tibiofemoral joint by improving the congruency of the articular surfaces and increasing the area of joint contact.[12] The medial meniscus transmits 50% of the load in the medial compartment, and the lateral meniscus transmits 70% of the load in the lateral compartment. They also act as important shock absorbers by virtue of their viscoelastic properties.[13] The medial meniscus also provides stability to the knee by acting as a secondary restraint to anterior tibial translation.[14,15] In addition, the menisci assist in joint lubrication and articular cartilage nutrition by maintaining a synovial fluid film over the articular surfaces compressing the synovial fluid into the articular cartilage. Nerve endings in the menisci are thought to provide proprioception input when stimulated by motion and deformation.

Mechanism of Injury

A combination of torsional and axial loading appears to underlie many meniscal injuries. If intrinsic degeneration of the meniscus is present, minimal trauma may cause tearing. Meniscal degeneration, as evidenced by an abnormal magnetic resonance imaging (MRI) signal, has been found in the asymptomatic contralateral knee of patients with a torn

meniscus.[16] This indicates that some patients who have meniscal degeneration are probably predisposed to meniscal tears. Meniscal injuries are common in the anterior cruciate ligament (ACL)–deficient knee, as a result of abnormal tibial translation.[17] Lateral meniscal injury is usually associated with an acute ACL tear, whereas medial meniscal tears occur more often in persons with chronic ACL insufficiency.[18,19]

Types of Tears

Acute meniscal tears are usually caused by trauma. Damage may take the form of vertical longitudinal tears, radial split tears, or flap tears (Figure 18-3). The often described bucket handle tear is a vertical longitudinal tear, with displacement of the inner meniscal segment (this is the handle fragment).

Vertical longitudinal tears tend to occur in an otherwise normal meniscus. Atraumatic horizontal cleavage, flap, and radial split tears are more common in older patients who have underlying meniscal degeneration. A combination of these injuries constitutes a complex meniscal tear.

Healing

The healing process begins with the formation of a fibrin clot, which acts as a scaffold for subsequent repair. Meniscal and synovial cells migrate into the fibrin clot, and vessels from the capillary plexus and vascular synovial fringe grow into the fibrin clot.[20] The lesions heal by formation of fibrovascular scar tissue, which in the canine model occurs by the tenth week.[20,21]

Several methods have been developed to enhance the healing response of the meniscus. These include application of an exogenous fibrin clot, abrasion of the synovial fringe to create a vascular pannus, placement of vascular channels or trephination to connect the tear to the vascular periphery, and the placement of pedicle synovial grafts over the meniscal tear.[22] In the future, application of cytokines and growth factors may have a role in augmenting healing.[6,23]

CLINICAL EVALUATION

Symptoms

Patients who sustain a traumatic tear may have mechanical symptoms of catching and/or locking. Pain and swelling, along with an effusion, may be present, with the pain being most noticeable when the knee is hyperflexed, such as when squatting. Some patients may have concomitant instability that is related to an associated ligamentous injury, such as an ACL disruption. Pain is more common than mechanical symptoms, as the presenting complaint in persons who have endured an atraumatic tear. A small effusion may also be present.[24]

Physical Examination

Signs suggestive of meniscal injury include joint line tenderness, a small effusion, clicking elicited by the combination of axial load plus rotational torque of the knee, and pain when the knee is flexed. During the physical examination, it is important to assess the axial alignment of the limp (by obtaining standing radiographs) as well as the stability of the ligaments. Other common potential sources of knee pain to rule out include intraarticular and extraarticular problems, such as arthrosis and tendopathy, respectively. The McMurray and Steinmann tests are the most commonly used clinical tests for meniscal pathology and have been described in Chapter 4.

Imaging

Radiographs

Plain radiographs should be the first films to be obtained. The standard series includes a standing (weight-bearing) anteroposterior view during extension, a lateral view, and a Merchant view. A standing posteroanterior view at 45 degrees of flexion demonstrates posterior compartment narrowing and is appropriate when the clinician suspects early joint degeneration. Standing radiographs from hip to ankle allow assessment of limb alignment. Examination of alignment is important, because atraumatic meniscal tears occur in knees with varus deformity, a configuration that increases stresses on the medial meniscus.[25]

Additional Imaging Studies

MRI is the gold standard for meniscal imaging. For greatest accuracy, multiplanar studies are obtained in the axial, sagittal, and coronal planes. MRI is not indicated if the results will not change the management of the injury and may not be useful if only conservative management is planned.[26]

Normal meniscal fibrocartilage has a low signal intensity on all pulse sequences. An abnormal signal and/or morphology indicates meniscal pathology. Areas of high signal intensity correlate with tears and/or intrinsic meniscal degeneration. Frequency-selective fat suppression techniques are useful for evaluating meniscal healing after repair and may be more accurate.[27,28]

In addition to showing meniscal tears, MRI demonstrates associated meniscal cysts and allows for assessment of adjacent articular cartilage, ligaments, and capsular attachments of the meniscus. MRI can also rule out lesions that simulate a meniscal tear—chondral injury or avascular necrosis, for example. Arthrography, with or without computed tomography (CT) scanning, is recommended for patients who cannot undergo MRI. Patients who have pacemakers or are claustrophobic are candidates for arthrography.[29,30]

MANAGEMENT

In general, management is based on the patient's symptoms, as well as age and functional expectations. Concomitant injuries, such as an ACL tear, need to be identified and may require treatment. It is important to rule out any associated arthritis, because a degenerative tear may occur in a knee that has articular cartilage degeneration. It may be difficult to distinguish the source of symptoms in an arthritic knee. Some tears that are noted during arthroscopy may not require treatment. These include vertical longitudinal tears, usually less than 1 cm long, that are stable to probing. A small radial split tear occurring at the posterior horn of the lateral meniscus and ACL-injured knees, partial thickness tears, and shallow radial tears less than 3 mm deep do not warrant any intervention.[31]

Nonoperative Tears

Indications for conservative management include absence of symptoms, horizontal cleavage (degenerative) tear in a knee with degeneration, and small separations in the meniscal capsular region (between the deep medial collateral ligament and the medial meniscus). Stable vertical longitudinal tears also appear to respond well to conservative treatment.[32] Radial tears are much less likely to heal with conservative intervention. The long-term implications of an unhealed radial tear are unknown.

Ice, moist heat, compression, wrapping, and nonsteroidal antiinflammatory drugs are cornerstones of nonoperative care. The best results are achieved when these are supplemented with physical therapy to improve range of motion

(ROM) and muscular strength. Injections of corticosteroids do not affect a tear and may even interfere with healing. The patient can be encouraged to gradually resume activities but should be careful to avoid cutting and pivoting maneuvers as well as knee hyperflexion for as long as symptoms are present. Complications of nonoperative treatment include progression of the tear and progressive joint degeneration, especially if there is significant loss of meniscal function.

Surgical Treatment

Absolute indications for surgery are tears that are displaced and occur in young patients. The fragment from a displaced tear, such as a bucket handle tear, can cause a locked knee or inability to achieve full extension. Relative indications for surgery include persistent symptoms, such as catching, locking, pain and swelling, and persistent problems after 6 to 12 weeks of conservative treatment.[33]

The goal of surgical intervention is to maximally preserve and stabilize the meniscus. Procedures available to restore meniscal function include partial meniscectomy, vascular stimulation to promote tear healing, meniscal repair, and meniscal replacement.[34] Open meniscectomy was the standard of care for meniscal tears for many years, beginning in the earlier part of the century. Fairbank reported that significant changes occur in the knee after meniscectomy.[35] Fairbank's changes include squaring of the condyles, osteophyte formation, and decreasing of the joint space. Despite Fairbank's findings, open complete meniscectomies were performed well into 1970s.[36] Partial meniscectomies (open technique) began to become popularized in the 1970s because of the realization of the consequences of total meniscectomy. Arthroscopic partial meniscectomies were popularized in the early 1980s and in the 1990s, and in the present day arthroscopic repairs have become popular. The first reported repair is credited to Anandale in 1885, when he performed an open meniscal repair. Given this evolution of meniscal surgery, the present day surgeon's armamentarium includes partial meniscectomy, meniscal repair, either with suture technique or with an implant, and meniscal transplantation.

Partial Meniscectomy

This approach is indicated for flap tears, radial tears in the inner or avascular area, and horizontal cleavage tears. During partial meniscectomy, the unstable, torn fragment is removed and the remaining tissue is resected, to promote stabilization. Meniscectomy can be achieved arthroscopically with cutting instruments, a motorized shaver, or an electrothermal device, such as a laser or radiofrequency probe. Studies demonstrate that results are satisfactory in 90% of knees without articular degeneration and in 60% to 70% of knees with concomitant degenerative joint disease.[37] Complications of partial meniscectomy include recurrent tearing (uncommon), injury to articular surface resulting from the use of rigid instruments,

and the risk of avascular necrosis of the underlying tibia (rare; occurs only with the use of electrothermal devices).[38]

Meniscal Repair

There are several techniques for meniscal repair. Taken broadly, there are two categories of repairs: suture repair and repair with an implant.

Suture Repair

There are two techniques for suture repair available to the present day surgeon: the outside-in technique, and the inside-out technique. A third, all-inside suture technique is possible now because of the development of a specialized implant; this technique is discussed in the section on the implant type of repair.

Outside-In Technique   The outside-in technique of arthroscopic meniscal repair was developed by Rodeo[39] and Warren[40] as a method to decrease the risk of injury to the peroneal nerve during arthroscopic lateral meniscal repair. Peroneal nerve injury is easily avoided during lateral meniscal repair by controlling the starting point for needle entry. The outside-in technique can be used for repair of most meniscal tears. Repairs in the anterior portion of the meniscus are easily accessed with this technique. In repairs of the posterior portion of the meniscus, it may be difficult to start far enough posteriorly, therefore resulting in oblique suture orientation across the tear. In this setting the inside-out technique with a posterior incision may be preferable.

The technique for outside-in repair requires only an 18-gauge spinal needle, an arthroscopic grasper, and suture material. Special instruments are also available, such as a K-cable loop for suture retrieval. To perform the outside-in meniscal repair, the knee is placed into approximately 10 degrees of flexion for a medial meniscal repair and 90 degrees of flexion for a lateral meniscal repair, to avoid peroneal nerve injury. While viewing the meniscus arthroscopically, the surgeon places the needle across the tear site from the outside. The starting point is located by palpation and by using topographic landmarks. Transillumination may also be used to identify small cutaneous nerves and veins. The needle passes across the tear in the meniscus and penetrates the inner segment of the meniscus. The needle then enters the joint on either the superior (femoral) or inferior (tibial) surface of the inner segment of the meniscus. A small skin incision is made, and the subcutaneous tissue is spread down to the capsule. It is important to identify and protect the saphenous nerve and vein on the medial side. A second needle is then passed, emerging from the meniscus, adjacent to the first needle, to achieve proper suture orientation. The second needle can be placed to create either a vertical or horizontal mattress across the tear. It is thought that a vertical suture orientation more effectively captures the circumferentially oriented collagen fibers of the meniscus. Usually #0 PDS suture is used for the repair. PDS suture is used because it is rigid enough to push through the needles. The suture is passed into each of the needles, grasped inside the joint, and pulled out of the anterior portal.

There are two ways to complete the repair. A knot may be made in the end of a suture, with three or four throws in a standard square knot fashion. The knot is then pulled back into the joint against the meniscus and maintains the tear in a reduced position. Adjacent sutures have been tied together subcutaneously over the capsule. An alternative way to complete the repair is to tie adjacent sutures together outside the anterior portal, using a standard square knot. The knot is then pulled through the meniscus, and adjacent sutures are tied together subcutaneously over the capsule. This technique allows creation of a mattress suture. This may be facilitated by placing a smaller dilator knot in front of the knot holder, holding the two ends together, then pulling the sutures so that the dilator knot passes through the meniscus before the larger knot. The dilator knot is a square knot made with only two throws. Another method for passing the suture after the needles are placed across the tear site is to pass a wire loop cable, place the suture through the other needle, then place the emerging suture into the wire loop. The suture has then been pulled through the meniscus, creating a horizontal mattress suture. The wire cable loop and cannulated needle are pulled out together, because the double suture may not easily fit into the 18-gauge spinal needle. The advantage of this method is that it eliminates the need to pull the sutures out through the anterior portal, where the sutures may entrap soft tissues unless a canula is used. This method also eliminates the need to pull the knot through the meniscus to make a mattress stitch.

It is also possible to use permanent, braided sutures with this technique. This is accomplished by passing a wire cable loop through the cannulated needle, then placing the end of the suture into the wire loop, using an arthroscopic grasper inserted through the anterior portal. The suture is then pulled through the meniscus, after which the process is repeated with the wire loop to pass the other end of the suture through the adjacent needle.

The use of permanent suture may be preferable for repair of tears with poor healing potential, such as those in older patients, chronic tears, or tears with marginal vascularity. The choice of permanent versus PDS suture for meniscal repair has been an area of debate. Barret and colleagues demonstrated that meniscus repair with permanent suture had a low incidence of clinical symptoms and a much lower failure rate.[41] This is thought to be because permanent sutures work for longer and more stable fixation, permitting more complete maturation and remodeling of the healing meniscus. PDS sutures have the longest reabsorption time and are rigid enough to push easily through the spinal needle.

The advantage of the outside-in technique is that sutures can be placed without the need for rigid cannulas for suture placement, as are used in many inside-out techniques.

Although there is a risk of causing minor damage to the articular surfaces when introducing needles from outside the joint, there is also risk of scraping the articular surface when using a rigid canula in the inside-out technique. The outside-in technique also allows precise suture placement in areas with limited access because only small needles are used instead of the larger cannulas or needle holders used in the inside-out technique. This can facilitate vertical suture placement. Except in very tight medial compartments, excellent visualization is possible, because there are no instruments between the meniscal tear and the arthroscopic view. Finally, the repair can be performed with small incisions, with less dissection than used with the inside-out technique.

There are very few reports of results of meniscal repair using the outside-in technique. Morgan and Casscells were the first to report the results of outside-in meniscal repair. They reported a 98% clinical healing rate, with a 2.8% complication rate with an 18-month follow up. Their evaluation was based on physical examination and symptoms only. This series included only acute tears in the outer third of the meniscus.[42] Mariani and co-workers reported good clinical results in 17 of 22 (77%) of patients undergoing outside-in repair of medial meniscal tears in conjunction with ACL reconstruction. These authors reported a 14% failure rate, using clinical criterion for meniscal retear. The authors reported that MRI demonstrated a gap larger than 1 mm at the repair site in those patients with clinical symptoms of meniscal retear.[43]

Nicholas and colleagues[44] used objective criteria to evaluate the outcome of outside-in meniscal repairs. Ninety patients were available for review, with a minimum follow up of 3 years. The patients were evaluated with physical examination, radiographs, and objective evaluation of the meniscus with CT arthrography, MRI, or arthroscopic inspection. Overall, 78 of 90 patients (87%) had a successful outcome. Twelve of the 90 patients (13%) had failure of healing. There was a significant difference in healing rate between patients with a stable knee and those with an ACL-deficient knee. The failure rate was 38% in unstable knees, 15% in stable knees, and only 5% in patients undergoing concomitant ACL reconstruction. (It is likely that hemarthrosis that occurs during ACL reconstruction provides factors that aid meniscal healing.)[44]

Inside-Out Technique The inside-out technique of meniscal repair was popularized by Henning in the early 1980s. This technique of repair uses double-armed sutures, with long flexible needles, which are placed into the meniscus arthroscopically and are directed by zone-specific cannulas. Medial or lateral incisions are required to retrieve the suture needles as they exit from the joint capsule. Appropriate positioning of the incisions and dissection down to the capsule are necessary to minimize risk of neurovascular injury. The advantage of this technique is that it provides excellent visualization for placement of the sutures very accurately, as well as the fact that this technique can be used for repair of menisci in any zone of the meniscus. The disadvantage is that it requires a large incision and there is a slightly increased risk of neurovascular injury. In general, the results are similar to those found using the outside-in technique.[45]

Meniscal Repair Using Implants

All-Inside Technique   The all-inside technique uses non-suture implants for the most part for performance of all inside meniscus repair. One particular implant that is currently available uses suture material. This implant is the FasT-Fix (Smith and Nephew, Inc. Memphis, TN). The other implants are usually a combination of polyester or polylactic acid implants. Their configuration varies from implants with hats to absorbable screws. In addition, there are also meniscal arrows, with barbs that prevent pull-out of the barb once inserted. Of all these implants, the FasT-Fix suture system affords the highest pull-out load, with a load failure of approximately 72 N.[46]

In general, for the all-inside technique the implant of choice is dependent on the surgeon's preference. All of these implants work quite well in the repair of menisci and have excellent track records.[47] The surgeon must be cognizant, however, of the potential for articular cartilage damage. Some of these implants tend to have a proud head once implanted, and this can lead to chondral injury. The results are similar to those obtained using the outside-in technique.

Meniscal Allograft Implantation

Currently meniscal allograft implantation (MAT) is an experimental, and for the most part a salvage, type of operation available for the completely meniscus-deficient knee. The ideal candidate for a meniscus allograft is a young, active individual with pain over a meniscus-deficient compartment. The general consensus is that the best results are obtained in a knee with little or no arthritic damage to the articular cartilage. Standing radiographs are important and should demonstrate acceptable limb alignment. Any malalignment should be addressed at the time of meniscal allograft transplantation. In addition, instability should also be addressed before or during meniscal allograft transplantation. Arnoczky and colleagues have demonstrated that the transplanted meniscus in a dog model demonstrates peripheral healing, as well as repopulation of the allograft with the host cells.[48] In a histologic analysis of human meniscal allograft, Rodeo and colleagues demonstrated that human meniscal allograft transplants are repopulated with cells that appear to be derived from the synovial membrane.[49] They also demonstrated low-level histologic evidence of an immune response, based on immunohistochemical studies that were performed on these human allograft specimens. However, this immune response did not correlate with the clinical outcome.[49,50] The longest-term results are reported by Wirth, Peters, and Milachowski, who originally described meniscal allograft

transplantation in 1989.[51,52] This group of authors followed the 23 patients for 14 years and reported in their clinical results that they had 100% follow-up rate. Lysholm score was 84 at 3 years after surgery and 75 at 14 years after surgery. They found that patients with deep frozen meniscal transplants generally had better results than patients with lyophilized meniscal transplants. MRI imaging revealed good preservation of the deep frozen meniscal transplant even after 14 years. In contrast, the lyophilized meniscal transplants were found to be reduced in size at second-look arthroscopy and as seen on MRI imaging.[52]

REHABILITATION

Rehabilitation after Partial Meniscectomy

Gaining immediate ROM and early ambulation are the critical factors involved after partial medial meniscectomy. The patient is allowed to walk as tolerated, and full weight bearing is encouraged immediately. Early ROM and return to weight bearing have been thought to decrease postoperative pain significantly (Box 18-1). Unfortunately, early supervised physical therapy has not been associated with better outcomes when compared with a home exercise program alone.[53] Nevertheless, data have shown significant isokinetic torque deficits of the knee extensor muscles for as long as 6 months after an arthroscopic meniscectomy.[54] Therefore, emphasis of the rehabilitation is to return normal bilateral strength to the quadriceps before competition. Patients routinely resume work after 1 to 2 weeks, resume activity after 2 to 4 weeks, and return to competition in 4 to 6 weeks.[55,56]

Rehabilitation after Meniscal Repair

Controversy exists among clinicians in the area of rehabilitation principles after meniscal repair. In the literature there seem to be two distinct rehabilitation approaches concerning weight bearing, early ROM, and the return to sports. The conservative guidelines limit weight bearing early and restrict full weight bearing until 4 weeks after surgery. In addition, these guidelines limit ROM to 90 degrees until 6 weeks after surgery and hold sports competition until 5 to 6 months after surgery.[45] In contrast, the accelerated guidelines allow full early weight bearing, unrestricted ROM, and no limitation of pivoting sports once clinical milestones have been met.[57,58] One study has evaluated the results of meniscal repair using an accelerated rehabilitation protocol.[59] This study demonstrated good meniscal healing rates and therefore does not support the need for activity restriction after meniscal repair. No difference in results was reported when comparing an accelerated rehabilitation protocol with a restricted standard rehabilitation protocol. Shelbourne and colleagues have also advocated an accelerated rehabilitation protocol and report no difference in meniscal healing rates between the accelerated and a conventional rehabilitation

BOX 18-1

Guidelines for Postoperative Rehabilitation after Meniscectomy

Phase I: Immediate Postoperative Phase (Postoperative Days 1-3)

Goals

Independent ambulation

Quadriceps activation

Decreased effusion

Wound healing

Restrictions

Weight bearing as tolerated (WBAT) with crutches as needed

No brace

Treatment

RICE (rest, ice, compression, elevation)

Gluteal sets

Quadriceps sets

Active assistive range-of-motion (AAROM) knee flexion

Clinical Milestones

Full extension present during gait

No limp

No increased effusion or edema

No increased pain

Phase II: Intermediate Postoperative Phase (1-3 Weeks)

Goals

Quadriceps control

Decreased pain

Normal gait

Normal patellar mobility

Increased range of motion (ROM)

Proximal strengthening initiated

Cardiovascular training initiated

Restrictions

Begin full weight bearing (FWB) without crutches

Treatment

Patellar mobility

Scar tissue mobilization

Pain management

Control of effusion

Neuromuscular re-education of quadriceps

Minisquats

Step-ups

Upper extremity reaches

ROM exercises

Flexibility exercises

Cardiovascular training

Clinical Milestones

Maximized ROM

Good quadriceps recruitment

Normal patellar mobility

Full passive extension

FWB

Phase III: Advanced Strengthening Phase (3-6 Weeks)

Goals

Normal quadriceps recruitment present

Full active ROM

Absence of pain

No effusion or edema

Isokinetics initiated

Restrictions

None

Treatment

Progression of quadriceps strengthening exercises

Standing balance training

Reduction of effusion or edema

Strengthening exercises

Upper extremity reaches

Leg presses

Step-downs

Endurance exercises

Proprioception exercises

Flexibility exercises

(continued)

program.[57] Similar results have also been reported by Mariani and co-workers.[43] It must be kept in mind, however, that in these studies meniscal healing was evaluated by clinical symptoms only, as opposed to objective evaluation using arthroscopy or MRI.

Before choosing a set of rehabilitation guidelines, it is important to understand the basic science of meniscal healing and how each of these areas may be affected. As previous described, the meniscus receives its blood supply from the superior, inferior, medial, and lateral geniculate arteries of the knee. Arnoczky and Warren have documented that there is ample blood supply to the peripheral 20% to 30% of the medial meniscus and 10% to 25% of the lateral meniscus to promote healing (Figure 18-4).[9,20] Because of poor blood supply in the inner two thirds of both menisci, nutrition is derived from the synovial fluid. Nevertheless, Cabaud and colleagues demonstrated that meniscal tears in monkeys could heal if a blood supply connection was established.[60] In both of these studies the animal limbs were free to move, thereby supporting unrestricted ROM after meniscal repair. After meniscal repair clinicians may be able to promote healing by using continuous ultrasound in an attempt to bring heat and increased blood supply to the healing meniscus during the immediate postoperative phase. In fact, the use of ultrasound treatment was found to increase ROM and decrease pain in a patient with an acute meniscal tear.[61] Our parameters are to use 1.5 W/cm^2 for 5 minutes after a cryotherapy treatment to decrease tissue resistance. The position of the knee differs for optimal medal and lateral meniscus ultrasound delivery. The position of the knee for the medial meniscus is in the figure-four position with the tibia in external rotation, as illustrated in Figure 18-5. For the lateral meniscus, the knee is flexed to 45 degrees and the tibia in internal rotation. Meniscal healing takes place over the course of 10 months in the canine model. At 2 weeks a fibrin clot is formed, and histologic evidence of meniscal regeneration

is evident at 5 weeks, followed by complete vascular healing at 10 weeks. However, remodeling of the scar may take up to 6 months.[20] It is on this basic science literature that we base our postoperative rehabilitation guidelines.

After meniscal repair surgery the immediate postoperative phase begins in the operating room with ice, compression, elevation, and rest in an effort to control postoperative effusion. Knee joint effusion and quadriceps contraction can be objectively quantified using the grading system proposed in Tables 18-1 and 18-2. Our guidelines instruct the patient in weight bearing as tolerated using bilateral axillary crutches with the knee braced in full extension (Box 18-2). With the knowledge that sheer stress is detrimental to the healing meniscus and may dislodge the fibrin clot, a rationale for full weight bearing can be made. With the knee in the fully extended position, the weight-bearing provides a hoop stress

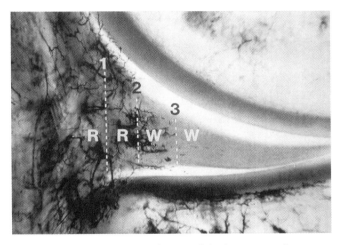

Figure 18-4: The microvasculature of the human meniscus. *(From Arnoczky SP, Warren RF: Microvasculature of the human meniscus, Am J Sports Med 10:90-95, 1982.)*

BOX 18-1

Guidelines for Postoperative Rehabilitation after Meniscectomy—cont'd

Clinical Milestones

Improved stability with unilateral stance

Minimal to no pain

Equal hip strength bilaterally

Isokinetic quadriceps strength <20% contralateral leg

Phase IV: Return to Activity Phase (6-8 Weeks)
Goals

Return to athletics

Restrictions

None

Treatment

Strengthening exercises

Endurance exercises

Agility drills

Plyometric training

Sport-specific drills

Clinical Milestones

Functional testing at least 90% of contralateral leg

Isokinetic testing at least 90% of contralateral leg

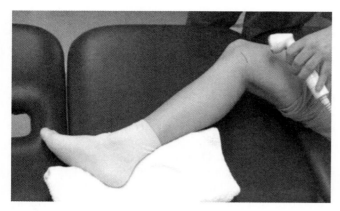

Figure 18-5: In this position of approximately 45 degrees of knee flexion and with the tibia in external rotation, the meniscus is maximally exposed.

TABLE 18-1

Objective Measurement of Knee Joint Effusion

KNEE JOINT EFFUSION GRADE	PALPATION END-FEEL
0	Bone on bone
1	Ability to milk fluid beneath patella but not visualize it
2	Ability to milk fluid beneath patella from one side and visualize it on the other side
3	A ballotable patella

TABLE 18-2

Objective Measurement of Vastis Medialis Oblique (VMO) Activity

VMO GRADE	OBSERVATION
Good	Ability to contract VMO and hold the contraction for as long as requested
Fair	Ability to contract VMO and hold the contraction for 3-5 seconds
Poor	Ability to contract the VMO (flicker)
Absent	No contraction present at all

to the meniscus and pushes the meniscus out to the periphery, thus approximating the repair and creating a stable environment. In fact, Morgan and colleagues identified on second-look arthroscopy that the most stable position for a meniscal repair is with the knee in full extension.[62] Motion after surgery can be handled in various ways ranging from restricted to no limitations.[62,63] Most authors agree that immobilization

of the leg after meniscal repair is detrimental to healing. In fact, several studies have evaluated the effects of immobilization and weight bearing from a basic science standpoint. Klein and colleagues showed that immobilization and non-weight bearing in a dog model resulted in significant atrophy of the soft tissues (lateral meniscus and ACL) as well as bone.[64] The same authors subsequently demonstrated that atrophy of ligaments and menisci can be prevented by active joint motion in a non–weight-bearing dog model.[65] Subsequently, Anderson and colleagues used a sheep model to demonstrate that the tensile properties of the menisci were not significantly affected, even if only limited joint motion was allowed.[66] Dowdy and co-workers have shown that prolonged immobilization leads to a decrease of collagen content within the healing meniscus, thus suggesting that patients undergoing isolated meniscal repair either be immediately mobilized after surgery or immobilized for short periods only.[67,68] In the early postoperative phase, ROM is progressed from 0 to 90 degrees. Early range-of-motion exercises are begun immediately, including full extension. Flexion is limited to 70 degrees during the first 4 weeks, to protect posterior horn repairs. The brace hinge is adjusted to allow ROM during ambulation, beginning at 4 weeks. Weight bearing out of the brace is allowed at 6 weeks. Running is begun at 3 to 4 months, with return to full athletic participation by 5 months. Squatting and hyperflexion are discouraged for up to 6 months after meniscal repair. Currently, the literature does not indicate a need to change rehabilitation guidelines based on the method and location of the repair.

In the setting of concomitant ACL reconstruction, the usual ACL rehabilitation protocol is used, because this provides appropriate protection for the healing meniscus. The typical ACL rehabilitation protocol includes immediate full weight bearing with full knee extension in a hinged brace. Progression to full ROM is allowed immediately as tolerated, with emphasis on early achievement of full extension. At 3 to 4 weeks the brace is unlocked to allow restoration of normal gait. Weight bearing out of the brace is allowed at 4 to 6 weeks. Closed kinetic chain strengthening exercises are begun in the second week and progress. Sport-specific activities are initiated 6 to 8 weeks for further development of strength and proprioception. Running is begun at 3 to 4 months, with return to full athletic participation by 5 months.

Rehabilitation after Meniscal Allograft Transplantation

Very little information is available in the literature to guide rehabilitation after meniscal allograft transplantation. However, the principles of basic science and biomechanics used for rehabilitation after meniscal repair can provide similar guidelines for determining the ideal program after meniscal transplantation. The biomechanical stresses on the healing meniscal allograft during rehab activities are unknown. Failure strength of meniscal sutures and of the

BOX 18-2
Postoperative Rehabilitation Guidelines after Meniscal Repair

Phase I: Immediate Postoperative Phase (Weeks 1-4)

Goals

Wound healing

Quadriceps activation

Decreased effusion

Restoration of full extension

Normal patella mobility

Initiation of proximal strengthening

Restrictions

WBAT with crutches with brace locked at 0

Brace locked at 0

ROM is limited to 0-70 for 4 weeks

Treatment

Ice, compression, elevation

Electrical muscle stimulation

Scar tissue mobilization

Active assisted ROM

Strengthening

Quadriceps isometrics

Hamstring isometrics

Hip abduction and adduction

Clinical Milestones

+1 effusion

Good quadriceps set

Good patella mobility

Absence of pain at rest

AROM 0-70 of flexion

Single limb stance

Phase II: Intermediate Postoperative Phase (Weeks 4-6)

Goals

WBAT with crutches with brace locked at 0-90

Progression to closed kinetic chain exercises

Patellar pain avoided

Restrictions

Gradual increase in flexion ROM based on pain assessment to 90

Flexion to 90

Treatment

Pain management

Control of effusion

Neuromuscular reeducation of quadriceps

Minisquats

Step-ups

Upper extremity reaches

ROM exercises

Flexibility exercises

Cardiovascular training

Toe raises

Cycling

Clinical Milestones

Full weight bearing (FWB)

Normal gait

AROM 0-90

Good quadriceps recruitment

Straight leg raise without lag

Normal patellar mobility

Phase III: Advanced Strengthening Phase (Weeks 6-10)

Goals

Increased strength, power, endurance

Normal knee ROM

Preparation of athlete for advanced exercises

Restrictions

Avoidance of pivoting

Flexion to 130

Treatment

Progression of quadriceps strengthening exercises

Standing balance training

Reduction of effusion and edema

Strengthening exercises

Upper extremity reaches

Lateral step-ups

Leg presses

Step-downs

(continued)

entire meniscal horn fixation to the tibia is also unknown, especially after repeated cyclic loading (Figure 18-6). It is thought that meniscal transplants are under higher stress in a joint with early degenerative changes. Therefore a more conservative protocol of rehabilitation is recommended.

Rodeo has recommended the following protocol.[50] A standard double upright-hinged knee brace is used for the first 6 weeks. Only toe-touch weight bearing with the knee in full extension is allowed for the first 4 weeks, with gradual progression to full weight bearing by 6 weeks postoperatively. Early ROM exercises are begun immediately, including full extension. As with meniscal repairs, flexion is limited to 90 degrees during the first 6 weeks, because progressive knee flexion subjects the meniscus to greater stress.[69] Morgan and co-workers contend that extension reduces the meniscus to the capsule, whereas flexion causes posterior horn tears to displace from the capsule.[62] Thompson and colleagues demonstrated that the menisci translate posteriorly with flexion.[70] However, meniscal movement was minimal below 60 degrees of flexion. No significant flexion limitations have occurred using this protocol.

Range of motion is progressed after 6 weeks. Closed kinetic chain strengthening exercises within the flexion limits are begun in the third week and then progressed (Figure 18-7). Fritz and co-workers suggested avoidance of

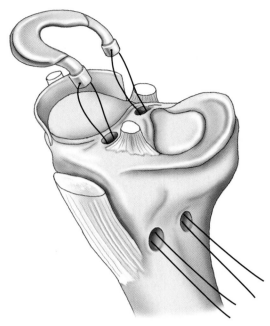

Figure 18-6: Meniscal transplant with bone plugs attached to the anterior and posterior horns. These bone plugs are transplanted into bone tunnels at the anterior and posterior horn attachment sites. *(From Rodeo SA: Meniscal allografts—where do we stand? Am J Sports Med 29:246-261, 2001.)*

BOX 18-2
Postoperative Rehabilitation Guidelines after Meniscal Repair—cont'd

Endurance exercises
Proprioception exercises
Flexibility exercises
Isokinetic exercises
Swimming
StairMaster
Minisquats
Cycling
NordicTrack

Clinical Milestones
Improved stability with unilateral stance
Minimal to no pain
Achievement of full ROM
Equal hip strength bilaterally
Isokinetic quadriceps strength <20% of contralateral leg

Phase IV: Return to Activity Phase (Weeks 11-16)
Goals
Increased power and endurance
Emphasis on return to skill activities
Preparation for return to full unrestricted activities

Restrictions
Avoidance of hyperflexion

Treatment
Strengthening exercises
Endurance exercises
Agility drills
Plyometric training
Sport-specific drills
Initiation of running program
Initiation of cutting program

Clinical Milestones
Full confidence in knee
Pain free activity at 5 months
Satisfactory clinical examination
Functional testing results at least 90% of contralateral leg
Isokinetic testing results at least 90% of contralateral leg

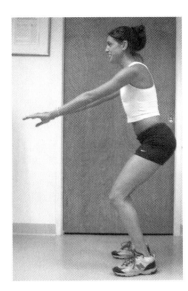

Figure 18-7: Minisquats can be an excellent closed kinetic chain strengthening exercise used within the flexion limits.

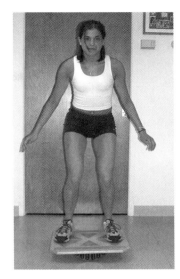

Figure 18-8: Balance board training can challenge the postoperative patient early to improve proprioception.

early open chain knee flexion exercises because of the attachment of the semimembranosus muscle on the medial meniscus and the popliteus muscle on the lateral meniscus.[71] Return to sport-specific activities is initiated after 4 months for further development of strength and proprioception (Figure 18-8). Running is not recommended for 6 months. Squatting and hyperflexion are discouraged for 6 months after meniscal transplantation. Return to high-load activities, involving cutting, jumping, and pivoting, is not currently recommended after meniscal transplantation. If there is concomitant ACL reconstruction, the usual ACL rehabilitation protocol is modified as previously described. Early full extension is emphasized. Concomitant procedures, such as cartilage resurfacing, may also require modification of the postoperative rehabilitation program.[72] Outcomes after meniscal transplantation are promising when expectations are reasonable (Box 18-3).[52,71,73] Overall, patients demonstrate a decrease in pain and increase in function and no signs of decreased joint space for up to 8 years after meniscal transplantation.[73] The retearing of the meniscal allograft seems to be the only limitation at this time. This procedure may prove to be a viable option for the athlete too young to consider an osteotomy or total knee replacement.

SUMMARY

The history of meniscal surgery is long and illustrious. Great advances have been made in the recent past, especially with regard to preserving menisci through repair. In addition, meniscus allograft transplantation has come into vogue for a select group of patients who are very carefully chosen for surgery. The indications for meniscal allograft transplantation continue to evolve. In the future, tissue engineering of menisci in vitro, with later implantation, is a possibility with the development of matrices, growth factors, and gene therapy. Rehabilitation protocols after meniscal surgery are also controversial and in some cases are evolving with more clinical experience as further observations are made after these innovative operations. Therefore the twenty-first–century surgeon and orthopedic sports physical therapist should be armed with the latest technologies and techniques to provide optimum care for the patients of the future.

BOX 18-3
Postoperative Rehabilitation Guidelines after Meniscal Transplantation

Phase I: Immediate Postoperative Phase (0-8 Weeks)

Goals

Protection of allograft fixation

Wound healing

Control of inflammation

Full knee extension

Prevention of adverse effects of immobilization

Regaining of quadriceps control

Restrictions

Postoperative day 1 to week 6: brace locked in extension for ambulation, sleeping

Weeks 6-8: discontinue brace for sleeping, unlock for controlled gait training

Toe-touch WB for 4 weeks

WBAT with bilateral crutches at 4 weeks

Active ROM 0-90

Avoid open chain knee flexion and extension

Treatment

Quadriceps sets, electrical stimulation as needed

Heel slides from 0-60 degrees of flexion

Ankle pumps, progressing to resistance

Scar tissue mobilization

Pain management

Control of effusion

Non–weight bearing, gastrocnemius and soleus, hamstring stretches

Straight leg raises (four ways)

Patellar mobilizations

Closed chain exercises at week 3

Aquatic therapy at 4 weeks

Clinical Milestones

Straight leg raise without extension lag

Full extension, 90 degrees of flexion

No signs of inflammation

Phase II: Intermediate Postoperative Phase (8-12 weeks)

Goals

Restore normal gait

Avoid overstressing the graft

Increase lower extremity strength, flexion ROM

Restrictions

Discontinue brace when patient has full extension, straight leg raise without extension lag, and nonantalgic gait pattern

FWB without assistive device if gait is normalized

No running, squatting or hyperflexion

Treatment

Continue straight leg raises, flexibility, aquatic exercises, and stationary bike

Closed kinetic chain exercises, 0-60 of flexion

Minisquats

Open kinetic chain knee extension, 45-90 of flexion

Toe raises

Balance exercises

Step-ups

Upper extremity reaches

Clinical Milestones

Normal gait without assistive device

Full extension, at least 100 of flexion

No patellofemoral joint complaints

Phase III: Advanced Strengthening Phase (3-9 Months)

Goals

Avoid overstressing the graft

Initiate isolated hamstring exercises

Improve strength, ROM, endurance, proprioception

Treatment

Continue flexibility program

Continue and advance closed kinetic chain activities

StairMaster, stationary bike, NordicTrack

Continue and advance balance exercises

Hamstring curls, 0-60 of flexion

Swimming—no breaststroke

Jogging in pool

Clinical Milestones

Necessary strength, ROM, endurance, proprioception for initiation of functional progression

(continued)

BOX 18-3
Postoperative Rehabilitation Guidelines after Meniscal Transplantation—cont'd

No patellofemoral complaints

Physician clearance for functional training

Phase IV: Return to Activity Phase (9 months+)

Goals

Maintain strength, endurance, and proprioception

Safe and gradual return to activity

Education regarding long-term activity modifications

Treatment

Continue strength, endurance, and proprioception program

Functional progression or work hardening as appropriate

Clinical Milestones

Functional testing results at least 90% of contralateral leg

Isokinetic testing results at least 90% of contralateral leg

References

1. Gupte CM, Smith A, McDermott ID, et al: Meniscofemoral ligaments revisited. Anatomical study, age correlation and clinical implications, *J Bone Joint Surg Br* 84:846-851, 2002.

2. Yamamoto M, Hirohata K: Anatomical study on the meniscofemoral ligaments of the knee, *Kobe J Med Sci* 37:209-226, 1991.

3. Rath E, Richmond JC: The menisci: basic science and advances in treatment, *Br J Sports Med* 34:252-257, 2000.

4. Seneviratne A, Rodeo S: Identifying and managing meniscal injuries, *J Musculoskelet Med* 10:690-697, 2000.

5. Rodkey WG: Basic biology of the meniscus and response to injury, *Instr Course Lect* 49:189-193, 2000.

6. Stone KR, Rodkey WG, Webber R, et al: Meniscal regeneration with copolymeric collagen scaffolds. In vitro and in vivo studies evaluated clinically, histologically, and biochemically, *Am J Sports Med* 20:104-111, 1992.

7. Bluteau G, Labourdette L, Ronziere M, et al: Type X collagen in rabbit and human meniscus, *Osteoarthritis Cartilage* 7:498-501, 1999.

8. Bessette GC: The meniscus, *Orthopedics* 15:35-42, 1992.

9. Arnoczky SP, Warren RF: Microvasculature of the human meniscus, *Am J Sports Med* 10:90-95, 1982.

10. Cooper DE, Arnoczky SP, Warren RF: Arthroscopic meniscal repair, *Clin Sports Med* 9:589-607, 1990.

11. Mine T, Kimura M, Sakka A, Kawai S: Innervation of nociceptors in the menisci of the knee joint: an immunohistochemical study, *Arch Orthop Trauma Surg* 120:201-204, 2000.

12. Rodeo SA, Warren RF: Meniscal repair using the outside-to-inside technique, *Clin Sports Med* 15:469-481, 1996.

13. Henning CE, Lynch MA: Current concepts of meniscal function and pathology, *Clin Sports Med* 4:259-265, 1985.

14. Thompson WO, Fu FH: The meniscus in the cruciate-deficient knee, *Clin Sports Med* 12:771-796, 1993.

15. Levy IM, Torzilli PA, Warren RF: The effect of medial meniscectomy on anterior-posterior motion of the knee, *J Bone Joint Surg Am* 64:883-888, 1982.

16. Negendank WG, Fernandez-Madrid FR, Heilbrun LK, Teitge RA: Magnetic resonance imaging of meniscal degeneration in asymptomatic knees, *J Orthop Res* 8:311-320, 1990.

17. Seitz H, Schlenz I, Muller E, Vecsei V: Anterior instability of the knee despite an intensive rehabilitation program, *Clin Orthop* 328:159-164, 1996.

18. Shelbourne KD, Nitz PA: The O'Donoghue triad revisited: combined knee injuries involving anterior cruciate and medial collateral ligament tears, *Am J Sports Med* 19:474-477, 1991.

19. Smith JP III, Barrett GR: Medial and lateral meniscal tear patterns in anterior cruciate ligament-deficient knees. A prospective analysis of 575 tears, *Am J Sports Med* 29:415-419, 2001.

20. Arnoczky SP, Warren RF: The microvasculature of the meniscus and its response to injury. An experimental study in the dog, *Am J Sports Med* 11:131-141, 1983.

21. Arnoczky SP, Warren RF, Kaplan N: Meniscal remodeling following partial meniscectomy—an experimental study in the dog, *Arthroscopy* 1:247-252, 1985.

22. Higuchi H, Kimura M, Shirakura K, et al: Factors affecting long-term results after arthroscopic partial meniscectomy, *Clin Orthop* 377:161-168, 2000.

23. Stone KR, Rodkey WG, Webber RJ, et al: Future directions. Collagen-based prostheses for meniscal regeneration, *Clin Orthop* 252:129-135, 1990.

24. Hede A, Hempel-Poulsen S, Jensen JS: Symptoms and level of sports activity in patients awaiting arthroscopy for meniscal lesions of the knee, *J Bone Joint Surg Am* 72:550-552, 1990.

25. Habata T, Ishimura M, Ohgushi H, et al: Axial alignment of the lower limb in patients with isolated meniscal tear, *J Orthop Sci* 3:85-89, 1998.

26. Magee T, Shapiro M, Williams D: MR accuracy and arthroscopic incidence of meniscal radial tears, *Skelet Radiol* 31:686-689, 2002.

27. van Trommel MF, Potter HG, Ernberg LA: The use of noncontrast magnetic resonance imaging in evaluating meniscal repair: comparison with conventional arthrography, *Arthroscopy* 14:2-8, 1998.

28. De Smet AA, Norris MA, Yandow DR, et al: MR diagnosis of meniscal tears of the knee: importance of high signal in the meniscus that extends to the surface, *Am J Roentgenol* 161:101-107, 1993.

29. Freiberger RH: Arthrography of the knee for diagnosis of torn meniscus, *J Sports Med* 1:24, 1972.

30. Ekstrom JE: Arthrography. Where does it fit in? *Clin Sports Med* 9:561-566, 1990.

31. Shelbourne KD, Johnson GE: Locked bucket-handle meniscal tears in knees with chronic anterior cruciate ligament deficiency, *Am J Sports Med* 21:779-782, 1993.

32. Weiss CB, Lundberg M, Hamberg P, et al: Non-operative treatment of meniscal tears, *J Bone Joint Surg Am* 71:811-822, 1989.

33. Stone KR: Current and future directions for meniscus repair and replacement, *Clin Orthop* 367(suppl):S273-S280, 1999.

34. Paessler HH, Franke K, Gladstone J: Moritz Katzenstein: the father of meniscus repair surgery, *Arthroscopy* 19:39e, 2003.

35. Fairbank TJ: Knee joint changes after meniscectomy, *J Bone Joint Surg Br* 30B:664-670, 1948.

36. Chatain F, Robinson AH, Adeleine P, et al: The natural history of the knee following arthroscopic medial meniscectomy, *Knee Surg Sports Traumatol Arthrosc* 9:15-18, 2001.

37. Schimmer RC, Brulhart KB, Duff C, Glinz W: Arthroscopic partial meniscectomy: a 12-year follow-up and two-step evaluation of the long-term course, *Arthroscopy* 14:136-142, 1998.

38. Osti L, Liu SH, Raskin A, et al: Partial lateral meniscectomy in athletes, *Arthroscopy* 10:424-430, 1994.

39. Rodeo SA: Arthroscopic meniscal repair with use of the outside-in technique, *Instr Course Lect* 49:195-206, 2000.

40. Warren RF: Arthroscopic meniscus repair, *Arthroscopy* 1:170-172, 1985.

41. Barret GR, Richardson K, Ruff CG, Jones A: The effect of suture type on meniscus repair: clinical analysis, *Am J Knee Surg* 10:2-9, 1997.

42. Morgan CD, Casscells SW: Arthroscopic meniscus repair: a safe approach to the posterior horns, *Arthroscopy* 2:3-12, 1986.

43. Mariani PP, Santori N, Adriani E, Mastantuono M: Accelerated rehabilitation after arthroscopic meniscal repair: a clinical and magnetic resonance imaging evaluation, *Arthroscopy* 12:680-686, 1996.

44. Nicholas SJ, Rodeo SA, Warren RF: Arthroscopic meniscus repair, using the outside-inside technique. Presented at annual meeting of the American Academy of Orthopaedic Surgeons (AAOS), Anaheim, CA, 1991.

45. Scott GA, Jolly BL, Henning CE: Combined posterior incision and arthroscopic intra-articular repair of the meniscus: an examination of factors affecting healing, *J Bone Joint Surg Am* 68:847-861, 1986.

46. Zantop T, Eggers AK, Musahl V, et al: A new rigid biodegradable anchor for meniscus refixation: biomechanical evaluation, *Knee Surg Sports Traumatol Arthrosc* 12:317-324, 2003.

47. Bohnsack M, Borner C, Schmolke S, et al: Clinical results of arthroscopic meniscal repair using biodegradable screws, *Knee Surg Sports Traumatol Arthrosc* 11:379-383, 2003.

48. Arnoczky SP, DiCarlo EF, O'Brien SJ, Warren RF: Cellular repopulation of deep-frozen meniscal autografts: an experimental study in the dog, *Arthroscopy* 8:428-436, 1992.

49. Rodeo SA, Seneviratne A, Suzuki K, et al: Histological analysis of human meniscal allografts: a preliminary report, *J Bone Joint Surg Am* 82:1071-1082, 2000.

50. Rodeo SA: Meniscal allografts—where do we stand? *Am J Sports Med* 29:246-261, 2001.

51. Milachowski KA, Weismeier K, Wirth CJ: Homologous meniscus transplantation: experimental and clinical results, *Int Orthop* 13:1-11, 1989.

52. Wirth CJ, Peters G, Milachowski KA, et al: Long-term results of meniscal allograft transplantation, *Am J Sports Med* 30:174-181, 2002.

53. Goodwin PC, Morrissery MC, Omar RZ, et al: Effectiveness of supervised physical therapy in the early period after arthroscopic partial meniscectomy, *Phys Ther* 83:520-535, 2003.

54. Gapejeva H, Paasuke M, Ereline J, et al: Isokinetic torque deficit of the knee extensor muscles after arthroscopic partial meniscectomy, *Knee Surg Sports Traumatol Arthrosc* 8:301-304, 2000.

55. Wheatley WB, Krome J, Martin DF: Rehabilitation programmes following arthroscopic meniscectomy in athletes, *Sports Med* 21:447-456, 1996.

56. Rangger C, Kathrein A, Klestil T, Glotzer W: Partial meniscectomy and osteoarthritis. Implications for treatment of athletes, *Sports Med* 23:61-68, 1997.

57. Shelbourne KD, Patel DV, Adsit WS, Porter DA: Rehabilitation after meniscal repair, *Clin Sports Med* 15:595-612, 1996.

58. Buseck MS, Noyes FR: Arthroscopic evaluation of meniscal repairs after anterior cruciate ligament reconstruction and immediate motion, *Am J Sports Med* 19:489-494, 1991.

59. Barber FA: Accelerated rehabilitation for meniscus repairs, *Arthroscopy* 10:206-210, 1994.

60. Cabaud HE, Rodkey WG, Fitzwater JE: Medical meniscus repairs. An experimental and morphologic study, *Am J Sports Med* 9:129-134, 1981.

61. Muche JA: Efficacy of therapeutic ultrasound treatment of a meniscus tear in a severely disabled patient: a case report, *Arch Phys Med Rehabil* 84:1558-1559, 2003.

62. Morgan CD, Wojtys EM, Casscells CD, Casscells SW: Arthroscopic meniscal repair evaluated by second-look arthroscopy, *Am J Sports Med* 19:632-637, 1991.

63. Miller DB Jr: Arthroscopic meniscus repair, *Am J Sports Med* 16:315-320, 1988.

64. Klein L, Player JS, Heiple KG, et al: Isotopic evidence for resorption of soft tissues and bone in immobilized dogs, *J Bone Joint Surg Am* 64:225-230, 1982.

65. Klein L, Heiple KG, Torzilli PA, et al: Prevention of ligament and meniscus atrophy by active joint motion in a non-weight-bearing model, *J Orthop Res* 7:80-85, 1989.

66. Anderson DR, Gershuni DH, Nakhostine M, Danzig LA: The effects of non-weight-bearing and limited motion on the tensile properties of the meniscus, *Arthroscopy* 9:440-445, 1993.

67. Dowdy PA, Miniaci A, Arnoczky SP, et al: The effect of cast immobilization on meniscal healing: an experimental study in the dog, *Am J Sports Med* 23:721-728, 1995.

68. Rodeo SA, Seneviratne AM: Arthroscopic meniscal repair using the outside-in technique—indications, technique and results, *Sports Med Arthrosc Rev* 7:20-27, 1999.

69. Walker PS, Erkman MJ: The role of the menisci in force transmission across the knee, *Clin Orthop* 109:184-192, 1975.

70. Thompson WO, Thaete FL, Fu FH, Dye SF: Tibial meniscal dynamics using three-dimensional reconstruction of magnetic resonance images, *Am J Sports Med* 19:210-215, 1991.

71. Fritz JM, Irrgang JJ, Harner CD: Rehabilitation following allograft meniscal transplantation: a review of the literature and case study, *J Orthop Sports Phys Ther* 24:98-106, 1996.

72. Kohn D, Aagaard H, Verdonk R, et al: Postoperative follow-up and rehabilitation after meniscus replacement, *Scand J Med Sci Sports* 9:177-180, 1999.

73. Rath E, Richmond JC, Yassir W, et al: Meniscal allograft transplantation: two- to eight-year results, *Am J Sports Med* 29:410-414, 2001.

CHAPTER 19

Complications of Meniscal Surgery

Robert E. Mangine, MEd, PT, ATC

W. Bays Gibson, PT

Marsha Eifert-Mangine, MEd, PT, ATC

Angelo J. Colosimo, MD

CHAPTER OUTLINE

THE SURGICAL MANAGEMENT AND SUB-SEQUENT rehabilitation of meniscal pathology has undergone substantial evolution in the past decades. This advancement is secondary to an increased knowledge of the anatomy, function, and healing capabilities of the meniscus. Surgical techniques have evolved from open total meniscectomy being the treatment of choice to allograft transplantations now being a viable intervention. Laboratory and clinical studies have laid the foundation for postoperative rehabilitation pathways. These advances have led to the shift toward preservation of the menisci as well as improved long-term functional outcomes, regardless of the specific procedure performed. Meniscal surgery is now among the most frequent surgical procedures performed by orthopedic surgeons, and those who undergo it constitute one of the patient populations most commonly seen by rehabilitation specialists. As surgical procedures are more widely performed on the meniscus, complications also occur at a more frequent rate. For successful postoperative management, it is imperative that each clinician fully understand the basic science of the meniscus, physiology of recovery, and potential complications. In this chapter the clinical implications of complications seen with meniscal surgery are discussed. The functional importance of the preserved meniscus is described, along with scientific rationale for current treatment of meniscal pathology. Complications encountered with meniscal surgery in general are discussed, as well as complications specific to meniscectomy, meniscal repair, and meniscal allograft transplantation.

FUNCTIONAL IMPORTANCE OF THE PRESERVED MENISCUS

Load Transmission

Although King[1] in 1936 demonstrated degenerative changes in the knees of canines after meniscectomy, it was Fairbank[2] who first suggested a direct load-bearing function of the meniscus. In this classic study, he documented the increased incidence of degenerative changes of the articular surface of meniscectomized knees. He argued that these changes were attributable chiefly to the loss of the load-bearing function of the meniscus. Since this early work, a number of clinical and biomechanical studies have supported Fairbank's thesis and further established the important role of the meniscus as a protective load-sharing structure.

The general response of the menisci-to-axial loading is the generation of circumferential "hoop" stresses as load bearing occurs.[1,3-5] Shrive and colleagues[3] estimated that 45% of the knee-joint load is carried by the meniscus. They also demonstrated that the load-bearing capability of the meniscus is greatly reduced after excision across the meniscus, rendering it unable to generate hoop stresses. The load-bearing capacity after radial excision is equivalent to that after complete meniscectomy.[3] Other authors have reported that the menisci transmit 70% to 99% of the joint load.[5-7] These authors state that after partial meniscectomy, as long as circumferential continuity is maintained, the remaining meniscus continues to transmit a significant proportion of the load.

Ahmed and Burke[5] determined that 50% of the body's weight is transmitted through the menisci in knee extension, and 85% is transmitted at 90 degrees of knee flexion. As little as 15% to 34% resection of the meniscus increases contact pressure by more than 350%.[8] After total meniscectomy the peak local contact stress is increased 235% because the tibiofemoral contact area decreases up to 75% of normal.[9] When partial meniscectomy is performed decreasing the contact area by only 10%, there is a 65% increase in peak load stress.[9] Such significantly increased compressive stress across the joint causes articular cartilage damage and degeneration. Even a partial loss of normal meniscal function affects the transmission of loads across the knee. Recently, studies have demonstrated improved contact areas and decreased contact pressures after meniscal allograft transplantation.[10,11]

Shock Absorption

The menisci exhibit viscoelastic properties that attenuate impacts sustained with loading of the knee.[4,12,13] As the joint compresses, the meniscus receives the load by extruding outward. This displacement is resisted by its anterior and posterior attachments, thus generating the hoop tension of the meniscus. It is the microstructure of the meniscus that provides its mechanical properties. The extracellular matrix of the meniscus is composed of water, collagen, fibrochondrocytes, and proteoglycans. Water represents 70% of the total weight of the meniscus, and collagen represents 70% of the dry weight.[4,14,15] The predominance of Type I collagen in the meniscus is the major difference between it and hyaline, or articular, cartilage, which is composed largely of Type II collagen. Fibrochondrocytes synthesize and maintain the extracellular matrix, especially collagen.[16] The menisci bear weight circumferentially because of the unique orientation of collagen fibers (Figure 19-1). These collagen fibers convert compressive loads into circumferential stresses. Thus, the meniscus absorbs energy and reduces the shock that the underlying cartilage and subchondral bone would receive.[17] Glycosaminoglycans (GAGs) constitute only 1% of the wet weight of the meniscus but contribute most to its material properties, such as hydration, compressive stiffness, and elasticity.[16] The GAGs, in combination with collagen orientation, are what give the menisci their compressive stiffness. The shock absorption capacity of the knee is reduced 20% by meniscectomy.[13]

Congruity and Stability

The articular surfaces of the tibiofemoral joint are noncongruous. The superior concave and inferior flat surfaces of the meniscus conform to the femoral and tibial condyles, respectively, and the wedge shape of the meniscus contributes to its function in joint stabilization.[18] The menisci deform and

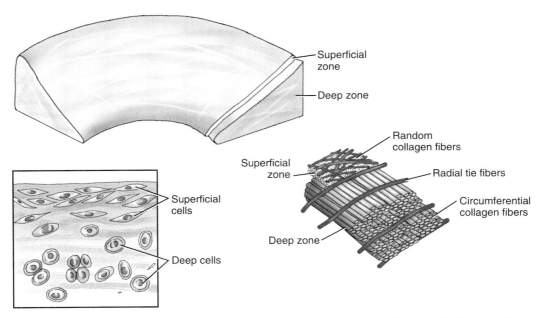

Figure 19-1: Collagen orientation and cell types in the meniscus. *(From Kawamura S, Lotito K, Rodeo SA: Biomechanics and healing response of the meniscus, Op Tech Sports Med 11:68-76, 2003.)*

change their radius at different angles of flexion, maintaining congruency.[19,20]

Meniscectomy has little effect on anteroposterior motion in the knee with an intact anterior cruciate ligament (ACL). In the ACL-deficient knee, however, medial meniscectomy results in a significant increase in laxity and anterior tibial translation of up to 58% at 90 degrees of flexion.[18] ACL deficiency increases anterior motion, allowing the meniscus to wedge between the femur and tibia, thus restraining the tibia from further displacement (Figure 19-2).[21-27] Allen and colleagues[24] showed that the resultant force on the medial meniscus in an ACL-deficient knee increases 52% in full extension and 197% at 60 degrees of flexion under a 134 N load. Because of these factors the medial meniscus is exposed to increased shear forces, predisposing the meniscus to damage.[21] Medial meniscectomy has also been shown to produce an increased force on an ACL graft.[25] This supports the belief that medial meniscus transplantation should be performed concurrently at the time of ACL reconstruction in the meniscus-deficient knee.

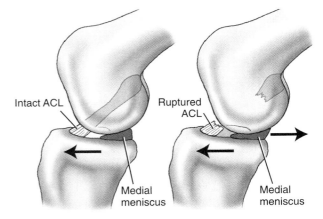

Figure 19-2: The medial meniscus acts as a restraint to anterior tibial translation in the ACL-deficient knee. *(From Levy IM, Torzilli PA, Gould JD: The effect of medial meniscectomy on anterior-posterior motion of the knee, J Bone Joint Surg 64A:883-888, 1982.)*

Proprioception

The menisci of the knee do not provide only passive stabilization. Histologic studies have identified the presence of neurologic receptors within the meniscus.[26-29] These neural elements contribute to the functional stability of the knee.[8,26-31] Four types of afferent mechanoreceptors have been classified and are present in noncontractile, capsular, and ligamentous structures in human joints. These same mechanoreceptors can be found in the anterior and posterior

horns of the meniscus and in the outer two thirds of the body of the meniscus (Table 19-1).[26-31]

Type I or Ruffini receptors are low-threshold, slow-adapting mechanoreceptors. These receptors are always active and categorized as both a static and dynamic receptor. Ruffini receptors respond to static and changing mechanical stresses signaled by static joint position, intraarticular pressure changes, and the direction, amplitude, and velocity of joint movements. Type I receptors allow the body to receive information about limb position constantly.

Type II mechanoreceptors or Pacinian receptors are considered to be dynamic mechanoreceptors. They are low-threshold, rapidly adapting receptors that respond to acceleration, deceleration, and passive joint movement. Type II receptors are silent during inactivity.

Type III or Golgi tendon organ–like mechanoreceptors have also been found in the menisci of the knee. These type III receptors are slow-adapting, high-threshold receptors that are inactive in immobile joints. They function as do the Golgi tendon organs of tendons in that they become active toward the extreme ends of range of motion or during considerable stress.

The final receptor found in the menisci is the type IV receptor or free nerve ending. Type IV receptors function as the pain receptor or nociceptive system of the meniscus. These receptors are small unmyelinated nerve fibers and are inactive under normal circumstances. Free nerve endings are activated by marked mechanical deformation or chemical irritation resulting from an inflammatory response.

All four mechanoreceptors of the menisci play a role in the proprioceptive feedback and neuromuscular control necessary for normal knee function. As stated previously, the neural elements of the menisci are most abundant in the outer two thirds of the body of the menisci and anterior and posterior horns. The inner third of the menisci lacks innervation.[29-31] Innervation only in the outer portion suggests the need for joint and biomechanical realignment; this occurs only when pressure is placed too far laterally.[31] Normal mechanics and pressure on the inner portion of the menisci would need no correction.[31] The anterior and posterior horns have a much denser population of mechanoreceptors than does the body of the meniscus.[26,29-31] During extremes of flexion and extension the meniscal horns become more taut, thus activating a greater concentration of mechanoreceptors. It is theorized that the need for afferent input is greatest at these extreme positions.[29,31]

Based on the evidence of mechanoreceptor innervation of the meniscus, it can be theorized that when damage to or excision of part or all of the meniscus occurs, diminished proprioceptive acuity and neuromuscular control results. Injuries to the menisci have been shown to significantly reduce position sense and proprioception of the knee.[32,33] Furthermore, decreased proprioceptive input secondary to meniscal injury can result in instability and accelerated degenerative changes because of repeated microtraumas.[32,33] Surgical preservation of the meniscus along with a rehabilita-

TABLE 19-1

Mechanoreceptor Innervation of the Human Meniscus

TYPE	FUNCTION	THRESHOLD	RESPONSE	ACTIVITY
Type I, Ruffini corpuscle	Provides central nervous system with information about static joint position, intraarticular pressure changes, and changes in the direction, amplitude, and velocity of joint motion	Low	Slow adapting	Always active Static and dynamic Activated at rest and with motion
Type II, Pacinian corpuscle	Signal information regarding joint acceleration and deceleration	Low	Rapid adapting	Dynamic only Activated at the onset of joint movement or changes in direction or acceleration with active and passive movements
Type III, Golgi tendon organ	Produces a protective reflex inhibition during tensioning	High	Slow adapting	Dynamic Active at end-range motion and with stress
Type IV, free nerve ending	Functions as part of the pain or nociceptive system	High	Slow adapting	Trauma Active in response to marked mechanical deformation and chemical irritation (inflammation)

tion program involving balance, coordination, and stability should be implemented because of the interruption of the mechanoreceptor system.

GENERAL COMPLICATIONS OF MENISCAL SURGERY

Meniscal surgery, although often a minimally invasive procedure, is not without risk of complications. DeLee reported the overall complication rate of arthroscopic knee procedures to be 0.8% in a study involving 118,000 cases.[34] A larger retrospective study by Small investigated the complication rate associated in 375,069 knee arthroscopies. An overall complication rate of 0.56% was reported with a 2.5% complication rate after meniscal repair.[35] Small subsequently described the complications encountered by 21 highly experienced arthroscopists over a 19-month period. The specific complications were similar to those reported previously, with the complication rate for all knee arthroscopies being 2%. The complication rate for meniscectomy was 1.69% (1.5% for lateral meniscectomy and 1.7% for medial meniscectomy) versus a rate of 1.29% reported for meniscal repair.[36] The consensus of these reports was that there is an acceptably low risk of complications associated with meniscal surgery, although arthroscopic meniscal surgery, despite being minimally invasive with generally low morbidity, is not free of complications.

Infection

The rate of infection after arthroscopic knee surgery is relatively low; however, serious sequelae can and do occur. Inherently, the risk of infection increases with open-meniscal procedures associated with specific repairs and allograft transplantations. Postarthroscopic rates have been reported to range from 0.03% to 0.42%.[34-38] The most commonly acquired infections after arthroscopy involve *Staphylococcus* and *Streptococcus* species. If left untreated, infection of the knee can result in septic arthritis, joint destruction, and osteomyelitis. Diagnosis of knee infection on physical examination is made from both subjective and objective data. The most common early symptoms are fever, chills, malaise, and associated joint pain. Joint effusion may be present, along with redness and an increased temperature of the knee. Purulent exudate from an incision site may be another indication of infection. If infection is suspected, a referral to a physician is warranted for proper diagnosis and treatment.

Deep Venous Thrombosis

Deep venous thrombosis (DVT) is the most potentially life-threatening complication after knee arthroscopy. Thrombophlebitis is a partial or complete occlusion of a vein by a thrombus, causing a secondary inflammatory reaction in the wall of the vein. It may affect the deep veins of the lower extremity or the superficial veins, most commonly the saphenous vein. Pulmonary embolism (PE) as a result of DVT is a potentially fatal development postoperatively if proper diagnosis and treatment do not occur. Although the incidence of DVT after arthroscopic knee surgery is low, it is important for health care practitioners to be aware of risk factors and signs and symptoms associated with DVT.

Recognized risk factors for the development of DVT include the use of contraceptives, smoking, cardiac insufficiency, obesity, clotting abnormalities, and varicosities. Risk factors specific to meniscal surgery include blood stasis caused by immobilization and decreased active muscle activation, both of which decrease circulation. In the early stages, patients with a DVT may have no signs or symptoms in the affected extremity.[39] A DVT may manifest up to 2 weeks postoperatively, with the chief complaints being a dull ache or pain, a feeling of tightness, or tenderness in the calf.[39] Signs are also frequently absent and unreliable and may consist of increased edema and temperature changes; if obstruction is severe, the skin may appear cyanotic. Signs and symptoms of PE are diffuse chest discomfort, tachypnea, tachycardia, dyspnea, hemoptysis, persistent cough, and, in rare instances, instant death.

History, physical examination, clinical assessment, and diagnosis of DVT are neither sensitive nor specific, and findings are notoriously inaccurate. Homans' sign is commonly assessed; however, this test has been found to be insensitive and nonspecific for the detection of a DVT.[39] Referral to a physician for objective diagnostic testing and treatment is warranted if the presence of a DVT is suspected.

During postoperative rehabilitation the risk for DVT development is profoundly decreased by immediate motion, decreased immobilization time, and active exercise occurring as soon as indicated. Each of these factors aids in decreasing venous stasis, thus decreasing the likelihood for DVT formation. Again, if DVT is suspected, immediate referral to a physician is warranted.

Reflex Sympathetic Dystrophy

Reflex sympathetic dystrophy (RSD) is now considered to be among the spectrum of disorders known as *complex regional pain syndrome* (CRPS). There is wide variability in the clinical presentation of this condition, with no consensus on its exact pathophysiology or treatment.[34,40-47] Many reports in the literature describe various possible pathophysiologic mechanisms of RSD.[43-47] O'Brien and colleagues found that arthroscopic procedures were the most common events precipitating RSD.[42] The wide array of clinical presentations, along with the absence of an accurate diagnostic test, makes this condition an enigma for treating clinicians. Often multiple surgical procedures are performed that fail to relieve pain secondary to incorrect diagnosis.[42] Success rates are higher when the diagnosis and treatment occur within the first 6 months of treatment.[44,47] This reinforces the importance of early detection and treatment.

Although there are autonomic abnormalities, trophic changes, and vasomotor disturbances, the outstanding characteristic of RSD is intense, prolonged pain out of proportion to physical findings and without discernible nerve injury.[42,44-47] Often, pain is associated with the saphenous nerve and localized to the medial knee. Hypersensitivity, cold intolerance, and muscular weakness and atrophy are also common findings. After accurate diagnosis, treatment often consists of lumbar sympathetic blockade, pharmacologic treatment, and a nonaggressive rehabilitation program. Although uncommon sequelae of arthroscopic meniscal surgery, RSD and CRPS can cause great morbidity in the affected patient.

Chronic Effusion

Surgery should be thought of as a controlled trauma to a tissue or joint. Therefore, the principles of the body's physiologic response to that trauma should be applied. Inflammation is the body's response to injury, which can result in undesired effects on healing tissue if not resolved in a normal 6-week time period. After an intraarticular surgical procedure, as with meniscal surgery, joint effusion is a common occurrence. Often before surgery, patients with both acute and chronic meniscal tears (often accompanied by degenerative joint changes) have synovial irritation, further complicating postoperative resolution. The effects of joint effusion and its relationship to functional stability of the knee have been well documented. Effusion leads to capsular distension, causing reflex inhibition of the quadriceps musculature by way of the mechanoreceptor system.[27,48,49] Hemarthrosis may occur in the early postoperative period and has a deleterious effect on articular cartilage.[50] Excessive synovial fluid may degrade the cartilage matrix as well. Persistent postoperative effusion may also represent synovitis, infection, or other intraarticular pathology. Often a patient's chief complaint, both preoperative and postoperative, is the feeling of instability or "giving way," rather than pain. These symptoms are in direct correlation with increased joint effusion. The early reduction of postoperative joint effusion is paramount to successful rehabilitation and quicker return to functional activities. Nonsteroidal antiinflammatory medications may be used early in the postoperative period to aid in controlling effusion. If a large amount of effusion persists, then aspiration of the joint may be indicated.

Intraoperative and Other Complications

Various iatrogenic complications have been reported to occur during meniscal surgery. Often these intraoperative complications are reported in large surveys or in case reports.[34-36,51] Many of the intraoperative complications can result in severe functional disability. Of particular concern intraoperatively is the risk to neurovascular structures. Rehabilitation specialists have to be conscious of their occurrence, particularly in the initial postoperative visit when many signs and symptoms may be first discovered.

Injury to the neurovascular structures can occur during meniscal surgery. Damage to the vasculature around the knee can be a serious and devastating injury. Injury to blood vessels occurs at the time of surgery from direct penetration or laceration; however, its occurrence is very low.[52-57] The popliteal artery and vein as well as the genicular arteries are the vascular structures most commonly injured during arthroscopic surgery.[34-36,52] Small found only 12 vascular injuries in his report of more than 375,000 knee arthroscopies.[35] Multiple case reports have described the vascular injuries occurring after meniscectomy[56-58] and meniscal repair.[54]

Compartment syndrome also occurs and can be detected in the early postoperative period. Clinicians must differentiate signs and symptoms of compartment syndrome, as its rapid recognition and treatment are paramount. Patients may have diminished peripheral pulse, hypesthesia, swelling, and often motor weakness. A tense or tight compartment is often the earliest finding, along with pain. Severe intracompartmental pressures require immediate fasciotomy to avoid tissue death.

The neural structures at greatest risk for iatrogenic injury are the peroneal nerve and saphenous nerve. Large retrospective analyses of the literature have found the risk of neurologic injury to be approximately 0.01% to 2.5%.[34-36,59,60] Small reported that nerve injuries constitute 50% of all complications and that the saphenous nerve is involved more often than the peroneal nerve.[35] The infrapatellar branch of the saphenous nerve is the most frequently injured branch of the saphenous nerve. It provides purely cutaneous sensation to the anterior knee and is injured when the anteromedial arthroscopy portal is made. Complications as a result of injury to the infrapatellar branch have been reported in the literature. A further description of the presentation and implications of neural injuries is provided in the discussion of complications of meniscal repair, where they occur most frequently.

COMPLICATIONS OF MENISCECTOMY

Open total meniscectomy was once the standard treatment for all types of meniscal tears. The meniscus is now known to be vital to proper knee function. Surgical preservation of meniscal tissue should be performed if at all possible, as indicated by the deleterious long-term effects of total meniscectomy. The advent in the 1980s of arthroscopy as a popular technique for meniscectomy has radically changed the way meniscal tears and pathology are treated. Although preservation of normal meniscal anatomy by way of arthroscopic partial meniscectomy has many advantages, all the complications attributed to knee arthroscopy in general can occur.

Degenerative Joint Changes

Of particular concern after meniscectomy is the occurrence of degenerative joint disease. Total meniscectomy is now rarely indicated because of advanced procedures, knowledge of menisci healing capabilities, and the known deleterious sequelae of complete meniscectomy. Arthroscopic partial meniscectomy should be performed when excision is required. Arthroscopic partial meniscectomy is now the procedure of choice because of the low morbidity, improved cosmesis, quicker return to function, and ability to preserve the greatest possible amount of normal meniscus. All meniscal tears requiring surgical intervention that are not suitable for repair should be treated by partial meniscectomy, leaving the greatest amount of residual meniscal tissue intact.

In 1948 Fairbank described the degenerative radiographic changes occurring in the knee after meniscectomy.[2] In his report three significant changes were noted: (1) narrowing of the joint space, (2) flattening of the outer edges of the femoral articular surface, and (3) formation of an anterior-posterior ridge projecting downward over the meniscal site. Since that time the late effects of meniscectomy have been well established, leading to the present trend of meniscal preservation. Baratz and colleagues showed that after total meniscectomy the peak local contact stress is increased 235%.[9] Baratz also showed that when partial meniscectomy was performed, the peak local contact stress was increased 65%.[9] Many other studies have confirmed the role of the menisci in load transmission after partial and total meniscectomy and the development of degenerative changes.[61-67] Roos and colleagues suggested that postmeniscectomy patients may develop premature arthritis 10 to 20 years earlier than patients who experience primary osteoarthritis.[66] Clinical studies have found that these osteoarthritic changes, ligamentous laxity, persistent pain and effusion, gait abnormalities, and varus angulation all continue to worsen with increased time after meniscectomy.[62,63,67-69] Although partial meniscectomy provides better clinical outcomes than total meniscectomy, long-term degenerative changes still occur,[70] and these changes correlate with the amount of meniscal tissue removed.[71] Despite these well-known risks and complications after meniscectomy, meniscal repair often remains unfeasible, and in these instances, partial meniscectomy is almost always preferred over total meniscectomy.

COMPLICATIONS OF MENISCAL REPAIR

Documentation of the consequences of meniscus loss has led to a more aggressive approach to meniscal preservation. Arthroscopic repair techniques were developed in the 1980s and continue to gain widespread attention and acceptance. As surgical repair techniques have advanced, so has subsequent rehabilitation. Critical to the success of meniscal repair is the careful implementation of a postoperative rehabilitation regimen. Just as there are numerous repair techniques performed (e.g., inside-out, outside-in, all-inside, and open repair), there is also a wide variety of rehabilitation protocols after meniscal repair. The evolutions in repair techniques have been made primarily to avoid complications. For the purpose of this discussion, complications of all techniques and rehabilitation protocols will be discussed as a whole.

With meniscal repair being more frequently performed, it is imperative that all clinicians have a fundamental understanding of the potential complications seen with meniscal repairs.

Failure of Repair

Of particular concern in the postoperative rehabilitation phase after meniscal repair is the possibility of retear or failure of the repair to heal. The reported rates of retear or failure may be somewhat misleading because "failure" has multiple definitions in the literature. Meniscal repair failure can be defined by clinical examination, based on imaging results, or second-look arthroscopic findings. Failure of repair has also been a topic of controversy as it relates to technique, repair devices, and rehabilitation pathways. The main concerns with rehabilitation involve weight bearing, range of motion, and return to sport. Improved understanding of meniscal healing after repair continues to support progression toward a more accelerated rehabilitation.

Numerous techniques and devices have been developed for meniscal repair. There have been reports of failure and complications associated with many of them. For the purposes of this section, only general statements will be made regarding them. Multiple repair devices, absorbable and nonabsorbable, have been developed for meniscal repair. These include but are not limited to arrows, darts, screws, fasteners, sutures, and anchors. Several of these are rigid devices and lack the ability to deform with the meniscus with compressive loads (Figure 19-3). Secondarily, there have been multiple reports of chondral injuries caused by rigid devices.[72-76] In several of these reports patients had joint effusions and/or pain months after the initial repair. Repeat arthroscopy showed osteochondral lesions of the femoral condyles.[72-80] Two case reports have actually reported the migration of meniscal arrows through the skin.[81,82]

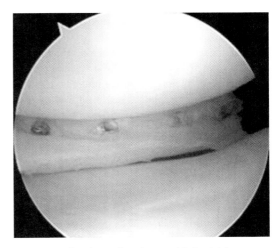

Figure 19-3: Meniscal repair using multiple rigid arrows.

Arthrofibrosis

Arthrofibrosis is another potential complication of meniscal repair. Immobilization of a joint for a prolonged period of time is the most recognized risk factor for the development of arthrofibrosis. Because of the protection of the repaired meniscus and gradual progression of range of motion, meniscal repair itself is a risk factor for arthrofibrosis. Austin and Sherman reported an arthrofibrosis rate of 1% to 2% in isolated ACL reconstruction and 10% for both ACL reconstruction and meniscal repair.[76] This complication can be prevented by early motion and decreased immobilization times.

Neurologic Injury

Injury to the saphenous nerve is the single most common complication after meniscal repair.[35,59,76,77] The infrapatellar branch is the most often injured branch of the saphenous nerve, and the injury occurs at the anteromedial arthroscopy portal. Stone and Miller reported saphenous nerve neurapraxia in 28% of all meniscal repairs. Forty-three percent of all medial meniscal repairs demonstrated saphenous neurapraxia, with only 8% remaining symptomatic at follow-up.[77] Neurapraxic injuries of this sort are thought to be transient and recover spontaneously within 2 to 3 months.[78] Several authors have cited saphenous neuropathy as a complication of meniscal repair and stated that it is an acceptable, transient, and often unavoidable sequela.[36,76,79,83,84] Injury to the infrapatellar branch of the saphenous nerve, although quite common, causes no functional limitation to the patient.

On the lateral side of the knee, the peroneal nerve is at risk for injury during meniscal repair. Trauma to the nerve can result from neurapraxia, suturing of the nerve (Figure 19-4), and direct puncture or laceration. Fortunately, peroneal nerve injury is rare. Injury to the peroneal nerve is generally more severe than that of the saphenous nerve because it can lead to motor dysfunction. This is of particular concern to the rehabilitation specialist. During early postoperative rehabilitation the presence of motor dysfunction, specifically with dorsiflexion and eversion, may first be recognized. When peroneal nerve injury is suspected, electrodiagnostic testing is indicated to determine the location, severity, and prognosis of injury to assist in its management. Recovery depends on the severity of damage. Neurapraxia, axonotmesis, and the most severe condition, neurotmesis, are the classifications and gradations of nerve injury.[85] Lesions to neural tissue may heal gradually or, if severe enough, may require surgery. Again, complications involving the peroneal nerve do not frequently occur. However, failure to recognize, document, and address injury in an appropriate and timely manner could prove devastating for the patient. Referral to a physician is critical if signs and symptoms of nerve damage are discovered.

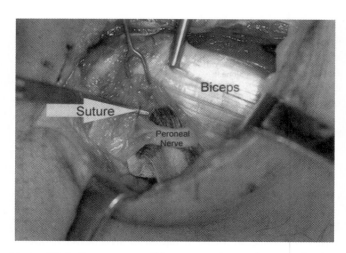

Figure 19-4: Entrapment of the peroneal nerve by a meniscal repair suture. *(From Kline AJ, Miller MD: Complications in meniscal surgery, Op Tech Sports Med 11:134-143, 2003.)*

COMPLICATIONS SPECIFIC TO MENISCAL ALLOGRAFT TRANSPLANTATION

Meniscal transplantation remains in its infancy. Therefore large clinical trials on long-term outcomes and objective data have been limited to date. Only long-term follow-up will determine whether meniscal transplantation can prevent or delay the progression of degenerative changes.

There are four clinical situations in which meniscal transplantation is currently indicated. The most common indication is in the symptomatic meniscus-deficient knee, to avoid the progression of degeneration (Figure 19-5). However, in the presence of advanced joint degeneration, results of meniscal transplantation have been poor, and it is therefore contraindicated.[86,87] Osteotomy performed with meniscal transplantation is also a current indication. This is typically performed in the younger, active patient with varus or valgus deformity and unicompartmental degeneration of the tibiofemoral joint. Concomitant meniscal transplantation could enhance the effects of osteotomy and delay the recurrent deformity and progressive arthrosis that is known to occur after osteotomy.[88] Transplantation has also been indicated during ACL reconstruction to provide additional stabilization, protection of the ACL graft, and avoidance of potential shear loading of the articular surfaces. Lastly, meniscectomy may be the most opportune time for transplantation, to avoid the future complications of meniscectomy previously discussed. This prophylactic transplantation may be indicated when there is irreparable pathology of the meniscus.

Since the effects of meniscal transplantation remain investigational, few postoperative complications have been reported in the literature. However, there are potential pitfalls seen with the procedure. An obvious complication with

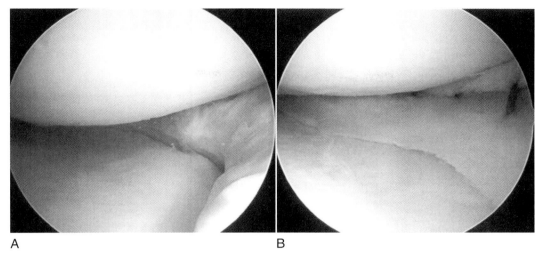

Figure 19-5: A, Arthroscopic view of meniscus-deficient knee. **B,** Arthroscopic view of same knee after meniscus allograft transplantation.

the use of allograft tissue is the risk of disease transmission. Currently the risk of viral transmission through allograft tissue is extremely low.[89,90] The risk of HIV transmission is estimated at one in one million.[90] Frank immune rejection of the graft does not appear to occur. Microscopic evidence of an immune response against the transplant has been reported and may contribute to persistent effusion and symptoms often reported.[91]

Allograft size mismatching can inevitably lead to transplant failure. Graft selection should be specific to the compartment being transplanted. Appropriate size matching is critical for optimal mechanical function. Currently, there is no agreement as to which preoperative imaging modality is most effective (i.e., plain radiography, magnetic resonance imaging, computed tomography).[92] Another potential complication is that transplanted meniscal allografts have been found to undergo shrinkage. This has been shown to be associated with lyophilized, or freeze-dried, meniscal grafts. Fresh and cryopreserved allografts may contain viable cells through preservation of the extracellular matrix, whereas fresh-frozen and lyophilized grafts are acellular. Nonanatomic placement of meniscal allografts has been shown to cause increased contact pressures within the knee joint.[11] Meniscal allografts have been proven to increase contact areas and decrease contact pressures.[10,11]

Loss of fixation, either at the periphery of the meniscus or at the bone plug insertion site, is a possible complication of allograft transplantation.[93,94] This extrusion of the meniscal allograft is likely to cause mechanical symptoms of locking, constant pain, and recurrent effusions. Soft-tissue fixation alone is insufficient and does not provide adequate strength, which leads to extrusion of the graft during weight bearing.[92] Fixation via bone plugs is more secure but also has the potential for failure. Paletta and colleagues demonstrated the importance of securely fixating the anterior and posterior

horns of the meniscus. They showed that contact pressures with allografts were equal to contact pressures in meniscectomized knees when both horns are released.[10]

SUMMARY

A thorough understanding of the functional importance of the meniscus is necessary to successfully treat its pathology, both surgically and during the postoperative rehabilitation process. A thorough knowledge of possible complications as well as the ability to recognize them during the postoperative period lead to decreased morbidity for the affected patient.

References

1. King D: The function of semilunar cartilages, *J Bone Joint Surg* 18:1069-1076, 1936.
2. Fairbank TJ: Knee joint changes after meniscectomy, *J Bone Joint Surg Br* 30:664-670, 1948.
3. Shrive NG, O'Connor JJ, Goodfellow JW: Load bearing in the knee joint, *Clin Orthop* 131:279-287, 1978.
4. Fithian DC, Kelly MA, Mow VC: Material properties and structure-function relationships in the menisci, *Clin Orthop* 252:19-31, 1990.
5. Ahmed AH, Burke DL: In-vitro measurement of static pressure distribution in synovial joints—Part 1: tibial surface of the knee, *J Biomech Eng* 105:216-225, 1983.
6. Seedholm BB: Transmission of the load in the knee with special reference to the role of the menisci. Part 1. *N Engl J Med* 8:207-218, 1978.
7. Seedholm BB, Hargreaves DJ: Transmission of the load in the knee joint with special reverence to the role of the menisci. Part II. *N Engl J Med* 8:220-228, 1979.
8. Arnoczky SP, McDevitt CA: The meniscus: structure, function, repair, and replacement. In Buckwalter JA, Einhorn TA, Simon SR, editors: Orthopaedic basic science. Rosemont, IL, 2000, American Academy of Orthopedic Surgeons.

9. Baratz ME, Fu FH, Mengato RL: The effect of meniscectomy and of repair on intra-articular contact areas and stress in the human knee, *Am J Sports Med* 14:270-275, 1986.

10. Paletta GA, Manning T, Snell E, et al: The effect of meniscal replacement on intraarticular contact area and pressures in the human knee: A biomechanical study, *Am J Sports Med* 25:692-698, 1997.

11. Hyang A, Hull ML, Howell SM: The level of compressive load affects conclusions from statistical analyses to determine whether a lateral meniscal autograft restores tibial contact pressure to normal. A study in human cadaveric knees, *J Orthop Res* 21:459-464, 2003.

12. Anderson DR, Woo SL-Y, Kwan MK, Gerstais DH: Viscoelastic shear properties of the equine medial meniscus, *J Orthop Res* 9:550-558, 1991.

13. Voloshin AS, Wosk J: Shock absorption of meniscectomized and painful knees: a comparative in-vivo study. *J Biomed Eng* 5:157-161, 1983.

14. McDevitt CA, Webber RJ: The ultrastructure and biochemistry of meniscal cartilage, *Clin Orthop* 252:8-18, 1990.

15. Mow VC, Ratcliffe A, Chern KY, Kelly MA: Structure and function relationships on the menisci of the knee. In Mow VC, Arnoczky SP, Jackson DW, editors: *Knee meniscus: basic and clinical foundations*, New York, 1992, Raven Press.

16. Adams ME, Hukins WL: The extracellular matrix of the meniscus. In Mow VC, Arnoczky SP, Jackson DW, editors: *Knee meniscus: basic and clinical foundations*, New York, 1992, Raven Press.

17. Bullough P, Munuera L, Murphy J, Weinstein AM: The strength of the menisci of the knee as it relates to their fine structure, *J Bone Joint Surg Br* 52:564-570, 1970.

18. Levy IM, Torzilli PA, Gould JD: The effect of medial meniscectomy on anterior-posterior motion of the knee, *J Bone Joint Surg* 64A:883-888, 1982.

19. Fu FH, Thompson WO: Motion of the meniscus during knee flexion. In Mow VC, Arnoczky SP, Jackson DW, editors: *Knee meniscus: basic and clinical foundations*, New York, 1992, Raven Press.

20. Thompson WO, Thaete FL, Fu FH: Tibial meniscal dynamics using three-dimensional reconstruction of magnetic resonance images, *Am J Sports Med* 19:210-216, 1991.

21. Levy IM, Torzilli PA, Fisch ID: The contribution of the meniscus to the stability of the knee. In Mow VC, Arnoczky SP, Jackson DW, editors: *Knee meniscus: basic and clinical foundations*, New York, 1992, Raven Press.

22. Shoemaker SC, Markolf KL: The role of the meniscus in the anterior-posterior stability of the loaded anterior cruciate ligament deficient knee, *J Bone Joint Surg* 68A:71-79, 1986.

23. Markolf KL, Mensch JS, Amstutz HC: Stiffness and laxity of the knee: the contributions of the supporting structures, *J Bone Joint Surg* 58A:583-593, 1976.

24. Allen CR, Wong EK, Levesay GA: Importance of the medial meniscus in the anterior cruciate ligament–deficient knee, *J Orthop Res* 18:109-115, 2000.

25. Papageorglou CD, Gill JE, Kanamori A: The biomechanical interdependence between the anterior cruciate ligament replacement graft and the medial meniscus, *Am J Sports Med* 29:226-231, 2001.

26. Day B, Mackensie WG, Shimn SS, Leung G: The vascular and nerve supply of the human meniscus, *Arthroscopy* 1:58-62, 1985.

27. Kennedy JC, Alexander IJ, Hayes KL: Nerve supply of the human knee and its functional importance, *Am J Sports Med* 10:329-335, 1982.

28. Wilson AS, Legg PG, McNeur JC: Studies on the innervation of the medial meniscus in the human knee joint, *Anat Rec* 165:485-492, 1969.

29. Zimny ML: Mechanoreceptors in articular tissues, *Am J Anat* 182:16-32, 1998.

30. Assimakopoulus AP, Katonis PG, Agapitos MV, Exarchov EL: The innervation of the human medial meniscus, *Clin Orthop* 75:232-236, 1992.

31. Zimny ML, Albright DJ, Dabezies E: Mechanoreceptors in the human medial meniscus, *Acta Anat* 133:35-40, 1988.

32. Jerosch J, Prymka M: Proprioception and joint stability, *Knee Surg Traumatol Arthrosc* 4:171-179, 1996.

33. Jerosch J, Prymka M, Castro WHM: Proprioception of the knee joint with a lesion of the medial meniscus, *Acta Orthop Belgica* 62:41-45, 1996.

34. DeLee JC: Complications of arthroscopy and arthroscopic surgery: results of a national survey, *Arthroscopy* 1:204-220, 1985.

35. Small NC: Complications in arthroscopy: The knee and other joints. Committee on Complications of the Arthroscopy Association of North America, *Arthroscopy* 2:253-258, 1986.

36. Small NC: Complications in arthroscopic surgery performed by experienced arthroscopists, *Arthroscopy* 4:215-221, 1988.

37. Armstrong RW, Bolding F, Joseph R: Septic arthritis following arthroscopy: clinical syndromes and analysis of antibiotic prophylaxis, *Arthroscopy* 4:10-14, 1988.

38. Keiser CH: A review of the complications following arthroscopic knee surgery, *Arthroscopy* 8:79-83, 1992.

39. Goodman CC, Boissonnault WG, Fuller KS: *Pathology. Implications for physical therapists*, ed 2, Philadelphia, 2003, Saunders.

40. Amadio PC: Pain dysfunction syndromes, *J Bone Joint Surg* 77A:944-949, 1988.

41. Campa JA, Broadnax W, Broderick J, et al: Neuropathic and sympathetically maintained pain complicating trauma or surgery to the knee, *Neurology* 41:165, 1991.

42. O'Brien SJ, Ngeow J, Gibney MA, et al: Reflex sympathetic dystrophy of the knee: causes, diagnosis, and treatment, *Am J Sports Med* 23:655-659, 1995.

43. Tietjen R: Reflex sympathetic dystrophy of the knee, *Clin Orthop* 209:234-243, 1986.

44. Ogilvie-Harris DJ, Roscoe M: Reflex sympathetic dystrophy of the knee, *J Bone Joint Surg* 69B:804-806, 1987.

45. Seale KS: Reflex sympathetic dystrophy of the lower extremity, *Clin Orthop* 243:80-85, 1989.

46. Katz MM, Hungerford DS: Reflex sympathetic dystrophy affecting the knee, *J Bone Joint Surg* 69B:797-803, 1987.

47. Cooper DE, DeLee JC, Ramamurthy S: Reflex sympathetic dystrophy of the knee. Treatment using continuous epidural anesthesia, *J Bone Joint Surg* 71A:365-369, 1989.

48. de Andrade JR, Grant C, Dixon A: Joint distension and reflex muscle inhibition, *J Bone Joint Surg* 2A:313-322, 1965.

49. Spencer JD, Hayes KC, Alexander IJ: Knee joint effusion and quadriceps reflex inhibition in man, *Arch Phys Med Rehabil* 65:171-177, 1984.

50. Hoaglund FJ: Experimental hemarthrosis effect on articular cartilage, *J Bone Joint Surg* 49A:285, 1967.

51. Sherman OH, Fox JM, Snyder SJ, et al: Arthroscopy—"no-problem surgery." An analysis of complications in two thousand six hundred and forty cases, *J Bone Joint Surg* 68A:256-265, 1986.

52. Kim TK, Savino RM, McFarland EG, Cosgarea AJ: Neurovascular complications of knee arthroscopy, *Am J Sports Med* 30:619-629, 2002.

53. Tawes RL, Etheredge SN, Webb RL, et al: Popliteal artery injury complicating arthroscopic meniscectomy, *Am J Surg* 156:136-138, 1988.

54. Casscells SW: Injury to the popliteal artery as a complication of arthroscopic surgery. A report of two cases, *J Bone Joint Surg* 70A:150, 1988.

55. Furie E, Yerys P, Cutcliffe D, et al: Risk factors for arthroscopic popliteal artery laceration, *Arthroscopy* 11:324-327, 1995.

56. Jeffries JT, Gainor BJ, Allen WC, et al: Injury of the popliteal artery as a complication of arthroscopic surgery. A report of two cases, *J Bone Joint Surg* 69A:783-785, 1987.

57. Potter D, Morris-Jones W: Popliteal artery injury complication arthroscopic meniscectomy. Case Report, *Arthroscopy* 11:723-726, 1995.

58. Ritt MJ, Te Slaa RL, Koning J, et al: Popliteal pseudoaneurysm after arthroscopic meniscectomy. A report of two cases, *Clin Orthop* 295:198-200, 1993.

59. Small NC: Complications in arthroscopic meniscal surgery, *Clin Sports Med* 9:609-617, 1990.

60. Small NC, Farless BL: Avoiding complications in meniscal repair, *Tech Orthop* 8:70-75, 1993.

61. Krause WR, Pope MH, Johnson RJ, et al: Mechanical changes in the knee after meniscectomy, *J Bone Joint Surg Am* 58:599-604, 1976.

62. Jackson JP: Degenerative changes in the knee after meniscectomy, *Br Med J* 2:525-527, 1968.

63. Johnson RJ, Kettlecamp DB, Clark W, et al: Factors affecting late results after meniscectomy, *J Bone J Surg Am* 56:719-729, 1974.

64. Gear MW: The late results of meniscectomy, *Br J Surg* 54:270-277, 1967.

65. Allen PR, Denham RA, Swan AV: Late degenerative changes after meniscectomy. Factors affecting the knee after operation, *J Bone Joint Surg Br* 66:666-671, 1984.

66. Roos H, Lauren M, Adalberth T, et al: Knee osteoarthritis after meniscectomy. Prevalence of radiographic changes after twenty-one years, compared with matched controls, *Arthritis Rheum* 41:687-693, 1998.

67. Appel H: Late results after meniscectomy in the knee joint. A clinical and roentgenographic follow-up investigation, *Acta Orthop Scand* 133(suppl):1-111, 1970.

68. Jones RE, Smith EC, Reisch JS: Effects of medial meniscectomy in patients older than forty years, *J Bone Joint Surg* 60A:783-786, 1978.

69. Tapper EM, Hoover NW: Late results of meniscectomy, *J Bone Joint Surg* 51A:517-526, 1969.

70. Scheller G, Sobau C, Bulow J: Arthroscopic partial lateral meniscectomy in an otherwise normal knee. Clinical, functional, and radiographic results of a long-term follow-up study, *Arthroscopy* 17:946-952, 2001.

71. Cox JS, Nye CE, Shaeffer WW, Woodstein IJ: The degenerative effects of partial and total resection of the medial meniscus in dogs' knees, *Clin Orthop* 109:178-183, 1975.

72. Ross G, Grabill J, McDevitt E: Chondral injury after meniscal repair with bioabsorbable arrows, *Arthroscopy* 16:754-756, 2000.

73. Schultz WR, Carr CF: Femoral osteochondral lesion resulting from meniscus arrow repair, *Arthroscopy* 16:1-3, 2000.

74. Seil R, Rupp S, Dienst M, et al: Chondral lesions after arthroscopic meniscus repair using meniscus arrows, *Arthroscopy* 16E:1-4, 2000.

75. Tingstad EM, Teitz CC, Simonian PT: Complications associated with the use of meniscal arrows, *Am J Sports Med* 29:96-98, 2001.

76. Austin KS, Sherman OH: Complications of arthroscopic meniscal repair, *Am J Sports Med* 21:864-868, 1993.

77. Stone RG, Miller GA: A technique of arthroscopic suture of torn menisci, *Arthroscopy* 1:226-232, 1985.

78. Wilbourn AJ: Iatrogenic disorders. Iatrogenic nerve injuries, *Neurol Clin* 16:55-82, 1998.

79. Barber FA: Meniscus repair. Results of an arthroscopic technique, *Arthroscopy* 3:25-30, 1987.

80. Stone RG, VanWinkle GN: Arthroscopic review of meniscal repair. Assessment of healing parameters, *Arthroscopy* 2:77-81, 1986.

81. DeHaven KE, Black KP, Griffiths HJ: Open meniscus repair, *Am J Sports Med* 17:788-795, 1989.

82. Seddon HJ: Three types of nerve injury, *Brain* 66:237-288, 1943.

83. Garrett JC: Meniscal transplantation. A review of 43 cases with 2-7 year follow-up, *Sports Med Arthrosc Rev* 1:164-167, 1993.

84. van Arkel ERA, de Boer HH: Human meniscal transplantation. Preliminary results at 2- to 5-year follow-up, *J Bone Joint Surg* 77B:589-595, 1995.

85. Holden DL, James SL, Larson RL, et al: Proximal tibial osteotomy in patients who are fifty years old or less. A long-term follow-up study, *J Bone Joint Surg* 70A:977-982, 1988.

86. Nemzek JA, Arnoczky SA, Swenson CL: Retroviral transmission by the transplantation of connective-tissue allografts, *J Bone Joint Surg* 76A:1036-1041, 1994.

87. Buck BE, Malinin TI, Brown MD: Bone transplantation and human immunodeficiency virus. An estimate of risk of acquired immunodeficiency syndrome (AIDS), *Clin Orthop* 240:129-136, 1989.

88. Shaffer B, Kennedy S, Klimkiewicz J, Yao L: Preoperative sizing of meniscal allografts in meniscus transplantation, *Am J Sports Med* 28:524-533, 2000.

89. Shelton WR, Dukes AD: Meniscus replacement with bone anchors. A surgical technique, *Arthroscopy* 10:324, 1994.

90. de Boer HH, Koudstaal J: Failed meniscus transplantation. A report of three cases, *Clin Orthop* 306:155-162, 1994.

91. Rodeo SA, Seneviratne A, Suzuki K, et al: Histological analysis of human meniscal allografts. A preliminary report, *J Bone Joint Surg* 82A:1071-1082, 2000.

92. Johnson DL, Bealle D: Meniscal allograft transplantation, *Clin Sports Med* 18:1-16, 1999.

93. Jones HP, Lemos MJ, Wilk RM, et al: Two-year follow-up of meniscal repair using a bioabsorbable arrow, *Arthroscopy* 18:64-69, 2002.

94. Oliverson TJ, Lintner DM: Biofix arrow appearing as a subcutaneous foreign body, *Arthroscopy* 16:652-655, 2000.

Rehabilitation after Articular Cartilage Repair: Chondroplasty, Abrasion Arthroplasty, and Microfracture

John T. Cavanaugh, MEd, PT/ATC
Nicholas A. Sgaglione, MD

ADVANCES IN THE UNDERSTANDING OF

structure and function of articular cartilage, as well as improved imaging and arthroscopic surgical techniques, have contributed to an evolution in guidelines for rehabilitation after articular cartilage repair.

Articular cartilage plays a critical role in the function of the musculoskeletal system by permitting nearly frictionless motion to occur between the articular surfaces of synovial joints.[1] The distinctive structure of articular cartilage allows for the withstanding of high compressive and shear loads during functional activities over a lifetime. Injury to the articular cartilage in the knee decreases mobility and frequently causes pain with movement and may progress to deformity and constant pain.[2]

Articular cartilage is avascular and aneural and therefore has a minimal potential to regenerate after injury.[3] Therefore the treatment of symptomatic articular cartilage lesions of the knee in active individuals remains a significant challenge for rehabilitation specialists and orthopedic surgeons alike. Nonsurgical treatment for many patients remains effective, particularly in the short term; however, recent advances in the surgical approach to knee chondral pathology, as well as a greater understanding of the long-term natural history of these lesions to go on to degenerative arthritis, has heightened the interest in surgical solutions to this problem.[4] Modern operative procedures can include: (1) arthroscopic debridement or chondroplasty, (2) marrow stimulation techniques including abrasion arthroplasty or microfracture procedures, (3) periosteal and perichondral grafting, (4) osteochondral autograft transplantation, and (5) autologous chondrocyte transplantation. In this chapter we will discuss the postoperative rehabilitation programs that follow these surgical procedures (chondroplasty, abrasion arthroplasty, and microfracture).

BASIC SCIENCE REVIEW

Articular cartilage lesions are challenging to treat, in part because of the distinctive structure and remarkable function of hyaline cartilage.[1,2,5,6] The unique architecture and ultrastructure is based on the complex interaction of water, chondrocytes, negatively charged matrix proteoglycan macromolecules or aggrecans, and type 2 collagen fibril meshwork. The extracellular matrix is synthesized and maintained by the chondrocytes. These metabolically active chondrocytes are distinctive in that they have a relatively low turnover rate and are sparsely dispersed within the surrounding matrix, maintaining minimal cell-to-cell contact. The interaction among the cells, collagen framework, aggrecans, and retained fluid is responsible for the complex biomechanical profile and superior loading characteristics of hyaline cartilage that make it difficult to replace or reproduce.[1,7]

Biomechanically, hyaline cartilage consists of two phases: a fluid phase composed of water and electrolytes, and a solid phase consisting of collagen, proteoglycans, and other glycoproteins.[8,9] Under compression, interstitial fluid flows out of the permeable collagen-proteoglycan matrix, and when the joint is unloaded, fluid flows back into the tissue. The low permeability of articular cartilage prevents fluid from being quickly compressed out of the matrix. This allows the fluid phase to shield the solid phase of articular cartilage from the deleterious effects of high impact-rapid loading.[8,10] The interaction between the solid and fluid phases also is responsible for carrying nutrients from the synovial fluid into the matrix and conveying metabolites away.[10] Joint movement also assists in articular cartilage nutrition in keeping synovial fluid viable.[11]

Mechanisms of articular cartilage breakdown involve multiple factors and imbalance between extracellular matrix degradation and synthesis.[12] Mechanisms can include direct trauma, indirect compressive impact loading, torsional loading, or shear mechanisms across the knee joint. Articular cartilage is also susceptible to abnormal unloading. If deprived of the mechanical stimulus of load, cartilage becomes less stiff and is more vulnerable to injury.[12,13] Secondary to its poor healing capacity, articular cartilage lesions may become problematic, resulting in pain, mechanical symptoms, and effusion, which can interfere with an individual's normal activities of daily living and participation in sports activity.

INCIDENCE

During the past few decades the recognition of acute lesions of the articular surfaces of the knee has increased as a result of the advances in arthroscopic surgery and magnetic resonance imaging (MRI). In a retrospective review of 31,516 knee arthroscopies, Curl and colleagues[14] noted a 63% incidence of hyaline cartilage lesions. Patients under age 40 with a single grade IV chondral lesion accounted for 4% (1277). Several studies[14-16] have demonstrated the medial femoral condyle to be the most common location for full-thickness focal chondral defects. Maffulli and colleagues[17] reported that at least one articular cartilage lesion was present at arthroscopy in 157 of 378 (41.5%) skeletally mature anterior cruciate–deficient patients. A meniscal tear was associated with a greater degree of articular damage. Oeppen and colleagues[18] studied the prevalence of injuries of the articular cartilage and subchondral bone after acute trauma in skeletally immature knees using high-resolution MRI. Their results demonstrated that chondral lesions were the most prevalent knee injury, followed by meniscal and anterior cruciate ligament injuries.

ASSESSMENT

Diagnosis of articular cartilage pathology can now be more precise through the use of noninvasive cartilage-specific MRI. Potter and co-workers[19] have shown a significant degree of accuracy using high-resolution modified echo time fast spin sequence techniques to evaluate and predict lesion site, size, and depth (Figure 20-1).

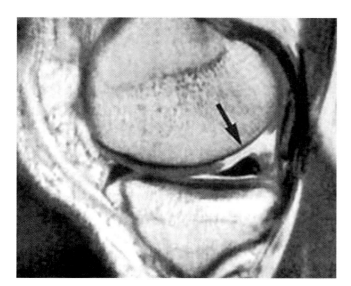

Figure 20-1: Magnetic resonance image of grade IV femoral condyle chondral defect.

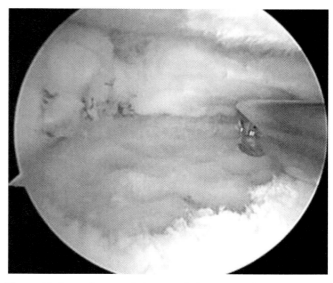

Figure 20-2: Arthroscopic image of abrasion arthroplasty.

Outerbridge[20] has developed a classification system whereby articular cartilage lesions are graded 0 to 4. Grade 0 is normal, grade 1 indicates softening, grade 2 indicates fibrillation, grade 3 indicates fissuring, and grade 4 indicates penetration to the depth of bone.

Grades 1 and 2 are considered partial lesions, whereas grades 3 and 4 are considered full-thickness lesions.

SURGICAL INTERVENTION

Arthroscopic joint debridement or chondroplasty is generally indicated for patients who have small articular cartilage lesions (<1 cm^2). Surgical technique involves arthroscopic debridement of the chondral surface in order to achieve a smooth stable surface. Concomitant procedures may include resection of meniscus, removal of loose bodies and osteophytes, partial synovectomy, or lavage. Jackson and colleagues[21] reported that 88% of 137 patients undergoing this procedure reported some initial improvement, but by 3 years only 68% maintained their satisfaction. In a retrospective review of 204 knees with osteoarthritis that were treated with arthroscopic debridement, Harwin[22] reported that 63% of the patients reported that their knees were better at a mean follow-up of 7.4 years. Analysis concluded that patients with minimal malalignment, ages <65 years, and no prior surgery achieved more favorable outcomes.

Several surgical techniques have been developed to improve on the results and longevity of debridement.[23-25] These techniques are directed toward bone marrow stimulation for a classic healing response to include a fibrin clot, blood and marrow cells, cytokines, growth factors, and vascular invasion for eventual differentiation into a fibrocartilage repair.[26,27] In 1959 Pridie[23] was the first to describe

drilling of denuded areas of articular cartilage to evoke such a response.

Advances in arthroscopic surgery led Johnson[24] in 1986 to introduce an abrasion arthroplasty procedure. Abrasion arthroplasty is performed by first debriding the damaged articular cartilage remnants and any fibrous tissue within the defect back to the demarcation of the surrounding healthier cartilage to allow clot binding to the edges of the normal remaining cartilage. The surface of the exposed subchondral bone is then abraded with an arthroscopic burr to create a bleeding bony surface (Figure 20-2). Clinical results have been varied.[28-31] In a study of almost 400 patients with an average age of 60 years, Johnson[28] reported that only 12% were asymptomatic, whereas 66% continued to experience pain. Bert and Maschka[29] in a retrospective study of 126 patients with an average follow-up of 5 years compared abrasion arthroplasty with debridement alone. The abrasion group reported results of 51% good to excellent, 16% fair, and 33% poor. The debridement-alone group reported results of 66% good to excellent, 13% fair, and 21% poor. Outcomes when abrasion arthroplasty is used appear to be better in younger patients.[29-31]

MICROFRACTURE

More recently, Steadman and colleagues[25] introduced the technique of microfracture chondroplasty. Indications for this procedure most commonly include a full-thickness articular cartilage lesion on either a weight-bearing surface (femur or tibia) or a contact lesion on either the patella or trochlear surfaces of the patellofemoral joint.[25,32,33] Other indications include unstable cartilage overlying subchondral bone and degenerative changes in knees that present with normal axial

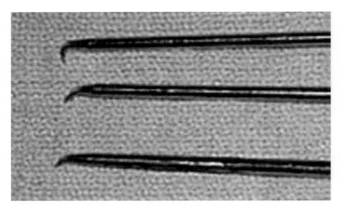

Figure 20-3: Microfracture arthroscopic awls.

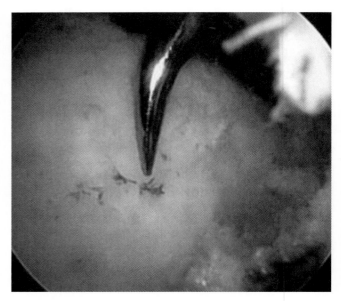

Figure 20-4: Microfracture technique of subchondral bone perforation.

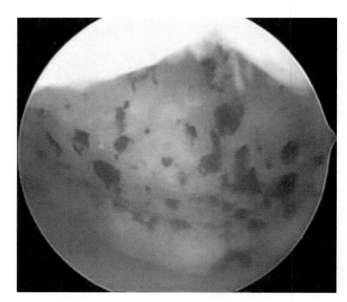

Figure 20-5: Postmicrofracture marrow stimulation and bleeding.

alignment. Age and activity level should also be considered for optimal outcome. Contraindications to this procedure include axial malalignment, low rehabilitation potential, partial thickness defects, any systemic immune-mediated disease, disease-induced arthritis, or cartilage disease.[34] The surgical procedure begins with an arthroscopic assessment of the articular cartilage defect. A debridement of the base of the defect is then performed to fully expose the subchondral bone with a standard arthroscopic shaver or a curved curette. Any unstable cartilage is removed, particularly the calcified cartilage layer, and a stable perimeter boundary is defined. The walls of the perimeter of the defect should be perpendicular to the subchondral plate so that the marrow elements to follow will be optimally contained within the defect.[35] Arthroscopic angled awls are then used to make multiple perforations, or microfractures, in the exposed subchondral plate. These awls produce essentially no thermal necrosis of the bone compared with hand-driven or motorized drills. The microfracture holes are approximately 3 to 5 mm apart and are typically made to a depth of 3 to 4 mm.[34,35] These perforations serve as an access channel for blood and mesenchymal stem cells from cancellous bone and the marrow cavity to migrate into the prepared defect, resulting in a reparative granulation superclot. The eventual goal of the procedure is to establish this superclot and have it proliferate and differentiate into a fibrous or fibrocartilage mosaic repair tissue (Figures 20-3 to 20-5).[7,34] Outcomes after microfracture surgery have been favorable.[36-38] Passler[36] in 2000 reported that 78% of the 162 patients on whom he performed a microfracture procedure had less pain at a mean follow-up of 4.4 years than before surgery. Steadman and colleagues[37] reported on a series of 72 patients with an average follow-up of 11.3 years who underwent the microfracture procedure for full-thickness chondral defects, without associated meniscus or ligament pathology. These patients indicated that they had less pain and reported statistically significant improvement in function. Recently in a prospective study Gobbi and colleagues[38] followed up on 53 athletes with an average age of 38 years who were treated with the microfracture technique.

At an average follow-up of 6 years, 70% reported decreased pain and swelling as well as having a normal hop test.

REHABILITATION PRINCIPLES

Rehabilitation of the patient after an articular cartilage procedure presents a challenging task for the rehabilitation specialist. The rehabilitative process is typically long, especially after microfracture or abrasion chondroplasty surgery.

Respect for the healing response is crucial. A progressive program for restoration of lower extremity range of motion (ROM), flexibility, strength, and proprioception is crucial to optimize the results of the surgery. In order to achieve an optimal outcome, certain principles should be adhered to (Box 20-1).

Communication with the Surgeon

Ascertain the size and location of the articular cartilage lesion, as this information will have a direct impact on the rehabilitation program. The rehabilitation specialist will then avoid any exercises or activities that could hinder the healing process by producing a shear and/or compressive force. Femoral condyle lesions are commonly found in the area that contacts the tibia at between 30 and 70 degrees of flexion.[39] A rehabilitation guideline after surgery to address a lesion in this area will differ from a program designed for lesions on a non–weight-bearing femoral surface or patellofemoral defect. The rehabilitation specialist should also look to the surgeon for the direction of the rehabilitation program—that is, weight-bearing progression, ROM limitations, criteria for return to sport. Patient progress and symptoms should also be conveyed, as these findings will directly affect the progression and direction of the rehabilitation program.

Evidence-Based Practice

Therapeutic interventions previously anecdotal have evolved into treatment with sound biomechanical foundations. Many treatment strategies used today, however, remain theoretic. Continued research and outcome studies are needed to substantiate treatment rationale.

Maintenance of a Safe Environment

After an articular cartilage procedure, the rehabilitation program is designed to promote the ideal physical environment in which an articular cartilage lesion can heal. The rehabilitation specialist needs to apply a working knowledge of the function, structure, and biomechanics of articular cartilage into the rehabilitation program. This understanding,

combined with an appreciation of the forces induced on the articular surfaces of the knee joint during specific exercises and activities, will permit the clinician to protect and progress the patient toward an optimal outcome.

Examples of this principle include maintenance of weight-bearing status after a surgical procedure and limiting the arc of motion on a progressive resistance machine so as to not subject a healing articular cartilage site to shear or compressive force.

Criteria-Based Progression

Rehabilitation programs, particularly those after articular cartilage procedures, should follow a progression less structured than the "protocols" of yesteryear. Postoperative "guidelines" should be individualized to each patient. Surgical technique, size and location of the lesion, and physical condition of the patient should be considered. Subjective and objective findings demonstrated throughout the rehabilitative course should correlate to a progression that is criteria based. Each patient will progress at a different pace. A "cookbook" approach to treatment (protocol) can accelerate a program too quickly for the patient whose progress is delayed and can impede the patient who is progressing very well. Therefore, guidelines should incorporate flexible time frames in their progression, to allow the individual patient to meet certain criteria—for example, "Week 6 to 8: Discontinue crutches when nonantalgic gait is demonstrated" versus "Week 6: Discontinue crutches for ambulation." An essential component of a criteria-based progression of therapeutic exercise is that the progression be functional. Kegerreis[40] defined a functional progression as an ordered sequence of activities enabling the acquisition or reacquisition of skills required for the safe, effective performance of athletic endeavors. The patient should therefore master a simple activity before advancing to a more demanding activity. A typical functional progression for postoperative knee patients would be to first demonstrate quadriceps control by performing a straight leg raise without pain or an extensor lag followed by the ability to ambulate with a normal gait pattern without deviations. As ROM and muscle strength continue to improve, the patient should demonstrate the ability to ascend stairs, followed by the ability to descend stairs. Having met set criteria with the additional evidence of improved flexibility and balance, the patient would then initiate a running program followed by agility-related, plyometric, and sport-specific activities.[41]

Continual reassessment of the patient is vital to ensure a consistent and safe treatment progression. Therapeutic exercise programs often need to be modified based on daily evaluations. Too rapid a progression in therapy and/or normal functional activities of daily living will be demonstrated by increased effusion and pain. This is most likely related to muscular fatigue, which leaves the articular surfaces unprotected against compressive forces.

BOX 20-1
Rehabilitation Principles

Communication with the surgeon
Evidence-based practice
Maintenance of a safe environment
Criteria-based progression
Patient compliance

Patient Compliance

Just as the surgeon and rehabilitation specialist have important responsibilities, the patient plays an important role in the rehabilitative process as well. Rehabilitation after articular cartilage surgery is a long and tedious process. Muscular atrophy from preoperative disuse combined with an extensive limited weight-bearing period leads to significant strength deficits that can routinely take several months (6 to 12) to reestablish. The patient should adhere to the recommendations given by the surgeon and rehabilitation specialist. Compliance with prescribed home therapeutic exercises and activity modifications in daily routines is essential for consistent progress and progression. Given that there are 168 hours in a week, a patient may be under the supervision of a rehabilitation specialist only 2% of the time—three times per week for 1 hour per treatment session, for a total of only 3 hours per week (2%). This leaves the patient responsible for his or her own care for 165 hours per week (98%) (Figure 20-6).[41] A compliant patient, therefore, is imperative to a successful outcome.

POSTOPERATIVE REHABILITATION

Rehabilitation after Arthroscopic Joint Debridement or Chondroplasty

Postoperatively after arthroscopic debridement or chondroplasty of the knee, the patient is instructed to perform a postsurgical exercise program consisting of quadriceps setting, straight leg raising, and active-assisted ROM (AAROM) exercises (Figure 20-7). Cryotherapy application is encouraged to control postoperative pain and swelling. The patient is instructed to use crutches and to bear weight as tolerated. The patient is encouraged to limit the amount of ambulation for several days. Crutches may be discontinued on adequate demonstration of quadriceps control (ability to perform straight leg raise without a quadriceps lag), ROM 0 to 100 degrees, and a nonantalgic gait. Full ROM is expected to be attained by 8 weeks after the surgical procedure. The goals of the rehabilitation program that follow are to achieve full ROM and to maximize muscle strength and flexibility throughout the involved lower extremity so as to meet the demands of activities of daily living. The rehabilitation specialist should select therapeutic exercises that do not engage the articular cartilage lesion during the early stages of rehabilitation. Early strengthening strategies emphasize closed kinetic chain (CKC) exercises inside a protected arc of motion. Isolated quadriceps strengthening using isotonic and isokinetic training are included later in the rehabilitation program as a sufficient strength base is developed and symptoms allow. Careful attention is paid to surgically addressed patellofemoral lesions. Treatment should advance via a functional progression (as mentioned previously) based on achieved criteria. The rehabilitation guidelines for this procedure are detailed in Box 20-2.

Rehabilitation after Microfracture and Abrasion Chondroplasty Procedures

Phase I: Immediate Postoperative Phase (0 to 6 Weeks)

Maximum protection is provided during this first of four phases after a microfracture or abrasion chondroplasty procedure on the knee. A healing environment is established by limiting weight bearing to toe touch (<5 lb) with crutches for those patients with femoral or tibial focal lesions. For patients having undergone the procedure for a patellofemoral

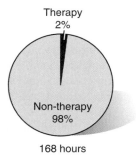

Figure 20-6: Diagram demonstrates the number of hours in a week (168 hours) and the percentage of time that a patient spends under rehabilitation supervision and the time spent away from therapy. *(Adapted from Cavanaugh JT: Rehabilitation for nonoperative and operative management of knee injuries. In: Callaghan J, Simonian P, Wickiewicz T, editors: The adult knee, Philadelphia, 2003, Lippincott, Williams & Wilkins.)*

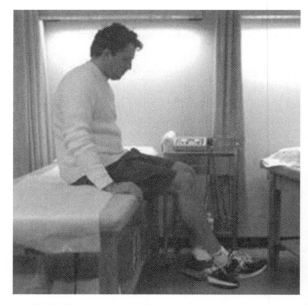

Figure 20-7: The patient performs active-assisted flexion and extension of the surgical knee using the contralateral extremity for support.

BOX 20-2

Arthroscopic Joint Debridement or Chondroplasty Rehabilitation Guidelines

Phase I: Immediate Postoperative Phase (Weeks 0-4)

Goals

Control postoperative pain and swelling

Achieve range of motion (ROM) 0 → 130 degrees

Restore normal gait

Prevent quadriceps inhibition

Normalize proximal musculature muscle strength

Achieve independence in home therapeutic exercise program

Precautions

Avoid ascending and descending stairs reciprocally until adequate quadriceps control and lower extremity alignment are demonstrated

Avoid pain with therapeutic exercise and functional activities

Treatment Strategies

Active-assistive ROM exercises (pain-free ROM)

Towel extensions

Patellar mobilization

Progressive weight bearing as tolerated; ambulation with crutches (discontinue [D/C] crutches when gait is nonantalgic)

Quadriceps reeducation (quadriceps sets with electrical muscle stimulation [EMS] or electromyography [EMG])

Multiple-angle quadriceps isometrics (bilaterally—submaximal) (tibiofemoral lesions)

Short crank ergometry → Standard ergometry

SLRs (all planes)

Leg presses 60- → 0-degree arc (avoid lesion)

Hip progressive-resisted exercises

Underwater treadmill system (gait training) if incision benign

Calf raises (bilateral)

Proprioception and balance training (bilateral) (proprioception board or balance systems)

Lower extremity flexibility exercises

Upper extremity cardiovascular exercises as tolerated

Cryotherapy

Home therapeutic exercise program: evaluation based

Emphasize patient compliance with home therapeutic exercise program and weight-bearing restrictions

Criteria for Advancement

ROM 0 → 130 degrees

Proximal muscle strength 5/5

Phase II: Intermediate Postoperative Phase (Weeks 4-8)

Goals

ROM 0 → within normal limits (WNL)

Normal patellar mobility

Ascend 8-inch stairs with good control without pain

Precautions

Avoid descending stairs reciprocally until adequate quadriceps control and lower extremity alignment are demonstrated

Avoid pain with therapeutic exercise and functional activities

Treatment Strategies

Active-assisted ROM (AAROM) exercises

Leg presses (pain-free arc)

Minisquats 60- → 0-degree arc (avoid lesion)

Retrograde treadmill ambulation

Proprioception and balance training: (bilateral → unilateral)

Proprioception board, contralateral Thera-Band exercises, balance systems

Initiate forward step-up program

StairMaster

SLRs (progressive resistance)

Hamstring curls, progression of proximal strengthening

Lower extremity flexibility exercises

Multiple-angle quadriceps isometrics (bilaterally—submaximal) (patellofemoral lesions—avoiding lesion)

Open kinetic chain (OKC) knee extension to 40 degrees (tibiofemoral lesions); closed kinetic chain (CKC) exercises preferred

Initiate forward step-down program

Home therapeutic exercise program: evaluation based

Criteria for Advancement

ROM 0 → WNL

Normal patellar mobility

(continued)

BOX 20-2
Arthroscopic Joint Debridement or Chondroplasty Rehabilitation Guidelines—cont'd

Demonstrate ability to ascend 8-inch step

Muscle strength 5/5 throughout involved lower extremity

Phase III: Advanced Strengthening Phase (Weeks 8-12)
Goals

Demonstrated ability to descend 8-inch stairs with good leg control without pain

85% limb symmetry on isokinetic testing (tibiofemoral lesions) and forward step-down test

Return to normal activities of daily living (ADL)

Improved lower extremity flexibility

Precautions

Avoid pain with therapeutic exercise and functional activities

Avoid running until strength development is adequate and physician has approved

Treatment Strategies

Progressive squat program (progressive resistive exercise [PRE]/pain-free arc)

Leg presses (emphasizing eccentrics)

OKC knee extensions (pain-free arc)

Isokinetic training (high velocities)

Advanced proprioception training (perturbations)

Elliptical trainer

Retrograde running

Lower-extremity stretching

Forward step-down test (NeuroCom)

Isokinetic testing

Initiation of forward running

Agility exercises (sport cord)

Home therapeutic exercise program: evaluation based

Criteria for Advancement

Ability to descend 8-inch stairs with good leg control without pain

85% limb symmetry on isokinetic testing (tibiofemoral lesions) and forward step-down test

Phase IV: Return to Activity Phase (Weeks 12-16)
Goals

Lack of apprehension with sport-specific movements

Strength and flexibility maximized to meet demands of individual's sport activity

Hop test >85% limb symmetry

Isokinetic testing (patellofemoral lesions) >85% limb symmetry

Precautions

Avoid pain with therapeutic exercise and functional activities

Avoid sport activity until strength development is adequate and physician has cleared

Treatment Strategies

Continue to advance lower extremity (LE) strengthening, flexibility, and agility programs

Advance forward running program

Begin plyometric program

Perform functional testing (hop test)

Perform isokinetic testing

Monitor patient's activity level and volume of therapeutic exercise

Reassess patient's complaints (e.g., pain or swelling daily); adjust program accordingly

Encourage compliance with home therapeutic exercise program

Home therapeutic exercise program: evaluation based

Criteria for Discharge

Hop test and isokinetic test (patellofemoral lesions) >85% limb symmetry

Lack of apprehension with sport-specific movements

Flexibility to acceptable levels for sport performance

Independence with gym program for maintenance and progression of therapeutic exercise program at discharge

defect, weight bearing is initiated at 50% and is then gradually progressed as tolerated. A double-upright knee brace is used. A femoral or tibial lesion is braced with the involved extremity in full extension. A patellofemoral lesion is braced allowing for a 0- to 20-degree ROM allowance. This is to prevent placing excessive shear force on the maturing marrow clot and to prevent flexion past the point at which the median ridge of the patella engages the trochlear groove.[34]

Mobilization of the surgical knee is encouraged immediately after the microfracture procedure, to achieve motion, diminish adhesion formation, and reduce pain. A goal of 0 to 120 degrees of knee motion or greater should be achieved by 6 weeks after microfracture. Research has supported early controlled motion after articular cartilage injury.[11,33,42,43] Controlled joint motion after articular cartilage injury may facilitate healing as long as shear forces are minimized.[43] Excessive shear loads therefore should be avoided during ROM activities while the knee joint is under compression. The use of continuous passive motion (CPM) and unloaded AAROM exercises are used as treatment strategies. CPM is applied immediately after surgery (Figure 20-8). ROM is begun in the 0- to 45-degree range and progressed as tolerated. Rodrigo and colleagues[33] concluded that CPM for 6 hours daily for 8 weeks after microfracture for full-thickness cartilage defects in the knee appears to result in better gross healing of the lesion when evaluated by arthroscopic visualization compared with the same treatment without CPM. In conjunction with the use of CPM, the patient is instructed to perform AAROM exercises several times per day. The achievement of full passive extension is a critical early goal of this first postoperative phase, as the development of a flexion contracture will result in gait abnormalities with resultant patellofemoral symptoms.[44-46] Towel extensions are performed as the patient sits or lies with a towel under the heel, allowing gravity to apply a low-load prolonged stretch into extension (Figure 20-9). The patient is instructed to perform this activity several times per day. It can be discontinued on achievement of full passive extension. Patellar

mobilization should be performed by the rehabilitation specialist to assist in reestablishing normal patellar mobility. Superior mobility of the patella is required for complete knee extension. Inferior glide mobility of the patella is necessary for full knee flexion.[47] The patient is educated to incorporate this activity into the daily home exercise program.

Muscle strengthening during this phase is initiated by having the patient perform isometric quadriceps setting exercises. Knee position should be close to full extension, as most articular cartilage lesions will not be engaged in this range. A submaximal effort is encouraged, and a rolled towel can be used for feedback and comfort. If a patient has difficulty eliciting a quadriceps contraction, a biofeedback unit or an electrical muscle stimulator can be used in conjunction with the quadriceps setting exercise to better facilitate quadriceps reeducation (Figure 20-10).

As ROM improves, multiple angle quadriceps isometric exercises may be added later in this phase. The rehabilitation specialist should be careful to avoid angles that directly

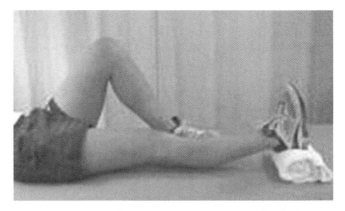

Figure 20-9: Passive knee extension using a towel rolled up under heel to promote early full extension.

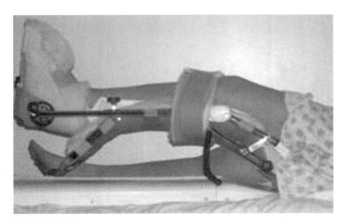

Figure 20-8: Continuous passive motion (CPM) machine is applied immediately after surgery.

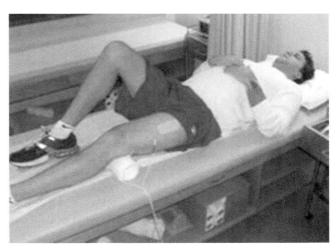

Figure 20-10: Quadriceps reeducation using an electrical stimulation device.

engage the articular cartilage lesion addressed during surgery. This understanding is especially important during this exercise for patients having undergone a patellofemoral microfracture procedure. Multiple plane straight leg raises are begun during this phase and progressed via a progressive-resistance approach. Proximal strengthening may also be facilitated by the use of progressive resistive exercise (PRE) equipment (Figure 20-11).

As knee ROM approaches 85 degrees, stationary bicycling can be performed by using a short crank (90 mm) ergometer.[48] As knee flexion improves to 110 to 115 degrees, a standard ergometer can be employed. Deep water exercises including use of a kick board and a flotation vest for deep water running may be initiated at 2 to 3 weeks after surgery as quadriceps muscle control and ROM improvement are demonstrated.

Flexibility exercises for calf and hamstring musculature are integrated into the therapeutic exercise program. Cryotherapy and transcutaneous electrical neuromuscular stimulation (TENS) may be used for pain control. Home therapeutic exercise programs are continually updated. Uniform compliance is strongly encouraged.

Phase II: Intermediate Postoperative Phase (Postoperative Weeks 6 to 12)

Phase II of the postoperative rehabilitation program after microfracture or abrasion chondroplasty is dedicated to the restoration of normal ROM and gait.

As quadriceps control is demonstrated (SLR without pain or lag), the double-upright knee brace is discontinued and the patient is placed in a patella sleeve for activities of daily living. For patients with patellofemoral lesions, the postoperative brace is opened gradually before it is discontinued. For patients with an excessive varus or valgus malalignment an unloader brace is prescribed.

Weight-bearing progression may vary as the size, location, and nature of the lesion may dictate a more or less aggressive treatment strategy. Typically at 6 weeks after surgery fibrocartilage should have begun to fill in the articular defect, and a progressive weight-bearing period is inaugurated. A computerized force plate system is used to assist the patient in the gradual loading of the involved extremity (Figure 20-12). During this activity the patient gradually loads the involved limb to the prescribed percentage of body weight, receiving visual feedback. This awareness is carried over into the progressive weight-bearing component of gait training during this phase. Treatment strategies using an underwater treadmill (Figure 20-13) and/or a deweighting system (Figure 20-14) are therapeutic as load is gradually introduced to the healing lesion. Walking in chest-deep water results in a 60% to 75% reduction in weight bearing, whereas walking in waist-deep water results in a 40% to 50% reduction in weight bearing.[49,50] Crutches are discontinued as a normal gait pattern without deviations is established. Patients should be treated individually during this progression. Demonstration of a normal gait pattern can take several weeks to achieve.

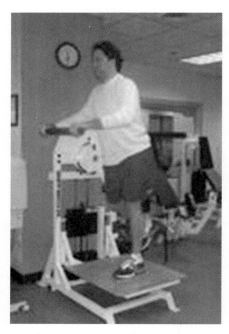

Figure 20-11: Hip extensor strengthening using progressive resistive exercise equipment.

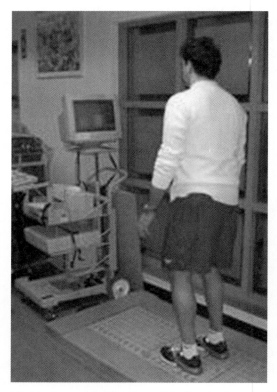

Figure 20-12: Progressive loading of the involved extremity is performed using the NeuroCom Balance Master (NeuroCom International, Clackamas, OR).

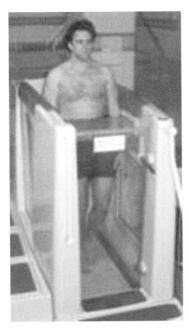

Figure 20-13: Gait training using an underwater treadmill system.

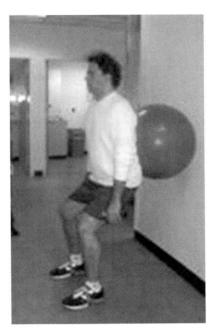

Figure 20-15: Minisquats inside a 45- to 0-degree arc of motion using a Physioball for support.

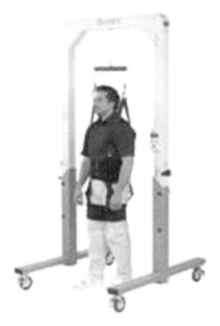

Figure 20-14: Biodex Unweighing System (Biodex, Inc., Shirley, NY).

AAROM exercises are progressed to tolerance, avoiding pain with the goal of achieving full ROM by 12 weeks postoperatively.

Strength development is crucial in promoting a safe progression and optimal functional outcome. A strong muscle-tendon unit may dissipate compressive force and absorb shock from the articular surface. The rehabilitation specialist is to avoid exercises that induce shear in conjunction with compression forces in the range in which the healing defect is articulating with the opposing joint surface.

The understanding of specific compressive and shear forces induced on articular cartilage during common therapeutic strengthening exercises is limited. Research does, however, support using a combination of open kinetic chain (OKC) and CKC strengthening exercises in ranges that do not high-load lesion site(s).[51-55] During OKC knee extension, an arc of motion from 60 to 90 degrees appears to provide the greatest amount of compressive loading at the knee joint, whereas the greatest amount of shear appears in the 40- to 0-degree range.[55] During CKC exercises a 60- to 100-degree arc of motion appears to produce the greatest amount of shear and compression.[51,55] Palmitier and colleagues,[53] in a biomechanical model of the lower extremity, demonstrated reduced tibiofemoral shear force when a compressive force is applied to the knee joint. Therefore an emphasis on CKC activities is used for muscle strengthening during this phase. A leg press is used inside a 60- to 0-degree arc of motion. A high-repetition, low-load approach is used during this phase, using bilateral lower extremities. ROM and weight are gradually increased. Minisquats inside a 45- to 0-degree range are added using a Physioball for proper technique (Figure 20-15). A PRE approach is gradually incorporated. Using a medial or lateral wedge under the involved extremity during the squatting exercise may protect the healing defect by creating a valgus or varus moment at the knee joint, thereby unloading the involved compartment from compressive force. A graduated forward step-up program is introduced, beginning with a 4-inch step height and progressing to an 8-inch step height.

OKC knee extension exercise is used judiciously during this phase, avoiding engagement of the articular cartilage lesion. Escamilla and colleagues have demonstrated that OKC extension exercise produces significantly greater patellofemoral forces than CKC activities at knee angles less than 57 degrees.[51] For patients having undergone microfracture procedure for patellofemoral lesions, OKC knee extensions are withheld from the program until 3 months postoperatively.

Proprioceptive and balance training is initiated as soon as the patient demonstrates the ability to bear 50% weight. A rocker board in sagittal and coronal planes, maintaining even weight distribution, is initiated, advancing to dynamic stabilization activity on a balance system (Figure 20-16). As strength and balance demonstrate improvement, the patient is advanced to unilateral balance and strengthening by performing contralateral elastic band exercises (Figure 20-17).

Retrograde treadmill ambulation on progressive percentage inclines is used to facilitate quadriceps strengthening[56] (Figure 20-18).

Flexibility exercises throughout the involved lower extremity are continued. The addition of quadriceps stretching is added as knee ROM demonstrates improvement (Figure 20-19).

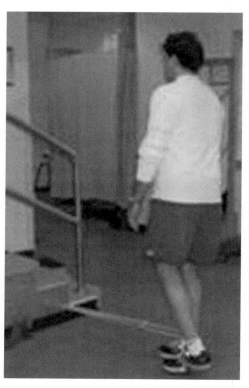

Figure 20-17: Contralateral elastic band exercise. The patient stands and balances on the involved extremity as the noninvolved extremity performs movement in the frontal plane.

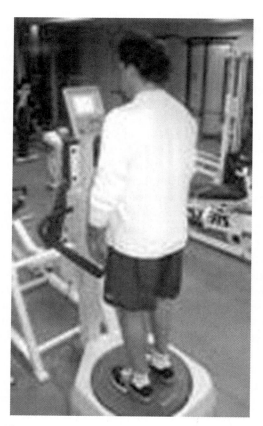

Figure 20-16: Dynamic stabilization training using Biodex Balance System (Biodex, Inc., Shirley, NY).

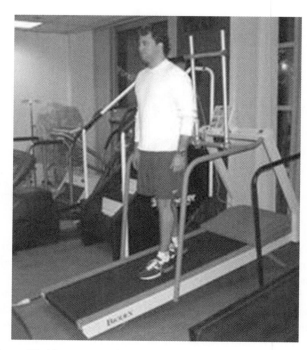

Figure 20-18: Retrograde treadmill ambulation on an incline.

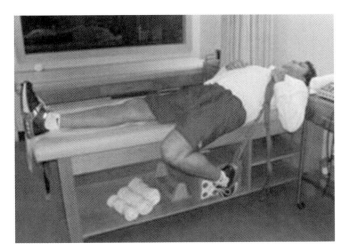

Figure 20-19: Quadriceps stretching.

Phase III: Advanced Strengthening Phase (Postoperative Weeks 12 to 18)

The third postoperative phase after microfracture or abrasion arthroplasty surgery is dedicated toward the restoration of the strength required for normal functional activities.

Treatment strategies initiated in the previous phase are advanced. Closed chain activities are now performed through a greater ROM (e.g., leg presses and squatting 0 to 80 degrees) A step-down program is begun, starting with a 4-inch step and progressing to an 8-inch step as symptoms allow. Quality and control of lower extremity movement are monitored before advancement. OKC knee extension exercise is added in a ROM that does not engage the lesion site. Signs of pain and/or crepitus are closely monitored. A 90- to 40-degree arc of motion is used initially, progressing to full arc exercise. For patients having undergone a patellofemoral articular cartilage procedure, this exercise is supervised very closely. Hamstring curls (PRE) are introduced, and proximal strengthening is progressed.

Balance and proprioception activities are progressed to include activities on multiplane support surfaces (e.g., foam rollers, rocker boards) (Figure 20-20) and perturbation training.

As strength development is demonstrated by involved lower extremity control during a step-down exercise, impact is introduced to the program by progressing retrograde walking to retrograde running for 30 to 60 seconds based on patient feedback on a treadmill. A greater emphasis is placed on lower extremity flexibility exercises in this phase, as advanced functional activities are soon to follow.

At 4 months after surgery, strength is assessed using a functional forward step-down test[57] (Figure 20-21) and an isokinetic test. Test speeds of 180 and 300 degrees/second are selected for the isokinetic test, as these velocities have been shown to produce less compressive and shear forces than slower speeds.[58,59] The goal for both tests is 85% limb symmetry.

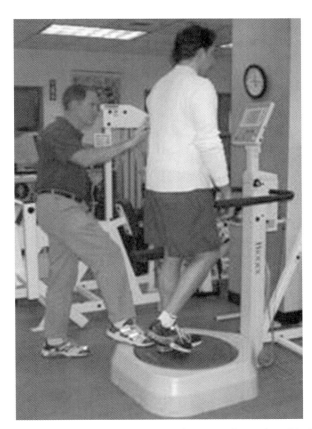

Figure 20-20: Perturbation training being performed on Biodex Balance System.

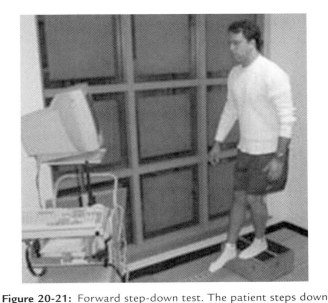

Figure 20-21: Forward step-down test. The patient steps down an 8-inch step onto a forceplate (NeuroCom Balance Master System) as slowly and in as controlled a manner as possible on each leg. Three trials are recorded. Mean impact and limb symmetry scores are calculated. Lower extremity control is observed for deviations. Normative data have established a mean impact of 10% body weight and limb symmetry of 85%.

The patient's individual goals are considered in the further direction of the rehabilitation program. If full ROM and a satisfactory strength assessment have been achieved, the patient is discharged from formal rehabilitation to a gym and home program. Should the patient's aspirations include a return to sport activity, participation in the last phase of rehabilitation is recommended.

Phase IV: Return Activity Phase (Postoperative Week 18+)

This final phase of rehabilitation after microfracture or abrasion chondroplasty surgery is geared toward preparing the patient-athlete for the return to individual sporting activities. As strength (functional and isokinetic) proves better than or equal to an 85% limb symmetry, a forward running program is initiated on a treadmill. Short distances, with speed development, rather than longer, slower distance running are emphasized. Plyometric activities are added specific to the individual patient's desired sport. Advanced neuromuscular training activities to include deceleration and cutting maneuvers are added to simulate game or practice conditions. Single-leg hop test and cross-over hop tests are administered with the goal of achieving an 85% limb symmetry score.[60,61] Apprehension during functional sport-specific movements and testing are closely monitored. These observations, along with any other pertinent clinical findings, are presented to the referring orthopedic surgeon for the final determination with regard to a return to sports. The rehabilitation guidelines for these procedures are detailed in Box 20-3.

BOX 20-3
Microfracture and Abrasion Chondroplasty Procedures—Rehabilitation Guidelines

Phase I: Immediate Postoperative Phase (Weeks 0-6)

Goals

Control postoperative pain and swelling

Range of motion (ROM) 0 → 120 degrees

Prevent quadriceps inhibition

Normalize proximal musculature muscle strength

Achieve independence in home therapeutic exercise program

Precautions

Maintain weight-bearing restrictions: postoperative brace locked at 0 degrees, 0 → 20 degrees for patellofemoral lesion

Avoid neglect of ROM exercises

Treatment Strategies

Continuous passive motion (CPM)

Active-assistive ROM exercises (AAROM) (pain-free ROM)

Towel extensions

Patellar mobilization

Toe-touch weight bearing with brace locked at 0 degrees with crutches

Partial weight bearing progressing to weight bearing as tolerated, brace 0 → 20 degrees for patellofemoral lesions

Quadriceps reeducation (quadriceps sets with electrical muscle stimulation [EMS] or electromyography [EMG])

Multiple-angle quadriceps isometrics (bilaterally—submaximal) (tibiofemoral lesions)

Short crank ergometry → standard ergometry

Straight leg raises (SLRs) (all planes)

Hip progressive resistive exercises

Pool exercises

Plantar flexion Thera-Band

Lower extremity flexibility exercises

Upper extremity cardiovascular exercises as tolerated

Cryotherapy

Home therapeutic exercise program: evaluation based

Emphasize patient compliance with home therapeutic exercise program and weight-bearing restrictions

Criteria for Advancement

Physician direction for progressive weight bearing (week 6)

ROM 0 → 120 degrees

Proximal muscle strength 5/5

SLR (supine) without extension lag

Phase II: Intermediate Postoperative Phase (Weeks 6-12)

Goals

ROM 0 → within normal limits (WNL)

Normal patellar mobility

Restoration of normal gait

Ascension of 8-inch stairs with good control without pain

(continued)

BOX 20-3
Microfracture and Abrasion Chondroplasty Procedures—Rehabilitation Guidelines—cont'd

Precautions

Avoid descending stairs reciprocally until adequate quadriceps control and lower extremity alignment are demonstrated

Avoid pain with therapeutic exercise and functional activities

Treatment Strategies

Progressive weight bearing and gait training with crutches

Discontinue (D/C) crutches when gait is nonantalgic

Postoperative brace discontinued as good quadriceps control (ability to perform SLR without lag or pain) is demonstrated

Unloader brace or patella sleeve per physician preference

Computerized forceplate (NeuroCom) for weight-bearing progression and patient education

Underwater treadmill system (gait training) if incision benign

Gait unloader device

AAROM exercises

Leg presses (60- → 0-degree arc)

Minisquats and weight shifts

Calf raises (bilateral)

Retrograde treadmill ambulation

Proprioception and balance training: proprioception board, contralateral Thera-Band exercises, balance systems

Initiate forward step-up program

Stairmaster

SLRs (progressive resistance)

Lower extremity flexibility exercises

Open kinetic chain (OKC) knee extension to 40 degrees (tibiofemoral lesions); closed kinetic chain (CKC) exercises preferred

Home therapeutic exercise program: evaluation based

Criteria for Advancement

ROM 0 degrees → WNL

Normal patellar mobility

Normal gait pattern

Demonstrate ability to ascend 8-inch step

Phase III: Advanced Strengthening Phase (Weeks 12-18)

Goals

Demonstrate ability to descend 8-inch stairs with good leg control without pain

85% limb symmetry on isokinetic testing (tibiofemoral lesions) and forward step-down test

Return to normal activities of daily living (ADLs)

Improve lower extremity flexibility

Precautions

Avoid pain with therapeutic exercise and functional activities

Avoid running until strength development is adequate and physician has cleared

Treatment Strategies

Progress squat program

Initiate step-down program

Leg presses (emphasizing eccentrics)

OKC knee extensions 90 → 40 degrees (CKC exercises preferred)

Advanced proprioception training (perturbations)

Agility exercises (sport cord)

Elliptical trainer

Retrograde treadmill ambulation and running

Hamstring curls and proximal strengthening

Lower extremity stretching

Forward step down test (NeuroCom) at 4 months

Isokinetic testing at 4 months

Home therapeutic exercise program: evaluation based

Criteria for Advancement

Ability to descend 8-inch stairs with good leg control without pain

85% limb symmetry on isokinetic testing (tibiofemoral lesions) and forward step-down test

Phase IV: Return to Activity Phase (Week 18+)

Goals

Lack of apprehension with sport-specific movements

Maximize strength and flexibility as to meet demands of individual's sport activity

(continued)

SUMMARY

The knowledge of the response of articular cartilage to loading and to mechanical stress continues to evolve. The rehabilitation specialist needs to keep current with the advances being made in the areas of basic science, imaging, and orthopedic surgery to achieve favorable outcomes. Rehabilitation after articular cartilage surgery can be a lengthy process. The clinician should make every attempt to make the rehabilitation process interesting by being aggressive where appropriate and adding new activities when warranted to the rehabilitation program. Care must be given to avoid exercises or activities that provide excessive shear stress while the knee joint is under compression. This is particularly critical during the early stages of rehabilitation. Criteria should be used in order to ensure a safe, progressive advancement through the rehabilitative course. Communication between the referring orthopedic surgeon and the rehabilitation specialist is crucial not only in the early stages of postoperative rehabilitation but throughout the successive phases as well. Last, but most important, the patient must be an active participant in the rehabilitation program.

References

1. Buckwalter JA, Mankin HJ: Articular cartilage I. Tissue design and chondrocyte-matrix interactions, *J Bone Joint Surg* 79A:600-611, 1997.

2. Buckwalter JA, Mankin HJ: Articular cartilage II. Degeneration and osteoarthritis, repair, regeneration and transplantation, *J Bone Joint Surg* 79A:612-632, 1997.

3. Mankin HJ: The response of articular cartilage to mechanical injury, *J Bone Joint Surg* 64A:460-466, 1982.

4. Messner K: The long-term prognosis for severe damage to weight-bearing cartilage in the knee. A 14-year clinical and radiographic follow-up in 28 young athletes, *Acta Orthop Scand* 67:165-168,1996.

5. O'Driscoll S: The healing and regeneration of articular cartilage, *J Bone Joint Surg* 80A:1795-1807, 1998.

6. Newman AP: Articular cartilage, *Am J Sports Med* 2:309-324, 1998.

7. Sgaglione NA, Miniaci A, Gillogly SD, et al: Update on advanced surgical techniques in the treatment of traumatic focal articular cartilage lesions in the knee, *Arthroscopy* 18(suppl 2):9-32, 2002.

8. Mow VC, Ateshian GA, Ratcliffe A: Anatomic form and biomechanical properties of articular cartilage of the knee joint. In Finerman GAM, Noyes FR, editors: *Biology and biomechanics of the traumatized synovial joint: the knee as a model.* Rosemont, IL, 1992, American Academy of Orthopaedic Surgeons (AAOS).

9. Mow VC, Holmes MH, Lai WM, et al: Fluid transport and mechanical properties of articular cartilage: a review, *J Biomech* 17:377-394, 1984.

10. Mow VC, Rosenwasser M: Articular cartilage: biomechanics. In Woo SL-Y, Buckwalter JA, editors: *Injury and repair of the musculoskeletal soft tissues.* Park Ridge, IL, 1988, AAOS.

11. Buckwalter JA: Effects of early motion on healing of musculoskeletal tissues, *Hand Clin* 12:13-24, 1996.

BOX 20-3

Microfracture and Abrasion Chondroplasty Procedures—Rehabilitation Guidelines—cont'd

Hop test >85% limb symmetry

85% limb symmetry on isokinetic testing (patellofemoral lesions)

Precautions

Avoid pain with therapeutic exercise and functional activities

Avoid sport activity until strength development is adequate and physician has cleared

Treatment Strategies

Continue to advance LE strengthening, flexibility, and agility programs

Forward running

Plyometric program

Brace for sport activity (physician's preference)

Monitor patient's activity level throughout course of rehabilitation

Reassess patient's complaints (e.g., pain and swelling daily); adjust program accordingly

Encourage compliance with home therapeutic exercise program

Functional testing (hop test)

Isokinetic testing

Home therapeutic exercise program: evaluation based

Criteria for Discharge

Hop test >85% limb symmetry

85% limb symmetry on isokinetic testing (patellofemoral lesions)

Lack of apprehension with sport-specific movements

Flexibility to acceptable levels for sport performance

Independence with gym program for maintenance and progression of therapeutic exercise program at discharge

12. Walker JM: Pathomechanics and classification of cartilage lesions, facilitation of repair, *J Orthop Sports Phys Ther* 28:216-231, 1998.

13. Palmoski MJ, Colyer RA, Brandt KD: Joint motion in the absence of normal loading does not maintain normal articular cartilage, *Arthritis Rheum* 23:325-334, 1980.

14. Curl WW, Krome J, Gordon ES, et al: Cartilage injuries: a review of 31,516 knee arthroscopies, *Arthroscopy* 13:456-60, 1997.

15. Hjelle K, Ausigulen O, Muri R, et al: Full-thickness chondral defects: a prospective study of 1000 knee arthroscopies. Paper presented at Third International Cartilage Repair Society Symposium, Gothenburg, Sweden, April 27-29, 2000.

16. Terry GC, Flandry F, Van Manen JW, et al: Isolated chondral fractures of the knee, *Clin Orthop* 234:170-177, 1988.

17. Maffulli N, Binfield PM, King JB: Articular cartilage lesions in the symptomatic anterior cruciate ligament-deficient knee, *Arthroscopy* 19:685-690, 2003.

18. Oeppen RS, Connolly SA, Bencardino JT, et al: Acute injury of the articular cartilage and subchondral bone: a common but unrecognized lesion in the immature knee, *Am J Roentgenol* 182:111-117, 2004.

19. Potter HG, Linklater JM, Allen AA, et al: Magnetic resonance imaging of articular cartilage in the knee. An evaluation with use of fast-spin-echo imaging, *J Bone Joint Surg Am* 80:1276-1284, 1998.

20. Outerbridge RE: The etiology of chondromalacea patellae, *J Bone Joint Surg* 43B:752-767, 1961.

21. Jackson R, Marans H, Silver R: Arthroscopic treatment of degenerative arthritis of the knee, *J Bone Joint Surg* 70B:332, 1988 (abstract).

22. Harwin SF: Arthroscopic debridement for osteoarthritis of the knee: predictors of patient satisfaction, *Arthroscopy* 15:142-146, 1999.

23. Pridie AH: The method of resurfacing osteoarthritic joints, *J Bone Joint Surg* 41B:618-623, 1959.

24. Johnson L: Arthroscopic abrasion arthroplasty historical and pathologic perspective: present status, *Arthroscopy* 2:54-69, 1986.

25. Steadman JR, Rodkey WG, Singleton SB, et al: Microfracture technique for full-thickness chondral defects: technique and clinical results, *Oper Tech Orthop* 7:300-304, 1997.

26. Shapiro F, Koide S, Glimcher MJ: Cell origin and differentiation in the repair of full-thickness defects of articular cartilage, *J Bone Joint Surg* 75A:532-553, 1993.

27. Gillogly SD, Voight M, Blackburn T: Treatment of articular cartilage defects of the knee with autologous chondrocyte implantation, *J Orthop Sports Phys Ther* 28:241-251, 1998.

28. Johnson L: Arthroscopic abrasion arthroplasty. In McGinty JB, editor: *Operative arthroscopy*, New York, 1991, Raven Press.

29. Bert J, Maschka K: The arthroscopic treatment of unicompartmental gonarthrosis: a five year follow-up study with abrasion arthroplasty plus arthroscopic debridement and arthroscopic debridement alone, *Arthroplasty* 5:25-32, 1989.

30. Friedman M, Berasi C, et al: Preliminary results with abrasion arthroplasty in the osteoarthritic knee, *Clin Orthop* 182:200-205, 1984.

31. Rand J: Role of arthroscopy in osteoarthritis of the knee, *Arthroscopy* 7:358-363, 1991.

32. Blevins FT, Steadman JR, Rodrigo JJ, et al: Treatment of articular cartilage defects in athletes: an analysis of functional outcome and lesion appearance, *Orthopedics* 21:761-768, 1998.

33. Rodrigo JJ, Steadman JR, Silliman JF, et al: Improvement of full-thickness chondral defect healing in the human knee after debridement and microfracture using continuous passive motion, *Am J Knee Surg* 7:109-116, 1994.

34. Steadman JR, Rodkey WG, Rodrigo JJ: Microfracture: surgical technique and rehabilitation to treat chondral defects [review], *Clin Orthop* Oct(391 suppl):S362-S69, 2001.

35. Wright JM, Millett PJ, Steadman JR: Osteochondral injury: acute management. In: Callahan J, Rosenberg AG, Rubash HE, et al, editors: *The adult knee,* Philadelphia, 2003, Lippincott Williams & Wilkins.

36. Passler HH: Microfracture for treatment of cartilage detects, *Zentralbl Chir* 125:500-504, 2000.

37. Steadman JR, Briggs K, Rodrigo J, et al: Outcomes of microfracture for traumatic chondral defects of the knee: average 11-year follow-up, *Arthroscopy* 19:477-484, 2003.

38. Gobbi A, Nunag P, Malinowski K: Treatment of full thickness chondral lesions of the knee with microfracture in a group of athletes, *Knee Surg Sports Traumatol Arthrosc* 13:213-221, 2005.

39. Rosenberg TD, Paulos LE, Parker RD, et al: The forty-five degree posteroanterior flexion weightbearing radiograph of the knee, *J Bone Joint Surg* 70A:1479-1483, 1988.

40. Kegerreis S: The construction and implementation of a functional progression as a component of athletic rehabilitation, *J Orthop Sports Phys Ther* 5(1):14-19, 1983.

41. Cavanaugh JT: Rehabilitation for nonoperative and operative management of knee injuries. In Callahan J, Rosenberg AG, Rubash HE, et al, editors: *The adult knee,* Philadelphia, 2003, Lippincott Williams & Wilkins.

42. Salter RB, Simmonds DF, Malcolm BW, et al: The biological effect of continuous passive motion on the healing of full-thickness defects in articular cartilage. An experimental investigation in the rabbit, *J Bone Joint Surg Am* 62:1232-1251, 1980.

43. Suh J, Aroen A, Mozzonigro T, et al: Injury and repair of articular cartilage: related scientific issues, *Oper Tech Orthop* 7:270-278, 1997.

44. Benum P: Operative mobilization of stiff knees after surgical treatment of knee injuries and posttraumatic conditions, *Acta Orthop Scand* 53:625-631, 1982.

45. Matsusue Y, Yamamuro T, Hama H: Arthroscopic multiple osteochondral transplantation to the chondral defect in the knee associated with anterior cruciate ligament disruption, *Arthroscopy* 9:318-321, 1993.

46. Perry J, Antonelli D, Ford W: Analysis of knee-joint forces during flexed-knee stance, *J Bone Joint Surg* 57A:961-967, 1975.

47. Fulkerson JP, Hungerford D: *Disorders of the patellofemoral joint,* ed 2, Baltimore, 1990, Lippincott Williams & Wilkins.

48. Schwartz RE, Asnis PD, Cavanaugh JT, et al: Short crank cycle ergometry, *J Orthop Sports Phys Ther* 13:95, 1991.

49. Bates A, Hanson N: The principles and properties of water. In *Aquatic Exercise Therapy*, Philadelphia, 1996, Saunders.

50. Harrison RA, Hilman M, Bulstrode S: Loading of the lower limb when walking partially immersed: implications for clinical practice, *Physiotherapy* 78:164, 1992.

51. Escamilla RF, Fleisig GS, Zheng N, et al: Biomechanics of the knee during closed kinetic chain and open kinetic chain exercises, *Med Sci Sports Exerc* 30:556-569, 1998.

52. Lutz GE, Palmitier RA, An KN, Chao EY: Comparison of tibiofemoral joint forces during open kinetic chain and closed kinetic chain exercises, *J Bone Joint Surgery* 75A:732-739, 1993.

53. Palmitier RA, An KN, Scott SG, Chao EYS: Kinetic chain exercises in knee rehabilitation, *Sports Med* 11:402-413, 1991.

54. Steinkamp LA, Dillingham MF, Markel MD, et al: Biomechanical considerations in patellofemoral joint rehabilitation, *Am J Sports Med* 21:438-444, 1993.

55. Wilk KE, Escamilla RF, Fleisig GS, et al: A comparison of tibiofemoral joint forces and electromyographic activity during open

and closed kinetic chain exercises, *Am J Sports Med* 24:518-527, 1996.

56. Cipriani DJ, Armstrong CW, Gaul S: Backward walking at three levels of treadmill inclination: an electromyographic and kinematic analysis, *J Orthop Sports Phys Ther* 22:95-102, 1995.

57. Cavanaugh JT, Stump TJ: Forward step down test, *J Orthop Sports Phys Ther* 30:A-46, 2000.

58. Nisell R, Ericson MO, Nemeth G, et al: Tibiofemoral joint forces during isokinetic knee extension, *Am J Sports Med* 17:49-54, 1989.

59. Kaufman KR, An KN, Litchy WJ, et al: Dynamic joint forces during knee isokinetic exercise, *Am J Sports Med* 19:305-316, 1991.

60. Daniel DM, Malcolm L, Stone ML, et al: Quantification of knee stability and function, *Contemp Orthop* 5:83-91, 1982.

61. Barber SD, Noyes FR, Mangine RE, et al: Quantitative assessment of functional limitations in normal and anterior cruciate ligament deficient knees, Clin Orthop 255:204-214, 1990.

Rehabilitation after Articular Cartilage Repair Procedures: Osteochondral Autograft Transplantation and Autologous Chondrocyte Implantation

Michael M. Reinold, DPT, ATC, CSCS

Leonard C. Macrina, MSPT, CSCS

Roger V. Ostrander, MD

E. Lyle Cain, MD

Jeffrey R. Dugas, MD

CHAPTER OUTLINE

ARTICULAR CARTILAGE DEFECTS OF

the knee are a common cause of pain and functional disability in orthopedics and sports medicine. The avascular nature of articular cartilage predisposes the individual to progressive symptoms and degeneration because of the extremely slowness of healing and often the inability to heal. Traditional methods of treating these lesions have led to unfavorable results, stimulating the need for newer surgical procedures designed to transplant cartilage, such as osteochondral grafting and chondrocyte implantation. Postoperative rehabilitation programs will vary greatly among patients and are individualized based on lesion specifics (size, depth, location, quality of tissue), patient specifics (age, activities, goals, quality of tissue), and surgical specifics (procedure, concomitant surgeries). These programs are designed based on knowledge of the basic science, anatomy, and biomechanics of articular cartilage as well as the natural course of healing after surgery. The goal is to restore full function in each patient as quickly as possible without overloading the healing articular cartilage. This chapter will briefly describe the basic science of articular cartilage, principles of articular cartilage rehabilitation, and the surgical procedures and rehabilitation guidelines for osteochondral autograft transplantations (OATs) and autologous chondrocyte implantation (ACI).

BASIC SCIENCE AND PATHOMECHANICS OF ARTICULAR CARTILAGE

Articular cartilage provides a low-friction, resilient, weight-bearing joint surface that helps to absorb mechanical shock by dampening the force to the underlying subchondral bone. Cartilage has truly unique features; however, no synthetic material to date has been able to duplicate these properties, facilitating the desire to repair or regenerate the patient's own articular cartilage. Cartilage has a coefficient of friction that is 15 times less than that of ice on ice even while supporting loads of several times body weight.[1] This coefficient of friction is an order of magnitude lower than that of any combination of synthetic materials.

Articular cartilage is composed of an extracellular matrix (ECM) with a small number of highly specialized cells known as *chondrocytes*. The formation and maintenance of cartilage depends on the chondrocytes, although they account for only approximately 10% of the cartilage by volume. Cartilage is an avascular tissue, and this lack of blood supply limits oxygen delivery to the chondrocytes. For this reason, chondrocytes rely principally on the anaerobic pathway for energy production.

Because chondrocytes occupy only a small proportion of the total volume of the tissue, cartilage composition is determined primarily by the matrix. Water is the most abundant component of the matrix, accounting for 65% to 80% of its wet weight. The water content of cartilage is not uniform and varies throughout the cartilage depth. It makes up 80% of the matrix at the cartilage surface and 65% in the deeper

zones. Two classes of structural macromolecules, collagen and proteoglycan, are the other two major matrix components. There are several other minor matrix molecules that combine to make up less than 5% of the cartilage wet weight. The function of many of these minor components has not been clearly established.

Cartilage has an affinity for water because of the hydrophilic (water-loving) nature of the proteoglycan molecules. Water rests in pores in the cartilage matrix that have a high resistance to water flow. This resistance to water flow and the resulting pressure generated during water movement allow cartilage to support very high joint loads. The flow of water also allows the transport of nutrients through the tissue to the chondrocytes through diffusion.

Collagen is the major structural macromolecule of the ECM, making up 50% of cartilage dry weight. Collagen is responsible for the tissue's tensile and shear properties. At least 20 distinct collagen types are found in nature. Types II, V, VI, IX, X, and XI are found in articular cartilage, but type II collagen predominates, representing 95% of the total collagen in cartilage. Collagen is composed of three polypeptide chains, or alpha chains, made up of repeating triplets of amino acid residues. Hydrogen bonds, the stabilizing force of the triple helix chains, are incredibly strong, resulting in tensile strength that is greater than that of steel wire across an equal cross section. Collagen fiber formation takes place within the chondrocyte and the surrounding matrix.

The final major component of the ECM is proteoglycan. Proteoglycans are complex macromolecules composed of a protein core and covalently bound glycosaminoglycan (GAG) chains. Three major types of GAG chains have been found in articular cartilage proteoglycans: chondroitin sulfate (types 4 and 6), keratin sulfate, and dermatan sulfate. Hyaluronic acid is an important component of proteoglycan molecules and the cartilage matrix—hence the use of hyaluronic acid injections for degenerative cartilage diseases (arthritis). Proteoglycan molecules have an affinity for water. The GAG chains have negatively charged carboxyl and sulfate groups that attract free–floating positive ions such as Na^+ and Ca^+. The presence of these ions results in an osmotic pressure effect, drawing in water. It is the presence of these negative charges and the attraction to water that accounts for the compressive qualities of cartilage. Cartilage is able to attract and hold large amounts of water (or swell) when loaded in compression.

Cartilage has a highly organized architecture, and its structure and composition vary throughout its depth. Cartilage has been divided into four zones (Figure 21-1). The superficial zone is made up of two components. The most superficial layer is an acellular, fine, fibrillar gliding surface known as the *lamina splendens*. Beneath the lamina splendens is a thin layer of flattened cells and collagen fibers oriented parallel to the cartilage surface. This zone has high collagen content and low proteoglycan content, which allows it to resist high shear stresses. The middle zone possesses larger, more rounded cells and large diameter, obliquely oriented

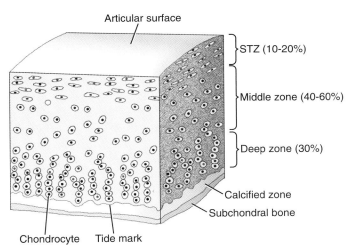

Articular surface

STZ (10-20%)

Middle zone (40-60%)

Deep zone (30%)

Calcified zone

Subchondral bone

Chondrocyte   Tide mark

Figure 21-1: The four histologic zones of cartilage. *STZ,* Superficial zone.

collagen fibers. The deep zone has large cells arranged in a columnar pattern perpendicular to the cartilage surface. This zone has the highest concentration of proteoglycan and the lowest water content. The collagen fibers are large and are oriented perpendicular to the joint surface. The calcified zone is the deepest zone and connects the hyaline cartilage to the underlying subchondral bone. It is composed of mineralized, calcified matrix as the cartilage connects to the subchondral bone layer.

Most tissues rely on a vascular supply for delivery of nutrients to cells. However, cartilage is an avascular tissue. The delivery of nutrients is achieved by the process of diffusion from synovial fluid. In immature cartilage the chondrocytes get nutrition by diffusion of substances from the permeable underlying subchondral bone as well as from the synovial fluid. In adult tissue, once the physeal plate has closed, the majority of nutrition comes from the synovial fluid. Animal studies have confirmed the importance of synovial fluid for chondrocyte health. If you deprive cartilage of synovial fluid (e.g., by immobilizing a joint), it will degenerate.[2-4]

The biomechanical properties of cartilage are best understood when the tissue is viewed as a biphasic material, composed of a solid phase and a fluid phase. The solid phase is made up of the structural molecules such as collagen and proteoglycan. The solid phase of the matrix is strong, fatigue resistant, and tough. However, it is also porous, somewhat permeable, and soft. The fluid phase is water, which resides in the microscopic pores of the matrix. It flows through the matrix by pressure gradients or matrix compaction. Articular cartilage is considered to be a viscoelastic material, exhibiting both viscous and elastic behavior. The characteristic feature of a viscoelastic material is that its deformation depends on the load and the rate of load application. The faster a load is applied, the more elastic the behavior. In simpler terms, viscoelastic materials are stronger and stiffer at higher rates of load application and more deforming and softer at low rates of loading.

Joint loading and motion are both important to cartilage health and are required to maintain normal cartilage composition, structure, and mechanical properties. Animal studies have shown that immobilization of a joint results in atrophy or degeneration of the cartilage.[2-4] Changes that occur include cartilage fibrillation, altered aggregate structure, and decreased proteoglycan synthesis and content. Some of this change is reversible. The exact mechanism is unknown, although various mechanical, physiochemical, and electrical transduction theories have been proposed. Chondrocytes respond to a variety of different stimuli including mechanical loads and hydrostatic pressure changes. When stimuli are removed by immobilizing a joint, chondrocyte metabolism may be altered. Fluid flow is also important for chondrocyte nutrition. When joint movement or loading is stopped, alterations in fluid flow and changes in nutrient delivery to chondrocytes will occur. It is for these reasons that continuous passive motion (CPM) machines are often used after cartilage procedures and why it is often desired to avoid prolonged joint immobilization or limited weight bearing.

The unique properties of cartilage account for its remarkable durability. Despite this durability, articular cartilage is frequently vulnerable to traumatic or degenerative conditions that may cause pain and can lead to the development of osteoarthritis. Cartilage has limited ability for repair or regeneration. The limited healing potential of cartilage is related to a number of factors. Cartilage is a hypocellular tissue with few cells available to participate in a repair response. Additionally, the few cells that are available are "imprisoned" within a tough matrix and are unable to migrate to the site of repair. As mentioned earlier, cartilage is an avascular tissue in addition to being alymphatic and aneural (it has no blood, lymph, or nerve supply). Therefore the vascular, lymphatic, and nervous systems cannot help import cells from other areas to participate in the healing response. This is a particular problem with younger, more active patients because total joint arthroplasty results in a high rate of failure.[5,6] For these reasons a biologic solution to the repair of clinically significant articular cartilage defects is appealing.

Few studies document the true incidence of cartilage lesions, but it is believed to be high, especially in sports-related injuries. Trauma is the most common cause of chondral (cartilage alone) or osteochondral (bone and cartilage) injuries. Other etiologies include osteochondritis desiccans, avascular necrosis, and developmental dysplasias of the joint and cartilage. Two major types of cartilage injury, partial-thickness defects and full-thickness defects, must be considered separately because of the difference in healing response. Partial-thickness injuries result in disruption of the cells and matrix. The lesion is limited to the cartilage layer itself and does not extend into the underlying subchondral bone. Full-thickness wounds extend through the entire depth of the cartilage and into the underlying vascular subchondral bone. The body's biologic responses to these two types of wounds are quite different.

Partial-thickness lacerations of the articular cartilage create necrosis in the area of the wound, with disruption of the matrix and death of chondrocytes. There is no significant inflammatory response, because this is mediated by the vascular system, which is absent in articular cartilage. In the absence of vessels there is no development of a fibrin clot, no infusion of reparative stem cells or growth factors, and no angiogenesis to support the metabolic demands of repair tissue. In effect, there is no repair response. Fortunately, these types of lesions are usually of little concern, because a portion of the protective chondral surface remains. If the lesion is located in a mechanically neutral (unloaded) area of the joint, there tends to be no progression with time.[7,8]

Unlike partial-thickness wounds, full-thickness wounds do initiate the typical injury response with necrosis, inflammation, and repair.[9] After penetration of the vascular subchondral bone, a fibrin clot is formed. Undifferentiated mesenchymal cells migrate into the clot from the underlying marrow. Blood vessels then begin to grow into the defect. As the blood clot is resorbed the mesenchymal cells lay down fibrovascular scar with the development of fibrinous arcades. Osteoblasts in the depths of the lesion begin the synthesis of new subchondral bone. The mesenchymal cells then differentiate into cells with a chondrocyte phenotype and begin laying down new matrix. The fibrovascular scar is ultimately converted into "hyaline neocartilage" or "fibrocartilage," similar to that mechanically produced using an abrasion or microfracture surgical technique.

The resultant fibrocartilage repair tissue has different biochemical and biomechanical properties than normal cartilage does. The collagen makeup is altered, with the production of both type I and type II collagen. Type I collagen, primarily found in bone, is not a normal constituent of articular cartilage. Although type II collagen is produced, its amount is reduced. The proteoglycan content of fibrocartilage is also lower than normal. Biomechanically, this fibrocartilage repair tissue is inferior to normal articular cartilage and tends to degenerate with time.[9,10]

There are a number of classification schemes used to describe articular cartilage lesions. Most are based on the depth of cartilage abnormality as initially described by Outerbridge. The International Cartilage Repair Society (ICRS) classification system is one of the systems most commonly used by knee surgeons and is frequently cited in the scientific literature (Figure 21-2). Grade I lesions are nearly normal, with soft indentation or superficial fissures on palpation, but the cartilage surface is intact. Grade II lesions demonstrate cartilage injury, with lesions extending less than 50% of the cartilage depth. With grade III lesions, there is fissuring or cracking that extends through the full thickness of the cartilage to bone, but not through the subchondral

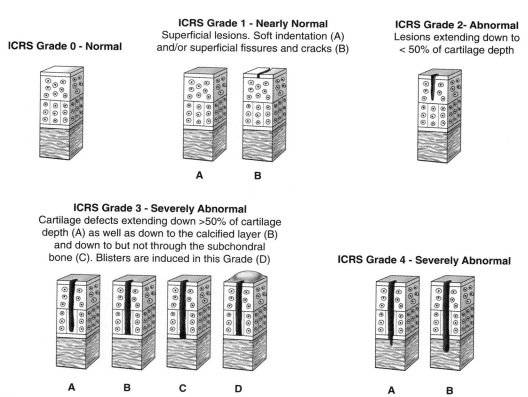

Figure 21-2: The International Cartilage Repair Society (ICRS) classification system for articular cartilage lesions. (*Reprinted with permission from the International Cartilage Repair Society.*)

bone. Grade IV lesions are full-thickness lesions with exposed bone involvement.

The size of the lesion is also important in terms of prognosis. Smaller lesions that are well shouldered by a surrounding rim of normal cartilage may not progress or cause symptoms. When larger lesions result in incongruous opposing surfaces (two opposing rough surfaces), there are changes in biomechanics that can lead to progression of the lesion and degeneration of both cartilage surfaces. Lesions smaller than $2\,cm^2$ are considered small. Those from 2 to $10\,cm^2$ are considered medium. Defects larger than $10\ cm^2$ are considered large.

Trauma, osteochondritis dissecans (OCD), osteonecrosis, osteochondroses, and hereditary epiphyseal abnormalities may cause osteochondral lesions in the knee joint. When a chondral or osteochondral defect persists in a weight-bearing portion of the knee joint, progressive wear and thinning with eventual degenerative arthritis may result. Treatment of osteochondral injuries and OCD is quite controversial and has received enormous attention recently in the orthopaedic literature. The spectrum of pathology ranges from the young child with open physes and an OCD lesion to the middle-age athlete with an osteochondral fracture resulting from trauma.

PRINCIPLES OF ARTICULAR CARTILAGE REHABILITATION

There are several key principles involved when designing rehabilitation programs for use after articular cartilage procedures. These key principles have been designed based on our understanding of the basic science and mechanics of articular cartilage. The principles include creating a healing environment, understanding the biomechanics of the knee, restoring soft tissue balance, reducing pain and effusion, restoring muscle function, gradually progressing applied loads, and emphasizing team communication. We will briefly describe each one as it relates to the rehabilitation program.

Create a Healing Environment

The first principle of articular cartilage rehabilitation involves creating an environment that facilitates the repair process while avoiding potentially deleterious forces on the repair site. This involves a thorough knowledge of the physiologic repair process after surgery. Through animal studies, as well as by closely monitoring the maturation of the OATS and ACI repair tissue in human patients via arthroscopic examination, the biologic phases of maturation have been identified.[11-15]

Knowledge of the healing and maturation process that follows these procedures will assure that the repair tissue is gradually loaded and that excessive forces are not introduced too early in the repair process. The specific phases of healing and rehabilitation that follow the OATS and ACI procedures will be discussed in later sections of this chapter.

As mentioned previously, immobilization and unloading have been shown to be deleterious to articular cartilage, resulting in proteoglycan loss and gradual weakening. Therefore controlled weight bearing and motion are essential to facilitate healing and prevent degeneration. This gradual progression has been shown to stimulate matrix production and improve the tissue's mechanical properties.[16-18]

Controlled compression and decompression forces observed during weight bearing may provide the signals to the repair tissue to produce a matrix that will match the environmental forces. A progression of partial weight bearing with crutches is used to gradually increase the amount of load applied to the weight-bearing surfaces of the joint. The use of a pool or aquatic therapy may be beneficial to initiate gait training and lower extremity exercises. The buoyancy of the water has been shown to decrease the amount of weight-bearing forces to approximately 25% body weight with a water depth to the axilla and 50% with a water depth to the waist.[19] Therefore the pool may be used during early phases of rehabilitation to perform limited weight-bearing activities.

Passive range-of-motion (PROM) activities, such as use of CPM machines, are also performed immediately after surgery to nourish the healing articular cartilage and prevent the formation of adhesions. Motion exercises may assist in creating a smooth low frictional surface by sliding against the joint's articular surface. The use of CPM has been shown to enhanced cartilage healing and long-term outcomes after articular cartilage procedures.[20,21]

Biomechanics of the Knee

The next rehabilitation principle involves understanding the biomechanics of the tibiofemoral and patellofemoral joint during normal joint articulation.

Articulation between the femoral condyle and tibial plateau is constant throughout knee range of motion (ROM). The anterior surface of the femoral condyles is in articulation with the middle aspect of the tibial plateau near full knee extension. With weight bearing, as the knee moves into greater degrees of knee flexion, the femoral condyles progressively roll posteriorly and slide anteriorly causing articulation to shift posteriorly on the femoral condyle and tibial plateaus.[22,23]

Articulation between the inferior margin of the patella and the trochlea begins at approximately 10 to 20 degrees of knee flexion.[24] As the knee proceeds into greater degrees of flexion, the contact area of the patellofemoral joint moves proximally along the patella. At 30 degrees the area of patellofemoral contact is approximately $2\,cm^2$.[24] The area of contact gradually increases as the knee is flexed. At 90 degrees of knee flexion, the contact area increases up to $6\,cm^2$.[24]

Using this knowledge of joint arthrokinematics, the clinician can progress the rate of weight bearing and PROM based on the exact location of the lesion. For example, a lesion on the anterior aspect of the femoral condyle may be progressed into deeper degrees of passive knee flexion without causing articulation at the repair site. Conversely, lesions on the posterior condyle may require a slower rate of PROM progression because of the progressive rolling and sliding component of articulation during deeper knee flexion. Furthermore, lesions on a non–weight-bearing surface, such as the trochlea, may include immediate partial weight bearing with a brace locked in full knee extension without causing excessive compression on the repair site.

Rehabilitation exercises are also altered based on the biomechanics of the knee to avoid excessive compressive or shearing forces. Open kinetic exercises, such as knee extension, are commonly performed from 90 to 40 degrees of knee flexion. This ROM provides the least patellofemoral joint reaction force while exhibiting the greatest patellofemoral contact area.[24-26] Closed kinetic chain exercises such as leg presses, vertical squats, lateral step-ups, and wall squats are performed initially from 0 to 30 degrees and then progressed to 0 to 60 degrees when tibiofemoral and patellofemoral joint reaction forces are lowered.[24-26] As the repair site heals and the patient's symptoms subside, the ranges of motion that are performed are progressed to allow greater muscle strengthening in larger ranges. Exercises are progressed based on the patient's subjective reports of symptoms and the clinical assessment of swelling and crepitation.

Restoration of Soft Tissue Balance

One of the most important aspects of articular cartilage rehabilitation involves the avoidance of arthrofibrosis, particularly in the OATS and ACI procedures because of the large open incision. This is achieved by focusing on the restoration of full passive knee extension, patella mobility, and soft tissue flexibility of the knee and entire lower extremity. The inability to fully extend the knee results in abnormal joint arthrokinematics and subsequent increases in patellofemoral and tibiofemoral joint contact pressure, strain on the quadriceps muscle, and muscular fatigue.[27] Several authors have reported that immediate motion is essential to avoid ROM complications and minimize poor functional outcomes.[28,29] Therefore a drop-lock postoperative knee brace locked into 0 degrees of extension is used, and CPM and PROM out of the brace are performed immediately after surgery.

The goal is to achieve at least 0 degrees of knee extension the first few days postoperatively. Specific exercises used include manual PROM exercises performed by the rehabilitation specialist, supine hamstring stretches with a wedge under the heel, and gastrocnemius stretching with a towel. Overpressure of 6 to 12 lb may be used for a low-load long-duration stretch as needed to achieve full extension.

Patients will often exhibit a certain amount of hyperextension preoperatively or in the uninvolved knee. For patients with significant hyperextension of the uninvolved extremity, we suggest regaining approximately 5 to 7 degrees of hyperextension through stretching techniques in the clinic. The remaining hyperextension may be achieved through functional activities. We believe this allows the patient to gain a greater degree of neuromuscular control at the end range of extension and avoids uncontrolled and unexpected hyperextension movements.

The loss of patellar mobility after surgery may have various causes, including excessive scar tissue adhesions from the incision anteriorly, as well as along the medial and lateral gutters. The loss of patellar mobility may result in ROM complications and difficulty recruiting quadriceps contraction. Patellar mobilizations in the medial-lateral and superior-inferior directions are performed by the rehabilitation specialist and independently by the patient during the home exercise program.

Soft tissue flexibility and pliability are also important for the entire lower extremity. Soft tissue massage and scar management are performed to prevent adhesion development around the anterior, medial, and lateral aspects of the knee. In addition, flexibility exercises are performed for the entire lower extremity, including the hamstrings, hip, and calf musculature. As ROM improves and the lesion begins to heal, quadriceps stretching may also be performed as tolerated by the patient.

Reduction of Pain and Effusion

Numerous authors have studied the effect of pain and joint effusion on muscle inhibition. A progressive decrease in quadriceps activity has been noted as the knee exhibits increased pain and distention.[30,31] Therefore the reduction in knee joint pain and swelling is crucial to restore normal quadriceps activity.

Treatment options for reduction of swelling include cryotherapy, high-voltage stimulation, and joint compression through the use of a knee sleeve or compression wrap. Patients with chronic joint effusion may also benefit from a knee sleeve or compression wrap to apply constant pressure during everyday activities in an attempt to minimize the development of further effusion.

Pain can be reduced passively through the use of cryotherapy and analgesic medication. Immediately after injury or surgery, the use of a commercial cold wrap can be extremely beneficial. PROM may also provide neuromodulation of pain during acute or exacerbated conditions.[32]

Restoration of Muscle Function

The next principle involves restoring muscle function of the lower extremity. Inhibition of the quadriceps muscle is a common clinical enigma in the presence of pain and effusion during the acute phases of rehabilitation immediately after the OATS or ACI procedure. Electrical muscle stimulation and biofeedback are often incorporated with therapeutic exercises to facilitate the active contraction of the quadriceps musculature.

The use of electrical stimulation and biofeedback on the quadriceps musculature appears to facilitate the return of muscle activation and may be valuable additions to therapeutic exercises.[33,34] Clinically, we use electrical stimulation immediately after surgery while performing isometric and isotonic exercises such as quadriceps sets, straight leg raises, hip adduction and abduction, and knee extensions (Figure 21-3). Electrical stimulation is used before biofeedback when the patient presents acutely with the inability to activate the quadriceps musculature. Once independent muscle activation is present, biofeedback may be used to facilitate further neuromuscular activation of the quadriceps. The patient must concentrate on neuromuscular control to independently activate the quadriceps during rehabilitation.

Exercises that strengthen the entire lower extremity, such as machine weights and closed kinetic chain exercises, must be included as the patient progresses to more advanced phases of rehabilitation. It is important that total leg strength be emphasized rather than concentrating solely on the quadriceps. Training of the hip and ankle located proximally and distally along the kinetic chain is emphasized to assist in controlling the production and dissipation of forces in the knee. In addition, the hip and ankle assist in controlling abduction and adduction moments at the knee joint.

Proprioceptive and neuromuscular control drills of the lower extremities should also be included to restore dynamic stabilization of the knee joint postoperatively. Specific drills initially include weight shifting side to side, weight shifting diagonally, mini-squats, and mini-squats on an unstable surface such as a tilt board. Perturbations can be added to challenge the neuromuscular system, as can additional exercises including lateral lunges onto unstable surfaces and balance beam walking.

Gradual Progression of Applied Loads

The next principle of rehabilitation involves gradually increasing the amount of stress applied to the injured knee as the patient returns to functional activities. The rehabilitation process involves a progressive application of therapeutic exercises designed to gradually increase function in the postoperative knee. This progression is used to provide a healthy stimulus for healing tissues while assuring that forces are gradually applied without causing damage. The rehabilitation progression is designed based on the four biologic phases of cartilage maturation.[11-15, 35-37]

The first phase is the proliferation phase, which typically involves the first 4 to 6 weeks after surgery. During this phase, the initial healing process begins. It is imperative to decrease swelling, restore full PROM, and enhance volitional control of the quadriceps during the early phases of rehabilitation.

During this initial phase, controlled active and passive ROM and a gradual weight-bearing progression are critical components of the rehabilitation process. As previously discussed, PROM and controlled partial weight bearing will help to promote the nurturing of the cartilage through the synovial fluid diffusion as well as provide the proper stimulus for the cells to produce specific matrix markers. A progression of partial weight bearing with crutches and progressive loading exercises (Figure 21-4) are used to gradually increase the amount of load applied to the weight-bearing surfaces of the joint. The use of a pool or aquatic therapy may be beneficial to begin gait training and lower extremity exercises.

PROM actives, such as use of CPM machines, are also performed immediately after surgery to nourish the healing articular cartilage and prevent the formation of adhesions.

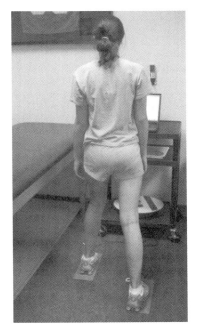

Figure 21-4: Weight-shifting proprioceptive exercises using a force platform to monitor the amount of weight distribution between limbs. The patient is able to visualize the weight distribution between both legs. (*Uni-Cam Balance Trainer, Uni-Cam Corporation, Ramsey, NJ.*)

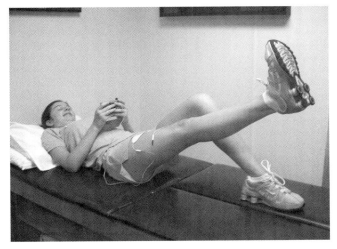

Figure 21-3: Neuromuscular electrical stimulation of the quadriceps during straight leg raises. (*Empi 300 PV, Empi Corporation, St. Paul, MN.*)

CPM typically begins 6 to 8 hours after surgery and is performed for at least 2 to 3 weeks, with recommendations of up to 6 to 8 weeks. Motion exercises may assist in creating a smooth, low-friction surface by sliding against the joint's articular surface.

The second phase is the transitional phase and typically includes weeks 4 through 12. The repair tissue at this point is gaining strength, which will allow for the progression of rehabilitation exercise. During this phase the patient progresses from partial weight bearing to full weight bearing, and full ROM and soft tissue flexibility are achieved. Continued maturation of the repair tissue is fostered through higher-level functional and motion exercises. It is during this phase that patients typically resume most normal activities of daily living. The rehabilitation program will gradually progress strengthening activities to include machine weights and closed kinetic chain exercises as the patient's weight-bearing status returns to normal.

At this time the rehabilitation process involves a progressive application of therapeutic exercises designed to gradually increase function in the postoperative knee. The progression of weight bearing and ROM restoration, as previously discussed, involves a gradual advancement to assure that complications such as excessive motion restrictions or scar tissue formation are avoided while progressing steadily to avoid overstressing the healing graft site. An overaggressive approach early in the rehabilitation program may result in increased pain, inflammation, or effusion, as well as graft damage. This simple concept may be applied to the progression of strengthening exercises, proprioception training, neuromuscular control drills, and functional drills. For example, exercises such as weight shifts and lunges are progressed from straight plane anterior-posterior or medial-lateral directions to involve multiplane and rotational movements. Exercises using two legs, such as leg presses and balance activities, are progressed to single-leg exercises. Thus the progression through the postoperative rehabilitation program involves a gradual progression of applied and functional stresses. This progression is used to provide a healthy stimulus for healing tissues while assuring that forces are gradually applied without causing damage.

The third phase is known as the *remodeling phase* and occurs from 12 weeks through 32 weeks postoperatively. During this phase there is a continuous remodeling into a more organized structural tissue. The tissue at this point is beginning to increase in strength and durability. As the tissue becomes more firm and integrated, it allows for more functional training activities to be performed. At this point the patient typically notes improvement of symptoms and has normal motion. The patient is encouraged to continue with the rehabilitation program to maximize strength and flexibility. Low- to moderate-impact activities such as bicycle riding, golfing, and recreational walking may be gradually incorporated.

The final phase is known as the *maturation phase* and can last up to 15 to 18 months depending on the type of surgery and the size and location of the lesion. It is during this phase that the repair tissue reaches its full maturation. The duration of this phase varies based on the several factors such as lesion size and location. The patient will gradually return to full premorbid activities as tolerated.

In addition, patients may benefit from use of orthotics, insoles, and bracing to alter the applied loads on the articular cartilage during functional activities. These devices are used to avoid excessive forces by unloading the area of the knee in which the implantation is located. Unloader braces are often used for patients with subtle uncorrected abnormal alignments (genu varum) or large or uncontained lesions, as well as in the presence of concomitant osteotomies and meniscal allografts (Figure 21-5).

Team Communication

The last principle of rehabilitation involves a team approach; the team consists of the surgeon, physical therapist, and patient. Communication between the surgeon and therapist is essential to determine the accurate rate of progression based on the location of the lesion, size of the lesion, tissue quality of the patient, and addition of concomitant surgical procedures. Also, communication between the medical team

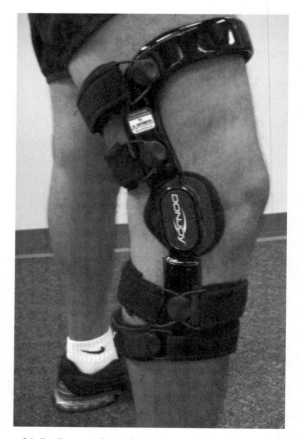

Figure 21-5: Osteoarthritic knee brace designed to unload the medial compartment of the knee. (*DonJoy OA Defiance, DonJoy Corporation, Vista, CA.*)

and patient is essential to provide patient education regarding the avoidance of deleterious forces as well as compliance with precautions. Often a preoperative physical therapy evaluation may be useful to mentally and physically prepare the patient for the articular cartilage procedure and postoperative rehabilitation.

TREATMENT OPTIONS

Treatment options for restoration of joint congruity vary widely from nonoperative closed treatment to arthroscopic drilling, with or without fixation, to tissue transplantation or reconstructive procedures. Several new techniques have been developed in recent years to replace or regenerate articular cartilage using autogenous tissue. The goal of these procedures is to replicate the biomechanics and durability of Type II hyaline articular cartilage as closely as possible. The following is an overview of the treatment options available for osteochondral defects in the knee involving the transplantation or replacement of articular cartilage; other techniques, such as abrasion chondroplasty and microfracture, will be discussed in Chapter 20. A sample treatment algorithm based on our current orthopedic practice can be found in Figure 21-6.

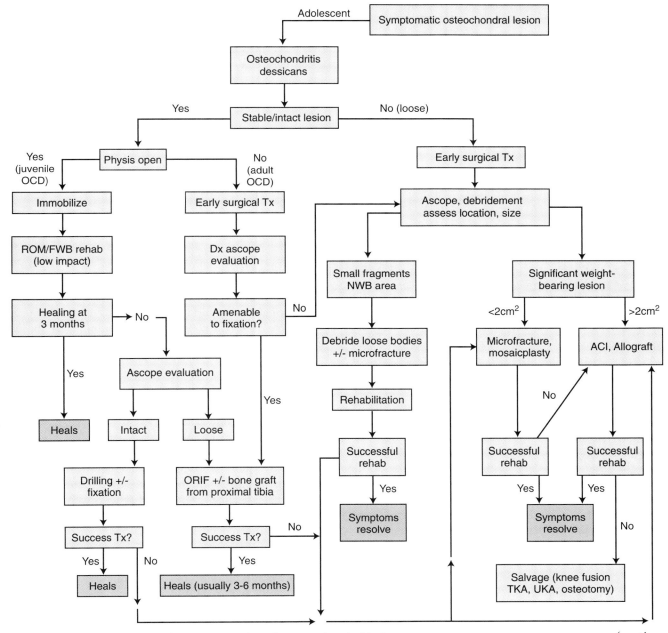

Figure 21-6: Sample algorithm of treatment options for osteochondral lesions.   (continued)

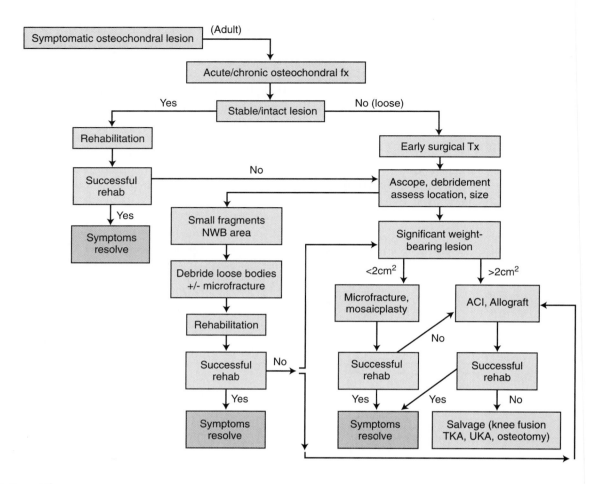

Figure 21-6: *cont'd.*

OSTEOCHONDRAL AUTOGRAFT TRANSPLANTATION

Transplantation of cylindric osteochondral plugs from non–weight-bearing areas of the knee into an osteochondral defect has become a popular articular reconstruction method (Figure 21-7). Hangody and colleagues of Hungary developed an osteochondral autograft technique called *mosaicplasty* (MP) in 1991 for focal osteochondral lesions in the knee or talus.[38]

In these types of procedures, plugs of bone with overlying articular cartilage are harvested from non–weight-bearing areas of the knee such as the proximal lateral trochlea or the interchondylar notch area. These plugs are round and range in size from 4.5 to 8.5 mm in diameter. Typically the depth of bone harvested is around 15 mm. The defect at the donor site reliably fills in with scar tissue consisting of fibrocartilage, similar to what occurs with marrow stimulation techniques.

The plugs that are harvested can then be implanted into holes drilled to accommodate the specifically sized graft (Figure 21-8). Several plugs of similar or varying size can be used with the purpose of obtaining as much fill of the defect as possible. Obtaining adequate fit of the plugs and seating them exactly at the level of the surrounding articular surface are of paramount importance.

Patients who are considered good candidates for MP procedures are typically healthy with no ligamentous instability and adequate alignment. Concomitant realignment or ligamentous stabilization can be performed. There is obviously a limit to how many plugs can be harvested, and therefore a limit to how large a defect can be for this procedure to be considered. Large defects (>6 cm²) can be considered; however, we prefer to use MP for defects less than 2 to 3 cm².

Although the age of patients undergoing this type of surgery has an upper limit of 50, studies have shown that the rate of success declines greatly with patients who are 35 years of age or older.[39] However, the reported success rate for MP is 92% with isolated femoral condylar lesions, 87% with tibial resurfacing, 79% with patellar and/or trochlear mosaicplasties, and 94% with talar procedures.[39]

Another concern with MP is the morbidity of the donor site. A recent biomechanical study demonstrated relatively high loading forces in the donor area but stated that to date there has been no evidence that graft harvest would result in degenerative changes.[40]

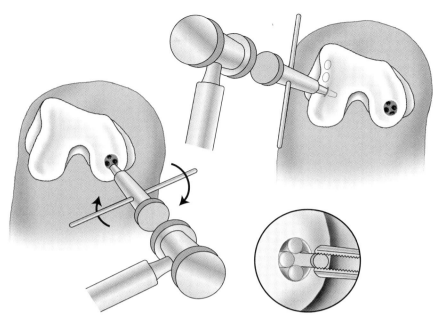

Figure 21-7: Osteochondral autograft transplantation. Cylindric plugs of exposed bone are removed from the defect, and plugs of normal cartilage and bone are harvested and placed into the defect. Plugs can be created in various sizes and geometrically placed to maximally fill the area. (*From Miller MD: Atlas of chondral injury treatment,* Oper Tech Orthop *4:289-293, 1997.*)

Although MP may be effective in treating knees with isolated cartilage lesions, it may be contraindicated in the knee with many degenerative cartilage lesions. Andres and colleagues[41] compared knees with isolated defects and knees with multiple lesions that were repaired using MP. It was reported that the group with isolated degenerative cartilage lesions had a significant decrease in pain and increase in function as compared with the group with multiple lesions.

The initial rehabilitation program progresses cautiously as the bone plugs unite with the subchondral bone at the graft site (Box 21-1). Whiteside and co-workers[42] have shown an initial 44% reduction in the pull-out and push-in strength at 7 days postoperatively in the porcine model. Initial union of the cancellous bone between the plugs occurs by 4 weeks postoperatively and continues to increase in strength from weeks 4 to 8, with fibrocartilage filling the gaps between plugs by 8 weeks postoperatively.[36] A recent study by Nam and colleagues[37] in the rabbit model has shown full subchondral integration at 6 weeks, with 50% of grafts showing evidence of articular cartilage bonding. Furthermore, after a 37% decrease in stiffness at 6 weeks, graft stiffness increased to 150% of the original stiffness by 12 weeks postoperatively.

Therefore early weightbearing activities are avoided, limiting the patient to non–weight-bearing ambulation for at least the first 2 weeks. As the plugs unite and begin to gain strength, partial weight bearing between 25% and 50% body weight is performed from 4 to 6 weeks postoperatively, progressing to full weight bearing around week 8 as full integration occurs. In the event that the OATS procedure is performed on the patella or trochlea, the patient is allowed to bear weight as tolerated immediately after surgery with a brace locked in full extension (Box 21-2).

Because the surgical procedure involves an open approach and subsequent soft tissue trauma, PROM is performed cautiously to not facilitate swelling. However, caution must be exercised to avoid loss of motion from soft tissue scarring. Therefore a gradual restoration of motion is used. Typical goals include 90 degrees of flexion at 1 week postoperatively, 105 degrees at week 2, 115 degrees at week 3, 125 degrees at week 4, and gradual progression to 135+ degrees after week 6.

Exercises are initially limited by the weight-bearing status, beginning with quadriceps setting and straight leg raise exercises and progressing to a full machine progressive resistive exercise and closed kinetic chain program by 8 weeks postoperatively. Early strength and proprioceptive exercises, such as weight shifts and mini-squats, are initially performed within the patient's limited weight-bearing status and gradually progressed to full weight bearing. For the patellofemoral lesion, caution is exercised with exercises that create shear across the graft, such as open kinetic chain knee extension. Low-impact activities are initiated at month 4 or 5, progressing to more moderate activities after 6 months postoperatively.

Results after the OATS procedure have been good. Hangody and Fules[39] reported the results of the first 10 years of OATS procedures in 831 patients. The authors report good to excellent results in 92% of femoral condyle lesions and 79% of patellar and trochlear lesions. Aubin and co-workers[43] have shown similar results with 85% graft

Text continued on p. 399

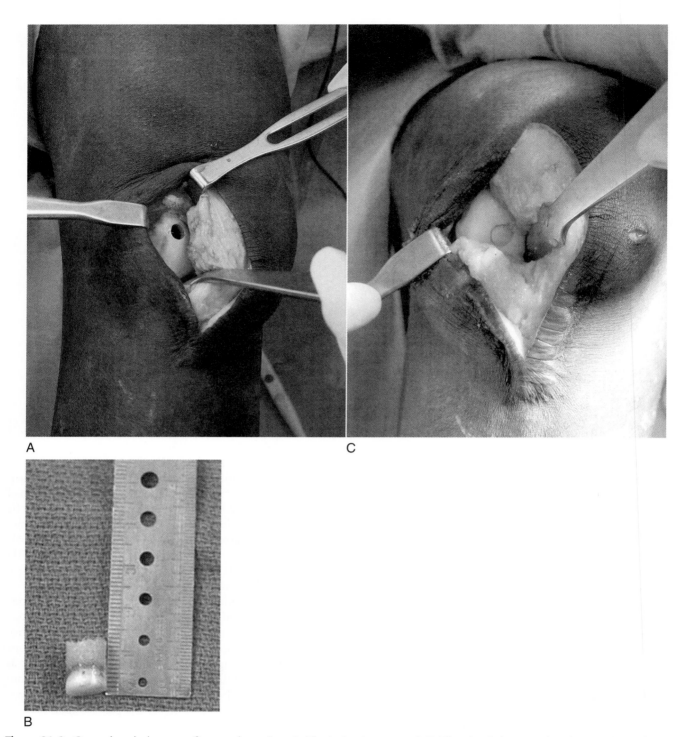

Figure 21-8: Osteochondral autograft transplantation. **A,** The lesion is prepared. **B,** The plug is harvested and, **C,** implanted into defect.

BOX 21-1

Osteochondral Autograft Transplantation: Femoral Condyle Rehabilitation Program

Phase I—Protection Phase (Weeks 0-6)

Goals

Protect healing tissue from load and shear forces

Decrease pain and effusion

Restore full passive knee extension

Gradually improve knee flexion

Regain quadriceps control

Brace

Locked at 0 degrees during weight-bearing (WB) activities

Sleep in locked brace for 2-4 weeks

Weight Bearing

Non–weight-bearing status for 2-4 weeks (physician direction)

If large lesion ($>5cm^2$) may need to delay WB up to 4 weeks

Toe-touch WB (approx. 20-30 lb) weeks 2-4

Partial WB (approximately 25%-50% body weight) at week 6

Range of Motion

Immediate motion exercise

Full passive knee extension immediately

Initiate continuous passive motion (CPM) day 1 for 8-12 hours/day (0-40 degrees) for 2-3 weeks

Progress CPM range of motion (ROM) as tolerated 5-10 degrees/day

May continue CPM for 6-8 hours/day for up to 6-8 weeks

Patellar and soft tissue mobilization (four to six times per day)

Passive knee flexion ROM two or three times daily

Passive knee flexion ROM goal is 90 degrees by 1-2 weeks

Passive knee flexion ROM goal is 105-115 degrees by 4 weeks and 120-125 degrees by week 6

Stretch hamstrings, calf, and quadriceps

Strengthening Program

Ankle pump using rubber tubing

Quadriceps setting

Multiangle isometrics (co-contractions quadriceps/hamstrings)

Active knee extension 90-40 degrees (if no articulation—no resistance)

Straight leg raises (four directions)

Stationary bicycle when ROM allows

Biofeedback and electrical muscle stimulation, as needed

Isometric leg press at week 4 (multiangle)

May begin use of pool for gait training and exercises week 6

Functional Activities

Gradual return to daily activities

If symptoms occur, reduce activities to reduce pain and inflammation

Extended standing should be avoided

Swelling Control

Ice, elevation, compression, and edema modalities as needed to decrease swelling

Phase II—Transition Phase (Weeks 6-12)

Goals

Gradually increase ROM and WB to full

Gradually improve quadriceps strength and endurance

Gradually increase functional activities

Criteria to Progress to Phase II

Full passive knee extension

Knee flexion to 120 degrees

Minimal pain and swelling

Brace

Discontinue brace at 6 weeks

Weight Bearing

Progress WB as tolerated

75% body weight with crutches at 8 weeks

Progress to full WB at 10-12 weeks

May need to delay full WB up to 14 weeks if large lesion or multiple plugs

Discontinue crutches at 10-12 weeks

(continued)

BOX 21-1

Osteochondral Autograft Transplantation: Femoral Condyle Rehabilitation Program—cont'd

Range of Motion

Gradual increase in ROM

Maintain full passive knee extension

Progress knee flexion to 125-135 degrees

Continue patellar mobilization and soft tissue mobilization, as needed

Continue stretching program

Strengthening Exercises

Initiate weight shifts weeks 6-8

Initiate mini-squats 0-45 degrees weeks 8-10

Closed kinetic chain (CKC) exercises (leg presses) weeks 8-10

Toe-calf raises weeks 10-12

Open kinetic chain knee extension, 1lb/week weeks 10-12

Stationary bicycle (gradually increase time)

Balance and proprioception drills

Initiate front and lateral step-ups

Continue use of biofeedback and electrical muscle stimulation, as needed

Continue use of pool for gait training and exercise

May need to delay CKC exercises up to 14 weeks if large lesion

Functional Activities

As pain and swelling (symptoms) diminish, gradually increase functional activities

Gradually increase standing and walking

Phase III: Maturation Phase (Weeks 12-26)

Goals

Improve muscular strength and endurance

Increase functional activities

Criteria to Progress to Phase III

Full ROM

Acceptable strength level

Hamstrings within 10% of contralateral leg

Quadriceps within 10%-20% of contralateral leg

Balance testing within 30% of contralateral leg

Ability to bike for 30 minutes

Range of Motion

Patient should exhibit 125-135 degrees of flexion; no restrictions

Exercise Program

Leg presses (0-90 degrees)

Bilateral squats (0-60 degrees)

Unilateral step-ups progressing from 2 to 8 inches

Forward lunges

Begin walking program on treadmill

Open kinetic chain knee extension (0-90 degrees)

Bicycle

StairMaster

Swimming

NordicTrack or elliptical training

Functional Activities

As patient improves, increase walking (distance, cadence, incline, etc.)

Maintenance Program

Initiate at weeks 16-20

Bicycle—low resistance

Progressive walking program

Pool exercises for entire lower extremity

Straight leg raises into flexion

Leg presses

Wall squats

Hip abduction or adduction

Front lunges

Stretch quadriceps, hamstrings, gastrocnemius

Phase IV—Functional Activities Phase (Weeks 26-52)

Goals

Gradual return to full unrestricted functional activities

Criteria to Progress to Phase IV

Full nonpainful ROM

Strength within 90% of contralateral extremity

Balance and/or stability within 75% of contralateral extremity

No pain, inflammation, or swelling

(continued)

BOX 21-1

Osteochondral Autograft Transplantation: Femoral Condyle Rehabilitation Program—cont'd

Exercises

Continue maintenance program progression three or four times per week

Progress resistance as tolerated

Emphasize entire lower extremity strength and flexibility

Progress agility and balance drills

Impact loading program should be specialized to the patient's demands

Progress sport programs depending on patient variables

Functional Activities

Patient may return to various sport activities as progression in rehabilitation and cartilage healing allows. Generally, low-impact sports such as skating, rollerblading, and cycling are permitted at approximately 6-8 months. Higher-impact sports such as jogging, running, and aerobics may be performed at 8-10 months. High-impact sports such as tennis, basketball, football, and baseball are allowed at 9-12 months for small to medium lesions; however, for larger lesions these activities may be delayed up to 18 months.

BOX 21-2

Osteochondral Autograft Transplantation: Patella and Trochlea Rehabilitation Guidelines

Phase I—Protection Phase (Weeks 0-6)

Goals

Protect healing tissue from load and shear forces

Decrease pain and effusion

Restore full passive knee extension

Gradually improve knee flexion

Regain quadriceps control

Brace

Locked at 0 degrees during ambulation and WB activities

Sleep in locked brace for 4-6 weeks

Weight-Bearing

Immediate toe-touch WB at 25% body weight with brace locked in full extension

50% body weight week 2 in brace

75% body weight weeks 3-4 in brace

Range of Motion

Immediate motion exercise days 1-2

Full passive knee extension immediately

Initiate continuous passive motion (CPM) day 1 for total of 8-12 hours/day (0-60 degrees; if lesion >6 cm^2 0-40 degrees) for first 2-3 weeks

Progress CPM range of motion (ROM) as tolerated 5-10 degrees/day

May continue use of CPM for total of 6-8 hours/day for 6 weeks

Patellar and soft tissue mobilization (four to six times per day)

Motion exercises throughout the day

Passive knee flexion ROM 2-3 times daily

Passive knee flexion ROM goal is 90 degrees by 2-3 weeks

Passive knee flexion ROM goal is 105 degrees by 3-4 weeks and 120 degrees by week 6

Stretch hamstrings, calf

Strengthening Program

Ankle pump using rubber tubing

Quadriceps setting

Straight leg raises (four directions)

Toe-calf raises week 2

Stationary bicycle when ROM allows

Biofeedback and electrical muscle stimulation, as needed

Isometric leg press at week 4 (multiangle)

Initiate weight shifts week 4

May begin pool therapy for gait training and exercise week 4

Functional Activities

Gradual return to daily activities

If symptoms occur, reduce activities to reduce pain and inflammation

(continued)

BOX 21-2

Osteochondral Autograft Transplantation: Patella and Trochlea Rehabilitation Guidelines—cont'd

Extended standing should be avoided

Swelling control

Ice, elevation, compression, and edema-control modalities as needed to decrease swelling

Criteria to Progress to Phase II

Full passive knee extension

Knee flexion to 115-120 degrees

Minimal pain and swelling

Voluntary quadriceps activity

Phase II—Transition Phase (Weeks 6-12)

Goals

Gradually increase ROM

Gradually improve quadriceps strength and endurance

Gradually increase functional activities

Brace

Discontinue brace at 6-8 weeks

Weight Bearing

Progress WB as tolerated

Progress to full WB at 6-8 weeks

Discontinue crutches at 6-8 weeks

Range of Motion

Gradual increase in ROM

Maintain full passive knee extension

Progress knee flexion to 120-125 degrees by week 8

Continue patellar mobilization and soft tissue mobilization, as needed

Continue stretching program

Strengthening Exercises

Closed kinetic chain exercises (leg presses 0-60 degrees) week 8

Initiate mini-squats 0-45 degrees week 8

Toe-calf raises

Open kinetic chain knee extension without resistance

Begin knee extension 0-30 degrees, then progress to deeper angles

Stationary bicycle (gradually increase time)

StairMaster at week 12

Balance and proprioception drills

Initiate front and lateral step-ups

Continue use of biofeedback and electrical muscle stimulation, as needed

Larger lesions or lesions with multiple plugs may need to be delayed 2-4 weeks per physician

Functional Activities

As pain and swelling (symptoms) diminish, the patient may gradually increase functional activities

Gradually increase standing and walking

Criteria to Progress to Phase III

Full ROM

Acceptable strength level

- Hamstrings within 10%-20% of contralateral leg
- Quadriceps within 20%-30% of contralateral leg

Balance testing within 30% of contralateral leg

Able to walk 1-2 miles or bike for 30 minutes

Phase III: Remodeling Phase (Weeks 13-32)

Goals

Improve muscular strength and endurance

Increase functional activities

Range of Motion

Patient should exhibit 125-135 degrees of flexion

Exercise Program

Leg presses (0-60 degrees; progress to 0-90 degrees)

Bilateral squats (0-60 degrees)

Unilateral step-ups progressing from 2 to 6 inches

Forward lunges

Walking program on treadmill

Open kinetic chain knee extension (90-40 degrees); progress 1 lb every 10-14 days if no pain or crepitation; must monitor symptoms; may delay heavy resistance for up to 6 months

Bicycle

StairMaster

Swimming

NordicTrack or elliptical training

(continued)

survival at 10 years and 74% graft survival at 15 years postoperatively.

AUTOLOGOUS CHONDROCYTE IMPLANTATION

ACI was first reported in 1994 by Brittberg and colleagues for treatment of symptomatic full-thickness weight-bearing chondral injuries in the young compliant patient (Figure 21-9).[11]

This is accomplished by harvesting small full-thickness pieces of cartilage from non–weight-bearing areas of the knee. The cartilage is then transported in a nutrient medium to a laboratory where the cartilage is denatured into chondrocytes (cartilage cells) and matrix (fibrous tissue produced by chondrocytes). The chondrocytes can then be grown and multiplied to a volume necessary to reimplant into the knee defect of the donor patient. The harvest of the cartilage is carried out arthroscopically. Several weeks are necessary for the cells to

be adequately isolated and multiplied. The cells are then returned to the surgeon on the day of implantation.

The implantation of chondrocytes is accomplished via an open arthrotomy of the knee. The location of the arthrotomy depends on the location of the lesion. For a medial femoral condyle lesion, a medial parapatellar arthrotomy is commonly used. Once exposed, the lesion is then debrided until a well-circumscribed area with sharp edges is created. Generally, contained defects are considered optimal, although there are alternatives for uncontained defects. Once prepared, the tourniquet is released to ensure that no bleeding occurs from the bony bed. This is of particular importance since we know from marrow stimulation techniques that bleeding onto the subchondral bone will produce fibrocartilage. Once hemostasis has been achieved, a patch of periosteum is harvested from the medial border of the midshaft of the tibia, sized to cover the defect. The periosteum is then sewn over the defect with the cambium layer down. Absorbable 6-0 braided suture is used to sew the patch down at 3 to 5 mm intervals. Once

---

BOX 21-2

Osteochondral Autograft Transplantation: Patella and Trochlea Rehabilitation Guidelines—cont'd

Functional Activities

As patient improves, increase walking (distance, cadence, incline, etc.)

Light running can be initiated toward end of phase, based on physician decision

Maintenance Program

Initiate at weeks 16-20

Bicycle—low resistance, increase time

Progressive walking program

Pool exercises for entire lower extremity

Straight leg raises

Leg presses

Wall squats

Hip abduction and adduction

Front lunges

Step-ups

Stretch quadriceps, hamstrings, calf

Criteria to Progress to Phase IV

Full nonpainful ROM

Strength within 80%-90% of contralateral extremity

Balance and/or stability within 75% of contralateral extremity

No pain, inflammation, or swelling

Phase IV—Maturation Phase (8-15 Months)

Goals

Gradual return to full unrestricted functional activities

Exercises

Continue maintenance program progression three or four times per week

Progress resistance as tolerated

Emphasize entire lower extremity strength and flexibility

Progress agility and balance drills

Progress walking program as tolerated

Impact loading program should be specialized to the patient's demands

No jumping or plyometric exercise for 12 months

Progress sport programs depending on patient variables

Functional Activities

Patient may return to various sport activities as progression in rehabilitation and cartilage healing allows. Generally, low-impact sports such as swimming, skating, rollerblading, and cycling are permitted at approximately 6 months. Higher-impact sports such as jogging, running, and aerobics may be performed at 8-9 months for small lesions or 9-12 months for larger lesions. High-impact sports such as tennis, basketball, football, and baseball are allowed at 9-12 months for small to medium lesions; however, for larger lesions such activities may be delayed up to 18 months.

the patch is in place, a fibrin glue is used to seal the edges of the patch to create a watertight seal. Saline is injected under the patch to ensure that no fluid leaks out. Once the patch has been secured and sealed, the chondrocytes and the liquid medium that are shipped in are drawn into a syringe and injected beneath the patch (Figure 21-10). The site of the injection is then sealed with more sutures and fibrin glue.

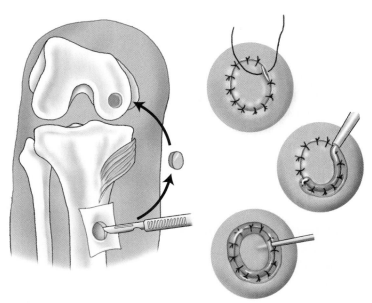

Figure 21-9: Autologous chondrocyte implantation. Periosteum is harvested and sewn into the prepared defect with the cambium layer facing inward. The patch is stitched into the surrounding articular cartilage. Fibrin glue is used to seal the patch. The chondrocytes are then implanted beneath the patch. (*From Miller MD: Atlas of chondral injury treatment,* Oper Tech Orthop 4:289-293, 1997.)

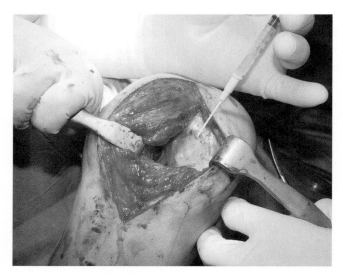

Figure 21-10: Autologous chondrocyte implantation. The chondrocytes are being injected underneath the periosteal patch.

The arthrotomy is then closed with careful attention to protect the area of implantation.

The live chondrocytes begin to adhere to the underlying bone within the first 4 hours after implantation. Over the next several months the chondrocytes produce the matrix material, forming a hyaline-like articular cartilage surface in the area where full-thickness cartilage loss had previously existed.

The major advantage of ACI is that follow-up arthroscopy and biopsies have shown living hyaline-like cartilage repair tissue.[44,45] Initial histopathologic analyses of the ACI procedure by Peterson and colleagues[13] have shown the regeneration of the type II hyaline cartilage in greater than 80% of grafts. A more recent study by Roberts and co-workers[46] has also shown that a greater amount of hyaline tissue is present as the graft matures. The authors note that some ACI biopsies revealed fibrocartilage at 12 months postoperatively; however, the majority of grafts matured to hyaline cartilage by 20 months postoperatively.

Disadvantages of ACI include the cost of cartilage cell culture, multiple surgical procedures, and tenuous fixation of periosteum to the chondral surface. ACI may be indicated for medium or large lesions (2 cm to >10 cm), although deep (>8 mm) bone defects may require bone grafting or an additional staged procedure to recreate the native subchondral bone layer.

Candidates for ACI are young (<50 years old) with no instability or malalignment. Also, the meniscus in the affected compartment should be predominantly intact, and the opposing joint surface should be unaffected. Therefore concomitant or staged procedures must be performed to address ligamentous instability, malalignment, or meniscal deficiency. Nonsmokers are preferred and also tend to have more robust periosteum. Although appropriate for lesions as small as 2 cm^2, there is no real upper limit to the area that can be treated, because an unlimited number of chondrocytes can be obtained. It is therefore possible to treat multiple lesions in the same knee in various locations. For larger lesions that may not be amenable to MP or marrow stimulation, ACI is an excellent option. Although the rehabilitation and healing process is longer than with other treatment options such as microfracture and MP,[47] the patient returns to functional activities within a similar time frame.

Many studies have recommended reserving ACI as a first-line treatment for patients with large defects (>2 cm^2) and for revision therapy in patients who have failed other surgical techniques.[48-50]

The rehabilitation program that follows chondrocyte implantation is vital to the success and long-term outcomes of patients. Early controlled ROM and weight bearing are necessary to stimulate chondrocyte development, although caution is exercised with overaggressive activities that may result in cell damage or graft delamination (Box 21-3).

Knowledge of the biologic healing response is vital for the development of appropriate rehabilitation guidelines. The first phase is the proliferation phase, which involves the first

BOX 21-3

Autologous Chondrocyte Implantation: Femoral Condyle Rehabilitation Guidelines

Phase I: Protection Phase (Weeks 0-6)

Goals

Protect healing tissue from load and shear forces

Decrease pain and effusion

Restore full passive knee extension

Gradually improve knee flexion

Regain quadriceps control

Brace

Locked at 0 degrees during WB activities

Sleep in locked brace for 2-4 weeks

Weight Bearing

Non–WB status for 1-2 weeks, may begin toe-touch WB immediately per physician if lesion is small

Toe-touch WB (approximately 20-30 lb) weeks 2-3

Partial WB (approximately 25% body weight) at week 4

Range of Motion

Immediate motion exercise

Full passive knee extension immediately

Initiate continuous passive motion (CPM) day 1 for total of 8-12 hours/day (0-40 degrees) for 2-3 weeks

Progress CPM range of motion (ROM) as tolerated 5-10 degrees/day

May continue CPM for total of 6-8 hours/day for up to 6 weeks

Patellar mobilization (four to six times per day)

Motion exercises throughout the day

Passive knee flexion ROM two or three times daily

Knee flexion ROM goal is 90 degrees by 1-2 weeks

Knee flexion ROM goal is 105 degrees by 3-4 weeks and 120 degrees by weeks 5-6

Stretch hamstrings and calf

Strengthening Program

Ankle pump using rubber tubing

Quadriceps setting

Multiangle isometrics (co-contractions quadriceps/hamstrings)

Active knee extension 90-40 degrees (no resistance)

Straight leg raises (four directions)

Stationary bicycle when ROM allows

Biofeedback and electrical muscle stimulation, as needed

Isometric leg presses at week 4 (multiangle)

May begin use of pool for gait training and exercises week 4

Functional Activities

Gradually return to daily activities

If symptoms occur, reduce activities to reduce pain and inflammation

Extended standing should be avoided

Swelling Control

Ice, elevation, compression, and edema modalities as needed to decrease swelling

Criteria to Progress to Phase II

Full passive knee extension

Knee flexion to 120 degrees

Minimal pain and swelling

Voluntary quadriceps activity

Phase II—Transition Phase (Weeks 6-12)

Goals

Gradually increase ROM

Gradually improve quadriceps strength and endurance

Gradually increase functional activities

Brace

Discontinue brace at week 6

Consider unloading knee brace

Weight Bearing

Progress WB as tolerated

50% body weight with crutches at 6 weeks

Progress to full WB at 8 weeks

Discontinue crutches at 8 weeks

May delay full WB 1-2 weeks if lesion is large or uncontained

(continued)

BOX 21-3

Femoral Condyle Rehabilitation Guidelines—cont'd

Range of Motion

Gradual increase in ROM

Maintain full passive knee extension

Progress knee flexion to 125-135 degrees

Continue patellar mobilization and soft tissue mobilization, as needed

Continue stretching program

Strengthening Exercises

Initiate weight shifts week 6

Initiate mini-squats 0-45 degrees

Closed kinetic chain exercises (leg presses)

Toe-calf raises

Open kinetic chain knee extension (progressive resistive exercise), 1 lb/week

Stationary bicycle, low resistance (gradually increase time)

Treadmill walking program

Balance and proprioception drills

Initiate front and lateral step-ups

Continue use of biofeedback and electrical muscle stimulation, as needed

Continue use of pool for gait training and exercise

Functional Activities

As pain and swelling (symptoms) diminish, gradually increase functional activities

Gradually increase standing and walking

Criteria to Progress to Phase III

Full ROM

Acceptable strength level

• Hamstrings within 10%-20% of contralateral leg

• Quadriceps within 20%-30% of contralateral leg

Balance testing within 30% of contralateral leg

Able to walk 1-2 miles or bike for 30 minutes

Phase III: Maturation Phase (Weeks 12-26)

Goals

Improve muscular strength and endurance

Increase functional activities

Range of Motion

Patient should exhibit 125-135 degrees of flexion

Exercise Program

Leg presses (0-90 degrees)

Bilateral squats (0-60 degrees)

Unilateral step-ups progressing from 2 to 8 inches

Forward lunges

Walking program

Open kinetic chain knee extension (0-90 degrees)

Bicycle

StairMaster

Swimming

NordicTrack or elliptical

Functional Activities

As patient improves, increase walking (distance, cadence, incline, etc.)

Maintenance Program

Initiate at weeks 16-20

Bicycle—low resistance, increase time

Progressive walking program

Pool exercises for entire lower extremity

Straight leg raises

Leg presses

Wall squats

Hip abduction and adduction

Front lunges

Step-ups

Stretch quadriceps, hamstrings, calf

Criteria to Progress to Phase IV

Full, nonpainful ROM

Strength within 80%-90% of contralateral extremity

Balance and/or stability within 75% of contralateral extremity

No pain, inflammation, or swelling

Phase IV—Functional Activities Phase (Weeks 26-52)

Goals

Gradual return to full unrestricted functional activities

(continued)

6 weeks after cell implantation. During the first 24 hours after cell implantation, the cells line the base of the lesion and multiply several times to produce a matrix that will fill the defect with a soft repair tissue up to the level of the periosteal cover. PROM and controlled partial weight bearing will help to promote the nurturing of the cells through the synovial fluid diffusion as well as provide the proper stimulus for the cells to produce specific matrix markers. During this initial phase, controlled PROM and a gradual weight-bearing progression are the two components critical to the rehabilitation process.

Immediate toe-touch weight bearing is performed, progressing to 25% at week 2, 50% at weeks 4 to 5, and finally full weight bearing at week 8. This progression may be delayed approximately 2 weeks, with 2 weeks of non–weight bearing, if the lesion is large, deep, or uncontained. For lesions within the patella or trochlea, the patient is allowed to bear weight as tolerated immediately after surgery with a brace locked in full extension. ROM is progressed cautiously to avoid swelling as with the OATS procedure, with at least 90 degrees of flexion at week 1, 105 degrees at week 2, 115 degrees at week 3, and 125 degrees at week 4 (Box 21-4).

BOX 21-3

Femoral Condyle Rehabilitation Guidelines—cont'd

Exercises

Continue maintenance program progression three or four times per week

Progress resistance as tolerated

Emphasis on entire lower extremity strength and flexibility

Progress agility and balance drills

Impact loading program should be specialized to the patient's demands

Progress sport programs depending on patient variables

Functional Activities

Patient may return to various sport activities as progression in rehabilitation and cartilage healing allows. Generally, low-impact sports such as swimming, skating, rollerblading, and cycling are permitted at approximately 6 months. Higher-impact sports such as jogging, running, and aerobics may be performed at 8-9 months for small lesions or 9-12 months for larger lesions. High-impact sports such as tennis, basketball, football, and baseball are allowed at 9-12 months for small to medium lesions; however, for larger lesions these activities may be delayed up to 18 months.

BOX 21-4

Autologous Chondrocyte Implantation: Patella and Trochlea Rehabilitation Guidelines

Phase I—Protection Phase (Weeks 0-6)

Goals

Protect healing tissue from load and shear forces

Decrease pain and effusion

Restore full passive knee extension

Gradually improve knee flexion

Regain quadriceps control

Brace

Locked at 0 degrees during ambulation and WB activities

Sleep in locked brace for 4 weeks

Weight Bearing

Immediate toe-touch WB, 25% body weight with brace locked in full extension

50% body weight week 2 in brace

75% body weight weeks 3-4 in brace

Range of Motion

Immediate motion exercise days 1-2

Full passive knee extension immediately

Initiate continuous passive motion (CPM) day 1 for total of 8-12 hours/day (0-60 degrees; if lesion >6 cm^2 0-40 degrees) for first 2-3 weeks

Progress CPM ROM as tolerated 5-10 degrees per day

May continue use of CPM for total of 6-8 hours/day for 6 weeks

Patellar mobilization (four to six times per day)

Motion exercises throughout the day

Passive knee flexion ROM two or three times daily

Knee flexion ROM goal is 90 degrees by 2-3 weeks

Knee flexion ROM goal is 105 degrees by 3-4 weeks and 120 degrees by week 6

Stretch hamstrings, calf

(continued)

BOX 21-4

Patella and Trochlea Rehabilitation Guidelines—cont'd

Strengthening Program

Ankle pump using rubber tubing

Quadriceps setting

Straight leg raises (four directions)

Toe-calf raises week 2

Stationary bicycle when ROM allows

Biofeedback and electrical muscle stimulation, as needed

Isometric leg press at week 4 (multiangle)

Initiate weight shifts week 4

May begin pool therapy for gait training and exercise week 4

Functional Activities

Gradually return to daily activities

If symptoms occur, reduce activities to reduce pain and inflammation

Extended standing should be avoided

Swelling Control

Ice, elevation, compression, and edema-control modalities as needed to decrease swelling

Criteria to Progress to Phase II

Full passive knee extension

Knee flexion to 115-120 degrees

Voluntary quadriceps activity

Phase II—Transition Phase (Weeks 6-12)

Goals

Gradually increase ROM

Gradually improve quadriceps strength and endurance

Gradually increase functional activities

Brace

Discontinue brace at 6 weeks

Weight Bearing

Progress WB as tolerated

Progress to full WB at 6 weeks

Discontinue crutches at 6 weeks

Range of Motion

Gradual increase in ROM

Maintain full passive knee extension

Progress knee flexion to 120-125 degrees by week 8

Continue patellar mobilization and soft tissue mobilization as needed

Continue stretching program

Strengthening Exercises

Closed kinetic chain exercises (leg presses 0-60 degrees) week 8

Initiate mini-squats 0-45 degrees week 8

Toe-calf raises

Open kinetic chain knee extension without resistance

Begin knee extension at 0-30 degrees, then progress to deeper angles

Stationary bicycle (gradually increase time)

StairMaster at week 12

Balance and proprioception drills

Initiate front and lateral step-ups

Continue use of biofeedback and electrical muscle stimulation, as needed

Functional Activities

As pain and swelling (signs and symptoms) diminish, gradually increase functional activities

Gradually increase standing and walking

Criteria to Progress to Phase III

Full ROM

Acceptable strength level

• Hamstrings within 10%-20% of contralateral leg

• Quadriceps within 20%-30% of contralateral leg

Balance testing within 30% of contralateral leg

Able to walk 1-2 miles or bike for 30 minutes

Phase III: Remodeling Phase (Weeks 13-32)

Goals

Improve muscular strength and endurance

Increase functional activities

Range of Motion

Patient should exhibit 125-135 degrees of flexion

(continued)

Early strength and proprioceptive exercises are performed according to the patient's weightbearing status.

The second phase is the transitional phase and includes weeks 7 through 12. The repair tissue at this point is spongy and compressible with little resistance. On arthroscopic examination the tissue may, in fact, have a wavelike motion to it when a probe is slid over the tissue. During this phase the patient achieves full ROM and progresses from partial weight bearing to full weight bearing. Continued maturation of the repair tissue is fostered through higher-level functional and motion exercises. Closed kinetic chain exercises, such as front lunges, step ups, and wall squats, are performed as well as machine exercises for the entire lower extremity. Again,

caution should be used with exercises that produce sheer in patients with patellofemoral lesions.

The third phase is known as the *remodeling-functional phase* and occurs from 12 weeks through 32 weeks postoperatively. During this phase there is a continuous produciton of matrix with further remodeling into a more organized structural tissue. The tissue at this point has the consistency of soft plastic on probing. As the tissue becomes more firm and integrated, it allows for more functional training activities to be performed.

The final phase is known as the *maturation and optimizing phase* and can last up to 15 to 18 months depending on the size and location of the lesion. It is during this phase that the

---

BOX 21-4

Patella and Trochlea Rehabilitation Guidelines—cont'd

Exercise Program

Leg presses (0-60 degrees; progress to 0-90 degrees)

Bilateral squats (0-60 degrees)

Unilateral step-ups progressing from 2 to 6 inches

Forward lunges

Walking program on treadmill

Open kinetic chain knee extension (90-40 degrees); progress 1 lb every 10-14 days if no pain or crepitation is present; must monitor symptoms

Bicycle

StairMaster

Swimming

NordicTrack or elliptical training

Functional Activities

As patient improves, increase walking (distance, cadence, incline, etc.)

Light running can be initiated toward end of phase based on physician decision

Maintenance Program

Initiate at weeks 16-20

Bicycle—low resistance, increase time

Progressive walking program

Pool exercises for entire lower extremity

Straight leg raises

Leg presses

Wall squats

Hip abduction and adduction

Front lunges

Step-ups

Stretch quadriceps, hamstrings, calf

Criteria to Progress to Phase IV

Full nonpainful ROM

Strength within 80%-90% of contralateral extremity

Balance and/or stability within 75% of contralateral extremity

No pain, inflammation, or swelling

Phase IV—Maturation Phase (8-15 Months)

Goals

Gradual return to full unrestricted functional activities

Exercises

Continue maintenance program progression three or four times per week

Progress resistance as tolerated

Emphasis on entire lower extremity strength and flexibility

Progress agility and balance drills

Progress walking program as tolerated

Impact loading program should be specialized to the patient's demands

No jumping or plyometric exercise for 12 months

Progress sport programs depending on patient variables

Functional Activities

Patient may return to various sport activities as progression in rehabilitation and cartilage healing allows. Generally, low-impact sports such as swimming, skating, rollerblading, and cycling are permitted at approximately 6 months. Higher impact sports such as jogging, running, and aerobics may be performed at 8-9 months for small lesions or 9-12 months for larger lesions. High-impact sports such as tennis, basketball, football, and baseball are allowed at 9-12 months for small to medium lesions; however, for larger lesions such activities may be delayed up to 18 months.

repair tissue reaches its full maturation. The stiffness of the cartilage resembles that of the surrounding tissue. The duration of this phase varies, based on several factors such as lesion size and location.

These basic science studies have shown that it may take up to 6 months for the graft site to become firm and at least 9 months to become as durable as the surrounding healthy articular cartilage.[13,15] Therefore low-impact activities are initiated by months 5 to 6 and progressed to moderate-impact activities from months 7 to 9 as tolerated.

Long-term outcome studies after ACI have also shown favorable outcomes.[11,13,15] Peterson and colleagues[15] have followed the first 61 patients for up to 11 years postoperatively. The authors report good to excellent results in 89% of femoral condyle lesions, 86% of OCD lesions, and 79% of patellar lesions (with concomitant realignment procedures). Furthermore, graft survival and durability in patients with good to excellent results at 2 years after surgery was 100% at second follow-up of up to 11 years. These results are similar to those of Minas and Peterson[44] and Gillogly,[51] who have continued to show a gradual improvement in subjective and functional scores each year after implantation.

SUMMARY

The treatment of articular cartilage lesions of the knee continues to evolve in an attempt to regenerate healthy cartilage tissue and allow return to asymptomatic functional activities. Several new procedures, including OAT and ACI, have been developed. The rehabilitation program is based on several key principles and is individualized based on lesion, patient, and surgical variables. Rehabilitation is vital to the overall success of these procedures and must facilitate a healing environment by gradually applying and controlling forces while avoiding overloading of the healing tissue.

References

1. Minas T, Nehrer S: Current concepts in the treatment of articular cartilage defects, *Orthopedics* 20:525-538, 1997.
2. Behrens F, Draft E, Oegema T: Biochemical changes in articular cartilage after joint immobilization by casting or external fixation, *J Orthop Res* 7:335-343, 1989.
3. Haapala J, Arokoski J, Pirttimaki J, et al: Incomplete restoration of immobilization induced softening of young beagle knee articular cartilage after 50-week remobilization, *Int J Sports Med* 21:76-81, 2000.
4. Vanwanseele B, Lucchinetti E, Stussi E: The effects of immobilization on the characteristics of articular cartilage: current concepts and future directions, *Osteoarthritis Cartilage* 10:408-419, 2002.
5. Chandler HP, Reineck FT, Wixson RL, McCarthy JC: Total hip replacement in patients younger than 30 years old: a five year follow-up study, *J Bone Joint Surg* 63A:1426-1434,1981.
6. Dorr LD, Takei GK, Conaty JP: Total hip arthroplasties in patients less than forty-five years old, *J Bone Joint Surg* 65A:474-479,1983.
7. Buckwalter JA, Rosenberg LC, Hunziker EB: Articular cartilage: composition, structure, response to injury, and methods of facili-

tating repair. In Ewing JW, editor: *Articular cartilage and knee joint function: basic science and arthroscopy*, New York, 1990, Raven Press.
8. Mankin H: The response of articular cartilage to mechanical injury, *J Bone Joint Surg* 64A:460-466,1982.
9. Shapiro F, Koide S, Glimcher MJ: Cell origin and differentiation in the repair of full-thickness defects of articular cartilage, *J Bone Joint Surg* 75A:532-553,1993.
10. Convery FR, Akeson WH, Keown GH: The repair of large osteochondral defects: an experimental study in horses, *Clin Orthop* 82:253-262, 1972.
11. Brittberg M, Lindahl A, Nilsson A, et al: Treatment of deep cartilage defects in the knee with autologous chondrocyte transplantation, *N Engl J Med* 331:889-895, 1994.
12. Brittberg M, Nilsson A, Lindahl A, et al: Rabbit articular cartilage defects treated with autologous cultured chondrocytes, *Clin Orthop* 326:270-283, 1996.
13. Peterson L, Minas T, Brittberg M, et al: Two- to 9-year outcome after autologous chondrocyte transplantation of the knee, *Clin Orthop* 374:212-234, 2000.
14. Grande DA, Pitman MI, Peterson L, et al: The repair of experimentally produced defects in rabbit articular cartilage by autologous chondrocyte implantation, *J Orthop Res* 7:208-218, 1989.
15. Peterson L, Brittberg M, Kiviranta I, et al: Autologous chondrocyte transplantation: biomechanics and long-term durability, *Am J Sports Med* 30:2-12, 2002.
16. Buckwalter JA, Mankin HJ: Articular cartilage. Tissue design and chondrocyte matrix interactions, *J Bone J Surg Am* 79(A):600-611, 1997.
17. Buckwalter JA: Articular cartilage: injuries and potential for healing, *J Orthop Sports Phys Ther* 28:192-202, 1998.
18. Waldman SD, Spiteri CG, Grynpas MD, et al: Effect of biomechanical conditioning on cartilaginous tissue formation in vitro, *J Bone Joint Surg Am* 85-A(suppl 2):101-105, 2003.
19. Harrison RA, Hillman M, Bulstrode S: Loading of the limb when walking partially immersed, *Physiotherapy* 78:1992.
20. Salter RB: The biological concept of continuous passive motion of synovial joints: the first 18 years of basic research and its clinical application. In Ewing JW, editor: *Articular cartilage and knee joint function*, New York, 1990, Raven Press.
21. Rodrigo JJ, Steadman JR, Sillman JF, et al: Improvement of full-thickness chondral defect healing in the human knee after debridement and microfracture using continuous passive motion, *Am J Knee Surg* 7:109-116, 1994.
22. Iwaki H, Pinskerova V, Freeman MAR: Tibiofemoral movement 1: the shapes and relative movements of the femur and tibia in the unloaded cadaver knee, *J Bone Joint Surg* 82B:1189-1195, 2000.
23. Martelli S, Pinskerova V: The shapes of the tibial and femoral articular surfaces in relation to tibiofemoral movement, *J Bone Joint Surg* 84B:607-613, 2002.
24. Hungerford DS, Barry M: Biomechanics of the patellofemoral joint, *Clin Orthop* 144:9-15, 1979.
25. Huberti HH, Hayes WC: Patellofemoral contact pressures, *J Bone Joint Surg* 66A:715-724, 1984.
26. Steinkamp LA, Dillingham MF, Markel MD, et al: Biomechanical considerations in patellofemoral joint rehabilitation, *Am J Sports Med* 21:438-444, 1993.
27. Perry J, Antonelli D, Ford W: Analysis of knee-joint forces during flexed-knee stance, *J Bone Joint Surg* 57:961-967, 1975.
28. Millett PJ, Wickiewicz TL, Warren RF: Motion loss after ligament injuries to the knee: Part I: Causes, *Am J Sports Med* 29:664-675, 2001.

29. Shelbourne KD, Wilckens JH, Mollabashy A, et al: Arthrofibrosis in acute anterior cruciate ligament reconstruction. The effect of timing of reconstruction and rehabilitation, *Am J Sports Med* 19:332-336, 1991.

30. Spencer JD, Hayes KC, Alexander I: Knee joint effusion and quadriceps reflex inhibition in man, *Arch Phys Med Rehabil* 65:171-177, 1984.

31. Young A, Stokes M, Shakespeare DT, Sherman KP: The effect of intra-articular bupivacaine on quadriceps inhibition after meniscectomy, *Med Sci Sports Exerc* 15:154, 1983.

32. Salter RB, Hamilton HW, Wedge JH: Clinical application of basic science research on continuous passive motion for disorders of injuries and synovial joints, *J Orthop Res* 1:325-333, 1984.

33. Delitto A, Rose SJ, McKowen LM, et al: Electrical stimulation versus voluntary exercise in strengthening thigh musculature after anterior cruciate ligament surgery, *Phys Ther* 68:660-663, 1988.

34. Snyder-Mackler L, Delitto A, Bailey SL, Stralka SW: Strength of the quadriceps femoris muscle and functional recovery after reconstruction of the anterior cruciate ligament. A prospective, randomized clinical trial of electrical stimulation, *J Bone Joint Surg Am* 77:1166-1173, 1995.

35. Frisbie DD, Oxford JT, Southwood L, et al: Early events in cartilage repair after subchondral bone microfracture, *Clin Orthop* 407:215-227, 2003.

36. Hangody L, Kish G, Karpati Z, et al: Autogenous osteochondral graft technique for replacing knee cartilage defects in dogs, *Orthopedics* 5:175-181, 1997.

37. Nam EK, Makhsous M, Koh J, et al: Biomechanical and histological evaluation of osteochondral transplantation in a rabbit model, *Am J Sports Med* 32:308-316, 2004.

38. Hangody L, Kish G, Karpati Z, et al: Osteochondral plugs: autogenous osteochondral mosaicplasty for the treatment of focal chondral and osteochondral articular defects, *Oper Tech Orthop* 7:312, 1997.

39. Hangody L, Fules P: Autologous osteochondral mosaicplasty for the treatment of full-thickness defects of weight-bearing joints; ten years of experimental and clinical experience, *J Bone Joint Surg* 85-A:25-32, 2003.

40. Simonian P, Sussman P, Wickiewicz T, et al: Contact pressures at osteochondral donor sites in the knee, *Am J Sports Med* 26:491-494, 1998.

41. Andres B, Mears S, Somel D, et al: Treatment of osteoarthritic cartilage lesions with osteochondral autograft transplantation, *Orthopedics* 26:11:1121-1126, 2003.

42. Whiteside RA, Bryant JT, Jakob RP, et al: Short-term load bearing capacity of osteochondral autografts implanted by the mosaicplasty technique: an in vitro porcine model, *J Biomech* 36:1203-1208, 2003.

43. Aubin PP, Cheah HK, Davis AM, Gross AE: Long-term followup of fresh femoral osteochondral allografts for posttraumatic knee defects, *Clin Orthop* 391(suppl):S318-S327, 2001.

44. Minas T, Peterson L: Advanced techniques in autologous chondrocyte transplantation, *Clin Sports Med* 18:13, 1999.

45. Minas T, Peterson L: Chondrocyte transplantation, *Oper Tech Orthop* 7:323, 1997.

46. Roberts S, McCall IW, Darby AJ, et al: Autologous chondrocyte implantation for cartilage repair: monitoring its success by magnetic resonance imaging and histology, *Arthritis Res Ther* 5:R60-R73, 2003.

47. Horas U, Pelinkovic D, Herr G, et al: Autologous chondrocyte implantation and osteochondral cylinder transplantation in cartilage repair of the knee joint, *J Bone Joint Surg* 85:185-192, 2003.

48. Mandelbaum B, Browne J, Fu F, et al: Articular cartilage lesions of the knee, *Am J Sports Med* 26:853-861, 1998.

49. Minas T: The role of cartilage repair techniques, including chondrocyte transplantation, in focal chondral knee damage, *Instr Course Lect* 48:629-643, 1998.

50. Minas T, Nehrer S: Current concepts in the treatment of articular cartilage defects, *Orthopedics* 20:525-538, 1997.

51. Gillogly SD: Treatment of large full-thickness chondral defects of the knee with autologous chondrocyte implantation, *Arthroscopy* 19(suppl 1):147-153, 2003.

CHAPTER 22

Salvage of Failed Knee Chondroplasty Using Articular Cartilage Paste Grafting

Kevin R. Stone, MD
Ann W. Walgenbach, RNNP, MSN
Laura E. Keller, MPT
Brandon Smetana

CHAPTER OUTLINE

DAMAGE TO ARTICULAR CARTILAGE

often leads to pain and swelling. Successful treatment of the signs and symptoms by arthroscopic methods has led to variable outcomes. When the treatments fail, the alternatives are few, and often the patient is left waiting for artificial joint arthroplasty.

This chapter discusses our method of salvaging failed chondroplasties with a technique called *articular cartilage paste grafting*. We present the technique and discuss the outcomes with case study examples from efforts to salvage a failed microfracture, a failed primary fixation for a large osteochondritis dissecans (OCD) lesion, and a failed osteochondral autograft transfer (OAT) procedure and to treat traumatic arthritis. We also present the rehabilitation program that has successfully returned these patients to sports performance.

ARTICULAR CARTILAGE PASTE GRAFTING TECHNIQUE

History of Procedure

Articular cartilage lesions in the knee joint encountered at arthroscopy appear on a continuum from fibrillation or a "crabmeat" appearance of the cartilage surface to fragmentation with exposed bone. The appearance of the lesions is often deceiving because more of the surrounding articular cartilage is often involved than appears from the surface appearance. When the cartilage is damaged, it loses the viscoelasticity that permits shock absorption. After damage the underlying bone becomes diseased or sclerotic from the abnormal forces applied to it. High-field magnetic resonance imaging can reveal the extent of the associated damage to the surgeon more than arthroscopic surface viewing. However, treatments for articular cartilage lesions have been primarily focused on mechanical removal of fragmented cartilage by shaving or debridement of the chondral lesions. By removing damaged cartilage, the surgeon hopes to reduce cartilage fragmentation into the joint, thereby reducing the inflammation of the synovium. Although diseased cartilage is removed, there is no stimulation for new cartilage to form. Cartilage stimulation methods were developed such as drilling and microfracture in an effort to stimulate a repair process. The blood from the marrow provides pluripotential cells to the damaged surface and forms cartilage repair tissue. The variable quality of the repair tissue leads to variable outcomes. In an effort to grow hyaline-like cartilage from chondrocytes, cartilage cellular regrowth methods are used; these are discussed in other chapters. Lastly, complete plugs of intact articular cartilage are being tried with the "rob Peter to pay Paul" approach of taking healthy cartilage surfaces from one part of the knee and transplanting them to another. Although each of these methods has resulted in some success, none of these methods have been indicated in the setting of arthritis, and none have been designed as a salvage procedure.

We noticed that when a notchplasty is performed to reconstruct the anterior cruciate ligament (ACL), the notch frequently grows back. In addition, we noted in our skiing population that larger intraarticular fractures often stimulated an exuberant healing process. From this observation we speculated cartilage regeneration in arthritic lesions may be possible by providing a similarly favorable environment. We believe that for this to occur, chronic arthritic lesions of dead bone should be converted into fresh fractures by morselizing the entire lesion with a fracture awl. Evolving from the principles of microfracture, in which the structure and subchondral bone are preserved but perforated, our intention was to completely fracture the surface and the subchondral bone to stimulate the largest possible fracture repair stimulation model. We then hypothesized that live articular cartilage cells could be harvested from the intercondylar notch with underlying cancellous bone and smashed into a paste that would contain both the cells and the stimulating factors found in the extracellular matrix of cartilage combined with the support of a bony matrix. This paste could then be impacted into the fracture bed, allowing for a single-step arthroscopic cartilage transplantation and joint surface reconstruction. We have observed that only a small amount of the paste is needed within the prepared fracture site to stimulate a repair response. This response can lead to hypertrophy of the repair lesion, which is most likely a result of the stimulation of the repair process by the pluripotential marrow cells and growth factors mixing with the transplanted chondrocytes and matrix of the paste in the fracture site.

As of 2005 we have performed this paste graft technique in more than 210 patients. This chapter presents the technique and focuses on examples of patients who have failed other chondroplasty methods.

UNDERGOING THE ARTICULAR CARTILAGE PASTE GRAFTING SURGICAL TECHNIQUE

The workup of the failed chondroplasty is as important as the surgical treatment. The first goal is to identify what failure means to the patient. If pain at the site of the treated lesion is the primary problem, salvage treatment has a chance. However, if there are significant biomechanical abnormalities such as axis deviation into varus or valgus with posterior medial or lateral thrust in gait, any biologic procedure will be doomed to fail earlier than expected. As we tell our patients, "Bad biomechanics kills good biology any day of the week."

A patient coming to our clinic will first undergo a careful history assessment by the nurse practitioner or physician's assistant, independent of the surgeon, to identify the site, cause, and frequency of the symptoms. Standardized outcome forms including International Knee Documentation Committee (IKDC), Tegner activity, and SF-36 are completed by the patient. The surgeon repeats the history assessment and performs a manual examination of the knee to identify the source of pain. Remarkable amounts of different information are obtained through this process, and odd symptoms or expectations can be identified to prevent surgical disappointment. A gait analysis by the orthopedic surgeon and subsequently by the physical therapy team is performed, in combination with radiographic images including standing posteroanterior (PA) flexion, anteroposterior (AP), skyline, and long leg views. A high-field magnetic resonance imaging (MRI) (ONI, Wilmington, MA) scan is obtained to evaluate the joint. We review surgical images and reports from any previous procedures. A functional physical therapy examination is undertaken to identify core weaknesses and functional restrictions that might be increasing joint pain. Finally, the therapy team assists in determining the patient's willingness to comply with the detailed rehabilitation program required to obtain the best outcome.

With this information the surgeon sits down with the patient to review all the data obtained at the office, including the MRI scan and radiographs. If the patient, the surgeon, the nurse, and the rehabilitation team are all in agreement that the arthritic lesion and the patient can be successfully treated, and if the patient agrees to participate in a detailed rehabilitation program, a surgical date is scheduled.

Preoperative Physical Therapy Evaluation

Physical therapy for a preoperative articular cartilage patient varies case by case, as multiple factors determine what exercises and treatments will help relieve pain preoperatively and postoperatively. These factors include location of injury (medial, lateral, etc.), extent of general pain, activities that induce pain, and overall fitness level. Although each patient's preoperative physical therapy is unique, several general guidelines and exercises are followed that have been proven to reduce signs and symptoms.

Activity Modification

It is essential to modify activities that increase symptoms. "Listening" to a patient's body and finding the level of activity the injured knee can tolerate with given activities will help in making the time spent performing them more comfortable.

Shoe Wear

Wearing shock-absorbing insoles and/or cushioned shoes will help reduce daily pounding to the joint. The less often the joint is stressed repetitively, the less overall damage it incurs in the long run.

Unloading Wedges

Using unloading wedges in a patient's shoe will help take stress off the involved side of the injured joint, distributing it more evenly onto the knee. This not only aids in pain relief, but also in decreasing wear to the joint.

Glucosamine

Glucosamine sulfate is a substance synthesized by the body and naturally present in cartilage. It stimulates cartilage cells to produce certain compounds that are the building blocks of articular cartilage. A daily dose of 1500 mg of glucosamine has been found to be most effective. Glucosamine can be obtained at most stores in pill form or in the liquid form (Joint Juice).

Pain Management

Moist heat packs, warm baths, and Jacuzzis will help relax sore muscles and relieve tightness and soreness. Using a cold pack for 15 minutes when the knee feels acutely irritated or inflamed will reduce pain. Taking nonsteroidal antiinflammatory medications (NSAIDs) can help diminish pain and swelling.

Exercise

Maintaining or improving physical fitness during injury is essential and is accomplished through safe cardiovascular activity, stretching, and strengthening of the muscles surrounding the injury and by altering everyday routines. A healthy body weight helps relieve stress on the joint and is accomplished through regular exercise, good dietary intake, and a healthful lifestyle. Exercise is a critical component in the treatment of a patient undergoing an articular cartilage paste graft. Exercise strengthens the muscles surrounding the joint and improves stability, joint flexibility with decreased pain, and shock absorption. Nonpounding exercises are used to work, stretch, and strengthen the muscles surrounding the injured joint. Such exercises include the stationary bike with light or no resistance, stretching of the entire lower extremity (hamstring, gluteus, quadriceps, and calf), and muscle strengthening by single leg bridging (Figure 22-1). Refer to www.stoneclinic.com for further physical therapy stretching and strengthening exercises.

Technique of Articular Cartilage Paste Grafting for Failed Chondroplasty

The surgical technique includes a complete arthroscopy of the joint, with removal of scar tissue typically found in the suprapatellar pouch and at the patellar tendon tibial interval.

The previously treated lesion is debrided with a shaver, and fragments of bone and cartilage are removed to create a fresh bed (Figure 22-2).

The underlying bone is fractured with an awl to ensure bleeding and fragmentation of the entire subchondral bone area (Figure 22-3).

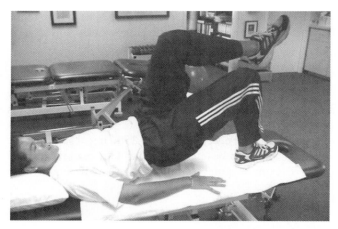

Figure 22-1: Single leg bridge. On the table or floor, start with the knees bent and both feet flat. Bridge up with both feet, and hold with the abdominals tight. Shift weight to the involved side, and lift the opposite leg. Maintain level hips, and press through the heel on the floor. Drop the hips down, then push back to starting position. If any discomfort is felt in the back, do double leg bridges. Three sets of 15 are performed. *(From Stone KR, Walgenbach AW: Surgical technique for articular cartilage transplantation to full thickness cartilage defects in the knee joint, Oper Tech Orthop 7:305-311, 1997.)*

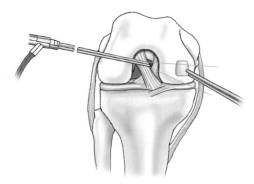

Figure 22-2: Articular cartilage defect site. *(From Stone KR, Walgenbach AW: Surgical technique for articular cartilage transplantation to full thickness cartilage defects in the knee joint, Oper Tech Orthop 7:305-311, 1997.)*

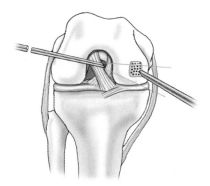

Figure 22-3: Morselization of the articular cartilage lesion. *(From Stone KR, Walgenbach AW: Surgical technique for articular cartilage transplantation to full thickness cartilage defects in the knee joint, Oper Tech Orthop 7:305-311, 1997.)*

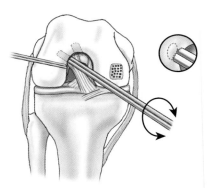

Figure 22-4: Harvesting of the articular cartilage and bone. *(From Stone KR, Walgenbach AW: Surgical technique for articular cartilage transplantation to full thickness cartilage defects in the knee joint, Oper Tech Orthop 7:305-311, 1997.)*

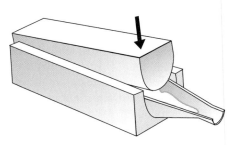

Figure 22-5: Manual crusher used to make the paste graft. *(From Stone KR, Walgenbach AW: Surgical technique for articular cartilage transplantation to full thickness cartilage defects in the knee joint, Oper Tech Orthop 7:305-311, 1997.)*

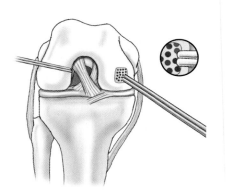

Figure 22-6: Impacting the paste graft into the morselized defect.

The intercondylar notch is approached with a 10 mm trephine. The edge of the trephine captures 3 to 4 mm of articular cartilage and is buried into the bone for a distance of 15 mm (Figure 22-4).

The core of bone and cartilage is placed into a graft impactor and smashed into a paste (Figure 22-5).

The harvesting step is repeated until enough graft is captured to fill the base of the lesion. At the end of the case the graft is impacted into the lesion with the arthroscopy fluid at a very low level (Figure 22-6).

Marcaine is instilled, and the patient is returned to the recovery room.

PATIENT EXAMPLES: ARTICULAR CARTILAGE PASTE GRAFTING EXPERIENCES OF PATIENTS WHO HAVE FAILED OTHER CHONDROPLASTY METHODS

Patient #1: Failed Microfracture Requiring an Articular Cartilage Paste Graft

Patient #1 was a 28-year-old male who injured his knee. After approximately 1 year of conservative care, he underwent a microfracture procedure in April 1999 for a medial femoral condyle defect (Figures 22-7 and 22-8).

After surgery and a course of physical therapy he continued to have pain at the medial joint line. His MRI scan demonstrated irregularity at the medial femoral condyle and mild osteopenia (Figure 22-9). He rated his knee as abnormal and had difficulty descending stairs. He had pain with standing, and he rated his knee as greatly worse than before surgery, with pain at 7 on a scale of 1 to 10 often occurring.

The patient underwent physical therapy following the microfracture procedure and was non–weight bearing for 2 months after the procedure. In January of 2000, he requested arthroscopic intervention due to failure of the microfracture procedure to afford relief.

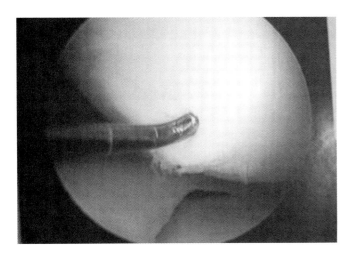

Figure 22-7: Articular cartilage lesion marked.

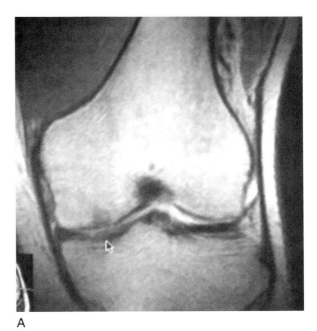

A

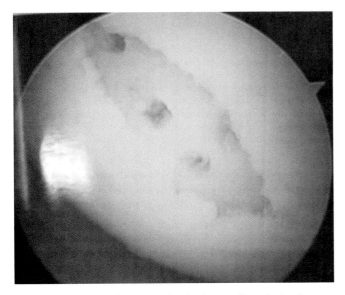

Figure 22-8: Microfracture of articular cartilage lesion by probe.

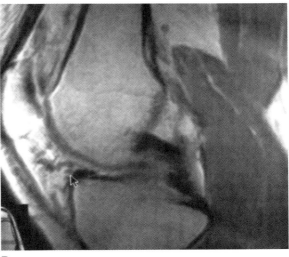

B

Figure 22-9: Magnetic resonance imaging scans indicating irregularity at the medial femoral condyle *(arrows)* and mild osteopenia.

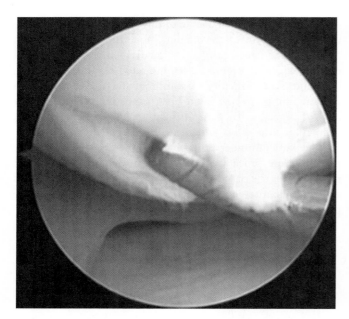

Figure 22-10: Chondral flap of previous medial femoral chondral drilling.

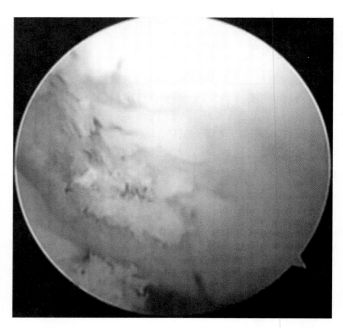

Figure 22-12: Articular cartilage paste grafting, medial femoral condyle.

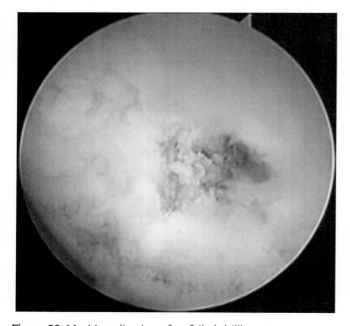

Figure 22-11: Morselization after failed drilling.

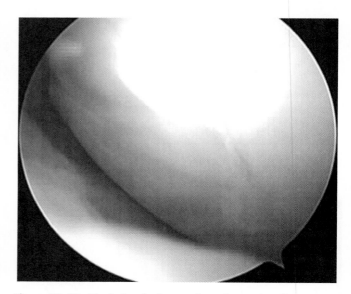

Figure 22-13: Healed articular cartilage 8 months after paste grafting.

The arthroscopic evaluation revealed apparent healing over the microfracture site. However, there was a chondral flap in the central aspect of the site (Figure 22-10), which on probing, continued down to eburnated bone (Figure 22-11). An articular cartilage paste grafting procedure was performed (Figure 22-12).

Before the second surgery a preoperative MRI scan documented an osteochondral defect in the medial femoral condyle, with abnormal bone signal in the femoral compartment of the femur. After 1 month of non–weight bearing,

continuous passive motion (CPM) for 6 hours a night, and a careful rehabilitation program, he did well until 8 months later, when he developed catching at the site of his cartilage grafting.

A MRI scan documented hypertrophy of the cartilage grafting. Repeat arthroscopic intervention was carried out (Figures 22-13 and 22-14). Approximately 21 months after surgery he had returned to bicycling and weight lifting and noted that his knee was generally improving all the time.

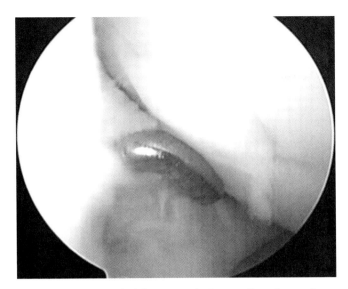

Figure 22-14: Chondral flap on articular cartilage 8 months after paste grafting.

Patient #2: Failed Primary Fixation for Large Osteochondritis Dissecans Lesion Requiring an Articular Cartilage Paste Graft

Surgical procedures to treat OCD lesions have included open or arthroscopic drilling, debridement, reduction and fixation with Smillie pins or Herbert screws, bone grafting, autologous chondrocyte implantation, osteochondral autografts, periosteal and perichondral autografts, and osteochondral allografts.

If treatment fails, an even larger lesion may be the result. Orthopedists are then faced with difficult questions regarding future therapy. Their choices may include attempting another trial of the surgical treatments listed previously or possibly a total or partial knee replacement. Because many of these patients are young, and because knee replacements need replacing every 10 to 20 years, knee replacement is a less desirable option.

Patient #2 was a 25-year-old athletic male in whom Herbert screw fixation of a large OCD lesion had failed. He had injured his knee at age 12 and developed progressive knee pain, such that by his junior year in high school he had to hold onto walls to walk. In 1990, when he was age 18, x-ray films revealed a large OCD lesion involving the weight-bearing surface of the medial femoral condyle. It was believed that the OCD lesion was separating at that point in time, and the patient subsequently underwent a knee arthrotomy (open knee surgery) with elevation of the articular cartilage flap, debridement of the crater, and flap fixation with two Herbert screws. He continued to have pain and popping. Arthrograms and radiographs appeared to show good position of the screws and the fragment. In October 1992, computed tomography (CT) reportedly revealed a nonunion of the fracture fragment, and in April 1993 at diagnostic arthroscopy, one of the Herbert screws was noted to be

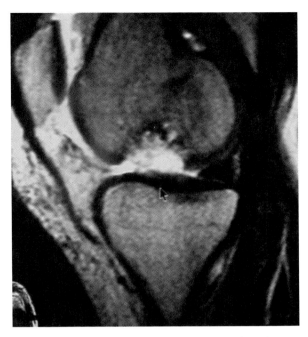

Figure 22-15: Preoperative magnetic resonance imaging scan indicating the osteochondritis dissecans lesion.

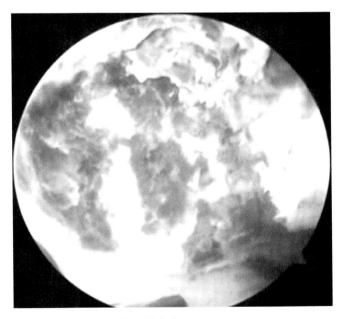

Figure 22-16: Osteochondritic lesion.

slightly loose and the screw was tightened. The pain progressed, and at arthroscopy in January 1998, the screws and the unstable OCD lesion were removed, and he was referred for articular cartilage paste grafting.

Preoperative radiographs and MRI scan revealed a large OCD lesion with underlying avascular necrosis involving a large portion of the femoral condyle (Figure 22-15).

At arthroscopy, a lesion measuring approximately 35 mm × 40 mm × 30 mm was found (Figure 22-16).

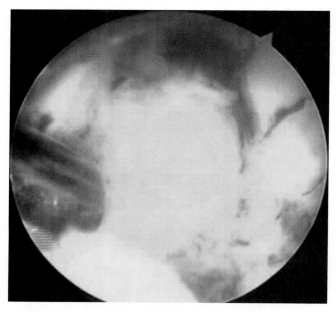

Figure 22-17: Articular cartilage paste grafting, medial femoral condyle, osteochondritis dissecans lesion.

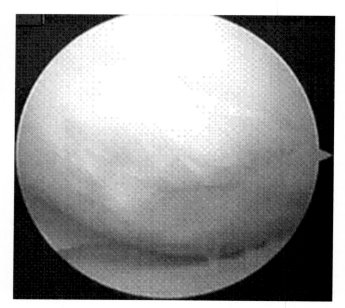

Figures 22-18: Surgical appearance of osteochondritis dissecans lesion 8 months after articular cartilage paste grafting.

The base was hard and sclerotic. The articular cartilage paste grafting procedure previously described was used. The base of the lesion was morselized until bleeding occurred. Articular cartilage and cancellous bone were harvested from a non–weight-bearing region of the knee. The articular cartilage and cancellous bone were smashed to form a paste in a bone graft crusher and were arthroscopically impacted into the lesion (Figure 22-17).

Postoperatively, the patient was kept non–weight bearing for 4 weeks, using crutches. A CPM unit was used in a range of motion from 0 to 75 degrees for 6 hours each night for 4 weeks. Bike and pool exercises with minimal resistance were started at 2 weeks. Impact sports were started after 3 months (See complete rehabilitation program at the end of this chapter).

The patient noted immediate pain relief. He stated that he had not been pain free since he was 12 years old. At the 8-month follow-up he graded his knee as normal in activities of daily living including walking, stairs, and squatting and kneeling, and he water-skied regularly.

Arthroscopy revealed a healed OCD lesion with a full fibrous covering (Figures 22-18 and 22-19). At 20 months after the original graft was placed he rated his knee as having no pain with all activities on the WOMAC Osteoarthritis Index.

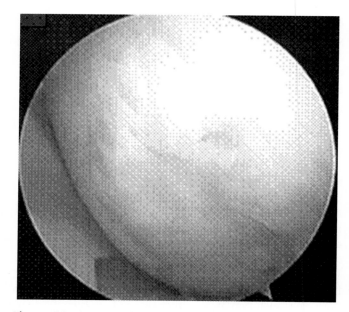

Figures 22-19: Surgical appearance of osteochondritis dissecans lesion 8 months after articular cartilage paste grafting.

Patient #3: Failed Osteochondral Autograft Transfer Procedure Requiring an Articular Cartilage Paste Graft

Patient #3, a 39-year-old engineer, experienced failure of an osteochondral autograft transplantation and fixation proce-

dure to an OCD lesion located at the weight-bearing surface of the medial femoral condyle (Figure 22-20).

He reportedly grew 5 inches in 4 to 5 months at approximately age 15 and developed the knee pain around that time. Beginning around age 18 he underwent three surgical debridements in 1978, 1985, and 1986. Although the operative reports were not available, it was speculated that the second surgery might have consisted of an abrasion chondroplasty to the lesion. In April 1998 an OATS procedure (a

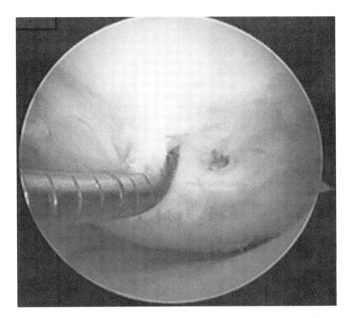

Figure 22-20: Retained hardware in medial femoral condyle 7 months after failed osteochondral autograft transfer procedure.

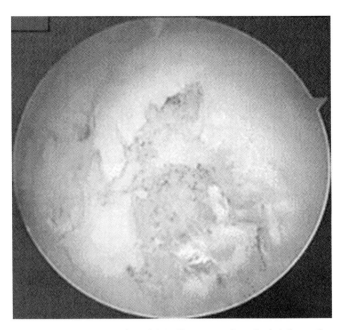

Figure 22-22: Osteochondritis dissecans chondral defect after debriding.

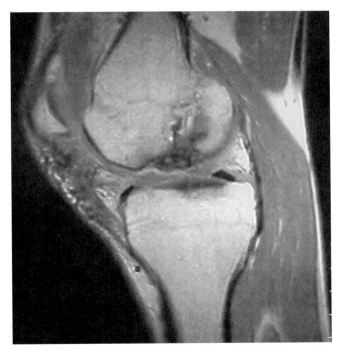

Figure 22-21: Preoperative magnetic resonance imaging scan of the osteochondritis dissecans lesion with failed osteochondral autograft transfer and pin fixation.

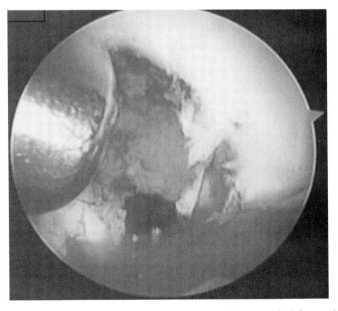

Figure 22-23: Articular cartilage paste grafting, medial femoral condyle, osteochondritis dissecans lesion.

type of osteochondral autografting) was performed by his private physician at the central aspect of the lesion while a portion of the OCD lesion was stabilized using absorbable screws. The patient was pain free until October 1998, and an MRI scan (Figure 22-21) was obtained, revealing a possible large chondral defect and an apparent loose body.

The resorbable pins were removed at arthroscopy in November 1998 and an articular cartilage paste graft was placed (Figures 22-22, 22-23, and 22-24). The paste graft was applied to the 20 × 25 × 25 mm depth lesion at the medial femoral condyle using the same technique as previously described.

The patient was non–weight bearing using crutches and a CPM machine for 4 weeks. He eventually returned to full sports and rated his knee as greatly improved.

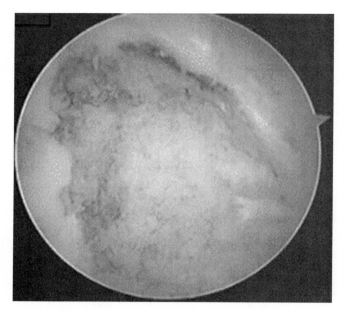

Figure 22-24: Osteochondritis dissecans cartilage defect after paste grafting.

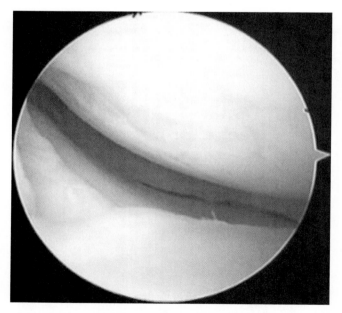

Figure 22-25: Appearance of the medial femoral condyle 14 months after articular cartilage paste grafting of the osteochondritis dissecans lesion.

While rollerblading in December 1999 he crashed onto the surgical knee. By February 2000 he developed increasing pain, catching, and limping. At arthroscopy, 14 months after the articular cartilage graft was placed, the condyle appeared well healed with a thickened fibrous cover (Figure 22-25). He is now without pain or swelling. He has been able to ski, golf, and Jet Ski without complaint.

These patients had large defects on the weight-bearing surfaces of the medial femoral condyle and pain that had been refractory to prior treatment. Through articular cartilage paste grafting, these patients were successfully treated and reported dramatic pain relief.

ARTICULAR CARTILAGE TRANSPLANTATION REHABILITATION GOALS

The desired outcome of a successful rehabilitation program is that the patient is discharged fitter, faster, and stronger than before any given procedure. To accomplish this, the clinician must address all aspects of the rehabilitation process, including good preoperative education and utmost compliance with each of the phases of the physical therapy postoperative protocol.

Primary goals for those who receive articular cartilage transplantation (paste graft) include full and pain-free restoration of movement and strength, a smooth and restored articular surface, a return to all activities of daily living, and a return to all athletic endeavors. These goals are achieved through good preoperative and postoperative teamwork among the patient, the doctor, and the physical therapist. Full analysis by the rehabilitation specialist of gait and mechanics must be performed on an ongoing basis, and any compensatory patterns should be identified to prevent any comorbidities to a healthy joint. During the rehabilitation patients should be placed on a whole-body fitness program, including a cardiovascular regimen, strengthening of the unaffected limbs, and a special emphasis on core (abdominal and gluteal) strengthening. If the patient is physically fit despite the precautions needed for the paste graft, he or she will be able to return to athletic activities at a higher level of function when the graft is ready.

Long-term care of the articular cartilage transplantation rests in the hands of the patient. Such patients must know that they are never officially "discharged" from their home exercise programs. Patient education must include everything from proper shoe wear to the knowledge that he or she must keep body weight down, take 1500 mg of glucosamine each day, stay flexible and strong, and limit the overall amount of time spent in high-impact activities. The patient will have follow-up visits at 1, 5, and 10 years, with the doctor to evaluate the longevity of the procedure. At these visits, sports tests will also be conducted to make sure the patient is able to maintain the physical regimen for proper care of the graft.

Preoperative Phase

Ideally, a preoperative joint would be one that is not inflamed, painful, or lacking in range of motion or strength. However, this is seldom the case when patients are considering articular cartilage transplantation. Those with articular cartilage injuries will have chronic edema, pain, loss of motion, crepitus in the joint with movement, and in some cases, bone deformity. It is the goal preoperatively to restore as much normal function as possible.

Treatment includes techniques for edema control such as soft tissue mobilization, compression, ice, and elevation. An exercise program is established that will facilitate muscle recruitment and joint range of motion without exacerbating any symptoms of swelling or pain. At this time, the patient will also be started on a strong abdominal program, as well as continuing with resistance training of the uninjured limbs.

The general considerations discussed with the patient are as follows:

- Non–weight-bearing status will be required for 4 weeks after surgery (resting foot on floor and driving are acceptable).
- Most patients will be in a hinged neoprene brace for support and to serve as a reminder not to bear any weight on the limb. The patient may wear an unloading brace once swelling is reduced enough for proper fit.
- Depending on the location of the articular cartilage defect and subsequent graft, patients may have active and/or passive range of motion restrictions (this will be noted on the prescription); otherwise, push for full hyperextension equal to the opposite side.
- Regular manual treatment should be conducted to the patella and all incisions, with particular attention to the anterior medial portal, to decrease the incidence of fibrosis.
- Light to no resistance stationary cycling is begun 3 weeks *after* surgery.
- Early recruitment of the vastus medialis muscle will speed recovery. Neuromuscular electrical stimulation may be used for facilitation if the patient is having difficulty with recruitment.
- No resisted leg extension machines (isotonic or isokinetic) can be used at any point.
- Low-impact activities are to be performed for 3 months after surgery.
- 1500 mg of glucosamine sulfate is to be taken daily.
- Soft Sole insole or equivalent is worn for shock absorption in shoes.
- The CPM machine is used for 6 hours a day for 4 weeks.

Preoperative training also includes addressing the psychologic factors of apprehension and fear of the upcoming procedure. Patients who are well informed about each step of the surgery and subsequent rehabilitation do better than those who are uninformed. The patient should have a good support system at home, all doctor and physical therapy appointments should be scheduled, and a short leave of absence should be taken from work. If steps are taken to eliminate stress from recovery, the outcome is typically better.

Postoperative: Protective Phase (4 weeks)

Initial Postoperative Rehabilitation (Week 1)

The first 5- to 7-day period after surgery is perhaps the most important time for healing. At this time the graft is a soft paste made of articular cartilage and the underlying cancellous bone taken from the intercondylar notch and is being held in place only from the clotting reaction that occurs from bloodying the base of the lesion. As such, it needs to be protected and given the best environment for healing.

This phase is dedicated to controlling pain and inflammation. The body does not distinguish between a surgery that will help the joint and a trauma to the joint. The natural response is to create a chemical reaction that stimulates painful nerve endings and swelling and that inhibits muscle firing. This results in guarding, loss of function, and the promotion of scar tissue. To prevent this, manual therapy techniques are used by the physical therapist and the patient is given specific early postoperative guidelines (Box 22-1).

Early Rehabilitation (Weeks 2 to 4)

A visit with the surgeon is required at 8 to 10 days postoperatively for suture removal and check-up. During this remaining 3 weeks of the protective phase the physical therapy treatment will continue with pain control, range of motion exercises, soft tissue treatments, and modalities. The therapist will perform manual resistance (proprioceptive neuromuscular facilitation [PNF] patterns) to the hip, ankle, and foot of the involved leg. The patient will also be challenged with an upper extremity strengthening program and a core stabilization program using gym balls (Figures 22-26 and 22-27).

After the third week the patient may initiate bilateral cycling with light to no resistance. This is allowable only if there is no pain or resistance with the cycling and if there is no latent swelling after any of the exercises up to this point. At such a low level of cycling, there will be minimal cardiovascular benefit, so the patient is encouraged to continue with non–weight-bearing aerobic activities (e.g., aggressive unilateral cycling, upper body ergometer [UBE], and swimming).

By the end of the protective phase the patient will have full extension and flexion nearly equal to the opposite side, no persistent swelling, good patellar and scar mobilization, and minimal to no pain. If the clinical presentation is appropriate, then the patient may progress to the next phase.

Functional Phase (Weeks 4 to 8)

The patient will visit the surgeon for the 1-month follow-up appointment. The doctor will examine the knee and determine the smoothness of the articular surface. Along with the examination and the physical therapy progress report, the decision to progress to full weight bearing will be made. The progression from partial weight bearing to full weight

BOX 22-1
Early Postoperative Guidelines

Icing and Elevation

- As much as able for the first 3-4 days. After that, any time the knee feels inflamed, swollen, or irritated.
- If using a cryotherapy unit, it is best if on for an hour and off for an hour. If using ice wraps or bags, 20-30 minutes every hour. Always make sure to have a barrier between the cuff or wrap and the skin.
- Elevation above the level of the heart as high and as often as tolerated. Also to be performed with periodic sets of ankle pumps (50 reps hourly).

Extension Stretch

- If no ROM restrictions, then sit on floor with heel on a pillow, let the leg relax into *full* extension. Hold for 30 seconds, repeat 10 times/10 times a day.

Flexion Stretch

- If no ROM restrictions, slide heel along the floor toward you into a flexed position until the knee gets tight. Hold 30 seconds, repeat 10 times/10 times a day. This can be alternated with the extension stretch.

Quadriceps Sets

Tighten the muscles on the front of the thigh, focusing on the inner thigh muscle, and hold for 5 seconds. Repeat 10-20 times/10 times a day.

Leg Raises

- Lying back on elbows with uninvolved knee bent, tighten the thigh muscle and lift leg up in front from the hip to the level of the other knee.
- Lying on stomach with the involved knee lying comfortably, tighten the gluteal muscles and lift the leg up behind you from the hip without arching back.
- Lying on uninvolved side, tighten the thigh muscle and lift the leg out to the side, keeping it horizontal to the ground.
- Lying on involved side, step the uninvolved leg over so the foot is flat on the ground just in front of the surgical leg, tighten thigh, and lift involved leg up.
- Start with sets of 10, and work up to four sets of 25 reps.

Activities

- Swimming and deep-water workouts as soon as incisions are healed. Stationary bike with nonsurgical leg is acceptable immediately postoperatively, and two-legged cycling may be begun after 3 weeks, with light to no resistance.

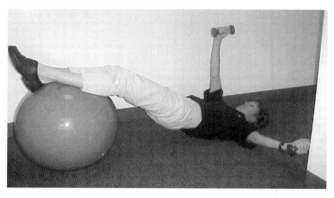

Figure 22-26: Feet on ball bridge. Start with calves on ball, legs straight. Tighten abdominal muscles and gluteals to then lift hips off of the floor. Keep the pelvis level, and hold the plank position. The position is stabilized while hand weights are alternated from side to side.

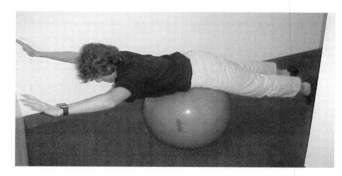

Figure 22-27: Prone on ball (Superman). Start prone over the ball with legs out straight, hands and toes touching down. Squeeze the gluteals and raise the upper body in line with the legs. Without arching the back, slowly straighten arms until they are out in front. Return to the starting position.

bearing is done gradually over the next 5 to 7 days, weaning down to one crutch or cane, to no assistive device. If pain or swelling is associated with the weight bearing, the progression will be slowed down until signs and symptoms no longer occur. Gait analysis is done to ensure there are no gait abnormalities with full weight bearing. If the patient is not able to normalize the gait, he or she must continue using a cane or a single crutch in order to prevent hip and/or lower back compensation.

At this point, the therapist will start to integrate functional exercises, with emphasis on closed chain movements now that open chain exercises are no longer the default (Box 22-2). Balance and proprioceptive exercises are added, as well as a return to road cycling and walking on a treadmill. The initial introduction of these exercises must be at a low level, and the progression must be based only on good clinical findings.

Increasing the resistance of the exercises beyond body weight and gravity will begin in the sixth week. It is also

BOX 22-2
Functional Phase

Week 5

Bilateral leg biking, light to no resistance

Upper body and trunk training

Gait training to normalize patterns

Standing calf raises

Weight shift in multiple planes

Seated or standing trunk mobility exercises (trunk rotation, side-bending)

Single leg balancing

Bridging

Weeks 6-7

Mini-squats and split squats

Wide-based walks with Thera-band loop around ankle ("monster walks")

2-legged stationary biking with light resistance

Mini step-ups with perfect knee biomechanics

Single leg balancing with perturbation

Deep-water workouts; flutter kicks

Elliptical cardiovascular machine (light resistance, no more than 20 minutes)

Week 8

Low-impact lateral agility work

Functional squatting and lunging

Outdoor road biking—avoid steep hills

Moderate step-ups

Train for components of sport-specific activities (e.g., lateral lunges for skiers)

Progress intensity of exercises per patient and symptom tolerance

Versa climber cardiovascular machine

Beyond Week 8

Progressive return to sports activities

Avoid cutting and pivoting until week 12

during this time that the therapist may add lateral training exercises. By the end of the functional phase (week 8), all gait abnormalities should be cleared, flexion should be to end range, and activities of daily living should be accomplished without difficulty (with the exception of lifting or pushing heavy items).

Advanced Functional Phase (Weeks 8 to 12)

During this last phase of rehabilitation, the emphasis is on achieving functional and athletic goals through continued strengthening. Attention is still paid to the soft tissue if needed for manual stretching and to make sure that no patellar symptoms arise. If compensations are not caught, strain to the low back and hips may occur as the exercises are advanced.

Low-impact activities are allowed through this phase, including road cycling, elliptical machines, walking on a treadmill, and cross-country skiing. Lateral movements are also incorporated, with exercises geared toward the desired sport.

SUMMARY

Cartilage lesions that have failed previous surgery are not necessarily end-stage lesions for many patients. The opportunity to refracture the arthritic lesion, stimulate a new healing bed, and provide pluripotential cells to a stimulatory matrix of paste graft permits the hope for successful healing.

A successful rehabilitation program after articular cartilage transplantation results in a patient who is fitter, faster, and stronger than before surgery. We hope to return the patient to most recreational sporting activities. Caution is exercised with the patient when discussing return to any high-impact sport or activity. The longevity of the new cartilaginous matrix is still unknown, so we believe that the less abuse to the new material, the longer it will last. Rather than having the patient return to running for a cardiovascular program, we encourage the patient to progressively challenge himself or herself with nonimpact activities.

The combination of surgical stimulation, natural regeneration matrices of cartilage and bone in a paste, inspiring rehabilitation, and a motivated patient is our formula for success.

CHAPTER 23

Proximal and Distal Realignment Procedures

Janice K. Loudon, PhD, PT, ATC

PATELLOFEMORAL PAIN SYNDROME

(PFPS) can be defined as anterolateral knee pain that is associated with excessive compression between the patella and the lateral femoral condyle. In a typical sports medicine practice, it has been reported that PFPS affects anywhere from 21% to 40% of patients seen.[1] It is estimated that 7% to 15% of the general population have some sort of anterior knee pain.[2-4] Females are typically more affected by PFPS than males.[5,6] PFPS is typically activity induced and aggravated by functional activities such as stair climbing, walking, running, and squatting.[7] The major complaints of patients with PFPS are diffuse knee pain, patellar crepitus, knee joint stiffness, and decreased activity levels.[8-12] Onset of symptoms is usually insidious and may occur bilaterally. Suggested causative factors include lower extremity weakness, especially the quadriceps muscle, increased Q angle, faulty lower extremity mechanics, overuse, and lateral retinaculum tightness.[6,13,14] Nonsurgical care is preferred, but if conservative measures fail then surgery may be indicated.

ANATOMIC REVIEW

The patellofemoral joint is a synovial gliding articulation between the patella and trochlear groove of the femur. The patella is the largest sesamoid bone in the body. Geometrically, the patella is shaped like an upside-down triangle that sits distal to the muscle bulk of the quadriceps within the patellar retinaculum that distally forms the patellar tendon. The average patella is 4 to 4.5 cm in length, 5 to 5.5 cm in width, and 2 to 2.5 cm thick.[15]

The patella consists of a trabecular core that is covered with a thin cortical shell. The underside of the patella is the articulating surface, which is covered with a thick layer of articular cartilage (4 to 7 mm). A major vertical ridge divides this surface into medial and lateral halves. The two ridges can be further divided into seven facets: three horizontal pairs—proximal, middle, and distal—and an odd facet that is located on the far medial, posterior aspect of the patella. The patellar facets are convex in order to accommodate the concave femoral surface, with the lateral side wider to help maintain patellar position.

The inverted U–shaped intercondylar groove of the femur forms a concave lateral and medial facet. As with the patella, the lateral facet of the femur is larger and extends more proximally to provide a bony buttress for the patella. A common synovial capsule exists between the patella and the medial and lateral tibiofemoral articulation. Anteriorly, the capsule inserts around the border of the patella.

The stability of the patellofemoral joint is dependent on proper alignment and static and dynamic stabilizers that surround the joint. The alignment of the patella is related to the depth of the femoral sulcus, height of the lateral femoral condyle wall, and the shape of patella. The patella should sit midway between the two condyles when the knee is flexed to 20 degrees. A 5-mm lateral displacement of the patella has been shown to cause a 50% decline in vastus medialis oblique

(VMO) tension in vitro.[16] With the knee flexed to 90 degrees the inferior pole should maintain alignment with the tibial tubercle. An angle greater than 10 degrees is indicative of pathology.[17] Clinically the Q angle is commonly used as a determining factor for proper patellar alignment. The Q angle is the angle between the line of pull of the quadriceps and a line connecting the center of the patella with the tibial tuberosity. The normal Q angle is 13 degrees for males and 18 degrees for females.[17] An increased Q angle is associated with patellofemoral dysfunction. The A angle is another clinical measurement that has been described in the literature.[18] The A angle is the angle formed by the intersection of the line that intersects the patella longitudinally and the line drawn from the inferior pole of the patella to the tibial tubercle. An increased A angle is also related to PFPS.[19,20]

In the tranverse plane the patella should lie horizontally such that the medial and lateral borders are equidistant from the femur (Figure 23-1). A lateral tilt, in which the medial border is higher than the lateral border, can lead to lateral patellofemoral compression syndrome (LPFCS).[15] In the sagittal plane the patella should be lined up so that the superior and inferior borders are equidistant from the femur. A posterior displacement of inferior pole commonly results in fat pad irritation. Ideally the inferior pole lies parallel to the long axis of the femur.

The shape of the patella has also been discussed as a contributing factor to patellar stability. Wiberg devised a classification system based on the articular facet shape of the patella.[21] However, the various shapes are hard to identify on radiographs and may not be as helpful as Wiberg proposed. Different forms of dysplastic patellae are associated with subluxation and dislocation and are easier to identify on x-ray films. Examples of dysplastic patellae include alpine hunter's cap, pebble, patella magna, and patella parva.[22]

Soft tissue structures such as the patellar tendon, capsule, and ligamentous structures also influence the static stability of the patellofemoral joint. The joint must rely on the medial and lateral retinaculum and joint capsule with less than 20 to 30 degrees of flexion because there is no bony stability. The medial structures become important in minimizing lateral translation, and the primary structure to lateral restraint is the medial patellofemoral ligament (MPFL). This ligament runs from the adductor tubercle to the medial border of the patella. Desio and colleagues describe the MPFL as providing 60% total restraint at 20 degrees of knee flexion.[23,24] Secondary restraints include the medial meniscopatellar ligament, which originates from the anterior aspect of the menisci and inserts into the inferior one third of the patella, and the medial retinaculum, with superficial fibers that interdigitate with the medial collateral ligament and the medial patellar tendon.[23]

On the lateral side of the patellofemoral joint, the following structures aid in stability: lateral patellofemoral ligament, capsule, iliotibial band (ITB), and lateral retinaculum (Figure 23-2). The lateral retinaculum consists of a thinner superficial layer that extends from the ITB to the patella and

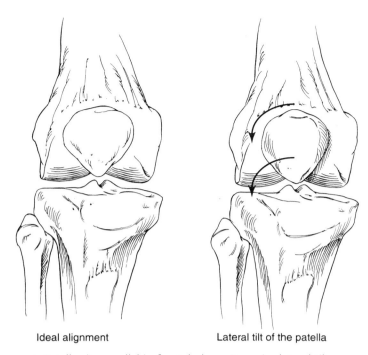

Ideal alignment   Lateral tilt of the patella

Figure 23-1: Ideal patellar alignment. Patella sits parallel in frontal plane. Excessive lateral tilt can cause increased patellar compression. (*From Zachazewski JE, Magee DJ, Quillen WS, editors:* Athletic injuries and rehabilitation, *Philadelphia, 1996, Saunders.*)

quadriceps expansion and a thicker deep layer that interdigitates with the vastus lateralis (VL), patellofemoral ligament, and patellotibial ligament.[25,26]

Dynamically, the contractile structure of the quadriceps, pes anserine muscle group, and biceps femoris muscle help to maintain patellar alignment (Figure 23-3). The importance of the VMO has been discussed extensively in the literature.[27-35] The VMO attaches to the midportion of patella, the MPFL, and the adductor magnus tendon. Its more oblique alignment (as compared with the vastus medialis lateral) provides mechanical advantage to promote medial stabilizing force to the patella.[36,37] The rectus femoris inserts on the anterior portion of superior aspect of the patella.[37] The vastus intermedius inserts posteriorly in the base of patella. Contraction of the quadriceps creates compressive forces on the joint. The VL provides lateral dynamic reinforcement in conjunction with the ITB and the patellar tendon to form the superficial oblique retinaculum.[38] Tightness in the ITB can cause the patella to glide and/or tilt laterally.

BIOMECHANICS

Patellofemoral mechanics are influenced by the quadriceps muscle, shape of the trochlear sulcus, patellar shape, and soft tissue restraints. The mechanical function of the patella is to increase the distance between the quadriceps tendon and the joint axis in order to improve muscle force production. This effect changes throughout the range of knee motion. In addition, the patella transmits compressive forces from the quadriceps tendon and acts as a bony shield for the trochlea (Figure 23-4).[39,40]

In full knee extension the patella lies proximal to the trochlea of the femur, resting on the suprapatellar fat pad and suprapatellar synovium. Its position is slightly lateral because of the external rotation of the tibia. As the knee flexes, the patella glides inferiorly and enters the trochlea from the lateral side. The patella is in contact with one fifth of the articular surface by 20 degrees and moves medially. Between 20 and 90 degrees of flexion the entire surface of patella is in contact with the trochlea, excluding the odd facet. After 90 degrees and until full flexion, the odd facet is the only articulating contact between the patella and the lateral surface of the medial femoral condyle. It is important to note this lateral-medial-lateral tracking of the patella from extension to flexion when examining this joint.[41,42]

Arthrokinematically, the patella should glide superiorly with knee extension. With a quadriceps set the patella should migrate 10 mm superiorly.[43,44] According to Huberti and Hayes the patella is critical in the last 30 degrees of knee extension.[45] At full knee extension the patella provides 31% of total knee extension torque; between 90 and 120 degrees of flexion it provides only 13% (Figure 23-5).

The greater the contact area between the surface of the patella and femur, the less stress is placed on the articular tissue.[42] In non–weight bearing, the contact area between the patella and trochlea increases as the knee flexes from 0 to 90

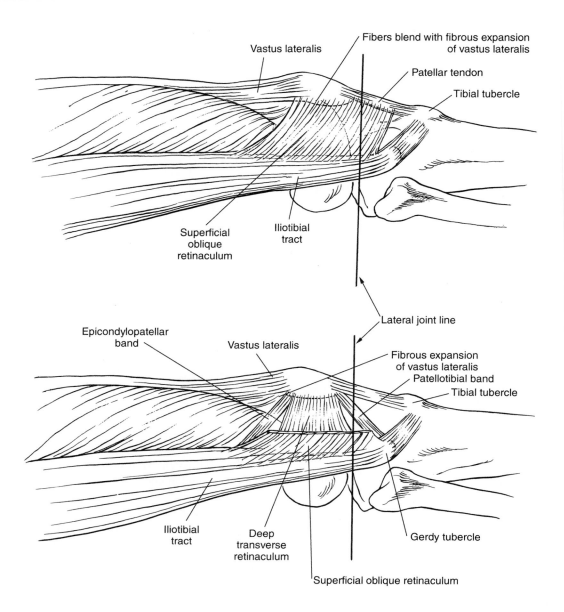

Figure 23-2: Anatomy of the lateral knee. (*From Zachazewski JE, Magee DJ, Quillen WS, editors:* Athletic injuries and rehabilitation, *Philadelphia, 1996, Saunders.*)

degrees, and therefore less stress is placed on this joint as knee flexion increases. However, when the foot is fixed, the patellofemoral joint forces increase from 0 to 90 degrees of knee flexion. Joint forces on the patellofemoral joint are presented in Table 23-1.

PATHOPHYSIOLOGY AND RATIONALE FOR SURGICAL TREATMENT

Conservative rehabilitation, including quadriceps strengthening, stretching, taping, and bracing, is often effective in pain relief and improved function in individuals with PFPS. However, there are circumstances in which patients do not respond to conservative physical therapy. Commonly in these

instances a severe mechanical disorder exists that requires surgical intervention. Examples include severe posttraumatic chondrosis-arthrosis, persistent patellar tilt, pathologic plica, infrapatellar contracture, and recurrent dislocation. Surgery for vague patellofemoral pain has a poor outcome and often leads to a vicious cycle of pain and further surgery. Before surgery there should be clear criteria for patellar surgery.

REHABILITATION

Patellar Taping

Patellar taping can be used as an adjunct to exercise after patellar surgery. Developed by Jenny McConnell, patellar taping attempts to correct patellar malalignments such as a

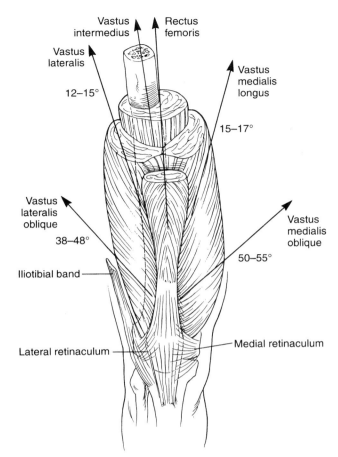

Figure 23-3: Components of the quadriceps femoris complex. (*From Zachazewski JE, Magee DJ, Quillen WS, editors:* Athletic injuries and rehabilitation, *Philadelphia, 1996, Saunders.*)

lateral glide, lateral tilt, inferior tilt, and rotation.[46-48] The use of taping after surgery is most likely beneficial for reducing joint load and improving muscle recruitment. Several studies investigating the effect of patellar taping on patellar mechanics have found no evidence that taping changes patellofemoral incongruence, although it does seem beneficial in symptom reduction.[20,49-52]

The clinician should select an aggravating activity (comparable sign) that will reproduce the patient's patellofemoral pain or symptoms. Commonly a single-leg squat or stepdown will be used. Once the comparable sign is identified, the tape is applied. First, the skin should be cleaned and free of hair. Shaving should occur, if possible, 24 hours in advance of the taping. A lubricant such as SkinPrep or Milk of Magnesia can be applied to the skin as a protectant. Next, the tape should be applied to correct the most significant problem first. Brown strapping tape is used in conjunction with a protective undercoat tape. The symptom-producing activity should be reassessed. Immediate improvement (50% decline in symptoms) should be found if the tape is applied appropriately for the patient. It may be necessary to add more tape

to correct a second fault. However, if one component of correction alleviates the patellofemoral joint pain, then continue with that one component.

The lateral tilt is corrected by placing a piece of tape from the midline on the patella crossing over to the medial femoral condyle (Figure 23-6). This tape application should lift the lateral border of the patella and therefore alleviate the lateral compression. In addition, it applies a prolonged, low-load, long-duration stretch on the lateral retinaculum and/or ITB.

A taping procedure that adds both an internal and an external rotation component to stabilize the patella is recommended for acute lateral retinaculum release (Figure 23-7). The tape should help minimize pain during knee flexion and extension and should aid in decreasing effusion.

Unloading the lateral soft tissue structures is achieved with two straps of tape. One piece extends from the posterior aspect of the lateral joint line down to the tibial tubercle and a second strap from the posterior lateral joint line to the distal mid thigh. Unloading the lateral retinaculum may help reduce symptoms (Figure 23-8).

The tape is kept on all day and may be used for several weeks until muscle activation is achieved. Crossley and colleagues[53] suggest the following progression of weaning from tape use.

The patient should be able to perform the following activities without symptoms:

1. Five sets of 10 steps (8-inch step) performed slowly and in a controlled manner with a 10-second rest between sets

2. 1 minute quarter squat against the wall

3. 1 minute half squat against the wall

4. A further five sets of 10 continuous steps

In addition, the patient should wear the tape during sports for up to 1 month.

Skin irritation can occur with patellar taping. This may be a result of friction or allergic reaction. Caution is exercised with regard to signs of allergic reaction—redness and itchy rash; if these develop, the tape should be discontinued.

If taping is not an option, several types of patellar sleeves that promote a medially directed pull of the patella are on the market. The GenuTrain P3 by Bierdsdorf is one example that provides a lateral buttress with breathable material (Figure 23-9).

Strengthening

Strengthening is divided into four stages (Box 23-1). The first two stages are non–weight bearing and will be called *open chain exercises.* Open chain exercises are performed initially, because weight bearing is limited and isolated muscle contraction is warranted. Short arc motions, if performed, are done in a nonirritating range (90 to 60 degrees of flexion) and with minimal load. Stage 1 open chain exercises include quadriceps sets performed for 10-second holds and done hourly.

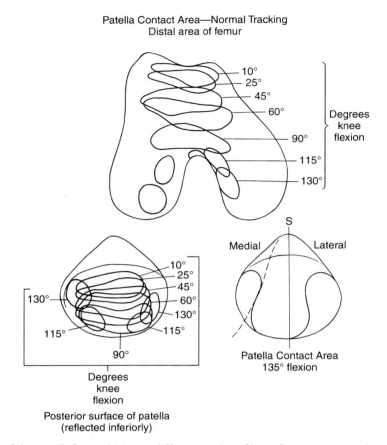

Figure 23-4: Contact areas of the patellofemoral joint at different angles of knee flexion. *(From Zachazewski JE, Magee DJ, Quillen WS, editors: Athletic injuries and rehabilitation, Philadelphia, 1996, Saunders.)*

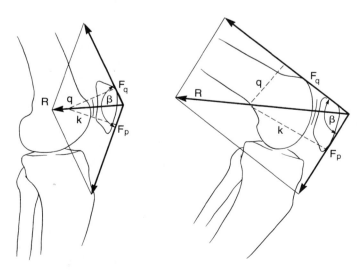

Figure 23-5: Effect of knee flexion on patellofemoral joint reaction force. *(From Zachazewski JE, Magee DJ, Quillen WS, editors: Athletic injuries and rehabilitation, Philadelphia, 1996, Saunders.)*

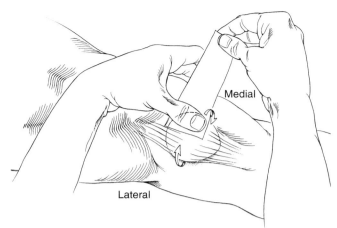

Figure 23-6: Correction of lateral tilt of patella. *(From Zachazewski JE, Magee DJ, Quillen WS, editors:* Athletic injuries and rehabilitation, *Philadelphia, 1996, Saunders.)*

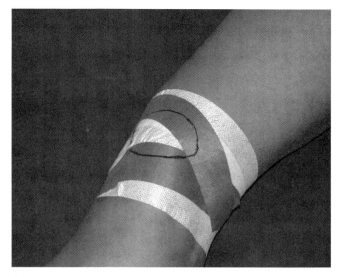

Figure 23-8: Taping to unload lateral tissue.

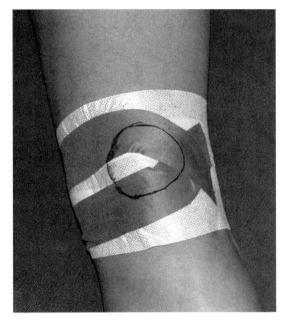

Figure 23-7: Stabilization taping of patella after lateral retinaculum release.

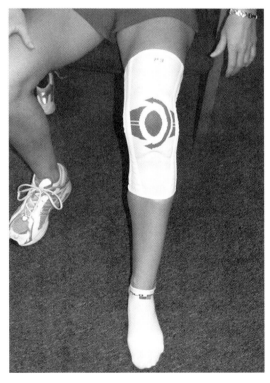

Figure 23-9: GenuTrain P3.

TABLE 23-1

Patellofemoral Joint Forces During Activity

0.5 × bw	Gait
3.3 × bw	Stair climbing
7.5 × bw	Deep squat
5.6 × bw	Running

bw, Body weight.

Electrical stimulation may be used in conjunction with the quadriceps sets to facilitate volitional contraction.[54-56] Straight leg raises (SLRs) are started to work the quadriceps isometrically at the knee. Initially the patient may not be able to fully extend the knee with the leg raises but is encouraged to achieve this within the first week after surgery. Some clinicians advocate adding internal rotation to the SLR to recruit the VMO, although recent research does not support that claim.[57,58]

Stage 2 open chain exercises continue where stage 1 ended. Additional planes are incorporated with the SLRs so that the patient is strengthening the entire hip. Isometric quadriceps at various knee angles are begun. Submaximal contractions in a range between 90 and 60 degrees of knee flexion are used because of the low patellofemoral joint reaction force (PFJRF).[40] As the patient tolerates, the contraction intensity and number of joint angles are increased. The use of selective VMO strengthening is debatable, and overall quadriceps strengthening is advocated throughout the full range of motion (ROM).[25,44,59,60] The posterior gluteus medius is commonly weak in patients with PFPS. Weakness may cause an increase in internal rotation, which provides advantage to the lateral quadriceps. A non–weight-bearing gluteus medius exercise is begun in the stage 2 open chain period (Figure 23-10).[61,62] Hip adductor isometrics are also begun because of the anatomic association between the adductors and the medial quadriceps.[63]

The next stage of strengthening begins with weight bearing or closed chain exercises. Closed chain exercises are more likely to produce VMO-VL synchrony.[64] The initial stage of closed chain exercises has minimal impact force on the patellofemoral and tibiofemoral joint. At angles less than 45 degrees of flexion, PFJRF is less than with leg extension exercises.[39,40] This phase includes leg presses, walk-stance position with quadriceps contraction (Figure 23-11), gluteus medius presses against the wall (Figure 23-12), wall squats to 90 degrees, backward and forward step-ups on a 2- to 4-inch step, mini-squats to 30 degrees, and low-resistance cycling.

BOX 23-1

Strengthening Exercises

Open-Chain Exercises

Stage 1

Quadriceps sets (electrical stimulation)—multiplane, 10-second hold, repeat 10 times, 10 times/day

Straight leg raises (flexion)—hold for 3 seconds at top, repeat sets of 10 reps

Stage 2

Straight leg raises: four planes—hold 3 seconds at top, repeat sets of 10 reps

Multiangle quadriceps isometrics

Adductor squeezes: ball or towel bolster between knees, hold 10 seconds, repeat 10 times

Clam exercise: repeat sets of 10 until fatigued

Closed-Chain Exercises

Stage 1

Leg press or Total Gym Stride, quadriceps contraction—10-second holds, 20 times for gluteus medius (press against the wall)

Wall squats

Step-ups (backward and forward), two sets of 25

Mini-squats

Cycling

Stage 2

Single-leg squats

Balance and reach

Step-downs (2 inches; progress to 8 inches)

Lunges: multiplane

Wall squats (with ball)

Lateral step-ups (2 inches to 8 inches)

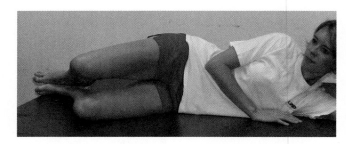

Figure 23-10: Non–weight-bearing posterior gluteus medius exercise.

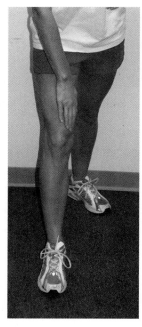

Figure 23-11: Walk-stance isometric quadriceps exercise.

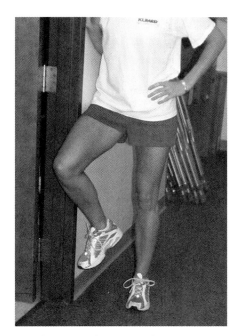

Figure 23-12: Gluteus medius strengthening against wall.

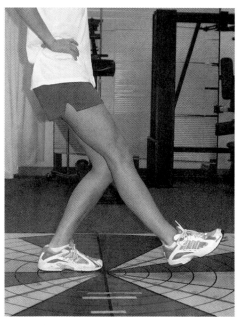

Figure 23-13: Balance and reach.

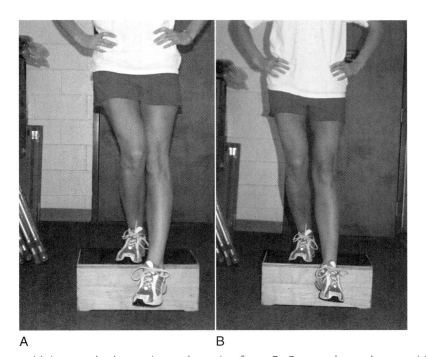

A   B

Figure 23-14: A, Step-down with increased valgus or internal rotation force. **B,** Corrected step-down position.

Stage 2 closed chain exercises challenge the neuromuscular system with optimal stimulus for regeneration of the connective tissue. This stage includes single-leg squats, balance and reach (Figure 23-13), step downs (Figure 23-14), multiplane lunges, wall squats, and lateral step-ups. Form is imperative during this phase. The knee should maintain good sagittal plane alignment and not deviate into a valgus or internal rotated position, and the knee should not move in front of toes.[61] In addition, balance exercises to improve the kinesthetic sense of the knee are instituted. Plyometric exercises can be incorporated specially for the athlete (Figure 23-15). A plyometric progression is included in Box 23-2.

Flexibility

Flexibility focuses on balance between agonist and antagonist muscles and side to side. The major tissues targeted include the ITB, anterior hip, rectus femoris, hamstrings, and gastrocnemius-soleus (Figure 23-16).[65] Stretches for each of these structures are found in Box 23-3.

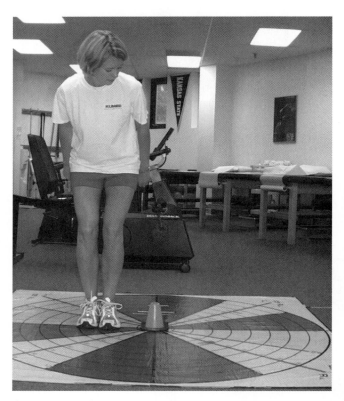

Figure 23-15: Plyometric cone hops.

FUNCTIONAL TESTING

We have developed five functional tests for patients with patellofemoral dysfunction.[66] These tests were developed to include weight-bearing stress with various knee flexion angles because these are common aggravating positions and require dynamic muscular control. The tests are time efficient, are simple to perform with minimal instruction needed, require minimal staff training, and are conducted within a clinical setting. A limb symmetry index of 90% has been established for each of the unilateral tests. The limb symmetry index is calculated as follows:

$$(\text{Involved/Uninvolved}) \times 100$$

Each test is described, and the reliability Intraclass Correlation Coefficient (ICC) value is presented.

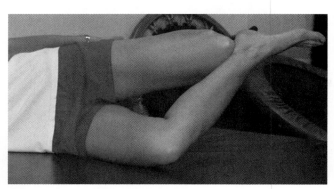

A

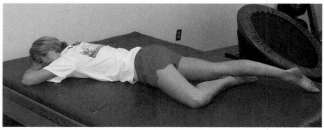

B

Figure 23-16: A, Iliotibial band stretch. **B,** Prone figure-4 stretch.

BOX 23-2

Plyometric Exercise Progression

Form is important, base strength established, soft landing with good lower extremity alignment

Squat catches

Bilateral jumps (horizontal, vertical)

Bilateral jumps (side to side, diagonal)

Jump and catch from 2- to 4-inch step—land bilaterally and progress to unilaterally

Jump 90 degrees, 180 degrees

Single-leg jumps on trampoline

Bounding for distance

Hops: forward, lateral cone hops

BOX 23-3

Flexibility

All stretches are held for 30 seconds and performed 3-5 times. Dynamic stretching may be more appropriate for presport warm-up.

Hamstrings

Gastrocnemius-soleus

Iliotibial band

Quadriceps

Prone figure-4 position

Anteromedial Lunge, Left and Right

The anteromedial lunge is performed by having the subject step forward with the uninvolved limb so that the front leg is bent to 90 degrees and crosses the midline. The subject must maintain good balance and an erect trunk posture. The greatest distance in three trials is recorded and marked. Eighty percent of this maximal distance is calculated and marked with a piece of tape. For the test the number of lunges the subject can perform in 30 seconds beyond the 80% mark is recorded. If the subject deviates from path of motion or takes an extra step, the lunge is not included in the count. The involved limb is then tested using the 80% mark from the uninvolved limb (Figure 23-17). The ICC is 0.90.

Step-Down Dip, Left and Right

The step-down is a unilateral test performed from a platform 8 inches high. Subjects step down to the floor with the heel touching the floor and then return to full knee extension. This counts as one repetition. The subject cannot use the down limb to accelerate return motion to the step. The number of repetitions the subject performs in 30 seconds is recorded. Both limbs are tested. The ICC is 0.92.

Total Gym Single-Leg Press

Subjects are positioned on the Total Gym at level 7, which is considered to be 50% of the subject's body weight. Subjects begin with the test knees in full extension. One repetition consists of a complete cycle of full knee extension to 90 degrees of knee flexion and return to full knee extension. The

number of unilateral squats completed in 30 seconds is recorded. Both limbs are tested. The ICC is 0.90.

Bilateral Squat

Subjects start this test in standing position with the knees in full extension, shoulder width apart, and with weight evenly distributed onto both limbs. Subjects lower their bodies to a knee position of 90 degrees of flexion and then return to full extension. One repetition consists of a complete cycle of straight standing to 90 degrees of knee flexion and return to straight standing. The number of bilateral squats completed in 30 seconds is recorded. The ICC is 0.90.

Balance and Reach

The balance and reach is performed by having the subject reach forward with the predetermined limb so that the heel touches the floor; the majority of the body weight remains on the back leg. The back leg is the test leg. The uninvolved limb is tested first. The greatest distance out of three trials is recorded and marked. Eighty percent of this maximal distance is calculated and marked with a piece of tape. For the test the number of touches beyond the 80% mark that the subject performs in 30 seconds is recorded. The involved limb is then tested using the 80% mark from the uninvolved limb (see Figure 12-13). The ICC is 0.80.

SPECIFIC SURGERIES

Arthroscopic Lateral Retinaculum Release

Chapter 24 of this text deals exclusively with arthroscopic lateral retinaculum release; please refer to that chapter for complete description of the surgery. Rehabilitation after arthroscopic lateral retinaculum release can be divided into four phases (Box 23-4). Phase I includes the period immediately after surgery up to 48 hours. The goals for this phase are to diminish pain and swelling, restore independent ambulation, begin ROM, restore patellar mobility, and begin quadriceps training. Research has demonstrated quadriceps inhibition with the presence of joint effusion.[67,68] Therefore effusion should be addressed immediately. The use of a compression wrap and ice is mandatory for effusion and edema control. The Cryotemp can be used during therapy for 20 minutes. In addition, ankle pumps performed every hour will help with venous flow.

Weight bearing begins immediately after surgery at ¼ weight bearing and progressing as tolerated. In addition, ROM begins with heel slides and wall slides. Manual therapy in the form of grade II joint mobilizations (Maitland) to the patella should be initiated with care. Primarily, a medial glide is performed (Figure 23-18). McConnell taping after a lateral release may help with pain and provide a continuous stress to the lateral retinaculum for mobilizing the healing tissue.[12,69] A second technique that unloads the lateral structures may

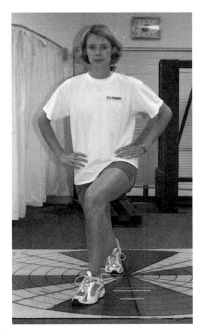

Figure 23-17: Anterior lunge.

BOX 23-4

Arthroscopic Lateral Retinaculum Release

Phase I: Immediate Postoperative Period (0-2 Days)

Goals

Diminish pain and swelling

Restore independent ambulation

Begin range-of-motion exercise

Restore patellar mobility

Begin quadriceps training

Weight bearing

¼ weight bearing

Range of Motion and Joint Mobilization

Heel slides

Wall slides

Gentle patellar mobilization

McConnell taping

Swelling

Compression wrap, full leg

Ice and elevation: three or four times per day for 20 minutes

Cryotemp

Ankle pumps: 50 every hour

Flexibility

Hamstrings

Gastrocnemius-soleus

Strengthening

Stage 1 open chain

Adjunct Exercise

Aerobic conditioning (single leg bicycle)

Phase II: Intermediate Phase (3 Days through 2 Weeks)

Goals

Minimize muscle atrophy

Restore range of motion

Resolve swelling

Achieve independent ambulation

Weight Bearing

Full weight bearing by week 2

Range of Motion

Active range of motion at least 0-120 degrees

Patella mobilization

Tibiofemoral mobilization for flexion and extension

Cycling for range of motion

Contract-relax for flexion

Swelling

Ice

Flexibility

Scar massage

Iliotibial band

Rectus femoris

Prone figure-4

Continue with hamstring, gastrocnemius-soleus

Strengthening

McConnell taping

Stage 2 open chain progressing to stage 1 closed chain

Adjunct Therapy

Biomechanical examination

Aerobic exercise

Upper extremity weightlifting

Phase III: Advanced Strengthening Phase (3-4 Weeks Postoperatively)

Goals

Improve muscular strength and endurance

Progress functional activity

Weight Bearing

Full weight bearing

Range of Motion

Full range of motion

Swelling

Absent

Flexibility

Continue flexibility exercises as with other phases

(continued)

help with joint effusion and pain. (See discussion of patellar taping.)

Stage 1 open chain exercises and flexibility training can begin in phase I. Adjunct treatment includes aerobic exercise. This may include an upper extremity ergometer or a single lower limb cycle.

The second phase of rehabilitation is the intermediate phase and lasts from 3 days after surgery to 3 weeks. The goals of this phase are to minimize muscle atrophy, restore ROM, resolve effusion, and achieve independent ambulation. Weight-bearing progression continues, and the patient should be fully weight bearing and without crutches by week 2. Joint effusion should be controlled. Application of ice should continue, especially after exercise. If joint effusion persists such that it limits ROM and quadriceps contraction,

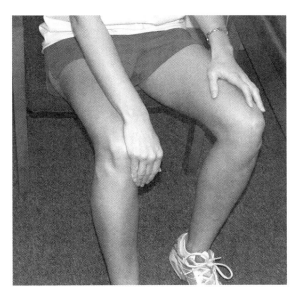

Figure 23-18: Manual passive mobilization of lateral retinaculum.

the physician should be contacted and the knee may require aspiration. Active ROM should progress to 120 degrees of flexion by the end of this phase. The patient is instructed to perform self-mobilization of the joint at home and to sit with the knee bent to approximately 60 degrees while applying a force on the medial half of the patella to create a medial patellar tilt. The patient should feel a slight stretch on the lateral side of the patella. The pressure is held for 10 seconds and performed 10 times, two or three times a day. Other manual techniques to improve ROM may include tibiofemoral glides, contract-relax, soft tissue mobilization, and low-resistance cycling. Flexibility issues are addressed fully in this phase. Common areas of tightness include the ITB, anterior hip, and rectus femoris. ITB tightness can have a dramatic effect on the patient with patellofemoral dysfunction secondary to its insertion on the lateral aspect of the patella.[70] For the anterior hip a prone figure-4 position (see Figure 23-16, *B)* can be easily incorporated into the home program. Specific scar massage may be needed along the surgical incision for the surgically altered tissue. Stage 2 open chain strengthening begins, and the patient should be able to progress quickly into stage 1 closed chain exercises. If the patient experiences pain with weight-bearing knee flexion, McConnell taping may be warranted. Once the patient's gait is normal, a thorough biomechanical examination should be performed. Increased pronation can cause increased internal rotation of the tibia, creating torsion and increased valgus at the knee.[71] At the other extreme, a rigid foot limits shock absorption of the foot and lower leg, creating more mechanical stress at the knee. In-shoe orthotics may be indicated to help neutralize the subtalar joint or provide some shock absorption.

The third phase after a lateral release is the advanced strengthening phase and encompasses weeks 3 and 4. Improvement in muscular strength and endurance is the emphasis during this phase. The patient should be weaned

---

BOX 23-4

Arthroscopic Lateral Retinaculum Release—cont'd

Strengthening

Stage 2 closed chain

Adjunct Therapy

Balance exercises: single-leg stance (eyes open/eyes closed); vestibular board

Continue aerobic exercise: cycling, swimming (avoid breaststroke), water walking, treadmill walking

Phase IV: Return to Activity (5 Weeks to Discharge)

Goals

Functional testing results within 90%

Flexibility

Continue flexibility exercises as with other phases

Strengthening, Endurance, and Agility

Continue stage 2 closed chain exercises

Plyometrics

Agility exercises

Adjunct Therapy

Aerobic exercise

from taping. Weight bearing and ROM should be full by this phase. Flexibility and aerobic training should continue.

Return to function is the last phase and lasts from week 5 until discharge. Therapy should focus on return to work or sport. Stage 2 closed chain exercises are emphasized, with increased load and planes of movement. Before discharge, functional testing should result in no less than 90% Limb Symmetry Index (LSI) between the involved and the uninvolved lower extremities.

Proximal Realignment (Insall Procedure)

The purpose of the proximal realignment is to alter the line of pull of the quadriceps muscle by rearranging the muscular attachments to the patella. Indications for this procedure are a deficient medial patellofemoral support structure, usually a result of recurrent lateral patellar subluxation or dislocation. Reefing the vastus medialis to a more central location on the patella or tightening the medial capsule allows a normal patellofemoral alignment to be restored. This is especially useful in the skeletally immature patient in whom a distal realignment may interfere with the tibial tubercle apophysis. The proximal realignment does not work well with patients who have primary patellofemoral pain, significant patellar hypoplasia, a large Q angle, or generalized ligament laxity.

The surgical procedure begins with a longitudinal skin incision over the center of the patella; the medial and lateral aspects of the extensor mechanism are exposed. Then a medial parapatellar capsular incision is made, extending from the upper edge of the vastus medialis into the quadriceps tendon around the patella and down to the tibial tubercle. Next, a lateral release is performed. Then the VMO is transferred from its normal proximal insertion distally into the patella (Figure 23-19). This increases the resting length of the VMO. Possible complications include VMO inhibition and possible entrapment of the saphenous nerve.

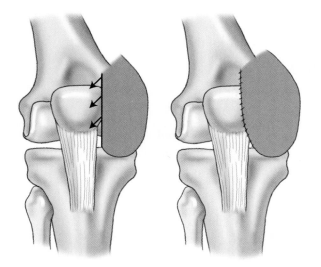

Figure 23-19: Insall procedure.

Physical therapy after proximal realignment surgery is slower than with an arthroscopic lateral release (Box 23-5). The first phase last 2 weeks. The goals of this phase are to diminish pain and swelling, begin safe non–weight-bearing ambulation, initiate ROM, maintain patellar mobility, and begin quadriceps training. Non–weight bearing is maintained for the first 2 weeks. A brace limited to 30 degrees is worn at all times but can be removed for ROM exercise. Gentle patellar glides are initiated, and knee flexion should be 90 degrees by week 3. Control of swelling is important as with the lateral release. Stage 1 open chain exercises can begin during phase I.

The second phase, the intermediate phase, lasts from weeks 3 to 6. During this phase ambulation begins at ¼ weight-bearing progression so that the patient should achieve full weight bearing by week 7. The patient continues to wear the ROM-limiting brace; flexion can be set to 60 degrees at week 3, to 90 degrees for weeks 4 through 6, then to full ROM. Flexibility issues should be addressed, and stage 2 open chain exercises are started. During the final week of phase II, stage 1 closed chain exercises can begin, keeping in mind the patient's weight-bearing status.

The advanced strengthening phase starts at week 6 and lasts for 6 weeks.

At this time the patient should have full ROM and near full weight bearing. By week 8 the brace is discharged. Emphasis is on strength and endurance. The patient progresses from stage 1 closed chain to stage 2 closed chain exercises.

Phase IV, return to activity, is similar to the lateral release rehabilitation program in that the emphasis is on closed chain exercises with increased loading and introduction of multiplane movements.

Distal Realignment Procedures

Distal realignments are used to correct extensor malalignment or reduce an excessive patellar Q angle. Lateral patellar malalignment can lead to chronic pain secondary to articular damage of the lateral facet of the patella. The distal realignment procedure involves transferring the patellar tendon and tibial tubercle anteriorly, medially, or both.

The original tubercle transfer was developed by Hauser in 1938.[72] This procedure repositions the patellar tendon, and a portion of the tibial tubercle is excised medially and distally. Unfortunately the results of the procedure create excessive tension on the patella and an unacceptable degree of long-term degenerative changes.[73] Since that time, several different distal realignments have been described.

Elmslie-Trillat Procedure

This procedure is performed through a lateral parapatellar skin incision. First, a lateral release is completed. Periosteal tissue is elevated from the anterior surface of the tibia. Next, the tibial tuberosity is transferred medially and supported with a thin wafer of bone (Figure 23-20). This surgery is an

BOX 23-5

Proximal Realignment

Phase I: Immediate Postoperative Period (0-2 weeks)

Goals

Diminish pain and swelling

Achieve safe non–weight-bearing ambulation

Begin range-of-motion (ROM) exercises

Achieve patellar mobility

Begin quadriceps training

Weight Bearing

Non–weight bearing

Range of Motion

Brace to limit ROM to 0-30 degrees

Patellar glides

90 degrees of knee flexion by week 3

Swelling

Compression wrap, full leg

Ice and elevation: three or four times per day for 20 minutes

Cryotemp

Ankle pumps: 50 every hour

Flexibility

Flexibility program as tolerated

Strengthening

Stage 1 open chain exercises

Phase II: Intermediate Phase (3-6 weeks)

Goals

Perform muscle activation exercises

Progressively improve ROM

Resolve swelling

Progressively improve ambulation

Weight Bearing

¼ weight-bearing progression over 4 weeks

Range of Motion

3 weeks: brace 0-60 degrees

4-6 weeks: protection brace, 0-90 degrees

Full ROM by week 6

Patellar mobilization

Swelling

Ice

Flexibility

Flexibility program

Strengthening

Stage 2 open chain exercises progressing to stage 1 closed chain as weight bearing permits

Adjunct Therapy

Gait training

Phase III: Advanced Strengthening Phase (6-12 weeks)

Goals

Improve muscular strength and endurance

Progressively improve functional activity

Weight Bearing

7-8 weeks: progress off crutches and discontinue brace

Range of Motion

Full ROM

Patellar mobilization

Swelling

Ice after exercise

Flexibility

Continue flexibility program

Strengthening

Stage 1 closed chain progressing to stage 2 closed chain exercises

Adjunct Therapy

Aerobic exercises

Biomechanical examination

(continued)

excellent option for correcting severe alignment and tracking problems, with good long-term results.

Fulkerson Procedure

Anteromedialization of the tibial tubercle was introduced by Dr. John P. Fulkerson in 1983.[74,75] This procedure involves both an anterior and a medial transfer of the tibial tuberosity. This procedure reduces articular stress by shifting the patellar contact area and improving patellar alignment.

The procedure involves a straight incision from the midlateral patella to a point approximately 5 cm distal to the tibial tuberosity. A lateral release is performed that includes the patellofemoral ligaments. A posterolateral oblique osteotomy of the anterior tibia is performed. This bone fragment is then transferred anteriorly and medially.

Anteromedial tibial tubercle transfer is most successful when lesions occur distally and/or laterally on the patellar articular surface. Less success was found with facet patellar articular lesions found proximal and medially.[76]

Maquet Procedure (Bandi Procedure)

Anterior elevation of tibial tuberosity increases the efficiency of the quadriceps by increasing the lever arm and at the same time decreasing the PFJRF. According to Maquet, a 2 cm elevation will decrease the patella compressive force by 50%.[77,78]

A lateral parapatellar skin incision is made, extending distally below the level of the tibial tubercle. Debridement of the patella is performed as necessary. Next, the tibial tubercle is split distally approximately 10 cm. The tubercle is levered forward and held by a bone graft taken from the iliac crest (Figure 23-21). Recent studies have reported less favorable results with the Maquet procedure.[79-82]

Roux-Goldthwait Procedure

Damage to the tibial tubercle apophysis is likely with most distal procedures. Therefore, a procedure that involves distal medialization is appropriate for the skeletally immature

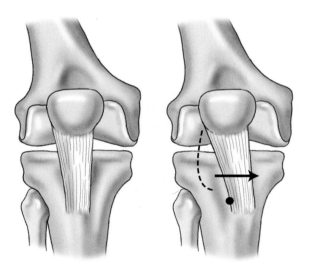

Figure 23-20: The Elmslie-Trillat surgery.

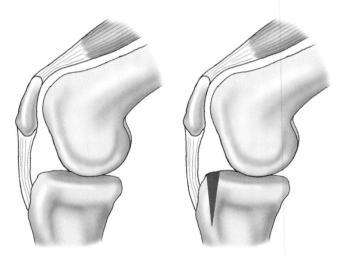

Figure 23-21: Maquet procedure.

BOX 23-5

Proximal Realignment—cont'd

Phase IV: Return to Activity (12 Weeks to Discharge)	*Swelling*
Goals	Resolved
90% score on functional test	
	Flexibility
Weight Bearing	Continue flexibility program
Full weight bearing	
	Strengthening
Range of Motion	Stage 2 closed chain
Full ROM	Sport-specific training; work conditioning

patient. In this procedure the lateral half of the patellar tendon is detached distally, passed behind the medial half of the tendon, and sutured to the pes anserinus insertion. The surgery is usually done in conjunction with a lateral release. One drawback of the procedure is the possibility of creating a lateral tilt of the patella.

Rehabilitation after distal realignment progresses more slowly than after proximal realignment (Box 23-6). Phase I is similar to proximal realignment with regard to weightbearing and limited ROM (60 degrees) in a controlled-motion brace. Strengthening is limited to isometric quadriceps exercises, starting at a submaximal level.

BOX 23-6
Distal Realignment

Phase I: Immediate Postoperative Phase (0-2 Weeks)

Goals

Diminish pain and swelling

Perform controlled ambulation

Begin range of motion exercises

Restore patellar mobility

Begin quadriceps training

Weight Bearing

Non–weight bearing

Range of Motion

Controlled-motion brace (0-60 degrees)

Swelling

Compression wrap, full leg

Ice and elevation: three or four times per day for 20 minutes

Cryotemp

Ankle pumps: 50 every hour

Flexibility

Gastrocnemius-soleus (if tolerated)

Strengthening

Isometric quadriceps (start submaximal)

Electrical stimulation

Phase II: Intermediate Phase (3-4 Weeks)

Goals

Minimize muscle atrophy

Restore range of motion (ROM)

Resolve swelling

Begin weightbearing ambulation

Weight Bearing

25% weight bearing at 3 weeks; progress to full weight bearing in 6-8 weeks

Range of Motion

0-90 degrees: week 3

0-110 degrees: week 4

Patellar mobilization

Swelling

Compression wrap, full leg

Ice and elevation: three or four times per day for 20 minutes

Cryotemp

Ankle pumps: 50 every hour

Flexibility

Flexibility program

Strengthening

Stage 1 open chain exercises progressing to stage 2 open chain exercises

Phase III: Advanced Strengthening Phase (5-10 Weeks)

Goals

Improve muscular strength and endurance

Achieve independent ambulation

Progress functional activity

Weight Bearing

Full weight bearing by week 8

Range of Motion

Full ROM by 6-8 weeks

(continued)

Phase II, the intermediate phase, encompasses weeks 3 and 4. Goals of phase II are to minimize muscle atrophy, restore ROM, resolve swelling, and begin weight-bearing ambulation. Weight bearing begins at ¼ weight bearing and progresses by 25% body weight per week until full weight bearing at approximately 4 weeks. Knee flexion reaches 90 degrees by week 3 and 110 degrees by week 4. Stage 1 open chain exercises, including SLRs, are begun and progressed to stage 2 open chain exercises by the end of week 4.

Flexibility exercises are prescribed as indicated.

The advanced strengthening phase begins at week 5 and lasts until week 10. Weight bearing and ROM are full by week 8. Strengthening, in the form of closed chain exercises, is progressed to stage 2.

The final phase of rehabilitation focuses on return to activity. Closed chain exercises are emphasized, with increased load and planes of movement. Depending on the need of the patient, this phase may include sport-specific drills or work-related ergonomics.

Autologous Chondrocyte Implantation

Chondral defects of the patella can be common after traumatic patellar dislocation. Beyond alignment procedures, patellar resurfacing may be indicated.

Human clinical trials to treat full-thickness chondral defects began in the late 1980s. Since that time results have been encouraging. This procedure requires two separate surgeries 1 to 3 months apart. The first surgery is an arthroscopic surgery in which healthy cartilage cells (200 to 300 mg) are removed from a non–weight-bearing femoral surface. The biopsied cells are transported to Genzyme Tissue Repair in Cambridge, MA, where the cells are cultured, leading to a tenfold increase in the number of viable autologous chondrocytes. The second operation involves implantation of the chondrocytes via an arthrotomy. Once the chondral defect is exposed, it is debrided down to the subchondral bone over the entire defect. The cartilage is then carefully excised with a curette. At this time a lateral release may be performed if indicated. Next, a second incision is made 1 cm distal to the inferior margin of the pes anserine. A periosteal graft the size of the chondral defect is removed from the tibia. The periosteal graft is then placed over the chondral defect and sutured into place. Fibrin glue is used to secure a watertight seal. A small opening at the superior portion of the defect is left open to allow injection of the autologous chondrocytes into the defect. The remaining opening is then sealed. The arthrotomy incision and wound are then closed in a routine fashion.

Rehabilitation after autologous chondrocyte implantation (ACI) is regimented based on connective tissue healing properties (Box 23-7). Patients' compliance is mandatory for a successful outcome. If abnormal lower extremity biomechanics or ligamentous instability exists, it should be corrected in conjunction with the ACI.

The first phase of rehabilitation is 6 weeks long. During this time the implanted cells are forming but are very fragile. Minimal to no stress should be applied to the proliferative cells. A continuous passive movement (CPM) device is used for 8 to 12 hours per day for cell stimulation. ROM is progressed slowly. Gentle patellar mobilization is started during

---

BOX 23-6
Distal Realignment—cont'd

Swelling	*Weight Bearing*
Resolved	Full weight bearing
Ice after exercise	
	Range of Motion
Flexibility	Full ROM
Flexibility program	
	Swelling
Strengthening	Ice after exercise
Stage 1 closed chain exercises progress to stage 2 closed chain exercises	
Balance exercises	*Flexibility*
	Flexibility program
Adjunct Therapy	
Assess foot biomechanics	*Strengthening*
	Stage 2 closed chain exercises
Phase IV: Return to Activity (20-24 Weeks)	Sport-specific exercises
Goals	Work conditioning
Functional testing at 90%	

BOX 23-7
Autologous Chondrocyte Implantation (Patellar Carticel)

Phase I: Protection Phase (0-6 Weeks)

Goals

Protect healing tissue from load and shear forces

Diminish pain and swelling

Restore independent ambulation

Begin range of motion (ROM) exercises, restore full passive knee extension

Begin quadriceps training

Weight Bearing

Weight bearing as tolerated (WBAT): Crutches with brace locked in full extension

Range of Motion

Heel slides

Wall slides

Gentle patellar mobilization

McConnell taping

Continuous passive motion (CPM): 8-12 hr/day, range does not exceed 90 degrees of flexion

Knee flexion: 90 degrees by 2 weeks

110 degrees by 4 weeks

120 degrees by 6 weeks

Swelling

Compression wrap, full leg

Ice and elevation: three or four times per day for 20 minutes

Cryotemp

Ankle pumps: 50 every hour

Flexibility

Flexibility program as tolerated

Strengthening

Stage 1 open chain exercises, progress to stage 2 open chain exercises

Phase II: Transition Phase (6-12 Weeks)

Goals

Minimize muscle atrophy

Restore ROM

Resolve swelling

Achieve independent ambulation

Weight Bearing

Full weight bearing

Range of Motion

Discontinue brace

Progress to full ROM

Patellar mobilization

Swelling

Ice after exercise

Flexibility

Flexibility program

Strengthening

Stage 2 open chain exercises; progress repetitions to stage 1 closed chain exercises (0-30 degrees)

Adjunct Therapy

Check lower extremity biomechanics

Perform balance exercises

Phase III: Maturation Phase (12-26 Weeks)

Goals

Improve muscular strength and endurance

Progress functional activity

Weight Bearing

Full weight bearing

Range of Motion

Full ROM

Swelling

Resolved

Ice after exercise

Flexibility

Flexibility program

(continued)

this phase. Patients are allowed to bear weight immediately in a locked postoperative brace. Patients may need crutches initially but should discard them by the first postoperative week.

Patients may return to sporting activities as progression and cartilage healing allow. Low-impact sports such as golf, swimming, skating, rollerblading, and cycling are permitted at approximately 6 months. Higher-impact sports such as jogging, running, and aerobics may be performed at 8 to 9 months. High-impact sports such as tennis, basketball, football, and baseball are allowed at 12 months.

SUMMARY

Treatment of individuals with patellofemoral dysfunction can be challenging for the orthopedic specialist. A course of conservative care is recommended initially; however, if unsuccessful, several surgical procedures are available that can improve biomechanical fault and/or instability. Rehabilitation after these procedures is critical and should be performed methodically in order for a return to full function to be achieved.

References

1. Chesworth BM, Culham EG, Tata GE, Malcolm P: Validation of outcome measures in patients with patellofemoral syndrome, *J Orthop Sports Phys Ther* 11:302-308, 1989.
2. Almedia SA, Trone DW, Leone DM, et al: Gender differences in musculoskeletal injury rates: a function of symptom reporting, *Med Sci Sports Exerc* 31:1807-1812, 1998.
3. Devereaux M, Lachmann S: Patellofemoral arthralgia in athletes attending a sports injury clinic, *Br J Sports Med* 18:18-21, 1984.
4. Malek MM, Mangine RE: Patellofemoral pain syndromes: a comprehensive and conservative approach, *J Orthop Sports Phys Ther* 2:108-116, 1981.
5. Reid DC: The myth, mystique, and frustration of anterior knee pain, *Clin J Sports Med* 3:139-143, 1993.
6. Thomee R, Renstrom P, Karlsson J, Grimby G: Patellofemoral pain syndrome in young women, II: muscle function in patients and healthy controls, *Scand J Med Sci Sports* 5:245-251, 1995.
7. Post MD, Fulkerson MD: Knee pain diagrams: correlation with physical examination findings in patients with anterior knee pain, *Arthroscopy* 10:618-623, 1994.
8. Ficat RP: Lateral fascia release and lateral hyperpressure syndrome. In Pickett JC, Radin EL, editors: *Chondromalacia of the patella*, Baltimore, 1983, Williams & Wilkins.
9. Greenfield MA, Scott WN: Arthroscopic evaluation and treatment of the patellofemoral joint, *Orthop Clin North Am* 23:587-600, 1992.
10. James SL: Chondromalacia of the patella in the adolescent. In Kennedy JC, editor: *The injured adolescent knee*, Baltimore, 1979, Williams & Wilkins.
11. Kannus P, Nittymaki S: Which factors predict outcome in the nonoperative treatment of patellofemoral pain syndrome? A prospective follow-up study, *Med Sci Sports Exerc* 26:289-296, 1994.
12. Radin EL: Does chondromalacia patella exist? In Pickett JC, Radin EL, editors: *Chondromalacia of the patella*, Baltimore, 1983, Williams & Wilkins.
13. Bennett JG, Strauber WT: Evaluation and treatment of anterior knee pain using eccentric exercise, *Med Sci Sports Exerc* 18:526-530, 1986.
14. Werner S, Eriksson E: Isokinetic quadriceps training in patients with patellofemoral pain, *Knee Surg Sports Traumatol Arthrosc* 1:162-168, 1993.
15. Fulkerson J, Hungerford D: *Disorders of the patellofemoral joint*, ed 2, Baltimore, 1990, Williams & Wilkins.
16. McConnell J, Fulkerson J: The knee: patellofemoral and soft tissue injuries. In Zachazewski JE, Magee DJ, Quillen WS, editors: *Athletic injuries and rehabilitation*, Philadelphia, 1996, Saunders.
17. Magee DM: *Orthopedic physical assessment*, ed 4, Philadelphia, 2002, Saunders.

BOX 23-7

Autologous Chondrocyte Implantation (Patellar Carticel)—cont'd

Strengthening

Stage 1 closed chain exercises (0-45 degrees)

Leg presses not to exceed body weight

Unilateral step-ups (2 to 8 inches)

Stage 2 closed chain exercises at weeks 16-20

Phase IV: Functional Activities (26-52 weeks)
Goals

Gradual return to full unrestricted activities

90% strength of contralateral extremity

Weight Bearing

Full weight bearing

Range of Motion

Full ROM

Swelling

Resolved

Ice after exercise

Flexibility

Flexibility program

Strengthening

Stage 2 closed chain exercises (0-45 degrees), sport-specific exercises

Work conditioning

18. Gerrard B: The patellofemoral complex. In Zuluaga M, Briggs C, Carlisle J, et al, editors: *Sports physiotherapy*, New York, 1995, Churchill Livingstone.

19. DiVeta JA, Vogelbach WD: The clinical efficiency of the A angle in measuring patellar alignment, *J Orthop Sports Phys Ther* 16:136-139, 1992.

20. Arno S: The A angle: a quantitative measurement of patella alignment and realignment, *J Orthop Sports Phys Ther* 12:237-242, 1990.

21. Wiberg G: Roentgenographic and anatomic studies of the femoropatellar joint, *Acta Orthop Scand* 12:319-410, 1941.

22. Ficat RP, Hungerford DS: *Disorders of the patellofemoral joint,* Baltimore, 1977, Williams & Wilkins.

23. Desio SM, Burks RT, Bachus KN: Soft tissue restraints to lateral patellar translation in the human knee, *Am J Sports Med* 26:59-65, 1989.

24. Reider B, Marshall J, Koslin B, et al: The anterior aspect of the knee joint, *J Bone Joint Surg* 63A:351-356, 1981

25. Mangine RE, Heckman TP, Eldridge VL: Muscle strengthening. In Scully RM, Barnes MR, editors: *Physical therapy*, Philadelphia, 1989, Lippincott.

26. Powers CM, Landel R, Perry J: Timing and intensity of vastus muscle activity during functional activities in subjects with and without patellofemoral pain, *Phys Ther* 76:946-966, 1996.

27. Powers CM: Rehabilitation of patellofemoral joint disorders: a critical review, *J Orthop Sports Phys Ther* 28:345-354, 1998.

28. Mariani PP, Caruso I: An electromyographic investigation of subluxation of the patella, *J Bone Joint Surg Br* 61:169-171, 1979.

29. Souza DR, Gross MT: Comparison of vastus medialis obliquus: vastus lateralis muscle integrated electromyographic ratios between healthy subjects and patients with patellofemoral pain, *Phys Ther* 71:310-316, 1991.

30. Voight ML, Wieder DL: Comparative reflex response times of vastus medialis obliquus and vastus lateralis in normal subjects and subjects with extensor mechanism dysfunction: an electromyographic study, *Am J Sports Med* 19:131-137, 1991.

31. Wise HH, Fiebert IM, Kates JL: EMG biofeedback as treatment for patellofemoral pain syndrome, *J Orthop Sports Phys Ther* 6:95-103, 1984.

32. Boucher JP, King MA, Lefebvre R, Pepin A: Quadriceps femoris muscle activity in patellofemoral pain syndrome, *Am J Sports Med* 20:527-532, 1992.

33. MacIntyre DL, Robertson GE: Quadriceps muscle activity in women runners with and without patellofemoral pain syndrome, *Arch Phys Med Rehabil* 73:10-14, 1992.

34. Powers CM, Landel R, Perry J: Timing and intensity of vastus muscle activity during functional activities in subjects with and without patellofemoral pain, *Phys Ther* 76:946-955, 1996.

35. Wild JJ, Franklin TD, Woods GW: Patellar pain and quadriceps rehabilitation: an EMG study, *Am J Sports Med* 10:12-15, 1982.

36. Goh JCH, Lee PYC, Bose K: A cadaver study of the function of the oblique part of vastus medialis, *J Bone Joint Surg* 77B:225-231, 1995.

37. Lieb F, Perry J: Quadriceps function: an anatomical and mechanical study using amputated limbs, *J Bone Joint Surg* 50A:1535-1548, 1968.

38. Terry GC, Hughston JC, Norwood LA: The anatomy of the iliopatellar band and iliotibial tract, *Am J Sports Med* 14:39-45, 1986.

39. Hungerford DS, Barry M: Biomechanics of the patellofemoral joint, *Clin Orthop* 144:9-15, 1979.

40. Steinkamp LA, Dillingham M, Markel M, et al: Biomechanical considerations in patellofemoral joint rehabilitation, *Am J Sports Med* 21:438-444, 1993.

41. Ahmed AM, Burke DL, Hyder A: Force analysis of the patellar mechanism, *J Orthop Res* 5:69-85, 1987.

42. Grelsamer RP, Klein JR: The biomechanics of the patellofemoral joint, *J Orthop Sports Phys Ther* 28:286-297, 1998.

43. Noyes FR, Wojtys EM, Marshall MT: The early diagnosis and treatment of the developmental patellar infra syndrome, *Clin Orthop* 265:241-252, 1991.

44. Mangine RE, Eifert-Mangine M, Burch D, et al: Postoperative management of the patellofemoral patient, *J Orthop Sports Phys Ther* 28:323-334, 1998.

45. Huberti HH, Hayes WC: Patellofemoral contact pressures: the influence of Q-angle and tendofemoral contact, *J Bone Joint Surg* 66A:715-724, 1984.

46. McConnell JS: The management of chondromalacia patellae: a long term solution, *Austr J Physiother* 32:215-225, 1986.

47. McConnell JS: Management of patellofemoral problems, *Man Ther* 1:60-66, 1996.

48. Hilyard A: Recent developments in the management of patellofemoral pain: the McConnell programme, *Physiotherapy* 76:559-565, 1990.

49. Crossley KM, Cowan SM, Bennell KL, et al: Patellar taping: is clinical success supported by scientific evidence? *Man Ther* 5:142-150, 2000.

50. Gigante A, Pasquinelli FM, Paladini P, et al: The effects of patellar taping on patellofemoral incongruence, *Am J Sports Med* 29:88-92, 2001.

51. Bockrathe K, Wooden C, Worrell T, et al: Effects of patella taping on patella position and perceived pain, *Med Sci Sports Exerc* 25:989-992, 1993.

52. Kowall MG, Kolk G, Nuber GW, et al: Patellar taping in the treatment of patellofemoral pain. A prospective randomized study, *Am J Sports Med* 24:61-66, 1996.

53. Crossley K, Bennell K, McConnell JS: Patellofemoral joint. In Kolt GS, Snyder-Mackler L, editors: *Physical therapies in sport and exercise*, London, 2003, Churchill Livingstone.

54. Kues JM, Mayhew TP: Concentric and eccentric force-velocity relationships during electrically induced submaximal contractions, *Physiother Res Int* 1:195, 1996.

55. Ingersoll CD, Knight KL: Patellar location changes following EMG biofeedback or progressive resistive exercise, *Med Sci Sports Exerc* 23:1122-1127, 1991.

56. Wise HH, Fiebert IM, Kates JL: EMG biofeedback as treatment for patellofemoral pain syndrome, *J Orthop Sports Phys Ther* 6:95-103, 1984.

57. Cerny K: Vastus medialis oblique/vastus lateralis muscle activity ratios for selected exercises in persons with and without patellofemoral pain syndrome, *Phys Ther* 75:672-682, 1995.

58. Mirzabeigi E, Jordan C, Gronley JK, et al: Isolation of the vastus medialis oblique muscle during exercise, *Am J Sports Med* 27:50-53, 1999.

59. Boucher JP, King MA, Lefebvre R, et al: Quadriceps femoris activity in patellofemoral pain syndrome, *Am J Sports Med* 20:527-532, 1992.

60. Grabiner MD, Koh TJ, Draganich LF: Neuromechanics of the patellofemoral joint, *Med Sci Sports Exerc* 261:10-21, 1994.

61. Mascal CL, Landel R, Powers C: Management of patellofemoral pain targeting hip, pelvis, and trunk muscle function: 2 case reports, *J Orthop Sports Phys Ther* 33:647-660, 2003.

62. Sahrmann S: *Diagnosis and treatment of movement impairment syndromes*, St. Louis, 2002, Mosby.

63. Hanten WP, Schulthies SS: Exercise effect on electromyographic activity of the vastus medialis oblique and vastus lateralis muscles, *Phys Ther* 70:561-565, 1990.

64. Gryzlo SM, Patek RM, Pink M, et al: Electromyographic analysis of knee rehabilitation exercises, *J Orthop Sports Phys Ther* 20:36-43, 1994.

65. Kaplan ED: The iliotibial tract, *J Bone Joint Surg Am* 40:817-832, 1958.

66. Loudon JK, Wiesner D, Goist-Foley HL, et al: Intrarater reliability of functional performance tests for subjects with patellofemoral pain syndrome, *J Athl Train* 37:256-261, 2002.

67. Spencer J, Hayes K, Alexander I: Knee joint effusion and quadriceps reflex inhibition in man, *Arch Phys Med Rehabil* 65:171-177, 1984.

68. Stratford P. Electromyography of the quadriceps femoris muscles in subjects with normal knees and acutely effused knees, *Phys Ther* 62:279-283, 1981.

69. Brooks AA, Farwell D: Arthroscopic lateral retinaculum release. In Maxey L, Magnusson J, editors: *Rehabilitation for the postsurgical orthopedic patient*, St. Louis, 2001, Mosby.

70. Punicello MS: Iliotibial band tightness and medial patellar glide in patients with patellofemoral dysfunction, *J Orthop Sports Phys Ther* 17:144-148, 1993.

71. Tiberio D: The effect of excessive subtalar joint pronation on patellofemoral mechanics: a theoretical model, *J Orthop Sports Phys Ther* 9:160-165, 1987.

72. Hauser EW: Total tendon transplant for slipping patella, *Surg Gynecol Obstet* 66:199-203, 1938.

73. DeCesare WF: Late results of Hauser procedure for recurrent dislocation of the patella, *Clin Orthop* 140:137-142, 1979.

74. Fulkerson JP: Anteromedialization of the tibial tuberosity for patellofemoral malalignment, *Clin Orthop* 177:176, 1983.

75. Fulkerson JP, Becker GJ, Meaney JA, et al: Anteromedial tibial tubercle transfer without bone graft, *Am J Sports Med* 18:490, 1990.

76. Pidoriano AJ, Weinstein RN, Buuck DA, et al: Correlation of patellar articular lesions and results from anteromedial tibial tubercle transfer, *Am J Sports Med* 25:533-537, 1997.

77. Maquet P: Advancement of the tibial tuberosity, *Clin Orthop* 115:225, 1976.

78. Maquet P: Mechanics and osteoarthritis of the patellofemoral joint, *Clin Orthop* 144:70, 1979.

79. Jenny JY, Sader Z, Henry A, et al: Elevation of the tibial tubercle for patellofemoral pain syndrome. An 8- to 15-year follow-up, *Knee Surg Sports Traumatol Arthrosc* 4:92-96, 1996.

80. Leach RE, Schepsis AA: Anterior displacement of the tibial tubercle: the Maquet procedure, *Contemp Orthop* 3:199-204, 1981.

81. Radin EL, Pan HQ: Long-term follow-up study on the Maquet procedure with special reference to the causes of failure, *Clin Orthop* 290:253-258, 1993.

82. Schepsis AA, DeSimone AA, Leach RE: Anterior tibial tubercle transposition for patellofemoral arthrosis: a long-term study, *Am J Knee Surg* 7:13-20, 1994.

CHAPTER 24

Arthroscopic Lateral Release

Chris Alford, PT, SCS, ATC, CSCS
Patrick Denton, MD

ARTHROSCOPIC LATERAL RELEASE HAS historically been used to manage patellofemoral pain syndrome (PFPS), which was unresponsive to traditional conservative intervention. Often, this approach led to unsatisfactory surgical outcomes. Today, the indications for lateral release surgery have been more clearly defined, leading to improved patient selection and subsequent improved outcomes. To grasp the history related to patellofemoral pain (PFP) and indications for subsequent arthroscopic lateral release, an overview of the anatomy and biomechanics of the complex patellofemoral joint (PFJ) must be given.

The PFJ has become increasingly recognized as a source of knee pain and disability in the athlete.[1] Early in the twentieth century, orthopedic surgeons viewed patellofemoral (PF) problems largely as a female problem and generally ignored the topic in literature that addressed typical male athletic injuries.[2] Individuals with PF instability problems were portrayed as "somewhat obese, knock-kneed, teenaged females."[3,4] These concepts and ideas continued into the 1950s and 1960s until Dr. Jack Hughston and others began describing PF dysfunction in all athletic populations.[5-8]

Today, PF dysfunction is recognized as the most common type of knee pain or disorder seen in clinical practice by orthopedic surgeons.[9-12] In fact, 25% of all knee patients evaluated in a sports-related clinic were diagnosed with PFP in a study by Devereaux and Lachmann.[13] Dersheid and Feiring[14] also found that PFP accounts for around 30% of all patients being evaluated at a sports medicine clinic.

Patellofemoral pain syndrome was the most common diagnosis reported in a survey of 2002 patients with running injuries, representing 17% of all diagnoses.[15] Even in the general population, it has been reported that PFP affects one in four individuals.[16] Women today are much more active in sports and have a higher incidence of PFPS than males.[17,18] Many reasons for the difference in incidence have been published, but the most common are related to the tendency of women to have a broader pelvis and more valgus at the tibiofemoral joint.[12] Even with these reasons being cited repeatedly in literature, the male athlete with "normal" lower extremity biomechanics can have PFP.

Chondromalacia patella (a pathologic state of softening of the cartilage accompanied by fibrillation, fissuring, or erosion on the posterior patella)[19] was presumed to be the primary source of anterior knee pain until the late 1960s. Büdinger,[20] in 1908, first described these PF cartilage changes. Most authors believed these cartilage changes were traumatic in nature,[21-26] although some authors cited PFJ morphology as the main contributing factor in progressive chondromalacia patella.[27,28] In fact, Wiles and colleagues[29] found that half of all patients older than 30 had chondromalacia at the PFJ. Heywood,[30] in 1961, was first to implicate abnormal patellar tracking as the cause of chondromalacia. Later, in 1968, Hughston[7] made a clear connection between patellar malalignment and anterior knee pain. He theorized that abnormal patellar tilt and increased subluxation could be the primary cause of anterior knee pain. By the 1970s, authors began to

notice that chondromalacia patella could be clinically asymptomatic.[31,32] Later in the same decade, authors began to encourage the use of "patellar pain syndrome" rather than "chondromalacia" to describe anterior knee pain.[7]

Today, classification systems for evaluation and treatment of the PFJ are numerous and contradictory in literature.[33] The extensive volume of information related to PF dysfunction indicates the lack of clear identification criteria and successful management. The confusion of PF dysfunction classification begins with the evaluation. Some methods are based exclusively on radiographic findings, whereas others are based solely on the physical examination and clinical findings.[34-37] The terms that describe abnormal biomechanics of the PFJ in literature can have a wide variety of meanings and interpretations. Some of the more common terms are *malalignment, subluxation, chondromalacia, lateral pressure syndrome, patella alta,* and even *patella tilt.*[36] Merchant[35] has advocated for development of standardized classification systems to assist the clinician in selecting the proper treatment and providing clearly defined diagnostic categories for accurate comparison of results.

The disorder and pain source remain unclear and confusing to clinicians and researchers. The currently accepted hypothesis is an "anatomic predisposition" or malalignment of the extensor mechanism. The malalignment, or patellar tracking problem, could arise from anatomic abnormalities, biomechanical alterations, soft tissue support problems, or malalignment of the extremity.[38] Patellar tracking malalignment has been implicated in increasing PFJ compression and subsequent articular cartilage wear.[30,39-42] Articular cartilage tissue is aneural, is largely avascular, and has been essentially ruled out as a source of pain and symptoms in the PFJ. Wearing of the articular cartilage may allow the endplate to be exposed, which could stimulate pain receptors in the subchondral bone.[19,27,43,44] The potential sources of PFPS include subchondral bone, synovium, and retinaculum.[19] When considering the pain sources involved with PFPS, it is crucial to review PF anatomy, biomechanics, and kinematics before developing rehabilitation programs for the postsurgical PF patient.[19]

ANATOMY

Powers[45] describes the knee as a "mobile adaptor between two long bones" that has tremendous forces placed on it proximally and distally. Therefore external influences on the extensor mechanism span from the hip to the foot, including both bony and soft tissue structures.[12] Patellofemoral anatomy can be divided into static and dynamic stabilizers.

Static Stabilizers

The patella has static osseous and soft tissue structures that assist with proper patellar tracking and biomechanical function. The static osseous components include the femur, patella, tibia, and subtalar joint.[46] The femoral anatomy is crucial to the function of normal and abnormal PF kinematics. The version angle of the femoral neck and head affects the patella's positioning on the femur. Galland and colleagues[47] used computed tomography to determine normal femoral head anteversion as 11 degrees with a standard deviation of 7 degrees. Abnormal increases in femoral head anteversion can cause the distal femoral trochlea to deviate more medially when the femoral neck assumes a neutral position in the hip.[47] Retroversion may cause the opposite effect. Torsional deformities can also affect trochlear orientation. If femoral neck anteversion and internal femoral torsion occur concurrently or independently, external tibial torsion may occur. The result can be lateral displacement of the patella.[12] Torsions such as these can cause lateral patellar tracking, subluxation, and even increased risk for lateral facet impingement syndrome. Therefore femoral anatomic predisposition can have a direct impact on PF biomechanics.

The patellar anatomy has been well described in the literature.[5,28,47-49] The patella is a sesamoid bone contained within the extensor or quadriceps mechanism. The shape of the patella can vary widely among individuals, but the clinical significance of this finding remains controversial. It is assumed that unusual patellar shapes predispose people to extensor mechanism dysfunction.[28,50] The patella is separated posteriorly into a medial facet and a lateral facet. The lateral facet is usually longer and more sloped to account for the larger lateral femoral condyle.[12] Hughston and colleagues[34] reported that the length ratio between the lateral facet and the medial facet is 3:2. A third facet that is situated along the medial portion of the medial facet has also been identified.[12] This area of the patella is in direct contact with the femur only during full knee flexion.[51-53] The patella contains a significant amount of articular cartilage and is in fact the thickest cartilage in the human body. The articular cartilage can be up to 7 mm thick near the midsagittal ridge.[50]

Tibial anatomy must also be considered when assessing PF biomechanics and kinematics. Tibial tuberosity placement influences the quadriceps angle (Q angle) of the knee[54] (Figure 24-1). The Q angle is produced by the intersection of a line drawn from the anterior superior iliac spine (ASIS) to the midpoint of the patella and a distal line drawn from the tibial tuberosity to the midpoint of the patella.[12,46] The Q angle typically increases with a valgus deformity or increased tibial external rotation. Schulthies and colleagues[55] found that a larger Q angle predisposes the knee to lateral patellar tracking when compared with a smaller Q angle. However, the literature connecting increased lateral patellar tracking and PFPS has been largely inconsistent.[54]

Excessive subtalar joint pronation has been theorized to produce abnormal PFJ biomechanics.[56] Increased foot pronation is associated with an increased Q angle and a laterally directed force on the patella resulting from the quadriceps and patellar tendon angle. Prolonged pronation could facilitate the femoral internal rotation when it would normally rotate externally.[56,57] The abnormal femoral internal rotation would allow for increased external tibial rotation during

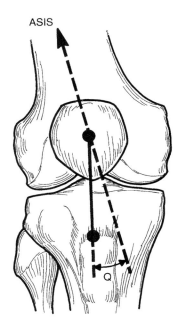

Figure 24-1: The Q angle. The angle is formed by a line drawn from the anterior superior iliac spine (ASIS) through the center of the patella and a second line from the center of the patella to the center of the tibial tubercle. *(From Merchant AC: Extensor mechanism injuries: classification and diagnosis. In Scott WN, editor:* The knee, *St Louis, Mosby, 1994.)*

weight bearing.[46] External tibial rotation can lead to compressive stress syndrome of PFJ or altered biomechanical tracking.[56]

Static soft tissue components affecting the PFJ include the patellar tendon, capsular and ligamentous structures such as the lateral retinaculum, iliotibial band (ITB), PF ligaments, patellotibial ligaments, and meniscopatellar ligaments. Many variations of these structures have been described in the literature, which provide direct restraint on medial and lateral patellar positioning.[48,49,58,59]

The patellar tendon originates at the inferior pole of the patella and attaches to the tibial tuberosity. A bursa (deep infrapatellar bursa) lies between the patellar tendon and the tibia, which reduces friction during use of the knee extensor mechanism. If scarring or inflammation in this area is present, alteration of proper gliding of the tibiofemoral joint may occur, causing PFP.[34]

The medial patellofemoral ligament (MPFL), which has been called the "primary restraint to lateral displacement of the patella," prevents lateral movement of the patella, originates from the adductor tubercle, and attaches to the medial border of the patella[12] (Figure 24-2). The vastus medialis oblique (VMO) interfaces with the MPFL, allowing for ligamentous tightening during VMO contraction.[44]

The lateral patellofemoral ligament, capsule, ITB, and lateral retinaculum provide lateral guiding and stabilization of the patella during knee motion. Many patients with PF

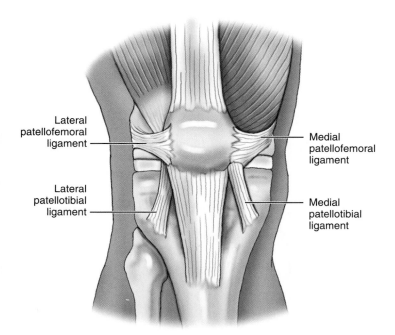

Figure 24-2: Patellofemoral and patellotibial ligaments: static stabilizers of the patella. *(From Walsh WM: Patellofemoral joint. In DeLee JC, Drez D, editors: Orthopaedic and sports medicine: principles and practice, Philadelphia, 1994, Saunders.)*

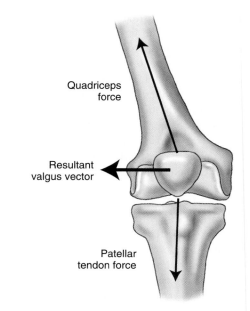

Figure 24-3: Patellofemoral valgus vector. A lateral force vector is produced by the angle of pull from the quadriceps and the patellar tendon. *(From Weber MD, Ware AN: Knee rehabilitation. In Andrews JR, Harrelson GL, Wilk KE, editors: Physical rehabilitation of the injured athlete, Philadelphia, 1994, Saunders.)*

complaints have an abnormally high insertion of the ITB on the patella, or a shortening of the lateral structures, which may laterally displace the patella, causing anterior knee pain.[60,61]

Dynamic Stabilizers

The relevant active or dynamic stabilizers of the PFJ include the quadriceps muscle group and the articularis genu.[12,44] The quadriceps muscle group consists of the rectus femoris, the vastus lateralis, the vastus intermedialis, and the vastus medialis. All of the quadriceps muscles except the rectus femoris originate on the proximal one third of the femur. The rectus femoris originates at the ASIS on the pelvis. Each muscle attaches distally to the patella at differing angles, creating vector forces on the patella and assisting with patellar stabilization[34,59,62] (Figures 24-3 and 24-4). The rectus femoris is believed to function as the "command post" for coordination of quadriceps activity as a whole.[34] The aponeurosis of the vastus medialis and lateralis are interwoven within the medial and lateral retinacula, which attach to the proximal tibia. Therefore the retinacula contain a dynamic component from quadriceps input, which assists in controlling the patella.[12]

The vastus lateralis has been implicated in displaying three variations in anatomic patterns. A unique oblique portion of the vastus lateralis has been described by Hallisey and colleagues.[63] This muscle strand, the vastus lateralis oblique (VLO), can originate from the lateral intermuscular

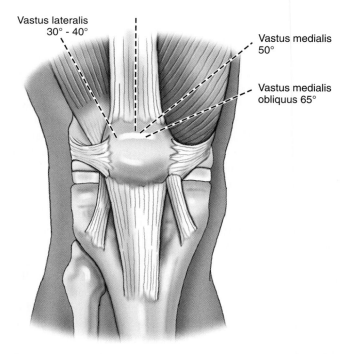

Figure 24-4: Angles of quadriceps insertion. The quadriceps muscles attach to the patella at different angles, creating stabilizing vector forces. *(From Walsh WM: Patellofemoral joint. In DeLee JC, Drez D, editors: Orthopaedic and sports medicine: principles and practice, Philadelphia, 1994, Saunders.)*

septum and insert in one of three distinct patterns, including the vastus lateralis itself, the lateral retinaculum, or the oblique fibers of the lateral retinaculum, in which the VLO intertwines together with the vastus lateralis muscle. Normally, the vastus lateralis longus has a 12- to 15-degree angulation,[59] but Hallisey and colleagues[63] found the VLO to insert at an average angle of 38 degrees in women and 48 degrees in men. The VLO provides a laterally directed force on the patella, in addition to assisting with knee extension. Consequently, the VLO may be specifically released from the patella without disrupting the vastus lateralis.[63]

Lieb and Perry[64] first drew attention to the VMO by describing the function of the distal third of the vastus medialis. The VMO's proximal attachment is located on the distal medial intermuscular septum and the adductor tubercle, and the distal attachment is normally near the proximal one third to one half of the medial patellar edge. They reported that the VMO did not function in knee extension from 30 to 0 degrees, but instead stabilized the patella medially, allowing for a delicate balancing against the significant lateral forces on the patella.[64] Since that publication over 30 years ago, the VMO has been implicated in literature as the primary dynamic stabilizer of the patella and a prime anatomic factor in PF disorders. More current findings suggest that patellar stabilization is much more complex than first believed.[10,11,46,56,57,64-69]

The articularis genu (AG), often called the "fifth quadriceps muscle," is clearly a muscular component affecting the PFJ.[70] It originates from the distal femur and attaches to the suprapatellar pouch. The AG functions to "pre-position" the patella in preparation for knee extension by retracting the suprapatellar pouch superiorly. Abnormalities such as scarring or inflammation of the suprapatellar plica have been implicated in preventing the AG from retracting the synovial fold properly, causing possible PFP.[34]

Patellofemoral Biomechanical Considerations

The patella functions to improve or maximize mechanical advantage of the knee extensor mechanism. The patella acts similarly to a pulley and a class I lever to redirect not only quadriceps force but also to change the magnitude of the force when moving the tibia.[50] With the knee in full extension, almost no PF contact exists.[52] As the knee moves from 0 to 60 degrees of flexion, the magnitude of PF contact area increases.[50] In regard to PF contact force, knee flexion past 60 degrees is more controversial. Some investigators have demonstrated that the contact area remains unchanged from 60 to 90 degrees of knee flexion,[71] whereas others see a reduction of force after 60 degrees, and still others report a rise in pressure after 90 degrees of flexion.[72] More research is needed to clarify PF contact forces at positions greater than 60 degrees of flexion as treatment for damaged articular cartilage continues to advance. Regardless, many clear and objective principles from the biomechanics currently understood can be applied to the rehabilitation program.

Closed Kinetic Chain (Weight Bearing)

In a closed kinetic chain (CKC) setting, the patellofemoral joint reaction force (PFJRF) increases as the knee flexion angle increases[73] (Figure 24-5). The PF contact area concurrently increases as the knee flexes from 0 to 90 degrees, but the change is reportedly less than the PFJRF change. With this information, it is clear that the net change in PF stress actually increases as knee flexion increases.[50] On the contrary, some investigators report a decrease in net PF stress as knee flexion moves from 90 to 120 degrees in a CKC position.[74] The increased PF contact area while in weight bearing allows for a subsequent decrease in shear force on PF articular cartilage. The CKC or weight-bearing position between 0 and 45 degrees of knee flexion has been suggested to be safer and more effective compared with open kinetic chain (OKC) or non–weight-bearing exercises for PF rehabilitation success.[53,74-77] Witvrouw and others[78] recently compared the clinical effectiveness of OKC versus CKC exercises for patients with PFP. Both groups significantly increased in overall functionality and had good-to-excellent functional results after a CKC or an OKC protocol. Both groups demonstrated similar reductions in pain and strength improvements during open chain isokinetic testing. They concluded that the CKC exercises are generally more effective in the treatment of PFP, but they now incorporate OKC and CKC exercises in their treatment program as a result of their study comparing the two groups. They further reported that the recommendation to totally avoid OKC exercises in the treatment of PFP is essentially unfounded because these exercises are effective for pain reduction and functional restoration.[78]

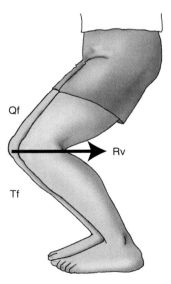

Figure 24-5: Patellofemoral joint reaction forces. As knee flexion increases, a posterior force is placed on the patellofemoral joint. *(From Weber MD, Ware AN: Knee rehabilitation. In Andrews JR, Harrelson GL, Wilk KE, editors: Physical rehabilitation of the injured athlete, Philadelphia, 1994, Saunders.)*

Open Kinetic Chain (Non–Weight Bearing)

The OKC form of exercise produces quite different effects on the PFJ biomechanically. During non–weight bearing, the forces across the patella are the lowest at 90 degrees of flexion and sharply increase as the knee actively moves toward full extension. The contact area also continues to decrease as the knee moves toward extension, producing a significant net increase in PF stress with OKC knee extension, specifically from 25 to 0 degrees.[50] Steinkamp and colleagues[76] calculated PFJ stress, PFJRF, and knee moment during the leg press and the leg extension exercise. Each parameter was significantly greater during the leg extension exercise compared with the leg press at 0 degrees and 30 degrees of knee flexion. The leg press produced higher PFJ stress and PFJRF at 60 degrees and 90 degrees of knee flexion. Steinkamp and colleagues[76] concluded that individuals with PFJ arthritis may tolerate resistive quadriceps exercises with the leg press during functional range of motion (ROM) (0 to 30 degrees of knee flexion) with less PFJ stress compared with the knee extension exercise. Witvrouw and colleagues[79] more recently investigated reflex response times of the vasti muscles in patients with anterior knee pain after performing a 5-week program of OKC or CKC exercises. The anterior knee pain decreased in both the OKC and CKC groups, and no statistically significant change was found in either group for reflex response time.[79]

Patellar Tracking Mechanics

Powers and colleagues[46,57] investigated PF kinematics using kinematic magnetic resonance imaging (KMRI) during weight-bearing and non–weight-bearing knee extension in persons with lateral subluxation of the patella. They demonstrated that the patella is displaced laterally during non–weight-bearing (OKC) knee extension between 30 and 12 degrees. No differences in lateral patellar tilt between the weight-bearing and non–weight-bearing positions were found. Lateral patellar rotation was significantly higher throughout the entire ROM during non–weight bearing as compared with weight bearing. During weight bearing the femur internally rotates as the knee is extended from 18 to 0 degrees. These findings support recent evidence and preliminary investigations indicating that during non–weight-bearing activities the patella rotates on the femur, and during weight bearing the femur rotates under the patella.[46,57]

The patella may be in a tilted position (lateral side down) during early knee flexion and full extension. If true malalignment is present, this tilt will be significant and manually difficult to manipulate.[50] Patel and associates[80] investigated whether patellar tilt at full knee extension was pathologic or simply a normal finding. Patellar position was assessed during various angles of knee flexion while in a modified CKC position. Using magnetic resonance imaging (MRI), lateral patellar tilt and subluxation occurred in normal knees at full extension, and the patella self-reduced in the trochlear groove at 30 degrees of knee flexion. The authors concluded that lateral patellar tilt and subluxation typically observed during arthroscopy, with the knee in full extension, may be normal and nonpathologic.[80] Consequently, although speculation and theories exist, more investigation is needed to clarify the origin of pain and pathologic biomechanics of the PFJ.

REVIEW OF TRADITIONAL CONSERVATIVE REHABILITATION

Conservative treatment for PFP and dysfunction has traditionally focused on normalizing abnormal patellar tracking through strengthening of the quadriceps muscle, specifically the VMO.[76,81-84] As previously mentioned, Lieb and Perry[64] first described the VMO as a medial patellar stabilizer, capable of balancing the significant lateral pull stemming from the vastus lateralis. Conservative clinical strengthening programs have focused on selectively recruiting the VMO to restore patellar tracking and the delicate balance of the PFJ.[12,19,73,85,86]

Recent investigative research has presented opposition to the typical clinical practice of selectively recruiting the VMO as the preferred rehabilitation technique for PFP. Powers and colleagues[60] found decreased recruitment of the entire quadriceps muscle group in individuals with PFP during gait activities. The reduced quadriceps activity was not statistically significant in the VMO versus the other vasti muscles.[60] Mirzabeigi and colleagues[87] also found no statistical difference between VMO and other quadriceps muscle activity during performance of nine different quadriceps exercises.

For years the standard evidence and available research have suggested that the main contributing factor in PFPS is an alteration of normal joint mechanics caused by weakness and insufficiency in the VMO.[64,76,81-84] Despite previous data supporting this position, more recent evidence suggests otherwise.[44,87,88] In fact, no sound evidence currently exists to support the VMO being selectively recruited during exercise activities. Attempts at selectively recruiting the VMO have often produced generalized quadriceps strengthening.[44,87,88] Cerny[88] investigated 22 different variations of commonly prescribed quadriceps exercises, including quadriceps sets, isometric holds with knee flexion, knee extension, wall slides, and others. No exercise produced greater VMO activity compared with the vastus lateralis.[88] Laprade and colleagues[89] found similar results in subjects with and without PFP. Witvrouw and associates[79] found no difference in reflex response times of the vasti muscles after 5 weeks of OKC or CKC exercise programs. Interestingly, both groups had a significant reduction in knee pain.[79]

Currently, the mechanism by which quadriceps strengthening reduces PFP is not fully understood, but it is believed to alter the muscle balance around the patella.[11,90] Research on traditional conservative management, including quadriceps strengthening, has demonstrated the reduction of pain

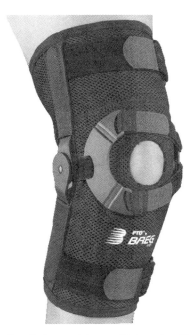

Figure 24-6: Patellofemoral brace. This style of brace allows for adjustable patellar compression while forming a comfortable lateral wall during knee flexion and extension. *(From Breg, Inc., 2611 Commerce Way, Vista, CA 92081.)*

and symptoms, despite no evidence of altered patellar tracking.[16,44,91,92] Evidence does suggest that bracing and external patella supports can reduce symptoms and offer pain relief, despite the controversy about whether the support changes patellar tracking.[11] Pain may contribute to inhibition of normal quadriceps activity; therefore pain reduction using an external brace or support may aid in recovery and speed the restoration of PF function preoperatively or postoperatively.[11] Many PF support braces are on the market. A brace that allows for variation in medial patellar pull and pressure is suggested. This type of brace is available in multiple types of breathable fabrics and is easy to apply (Figure 24-6). These types of braces are consistently improving, and many are clinically useful for pain control in conjunction with strengthening.

Taping for PFP, described by McConnell,[16] can be useful clinically during the nonoperative or postoperative rehabilitation program. Patellar taping has proven itself to be clinically useful for pain reduction.[16,93] In a randomized control trial, Wittingham and colleagues[94] demonstrated that the combination of patellar taping and exercise was superior to the use of exercise or taping alone in reducing pain and improving function. Controversy over whether external patellar supports actually change or alter patellar tracking remains unsettled. Bockrath and others[95] reported that patellar taping significantly reduced pain despite not changing the patella's position. Larsen and co-workers[96] demonstrated medial movement of the patella with patellar taping in a

static position; however, medial patellar positioning was absent after exercise was completed. Changes in neuromuscular recruitment of the VMO during step-up and step-down activities, accompanied by patellar taping or bracing, have been reported by Gilleard and colleagues,[97] but Cerny[88] reports no effect on VMO:vastus lateralis(VL) electromyogram ratio with PF taping. Powers[11] reports a theory that the external supports may increase the PF contact area with increased compression from the brace or tape, thereby reducing the contact stress and subsequent pain production. This theory is consistent with all of the available evidence, but more research will clarify why patellar bracing or taping reduces PFP.

Patients with PFP may benefit from the use of foot orthoses, but the evidence for such use is limited. Gross and Foxworth[56] provided a comprehensive literature review regarding the role of foot orthoses as an intervention for PFP. They concluded that patients with PFP may benefit from the use of foot orthoses if they concurrently have signs of excessive foot pronation or a lower extremity alignment profile that includes excessive lower extremity internal rotation during weight bearing and increased Q angle.[56] The authors further describe possible mechanisms for foot orthoses to facilitate pain reduction and functional improvement for patients with PFP. Possible mechanisms include a reduction in internal rotation of the lower extremity; a reduction in Q angle; reduced laterally directed soft tissue forces from the patellar tendon, the quadriceps tendon, and the iliotibial band; and reduced PF contact pressures and altered PF contact pressure mapping.[56] Sutlive and associates[98] recently investigated the use of foot orthosis and modified activity to reduce PFP. Results suggest that "patients with PFPS who have forefoot valgus alignment greater than 2 degrees, passive great toe extension less than 78 degrees, or minimal motion during the navicular drop test of less than 3 mm are most likely to respond favorably to intervention with an off-the-shelf foot orthosis and instruction in activity modification." They further suggest that clinicians should attempt the use of an off-the-shelf orthotic device if a patient has one or more of the previously identified characteristics.[98] Thus orthotics may be a significant pain-reducing option for certain patients who meet the criteria during screening. More research is needed to further investigate the use of foot orthoses for patients with PFP.

Research indicates that no one factor is the sole defining etiology for PFP production.[67] The PFJ is one of the most complex diarthrodial joints in the human body, and multiple compounding etiologic factors can lead to pathology. These factors should be considered for developing repair and rehabilitation strategies for the PFJ.[67]

After this thorough overview of conservative interventions for PFP, it is time to consider more aggressive treatment options, such as surgery. The most frequent surgical procedure used in patients with PFPS is the lateral retinacular release.[99,100]

SURGICAL INTERVENTION

History of Lateral Release

In 1891, Pollard[101] first described the lateral release surgical technique with trochlear groove chiseling to treat subluxation or dislocation of the patella. More recently, in 1970, Willner[102] also described the lateral retinacular release for surgical management of recurrent patellar dislocations. Four years later, Merchant and Mercer[103] published a report regarding the lateral release of the patella where the lateral retinaculum and capsule were released at the superior pole of the patella directed toward the quadriceps tendon. In 1981, McGinty and McCarthy[104] described a technique for endoscopic lateral release. Since Merchant and Mercer's preliminary report, there have been hundreds of reports on the use of lateral release for anterior knee pain. The specific criteria for surgical intervention using the lateral release have been poorly defined, leading to confusion and difficulty in assessing the surgical outcome and results. In addition, the varied evaluation techniques, classification of symptoms, and preoperative diagnoses further contribute to the confusion when discussing PFPS patients. The myriad of diagnoses may include chondromalacia patellae, osteoarthritis, recurrent subluxation, PF malalignment, patellar compression syndrome, excessive lateral pressure syndrome, PF stress syndrome, PFPS, patellar tendonitis, patellar tendinosus, plica syndrome, or simply anterior knee pain.[103-111]

Over the course of evolution of this surgical technique, the initial indication for performing the lateral release was PFPS that did not respond to conservative rehabilitation. Even today, there remains no clear consensus on inclusion criteria for lateral retinacular release surgery.[105,110,112-115] Some have attempted to clarify inclusion criteria by supporting the use of the lateral release in patients with pain but no instability; others use it in patients with instability but no pain; and still others use it with both types of syndromes.[12] In order for any surgical technique to be beneficial with predictable and reproducible outcomes, it must be applied to patients with specific parameters and symptoms. The paintbrush application of the lateral release to all patients with failed conservative management of anterior knee pain has led to highly variable and unpredictable surgical outcomes and even significant complications in some cases. A systematic evaluation of patients who have failed conservative treatment of anterior knee pain is critical to determine the cause of their PFP, as well as which signs and symptoms should be addressed surgically to eliminate pain and allow patients to continue their given level of activity.

HISTORY AND PHYSICAL EXAMINATION

A thorough medical history and physical examination are the core foundation to any investigation of PFP. The medical history should focus on the events surrounding the onset of the anterior knee pain. Was it a traumatic event? Has the patient experienced any patellar dislocations or subluxations? Are there any mechanical symptoms associated with the pain? Often patients report that the knee "gives way," which is a frequent complaint associated with multiple knee pathologies including ligamentous instability, patellar subluxation, or quadriceps weakness. Is crepitation a complaint? If so, at what degree of knee flexion does it occur? This information provides insight to the location of a chondral injury to the undersurface of the patella or the trochlea of the femur. In smaller degrees of flexion, the lesion is more likely to be near the inferior pole, and as flexion increases, the patellar location migrates more superiorly.

It is important for the patient to qualify the reported pain. Is it activity related? What activities and knee positions aggravate it? Is it bothersome going up or down stairs? Is any swelling associated with the complaints? If so, determine whether the swelling is from true joint effusion or extraarticular edema. Most often, the patient can point to a specific region of the knee as the source of pain. Be sure to document any other joints that are involved. Multiple joint complaints can be a sign of a systemic disease process, indicating the need for further investigation or possible referral to appropriate medical personnel.

The last important point on the medical history and systems review is to determine what previous treatments have been attempted. Most often, by the time the patient has reached an orthopedic surgeon's office, he or she has had some form of prior treatment. Inquire about any previous treatment, including medication, rehabilitation, or bracing. The previous treatment duration is significant to note, as well as whether it provided any relief, even if temporary. Any prior surgical intervention should be investigated and included in the medical history of symptoms.

PHYSICAL EXAMINATION

The physical examination for anterior knee pain includes a complete musculoskeletal evaluation of not only the knee joint but also both lower extremities, including the lumbar spine. As mentioned earlier, any malalignment of the hip, knee, or foot can have detrimental effects on the PFJ. The majority of today's physical examination knowledge on the PFJ can be accredited to Fulkerson,[116,117] Post,[118] and their colleagues. Initially, the patient's knee is observed for any evidence of swelling, skin color changes, atrophy, and any previous surgical scars. Any dystrophic changes or hypersensitivity may indicate reflex sympathetic dystrophy (RSD), which is now more commonly called complex regional pain syndrome (CRPS). Any suspicion of such should initiate a thorough CRPS evaluation, and any surgical options should be delayed.

An assessment of gait should be completed with any deviations noted. During ambulation, watch the progression of the patella through a knee flexion and extension cycle. Notice any varus/valgus alignment abnormalities. Does the patient have hyperpronation of the subtalar joint with ambulation?

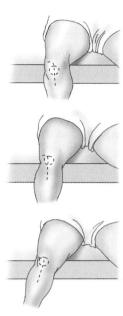

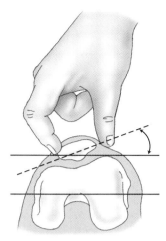

Figure 24-8: Passive patellar tilt test. The lateral border of the patella should rise to or above the horizontal plane. If this motion is not available, the lateral knee structure may be tight and subsequently cause lateral patellar compression syndrome. *(From Walsh WM: Patellofemoral joint. In DeLee JC, Drez D, editors: Orthopaedic and sports medicine: principles and practice, Philadelphia, 1994, Saunders.)*

Figure 24-7: J sign. Watch for the patella to take an inverted J-shaped course as the knee is actively extended from 90 degrees of flexion to full extension at 0 degrees. *(From Walsh WM: Patellofemoral joint. In DeLee JC, Drez D, editors: Orthopaedic and sports medicine: principles and practice, Philadelphia, 1994, Saunders.)*

Also, pay careful attention to hip rotation with the gait cycle.

With the patient sitting, thoroughly palpate the knee joint and associated structures. Note any tenderness over the lateral and medial retinaculum. Fulkerson and colleagues[119] have noted that the retinaculum is richly innervated with nerve endings and can be inflamed with tight lateral constraints. Document any knee effusions, which can indicate an intraarticular problem. All previous surgical scars should be palpated to ensure that there are no painful neuromas.

Next, have the patient flex and extend the knee while palpating and observing the tracking of the patella. All crepitance should be noted. When does the patella engage into the trochlea? Is this a smooth transition or does it jump? A sudden jump in the trochlea may be perceived by the patient as a subluxation. The J sign is the lateral tracking of the patella on terminal extension (Figure 24-7). Be sure to measure the Q angle, which is the angle of the quadriceps tendon and the patellar tendon.[12,46] An increased Q angle may allow for the lateral tracking of the patella, although the exact significance of the Q angle has been questioned.[118,120] With the patient in the supine position, palpate the iliotibial band and the medial structures. After an acute dislocation, the medial retinaculum and MPFL will be tender. Evaluate patellar stability and mobility. The patellar tilt test is performed by attempting to elevate the lateral border of the patella using the thumb and index finger (Figure 24-8). Normally, the lateral border of the patella should rise to or

above the horizontal plane. If it does not, tight lateral constraints are present, and the patient may have lateral patellar compression syndrome.[121] This condition can lead to pain and even to breakdown on the lateral facet of the patella.

Patellar glide is measured in full extension and in 20 to 30 degrees of knee flexion (Figure 24-9). The displacement of a medially and laterally directed force is measured in quadrants of the patella. A medial glide of 1 quadrant or less is consistent with tight lateral constraints. If the patella glides 3 quadrants or more laterally, medial structures are incompetent.[121] Any apprehension with the laterally directed force should be noted.

A complete evaluation also requires the patient to be examined in the prone position. In this position, the patient's femoral and tibial version can be documented. Flex both knees in the prone position, noting any quadriceps tightness.

RADIOGRAPHIC EVALUATION

Initial radiographic images of the knee should consist of a standard weight-bearing anteroposterior (AP) view and true lateral radiographs with a merchant view of bilateral knees. Plain films are a good screening tool for overall alignment, fractures, and bony lesions. The lateral view can provide an assessment of femoral trochlea depth and patellar rotation.[122]

The Merchant view allows for the measurement of patellar tilt and subluxation. When viewed on the Merchant radiograph, the congruence angle can be calculated. The central ridge of the patella should lie at or medial to the bisector of the trochlear angle.[117] Any lateral displacement

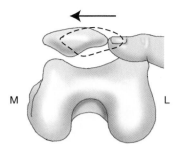

Figure 24-9: Patellar glide test. The test is performed with the knee in 20 to 30 degrees of flexion. *(From Fu FH, Maday MG: Arthroscopic lateral release and the lateral patellar compression syndrome,* Orthop Clin North Am *23[4]:601-611, 1992.)*

of the central ridge constitutes lateral subluxation or translation.

A more sensitive imaging modality is computed tomography (CT), which can demonstrate patellar alignment and intraosseous pathologic changes in the patella and trochlea.[123] The PFJ should be imaged at 15, 30, and 45 degrees of knee flexion with midtransverse patellar cuts. These images will demonstrate any subluxation abnormality that may be missed on a single-axial radiographic view.

Magnetic resonance imaging can be helpful in the evaluation of patellar instability, especially after an acute dislocation. With MRI, it is possible to see any acute bone bruises, chondral defects or injuries, and tears of the MPFL. Sallay and colleagues[124] demonstrated tears of the MPFL and vastus medialis muscle, along with associated bone bruises and osteochondral loose bodies.

INDICATIONS FOR LATERAL RELEASE

Previously, lateral release was the surgical treatment of choice for patients with anterior PFP that was resistant to conservative treatment protocols. Surgeons used lateral release to treat nonspecific anterior pain, patellar tilt, subluxation, and even patellar dislocations. Often this arbitrary use led to unpredictable outcomes that deteriorated with continued follow-up.[125] Kolowich and colleagues[33] looked at the lateral release patient population and determined specific positive predictors for good and excellent outcomes. A negative passive patellar tilt and a patellar glide of 2 quadrants or less were indications for lateral release. These physical examination findings are consistent with lateral patellar compression syndrome. These indications have been supported by several authors who believe that lateral release is the surgical treatment of choice for tight lateral constraints with minimal or absent malalignment.[117,121] Patients with significant malalignment or recurrent instability of the PFJ are better candidates for either proximal or distal realignment.[116]

SURGICAL TECHNIQUE

Any surgical procedure on the PFJ should be preceded by a thorough examination under anesthesia, followed by com-

plete diagnostic arthroscopic evaluation. The arthroscopic examination assesses the complete knee joint, including meniscal and ligamentous structures, as well as the chondral surfaces. Any articular surface injury is documented and graded according to the Outerbridge classification.[27] The location of any articular surface injury or wear in the PFJ can play a role in the surgical decision process. If a patient has significant wear in both facets of the patella, he or she may be better served with a distal anteriorization to unload the PFJ.[116,126] Any loose chondral flaps on the lateral facet can be debrided arthroscopically.

The superomedial portal can be used to watch patellar tracking while flexing and extending the knee. The lateral facet should engage and align itself with the trochlea by 20 to 25 degrees of knee flexion.[121] Any lateral overhang of the patella on the femoral condyle should be documented.

The lateral release can be performed open or arthroscopically. Both techniques provide similar results.[127] Currently, with the technology of arthroscopic electrocautery, a majority of releases are done arthroscopically. After the arthroscopic examination, the camera is placed in the anteromedial portal, and the electrocautery device is used from the superomedial and anterolateral portals to perform the release (Figures 24-10 and 24-11). The entire retinaculum is released approximately 7 to 10 mm from the border of the patella. Near the superior patella, the release should err to the posterior side, in order to avoid injury to the vastus lateralis. A release of the vastus lateralis tendon could cause medial subluxation of the patella.[121] If the procedure was performed with the tourniquet, it should be deflated to ensure that all bleeding has been addressed and that hemostasis is achieved. The patella should be inspected and the patellar tilt test performed. The patella should be able to tilt 70 to 90 degrees above the horizontal (see Figure 24-11).[128] If this angle is not achieved, any remaining tethers should be released. Instruments are then removed, and portal sites closed. A well-padded compression dressing is applied, as well as a cryotherapy pad. Routinely, no splint or immobilizer is used. The patient is given crutches and can be weight bearing as tolerated, provided he or she can ambulate with a proper gait pattern. Range-of-motion exercises can be started on the first postoperative day. The patient is discharged the same day.

COMPLICATIONS

Overall, when used with proper indications and technique, the lateral release procedure can produce successful outcomes. In reviewing the literature for lateral release, over two thirds of published reports describe more than 70% satisfactory results.[129] Lateral release, however, is not an innocuous procedure. In a review of the complications associated with 10,262 knee arthroscopies, Small[130] found 446 lateral releases with 32 complications for an overall complication rate of 7.2%. The lateral release procedure had the highest complication rate of all arthroscopic knee procedures.

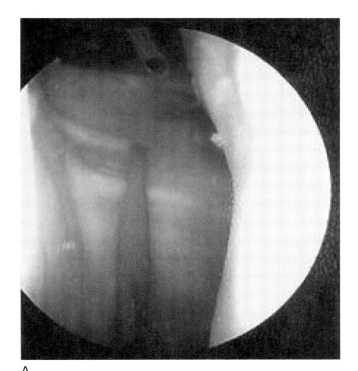

A

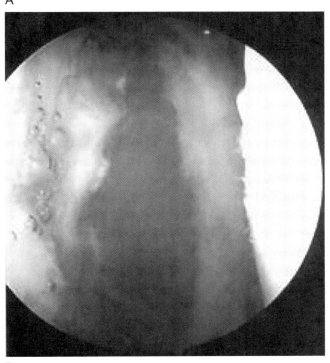

B

Figure 24-10: A, Arthroscopic view of the lateral retinaculum.
B, Complete lateral release using electrocautery.

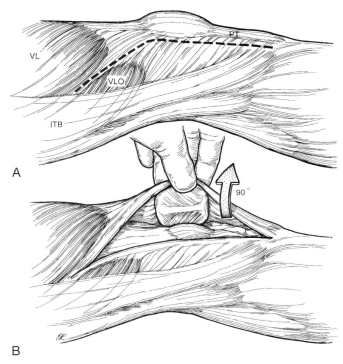

Figure 24-11: Complete lateral release. **A,** The *dashed line*
represents the recommended lateral release. The proximal
release is performed without involving the VLO or vastus
lateralis. **B,** Postoperatively, the patella should be able to tilt 70
to 90 degrees above the horizontal. *(From Post WR, Fulkerson JP:
Surgery of the patellofemoral joint: indications, effects, results, and
recommendations. In Scott WN, editor:* The knee, *St Louis, 1994,
Mosby.)*

The most common complication after lateral release is
hemarthrosis, accounting for 65% of all complications.[131]
The incidence of hemarthrosis appeared to be related to
tourniquet use, a subcutaneous technique, and the use of a
drain for more than 24 hours. Electrocautery and prolonged

hospital stay did not have an effect on the occurrence of
hemarthrosis. The presence of a hemarthrosis is not only
painful to the patient but also hinders postoperative
rehabilitation. The large effusion hampers postoperative
quadriceps function and ability to progress ROM. To
prevent quadriceps shutdown, it is recommended that a tourniquet, if used, be deflated immediately after the lateral
release and that electrocautery be administered to obtain
meticulous hemostasis. Most often the bleeding is from the
lateral superior genicular artery and its branches. If a drain
is used, it should only be in place for 2 to 3 hours and then
discontinued.[130]

The aggressiveness of the lateral release can predispose
patients to several complications, including medial subluxation of the patella, quadriceps tendon rupture, quadriceps
weakness, and patellar hypermobility.[132] Most of these complications are a result of an overzealous surgical release that
involves the vastus lateralis insertion.[133] Blasier and Ciullo[134]
reported a case in which a patient suffered a quadriceps
rupture following an arthroscopic release. In this case, the
extensor mechanism was injured proximal to the patella.
Hughston and Deese[135] found that 50% of patients who failed
to improve after arthroscopic lateral release had evidence of
medial patellar subluxation. Any patient who has had previ-

ous patellofemoral surgery should be screened for any evidence of medial patellar subluxation on physical and radiologic examination. Fulkerson and Hungerford[90] stated that all of the patients they had seen with medial subluxation had iatrogenic causes.

Excessive scarring can occur after lateral release, resulting in infrapatellar contracture and arthrofibrosis.[136] Infrapatellar contracture results from adhesions forming between the patellar tendon and the tibia. The adhesions, in turn, cause a functional shortening of the patellar tendon, thereby increasing PFJRF with knee flexion. Arthrofibrosis results in excessive scar formation intraarticularly and occasionally extraarticularly. The patient has decreased ROM, especially in knee flexion, and declining function. Kolowich and colleagues[33] reported that patients who developed arthrofibrosis, after a lateral release, may require a manipulation under anesthesia. The fundamental treatment for these complications is prevention. This approach includes early aggressive ROM, patellar mobilization exercises, and early swelling control.[129]

Less common complications include infection and CRPS. As with any surgical procedure, infection is a known risk and complication. Any suspicion of infection in the postoperative period should be aggressively investigated, including blood studies such as a complete blood count, erythrocyte sedimentation rate, and C-reactive protein. If there is a knee effusion, it should be aspirated and sent for culture, as well as sensitivity and Gram stain. Positive results necessitate incision and drainage followed by parenteral antibiotics.

Complex regional pain syndrome is fortunately an infrequent complication after knee surgery, but it is known to occur more frequently after PFJ surgery. In a review of a patient population with CRPS of the knee, Cooper and colleagues[137] found that of the 14 patients studied, 11 had had surgery of the PFJ. Initial symptoms include burning pain, hypersensitivity, skin color changes, an increase in skin temperature, and decreased ROM. Treatment for CRPS should include a multispecialty approach, including pain management, physical therapy, and possibly sympathetic neural blocks. The key to success is early recognition and treatment.

The intention of any PF surgery is to minimize any potential complications and to ensure maximum benefit to the patient. This goal can be accomplished by strict patient selection criteria, meticulous surgical technique, and a comprehensive rehabilitation program designed specifically for the postoperative goals associated with PF surgery. The postoperative rehabilitation program is as crucial to the overall outcome as the surgical procedure itself.

POSTOPERATIVE REHABILITATION

The lateral release has been called "one of the simplest procedures to manage" postoperatively.[44] This statement is true regarding the ease of healing and lack of extensive tissue disruption associated with lateral release surgery. Although these factors contribute to easy postoperative management, the disparity in positive outcomes following surgery poses some limitations in rehabilitation.[121] It is therefore difficult to determine exactly what percentage and type of patients benefit from the lateral release procedure. Because the criteria for needing this surgical procedure are vague and poorly defined, many patients come out of surgery with the same symptoms that they had preoperatively. Thus postoperative management is often an extension of their conservative treatment, with adequate consideration for postoperative soft tissue healing time frames.[44,138]

If appropriate orthopedic rehabilitation principles are implemented and reassessed by the rehabilitation specialist, the postoperative recovery should be fairly uneventful. Attention to detail is paramount to ensure that the lateral release procedure is managed well postoperatively.

Many different, and sometimes contradictory, suggestions have been given regarding the postoperative management of the patient following lateral release. Some authors advocate immediate immobilization with a knee immobilizer, whereas others advocate immediate movement and no use of a knee immobilizer.[12,44,121,139,140] Weight-bearing progression after a lateral release is also controversial in the literature. Some surgeons advocate immediate weight bearing as tolerated (WBAT), using a ROM-limiting brace. Others recommend crutches with partial weight bearing for 1 to 2 weeks postoperatively, until the immobilizer is discontinued.[12,44,121,139,140] Physical therapy is suggested to be initiated anywhere from 1 day to 2 weeks postoperatively, depending on the hemarthrosis and the particular surgeon's perspective.[12,44,121,139,140]

Mangine and others[44] described clinical pathways following lateral release (Box 24-1). The concept of using clinical pathways rather than a time-based protocol has many advantages in the rehabilitation setting. The primary benefit is that the patient's particular problem and changing needs can be the focus of treatment, rather than the limitation of a time-based protocol. Certainly, there are trends that commonly occur during the rehabilitation process, but specific intervention for a specific problem is more beneficial to facilitate the appropriate outcome. The terminology and conceptual design of this clinical pathway were derived from Mangine and colleagues[44] and the *Guide to Physical Therapist Practice*, second edition.[141]

Most orthopedists recommend that physical therapy/ rehabilitation begin 1 to 2 days postoperatively for assistance with reduction and control of the postoperative hemarthrosis and pain. Mangine and colleagues[44] suggest initiating physical therapy no later than 2 days postoperatively. Rehabilitation postoperatively may include many of the techniques and approaches used preoperatively. Frequently, PF bracing, taping, or even orthotics may be used to assist in a successful recovery process postoperatively. Rehabilitation guidelines and protocols are developed to reestablish function by restoring ROM, muscle strength, coordination, and dynamic function of the involved joint or joints.

BOX 24-1

Lateral Release Clinical Pathway

Phase I (Immediate Postoperative Phase)

Time Frame

1 day to 2 weeks postoperatively

Criteria to Enter Phase I

Successful lateral release surgery

Evaluation and Assessment for Phase I

Range-of-motion (ROM) assessment

Joint mobility assessment

Strength and muscle performance assessment

Pain assessment

Swelling and hemarthrosis assessment

Activities of daily living (ADLs) (gait assessment)

Interventions for Phase I

Therapeutic exercise

    Gentle ROM exercises (extension/flexion)

    Stretching of hamstrings, gastrocnemius/soleus in non–weight bearing

    Muscle reeducation—quadriceps set, straight leg raise (SLR), hip adduction, multiangle isometrics, ankle pumps, heel slides

Joint mobilization

    Patellar mobilization

Electrical stimulation

    Muscle reeducation setting (Russian, functional)

    Pain management (interferential/premodulated)

    Edema control (high volt)

Cryotherapy/compression

    Swelling/hemarthrosis control

Gait training—performance of ADLs

    Partial weight bearing; weight bearing as tolerated using crutches; normalization of gait pattern, full weight bearing

    Educate on heel strike and full knee extension just before heel strike

Goals for Phase I

1. Protect healing structures
2. Decrease hemarthrosis or postoperative swelling
3. Control pain and prevent exercise-induced inflammation

4. Restore PROM (0 to 90 degrees)
5. Obtain good quadriceps contraction (10 mm of superior patellar migration)
6. Ensure consistent home program performance
7. Increase weight-bearing status as appropriate, from partial weight bearing to weight bearing as tolerated to full weight bearing

Phase II (Intermediate Postoperative Phase)

Time Frame

Weeks 2 to 4

Criteria to Advance to Phase II

No signs of active inflammation, unusual redness, or pallor

Minimal pain with ADLs and rehabilitation

Full active/passive knee extension (at least 0 degrees)

Greater than 90 degrees of active knee flexion

Good active quadriceps set (with superior patellar migration)

Ambulation with full weight bearing

Evaluation and Assessment for Phase II

ROM assessment (0 to 90 degrees minimum—0 to 115 degrees by end of week 2)

Strength and muscle performance assessment (SLR with less than 5 degrees of quadriceps lag)

Pain assessment (minimal pain)

Swelling and hemarthrosis (joint and soft tissue)

Activities of daily living (gait assessment)

Interventions for Phase II

Therapeutic exercise

    Progressive knee flexion ROM exercises (if needed)

    Stretching of gastrocnemius-soleus/iliotibial band in weight bearing

    Stretching of hip flexors

    Strengthening—initiate more progressive closed chain exercises (wall slides, leg press, lateral step-ups, heel raises)

    Balance activities (weight shifts, tandem walking, braiding, etc.)

(continued)

BOX 24-1

Lateral Release Clinical Pathway—cont'd

Electrical stimulation

Pain management (interferential/premodulated)

Edema control (high volt)

Cryotherapy/compression

Postexercise only

Gait training—performance of ADLs; full weight bearing

Goals for Phase II

1. Progress flexion ROM to greater than 120 degrees[44]
2. Gain lower extremity strength and flexibility; normal SLR without a quadriceps lag
3. Normalize ADLs
4. Restore full weight bearing with normal gait pattern
5. Improve balance
6. Enhance proprioception

Phase III (Advanced Strengthening Phase)

Time Frame

Weeks 4 to 6

Criteria to Advance to Phase III

Normal active TKE (0 to 10 degrees or greater)

Greater than 120 degrees of knee flexion AROM/PROM

Pain produced only with specific activities

Complete basic balance and agility exercises

Normalized gait

Evaluation and Assessment for Phase III

Strength and muscle performance assessment (SLR with no quadriceps lag)

Balance and proprioception assessment

ADLs (gait assessment)

Aerobic endurance assessment

Interventions for Phase III

Therapeutic exercise

Advanced closed chain/weight-bearing exercises

Full body strengthening/conditioning (nontraditional hip/pelvic/trunk strengthening)

Comprehensive lower extremity flexibility program

Agility exercises—proprioception exercises (stationary hopping, single-leg stance exercises)

Aerobic exercises—StairMaster™, stationary bike, treadmill; jogging, with progression to running

Goals for Phase III

1. Restore normal bilateral knee ROM
2. Acquire 70% muscle strength
3. Prevent exercise-induced swelling
4. Obtain normal/full performance of ADLs (including steps, etc.)
5. Regain normal single-leg stance balance/proprioception

Phase IV (Return to Activity Phase)

Time Frame

Week 6 and beyond

Criteria to Advance to Phase IV

Equal/normal ROM bilaterally

70% quadriceps strength (isokinetic test)

85% performance with functional testing

Complete advanced balance and agility exercises

Total pain resolution

Evaluation and Assessment for Phase IV

Functional testing assessment (one-leg hop sequence)

Isokinetic test assessment (greater than 120 degrees per second)

Aerobic endurance assessment

Interventions for Phase IV

Therapeutic exercise

Functional testing activities

Sport-specific activities (cutting, running, light plyometrics) to meet sport demands

Clear home program for remaining deficit areas

Continue aerobic exercises, progressing toward more sport-specific activities; running restoration

Comprehensive training program

Goals for Phase IV

1. Achieve full resumption of sport-specific activity
2. Promote independence with final long-term maintenance program

The initial physical therapy examination includes safe passive range of motion (PROM) measurements of the knee (flexion and extension), assessment of accessory patellar mobility, assessment of fibular mobility, assessment of strength using a quad set and straight leg raise (SLR), assessment of pain, assessment of joint hemarthrosis/swelling, and gait assessment for both the involved and uninvolved knees.

EXAMINATION

Range of Motion

Knee extension PROM is taken using a standard large goniometer, preferably in the supine position with a towel or roll under the ankle to allow for full knee extension during examination. Most published resources suggest that 0 degrees is normal for knee extension,[73,142,143] but clinically, in an athletic population, 5 to 10 degrees of knee extension is commonly found.[144] It is imperative to assess the uninvolved knee's extension to establish a normal baseline and goal for the rehabilitation process. Knee extension restoration is the first ROM goal postoperatively. Periarticular tissue changes can occur rapidly after a surgical intervention, causing irreversible loss of joint motion. During postoperative immobilization, a decrease in collagen's water content and an increase in collagen cross-linkage can occur, causing abnormal scar tissue formation and loss of ROM.[145] Knee extension loss of motion usually occurs due to muscular tightness, capsular restrictions, or muscular guarding caused by pain. Muscular and capsular tightness both cause an abnormal firm end feel, whereas muscular guarding causes an empty end feel (Table 24-1).[146-148] The capsular and ligamentous restrictions may not respond to typical ROM exercises. Accessory joint mobilizations may be required to regain and restore full arthrokinematic motion and full functional ROM in the knee joint. Accessory joint motion is found between the patella and femur, tibia and femur, and tibia and fibula. Lack of accessory joint motion will impede the overall joint function and restrict appropriate progression during the rehabilitation process. Knee extension must be normalized rapidly, but knee flexion can be gained more slowly to allow for healing of anterior knee structures. Hamstring flexibility is also assessed in the supine position, with the hip in 90 degrees of flexion and the knee directed toward extension.

TABLE 24-1

End Feels of the Tibiofemoral Joint

DIRECTION	END FEEL	DESCRIPTION
Normal End Feels (Knee)		
Flexion	Soft	Normal soft tissue approximation; compression of posterior calf and thigh
Extension	Firm	Normal end-range of hamstrings and gastrocnemius muscles; usually found with limited amounts of hamstring tightness
	Firm	Normal end-range of posterior capsular structures; usually found with full 5-10 degrees extension PROM
Abnormal End Feels (Knee)		
Flexion	Soft	"Spongy," soft tissue edema, soft tissue adhesions
	Firm	Abnormal quadriceps tightness
		Abnormal ligamentous shortening
	Hard	"Bony block," internal derangement, osteoarthritis
	Empty	"Pain/guarding," no specific structural resistance
		Protective muscle guarding, acute inflammation, fracture, psychogenic
Extension	Firm	Abnormal hamstring/gastrocnemius tightness limiting normal physiologic ROM
	Firm	Abnormal posterior capsule tightness limiting normal physiologic ROM
	Hard	"Bony block, " internal derangement, osteoarthritis
	Empty	"Pain/guarding," no specific structural resistance
		Protective muscle guarding, acute inflammation, fracture, psychogenic

Knee flexion active range of motion (AROM)/PROM may be gently and slowly progressed in the early postoperative period.[139] Normal knee flexion is cited in literature as 130 degrees, but commonly in the athletic population, knee flexion can exceed 150 degrees.[142,143] Knee flexion PROM will likely progress without complication, but initial swelling and hemarthrosis may limit early advancement. Initially, it is suggested to measure knee ROM in a sitting position to allow the two-joint muscles of the hip and knee to remain in a relaxed state. This position also gives the patient full control of usually uncomfortable knee flexion. Flexion is progressed as tolerated, while obtaining 90 degrees within the first 5 to 7 days postoperatively.[149]

Other concurrent surgical procedures need to be considered when progressing knee flexion postoperatively, and clear communication with the surgeon is imperative for safe progression. Once knee flexion PROM is beyond 90 degrees, the measurement position should be changed to supine, allowing for increased flexion while maintaining shortened two-joint hip and knee musculature.

Joint Mobility Assessment

Most important after a lateral release, the patellar accessory motion must be considered. The patella must glide superiorly, inferiorly, medially, and laterally to facilitate normal knee function. Maintaining patellar mobility postoperatively is necessary to prevent scarring and tightness of released structures. Superior patellar glide is necessary for proper functioning of the knee extension mechanism.[150,151] Inferior patellar glide is needed during knee flexion. Medial glides and medial tilts are performed to restore appropriate length of lateral retinacular structures postoperatively. Overly aggressive patella mobilization may increase pain, inflammation, or joint swelling, which will slow the rehabilitation process or even contribute to the development of CRPS.[44,152] Most patellar motion problems occur after distal or proximal realignments, but they can develop after a lateral release. Patella infra or baja can develop and cause serious complications to appropriate progression postoperatively. The infrapatellar fat pad may contribute to inferior positional scarring, causing a decreased motion potential of the patellar tendon during knee extension.[150,151,153] The superior patellar glide is required for normalization of active terminal knee extension. Extensor lag may be caused by limited superior patellar mobility. This condition is demonstrated by full knee extension passively, with a 5- to 10-degree lack of active extension. Long-term patella infra may cause increased stress to the PF articular surface by facilitating shortening of the patellar tendon over time.[44,154] The tibiofemoral joint may be assessed for anterior and posterior glide if overall physiologic motion is limited. Proximal tibiofibular articulation may also be assessed for normal anterior glide of the fibula on the tibia.[147]

Strength and Muscle Performance

Muscle strengthening after a lateral release should be focused on reestablishing quadriceps strength during terminal knee extension. The hemarthrosis and pain often lead to quadriceps inhibition postoperatively.[44,152]

Spencer and colleagues[155] have demonstrated that joint effusion can cause quadriceps muscle shutdown. The decline in quadriceps performance was generally statistically equal across all quadriceps muscles. Merchant and Mercer[103] reported poor results in patients who could not maintain quadriceps strength after a lateral release. During a quadriceps set, the patella should migrate 10 mm superiorly. If accomplished, the extensor mechanism is functioning properly, and superior patellar mobility is adequate.[44,151,156] Isometric quadriceps sets and SLR have been advocated early in the rehabilitation phase but are discussed later in the intervention phase.[44,139]

Pain

Pain control is crucial after a lateral release and is an essential part of the rehabilitation process. Pain is described by the International Association for the Study of Pain as "an unpleasant sensory and emotional experience associated with actual or potential tissue damage, or described in terms of such damage."[157] Pain can be defined by the patient subjectively on a scale of 0 to 10, where 0 is no pain and 10 is the highest pain possible. Postoperative pain is usually controlled by oral analgesics, cryotherapy, and nonsteroidal antiinflammatories.[44] The rehabilitation specialist can assist with pain management by identifying the pain source and subsequently providing relief using appropriate physical agents and modalities. Although long-term outcomes for use of modalities in pain management have been questioned, it is important to note that a reduction in the athlete's perception of pain is as valuable as actually reducing the pain. Even temporary pain relief can be effective to assist in breaking the pain cycle. Pain perception may be influenced by anxiety, attention, depression, past pain experiences, and cultural influences.[158] Over-aggressive application of therapeutic exercise in the lateral release patient can increase pain and soreness and possibly contribute to development of CRPS. If undiagnosed pain persists, early recognition of CRPS is paramount for successful management. Noyes and colleagues[150,151] and Oglivie-Harris and Roscoe[154] reported that treatment of CRPS is most successful when treated within the first 2 to 3 weeks of onset. They recommended initially using oral steroids and progressing to a sympathetic neurologic blockade if symptoms do not improve. Pain can influence muscle function and impede postoperative progression, resulting in muscular weakness and shutdown through type IV pain receptors or mechanoreceptors with concurrent antagonistic muscle spasm. If the hamstrings spasm as a result of increased pain in the quadriceps muscle, the patient could begin to lose crucial knee extension PROM postoperatively.[44,158,159] Pain usually can be managed clinically with cryotherapy, compression, and electrical stimulation, even if it is only the patient's perception of pain that improves.

Swelling/Hemarthrosis

The most common postoperative complication following a lateral release is hemarthrosis.[130,131,160] The initial physical therapy examination must include girth measurements at reproducible anatomic sites around the knee. Having initial girth measurements allows the rehabilitation specialist to monitor and track the postoperative swelling and edema around the knee. This data will assist in directing treatment intervention and monitoring for signs of postoperative complications, such as an infection. Compression and cryotherapy usually are initiated postoperatively in the recovery room and continued until swelling has subsided. Some surgeons advocate the use of a cold therapy compression cuff device continuously for 48 hours postoperatively.[161] Irrgang[152] advocates using compression continuously until bleeding stops and using cryotherapy continuously until pain and inflammation subside. Appropriate exercise implementation is crucial to prevent increased hemarthrosis and swelling in the immediate postoperative phase. Overly aggressive patellar mobilization and ROM exercises can increase pain and swelling, thus impeding the appropriate postoperative progression.[152] Premature progression of weight bearing can be detrimental in the early phases of rehabilitation by increasing swelling, hemarthrosis, and hamstring muscle firing, leading to decreased knee extension ROM.

Activities of Daily Living—Gait Assessment

Weight-bearing status after lateral release is controversial, with no clear consensus on application and approach. Recommended weight-bearing status after lateral release varies from full weight bearing, to weight bearing as tolerated, to partial weight bearing. Various time frames are suggested for progression through the weight-bearing stages.[12,44,121,139,140]

Currently, many believe a criterion-based approach to progression with weight bearing and immobilization is clinically beneficial. Keeping the knee in extension during weight-bearing activities prevents abnormal hamstring firing and subsequent loss of knee extension. Partial weight bearing facilitates prevention of avoidable hemarthrosis postoperatively. It is suggested that patients ambulate with partial weight bearing or weight bearing as tolerated using crutches until they can perform a straight leg raise in supine without a quadriceps lag or until they can perform ambulation with a correct heel strike on initial contact.[161]

PHASE I (IMMEDIATE POSTOPERATIVE PHASE)—DAY 1 TO WEEK 2

Decreased Range of Motion—Phase I

Normalization of knee extension PROM and AROM is crucial after most knee surgical interventions. Without normal knee extension, functional ambulation is severely impaired and the ability to participate competitively in sports or similar activities is compromised. Restoration of knee extension is facilitated by passive stretching and active initiation of the quadriceps musculature. Passive stretching of the hamstrings and gastrocnemius muscles can be achieved through various means in a non–weight-bearing position during this phase. In the immediate postoperative phase, supine knee extension PROM is accomplished by placing a towel roll or small bolster under the ankle, allowing a low-load, long-duration stretch to be placed on the hamstrings (Figure 24-12, *A*). It may also be necessary to allow a small towel roll to be placed under the knee to facilitate a stretch without pain production. As the hamstrings and posterior capsular structures lengthen, the size of the folded towel is slowly reduced under the knee, allowing for a controlled low-load, long-duration stretch toward extension. Reasonable relaxation needs to be achieved during this position to allow for hamstring lengthening without producing a hamstring contraction that would inhibit passive extension ROM of the knee. Knee extension can also be achieved through the prone hang position (Figure 24-12, *B*). The prone hang can be very effective in achieving functional knee extension ROM, but two adaptations to the commonly practiced prone hang are suggested: (1) Place a towel roll superior to the patella to allow for decreased compressive forces on the patella and anterior knee structures. (2) Place a roll under the distal tibia that will allow for hamstring relaxation and subsequent hamstring stretching via a low-load, long-duration stretch. The towel roll under the tibia will be slowly reduced in size as more pain-free extension is gained. Hamstring stretching through other means is also recommended. The stretches are held for approximately 30 seconds each for 3 to 5 repetitions three times per day.[162] The gastrocnemius muscle is a two-joint muscle that can contribute to knee extension loss of motion. This muscle can initially be stretched using a towel to pull the ankle toward dorsiflexion while in full knee extension.

If complications develop in regaining knee extension ROM, an ERMI Knee Extensionator (ERMI, Inc., Decatur, GA) can be used clinically and in the home by the patient for more aggressive attempts at knee extension restoration (Figure 24-12, *C*).[163] This device allows for a slow, progressive stretch in a controlled setting that is safe and effective. Another commonly used device when knee extension is not progressing as expected is the Joint Active Systems (JAS) Knee (Joint Active Systems (JAS) Theratech Equipment, Inc., Effingham, IL) static stretch device. It also allows for a static stretch to be held in a comfortable position for an

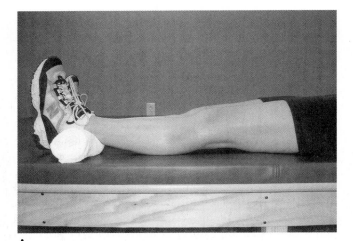

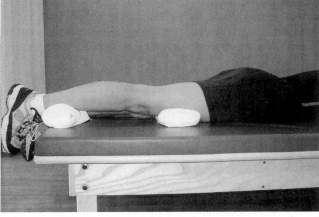

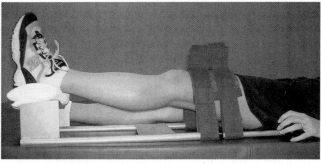

Figure 24-12: **A,** Supine knee extension stretch. Passive knee extension stretching in supine should be initiated at the first postoperative physical therapy visit. A towel can be placed under the knee (while maintaining a sufficient stretch), if needed, to allow for full relaxation. This position will facilitate the low-load, long-duration stretch principle that will be used throughout postoperative rehabilitation. **B,** Prone hang. The popular prone hang can be used to facilitate more force toward knee extension. A folded towel can be placed superior to the patella to decrease patellar compression during this stretch. Also, placing folded towels under the ankle to allow for full relaxation is paramount. The towel height can slowly be decreased, as needed, while maintaining a comfortable stretch. Increased force can be applied by placing a light weight on the ankle, if needed. **C,** The ERMI Knee Extensionator. This device can be used during phase II or III to assist with passive progressive knee extension. As the pressure cuff is inflated, the extension force is increased. NOTE: A patient after lateral release will rarely need to use the ERMI Knee Extensionator to assist with restoration of knee extension, but it can be an effective tool when indicated.

for restoration of knee flexion to 115 degrees at 1 to 2 weeks postoperatively for the lateral release patient. Phillips[139] reports that early knee flexion ROM tends to "spread the release," but does not clearly define appropriate flexion progression after surgery or give evidence of "spreading the release." He also reports that immobilization in extension for longer than 72 hours may allow the lateral release to adhere postsurgically.[139] Nevertheless, regaining functional knee flexion ROM after the lateral release is crucial. If flexion is not attained or progressively attempted, the lateral release and structures around the surgical site could build damaging lateral scar tissue, hindering a successful rehabilitation process.

Knee flexion in the immediate postoperative phase can be gained in the sitting position (Figure 24-13, *A*) to allow shortening of the rectus femoris and subsequent force transfer to the joint capsule and surrounding knee structures, which may develop adhesions. This position allows the patient to easily control active/passive stretching progression. It also allows for a low-load, long-duration stretch to be achieved and repeated by the patient in the home setting. This position is used until the patient reaches greater than 95 to 100 degrees of knee flexion, usually around 5 to 7 days postoperatively.

Once the knee can reach approximately 100 degrees, the position for stretching and ROM changes to the supine position. The patient can actively perform a heel slide or use a sheet passively to assist with progressive stretching (Figure 24-13, *B*). The stretches are held for 30 seconds to 2 minutes in a "stretching" but comfortable position.

Impaired Joint Mobility: Patellar Mobilization—Phase I

Patellar mobilization techniques are crucial to reestablishing normalized patellar mobility and preventing detrimental scar

extended period of time. These devices are only used in extreme cases where knee extension is not progressing as anticipated.

The secondary ROM goal is to slowly restore knee flexion without damaging released structures. The rate of knee flexion progression after a lateral release is controversial in the literature. Some surgeons and rehabilitation experts advocate for restoration of knee flexion to 90 degrees within 5 to 7 days.[149] Ford and Post[161] recommend early knee flexion emphasis to prevent scarring in the lateral release site. The protocol published by Mangine and colleagues[44] advocates

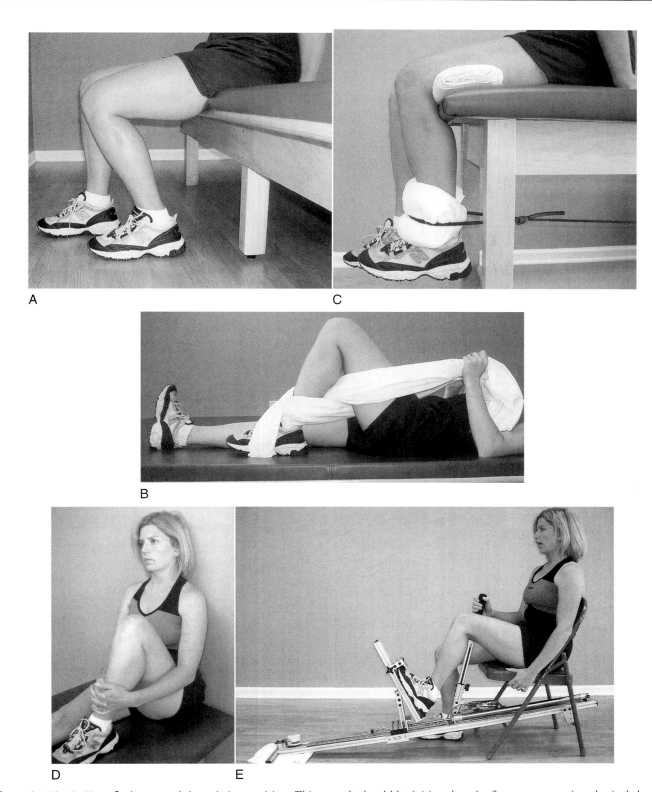

Figure 24-13: A, Knee flexion stretch in a sitting position. This stretch should be initiated at the first postoperative physical therapy visit and included in the home exercise program. This stretch position can be used until the patient achieves greater than 100 degrees of knee flexion. **B,** Supine heel slide with assistance. As knee flexion increases, the patient can perform self-PROM exercises using a sheet for assistance in the supine position. **C,** Knee flexion with resistive tubing. If passive knee flexion does not reach 115 degrees by postoperative week 3, resistive tubing can provide a progressive stretch over a longer period of time. **D,** Self-directed knee flexion stretch. This stretch can be used during late phase II and III if needed to regain terminal knee flexion. **E,** ERMI Knee Flexionator. This device can provide an avenue for slow progressive knee flexion, in a controlled fashion, where the patient increases the amount of force/ROM over time. The ERMI Knee Flexionator should only be used during phase II or III, when knee flexion remains limited and difficult to achieve.

tissue formation. Medial glides, superior glides, and medial tilts are performed clinically and are taught to the patient for immediate home program incorporation. The amount and intensity of patellar mobilization are graded according to the degree of pain and inflammation present.[152] Mangine and colleagues[44] recommend performing patellar mobilizations frequently each day for 5 to 10 minutes. They report that the mobilization techniques are frequently painful secondary to the retinacular incision, but patients need to have clear pain parameters established by the rehabilitation specialist to reduce tissue irritation with mobilization.[44]

Decreased Strength and Endurance—Phase I

Early strengthening after lateral release has been supported in the literature. Quadriceps strength restoration has been linked to a positive outcome after a lateral release. In fact, Merchant and Mercer[103] reported that patients who did not restore good quadriceps strength after a lateral release had a poor outcome. Micheli and Stanitski[114] report that the final result obtained after a lateral release is directly proportional to the time needed for quadriceps and hamstring strength restoration postoperatively.

Some authors advocate for quadriceps sets, SLRs, and co-contraction of quadriceps/hamstrings to be initiated in the recovery room as soon as the patient is conscious.[140,161]

The postoperative strengthening program is similar to the preoperative conservative program, with consideration given for soft tissue healing time frames, inflammation, and postoperative pain. Isometric quadriceps sets and SLRs toward flexion, adduction, and extension should begin as soon as possible postoperatively. Frequently, quadriceps muscle inhibition develops after the lateral release because of hemarthrosis, swelling, and pain. The patella should move superiorly during a quadriceps set (Figure 24-14, *A(1-2)*). If this cannot be accomplished early in the postoperative phase, the knee can be moved into approximately 5 to 10 degrees of flexion to assist with facilitation of a quadriceps set and initial "quad set" firing. Multiangle isometrics can be initiated soon postoperatively to assist with quadriceps strength restoration in conjunction with electrical stimulation for muscle reeducation. Various degrees are chosen based on the least amount of pain production with a quadriceps contraction between 90 and 0 degrees.[44] The SLR should be performed without a quadriceps lag (see Figure 24-14, *C*). If a quadriceps lag is present during an attempted SLR, the patient should be positioned with the heel on the wall and the hip at a 45- to 60-degree angle to decrease the difficulty level of performance (see Figure 24-14, *B(1-2)*). The patient will build strength and neuromuscular control to perform a standard SLR against full gravity. Ankle pumps (dorsiflexion/plantar flexion) are used in the immediate postoperative phase to assist with appropriate fluid movement toward the heart and prevention of a postsurgical deep vein thrombosis.

Closed chained exercises or weight-bearing exercises are initiated as soon as pain allows postoperatively. Resistance-free terminal knee extension (TKE), in standing, can be initiated soon after surgery as a preparatory exercise for normalizing gait and stimulating quadriceps strength recovery (see Figure 24-14, *D(1-2)*). Resistance can be added as pain allows with resistive tubing, a band, or a weight pulley system. Other CKC or weight-bearing exercises could include a mini-squat from 0 to 20 degrees performed without resistance in standing or using the wall slide at 0 to 20 degrees, if pain free. The Total Gym (EFI Sports Medicine, Inc., San Diego, CA) can also be used for a partial/controlled weight-bearing setting to perform a CKC mini-squat from 0 to 30 degrees.

Electrical stimulation for muscle reeducation may be selected to assist with recovery and retraining of quadriceps strength postoperatively. The quadriceps muscle group frequently "shuts down" postoperatively, as demonstrated by Spencer and colleagues,[155] and may require use of electrical stimulation to elicit a muscular response. The patient is given feedback by seeing and feeling the muscle contract, and then attempting to reproduce this action.[164] The criteria listed by Hooker[165] to accomplish muscle reeducation are important to acknowledge here:

1. Current intensity must be adequate for muscle contraction, but comfortable for the athlete.

2. Pulse duration must be set as close as possible to the duration needed for chronaxie of tissue to be stimulated. This setting is preset on most therapeutic devices.

3. Pulses per second should be high enough to give a tetanic contraction (20 to 40 pulses per second).

4. Interrupted or surged current must be used.

5. "On" time should be 1 to 2 seconds.

6. "Off" time should be 4 to 10 seconds.

7. The patient should be instructed to allow only the electricity to make the muscle contract, letting the patient feel and see the response desired. Next, the patient should alternate voluntary muscle contractions with current-induced contractions.

Figure 24-14: A (1-2), Quad set with superior patellar migration. The patella will migrate superiorly when the quadriceps are contracted. The superior migration of the patella can be palpated. **B (1-2),** Modified straight leg raise (mSLR). If a quadriceps lag is present during an attempted SLR, decrease the gravitational force by starting the exercise at approximately 45 to 60 degrees of hip flexion, while maintaining an extended knee. The patient will soon build enough neuromuscular control to perform a standard SLR without quadriceps lag. **C,** Straight leg raise: (1) SLR with an evident quadriceps lag and (2) SLR without a quadriceps lag.

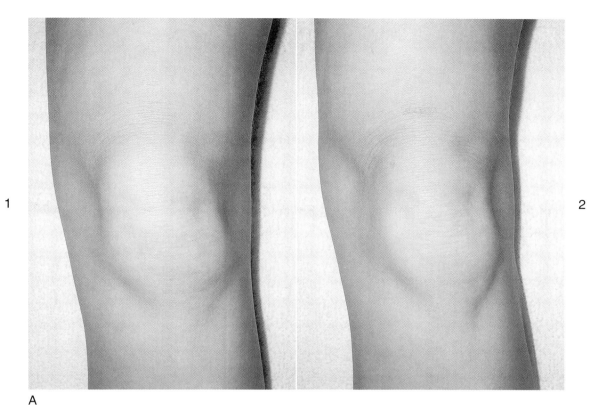

A

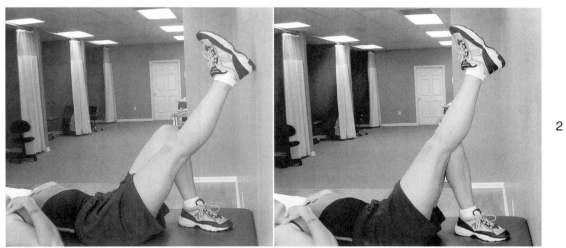

B

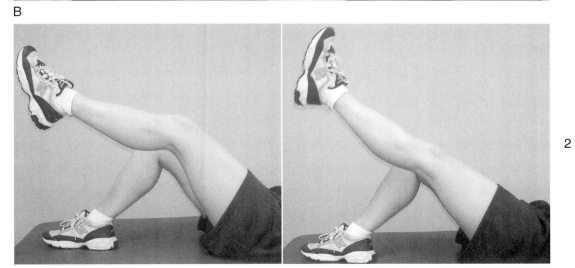

C

(continued)

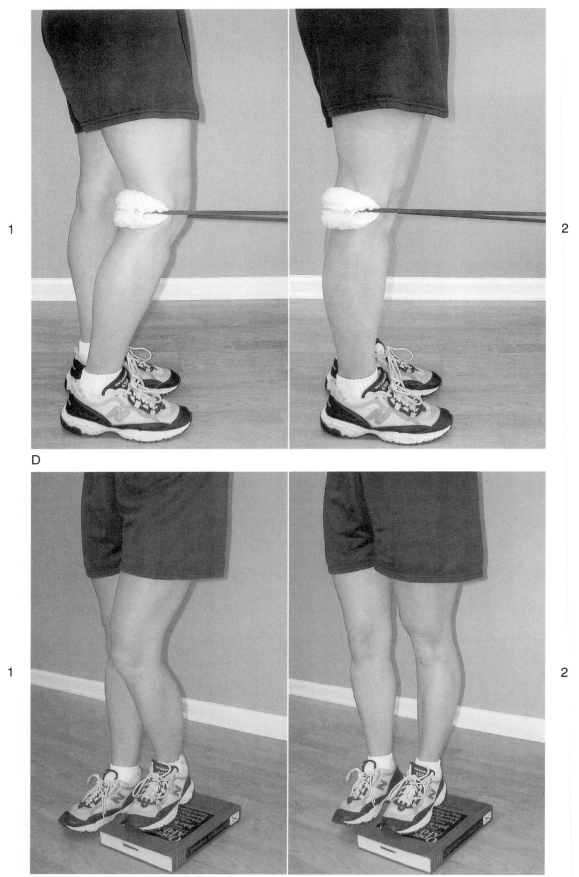

D

E

8. Total treatment time should be around 15 minutes, but this can be repeated several times daily.

9. High-voltage pulsed or medium-frequency alternating current may be most effective.

Robertson and Ward[166] recently published a case study supporting the use of aggressive electrical stimulation for muscle reeducation in a patient with poor progression 5 months after a lateral release. They reported that after only 8 days of electrical stimulation, the patient was able to ascend stairs unassisted and, after another 21 days, to hop unsupported. The functional recovery and pain reduction made during the 36 days exceeded all progression made during the previous 5-month period.[167]

Pain Control—Phase I

Mangine and colleagues[44] suggest that the management of postoperative pain is usually accomplished through oral analgesics, cryotherapy, and nonsteroidal antiinflammatories. These management strategies, as well as others, are addressed during the postoperative rehabilitation process. The surgeon often prescribes oral analgesics postoperatively to limit pain during the recovery process and may prescribe a nonsteroidal antiinflammatory. The pain can also be controlled with application of cryotherapy using one of many devices in which compression and cold are simultaneously placed on the knee and surrounding structures. These devices are usually used clinically, as well as in the home setting, during the immediate postoperative period. Clinically, cryotherapy, combined with elevation after each treatment session, has shown good results. The patient should be advised to use the device three to five times per day and as needed for pain control during the immediate postoperative period. If pain becomes a detriment to appropriate progression clinically, rehabilitation professionals can use electrical stimulation in many forms to attempt to control pain at the time of the clinical visit. Various electrical current modalities, including interferential, high-voltage, and premodulated current, may be useful to decrease pain clinically. Even though long-term outcomes regarding the use of electrical stimulation may be questionable, immediate reduction of pain can aid in the athlete's perception of pain and subsequent compliance with and participation in the rehabilitation process.

Figure 24-14, continued: D (1-2), Terminal knee extension (TKE) with resistance. Resistive tubing or band can be used to increase resistance during the TKE in standing. The TKE can also be performed early postoperatively, without resistance, to facilitate improved proprioception and quadriceps strengthening in weight bearing. **E (1-2),** Lateral step-up. This exercise is usually added during phase II and initiated with a 1- to 2-inch step or hardbound book, while in full weight bearing, maintaining balance on the involved extremity.

Prevention of pain can be assisted by appropriate progression of the exercise program during the rehabilitation process. Allowing proper healing of surrounding tissues during the postoperative phase is critical in preventing unusual swelling, hemarthrosis, and subsequent pain. Pain can be a useful guide during the progression in the postoperative period. Each individual has a unique physiologic response to surgical intervention and needs specific and appropriate progression according to the particular state of tissue postoperatively.

Swelling/Hemarthrosis—Phase I

Compression and cryotherapy are usually initiated in the postoperative recovery room. This technique can be administered with a cold compression. When the cold compression cuff is not donned, a device such as a compression bandage can be used to prevent unwarranted swelling and hemarthrosis from delaying usual progression. Mangine and colleagues[44] recommend using a horseshoe-shaped felt pad (one-half inch) under the compression wrap to assist with medialization of the patella and prevention of unwanted swelling. Electrical stimulation can also be used to assist with edema control postoperatively and minimize quadriceps shutdown.

Mangine and colleagues[44] further describe possible aspiration of joint effusion when loss of volitional muscle contraction remains after the first 2 weeks. Most patients return to functional activities within 2 weeks postoperatively whether hemarthrosis is present or not.[167]

Decreased Activities of Daily Living—Phase I

As mentioned during the examination portion of this chapter, a criterion-based approach to progression with weight bearing and immobilization can be beneficial. Keeping the knee in extension during early weight-bearing activities, with a correct heel strike on initial contact, is crucial to prevent abnormal loss of knee extension ROM. The simple criterion to ambulate with full weight bearing is the ability to perform a straight leg raise without a measurable quadriceps lag or full active knee extension with heel strike during gait.[161]

PHASE II (INTERMEDIATE POSTOPERATIVE PHASE)— WEEKS 2 TO 4

Rehabilitation during this phase should continue to address pain and inflammation/hemarthrosis if needed by appropriate means as addressed earlier during phase I.

Range of Motion—Phase II

Knee AROM should progress to greater than 0 to 115 degrees by the end of week 2. The therapeutic intervention may include activities and exercises that facilitate knee flexion. Examples of these have been mentioned earlier and could include heel slides with a sheet or self-directed manual knee flexion with back stabilized against a wall. In each of these examples, the stretch should be held for at least 30 seconds during each episode in a semicomfortable position to allow for slow progressive stretching and increased flexion ROM.

If complications develop during knee flexion progression, clinically, a low-load progressive stretch with tubing is used to assist with regaining knee flexion mobility. The patient sits at the end of a high plinth-style table, and tubing is placed on the ankle to facilitate a light progressive pull toward knee flexion (see Figure 24-13, *C*). The patient stays in this position for approximately 10 minutes. If 10 minutes cannot be achieved, the amount of tension may need to be adjusted to allow for appropriate relaxation during stretching. Knee flexion during this phase can also be progressed independently by the patient with the spine stabilized against the wall while sitting (see Figure 24-13, *D*). Another device produced by ERMI, Inc., can be of assistance clinically and in the home to restore appropriate knee flexion.[163] The Knee Flexionator (ERMI, Inc., Decatur, GA) allows for independent, controlled progression of knee flexion with static progressive holds for a low-load, long-duration stretch to be achieved (see Figure 24-13, *E*).[163] The JAS Knee brace (Theratech Equipment, Inc., Effingham, IL) can also be used if necessary to achieve a similar result. Restoration of flexion ROM is typically not a problem, but as in all rehabilitation programs, patients may have limitations and joint motion restrictions postsurgically. The skill, science, and art of therapeutic rehabilitation lie in achieving the desired outcome and goal despite being presented with a challenging and abnormal situation.

Restoration of ankle dorsiflexion by stretching the gastrocnemius-soleus complex can be initiated in a weight-bearing fashion using an angle board or a similar device. Patients are commonly taught to use a 2-inch hardbound book at home to facilitate this stretch. Iliotibial band and hip flexor stretching are also initiated during this phase to prevent further tightening of these structures during the period of decreased overall mobility in the recovery process.

Impaired Joint Mobility—Phase II

Patellar mobility should be normalized by the second phase of rehabilitation. If limited patellar mobility occurs, the home program for patellar mobilization needs to be re-addressed, and consistent clinical patellar mobilizations are indicated. No pain should be produced during patellar mobilizations. The surgeon needs to be aware of any problem that develops regarding patellar mobility. If PF motion is not established by 3 weeks, three options are available, according to Noyes and colleagues,[150] to regain functional patellar mobility:

1. Lateral and medial capsular releases
2. Continuous epidurals for 3 to 4 days
3. Gentle manipulation under anesthesia

Mangine and colleagues[44] emphasize that the ultimate effectiveness in management of patellar mobility problems depends on clear communication between the clinician and the surgeon to accurately determine the cause of the motion restriction and mechanism for loss of motion.

Decreased Strength and Endurance—Phase II

Strengthening during phase II of the rehabilitation program appropriately advances the CKC exercise program according to the functional strength restored at approximately 1 to 2 weeks postoperatively. All previously established exercises are continued during this phase. Wall slides may be initiated and performed from 0 to 45 degrees of knee flexion, with progression to standing mini-squats over time. If wall slides are not appropriate, continued progression on the Total Gym (EFI Sports Medicine, Inc., San Diego, CA) with increased weight bearing over time is indicated. The leg press (single and bilateral) can be initiated during this phase as a progressive CKC exercise. Resistance can be initiated using resistive tubing or a pulley-style resistive device during the standing terminal knee extension exercise. Active calf raises/heel raises can be initiated in full weight bearing. If greater than 110 degrees of knee flexion is present, the stationary bike could be a useful tool; however, progression to this activity is cautioned because of the repetitiveness of knee flexion/extension during the normal cycle motion. Use of the stationary bike needs to be judiciously applied based on the patient's ROM, pain, presurgical history, and effusion present.

Exercises to restore balance and proprioception become more important during this phase of rehabilitation. Examples of commonly used exercises include weight shifting, wall slides (0 to 20 degrees), lateral step-ups (see Figure 24-14, *E*), heel-to-toe ambulation, braiding, and bilateral balancing on a wobble board with assistance. Agility exercises are not usually initiated during this phase.

Swelling/Hemarthrosis—Phase II

Preventing postoperative swelling during phase II depends on appropriate exercise implementation through decreasing of the PF shear force during progressive strengthening activities. Closed chain or weight-bearing exercises decrease PF shear force and cause subsequent damage to articular cartilage. Open chain exercises from 20 to 0 degrees should be avoided in patients with known PF cartilage damage. The prevention of synovial joint effusion in patients with articular cartilage damage is crucial. Controlling edema therapeutically during this phase is similar to the previously discussed management options in phase I and phase II.

Decreased Activities of Daily Living—Phase II

Normal ambulation while fully bearing weight without crutches can begin if the following criteria are achieved: no extensor lag with SLR, full active knee extension, and knee flexion AROM of at least 90 to 100 degrees. If normal knee extension during heel strike or knee flexion during toe-off is absent, the use of a single crutch or cane may be indicated to allow for a smooth, nonantalgic gait pattern on all surfaces. The patient should achieve proper navigation of stairs during this phase. Treadmill ambulation may begin to fine-tune the gait pattern if all of the aforementioned criteria are met. Reverse treadmill ambulation can also be used as a progressive strengthening exercise in a weight-bearing position.

PHASE III (ADVANCED STRENGTHENING PHASE)—WEEKS 4 TO 6

Decreased Range of Motion—Phase III

Active and passive knee ROM should be accomplished by 4 weeks postoperatively. If full ROM is not attained, the rehabilitation specialist should immediately consult with the referring/surgical physician to develop an appropriate comprehensive plan for restoring ROM needed for an adequate and successful recovery. During this time frame, knee flexion is more frequently limited. Many options exist, ranging from more aggressive therapeutic interventions to surgical alternatives, depending on the cause, direction, and source of motion restriction. Therapeutic interventions can include use of a device that allows for a low-load, long-duration stretch, such as the ERMI Flexionator[163] (ERMI, Inc., Decatur, GA); the JAS Knee brace (Theratech Equipment, Inc., Effingham, IL); or a similar dynamic splint, as previously discussed. Manual joint mobilization (posterior tibial glides) can be included if a capsular restriction was implicated as the primary cause of limitation of knee flexion ROM.

More aggressive techniques have been recommended when postsurgical loss of ROM occurs at the knee, including medial or lateral capsular releases, continuous epidurals for 3 to 4 days, or manipulation under anesthesia.[150] It is highly rare and infrequent that these techniques need to be employed after a lateral release, but difficult and complicated cases do occur. In such events, an expedient implementation of proper treatment is paramount for a successful outcome.

Impaired Joint Mobility—Phase III

All accessory joint mobility should also be normalized during this time frame. Decreased patellar mobility can cause a loss of tibiofemoral joint motion toward flexion or extension.

Early, pain-free patellar mobilizations should be completed during the home exercise program in order to prevent prolonged patellar mobility restrictions. If patellar mobility is found to be restricted during this stage, clinical patellar mobilizations should immediately be initiated. Chronic synovial irritation can cause an abnormal pain production during attempted patellar mobilizations.[44] If significant pain is produced, use of grade I or II patellar joint mobilizations is indicated.

Decreased Strength and Endurance—Phase III

This phase of strength and endurance exercises typically includes appropriate OKC hip/pelvis/trunk strengthening exercises, advanced CKC strengthening exercises, proprioception exercises, a comprehensive lower extremity flexibility program, and initiation of endurance/aerobic conditioning exercises. All previous exercises for general strengthening and muscle recruitment are usually continued during phase III.

The OKC exercises or non–weight-bearing exercises initiated during this phase of rehabilitation are relatively new to the preferred approach to postoperative PF rehabilitation. Mascal and colleagues[69] recommended that comprehensive hip, pelvis, and trunk musculature be considered when treating PFP.

Hip and pelvic muscle weakness has been implicated in altering lower extremity kinematics enough to contribute to PFJ dysfunction.[46] The current theoretic perspective concludes that reduced strength of the hip abductors can allow for increased hip adduction/translation during weight-bearing activities.[46,69] Increased hip adduction may allow the femur to rotate under the patella, producing lateral patellar translation and subsequent PFP.[45,46,57] Because the postoperative strengthening program is similar in theory and practice to the conservative nonsurgical strengthening/rehabilitation program, it is warranted to add these recommended exercises. The marginal success rates of the lateral release procedure make it necessary to address biomechanical and strengthening concerns that may not have been covered preoperatively. These considerations are crucial during this phase, before returning to sport-specific activities.

The initial non–weight-bearing exercises targeting appropriate hip stabilization and strengthening are directed toward the gluteus medius and maximus. Mascal and colleagues[69] recommend teaching the patient to perform concurrent isometric contractions of the abdominals, gluteus medius, and gluteus maximus, before initiating the dynamic hip strengthening program. The patient is placed in a supine position, with knees bent to 90 degrees, while maintaining a stabilized pelvis. Concurrent hip and knee flexion with alternate legs is performed by the patient. Standard hip abduction in a side-lying position is also initiated during this phase, while maintaining a neutral pelvis. The gluteus medius is targeted in a side-lying position, with the hips and knees in slight flexion to decrease tensor fascia lata (TFL) recruitment (Figure 24-15, *A*). Gluteus maximus is strengthened by lying in a prone position with the knee flexed at 90 degrees and lifting the hip toward extension (keeping the leg relaxed to decrease hamstring recruitment), as recommended by Sahrmann.[168] To progress with treatment, the patient must be able to perform a specific exercise (or a 10-second isometric contraction), for two sets of 15 repetitions, while maintaining a neutral spinal position. The exercise would then be progressed by increasing resistance or starting weight-bearing exercises to target the same muscle groups.[69]

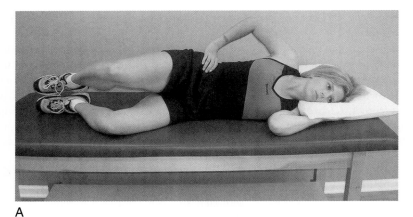

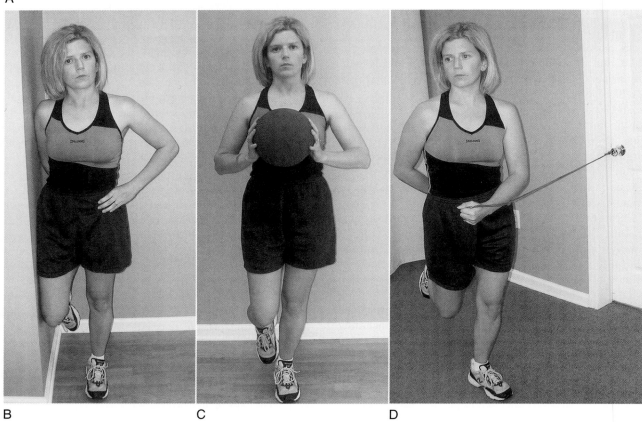

Figure 24-15: A, Modified side-lying hip abduction. The knees and hips are flexed to decrease tensor fascia lata (TFL) recruitment. **B,** Isometric hip external rotation. This exercise is performed in weight bearing with the contralateral knee flexed and placed against a wall. The transversus abdominis and gluteal muscles are isometrically contracted. The patient then performs isometric hip external rotation in the weight-bearing leg while continuing to push the contralateral limb into the wall. The pelvis is maintained in the neutral position during the entire exercise. The patient can be instructed to palpate the ASIS for feedback regarding pelvic positioning. **C,** Single-leg stance. This exercise requires contraction of the gluteus medius and TFL. The exercise is more challenging if a ball toss activity or circular motions of the contralateral limb are performed simultaneously. **D,** Resisted hip external rotation. The body is rotated medially while performing single-leg stance and holding resistive tubing. This position and movement allows for resisted external rotation of the hip in weight bearing.

Advanced CKC exercises are progressed as muscle strength and motor control improves. McConnell[169] has proposed the concept of "neutral lower extremity alignment," in which the ASIS and knee are positioned over the second toe, with the hip in approximately 10 degrees of external rotation during application of lower extremity CKC strengthening. These exercises are designed to increase dynamic strength, balance, and proprioception in the knee and involved lower extremity in preparation for more sport-specific activities during the next phase. All exercises should be performed without pain production. If pain is produced, alter the exercise to abolish pain, or remove the exercise entirely from the treatment regimen.

Traditional knee and lower extremity strengthening in weight bearing can be progressed while monitoring for pain during this phase. Closed kinetic chain exercises have been advocated for having a greater effect than joint isolation exercises alone in restoring function for patients with PFP.[170] Single- and double-limb mini-squats are continued and progressed using a device such as the Total Gym (EFI Sports Medicine, Inc., San Diego, CA) or Horizontal Leg Press (National Medical Alliance, Carmel, IN). The mini-squat is performed between 45 and 0 degrees, minimizing posterior PFJRF.[171] Stiene and colleagues[170] advocated for double-leg squats (0 to 45 degrees), 4-inch (10.2 cm) lateral step-ups, and reverse step-ups. They investigated three sets of 10 repetitions at 3 days per week for conservative management, but it is recommended that higher repetitions, in the 30-repetition range, be performed in the postsurgical lateral release patient, in order to produce muscular fatigue.[172] Initially, two sets of 15 repetitions are performed at the appropriate resistance level, while gradually working toward completion of 30 repetitions without rest. Once 30 repetitions without rest are achieved, resistance can be increased. Traditional lunges (0 to 45 degrees) with progressing resistance can also be initiated and advanced appropriately.[147]

Mascal and colleagues[69] again are cited for guidance in development of the nontraditional CKC strengthening program that addresses the pelvis and hip. Isometric hip abduction is performed with the patient standing next to a wall with the "stance limb furthest from the wall" (see Figure 24-15, B). The patient then contracts the transversus abdominis and gluteal muscles. The contralateral knee is flexed to 90 degrees. The hip is maintained in a neutral position while in single-limb stance. Once in this position, the patient then performs isometric external rotation of the stance limb, while abducting the bent leg into the wall. Pelvic stability is maintained during the exercise by self-monitoring, and feedback is provided with palpation of the ASIS. If the exercise can be performed for two sets of 15 repetitions for a 10-second hold with adequate control of the pelvis, various upper extremity exercises can be added while maintaining this position. Some suggested activities include ball throws against a wall, alternate bicep curls, and rowing exercises. Isolated single-leg stance can also be initiated and can also be performed concurrently with upper or lower extremity

activities (see Figure 24-15, C). As the ability to control the pelvis increases, in the weight-bearing position, resisted external rotation is performed in single-limb stance. This movement can be achieved by concurrently rotating the upper body and trunk medially against resistance with tubing (see Figure 24-15, D).[69]

More sport-specific functional exercises are initiated during the late portion of this phase and may typically include lateral slides facilitating hip adduction and abduction while maintaining a stabilized pelvis, lateral step-overs on a 4-inch step, and possibly stationary jumping in the pain-free ROM.

A comprehensive flexibility program is typically included in the next phase in preparation for return to sport-specific activities. This program can include flexibility exercises that target areas specific to the individual athlete's sport or his or her particular deficits found during evaluation and assessment. Commonly implemented flexibility exercises include hamstring stretching, gastrocnemius-soleus stretching, hip flexor stretching, ITB, trunk flexibility, and appropriate upper extremity flexibility, if needed during the patient's particular sport.

Aerobic conditioning exercises are also implemented during this phase and may include the Free Climber by StairMaster (StairMaster Health and Fitness Products, Inc., Kirkland, WA), reverse treadmill ambulation, or elliptical-style exercises.

Pain, joint swelling, and edema should be resolved before performance of many activities in the third phase of rehabilitation. Additionally, all activities of daily living should be normalized by 4 to 6 weeks postoperatively, including independent gait without the need for an assistive device.

PHASE IV (RETURN TO ACTIVITY PHASE)—WEEK 6 AND BEYOND
Evaluation for Progression to Phase IV

The evaluation and assessment criteria for entering phase IV include equal and normal ROM bilaterally, complete pain resolution, 85% functional testing when compared bilaterally, and 70% isokinetic testing when compared bilaterally.

Functional Testing

Functional testing provides objective data necessary to progress the patient through the rehabilitation process. It also guides appropriate decisions regarding return to activity or particular sports. The testing can demonstrate functional limitations that may not be clearly evident with isokinetic or manual muscle testing alone.[173] Mangine and associates,[44] Barber and colleagues,[174] and Noyes and co-workers[175] have investigated and developed the one-legged hop testing sequence. This testing sequence includes four hop tests to assess functional ability:

- One-leg hop for distance
- One-leg hop for time
- One-leg triple hop for distance
- One-leg crossover hop for distance

Mangine and colleagues[44] reported that the single-leg hop for distance or the timed hop tests on the involved extremity should produce no less than 85% of the results from the uninvolved extremity. They further explained that deficits higher than 15% would limit progression and delay functional return until strength is improved.[44] Booher and associates[176] reported the one-legged hop for distance to be the most reliable functional test at 0.99 intraclass correlation coefficient (ICC). They reported the single-leg 6-meter hop for time at an ICC of 0.77. Bolgla and Keskula[177] similarly reported very high reliability for single-hop, triple-hop, and crossover hop-for-distance tests, at ICC scores of 0.96, 0.95, and 0.96, respectively. This information indicates that functional performance testing can be used to obtain reliable measurements when determining an athlete's return-to-play status. Functional testing most closely duplicates future activities required during sport-specific performance in a CKC environment.[44]

Isokinetic Testing

Isokinetic testing has been advocated to assist in determining the readiness of an athlete to return to sport-specific activities.[44,178] The isokinetic test can provide useful data regarding specific muscle group strength.[178] Isokinetic testing is reliable for concentric and eccentric testing. Concentric testing reliability is higher (ICC at 0.99) compared with eccentric reliability (ICC at 0.58 to 0.99), but both remain acceptable clinical measures of strength.[179,180]

Steiner and associates[180] compared CKC and isokinetic joint isolation exercise in patients with PF dysfunction. They found that only the CKC group demonstrated significant improvement during CKC testing and subjective perceived functional status.[180] Lephart and associates[181] reported poor correlations between isokinetic tests and functional tests in individuals with ACL-deficient knees. The individuals who had higher scores on functional tests were more likely to return to their sport compared with individuals who demonstrated lower functional test scores.[181]

Mangine and colleagues[44] advise testing for muscle strength to be completed both functionally and isokinetically for patients recovering from PF surgery when determining return-to-play status. Weber and Ware[178] suggest that functional and isokinetic tests be completed before initiating sport-specific activities. When an isokinetic test is performed for assistance with muscle strength evaluation, Mangine and colleagues[44] and Weber and Ware[178] recommend at least 85% quadriceps strength compared with the uninvolved side before initiation of functional sporting activities.

Clinicians are cautioned in the use of isokinetic testing in recovery after a lateral release because of the documented PF compression forces during testing. The compression forces were reported to be as high as 5.1 times body weight at 70 to 75 degrees during concentric testing at 60 degrees per second in a study by Kaufman and associates.[182] Even at 180 degrees per second, the compressive forces were documented at 4.9 times body weight.[182] The use of isokinetic testing at lower speeds is contraindicated in postsurgical PF patients, and it is noted that even at higher speeds, the compressive forces are significant enough to seek other strengthening and testing measures. Isokinetic training and testing may not be the most appropriate manner to strengthen or functionally test for return-to-play status in patients recovering from PF dysfunction or specifically a lateral retinacular release.

INTERVENTIONS FOR IMPAIRMENTS: DECREASED STRENGTH AND ENDURANCE

Rehabilitation intervention during the fourth and final phase of rehabilitation is clearly dependent on the particular demands of the future sport and the patient's specific remaining deficits (if any). Many creative exercises have been advocated during this phase (Table 24-2). Mangine and colleagues[44] published late phase exercises and treatment for postoperative PF patients, including three categories: warm-up, lifting, and agility (Figure 24-16). The warm-up included jumping rope, stretching, sit-ups, and push-ups. The lifting or weight training component included reverse stomach flies, leg curls, toe raises, seated cable row, bench press with narrow grip, leg extension, squats, lunges, and tricep presses. The agility exercises included Plyoball sit-ups, Plyoball chest pass, dot drill, chest bands, and sit-ups with rotation.[44]

The rehabilitation specialist needs to biomechanically break down the demands of the particular sport or activity required and incorporate these component motions into the final phase of rehabilitation. A comprehensive and holistic strengthening and endurance program needs to be incorporated into the rehabilitation program to assist with full restoration of sports performance.

SUMMARY

The lateral retinacular release can be effective in reducing pathologic patellar tilt in patients with anterior knee pain. However, it is not generally effective in patients with significant patellar instability or patellar articular degeneration. Surgical intervention for PFPS should be used judiciously, and only after extensive conservative rehabilitation has failed. Each surgical procedure to the PFJ should attempt to address a specific cause of anterior knee pain.

The rehabilitation approach after a lateral retinacular release should follow a flexible but guided clinical pathway that allows the treatment to address specific problems. The high complication rate after the lateral retinacular release requires the rehabilitation specialist to deliver efficient and effective intervention strategies to facilitate appropriate progression. Communication with the surgeon is vital when postoperative complications are developing. Early intervention will improve recovery and minimize detrimental effects of the complications. The specific details of the clinical pathway will evolve over time as more biomechanical research on the PFJ and its relationship to the entire lower extremity becomes available. Understanding PFJ biomechanics will assist in developing the rehabilitation approach after a lateral retinacular release.

Acknowledgments

This chapter was completed with the assistance of many individuals and institutions. Chris Alford would like to specifically thank Jeanne Flowers at the Hughston Sports Medicine Foundation, Mercer University Medical Library, the staff at Twin Lakes Physical Therapy, and most of all Leslie, Nathan, and Justin, who sacrificed to allow completion of this chapter.

TABLE 24-2

Phase IV Comprehensive Exercise Program

General observation	No effusion; painless range of motion; joint stability	
	Performs activities of daily living and can complete previous protocol	
	Range of knee motion, 0–135°	
	Muscle tone minimal bilateral difference	
	PROCEDURES	EXPECTED OUTCOME
Evaluation	Biodex isometric test peak torque (% difference)	As previously defined, values within 15% bilateral
	Quadriceps	
	Hamstrings	
	Joint arthrometer (mm)	3 or 4
	Crepitus	
	Function tests	None/slight
	One-leg distance hop (% inv/unv)	85%
	One-leg timed hop	85%
	One-leg cross-over	85%
Treatment	Warm-up	
	Jump rope	3 × 30 seconds
	Stretch	10 minutes
	Sit-ups	20____20____20____
	Push-ups	20____20____20____
	Lifting	
	Reverse stomach flies	5____7____8____
	Leg curls	5____7____8____
	Toe raises	5____7____8____
	Seat cable row	5____7____8____
	Bench press narrow grip	5____7____8____
	Leg extension	5____7____8____
	Squats	5____7____8____
	Lunges	5____7____8____
	Triceps	5____7____8____
	Agility	
	Plyoball sit-ups	3 × 30 seconds
	Plyoball chest pass	3 × 30 seconds
	Dots	1 set of six cycles
	Chest bands	3 × 30 seconds
	Sit-up rotation	3 × 30 seconds
Goals	Increase function to full activity level	
	Establish maintenance program	
	Return to previous activity level	

From Mangine RE, Eifert-Mangine M, Burch D, et al: Postoperative management of the patellofemoral patient, *J Orthop Sports Phys Ther* 28(5):332, 1998.

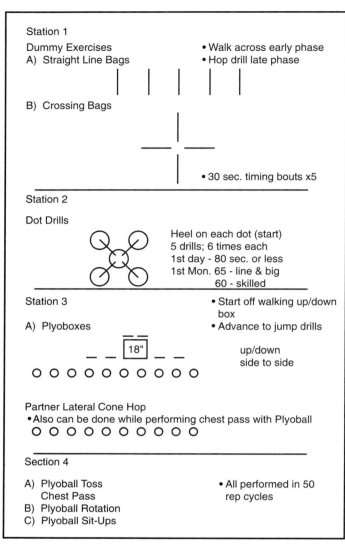

Figure 24-16: Progressive agility program. *(From Mangine RE, Eifert-Mangine M, Burch D, et al: Postoperative management of the patellofemoral patient,* J Orthop Sports Phys Ther 28[5]:332, 1998.)*

References

1. DeLee JC: Complications of arthroscopy and arthroscopic surgery: results of a national survey, Committee on Complications of Arthroscopy Association of North America, *Arthroscopy* 1:214-220, 1985.

2. O'Donoghue DH: *Treatment of injuries to athletes,* Philadelphia, 1962, Saunders.

3. Goldthwait JE: Permanent dislocation of the patella, *Ann Surg* 29:62, 1899.

4. Goldthwait JE: Slipping or recurrent dislocation of the patella: with the report of eleven cases, *Am J Orthop Surg,* vol 1, 85-A(12):293-308, 1903.

5. Hughston JC: Patellar subluxation: a recent history, *Clin Sports Med* 8:53-162, 1989.

6. Hughston JC: *Recurrent subluxation and dislocation of the patella.* Thesis presented to American Orthopaedic Association, 1962.

7. Hughston JC: Subluxation of the patella, *J Bone Joint Surg Am* 50A:1003, 1968.

8. Hughston JC, Stone MM: Recurring dislocations of the patella in athletes, *South Med J* 57:623-628, 1964.

9. Fox TA: Dysplasia of the quadriceps mechanism: hypoplasia of the vastus medialis muscle as related to the hypermobile patella syndrome, *Surg Clin North Am* 55:199-226, 1975.

10. Malek MM, Mangine RE: Patellofemoral pain syndrome: a comprehensive and conservative approach, *J Orthop Sports Phys Ther* 2(3):108-116, 1980.

11. Powers CM: Rehabilitation of patellofemoral joint disorders: a critical review, *J Orthop Sports Phys Ther* 28(5):345-354, 1998.

12. Walsh WM: Patellofemoral joint. In DeLee JC, Drez D, editors: *Orthopaedic sports medicine: principles and practice,* Philadelphia, 1994, Saunders.

13. Devereaux M, Lachmann S: Patellofemoral arthralgia in athletes attending a sports injury clinic, *Br J Sports Med* 18:18-21, 1984.

14. Dersheid GL, Feiring DC: A statistical analysis to characterize treatment adherence of the 18 most common diagnoses seen at a sports medicine clinic, *J Orthop Sports Phys Ther* 9:45, 1987.

15. Taunton JE, Ryan MB, Clement DB, et al: A retrospective case control analysis of 2,002 running injuries, *Br J Sports Med* 36(2):95-101, 2002.

16. McConnell J: The management of chondromalacia patellae: a long-term solution, *Aust J Physiother* 32:215-223, 1986.

17. Outerbridge R, Dunlop J: The problem of chondromalacia patella, *Clin Orthop* 110: 177-196, 1975.

18. Levine J: Chondromalacia patelle, *Phys Sportsmed* 7:41-49, 1979.

19. Kelly MA, Bullek DD: Nonoperative treatment of patellofomoral pain. In Scott WN: *The knee,* St Louis, 1994, Mosby.

20. Büdinger K: Ueber tramatische knorpeirisse im kniegelenk, *Dtsch Z Chir* 92:510, 1908.

21. Aleman O: Chondromalacia post-traumatic patellae, *Acta Chir Scand* 63:149, 1928.

22. Case EF, Rowe CR: The patella. Its importance in derangement of the knee, *J Bone Joint Surg Am* 32:542, 1950.

23. Chaklin UD: Injuries to the cartilage of the patella and the femoral condyle, *J Bone Joint Surg Br* 21:933, 1939.

24. Cox FF: Traumatic osteochondritis of the patella, *Surgery* 17:93, 1945.

25. Depalma AF, Sawyer B, Hoffman JD: Reconsideration of lesions affecting the patellofemoral joint, *Clin Orthop* 18:63, 1960.

26. Herzmark MH: Traumatic degenerative fibrillation of the patella, *J Bone Joint Surg Br* 24:1089, 1937.

27. Outerbridge RE: The etiology of chondromalacia patellae, *J Bone Joint Surg Br* 43B:752-757, 1961.

28. Wiberg G: Roentgenographic and anatomic studies on the femoropatellar joint. With special reference chondromalacia patellae, *Acta Orthop Scand* 12:319, 1941.

29. Wiles P, Andrews PS, Devas MB: Chondromalacia of the patella, *J Bone Joint Surg Br* 38-B(1):95-113, 1956.

30. Heywood AWB: Recurrent dislocation of the patella. A study of its pathology and treatment in 106 knees, *J Bone Joint Surg Br* 43B:508-517, 1961.

31. Abernathy PJ, Townsend PR, Rose RM, Radin EL: Is chondromalacia a separate clinical entity? *J Bone Joint Surg Br* 60B(2):205-210, 1978.

32. Emery IH, Meachim G: Surface morphology and topography of patellofemoral cartilage fibrillation in Liverpool necropsies, *J Anat* 116(1):103-120, 1973.

33. Kolowich PA, Paulos LE, Rosenberg TD, Farnsworth S: Lateral release of the patella: indications and contraindications, *Am J Sports Med* 18(4):359-365, 1990.

34. Hughston JC, Walsh WM, Puddu G: *Patellar subluxation and dislocation*, Philadelphia, 1984, Saunders.

35. Merchant AC: Classification of patellofemoral disorders, *J Arthrosc* 4(4):235-240, 1988.

36. Minkoff J, Fein L: The role of radiography in the evaluation and treatment of common anarthrotic disorders of the patellofemoral joint, *Clin Sports Med* 8(2):203-260, 1989.

37. Schutzer SF, Ramsby GR, Fulkerson JP: Computed tomographic classification of patellofemoral pain patients, *Orthop Clin North Am* 17:235-248, 1986.

38. Larson RL: Subluxation-dislocation of the patella. In Kennedy JC, editor: *The injured adolescent knee*, Baltimore, 1979, Williams & Wilkins.

39. Fulkerson JP, Shea KP: Mechanical basis for patellofemoral pain and cartilage breakdown. In Ewing JW, editor: *Articular cartilage and knee joint function: basic science and arthroscopy*, New York, 1990, Raven Press.

40. Grana W, Kriegshauser L: Scientific basis of extensor mechanism disorders, *Clin Sports Med* 4:247-257, 1985.

41. Insall J: "Chondromalacia patellae": patellar malalignment syndrome, *Orthop Clin North Am* 10(1):117-127, 1979.

42. Insall J, Falvo KA, Wise DW: Chondromalacia patellae: a prospective study, *J Bone Joint Surg* 58A:1-8, 1976.

43. Goodfellow J, Hungerford DS, Woods C: Patellofemoral joint mechanics and pathology: chondromalacia patellae, *J Bone Joint Surg* 58B:291-299, 1976.

44. Mangine RE, Eifert-Mangine M, Burch D, et al: Postoperative management of the patellofemoral patient, *J Orthop Sports Phys Ther* 28(5):323-334, 1998.

45. Powers CM: Influence of hip biomechanics on overuse injuries of the knee. Combined Sections Meeting—American Physical Therapy Association, Orthopaedic Section Programming, Nashville, TN, Feb 4-8, 2004.

46. Powers CM: The influence of altered lower-extremity kinematics on patellofemoral joint dysfunction: a theoretical perspective, *J Orthop Sports Phys Ther* 33(11):639-646, 2003.

47. Galland O, Walch G, Dejour H, Carret JP: An anatomical and radiological study of the femoropatellar articulation, *Surg Radiol Anat* 12:119-125, 1990.

48. Fulkerson JP, Gossling HR: Anatomy of the knee joint lateral retinaculum, *Clin Orthop* 153:183-188, 1980.

49. Kaplin EB: Some aspects of functional anatomy of the human knee joint, *Clin Orthop* 23:18-29, 1962.

50. Grelsamer RP, Klein JR: The biomechanics of the patellofemoral joint, *J Orthop Sports Phys Ther* 28(5):286-298, 1998.

51. Ficat RP, Hungerford DS: *Disorders of the patellofemoral joint*, Baltimore, 1977, Williams & Wilkins.

52. Goodfellow J, Hungerford DS, Zindel M: Patellofemoral joint mechanics and pathology. I. Functional anatomy of the patellofemoral joint, *J Bone Joint Surg* 58B:287-290, 1976.

53. Hungerford DS, Barry M: Biomechanics of the patellofemoral joint, *Clin Orthop* 144:9-15, 1979.

54. Livingston LA: The quadriceps angle: a review of the literature, *J Orthop Sports Phys Ther* 28:105-109, 1998.

55. Schulthies SS, Francis RS, Fisher AG, Van de Graaff KM: Does the Q angle reflect the force on the patella in the frontal plane? *Phys Ther* 75:24-30, 1995.

56. Gross MT, Foxworth JL: The role of foot orthoses as an intervention for patellofemoral pain, *J Orthop Sports Phys Ther* 33(11):661-670, 2003.

57. Powers CM, Ward SR, Fredericson M, et al: Patellofemoral kinematics during weight-bearing and non–weight-bearing knee extension in persons with lateral subluxation of the patella: a preliminary study, *J Orthop Sports Phys Ther* 33(11):677-685, 2003.

58. Reider B, Marshall JL, Koslin B, et al: The anterior aspect of the knee joint: an anatomical study, *J Bone Joint Surg* 63A:351-356, 1981.

59. Terry GC: The anatomy of the extensor mechanism, *Clin Sports Med* 8(2):163-177, 1989.

60. Powers CM, Landel R, Perry J: Timing and intensity of vastus muscle activity during functional activities in subjects with and without patellofemoral pain, *Phys Ther* 76(9):946-966, 1996.

61. Sakai N, Koshino T, Okamoto R: Patella baja after displacement of tibial tuberosity for patellofemoral disorders, *Bull Hosp Joint Dis* 53(3):25-28, 1993.

62. Lieb FJ, Perry J: Quadriceps function. An anatomical and mechanical study using amputated limbs, *J Bone Joint Surg* 50(8):1535-1548, 1968.

63. Hallisey MJ, Doherty N, Bennett WF, Fulkerson JP: Anatomy of the junction of the vastus lateralis tendon in the patella, *J Bone Joint Surg* 69A:545-549, 1987.

64. Lieb FJ, Perry J: Quadriceps function: an electromyographic study under isometric conditions, *J Bone Joint Surg* 53(4):749-758, 1971.

65. Ireland ML, Wilson JD, Ballantyne BT, Davis IM: Hip strength in females with and without patellofemoral pain, *J Orthop Sports Phys Ther* 33(1):671-676, 2003.

66. Karst GM, Willett GM: Onset timing of electromyographic activity in the vastus medialis oblique and vastus lateralis muscles in subjects with and without patellofemoral pain syndrome, *Phys Ther* 5(9):813-837, 1995.

67. Lee TQ, Morris G, Csintalan RP: The influence of tibial and femoral rotation on patellofemoral contact area and pressure, *J Orthop Sports Phys Ther* 33:686-693, 2003.

68. Lefebvre R, Boucher JP, King MA, Pepin A: Quadriceps femoris muscle activity in patellofemoral pain syndrome, *Am J Sports Med* 20(5):527-532, 1992.

69. Mascal CL, Landel R, Powers CM: Management of patellofemoral pain targeting hip, pelvis, and trunk muscle function: 2 case reports, *J Orthop Sports Phys Ther* 33(11):647-660, 2003.

70. Cummings G: Personal conversation/lecture in functional anatomy. Georgia State University, Department of Physical Therapy, 1995.

71. Ahmed AM, Burke DL: In vitro measurement of static pressure distribution in synovial joints. Part II. Retropatellar surface, *J Biomech Eng* 105:226-236, 1983.

72. Hehne HJ: Biomechanics of the patellofemoral joint and its clinical relevance, *Clin Orthop* 258:73-85, 1990.

73. Davis M, Prentice WE: Knee rehabilitation. In Prentice WE, editor: *Rehabilitation techniques in sports medicine*, St Louis, 1994, Mosby.

74. Huberti HH, Hayes WC: Patellofemoral contact pressures. The influence of Q-angle and tendofemoral contact, *J Bone Joint Surg* 66A:715-724, 1984.

75. Palmitier RA, An KN, Scott SG, Chao EY: Kinetic chain exercise in knee rehabilitation, *Sports Med* 11(6):402-413, 1991.

76. Steinkamp LA, Dillingham MF, Markel MD, et al: Biomechanical considerations in patellofemoral joint rehabilitation, *Am J Sports Med* 21(3):438-444, 1993.

77. Woodall W, Walsh J: A biomechanical basis for rehabilitation programs involving the patellofemoral joint, *J Orthop Sports Phys Ther* 11:535-542, 1990.

78. Witvrouw E, Lysens R, Bellemans J, et al: Open versus closed kinetic chain exercises for patellofemoral pain: a prospective, randomized study, *Am J Sports Med* 28(5):687-694, 2000.

79. Witvrouw E, Cambier D, Danneels L, et al: The effect of exercise regimens on reflex response time of the vasti muscles in patients with anterior knee pain: a prospective randomized intervention study, *Scand J Med Sci Sports* 13(4):251-258, 2003.

80. Patel W, Hall K, Ries M, et al: Magnetic resonance imaging of the patellofemoral kinematics with weight-bearing, *J Bone Joint Surg Am* 85A(12):2419-2424, 2003.

81. Doucette SA, Child DD: The effect of open and closed chain exercise and knee joint position on patellar tracking in lateral patellar compression syndrome, *J Orthop Sports Phys Ther* 23:104-110, 1996.

82. Hanten WP, Schulthies SS: Exercise effect on electromyographic activity of the vastus medialis oblique and the vastus lateralis muscles, *Phys Ther* 70:561-565,1990.

83. Kramer PG: Patella malalignment syndrome: rationale to reduce excessive lateral pressure, *J Orthop Sports Phys Ther* 8:301-309, 1986.

84. LeVeau BF, Rogers C: Selective training of the vastus medialis muscle using EMG biofeedback, *Phys Ther* 60:1410-1415, 1980.

85. Tria AJ, Palumbo RC, Alicea JA: Conservative care for patellofemoral pain, *Orthop Clin North Am* 23:545-553, 1992.

86. Davies GJ, Manske RC, Slamma K, et al: Selective activation of the vastus medialis obliquus. What does the literature really tell us? *Physiother Can* 53(2):136-151, 2001.

87. Mirzabeigi E, Jordan C, Gronley JK, et al: Isolation of the vastus medialis oblique muscle during exercise, *Am J Sports Med* 27(1):50-53, 1999.

88. Cerny K: Vastus medialis oblique/vastus lateralis muscle activity ratios for selected exercises in persons with and without patellofemoral pain syndrome, *Phys Ther* 75(8):672-683, 1995.

89. Laprade J, Culham E, Brouwer B: Comparison of five isometric exercises in the recruitment of the vastus medialis oblique in persons with and without patellofemoral pain, *J Orthop Sports Phys Ther* 27:197-204, 1998.

90. Fulkerson JP, Hungerford DS: *Disorders of the patellofemoral joint*, Baltimore, 1990, Williams & Wilkins.

91. DeHaven KE, Dolan WA, Mayer PJ: Chondromalacia patella in athletes: clinical presentation and conservative management, *Am J Sports Med* 7:5-11, 1979.

92. Whitelaw GP, Rullo DJ, Markowitz HD, et al: A conservative approach to anterior knee pain, *Clin Orthop* 246:234-237, 1989.

93. Gerrard B: The patellofemoral pain syndrome in young, active patients: a prospective study, *Clin Orthop* 179:129-133, 1989.

94. Wittingham M, Palmer S, Macmillan F: Effects of taping on pain and function in patellofemoral pain syndrome: a randomized controlled trial, *J Orthop Sports Phys Ther* 34(9):504-510, 2004.

95. Bockrath K, Wooden C, Worrell T, et al: Effects of patella taping on patella position and perceived pain, *Med Sci Sports Exerc* 25:989-992, 1993.

96. Larsen B, Andreasen E, Urfer A, et al: Patellar taping: a radiographic examination of the medial glide technique, *Am J Sports Med* 23:465-471, 1995.

97. Gilleard W, McConnell J, Parsons D: The effect of patellar taping on the onset of vastus medialis obliquus and vastus lateralis muscle activity in persons with patellofemoral pain, *Phys Ther* 78(1):25-32, 1998.

98. Sutlive TG, Mitchell SD, Maxfield SN, et al: Identification of individuals with patellofemoral pain whose symptoms improved after a combined program of foot orthosis use and modified activity: a preliminary investigation, *Phys Ther* 84(1):49-61, 2004.

99. Ceder LC, Larson RL: Z-plasty lateral retinacular release for the treatment of patellar compression syndrome, *Clin Orthop* 144:110-113, 1979.

100. Fredrico DJ, Reider B: Results of isolated patellar debridement for patellofemoral pain in patients with normal patellar alignment, *Am J Sports Med* 25(5):663-669, 1997.

101. Pollard B: Old dislocation of patella by inter-articular operation, *Lancet* 1(988):17-22, 1891.

102. Willner P: Recurrent dislocation of the patella, *Clin Orthop* 69:213-215, 1970.

103. Merchant AC, Mercer RL: Lateral release of the patella: a preliminary report, *Clin Orthop* 103:40-45, 1974.

104. McGinty JB, McCarthy JC: Endoscopic lateral retinacular release: a preliminary report, *Clin Orthop* 158:120-125, 1981.

105. Aglietti P, Pisaneschi A, Buzzi R, et al: Arthroscopic lateral release for patellar pain or instability, *Arthroscopy* 5(3):176-183, 1989.

106. Bigos SJ, McBride GG: The isolated lateral retinacular release in the treatment of patellofemoral disorders, *Clin Orthop* 186:75-80, 1984.

107. Chen SC, Ramanathan EB: The treatment of patellar instability by lateral release, *J Bone Joint Surg Br* 66(3):344-348, 1984.

108. Jackson RW, Kunkel SS, Taylor GJ: Lateral retinacular release for patellofemoral pain in the older patient, *Arthroscopy* 7(3):283-286, 1991.

109. Metcalf RW: An arthroscopic method of lateral release of the subluxating or dislocating patella, *Clin Orthop* 167:9-18, 1982.

110. Schonholtz GJ, Zahn MG, Magee CM: Lateral retinacular release of the patella, *Arthroscopy* 3(4):269-272, 1987.

111. Sherman OH, Fox JM, Sperling H, et al: Patellar instability: treatment by arthroscopic electrosurgical lateral release, *Arthroscopy* 3(3):152-160, 1987.

112. Bray RC, Roth JH, Jacobsen RP: Arthroscopic lateral release for anterior knee pain: a study comparing patients who are claiming worker's compensation with those who are not, *Arthroscopy* 3(4):237-247, 1987.

113. Lankenner PA, Micheli LJ, Clancy R, Gerbino PG: Arthroscopic percutaneous lateral retinacular release, *Am J Sports Med* 14(4):267-269, 1986.

114. Micheli LJ, Stanitski CL: Lateral retinacular disease, *Am J Sports Med* 9(5):330-336, 1981.

115. Schreiber SN: Arthroscopic lateral retinacular release using a modified superiomedial portal, electrosurgery, and postoperative positioning in flexion, *Orthop Rev* 17(4):375-380, 1988.

116. Fulkerson JP: Diagnosis and treatment of patients with patellofemoral pain, *Am J Sports Med* 30(3):447-456, 2002.

117. Fulkerson JP: Patellofemoral pain disorders: evaluation and management, *J Am Acad Orthop Surg* 2(2):25-134, 1994.

118. Post WR: Clinical evaluation of patients with patellofemoral disorders, *Arthroscopy* 15:841-851, 1999.

119. Fulkerson JP, Tennant R, Jaivin JS, Grunnet M: Histologic evidence of retinacular nerve injury associated with patellofemoral malalignment, *Clin Orthop* 197:196-205, 1985.

120. Dzioba RB: Diagnostic arthroscopy and longitudinal open lateral release: a four year follow-up study to determine predictor of surgical outcome, *Am J Sports Med* 18(4):343-348, 1990.

121. Fu FH, Maday MG: Arthroscopic lateral release and the lateral patellar compression syndrome, *Orthop Clin North Am* 23(4):601-611, 1992.

122. Grelsamer RP, Tedder JL: The lateral trochlear sign: femoral trochlear dysplasia as seen on a lateral view roentgenograph, *Clin Orthop* 281:159-162, 1992.

123. Fulkerson JP, Schutzer SF, Ramsby GR, Bernstein RA: Computerized tomography of the patellofemoral joint before and after a lateral release or realignment, *J Arthrosc* 3(1):19-24, 1987.

124. Sallay PI, Poggi J, Speer KP, Garrett WE: Acute dislocation of the patella: a correlative pathoanatomic study, *Am J Sports Med* 24:52-60, 1996.

125. Larson RL, Cabaud HE, Slocum DB, et al: The patellar compression syndrome: surgical treatment by lateral retinacular release, *Clin Orthop* 134:158-167, 1978.

126. Fulkerson JP, Schutzer SF: After failure of conservative treatment for painful patellofemoral malalignment: lateral release or realignment? *Orthop Clin North Am* 17(2):283-288, 1986.

127. Dandy DJ, Griffiths D: Lateral release for recurrent dislocation of the patella, *J Bone Joint Surg Br* 71(1):121-125, 1989.

128. Greenfield MA, Scott WN: Arthroscopic evaluation and treatment of the patellofemoral joint, *Orthop Clin North Am* 23(4):587-600, 1992.

129. Kunkle KL, Malek MM: Complications and pitfalls in lateral retinacular release in knee surgery. In Malek MM: *Complications, pitfalls, and salvage*, New York, 2001, Spinger-Verlag.

130. Small NC: An analysis of complications in lateral retinacular release procedures, *Arthroscopy* 5:282-286, 1989.

131. Small NC: Complications in arthroscopic surgery performed by experienced arthroscopists, *Arthroscopy* 4:215-221, 1988.

132. Evans IK, Paulos LE: Complications of patellofemoral joint surgery, *Orthop Clin North Am* 23(4):697-710, 1992.

133. Busch MT, DeHaven KE: Pitfalls of the lateral retinacular release, *Clin Sports Med* 8:279-290, 1989.

134. Blasier RB, Ciullo JV: Rupture of the quadriceps tendon after arthroscopic lateral release: a case report, *Arthroscopy* 2:262-263, 1986.

135. Hughston JC, Deese M: Medial subluxation of the patella as a complication of lateral retinacular release, *Am J Sports Med* 16:383-388, 1988.

136. Youmans WT: Surgical complications of the patellofemoral articulation, *Clin Sports Med* 8(2):331-342, 1989.

137. Cooper DE, DeLee JC, Ramamurthy S: Reflex sympathetic dystrophy of the knee, *J Bone Joint Surg Am* 71(3):365-369, 1989.

138. Shelton GL, Thigpen LK: Rehabilitation of patellofemoral dysfunction: a review of literature, *J Orthop Sports Phys Ther* 14:243-249, 1991.

139. Phillips BB: Arthroscopy of the lower extremity. In Canale ST, editor: *Campbell's operative orthopaedics*, Philadelphia, 2003, Mosby.

140. Shahriaree H: Malalignment syndrome. In Shahriaree H: *O'Connor's textbook of arthroscopic surgery*, Philadelphia, 1992, JB Lippincott.

141. *Guide to physical therapist practice*, ed 2, *Phys Ther* 81(1):9-744, 2001.

142. Clarkson HM, Gilewich GB: *Musculoskeletal assessment: joint range of motion and manual muscle strength*, Baltimore, 1989, Williams & Wilkins.

143. Norkin CC, White DJ: *Measurement of joint motion: a guide to goniometry*, Philadelphia, 1994, FA Davis.

144. Hammersly S: Complications after an anterior cruciate ligament reconstruction. Combined Sections Meeting—American Physical Therapy Association, Sports Physical Therapy Section, Complicated Patient Presentations, San Antonio, TX, 2001.

145. Jackson D, Drez D: *The anterior cruciate deficient knee*, St Louis, 1987, Mosby.

146. Gould J, Davies G: *Orthopaedic and sports physical therapy*, St Louis, 1990, Mosby.

147. Kisner C, Colby LA: *Therapeutic exercise: foundations and techniques*, Philadelphia, 1996, FA Davis.

148. Cyriax JH, Cyriax PJ: *Cyriax's illustrated manual of orthopaedic medicine*, Boston, 1993, Butterworth-Heinemann Ltd.

149. Ewing JW: Arthroscopic patellar shaving and lateral retinacular release. In McGinty JB, editor: *Operative arthroscopy*, New York, 1991, Raven Press.

150. Noyes FR, Mangine RE, Barber SD: The early treatment of motion complications following reconstruction of the anterior cruciate ligament, *Clin Orthop* 222:217-228, 1992.

151. Noyes FR, Wojitys EM, Marshall MT: The early diagnosis and treatment of the developmental patellar infera syndrome, *Clin Orthop* 265:241-252, 1991.

152. Irrgang JJ: Rehabilitation for nonoperative and operative management of knee injuries. In Fu FH: *Knee surgery*, Baltimore, 1994, Williams & Wilkins.

153. Akerson WH, Woo SLY, Amiel D, et al: The connective tissue response immobility. Biomechanical changes in periarticular connective tissue of the immobilized rabbit knee, *Clin Orthop* 93:356-362, 1973.

154. Oglivie-Harris DJ, Roscoe M: Reflex sympathetic dystrophy of the knee, *J Bone Joint Surg* 69B(5):804-806, 1987.

155. Spencer JD, Hayes KC, Alexander IJ: Knee joint effusion and quadriceps reflex inhibition in man, *Arch Phys Med Rehabil* 65:171-177, 1984.

156. Radin EL: The Maquet procedure—anterior displacement of the tibial tubercle, *Clin Orthop* 213:241-248, 1986.

157. Merskey H, Albe Fessard DG, Bonica JJ: Pain terms: a list with definitions and notes on usage, *Pain* 6:249-252, 1979.

158. Merskey H, Albe Fessard DG, Bonica JJ: Pain terms: a list with definitions and notes on usage, *Pain* 6:249-252, 1979.

159. Newton RA: Joint receptor contributions to reflexive and kinesthetic responses, *Phys Ther* 62:22-29, 1982.

160. Small NC: Complications in arthroscopy: the knee and other joints, *Arthroscopy* 4:253-258, 1986.

161. Ford DH, Post WR: Open or arthroscopic lateral release: indications, techniques, and rehabilitation; arthroscopic surgery. Part II. The knee, *Clin Sports Med* 16(1):29-49, 1997.

162. Bandy WD, Irion JM, Briggler M: The effect of time and frequency of static stretching on flexibility of the hamstring muscles, *Phys Ther* 77(10):1090-1096, 1997.

163. Branch TP, Karsch RE, Mills TJ, Palmer MT: Mechanical therapy for loss of knee flexion, *Am J Orthop* 4:195-200, 2003.

164. Benton LA, Baker LL, Bowman BR: *Functional electrical stimulation: a practical clinical guide*, Downey, CA, 1980, Rancho Los Amigos Hospital.

165. Hooker DN: Electrical stimulating currents. In Prentice WE: *Therapeutic modalities in sports medicine*, St Louis, 1994, Mosby.

166. Robertson VJ, Ward AR: Vastus medialis electrical stimulation to improve lower extremity function following a lateral patellar retinacular release, *J Orthop Sports Phys Ther* 32(9):437-443 (discussion, 443-446), 2002.

167. Krompinger WJ, Fulkerson JP: Lateral retinacular release for intractable lateral retinacular pain, *Clin Orthop Relat Res* 179:191-193, 1983.

168. Sahrmann S: *Diagnosis and treatment of movement impairment syndromes*, St Louis, 2002, Mosby.

169. McConnell J: Patellofemoral joint complications and considerations. In Ellenbecker TS, editor: *Knee ligament rehabilitation*, New York, 2000, Churchill Livingstone.

170. Stiene HA, Brosky T, Reinking MF, et al: A comparison of closed kinetic chain and isokinetic joint isolation exercise in

patients with patellofemoral dysfunction, *J Orthop Sports Phys Ther* 24(3):36-141, 1996.

171. Buff HU, Jones LC, Hungerford DS: Experimental determination of forces transmitted through the patello-femoral joint, *J Biomech* 21:17-23,1988.

172. Prentice WE: Impaired muscle performance: regaining muscular strength and endurance. In Prentice WE, Voight ML, editors: *Techniques in musculoskeletal rehabilitation*, New York, 2001, McGraw-Hill.

173. Tegner Y, Lysholm J, Lysholm M, Gillquist J: A performance test to monitor rehabilitation and evaluate anterior cruciate ligament injuries, *Am J Sports Med* 14:156-159, 1986.

174. Barber SD, Noyes FR, Mangine RB: Quantitative assessment of functional limitations in normal and anterior cruciate ligament–deficient knee, *Clin Orthop* 255:204-214, 1990.

175. Noyes FR, Barber SD, Mangine RE: Abnormal lower limb symmetry determined by function hop test after anterior cruciate ligament rupture, *Am J Sports Med* 19:513-518, 1991.

176. Booher LD, Hench KM, Worrell TW: Reliability of three single-leg hop tests, *J Sports Rehabil* 2:165-170, 1993.

177. Bolgla LA, Keskula DR: Reliability of lower extremity performance tests, *J Orthop Sports Phys Ther* 26(3):138-142, 1997.

178. Weber MD, Ware AN: Knee rehabilitation. In Andrews JR, Harrelson GL, Wilk KE: *Physical rehabilitation of the injured athlete*, Philadelphia, 1998, Saunders.

179. Perrin DH: *Isokinetic exercise and assessment*, Champaign, IL, 1993, Human Kinetics.

180. Steiner LA, Harris BA, Krebs DE: Reliability of eccentric isokinetic knee flexion and extension measurements, *Arch Phys Med Rehabil* 74(12):1327-1335, 1993.

181. Lephart SM, Perrin DH, Fu FH: Relationship between selected physical characteristics and functional capacity in the anterior cruciate ligament–insufficient athlete, *J Orthop Sports Phys Ther* 16:174-181, 1992.

182. Kaufman KR, An K, Litchy WJ, et al: Dynamic joint forces during knee isokinetic exercise, *Am J Sports Med* 19(3):305-316, 1991.

CHAPTER 25

Patellar and Quadriceps Tendon Rupture and Treatment

Lori A. Bolgla, PhD, PT, ATC
Terry R. Malone, PT, EdD, ATC, FAPTA
Scott D. Mair, MD

PATELLAR TENDON AND QUADRICEPS

tendon ruptures are relatively uncommon injuries.[1-4] A review of the literature reveals that these ruptures most often occur during a violent, eccentric action of the quadriceps muscles with the knee in a flexed position, which may occur during sporting activities or simply from a fall.[1,2,4-11] The estimated force required to disrupt either the patellar or quadriceps tendon is 17.5 times body weight, and injury may occur to the tendon itself (midsubstance), at the osteotendinous junction, or at the myotendinous junction.[11-14]

The pattern of tendon injury is age dependent in that patellar tendon injuries are more prominent in patients less than 40 years of age whereas quadriceps tendon injuries occur more frequently in older patients.[4,15] One reason for this trend may evolve from age-associated muscle fiber changes. Muscle tissue disperses forces transmitted through the lower extremities and often involves the activation of the large, fast-twitch muscle fibers. Because the central nervous system activates fast-twitch muscle fibers in response to high-velocity, excessive external loads, stronger muscles are more capable of attenuating these loads without injury.

Younger patients, typically those 20 to 40 years old, generally incur patellar tendon ruptures as the result of a severe overloading of the extensor mechanism on a flexed knee and planted foot, which may occur while playing basketball and soccer.[3,9] These patients are skeletally mature and exhibit a higher number (as a percent of the total muscle fibers) of fast-twitch fibers within the quadriceps muscle. A combination of a firm "anchor" (the tibial tuberosity) and strong quadriceps muscle commonly leads to a disruption at the midsubstance portion[12] of the patella tendon or at its osteotendinous junction (distal patellar pole).[10,15] In other words, the excessive force leads to failure at the knee structure's weakest point, which in these cases is the patellar tendon.

Alternatively, patients over 40 years of age tend to incur injury to the quadriceps tendon, typically at the bone-tendon junction.[16] Normal aging leads to a decrease in the number (as a percent of the total muscle fibers) of fast-twitch muscle fibers within the quadriceps muscle, and the quadriceps' inability to respond rapidly and strongly to an excessive force applied to the knee may lead to tissue failure. Furthermore, patients older than 35 years of age have demonstrated degenerative changes from chronic microtears, mucoid degeneration, or calcific tendinopathy that can also weaken tendons.[15,17] Together, muscle fiber type and degenerative changes lessen tissue strength, which reduces the amount of force needed to cause tendon rupture and increases the incidence of quadriceps tendon injury in older patient populations.

Researchers have reported cases of patellar and quadriceps tendon ruptures in patients with and without an evident underlying pathology. A review of the literature has revealed a higher incidence of such injury in patients diagnosed with renal disease, systemic lupus erythematosus, endocrine disorders such as hyperparathyroidism and diabetes, excessive anabolic steroid use, steroid injection, or obesity, who may sustain an injury simply from a fall on the knee or during routine ambulation.[10,18-24] Researchers believe that these conditions may lead to muscle fiber atrophy, decreased collagen content and vascular changes within the tendon, and diffuse fibrosis, all of which result in weaknesses at the osteotendinous junction.[10,16,17]

Researchers have also reported incidences of tendon ruptures in apparently healthy patients. These ruptures typically have occurred during sporting activities, with basketball being one of the most commonly reported sports.[2,3,5-7,25] Although many of these patients have no apparent underlying pathology, other precipitating factors may exist. For example, the inferior pole of the patella lacks a rich blood supply, which may lead to tissue vulnerability.[8] Kelly and colleagues[6] have also reported a strong correlation between patients with a history of patellar tendinosis ("jumper's knee") and patellar and quadriceps tendon ruptures. They believe that tendon degeneration occurred from repetitive microtrauma. The repetitive microtrauma, in combination with degenerative changes in collagen fibrils and a compromised vascular supply, can further promote tendon failure.

Health care providers can usually easily diagnose a patellar tendon or quadriceps tendon rupture solely on physical examination.[4] Patients usually complain of pain and swelling over the tendon and knee buckling during gait.[9] They lack complete active knee extension and often have a palpable defect (sulcus) over the ruptured tendon. McGrory[4] recommends that patients actively extend the knee while sitting over the side of an examination table to reduce the influence of an intact patellar retinaculum and iliotibial band that may enable a patient to perform a straight leg raise. He emphasizes that a patient should demonstrate full knee extension because some patients may partially extend the knee using other muscles.

Physicians may further determine superior or inferior migration of the patella following a patellar or quadriceps tendon rupture, respectively, by taking a lateral radiograph and calculating the Insall-Salvati ratio. They may calculate this ratio by dividing the length of the patella by the length of the patellar tendon. A ratio of less than 0.80 signifies a patella alta (high-riding patella) and may indicate a patellar tendon rupture.[3,5,8,9,25,26] A low-riding patella (Insall-Salvati ratio exceeding 1.20) or a forward tilting of the patella (due to tension from the intact patellar tendon) may indicate a quadriceps tendon rupture.[4,18,20,26,27]

The recommended treatment for complete patellar and quadriceps tendon rupture is early surgical repair for purposes of restoring normal extensor mechanism function.[3,4,8,28,29] A delay in surgery of greater than 2 weeks may lead to a retraction of tendon tissue and scar tissue formation, factors that may compromise a surgeon's ability to repair the tendon in an optimal anatomic position.[3,4] However, clinicians should also recognize the possibility of incomplete patellar tendon or quadriceps tendon tears. In these cases patients should follow a more conservative intervention that includes an initial 6-week immobilization period followed by knee range of motion (ROM) and quadriceps strengthening exercises.[16] Clinicians may vary the immobilization period based on the extent of injury and viability of the surrounding tissue. Because most tendon injuries of this nature require surgical repair, the remainder of this chapter addresses surgical techniques and postoperative care.

SURGICAL CONSIDERATIONS

The challenge confronting the surgeon is to approximate the torn or avulsed tissues and maintain their position to allow collagen deposition (healing), while attempting to provide the required function/mobility expected with activities of daily living (ADLs). Because these expectations and requirements are somewhat dichotomous, the surgeon often must attempt a compromise and convey this to the therapy personnel to enable optimal postoperative outcomes. An example of this process is in limiting early ROM and quadriceps activation when the surgeon is uncomfortable with fixation strength of the repaired tissues. Conversely, if good fixation and a protective restraint are present, the surgeon may allow early ROM and low-level (submaximal) quadriceps activation.

The surgery is typically performed relatively soon after the injury because retraction and muscle fiber shortening are detrimental to surgical approximation. The surgical techniques for quadriceps tendon are presented first, followed by patellar tendon techniques. A case study for each condition concludes the surgical section.

QUADRICEPS TENDON SURGERY

The typical patient is over age 40 with a history of falling backward over a fixed foot, thus driving the knee into flexion while weight bearing. A palpable gap is present above the patella with an inability to extend the knee against gravity. The patient has significant pain and often describes a tearing sensation during the injury. Patients are unable to walk because knee extension cannot be maintained. Surgeons rarely need significant diagnostic tests to determine patient status and typically schedule the surgery within a week whenever possible.[3,4]

Tendon ruptures are typically either within a degenerative (tendinotic) area of the tendon or at the quadriceps tendon–bony junction, more commonly the latter.[13,14] A variety of acute repair procedures/processes have been used to reapproximate the separated fibers. Typically, a midline incision is used to enable adequate exposure to the involved tissues. When an intratendinous lesion is seen, the tendon edges are debrided to the level of "good tissue" and approximated. An end-to-end repair is then performed using nonabsorbable suture. The surgeon also will repair the retinaculum in similar style.

When a rupture of the tendon-bone junction is present, direct tendon-bone approximation is performed. Sutures are woven into the tendon, using some form of locking stitch to prevent pull-out. The sutures are held to bone through drill holes or with suture anchors. The retinaculum is closed as in

the intratendinous lesion using nonabsorbable suture. Some surgeons add a pull-out wire or cable device to protect the repaired site from stress during the initial 6 weeks postoperatively. Such a device is passed through the tendon and around the patella to decrease forces on the repair with early ROM.[1,26,30,31] As stronger sutures have evolved, these wires are less commonly used.

Patients are commonly braced postoperatively, and allowable flexion is gradually increased over approximately 8 weeks, until full ROM is achieved. Quadriceps strengthening is then initiated.[27,32]

CASE STUDY 1

A 43-year-old surgeon was attending a soccer match when he attempted to jump over a water-filled ditch. On landing, his right foot sank into the mud and he fell awkwardly toward the ditch. He described a tearing sensation in his thigh just above his knee. He was unable to ambulate and needed assistance in moving from his semiseated position. Clinical examination exhibited an inability to ambulate; a significant, palpable gap between his patella and quadriceps tendon (Figure 25-1); inability to extend his knee; and significant pain. He underwent surgical repair the next day using a direct repair process. A 6-inch midline incision was made, exposing a complete disruption of the extensor mechanism. The hematoma was evacuating, allowing better delineation of the disruption. The failure was at the superior patellar insertion, although the deep portion of the vastus intermedius had torn more proximally. This was addressed using a modified Kessler stitch interweaving the medial and lateral portions through passing the stitch toward the proximal tendon. Four #5 Kessler stitches were used to approximate the extensor mechanism to the superior patella, and this was oversewn using #2 Tycron in a running baseball stitch. After superficial closure, a cylinder cast was applied to protect and

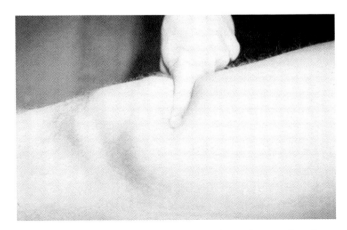

Figure 25-1: A palpable defect is seen above the patella when quadriceps tendon disruption is complete.

maintain knee extension for 2 weeks. He was to place his foot on the floor for balance using (touchdown weight-bearing) bilateral crutches in a comfortable fashion. He was to keep the leg elevated and use ice whenever possible.

Two days postoperatively, the patient complained of leg pain from cast compression and the cast was bivalved. Four days later, a DonJoy postoperative brace locked in extension was provided to the patient. Two weeks after surgery, a gentle, passive, 0- to 20-degree ROM program was initiated along with patellar mobility activities. The patient was instructed in the use of his thumb and index finger to passively move his patella from side to side gently to assist in maintenance of patellar mobility. He was allowed to increase his weight bearing but was to always have the brace locked in extension during ambulation. A gentle progression for increasing ROM was followed over the next few weeks, allowing 10- to 20-degree increases each week. The patient began an active quadriceps strengthening program (working around the 30-degree position) during postoperative weeks 6 to 8. He was full weight bearing but continued to use his immobilizer, keeping the knee in extension. He was to continue this until good quadriceps control was achieved. Eight weeks postoperatively, he had 45 to 50 degrees of active knee flexion and 60 degrees of passive knee flexion. A continuous passive motion (CPM) device was added to his program at this time to be used in the evenings in an attempt to achieve increasing ROM.

He started a formal physical therapy program for ROM and strengthening at this 8-week phase. Increases in ROM were enhanced and quadriceps strengthening quickly allowed improved ambulation. Three months after surgery, he was independent in ambulation and had approximately 80 to 90 degrees of active knee flexion. He continued to follow a strengthening and ROM program and had 130 degrees of flexion, full active extension, and good plus quadriceps function at the 5- to 6-month point. He continued to improve slowly and used a cycling program independently to assist with quadriceps strengthening. Interestingly, he demonstrated the normal frustration during the 6- to 12-month cycle (in keeping with our observations of these patients) as gains are very slow with the ultimate outcome still being a reduction in endurance and maximal strength. At this time, we introduced maximal eccentric strengthening as an emphasis, which included lunges and absorbing forms of exercise. This slow progression is true even in dedicated patients. He has returned to all ADLs but has been very cautious to return to aggressive sports activities.

PATELLAR TENDON SURGERY

The mechanism for patellar tendon rupture is the same as quadriceps rupture but frequently is in the younger, more fit population. Often the patient is landing from a jump or planting to enable him or her to change direction. The hallmark is a high-riding or floating patella. Muscle activation results in retraction of the patella without knee extension.

The surgeon wishes to operate relatively soon to avoid significant retraction and muscle adaptation.

Patellar Tendon Technique— Acute, High-Energy Injury

A straight midline incision is typically used with exposure demonstrating a disruption of the tendon-bone junction. The most common approach is to debride (creating a trough) the inferior patellar insertional area and the corresponding detached tendon to allow their approximation. A variety of nonabsorbable suture fixation techniques (Kessler stitch in tendon and bone tunnels or suture anchors in bone) can be used and are sometimes reinforced via wire, cable, or looped suture (Figures 25-2 and 25-3).[1,3,27,31,32] The associated retinacular tears are typically closed with absorbable suture. Many surgeons keep the knee in extension for a minimum of 3 weeks and immobilized (full extension) during ambulation for at least 6 weeks. Allowable flexion is gradually increased over 6 to 8 weeks. With strong fixation, it is typical to allow 0 to 45 degrees during the first 3 weeks and 0 to 90 degrees during weeks 4 through 6. If reinforcement was used, it is typically removed at the 4- to 6-week time frame. Quadriceps strengthening is begun approximately 6 weeks after surgery. As with case study 1, the rehabilitation progression is slow and long, with 4 to 6 months expected before normalization of gait and 1 year before higher-level activities are achieved.

When the patellar tendon rupture is associated with underlying preexisting conditions or is chronic in nature, surgical intervention frequently requires augmentation of the repair and special attention to gaining adequate displacement of the patella inferiorly to minimize quadriceps retraction.[28] Rehabilitation of these patients can be challenging because ROM can be decreased and functional levels impaired, even after lengthy rehabilitation.

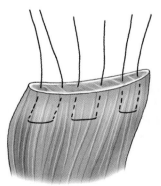

Figure 25-2: Nonabsorbable sutures using some type of technique to enhance holding capacity (Kessler, etc.) are inserted to the free tendon.

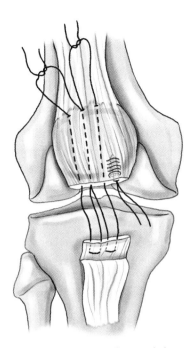

Figure 25-3: Interlocking sutures can be used through drill holes or suture anchors to enable approximation of the tendon to a bony trough.

CASE STUDY 2

A 22-year-old red-shirt junior football player suffered a complete right patellar tendon disruption that occurred as he attempted to plant his right foot and rotate to his left to receive a pass. He had a high-riding patella and a palpable defect below the patella. Interestingly, he had a several-month history of significant bilateral "jumper's knee" and a history of such symptoms recurrently over 5 years. He underwent a direct repair using three suture anchors with nonabsorbable suture and cerclage wire reinforcement. This was performed related to the large degenerative area seen at debridement. He was placed in an immobilizer (full extension) and used bilateral crutches weight bearing to comfort for 2 weeks. He was then permitted weight bearing to tolerance while immobilized. At that time he was allowed to initiate ROM from 0 to 15 degrees and increase to 40 degrees up through week 6. He was allowed to activate his quadriceps in the available ROM. His wire was removed at 6 weeks and ROM/strengthening activities increased. He was able to demonstrate 90 degrees of motion at 8 weeks and full active extension. He slowly improved both ROM and strength over the next 2 months. He demonstrated approximately 70% quadriceps strength at 5 months, allowing the initiation of a running program. He played football the following fall and experienced the same injury to his contralateral patellar tendon at midseason!

REHABILITATION PRINCIPLES

Historically, surgeons have immobilized patients who have undergone a patellar tendon or quadriceps tendon repair for a 6-week period.[10,24] The reason for immobilization has been to protect the tendon from tension that may disrupt the recently repaired/approximated tissue. Although tissue protection is an important consideration, prolonged immobilization can adversely affect tissue healing because it can lead to a decrease in the amount of collagen fibrils and the cross-sectional area of normal noninvolved ligaments and tendons. Lack of motion also decreases joint lubrication, which can adversely affect cartilage and tendon nutrition and lead to capsular contraction and joint stiffness.[13] Extended immobilization may also inhibit a patient's recovery of normal strength, ROM, and patellar position (often resulting in a patella baja) following the surgery.[3] Therefore postoperative rehabilitative care should minimize these detrimental effects while protecting the surgically repaired tissue.

A review of the literature has shown that surgeons have chosen both traditional and more progressive postoperative rehabilitation programs, generally with good functional outcomes.[10] Although both programs have resulted in acceptable functional outcomes, patients who follow a more progressive rehabilitation program have achieved full knee ROM and strength in a more timely fashion.[31] Many factors, such as the quality of the repaired tendon tissue and the patient's general health status, deserve consideration when choosing a specific protocol. The following sections include information regarding rehabilitation principles as related to traditional and more progressive rehabilitation postoperative care. Based on this review of the literature, we then present two different exercise protocols that clinicians may use to guide the decision-making process when designing, implementing, and individualizing a rehabilitation program.

General Exercise Considerations

Researchers have reported that patients with patellofemoral disorders can benefit from both open kinetic chain (OKC) and closed kinetic chain (CKC) exercises.[33] In designing a rehabilitation program, clinicians must consider the biomechanical influences of joint position and the effect on patellofemoral joint stresses because patellofemoral joint reaction forces are lessened at 0 to 40 degrees of knee flexion during CKC activities and at 40 to 90 degrees of knee flexion during OKC exercise.[34] Another key point is that patients perform all exercises in a pain-free manner.[35]

Choice of exercise parameters deserves further consideration. Before initiating active knee ROM exercises in this patient population, clinicians should discuss this progression with the surgeon. After receiving clearance for active knee extension, clinicians should employ relatively high-repetition, low-load therapeutic exercise sequences because this may facilitate joint lubrication, muscle endurance, and ROM while minimizing maximal loads to the repaired tissues. As patients demonstrate improved knee ROM and adequate quadriceps strength, they may initiate a more demanding strengthening exercise that incorporates lower-repetition, higher-load exercise. Typically, after 5 to 6 months, the introduction of eccentric exercises with higher demands is helpful in those individuals desiring a return to sporting activities. We cannot overemphasize the point that the rehabilitation professional discuss all exercise progression with the surgeon.

Traditional Rehabilitation Program

Many surgeons have immobilized patients in full knee extension for 6 weeks immediately following surgery in order to prevent excessive tension on the repaired tendon.[3,7,8,18-21,25,36] The majority of these patients wear a cylinder cast but ambulate without weight-bearing restrictions. After the immobilization period, they initiate a rehabilitation regimen to restore knee ROM and quadriceps strength; however, most authors have not provided specific detail regarding exercise type, parameters, or duration of rehabilitation.

Many reported cases exhibited similar patient characteristics, such as those who had underlying pathologic conditions such as diabetes, renal failure, anabolic steroid abuse, local steroid injection, or a diagnosed patellar tendinosis (jumper's knee). Based on these characteristics, the researchers implemented a more conservative postoperative care program to protect tissue having a preexisting "weakness." Ilan and colleagues[16] also recommended this type of intervention for patients diagnosed with an incomplete tendon tear. In summary, patients with either altered tendon tissue properties (from a disease process) or a less than optimal surgical fixation may benefit from a more traditional rehabilitation program (Table 25-1).

Progressive Rehabilitation Program

As mentioned previously, prolonged immobilization may have a detrimental effect on knee cartilage, ligament, and tendon tissue; therefore some surgeons have advocated earlier mobilization following a patellar tendon or quadriceps tendon repair than in the traditional 6-week pattern.[6,28,29,37,38] They believe that earlier mobilization minimizes or prevents potential impairments such as knee flexion limitations, patella immobility, and patella baja.[37] Although some surgeons use early mobilization for patients having tendon repairs without augmentation,[29,37] more surgeons have initiated a progressive program when repairing the tendon using augmentation from cerclage wiring,[1,26,39,40] neutralization wiring,[3] semitendinosus augmentation,[28] or a Dall-Miles cable.[31] Furthermore, Ravalin and colleagues[30] performed simulated surgical tendon repairs on cadaveric knees and reported that those repaired using augmentation (suture and Dall-Miles cable) more effectively resisted an externally applied cyclic load when compared with cadav-

eric knees repaired solely with suture material. They concluded that augmentation of patellar tendon repairs is appropriate when the surgeon wishes to initiate ROM early in the postoperative care. Overall, it appears that early ROM is becoming more common as stronger fixation has become available.

Patients following a progressive rehabilitation program typically begin passive range of motion (PROM) on the same day as surgery, beginning in a small arc of motion such as 0 to 30 degrees of knee flexion and progressing to 90 degrees over the next 4 to 6 weeks. A noteworthy point is that Shelbourne and colleagues[31] have successfully used higher PROM parameters. They studied 10 consecutive patients who underwent a patellar tendon repair (5 ruptures at the donor site of the ACL-reconstructed knee and 5 primary patellar tendon ruptures) and reported mean postoperative knee flexion of 88 degrees at 2 weeks, 112 degrees at 1 month, 133 degrees at 3 months, and 138 degrees at 6 months.

Surgeons advocating a progressive program also have allowed patients to begin gentle active knee flexion, quadriceps isometrics, and straight leg raise exercise under rehabilitation guidance during the first postoperative week. Although authors have not specifically described the position in which patients performed active knee flexion, we cannot overemphasize that the rehabilitation professional consider the effect of the rectus femoris, a muscle crossing both the knee and hip, when positioning patients for active ROM exercise.

Patients following a progressive program can ambulate safely without weight-bearing restrictions. All of the reported studies initially used bracing (with either a knee immobilizer or hinged knee brace) and allowed unrestricted ambulation once the patient achieved lower extremity control. Some patients wore a brace for as few as 2 weeks,[31] whereas others used a brace over a 6-week period.[1,37]

Researchers have initiated activities that are more demanding 6 weeks following surgery.[31,39,40] Examples of exercise include active knee extension, low-resistance cycling, and CKC activities. Most studies did not include specific information regarding the progression of exercise, but some stated that patients safely resumed light jogging activities and sport-specific drills 16 weeks after surgery.[1,37] In summary, research supports early mobilization of the knee following a patellar tendon or quadriceps tendon repair because controlled stress may facilitate tendon healing and prevent joint stiffness.[31] Before initiating early mobilization, clinicians must determine tissue viability, strength of the surgical fixation, and any other underlying contributing pathology that may adversely affect the tendon repair (Table 25-2).

SUMMARY

This chapter outlines the state of the art in patellar tendon and quadriceps rupture treatment. Earlier ROM and strengthening has become the rule as fixation of tissue has improved. This has enabled earlier return of motion and minimization of some deleterious effects associated with immobilization. However, the rehabilitation process is still lengthy and return to sporting activities challenging. A most difficult time frame is often approximately 4 to 6

months postoperatively as the patient begins to increase function. It is our recommendation that the addition of eccentric activities, including lunges and plyometric progressions for the quadriceps, is helpful for those desiring a return to sports.

TABLE 25-1

Traditional Rehabilitation Program

PHASE	WEEK	GOALS	ACTIVITY	EXPECTED OUTCOMES
Maximum protection	1–6	Maximal tissue protection	Weight bearing as tolerated (casted) Multiplane hip straight leg raises Standing heel raises Active ankle dorsiflexion	Independent ambulation with full weight bearing Independent with home exercise program
Moderate protection	7–10	Improve knee range of motion Normalize gait Improve quadriceps strength Enhance knee proprioception Pain control	Heel slides Gentle patellar glides Quadriceps isometrics Straight leg raises Midrange, short-arc quadriceps extension (30–60 degrees) Knee bends from 0–30 degrees Hamstring and triceps surae stretching High-repetition, low-load progressive resistance exercises (PREs) Single-leg stance balance activities Treadmill walking Modalities as indicated	Increase knee range of motion to 0–90 degrees Ambulate with normal gait pattern Perform a straight leg raise without an extensor lag Demonstrate normal hamstring and triceps surae flexibility
Minimum protection	11–20	Normalize knee range of motion Normalize knee strength Normalize knee proprioception	Cycling Lateral step-downs Quarter lunges/squats Prone quadriceps stretch (cautiously) Proprioception board Leg press (0–90 degrees) Full-arc knee extensions (0–90 degrees) Stair-stepping machine	Gain full knee range of motion Demonstrate quadriceps strength at 80% of normal Tolerate 45 minutes of aerobic activity Progression to light jogging program
Functional progression	21–24	Return to sporting activity	Supervised sport-specific drills	Return to sport participation

TABLE 25-2

Progressive Rehabilitation Program

PHASE	WEEK	GOALS	ACTIVITY	EXPECTED OUTCOMES
Maximum protection	1–2	Facilitate cartilage nutrition Minimize joint stiffness Pain control	Weight bearing as tolerated with brace in knee extension Multiplane hip straight leg raises Quadriceps isometrics Standing heel raises/active ankle dorsiflexion Continuous passive motion Hamstring and triceps surae stretching Modalities	Independent ambulation with full weight bearing Passive knee range of motion from 0–60 degrees Demonstrate normal hamstring and triceps surae flexibility
Submaximum protection	3–5	Improve knee range of motion Normalize gait Improve quadriceps activation Enhance knee proprioception	Heel slides Gentle patellar glides Straight leg raises Single-leg stance balance activities Slow-speed treadmill walking	Increase knee range of motion to 0–90 degrees Ambulate with normal gait pattern Perform a straight leg raise with less than 10 degrees of extensor lag
Moderate protection	6–8	Improve knee range of motion Improve quadriceps strength and endurance Enhance knee proprioception	Midrange, short-arc quadriceps extension (30–60 degrees) Knee bends from 0–30 degrees Lateral step-up (4-inch height) 0–40 degree wall slides High-repetition, low-load PREs Low-resistance cycling Proprioception board	Increase knee range of motion to 0–125 degrees Perform a straight leg raise without extensor lag
Minimum protection	9–16	Normalize knee range of motion Normalize knee strength Normalize knee proprioception	Quarter lunges/squats Prone quadriceps stretch (cautiously) Leg press (0–90 degrees) Full-arc knee extensions (0–90 degrees) Stair-stepping machine	Gain full knee range of motion Demonstrate quadriceps strength at 80% of normal Tolerate 45 minutes of aerobic activity Progression to light jogging program
Functional progression	17–24	Return to sporting activity	Supervised sport-specific drills	Return to sport participation

References

1. Enad JG, Loomis LL: Primary patellar tendon repair and early mobilization: results in an active-duty population, *J South Orthop Assoc* 10(1):17-23, 2001.

2. Shah M, Jooma N: Simultaneous bilateral quadriceps tendon rupture while playing basketball, *Br J Sports Med* 36:152-153, 2002.

3. Hsu K, Wang K, Ho W, Hsu RW: Traumatic patellar tendon ruptures: a follow-up study of primary repair and neutralization wire, *J Trauma* 36:658-660, 1994.

4. McGrory JE: Disruption of the extensor mechanism of the knee, *J Emerg Med* 24(2):163-168, 2003.

5. Ho HM, Lee WKE: Traumatic bilateral concurrent patellar tendon rupture: an alternative method, *Knee Surg Sports Trauma Arthrosc* 11(2):105-111, 2003.

6. Kelly DW, Carter VS, Jobe FW, Kerlan RK: Patellar and quadriceps tendon ruptures—jumper's knee, *Am J Sports Med* 12(5):375-380, 1984.

7. Kuechle DK, Stuart MJ: Isolated rupture of the patellar tendon in athletes, *Am J Sports Med* 22(5):692-695, 1994.

8. Podesta L, Sherman MF, Bonamo JR: Bilateral simultaneous rupture of the infrapatellar tendon in a recreational athlete, *Am J Sports Med* 19(3):325-327, 1991.

9. Rose PS, Frassica FJ: Atraumatic bilateral patellar tendon rupture, *J Bone Joint Surg* 83A(9):1382-1386, 2001.

10. Shah M: Simultaneous bilateral rupture of the quadriceps tendons: analysis of risk factors and associations, *South Med J* 95(8):860-866, 2002.

11. Whiting WC, Zernicke RF: *Biomechanics of musculoskeletal injury*, Champaign, IL, 1998, Human Kinetics.

12. Calvo E, Ferrer A, Robledo AG, et al: Bilateral simultaneous spontaneous quadriceps tendons rupture. A case report studied by magnetic resonance imaging, *Clin Imaging* 21:73-76, 1997.

13. Sandrey MA: Acute and chronic tendon injuries: factors affecting the healing response and treatment, *J Sport Rehabil* 12(1):70-91, 2003.

14. Kirkendall DT, Garrett WE: Function and biomechanics of tendons, *Scand J Med Sci Sports* 7:62-66, 1997.

15. Enad JG: Patella tendon ruptures, *South Med J* 92(6):563-566, 1999.

16. Ilan DI, Tejwani N, Keschner M, Leibman M: Quadriceps tendon rupture, *J Am Acad Orthop Surg* 11(3):192-200, 2003.

17. Kannus P, Jozsa L: Histopathological changes preceding spontaneous rupture of a tendon, *J Bone Joint Surg* 73A(10):1507-1525, 1991.

18. Bhole R, Johnson JC: Bilateral simultaneous spontaneous rupture of quadriceps tendon in a diabetic patient, *South Med J* 78(4):486, 1985.

19. Shah M: Simultaneous bilateral quadriceps tendon rupture in renal patients, *Clin Nephrol* 58(2):118-121, 2002.

20. Liow RYL, Tavares S: Bilateral rupture of the quadriceps tendon associated with anabolic steroids, *Br J Sports Med* 29(2):77-79, 1995.

21. Bhole R, Flynn JC, Marbury TC: Quadriceps tendon ruptures in uremia, *Clin Orthop* 195:200-206, 1985.

22. Clark SC, Jones MW, Choudhury RR, Smith E: Bilateral patellar tendon rupture secondary to repeated local steroid injections, *J Accident Emerg Med* 12:300-301, 1995.

23. Lombardi LJ, Cleri DJ, Epstein E: Bilateral spontaneous quadriceps tendon rupture in a patient with renal failure, *Orthopedics* 18(2):187-191, 1995.

24. Shah M: Outcomes in bilateral and simultaneous quadriceps tendon rupture, *Orthopedics* 26(8):797-798, 2003.

25. Kuo RS, Sonnabend DH: Simultaneous rupture of the patellar tendons bilaterally: case report and review of the literature, *J Trauma* 34(3):458-460, 1993.

26. Bhargava SP, Hynes MC, Dowell JK: Traumatic patella tendon rupture: early mobilization following surgical repair, *Injury* 35(1):76-79, 2004.

27. Scuderi GR: Quadriceps and patellar tendon disruptions. In Scott WN, editor: *The knee,* St Louis, 1994, Mosby.

28. Larson RV, Simonian PT: Semitendinosus augmentation of acute patellar tendon repair with immediate mobilization, *Am J Sports Med* 23(1):82-86, 1995.

29. Levy M, Goldstein J, Rosner M: A method of repair for quadriceps tendon or patellar ligament (tendon) ruptures without cast immobilization, *Clin Orthop Relat Res* 218:297-301, 1987.

30. Ravalin RV, Mazzocca AD, Grady-Benson JC, et al: Biomechanical comparison of patellar tendon repairs in a cadaver model. An evaluation of gap formation at the repair site with cyclic loading, *Am J Sports Med* 30:469-473, 2002.

31. Shelbourne KD, Darmelio MP, Klootwyk TE: Patellar tendon rupture repair using Dall-Miles cable, *Am J Knee Surg* 14(1):17-20, 2001.

32. Heiden EA: Tendinopathies about the knee. In Chapman MW, editor: *Chapman's orthopaedic surgery,* ed 3, Philadelphia, 2001, Lippincott Williams & Wilkins.

33. Witvrouw E, Lysens R, Bellemans J, et al: Open versus closed kinetic chain exercises for patellofemoral pain, *Am J Sports Med* 28(5):687-694, 2000.

34. Steinkamp LA, Dillingham MF, Markel MD, et al: Biomechanical considerations in patellofemoral joint rehabilitation, *Am J Sports Med* 21:438-446, 1993.

35. Malone TR, Davies GJ, Walsh WM: Muscular control of the patella, *Clin Sports Med* 21(3):349-362, 2002.

36. DeBaere T, Geulette B, Manche E, Barras L: Functional results after surgical repair of quadriceps tendon rupture, *Acta Orthop Belg* 68(2):146-149, 2002.

37. Marder RA, Timmerman LA: Primary repair of patellar tendon rupture without augmentation, *Am J Sports Med* 27:304-307, 1999.

38. Mandelbaum BR, Bartolozzi A, Carney B: Patellar tendon tears, *Clin Orthop Relat Res* 235:268-271, 1988.

39. Enad JG, Loomis LL: Patellar tendon repair: postoperative treatment, *Arch Phys Med Rehabil* 81(6):786-788, 2000.

40. DePalma MJ, Perkins RH: Patellar tendinosis: acute patellar tendon rupture and jumper's knee, *Phys Sports Med* 32(5):41-45, 2004.

Shoulder

Rehabilitation after Conservative and Operative Treatment of Acromioclavicular Joint Injuries

James W. Matheson, PT, DPT, MS, SCS, CSCS
Christopher R. Price, MD

CHAPTER OUTLINE

ACROMIOCLAVICULAR JOINT INJURIES

are common in today's athletic population. Young athletes who participate in such contact team sports as football, hockey, rugby, and soccer are at high risk for acromioclavicular joint injury. Furthermore, increased participation in noncontact recreational activities such as cycling, skiing, snowboarding, and skateboarding by "weekend warriors" has resulted in more individuals being susceptible to acromioclavicular joint injury.[1-8] Acromioclavicular joint injuries are five times more likely to occur in males than females and usually occur during the third decade of life.[9,10] The majority (2:1) of acromioclavicular injuries are incomplete rather than complete and, depending on the severity of the pathology, may be associated with significant pain, muscle weakness, and fatigue.[9,11] These are critical issues for sports medicine clinicians to consider when managing acromioclavicular joint injuries in all individuals, particularly those who participate in strenuous overhead athletic or work activities. Therefore physicians and rehabilitation professionals require a good understanding of the current operative techniques and rehabilitation concepts related to acromioclavicular joint pathology.

ANATOMY AND BIOMECHANICS OF THE ACROMIOCLAVICULAR JOINT

Osseous Anatomy

The acromioclavicular joint (Figure 26-1) is a diarthrodial synovial joint formed by the distal clavicle and the medial facet of the acromion. Together with the sternoclavicular joint, the acromioclavicular joint helps serve as the only true joint linkage between the upper extremity and the axial skeleton. The acromioclavicular joint articulation consists of the medial facet of the acromion and the distal end of the clavicle. The average articular surface has been described as being 9 by 19 mm in size[12] This is a relatively small area of contact when one considers the high forces placed on the joint during athletic activities such as throwing. The articular surfaces of the distal clavicle and the clavicular end of the acromion each undergo a change from hyaline cartilage to fibrocartilage around 17 and 23 years of age, respectively.[13] The joint congruency of the articular surfaces of the acromioclavicular joint varies significantly in the general population. Several different angles of joint inclination have been found in both the frontal and sagittal planes.[14] On examination of 100 random radiographs, Urist[15] found the clavicle to be in an overriding (49%), underriding (3%), vertical (27%), or incongruent (21%) orientation to the acromion. At present the research is limited on whether there is a relationship between joint inclination and disease.[16,17] Interposed inside the acromioclavicular joint is a fibrocartilaginous disk of variable size, shape, and completeness.[18-21] To observe the variation in disk morphology, Salter and colleagues[21] examined 53 acromioclavicular joints from 13 male and 14 female cadavers of individuals who died in their sixth or seventh decade of life. Their findings revealed 1 joint with a complete disk, 11 joints without disks, 16 joints with disk remnants, and 25 joints with meniscoid disks.[21] In general, it appears that the disk's function in the acromioclavicular joint is limited and that it undergoes rapid degeneration with aging.[18-21] This may be related to the fact that the acromioclavicular joint space itself is on average 1 to 3 mm in width and also decreases with age.[22]

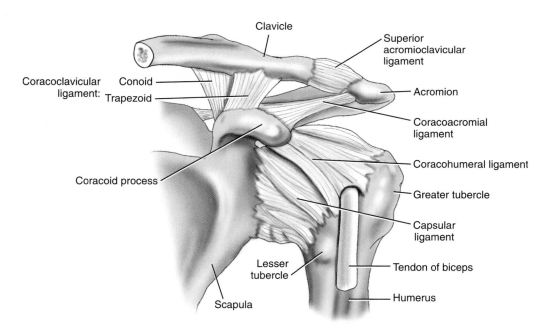

Figure 26-1: Anatomy of the acromioclavicular joint. *(From Gray H: Anatomy of the human body, Philadelphia, 1918, Lea & Febiger. Internet document available at www.bartleby.com [accessed 2000].)*

Stabilizing Structures of the Acromioclavicular Joint

The acromioclavicular joint is stabilized by both static and dynamic stabilizers. The static stabilizers consist of the acromioclavicular joint capsule, the acromioclavicular ligaments (superior, inferior, anterior, and posterior), the coracoclavicular ligaments (trapezoid and conoid), and the coracoacromial ligament. The middle deltoid and upper trapezius muscles provide dynamic stabilization of the acromioclavicular joint.

The joint capsule of the acromioclavicular joint is thin and is supported on all sides by the four acromioclavicular ligaments. This capsule-ligamentous complex is the primary restraint to posterior displacement and posterior axial rotation of the distal clavicle.[23] The inferior ligament is difficult to identify on cadaveric dissection and the superior ligament appears more pronounced and thicker.[21,24] Fibers from the superior ligament also tie directly into the fascia of the deltoid and trapezius muscles, adding to the stability of the acromioclavicular joint.[21] Klimkiewicz and colleagues[25] determined that the superior ligament contributes more than twice the resistance to posterior displacement of the distal clavicle as compared with the posterior ligament. When the integrity of the superior and posterior ligaments is disrupted, such as following injury or surgical resection, posterior restraint is lost and the posterolateral distal clavicle may abut against the anterior surface of the spine of the scapula.

The coracoclavicular ligament complex consists of the posteromedial conoid ligament and the anterolateral trapezoid ligament. These two ligaments provide vertical stability to the clavicle. Several studies have examined the insertion locations of these two ligaments on the distal clavicle.[24,26,27] Based on their results, it appears that the insertion of the trapezoid is variable and on average 9 to 16 mm from the articular surface of the distal clavicle.[24,26] This is important to consider when performing a lateral clavicle resection in the patient with acromioclavicular joint pathology. Excessive resection greater than 10 to 15 mm may violate the trapezoid ligament and lead to acromioclavicular instability. The trapezoid ligament prevents axial compression of the clavicle against the acromion with either high or low displacements of the distal clavicle. In contrast, the degree of anterior or superior clavicular restraint provided by the conoid ligament is displacement dependent. Fukuda and colleagues[23] have shown that with small displacements the conoid ligament acts as a secondary restraint to the acromioclavicular ligaments in resisting superior translation. However, with greater displacement of the clavicle, the conoid ligament becomes the primary restraint to superior and anterior displacement.[23] Recently, other researchers have demonstrated that one cannot consider the actions of the acromioclavicular and coracoclavicular ligaments in isolation.[23,28,29] It appears that the noncontractile stabilizers of the acromioclavicular joint act in a synergistic manner. Injury to one stabilizing structure will shift load onto another structure, which may or may not

be able to compensate. This concept is important to consider when determining surgical reconstruction and stabilization of the acromioclavicular joint.

Compared with the acromioclavicular joint capsule and the acromioclavicular and coracoclavicular ligaments, the coracoacromial ligament contributes little directly to the stability of the acromioclavicular joint. Salter and colleagues[21] demonstrated that the coracoacromial ligament was directly confluent with fibers of the inferior capsule of the acromioclavicular joint and therefore contributes indirectly to joint stability.[30] The coracoacromial ligament also serves as a secondary static glenohumeral joint stabilizer, limiting anterior and inferior motion of the humeral head in individuals with a history of chronic rotator cuff arthropathy.[21,30,31] As will be discussed later, the greatest contribution of the coracoacromial ligament to acromioclavicular joint instability has been the role it has played in surgical reconstructions of the acromioclavicular joint.[32]

Besides static ligamentous stabilization, the acromioclavicular joint receives dynamic stability from the middle deltoid and upper trapezius muscles. They contribute significantly to acromioclavicular joint stability via their attachments to the distal clavicle and superior capsuloligamentous complex. This is apparent in overhead activities, such as pitching, in which these muscles are active during the cocking phase.[33,34]

Motion at the Acromioclavicular Joint

In Inman and co-workers' classic article[35] on the biomechanics of the shoulder joint, it was determined that 40 to 50 degrees of upward rotation occurred at the clavicle during complete elevation of the shoulder. This was determined by the use of a percutaneous pin drilled into the clavicle of a volunteer. They also observed that when the pin was held manually, shoulder elevation was limited to 110 degrees. Inman and co-workers[35] concluded that rigid fixation of the acromioclavicular joint after dislocation would limit postoperative axial rotation. However, surgeons using rigid fixation methods to stabilize the acromioclavicular joint have reported greater than 165 degrees of elevation postoperatively.[9,36,37] To answer this question, Rockwood and colleagues[9,37] placed Kirschner wires into both the clavicle and acromion and repeated the original work of Inman and co-workers.[35] It was determined that the clavicular pin did indeed rotate 40 to 50 degrees; however, when observing the pins placed in the scapula, a relative difference of only 5 to 8 degrees of rotation occurred.[9,37] Clinically this implies that rigid fixation of the acromioclavicular joint may not cause a loss of shoulder range of motion (ROM). However, the 5 to 8 degrees of motion that remains may explain why, in some cases of rigid fixation, hardware migration or failure has occurred.[31,38,39] In addition one must consider that these in vivo studies were single-subject designs using two-dimensional radiographs for correlation. Recently, new technology allowing three-dimensional analysis of clavicular motion has demonstrated that a better understanding of clavicular kinematics is needed.[40]

MECHANISM OF ACROMIOCLAVICULAR JOINT INJURY

Acromioclavicular joint injury can be secondary to either direct or indirect trauma. The most common mechanism of injury is one of direct force (Figure 26-2, *A*). It is a result of the patient falling on the point of the shoulder onto the ground or a firm object with the arm in an adducted position. This is consistent with the typical mechanism of injury observed in hockey, football, and rugby players.[3] The direct-contact force drives the acromion medially and inferiorly in relation to the clavicle. If no fracture occurs, the clavicle remains in its normal anatomic position because of an interlocking of the sternoclavicular ligaments as described by Bearn.[41] As the scapula is driven further medially and inferiorly, an injury of propagation occurs. First the acromioclavicular ligaments and joint capsule are stretched and torn. If the downward force is large enough, the coracoclavicular ligaments stretch and tear, followed by damage to the deltoid and trapezius muscles, fascia, and overlying skin. Once the acromioclavicular and coracoclavicular ligaments are torn, the integrity of the structural suspension system of the upper extremity on the trunk is lost. The weight of the upper extremity pulls the shoulder downward and away from the distal end of the clavicle. This results in the visible step-off deformity observed during examination of the patient.

Indirect trauma, such as a fall on an outstretched arm or elbow, may also result in acromioclavicular injury (Figure 26-2, *B*). In this case an upward force is transmitted through the humeral head into the acromion process. This disrupts the acromioclavicular ligaments in isolation because the coracoclavicular ligaments are not under tension. With this mechanism of injury, fractures of the acromion and glenohumeral joint and rotator cuff pathology should be ruled out.[9]

CLASSIFICATION OF ACROMIOCLAVICULAR JOINT INJURIES

The pathoanatomy of acromioclavicular dislocation was first classified by Cadenat in 1917.[42] This system recognized two types of injuries, complete or incomplete, based on the integrity of the acromioclavicular and coracoclavicular ligaments. In the 1960s, Tossy and co-workers[43] and Allman[44] expanded this original system to include three categories of injury. This classification scheme divided Cadenat's incomplete classification into a type I and type II level of injury. In 1984, Rockwood and colleagues[37] expanded the Tossy and Allman type III classification into types III through VI based on the direction and amount of clavicular displacement (Figure 26-3). At present, this is the most accepted classification system in the literature. Table 26-1 describes each of the six types of injury in detail based on ligamentous and radiographic findings.[9,11,37,45,46]

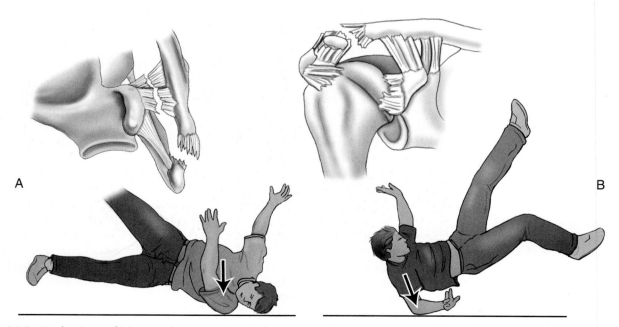

Figure 26-2: Mechanisms of injury to the acromioclavicular joint. **A,** Classic mechanism of direct downward force onto the point of the shoulder. **B,** An indirect force through an outstretched hand or elbow may also cause acromioclavicular joint injury. *(From Beim GM: Acromioclavicular joint injuries, J Athl Train 35[3]:261-267, 2000.)*

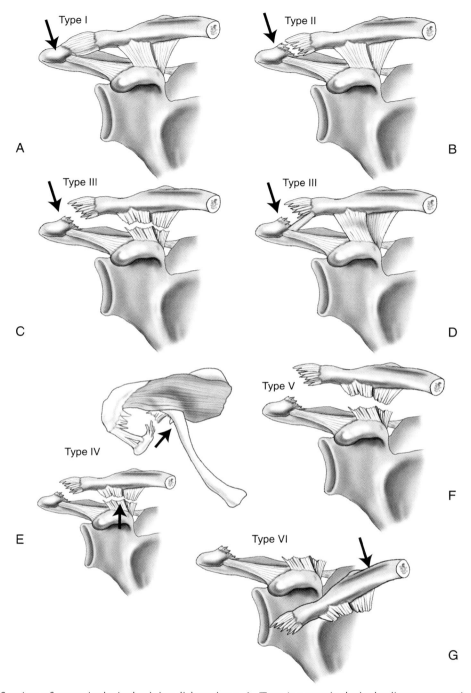

Figure 26-3: Classification of acromioclavicular joint dislocations. **A,** Type I: acromioclavicular ligament sprain. **B,** Type II: disruption of acromioclavicular joint capsule. **C,** Type III: disruption of both the acromioclavicular and coracoclavicular ligaments. **D,** Type III: displacement of the distal clavicle through a tear in the periosteal tube of the clavicle. This may occur in children. Note that the acromioclavicular and coracoclavicular ligaments are still attached to the periosteum. **E,** Type IV: disruption of the acromioclavicular and coracoclavicular ligaments with posterior displacement of the distal clavicle into the trapezius muscle fibers. **F,** Type V: disruption of the acromioclavicular and coracoclavicular ligaments with superior displacement of the distal clavicle. **G,** Type VI: disruption of the acromioclavicular and coracoclavicular ligaments with inferior displacement of the distal clavicle to the coracoid process. *(From Beim GM: Acromioclavicular joint injuries,* J Athl Train *35[3]:261-267, 2000.)*

TABLE 26-1

Descriptions of Acromioclavicular Joint Injury by Rockwood Classifications I through VI

TYPE	AC LIGAMENTS	CC LIGAMENTS	DELTOID AND TRAPEZIUS ATTACHMENTS	RADIOGRAPHIC FINDINGS		CLAVICULAR INSTABILITY
				WIDTH OF AC JOINT	WIDTH OF CC INTERSPACE	
Type I	Intact (sprain)	Intact	Intact	Normal	None	None
Type II	Torn	Intact (sprain)	Intact	Some widening Less than 4 mm or 40% difference	A downward displacement of scapula may be evident	Horizontal
Type III*	Torn	Torn	Detached from distal end of clavicle	Dislocated completely	CC space increases 25%-100%; clavicle may tent the skin	Horizontal and vertical
Type IV	Torn	Torn	Detached from distal end of clavicle	Dislocated completely	Clavicle is displaced posterior into or through trapezius muscle belly; therefore may appear equal to uninvolved shoulder	Horizontal and vertical
Type V	Torn	Torn	Detached from distal half of clavicle	Dislocated completely	CC space increases 100%-300%; clavicle may tent the skin	Horizontal and vertical
Type VI†	Torn	Torn in subcoracoid type and intact in subacromial type	Detached from distal clavicle	Dislocated completely	Clavicle displaced inferior to either acromion or coracoid process; CC interspace is reversed with subcoracoid type or decreased if subacromial type	May be lodged under coracoid

*Variants of type III may exist, including pseudodislocation through an intact periosteal tube of the clavicle, physeal injury, or fracture of the coracoid process.
†Extremely rare injury requiring severe trauma. Type VI dislocations are often associated with multiple fractures and brachial plexus injury.
AC, Acromioclavicular; *CC,* coracoclavicular.

EVALUATION OF THE PATIENT WITH ACROMIOCLAVICULAR JOINT INJURY

To be able to correctly classify the type of acromioclavicular injury, determine the appropriate course of nonoperative or operative management, and provide the patient with a prognosis, a thorough initial examination should be performed.

History and Examination

The initial interview with the patient should focus on the mechanism of injury. Was it a direct or an indirect force? Did the patient feel structures tear? Was there an audible pop? Does or could the patient have open growth plates? Has the patient injured this shoulder before? Is there a possibility of an associated head or cervical spine injury? Where is the pain located? Gerber and colleagues[47] mapped the pain referral pattern of the acromioclavicular joint by injecting subjects' acromioclavicular joints with a hypertonic saline solution. Subjects reported pain in the area directly over the acromioclavicular joint and also in the anterolateral neck, upper trapezius, and anterolateral deltoid.[47] Any reports of paresthesias or other neurologic symptoms should be addressed immediately. Neurovascular status may be compromised in type V and VI injuries. The patient's age, occupation, level of sports participation, and recreational activities are important aspects to consider when determining the appropriate interventions.

To best examine the patient, he or she should be placed in a seated position with clothing removed to completely expose both shoulders. The physical examination should begin with a visual inspection of both shoulders. Observations of the patient from superior, anterior, and lateral views are necessary to determine if a step-off deformity or posterior clavicular displacement is present. A neurovascular evaluation of the patient, including checking distal pulses at the wrist, capillary refill in the digits, and gross sensation testing, is performed. If neurovascular status is compromised, it represents a medical emergency and the patient should be transported to a medical facility immediately. Palpation of the bony structures, including the acromion, acromioclavicular joint, clavicle, sternoclavicular joint, and coracoid process, is necessary to test for fractures. Following bony palpation, palpation of both the contractile and noncontractile tissues near the acromioclavicular joint and coracoclavicular interspace should be carried out in order to inspect for swelling, tenderness, and tissue defects. If a dislocation of the acromioclavicular joint is apparent, gentle manual distal clavicular mobilization may be attempted in an effort to assess end feel and determine the degree of instability. This is performed by supporting the ipsilateral arm and manually depressing the distal clavicle.[11] In a type IV dislocation, the clavicle has perforated the deltotrapezial fascia and may be hooked or caught in the muscle fibers of the trapezius. In this case, manual reduction of the clavicle will not be possible. In addition, palpation, ROM assessment, and manual muscle testing of the cervical spine and distal upper extremity should be performed to rule out and clear these areas of involvement. Finally, depending on the acuteness and severity of the injury, ROM measurements and specific orthopedic special tests should be carried out. Acromioclavicular joint special tests that have been described in the literature include the cross-arm adduction stress test, O'Brien's active compression test, the Paxinos test, the acromioclavicular anterior-posterior shear test, and the acromioclavicular resisted extension test.[48-52] Recent research has examined the usefulness of these tests in assessing acromioclavicular joint pathology and has determined that a combination of several tests is more diagnostic than one special test used in isolation.[53]

Radiographic Evaluation of the Acromioclavicular Joint

Radiographs for evaluation of the injured acromioclavicular joint include anteroposterior, scapular Y, and lateral axillary views.[46,54] For anteroposterior views the subject should be standing with the injured arm resting at the side without support. If there are any doubts on the degree of injury, views of the uninjured shoulder could be easily obtained for normative comparison. If the acromioclavicular joint is superimposed on the spine of the scapula or the acromioclavicular radiograph is too dark, a Zanca view with reduced exposure (kilovoltage) is recommended.[9,11,31,46,55,56] The Zanca view involves taking a standing anteroposterior view with a 10- to 15-degree cephalic tilt of the radiograph beam.[56] Axillary lateral views are required to examine any posterior displacement of the clavicle. This view is taken with the arm abducted 70 to 90 degrees and the radiographic beam directed cranially. In the past, stress radiographs of the acromioclavicular joint have been described. However, investigators have determined that they are largely unnecessary and do not correlate with the surgeon's decision to perform a surgical reconstruction.[57-59] Therefore they are not routinely used in current practice. Other radiographic views may be necessary to adequately examine the patient with suspected acromioclavicular pathology. If the patient has a normal coracoclavicular interspace but a complete acromioclavicular dislocation, a fracture of the coracoid should be suspected. A Stryker notch view is recommended in this situation.[31,60] In addition, patients with open growth plates or individuals who have suffered severe or multiple trauma may require further imaging studies. In these cases and others, additional radiographic views, computed tomography, or magnetic resonance imaging may be necessary to rule out physeal injuries, occult fractures, and other soft tissue and bony lesions.[60,61]

Normal radiographic values vary significantly for the acromioclavicular joint. In his review of 1000 cases, Zanca[56] reported a variable acromioclavicular joint width of between 1 and 3 mm. However, because the joint width diminishes with age, a width of 0.5 mm in an individual greater than 60 years of age should be considered normal.[19] The coracoclavicular interspace also exhibits variability in the general population. The original work of Bosworth,[62] reporting a distance of 11 and 13 mm, is commonly cited in the literature. The variability in these joint and interspace numbers illustrates the importance of comparison with the contralateral acromioclavicular joint whenever possible.

TREATMENT OF ACROMIOCLAVICULAR JOINT INJURIES

Review of the current literature reveals that in most cases, type I and II injuries are treated conservatively and type IV, V, and VI injuries are treated operatively. Treatment of type III injuries remains controversial, and several opinions exist on whether immediate surgery, delayed surgery, or conservative treatment in type III injuries is appropriate. Detailed treatment interventions for each classification of acromioclavicular joint injury are described here. It is important to recognize that acromioclavicular injuries occur on a continuum and the severity of injury will vary within the six different Rockwood classifications.

Type I

Type I injuries involve minimal damage to the acromioclavicular joint and surrounding structures. They can be treated conservatively with a sling, cryotherapy, relative rest, and nonsteroidal antiinflammatory drugs (NSAIDs). The sling is used to reduce stress to the joint for several days; length of use is dictated by the patient's symptoms. Most athletes with type I acromioclavicular injuries return to full activities 2 weeks from the date of injury.[9,11,31] An over-the-counter orthosis (Figure 26-4) or a soft felt or gel doughnut pad may be used under shoulder pads in football or hockey players to

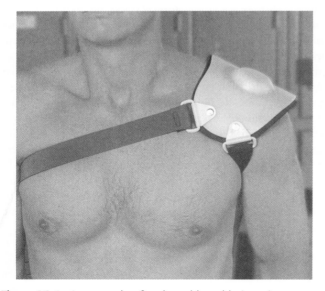

Figure 26-4: An example of pad used by athletic trainers to protect the acromioclavicular joint in contact sports. *(Photo of the IMPACT AC Pad was provided courtesy of Arthron, Inc., at www.sportsinjuries.com.)*

reduce the risk of reinjury from a second impact to the acromion.[54,63] Full pain-free active ROM, no joint tenderness with palpation, and strength within 10% of the uninvolved shoulder are criteria that may be used in the decision to return to sport activities. It is suspected that many athletes with type I injuries never seek medical attention.[64]

Refractory pain following type I acromioclavicular injuries is usually a result of degenerative changes within the joint. This may be a result of the most recent injury or a culmination of a history of minor injuries, physical labor, or sports participation. In any case, if pain remains after several weeks of analgesics and rest, a steroid injection into the acromioclavicular joint may reduce discomfort.[65] If physical therapy, steroid injections, and active rest fail to resolve the patient's pain and loss of function, a distal clavicle excision may be performed. The open distal clavicle resection originally described by both Mumford and Gurd over six decades ago has been the "gold standard" for surgical treatment of acromioclavicular joint pathology.[66-68] In the past two decades arthroscopic resection of the distal clavicle has also become popular and has been shown to have comparable outcomes.[69-74] Both open and closed procedures require adequate clavicle excision to decompress the acromioclavicular joint (4 to 10 mm) in order to avoid leaving bone to impact the joint or removing too much bone and risking joint instability.[68] The choice of an open or closed distal clavicle excision depends on the experience and training of the surgeon, as well as individual patient characteristics. Both arthroscopic resection and open resection of the distal clavicle have allowed patients to return to physically demanding occupations or sports with minimal loss of strength or upper extremity ROM.[63,75]

Type II

Type II injuries involve disruption of the acromioclavicular joint capsule and ligaments resulting in widening of the joint space and a downward displacement of the scapula (see Figure 26-3 and Table 26-2). The soft tissue trauma sustained in type II injuries is more extensive than in type I injuries. Therefore the initial time frame of immobilization and rest of the involved extremity is longer. As with a type I injury, initial treatment involves protection with a sling, relative rest, and analgesics.[9,32,37,44,64,76] Unlike type I injuries, type II injuries may demonstrate a visible step-off deformity and more degenerative changes because of the increased sagittal plane instability caused by disruption of the acromioclavicular capsuloligamentous complex.[76,77] A supervised rehabilitation program is necessary to ensure that goals of return to preinjury levels of strength and function are accomplished. Walsh and colleagues[78] noted that deficits in horizontal adduction strength may persist as late as 3 years following a type II injury. A supervised rehabilitation program with objective strength testing throughout the patient's rehabilitation may help prevent and measure objectively these types of chronic strength deficits.

TABLE 26-2

Nonoperative Rehabilitation Protocol for Type II and Type III Acromioclavicular Joint Injuries (Phases I and II)

	PHASE I: PROTECTION AND MOTION PHASE	PHASE II: INTERMEDIATE PHASE (INITIAL STRENGTHENING)
	WEEKS 1 TO 2 FOR TYPE II OR WEEKS 1 TO 3 FOR TYPE III*	WEEKS 3 TO 4 FOR TYPE II OR WEEKS 4 TO 6 FOR TYPE III
Goals (May not progress to next phase until goals are met)	Full pain-free scaption† AROM to approximately 140 degrees Equal lateral rotation ROM to contralateral side Measured in a seated position with arm in 30 degrees of abduction Minimal pain and tenderness with palpation of the AC joint Able to perform pain-free maximal multiangle (less than 90 degrees) isometric contractions in glenohumeral flexion, extension, abduction, adduction, medial rotation, and lateral rotation	Full pain-free AROM equal to the contralateral side No pain or tenderness with palpation Less than 25% deficit with handheld dynamometer testing of middle deltoid and upper trapezius Less than 10% deficit to contralateral shoulder with testing of medial and lateral rotators
Precautions	Avoid supine ROM (see text), No heavy lifting, pushing/pulling No contact sports No resisted overhead motion greater than 90 degrees Restrict horizontal extension and flexion ROM No PROM/AAROM/AROM into pain Avoid traction through upper extremity	Avoid supine exercises (see text) No heavy lifting, pushing/pulling No contact sports No resisted overhead motion greater than 90 degrees No resisted horizontal extension and flexion Avoid military or bench press Avoid traction through upper extremity
Interventions		
Protection	Fit with AC (Kenny-Howard) sling for comfort and to prevent downward displacement of scapula Taping for pain relief and protection (not done for anatomic reduction)	Wean from splint as tolerated Taping for pain relief and protection
Modalities	Cryotherapy Electrical stimulation modalities for pain control and neuromuscular reeducation	Cryotherapy following exercise Electrical stimulation modalities for pain control and neuromuscular reeducation May use heat for warm-up, stretching, and pain relief
ROM	Elbow and wrist AROM PROM in seated or side-lying position Begin AAROM exercises with wand or T-bar Begin gentle AROM exercises in pain-free ROM	Full AROM, all planes

TABLE 26-2

Nonoperative Rehabilitation Protocol for Type II and Type III Acromioclavicular Joint Injuries (Phases I and II)—cont'd

	PHASE I: PROTECTION AND MOTION PHASE	PHASE II: INTERMEDIATE PHASE (INITIAL STRENGTHENING)
	WEEKS 1 TO 2 FOR TYPE II OR WEEKS 1 TO 3 FOR TYPE III*	WEEKS 3 TO 4 FOR TYPE II OR WEEKS 4 TO 6 FOR TYPE III
Strengthening	Initiate trial of submaximal shoulder isometrics in all planes and at multiple angles at the beginning of week 2	Initiate trial of short-arc isotonic strengthening exercises
	Progress intensity of isometrics as tolerated by symptoms and visual analog scale pain rating less than 2/10 or 3/10	Progress ROM as tolerated by symptoms
	Forearm and hand intrinsic strengthening with putty or squeeze ball	Progress resistance as defined by symptoms, scapular control, and quality of motion
	Begin pain-free AAROM and AROM scapular retraction and protraction	Strengthening exercises should include the following exercises with individualized ROM modifications based on severity and irritability of patient's injury:
	May continue lower extremity and uninvolved upper extremity exercises	Seated chest press with plus (limit ROM)
	Initiate core trunk stability exercises	Seated row (limit ROM)
		Scaption limited to 90 degrees elevation
		Bent-over horizontal abduction (no resistance, AROM only)
		Shoulder flexion limited to 90 degrees elevation
		Shoulder shrugs (avoid traction force)
		Lateral and medial rotation strengthening
		Biceps and triceps strengthening (avoid traction force)
		Core trunk stability exercises
		With all dumbbell exercises, care should be taken to avoid traction force through upper extremity
Neuromuscular reeducation exercises	Submaximal rhythmic stabilizations	Progress side-lying rhythmic stabilizations in all planes of the scapula and up to 90 degrees scaption of the glenohumeral joint
	Slow speed	Moderate speed
	Known pattern	More random pattern
	Submaximal resistance	Moderate resistance
	Perform in side-lying position	
Assessment		
Clinical testing	Weekly AROM measurements	Weekly AROM measurements
	Seated isometric strength tests end of week 2 (type II) and end of week 3 (type III)	Strength testing at end of phase
		Isokinetic testing
		Handheld dynamometer testing

*The number of weeks suggested in this table is only a guideline. Determination of when to advance the patient to the next phase of the protocol is based on objective measurements and reported symptoms. Some patients may advance faster or slower than others. Quality of injured tissue, patient characteristics, and clinical testing and measurements should determine protocol advancement.
†Elevation in the plane of the scapula.
AAROM, Active-assistive range of motion; *AC,* acromioclavicular; *AROM,* active range of motion; *PROM,* passive range of motion; *ROM,* range of motion.

Immobilization, Strapping, and Bracing after Acromioclavicular Injury

A review of the literature reveals that nonoperative treatment of type II and III acromioclavicular joint injuries has involved two distinct treatment protocols.[9] The first protocol involves an attempted closed reduction of the distal clavicle using a sling and harness, adhesive strapping, crotch loops or casts, or plaster casts for a prolonged period of time. The purpose of these acromioclavicular braces is to maintain continuous pressure under the elbow and on the top of the distal clavicle for approximately 6 weeks to accomplish a closed reduction of the clavicular deformity. A current acromioclavicular sling, or Kenny-Howard sling, is shown in Figure 26-5. The difficulty with this type of prolonged bracing is twofold. First, compliance in wearing the orthosis is usually a problem. Second, authors have reported episodes of skin breakdown and nerve compression injuries from prolonged brace use.[79] In the second protocol, considered the standard of care today, closed anatomic reduction is not attempted. Instead, the residual deformity is ignored and short-term sling use and early ROM are recommended. This method has been referred to in the literature as one of "skillful neglect."[9,80,81] Acromioclavicular slings and taping may still be used in type II and III injuries following a "skillful neglect" protocol. Here the purpose of the acromioclavicular sling and taping becomes one of pain relief versus anatomic reduction. In addition to

bracing, taping may also help reduce the patient's symptoms. Shamus and Shamus[82] have described a taping technique that significantly reduced pain and improved function in two patients following acromioclavicular injury.

Type III

The management of type III acromioclavicular joints remains controversial. Type III injuries involve complete disruption of the acromioclavicular joint capsule and coracoclavicular ligaments. Instability is present in both the horizontal and vertical planes. It is also important to recognize that a type III classification is also the classification that represents a transition from conservative to surgical care. One hypothesis as to why the controversy exists is related to the sensitivity of the classification system. Perhaps subcategories of type III injuries need to be developed.

In 1974, Powers and Bach[83] documented surgical intervention in 92% of 116 Tossy type III injuries. The surgical procedure of choice was pin fixation of the acromioclavicular joint. In contrast, in 1992, a survey study by Cox[84] reported that 72% of residency chairpersons and 86% of professional team physicians were recommending nonoperative treatment in Rockwood type III injuries. Cox's survey also demonstrated that surgical fixation had also changed, with the majority of surgeons using fixation between the clavicle and coracoid. In 1998, Phillips and colleagues[85] performed a meta-analysis review of the literature. They found a total of 24 research studies that met their inclusion criteria. Only five of these studies involved a direct comparison of nonsurgical and surgical treatment. However, these studies are difficult to interpret because of the large number of different surgical interventions described and the differences in each study's postoperative protocol and long-term follow-up. Regardless, Phillips and colleagues[85] were able to review 1171 patients, 833 of whom underwent acromioclavicular surgery. They determined that in terms of overall satisfaction, ROM, and strength, conservative treatment is recommended over surgical management of type III injuries. The only advantage of surgery according to their report was the potential reduction of the clavicular step-off deformity.[85] Recently, Bradley and Elkousy[86] have written a concise review of the current literature surrounding this controversy. They reiterate that no perfect prospective randomized study currently exists that demonstrates the superiority of surgical or nonsurgical treatment. They, like Phillips and co-workers,[85] state the need for a large multicenter trial that has enough statistical power to resolve this continuing controversy.[85,86]

Other issues surrounding the decision for operative management include timing of the surgery and the patient's occupation or sport. Larsen and colleagues[87] found operative treatment to be best for patients who perform heavy physical work. Several authors have suggested that acute surgical treatment is warranted in cases where the injury involves the dominant arm of a professional pitcher.[9,37,63] On the other

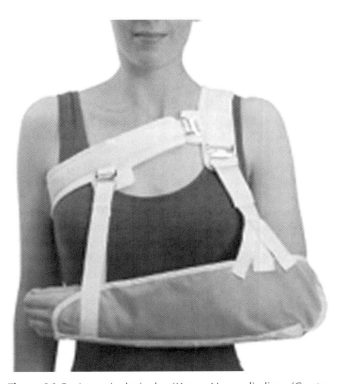

Figure 26-5: Acromioclavicular (Kenny-Howard) sling. *(Courtesy of dj Orthopedics, Inc., www.djortho.com/products/ProCare/details. asp?id=268.)*

hand, studies demonstrate that full return to sport in this elite population is possible following conservative treatment.[88,89] Timing of acromioclavicular surgery in type III injuries is also an important consideration.[90,91] Weinstein and colleagues[92] published a retrospective paper comparing early (less than 3 weeks) and late (greater than 3 weeks) surgical intervention in type III injuries. A modified Weaver-Dunn procedure using suture augmentation of the coracoclavicular interspace was the most common procedure used. Their results demonstrated a trend toward improved results in the early intervention group and a significant improvement in satisfaction when the early group was compared with patients who underwent surgery greater than 3 months after injury.[92]

In summary, the research literature has yet to provide sufficient evidence supporting the benefit of operative treatment over conservative treatment. However, general consensus appears to be that regardless of occupation or sport, conservative treatment is suggested for the first 12 weeks. If substantial disability, deformity, or loss of function is present at this time, surgical intervention is warranted.[86] Unlike a type II injury, in which distal clavicle excision is the standard of care, type III injuries also require stabilization of the distal clavicle. Occupation, sport, and surgical timing are other important variables to consider when making the decision to aggressively or conservatively manage these injuries.

Types IV, V, and VI

Because of the marked persistent displacement of the distal clavicle and clavicular stripping of the deltotrapezial fascia, operative intervention is generally recommended to a patient with a type IV, V, or VI injury.[9,31,37,64,92]

NONOPERATIVE MANAGEMENT OF ACROMIOCLAVICULAR JOINT INJURY

Conservative treatment of type II and III acromioclavicular injuries requires the patient's participation in a supervised rehabilitation program. The number of rehabilitation visits depends on the severity of the initial injury and the patient's ability to meet the rehabilitation goals.

A four-phase rehabilitation program for the nonoperative treatment of acromioclavicular joint injuries has been described by Gladstone and colleagues.[91] Phase I consists of pain control and immediate protected ROM. Isometrics are also initiated in this phase. During phase II, exercises are advanced with the addition of isotonic strengthening exercises. Phase III of the protocol initiates dynamic strengthening exercises to ensure the patient reaches goals of returning strength, power, endurance, and neuromuscular control to a preinjury level. Finally, phase IV returns the athlete or laborer to his or her prior sport or occupation with sport-specific drills.[91] The goals of any acromioclavicular rehabilitation

program are to achieve a pain-free shoulder with full ROM, full strength, and no functional limitations. However, one should realize that the demands placed on the rehabilitated shoulder after discharge from therapy will vary significantly from patient to patient. What is satisfactory for the sedentary 30-year-old computer programmer may not be a good outcome for the 60-year-old carpenter or the 22-year-old collegiate pitcher. Therefore rehabilitation protocols will have to be modified on an individual basis to best meet the needs of each patient. This illustrates the importance of determining and discussing the rehabilitation goals with the patient during his or her initial evaluation. A sample rehabilitation protocol for the nonoperative treatment of type II and III acromioclavicular joint injuries is shown in Tables 26-2 and 26-3.

Davies Resistive Exercise Continuum

The issue of determining when to progress the patient's ROM and strength training exercises is both an art and a challenge. All too often, clinicians rely solely on past experience and "cookbook"-type protocols when working with a patient. This type of method lacks significant evidence and objective measurement. To reduce the guesswork involved in progressing a patient through a resistive exercise program, Davies[93] has developed a resistive exercise continuum. This continuum can assist the rehabilitation professional in advancing the patient's exercise load and intensity in a logical, systematic manner (Figure 26-6).[93]

The patient's progression through the resistive exercise continuum is dictated by continual reassessment of the patient's subjective symptoms and objective measurements of ROM and strength.[93] Davies recommends continually monitoring these symptoms and measurements during the rehabilitation program. To advance a patient's program, a trial treatment of the desired exercise is administered. The following is an example of how the continuum might be used for a patient with an acromioclavicular injury. If the patient is able to complete 100% of his or her maximal external rotation isometrics on Monday without difficulty, on Wednesday a trial of 50% maximal isometrics and 50% short-arc isokinetics is performed. If isokinetic equipment is not available, a trial of short-arc isotonic exercise is performed instead. After this trial treatment the patient is reassessed using a subjective, objective, assessment, and plan (SOAP) format. If there is no increase in symptoms with the trial of short-arc isotonic external rotation, on Friday, during the patient's next visit, he or she will complete 100% of the external rotation exercise using the trial resistance and ROM from Wednesday's treatment. However, if the patient has any adverse effects during or after the new exercise, the patient continues his or her current exercise program at the prior level of intensity and load. The new exercise is withheld and not added until after the next successful trial.[93]

TABLE 26-3

Nonoperative Rehabilitation Protocol for Type II and III Acromioclavicular Joint Injuries (Phases III and IV)

	PHASE III: DYNAMIC STRENGTHENING PHASE	PHASE IV: RETURN TO ACTIVITY PHASE
	WEEKS 5 TO 6 FOR TYPE II OR WEEKS 6 TO 8 FOR TYPE III*	WEEKS 7 TO 8 FOR TYPE II OR WEEKS 8 TO 10 FOR TYPE III
Goals (May not progress to next phase until goals are met)	No pain or tenderness with palpation Less than 10% deficit with handheld dynamometer testing of deltoid and upper trapezius Ability to perform several repetitions of specific sport task without pain or instability No observed scapular dyskinesias	No functional deficits when compared with uninvolved extremity Isokinetic testing of medial and lateral rotation and horizontal flexion and extension within 10% of normative data and contralateral extremity Independent in home strengthening program Discharge from rehabilitation
Precautions	Avoid supine ROM (see text) Caution when performing military or bench press Suggest modifying ROM and arc of motion to limit AC joint stress Suggest alternative exercises No heavy lifting, pushing/pulling No contact sports Avoid traction through upper extremity	Avoid excessive traction through upper extremity with repetitive work or sport activity
Interventions		
Protection	Padding and protection for work or sport if necessary	Padding and protection for work or sport if necessary
Modalities	Cryotherapy as needed following exercise May use heat for warm-up, stretching, and pain relief	Cryotherapy as needed following exercise May use heat for warm-up, stretching, and pain relief
ROM	Begin some repetitive overhead motion without resistance (only if necessary for work tasks or sport) Establish home program of stretching if necessary to maintain ROM	No changes
Strengthening	Progress resistance and increase ROM of all exercises from phase II Progress to strengthening in all planes of motion based on symptoms Begin supervised horizontal extension and flexion resistance exercises Progress resistance based on trial treatments with short-arc isotonics Progress to overhead strengthening (90/90 position) based on trial treatments with short-arc isotonics	Continue with a core program based on specific demands of vocation or sport Use periodization principles

TABLE 26-3

Nonoperative Rehabilitation Protocol for Type II and III Acromioclavicular Joint Injuries (Phases III and IV)—cont'd

	PHASE III: DYNAMIC STRENGTHENING PHASE	PHASE IV: RETURN TO ACTIVITY PHASE
	WEEKS 5 TO 6 FOR TYPE II OR WEEKS 6 TO 8 FOR TYPE III*	WEEKS 7 TO 8 FOR TYPE II OR WEEKS 8 TO 10 FOR TYPE III
Neuromuscular reeducation exercises	Advance to diagonal (PNF) patterns of motion Increase speed and intensity of exercises Initiate submaximal upper extremity plyometrics using minimal resistance and control parameters of bilateral to unilateral, partial to full ROM, low to high speed, and low to high repetitions and resistance	Advance exercises from phase III by decreasing clinician control and increasing exercise intensity Advance plyometrics drills to incorporate demands of sport or work activity
Activity specific	Initiate work conditioning and simulated work tasks Perform work-site evaluation Initiate return to throwing program Initiate sport-specific drills Initiate preparation for closed kinetic chain upper extremity functional test	Sport-specific testing Trial return to sport or activity Continue return to throwing program
Assessment		
Clinical testing	Strength testing at end of phase Assessment of abilities or deficits with work or sport activities (these deficits will be focus of phase IV)	Closed kinetic chain upper extremity test (see text)

*The number of weeks suggested in this table is only a guideline. Determination of when to advance the patient to the next phase of the protocol is based on objective measurements and reported symptoms. Some patients may advance faster or slower than others. Quality of injured tissue, patient characteristics, and clinical testing and measurements should determine protocol advancement.
AC, Acromioclavicular; *PNF,* proprioceptive neuromuscular facilitation; *ROM,* range of motion.

Precautions during Rehabilitation of the Patient with Acromioclavicular Injury

Several precautions should be followed during the rehabilitation of a patient with an acute acromioclavicular injury or a patient following surgical reconstruction. The majority of these precautions are straightforward and are listed in Tables 26-2 through 26-5. However, two recommendations or clinical pearls specific to the patient with an acromioclavicular injury need to be explained in more detail.

Because of the "scapuloclavicular" coupled motion described earlier, active or passive ROM exercises with the patient in a supine position should be avoided. In supine, the patient's body weight prevents scapular motion. This results in greater clavicular rotation occurring at the acromioclavicular joint. Therefore it is suggested that all ROM activities

initially be performed in a side-lying, seated, or standing position.

The second recommendation involves the avoidance of allowing traction forces through the upper extremity. For example, during dumbbell shoulder shrugs to isolate the upper trapezius muscle, the patient will often let the dumbbell apply a distraction force through the upper extremity. Patients require verbal cues to isometrically set the muscles to support the weight before lifting it off the table or weight rack (Figure 26-7). Resting the weight on an adjustable high-low treatment table can also help the patient begin and end each repetition with the weight on the table to avoid the inferior traction force. The patient should also be discouraged from carrying the weight around between sets and allowing distraction forces on weight machines such as the lat pulldown or seated row machines.

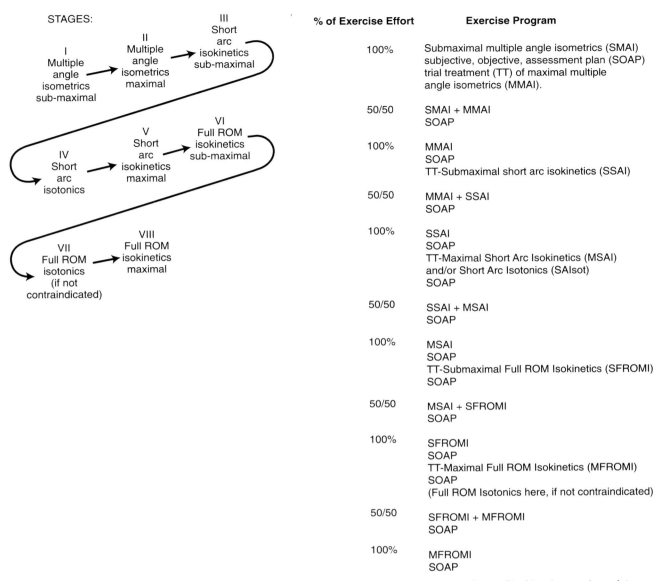

STAGES:	% of Exercise Effort	Exercise Program
	100%	Submaximal multiple angle isometrics (SMAI) subjective, objective, assessment plan (SOAP) trial treatment (TT) of maximal multiple angle isometrics (MMAI).
	50/50	SMAI + MMAI SOAP
	100%	MMAI SOAP TT-Submaximal short arc isokinetics (SSAI)
	50/50	MMAI + SSAI SOAP
	100%	SSAI SOAP TT-Maximal Short Arc Isokinetics (MSAI) and/or Short Arc Isotonics (SAIsot) SOAP
	50/50	SSAI + MSAI SOAP
	100%	MSAI SOAP TT-Submaximal Full ROM Isokinetics (SFROMI) SOAP
	50/50	MSAI + SFROMI SOAP
	100%	SFROMI SOAP TT-Maximal Full ROM Isokinetics (MFROMI) SOAP (Full ROM Isotonics here, if not contraindicated)
	50/50	SFROMI + MFROMI SOAP
	100%	MFROMI SOAP

Figure 26-6: The Davies resistive exercise progression continuum. *(From Davies GJ: A compendium of isokinetic exercise, ed 4, Onalaska, WI, 1994, S & S Publishing.)*

Return to Activity or Sport

When is the patient ready for the heavy demands of physical labor or sport? The requirements of the patient's occupation or sport should be considered early in the rehabilitation process. Knowing the repetitive physical demands that will be placed on the patient helps the physician and therapist determine when partial or full return to activity may occur. To decrease the risk of reinjury, a qualitative assessment of strength and function is required. Evaluation of strength and power may be completed using a handheld dynamometer or a computerized isokinetic dynamometer if available. With this instrumentation, measurements of isometric strength, peak torque, agonist/antagonist muscle ratios, and other strength-related criteria may be carried out. Comparison

with the contralateral upper extremity and with normative data from the current literature is used to interpret the results.[93-95] If the patient demonstrates minimal or no deficits with strength testing, he or she may advance to sport-specific testing.

Sport- or occupation-specific testing of the patient should include tests that simulate actual tasks that place the rehabilitated extremity in positions of stress. It is up to the clinician and physician to determine what sport-specific tests are appropriate, reliable, and valid for each individual patient. The closed kinetic chain upper extremity stability test originally described by Goldbeck and Davies[96] is an excellent example of a reliable clinical test that is appropriate for evaluation of patients following acromioclavicular joint injury and rehabilitation. The test involves placing two pieces of athletic

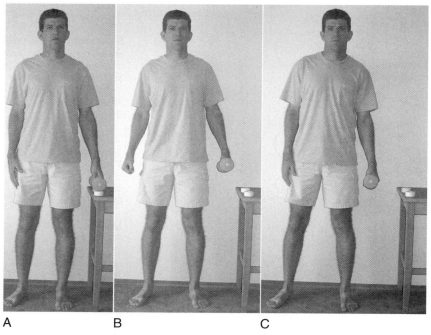

A   B   C

Figure 26-7: Example of upper trapezius exercise (shoulder shrug) performed with care being taken to avoid traction through upper extremity. **A,** Isometric contraction before lifting dumbbell off table. **B,** Maintaining isometric contraction during exercise. **C,** Picture showing improper form of allowing traction through upper extremity when weight is at side.

tape 3 feet apart on the floor. The subject assumes a push-up position with each hand placed on each piece of tape. Verbal cues are used to remind the subject to keep the legs and trunk as parallel to the floor as possible. The examiner shouts "Go!" and the subject, maintaining good posture, must remove one hand from the floor, cross midline to touch the opposite piece of tape, and then return the hand back to the original tape line (Figure 26-8). The other hand is then removed and the process is repeated. This alternate sequencing of horizontal extension and flexion is repeated for 15 seconds and the number of touches is recorded on a data sheet. Three trials with rest intervals of 45 seconds are performed. Goldbeck and Davies[96] retested the subjects a week apart and found a reliability interclass coefficient of 0.92. The subjects in this reliability study were 20-year-old collegiate football players who scored mean values of 27.8 and 27.9 touches on the test and retest, respectively. In contrast, Davies[97] has performed retrospective analyses of clinical data and found averages closer to 21 touches in males and 23 touches in females in the high school–age and college-age athletic populations following upper extremity rehabilitation (Figure 26-9). Females have higher scores because they were tested in a modified push-up position. Further studies are needed to establish normative data for different gender, age, occupational, and sport-specific groups. Because of the specific stresses this test applies to the acromioclavicular joint, qualitative assessment of the patient's confidence or apprehension during the test is as important to assess during testing as the patient's quantitative test score.

Serial strength and functional testing of the patient during the rehabilitation protocol is an important tool to determine when return to activity is safe and appropriate. This format also allows the patient to be part of the rehabilitation team because he or she knows from day 1 what must be accomplished in order for discharge from rehabilitation to occur.

OPERATIVE MANAGEMENT OF ACROMIOCLAVICULAR JOINT INJURY

The decision to proceed surgically must be carefully discussed with the patient. Surgical intervention is used when it demonstrates a superior clinical outcome to conservative treatment or when nonoperative treatment has been attempted and failed. Furthermore, once the decision to operate has been made, a specific procedure has to be chosen. Like the previous decision, this decision is based on many factors: the surgeon's expertise and preferences, the quality of the injured tissues, the patient's health status, the patient's ability to adhere to a supervised postoperative rehabilitation program, and the patient's anticipated activity level following surgery. This being said, one realizes that no single procedure is adaptable to fit all patients. Rather, the choice to pursue surgery and what procedure to perform is individualized.

Over 60 different surgical procedures have been described to correct acromioclavicular joint instability.[98] The goal of all these procedures has been to statically or dynamically reproduce or reconstruct the anatomic restraints of the acromioclavicular joint. To logically discuss the history, surgical

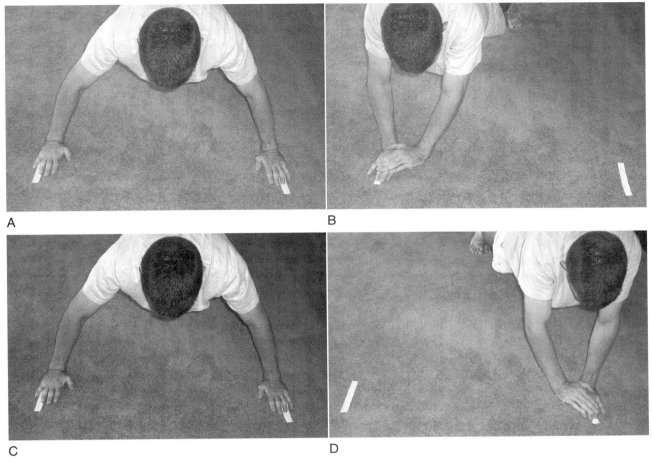

Figure 26-8: Illustration of closed kinetic chain upper extremity functional test. **A,** Start position with subject in push-up position. **B,** Subject crosses one arm over to touch opposite piece of tape. **C,** Return to start position. **D,** Subject crosses opposite arm over.

technique, and reported outcomes of these different procedures, they may be broadly categorized into three different types as described by Kwon and Lannotti.[99] These types are as follows: primary fixation across the acromioclavicular joint, dynamic stabilization of the joint via muscle transfer, and secondary stabilization of the acromioclavicular joint by re-creating the link between the distal clavicle and coracoid with autograft or synthetic materials. One should understand that these categories are not mutually exclusive. It is common to see procedures from one category combined with another in order to best reproduce the mechanical stability of the original structures.

Primary Fixation across the Acromioclavicular Joint

Historically, surgical fixation of the acromioclavicular joint has been performed with the use of Kirschner wires, Steinman pins, hook plates, screws, and other hardware.[100-107] Often this use of hardware to transfix the acromioclavicular joint was done in conjunction with repair of the superior acromioclavicular ligament.[108] Neviaser[107] stabilized the acromioclavicular joint with a pin and then detached the coracoacromial ligament from the coracoid and swung it up over the distal clavicle. A careful review of these studies reveals that no single fixation device has demonstrated superiority over another. Furthermore, all of the aforementioned papers report on relatively small numbers of subjects, and follow-up differs greatly between reports.[99] These fixation devices were placed either percutaneously or during an open procedure. The thin shape of the acromion and the curved clavicle also make this type of procedure technically demanding. In addition, migration of the pins or wires following surgical fixation may have disastrous and possibly fatal consequences.[38,39,55,109-111] Therefore in most cases the hardware is removed after 6 to 8 weeks of healing. Unfortunately, this means a second invasive procedure that can be extensive. Because of the potential risks of infection, hardware migration, and often the requirement of a second surgery, primary fixation of the acromioclavicular joint with pins or wires has fallen by the wayside with the development of other techniques, biodegradable fixation devices, and a greater emphasis on coracoclavicular ligament repair or reconstruction.

Closed Kinetic Chain Upper Extremity Stability Test

Patient Name: _____   DOB: _____

Clinician: _____   Date of Injury / Surgery: _____

Diagnosis: _____   Ht: _____ in   Wt: _____ lbs

Procedure:
1. Subject assumes push-up (male) or modified push-up (female) position.
2. Subject has to move both hands back and forth from each line as many times as possible in 15 sec. Lines are three feet apart.
3. Count the number of lines touched by both hands.
4. Begin with one submaximal warm-up. Repeat 3 times and average.
5. Normalize score by following formula:

$$\text{Score} = \frac{\text{Avg. \# of lines touched}}{\text{Height (in)}}$$

Determine power by using following formula:
(68% body weight = trunk, head and arms)

$$\text{Power} = \frac{68\% \text{ weight} \times \text{avg. \# of lines touched}}{15 \text{ sec}}$$

Data Collection Area

Date of Test:				
Trial	1	2	3	Mean
Touches:				
Score:				
Power:				

Date of Test:				
Trial	1	2	3	Mean
Touches:				
Score:				
Power:				

Date of Test:				
Trial	1	2	3	Mean
Touches:				
Score:				
Power:				

Date of Test:				
Trial	1	2	3	Mean
Touches:				
Score:				
Power:				

Date of Test:				
Trial	1	2	3	Mean
Touches:				
Score:				
Power:				

Normative Data		
	Males	Females
Average # of Touches	21.0 touches	23.0 touches

Figure 26-9: Data sheet for closed kinetic chain upper extremity stability test.

Dynamic Stabilization

Dynamic stabilization involves transferring a musculotendinous unit to the inferior surface of the distal clavicle. This results in the creation of force that dynamically depresses the clavicle.[112-116] This transfer is accomplished by removing the tip of the coracoid process with its attachments to the short head of the biceps tendon and coracobrachialis intact and fixing it to the bottom of the distal clavicle. Berson and colleagues[114] reported satisfactory results in 29 patients with both acute and chronic dislocations. Brunelli and Brunelli[116] have also reported good functional results in 51 patients following a dynamic transfer procedure in which the short head of the biceps tendon is transferred to the clavicle surface directly above the coracoid. Dynamic stabilization of the acromioclavicular joint remains an unpopular procedure. This is due to the concerns of whether the transferred musculotendinous unit can maintain the desired anatomic stability during rehabilitation and return to activity.[99] In addition, several incidents of transient injury to the musculocutaneous nerve have been documented.[117]

Secondary Stabilization

Secondary stabilization of the acromioclavicular joint is carried out by surgically reconstructing or re-creating the vertical restraint of the coracoclavicular ligaments. The incision required for surgical exposure during open coracoclavicular reconstruction is very similar to the incisions used for primary fixation of the acromioclavicular joint. The opening incision is made along Langer's line, but in the case of secondary stabilization, the incision is longer, extending from the posterior aspect of the distal clavicle down to the coracoid process (see Figure 26-10). The deltoid muscle is then released along its bony attachments as much as necessary to provide adequate visualization. Once this is completed, the anterior deltoid can be split parallel to the muscle fibers and the underlying bursal tissue removed. This results in exposure of the distal clavicle, coracoacromial ligament, and coracoid process. Clinicians involved in the patient's rehabilitation should be aware of how much the deltoid was taken down and the quality of the reattachment during closure. This is one of the most important factors in determining the initial intensity of the rehabilitation program and cannot be overemphasized.

Fixation of the clavicle to the coracoid process using a lag screw was originally described by Bosworth in 1941.[62] It is generally accepted that screw fixation be completed with surgical exposure. In 1989, Tsou[118] reported a 32% failure rate with percutaneous cannulated screw coracoclavicular fixation. Subsequent modifications have combined the screw fixation with open exploration and primary repair of the acromioclavicular and coracoclavicular ligaments.[9] Biomechanical studies have revealed that it is important that the lag screw purchase on the coracoid is bicortical. If the lag screw penetrates only the superior surface of the coracoid, the strength of this fixation method is significantly inferior to other forms of coracoclavicular fixation. However, if the lag screw is placed in a bicortical manner, the resultant fixation strength is significantly greater than that of the uninjured coracoclavicular ligaments.[119,120] The drawback of using a lag screw for fixation is that a secondary surgery for hardware removal is generally required after healing has occurred. Also, a recent study has shown that the fixation provided by the screw increases contact forces in the acromioclavicular joint by 200%.[121] Therefore use of a lag screw without distal clavicle excision is not recommended.

Coracoclavicular loops or slings also have been used to provide secondary stabilization of the acromioclavicular joint. Under tension the material is either looped or anchored between the coracoid and clavicle. These coracoclavicular cerclage or loop fixation techniques were used in isolation in the past.[101,122] However, today they are commonly used in combination with the modified Weaver-Dunn procedure

described later. Materials such as wire,[101] Dacron,[101,122,123] Merselene tape,[124,125] resorbable braided polydioxanonsulphate (PDS) bands,[124-127] Gore-Tex,[128,129] and tendon autografts[31,130-132] all have been used with success. Wire loops are no longer used in order to avoid the secondary surgery for hardware removal and limit the consequences of hardware migration. Some care needs to be taken when placing the suture or tendon loops around the coracoid process and the distal clavicle to achieve adequate reduction of the acromioclavicular joint. It is recommended that the inferior loop is placed around the absolute base of the coracoid process whereas the superior loop is passed through drill holes in the anterior one third of the distal clavicle.[99] There are some concerns about the technical difficulty and risk of neurovascular injury when passing the loop material around the base of the coracoid. To avoid this issue, some surgeons have reported success with the use of suture anchors instead of suture loops.[133,134] In all these coracoclavicular cerclage procedures there is a tendency for the clavicle to be displaced anteriorly relative to the acromion. This is because anatomically the clavicle does not set directly above the coracoid process. Baker and co-workers[135] examined three variations of clavicular drill hole placement and determined that joint congruity improved as the drill hole moved anteriorly on the clavicle. However, none of the three methods of coracoclavicular loop fixation restored full alignment.

Another method of obtaining fixation between the distal clavicle and the coracoid process is through transfer of the coracoacromial ligament.[32] In their widely cited article from 1972, Weaver and Dunn[32] describe a procedure in which the acromial end of the coracoacromial ligament is detached and the ligament is dissected free of the coracoid process. After excision of 2 cm of its lateral end, the clavicle is held in its anatomic position with traction applied to the coracoacromial ligament. The ligament is then cut for size and, with heavy nonabsorbable sutures, is secured through previously placed drill holes to the medullary canal of the clavicle. The deltoid and trapezius insertions are then restored.[32]

Since its initial publication, the use of the Weaver-Dunn procedure has gained widespread use and popularity. Multiple modifications of the original procedure have been developed with reported clinical success.[90,92,128,136,137] The procedure has been performed with or without distal clavicle excision, and the coracoacromial ligament may be transferred with or without a sliver of bone from the acromion. Theoretically, the concept of using a bone sliver attached to the ligament and a distal clavicle excision is ideal because it allows for bone-to-bone contact, which may accelerate healing and remodeling.[99]

Recently, Jari and co-workers[121] have examined the biomechanical function of the intact coracoclavicular ligaments in comparison with reconstruction methods using the Weaver-Dunn or coracoacromial ligament transfer, Rockwood lag screw, or coracoclavicular fixation with a suture or autograft tendon cerclage technique. They found that both primary translation and coupled translation in the anterior,

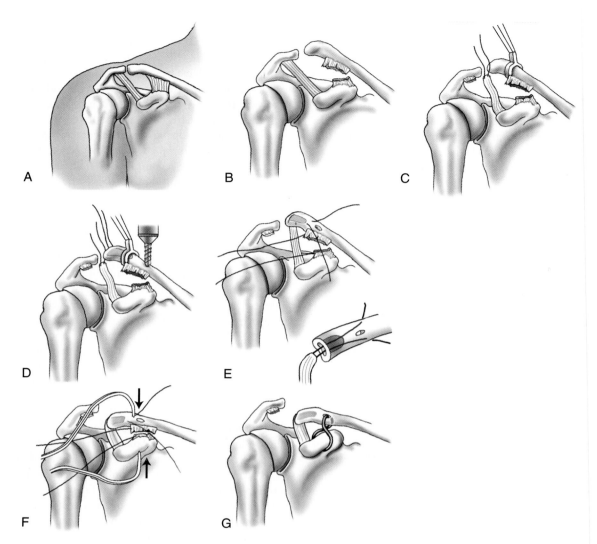

Figure 26-10: Pictorial and text description of a modified Weaver-Dunn surgical technique using tendon graft as material to reconstruct coracoclavicular ligaments. **A,** Saber-type incision (*dashed line*) starts slightly medially and posterior to the acromioclavicular joint and extended to just above the coracoid. This is accomplished after diagnostic glenohumeral arthroscopy and an arthroscopic distal clavicle excision have been performed. **B,** A horizontal incision is made in the deltoid trapezial fascia across the acromioclavicular joint. The joint is completely exposed with careful anterior and posterior subperiosteal dissection to assure full thickness of the flaps. **C,** The coracoacromial ligament is dissected off the acromion and a No. 2 permanent Ethibond suture is placed in a Krakow-type manner. The clavicle is secured. **D,** A curet is used to hollow out a trough for the coracoacromial ligament in the distal clavicle, and a large hole is made in the clavicle approximately 1 cm from the edge using a 4.5-mm drill. It is then made larger either with a curet or using the drill as a reamer. Two smaller holes are made on either side of this with a 3.2-mm drill. **E,** The two limbs of the Ethibond suture tied around the coracoacromial ligament are then placed through the small holes, and the ligament is placed into the bone tunnel. (*Inset* shows this with magnification.) Upward pressure is placed on the scapulohumeral complex to reduce the coracoclavicular distance. A suture can be placed around the coracoclavicular ligaments if possible. **F,** A tinaculum clamp is used to hold the reduction that has been accomplished with upper traction on the scapulohumeral complex. This facilitates easy and tight fitting of the coracoacromial ligament into its bone tunnel and passage of the semitendinosus graft. **G,** Shown is the placement of the semitendinous graft and the braided Ethibond suture in a figure-eight pattern around the base of the coracoid and through the large hole in the distal clavicle, with concomitant fixation of the coracoacromial ligament in the bone tunnel. Of note and not shown in these illustrations is repair of the deltotrapezial fascia with nonabsorbable sutures, which is extremely important. (*From Mazzocca AD, Sellards R, Garretson R, et al: Injuries to the acromioclavicular joint in adults and children. In DeLee J, Drez D, Miller MD, editors:* DeLee and Drez's orthopaedic sports medicine: principles and practice, *ed 2, Philadelphia, 2003, Saunders.)*

posterior, and superior planes were significantly higher in the Weaver-Dunn and coracoclavicular cerclage constructs compared with the native ligaments.[121] This study, along with others, has shown that although clinically good results are obtained, the anatomic reduction achieved during surgery is difficult to maintain once the patient returns to activity.[92] Therefore it has become popular to combine the aforementioned procedures into one that involves distal clavicular excision, transfer of the coracoclavicular ligament and fixation of the clavicle to the coracoid,[86,128,137-139] and repair of the deltotrapezial fascia. All of these procedures have been loosely referred to by some as "modified Weaver-Dunn" techniques. A detailed example of a modified Weaver-Dunn procedure is illustrated and described in Figure 26-10.[31]

The Future of Acromioclavicular Surgery

The future of acromioclavicular joint surgery is exciting. Although the conventional techniques available involve open surgeries, recent documentation of arthroscopic techniques has appeared in the literature.[140-143] Arthroscopic reconstruction of the acromioclavicular joint has the potential to be a less invasive method while simultaneously achieving cosmetic and clinical results of the open procedures. Further biomechanical studies and long-term clinical follow-up are necessary to determine whether arthroscopic reconstruction will be a viable alternative to the open procedures.

A new and novel technique that attempts to anatomically reconstruct both the acromioclavicular and the coracoclavicular ligaments has been suggested.[144] This technique is unique in that it attempts to place autogenous semitendinosus graft material into the exact anatomic footprint of the native coracoclavicular ligaments. Autograft tendon fixation is achieved with interference screw fixation to bone.[144] Long-term follow-up will determine if this new procedure will be more successful than the modified Weaver-Dunn. Nevertheless, it is hoped that this new procedure, as well as the recent modifications to the Weaver-Dunn procedure, will result in the number of surgical options available for acromioclavicular reconstruction being limited to several options. This will, it is hoped, allow for a greater number of prospective outcome studies and trials.

REHABILITATION FOLLOWING ACROMIOCLAVICULAR SURGERY

Following a modified Weaver-Dunn or similar surgical reconstruction technique, the patient, therapist, and physician need to follow a criterion-based rehabilitation protocol. This protocol must also incorporate the principles of exercise progression and serial testing that were described for nonoperative rehabilitation. However, because of the importance of protecting the fragile coracoacromial ligament transfer and clavicular reduction, a 4- to 6-week protective postoperative phase is required. During this phase, an acromioclavicular sling is used for support and to protect the surgical reconstruction. It is hoped that significant healing occurs during this protective time period. Once this protective phase is completed, the patient may be progressed according to the principles and exercises described for rehabilitation following nonoperative treatment as described previously. Tables 26-4 and 26-5 (pp. 512-515) illustrate a sample 24-week protocol for patients following modified Weaver-Dunn acromioclavicular reconstruction.

SUMMARY

Rehabilitation following conservative or operative acromioclavicular joint injury requires a team approach from the surgeon, physical therapist, and athletic trainer. All members of the rehabilitation team should have a thorough understanding of the anatomy and biomechanics of the acromioclavicular joint, the mechanisms of injury and initial examination and evaluation techniques, and the appropriate conservative and operative interventions for acromioclavicular joint injury. Successful outcomes for the patient depend on close communication among team members and objective documentation of patient progress.

References

1. Stuart MJ, Morrey MA, Smith AM, et al: Injuries in youth football: a prospective observational cohort analysis among players aged 9 to 13 years, *Mayo Clin Proc* 77(4):317-322, 2002.
2. Stuart MJ, Smith A: Injuries in junior A ice hockey. A three-year prospective study, *Am J Sports Med* 23(4):458-461, 1995.
3. Webb J, Bannister G: Acromioclavicular disruption in first class rugby players, *Br J Sports Med* 26(4):247-248, 1992.
4. Kocher MS, Dupre MM, Feagin JA Jr: Shoulder injuries from alpine skiing and snowboarding. Aetiology, treatment and prevention, *Sports Med* 25(3):201-211, 1998.
5. Kocher MS, Feagin JA Jr: Shoulder injuries during alpine skiing, *Am J Sports Med* 24(5):665-669, 1996.
6. Jeys LM, Cribb G, Toms AD, et al: Mountain biking injuries in rural England, *Br J Sports Med* 35(3):197-199, 2001.
7. Molsa J, Kujala U, Myllynen P, et al: Injuries to the upper extremity in ice hockey: analysis of a series of 760 injuries, *Am J Sports Med* 31(5):751-757, 2003.
8. Kelly BT, Barnes RP, Powell JW, et al: Shoulder injuries to quarterbacks in the national football league, *Am J Sports Med* 32(2):328-331, 2004.
9. Rockwood CA Jr, Williams GR, Young DC: Disorders of the acromioclavicular joint. In Rockwood CA Jr, Matsen FA III, editors: *The shoulder*, ed 2, Philadelphia, 1998, Saunders.
10. Williams GR, Rockwood CA Jr: Injuries to the acromioclavicular joint, sternoclavicular joint, clavicle, scapula, coracoid, sternum and ribs. In DeLee JC, Drez D, editors: *Orthopaedic sports medicine: principles and practice*, Philadelphia, 1994, Saunders.
11. Beim GM: Acromioclavicular joint injuries, *J Athl Train* 35(3):261-267, 2000.
12. Bosworth BM: Complete acromioclavicular dislocations, *N Engl J Med* 241:221-225, 1949.
13. Tyurina TV: Age-related changes characteristics of the human acromioclavicular joint, *Arkh Anat Gistol Embriol* 89:75-81, 1985.
14. DePalma AF: *Degenerative changes in the sternoclavicular and acromioclavicular joints in various decades*, Springfield, IL, 1957, Charles C Thomas.

TABLE 26-4

Postoperative Rehabilitation Protocol following Acromioclavicular Joint Reconstruction (Phases I and II)

	PHASE I: IMMEDIATE POSTOPERATIVE PHASE	PHASE II: INTERMEDIATE PHASE (INITIAL STRENGTHENING)
	WEEKS 1 TO 4*	WEEKS 5 TO 8
Goals (May not progress to next phase until goals are met)	Minimal pain and tenderness with palpation of AC joint Stable AC joint on clinical examination Able to perform submaximal lateral and medial isometric contractions in standing (30 degrees of abduction/scaption†) without pain	Full pain-free AROM Equal lateral rotation to contralateral side Measured in a seated position with arm in 30 degrees of abduction Minimal pain and tenderness with palpation of the AC joint Able to perform maximal isometric contractions pain free in all planes No observed scapular dyskinesias
Precautions	Avoid supine PROM (see text) No heavy lifting, pushing/pulling No contact sports No overhead motion greater than 90 degrees Restrict horizontal extension and flexion ROM No PROM/AAROM/AROM into pain Avoid traction through upper extremity	Avoid supine exercises (see text) No heavy lifting, pushing/pulling No contact sports No resisted overhead motion greater than 90 degrees No resisted horizontal extension and flexion Avoid military or bench press motions Avoid traction through upper extremity
Interventions		
Protection	Fit with AC (Kenny-Howard) sling for comfort and to prevent downward displacement of scapula Taping for pain relief and protection	Slowly wean from splint as tolerated weeks 5-6
Modalities	Cryotherapy Electrical stimulation modalities for pain control and neuromuscular reeducation	Cryotherapy following exercise Electrical stimulation modalities for pain control and neuromuscular reeducation May use heat for warm-up, stretching, and pain relief
ROM	Elbow and wrist AROM PROM in seated or side-lying position Begin AAROM exercises with wand or T-bar week 2 Begin gentle AROM exercises in pain-free ROM week 4	Full AROM all planes

TABLE 26-4

Postoperative Rehabilitation Protocol following Acromioclavicular Joint Reconstruction (Phases I and II)—cont'd

	PHASE I: IMMEDIATE POSTOPERATIVE PHASE	PHASE II: INTERMEDIATE PHASE (INITIAL STRENGTHENING)
	WEEKS 1 TO 4*	WEEKS 5 TO 8
Strengthening	Initiate trial of submaximal shoulder isometrics week 3	Initiate trial of short-arc isotonic strengthening exercises
	Isometrics in 30 degrees of abduction and scaption for shoulder flexion, medial rotation, and lateral rotation	Progress ROM as tolerated by symptoms
		Progress resistance as defined by symptoms, scapular control, and quality of motion
	Progress intensity of isometrics as tolerated by symptoms and visual analog scale pain rating less than 2/10 or 3/10	Strengthening exercises should include the following exercises with ROM modifications:
	Isometrics should all be performed below chest level	Seated chest press with plus
		Seated row
	Forearm and hand intrinsic strengthening with putty or squeeze ball	Scaption limited to 90 degrees of elevation
	Begin pain-free AROM scapular retraction and protraction week 2 in sling	Bent-over horizontal abduction (no resistance, AROM only)
	May continue lower extremity and uninvolved upper extremity exercises	Shoulder flexion limited to 90 degrees of elevation
	Initiate core trunk stability exercises	Shoulder shrugs (avoid traction force)
		Lateral and medial rotation strengthening
		Biceps and triceps strengthening
		Core trunk stability exercises
Neuromuscular reeducation exercises	Biofeedback to encourage correct arthrokinematics with standing or seated	Submaximal rhythmic stabilizations
		Slow speed
	AAROM (goal to facilitate inhibition of upper trapezius activity during activity)	Known pattern
		Submaximal resistance
Assessment		
Clinical testing	PROM measurements week 2	Perform in side-lying position
	AROM measurements week 4	Weekly AROM measurements

*The number of weeks suggested in this table is only a guideline. Determination of when to advance the patient to the next phase of the protocol is based on objective measurements and reported symptoms. Some patients may advance faster or slower than others. Quality of injured tissue, patient characteristics, and clinical testing and measurements should determine protocol advancement.
†Elevation in the plane of the scapula.
AAROM, Active-assistive range of motion; *AC,* acromioclavicular; *AROM,* active range of motion; *PROM,* passive range of motion; *ROM,* range of motion.

TABLE 26-5

Postoperative Rehabilitation Protocol following Acromioclavicular Joint Reconstruction (Phases III and IV)

	PHASE III: DYNAMIC STRENGTHENING PHASE	PHASE IV: RETURN TO ACTIVITY PHASE
	WEEKS 9 TO 15*	WEEKS 16 TO 24
Goals (May not progress to next phase until goals are met)	Full pain-free AROM equal to the contralateral side	No functional deficits when compared with uninvolved extremity
	No pain or tenderness with palpation	Isokinetic testing of medial and lateral rotation and horizontal flexion and extension within 10% of normative data and contralateral extremity
	Less than 25% deficit with handheld dynamometer testing of middle deltoid and upper trapezius	Independent in home strengthening program
	Less than 10% deficit to contralateral shoulder with testing of internal and external rotators	Discharge from rehabilitation
Precautions	Avoid supine ROM (see text)	Caution when performing military or bench press
	No heavy lifting, pushing/pulling	Suggest modifying ROM and arc of motion to limit AC joint stress
	No contact sports	Suggest alternative exercises
	No resisted overhead motion greater than 90 degrees	Avoid excessive traction through upper extremity with repetitive activity
	Restrict horizontal extension and flexion ROM	
	No PROM/AAROM/AROM into pain	
	Avoid traction through upper extremity	
Interventions		
Protection	Padding and protection for work or sport if necessary	Padding and protection for work or sport if necessary
Modalities	Cryotherapy following exercise	Cryotherapy as needed following exercise
	Electrical stimulation modalities for pain control and neuromuscular reeducation	May use heat for warm-up, stretching, and pain relief
	May use heat for warm-up, stretching, and pain relief	
ROM	Begin some repetitive overhead motion without resistance	No changes
	For endurance training	
	Avoid loss of scapular control or pain	
	Begin supervised horizontal extension and flexion resistance exercises	
	Progress resistance based on trial treatments with short-arc isotonics	
	Establish home program of stretching if necessary to maintain ROM	

TABLE 26-5

Postoperative Rehabilitation Protocol following Acromioclavicular Joint Reconstruction (Phases III and IV)—cont'd

	PHASE III: DYNAMIC STRENGTHENING PHASE	PHASE IV: RETURN TO ACTIVITY PHASE
	WEEKS 9 TO 15*	WEEKS 16 TO 24
Strengthening	Progress resistance and increase ROM of all exercises from phase II	Continue with a core program based on specific demands of vocation or sport
	Progress to strengthening in all planes of motion based on symptoms	Use periodization principles
	Week 12: carefully progress to overhead strengthening (90/90 position) based on trial treatments with short-arc isotonics	Initiate return to throwing program
Neuromuscular reeducation exercises	Advance to diagonal (PNF) patterns of motion	Advance exercises from phase III by decreasing clinician control and increasing exercise intensity
	Increase speed and intensity of exercises	Advance plyometrics drills to incorporate demands of sport or work activity
	Initiate submaximal upper extremity plyometrics using minimal resistance and control parameters of bilateral to unilateral, partial to full ROM, low to high speed, and low to high repetitions and resistance	
Activity specific	Initiate work conditioning and simulated work tasks	Sport-specific testing
	Perform work-site evaluation	Trial return to sport or activity
	Initiate sport-specific drills	Continue return to throwing program
	Initiate preparation for closed kinetic chain upper extremity functional test	
Assessment		
Clinical testing	Strength testing at end of phase	Closed kinetic chain upper extremity test (see text)
	Assessment of abilities or deficits with work or sport activities (these deficits will be focus of phase IV)	

*The number of weeks suggested in this table is only a guideline. Determination of when to advance the patient to the next phase of the protocol is based on objective measurements and reported symptoms. Some patients may advance faster or slower than others. Quality of injured tissue, patient characteristics, and clinical testing and measurements should determine protocol advancement.

AAROM, Active-assistive range of motion; *AC*, acromioclavicular; *AROM*, active range of motion; *PNF*, proprioceptive neuromuscular facilitation; *PROM*, passive range of motion; *ROM*, range of motion.

15. Urist MR: Complete dislocations of the acromioclavicular joint: the nature of the traumatic lesion and effective methods of treatments with an analysis of forty-one cases, *J Bone Joint Surg Am* 28:813-837, 1946.

16. Pettrone FA, Nirschl RP: Acromioclavicular dislocation, *Am J Sports Med* 6(4):160-164, 1978.

17. Pitchford KR, Cahill BR: Osteolysis of the distal clavicle in the overhead athlete, *Oper Tech Sports Med* 5(2):72-77, 1997.

18. Tillmann B, Peterson W: Clinical anatomy. In Fu FH, Ticker JB, Imhoff AB, editors: *Analysis of shoulder surgery*, Stamford, CT, 1998, Appleton & Lange.

19. Petersson C: Degeneration of the AC joint: a morphological study, *Acta Orthop Scand* 54:434-438, 1983.

20. DePalma AF, Callery G, Bennett G: Variational anatomy and degenerative lesions of the shoulder joint, *Instr Course Lect* 6:255-281, 1949.

21. Salter EJ, Nasca R, Shelley B: Anatomical observations on the AC joint and supporting ligaments, *Am J Sports Med* 15:199-206, 1987.

22. Bonsell S, Pearsall AW, Heitman RJ, et al: The relationship of age, gender, and degenerative changes observed on radiographs of the shoulder in asymptomatic individuals, *J Bone Joint Surg Br* 82(8):1135-1139, 2000.

23. Fukuda K, Craig EV, An KN, et al: Biomechanical study of the ligamentous system of the acromioclavicular joint, *J Bone Joint Surg Am* 68(3):434-440, 1986.

24. Renfree KJ, Wright TW: Anatomy and biomechanics of the acromioclavicular and sternoclavicular joints, *Clin Sports Med* 22(2):219-237, 2003.

25. Klimkiewicz JJ, Williams GR, Sher JS, et al: The acromioclavicular capsule as a restraint to posterior translation of the clavicle: a biomechanical analysis, *J Shoulder Elbow Surg* 8(2):119-124, 1999.

26. Boehm TD, Kirschner S, Fischer A, et al: The relation of the coracoclavicular ligament insertion to the acromioclavicular joint: a cadaver study of relevance to lateral clavicle resection, *Acta Orthop Scand* 74(6):718-721, 2003.

27. Harris RI, Vu DH, Sonnabend DH, et al: Anatomic variance of the coracoclavicular ligaments, *J Shoulder Elbow Surg* 10(6):585-588, 2001.

28. Debski RE, Parsons IM, Woo SL, et al: Effect of capsular injury on acromioclavicular joint mechanics, *J Bone Joint Surg Am* 83A(9):1344-1351, 2001.

29. Debski RE, Parsons IM, Fenwick J, et al: Ligament mechanics during three degree-of-freedom motion at the acromioclavicular joint, *Ann Biomed Eng* 28(6):612-618, 2000.

30. Lee TQ, Black AD, Tibone JE, et al: Release of the coracoacromial ligament can lead to glenohumeral laxity: a biomechanical study, *J Shoulder Elbow Surg* 10(1):68-72, 2001.

31. Mazzocca AD, Sellards R, Garretson R, et al: Injuries to the acromioclavicular joint in adults and children. In DeLee J, Drez D, Miller MD, editors: *DeLee and Drez's orthopaedic sports medicine: principles and practice*, ed 2, Philadelphia, 2003, Saunders.

32. Weaver JK, Dunn HK: Treatment of acromioclavicular injuries, especially complete acromioclavicular separation, *J Bone Joint Surg Am* 54(6):1187-1194, 1972.

33. Gowan ID, Jobe FW, Tibone JE, et al: A comparative electromyographic analysis of the shoulder during pitching. Professional versus amateur pitchers, *Am J Sports Med* 15(6):586-590, 1987.

34. Jobe FW, Moynes DR, Tibone JE, et al: An EMG analysis of the shoulder in pitching. A second report, *Am J Sports Med* 12(3):218-220, 1984.

35. Inman VT, Saunders JB, Abbott LC: Observations on the function of the shoulder joint, *J Bone Joint Surg Am* 26:1-30, 1944.

36. Kennedy JC, Cameron H: Complete dislocation of the acromioclavicular joint, *J Bone Joint Surg Br* 36:202-208, 1954.

37. Rockwood CA Jr, Williams GR, Young DC: Injuries to the acromioclavicular joint. In Rockwood CA Jr, Green D, editors: *Fractures in adults*, vol 1, ed 2, Philadelphia, 1984, JB Lippincott.

38. Falappa PG, Danza FM, Cotroneo AR, et al: Percutaneous removal of a Kirschner wire from the thoracic aorta, *Rays* 14(1):65-68, 1989.

39. Foster GT, Chetty KG, Mahutte K, et al: Hemoptysis due to migration of a fractured Kirschner wire, *Chest* 119(4):1285-1286, 2001.

40. Ludewig PM, Behrens SA, Meyer SM, et al: Three-dimensional clavicular motion during arm elevation: reliability and descriptive data, *J Orthop Sports Phys Ther* 34(3):140-149, 2004.

41. Bearn JG: Direct observations on the function of the capsule of the sternoclavicular joint in clavicle support, *J Anat* 101:159-170, 1967.

42. Cadenat FM: The treatment of dislocations and fractures of the outer end of the clavicle, *Int Clin* 1:145-169, 1917.

43. Tossy JD, Mead NC, Sigmond HM: Acromioclavicular separations: useful and practical classification for treatment, *Clin Orthop* 28:111-119, 1963.

44. Allman FL: Fractures and ligamentous injuries of the clavicle and its articulation, *J Bone Joint Surg Am* 49:774-784, 1967.

45. Turnbull JR: Acromioclavicular joint disorders, *Med Sci Sports Exerc* 30(4 suppl):S26-32, 1998.

46. Garretson RB, Williams GR Jr: Clinical evaluation of injuries to the acromioclavicular and sternoclavicular joints, *Clin Sports Med* 22(2):239-254, 2003.

47. Gerber C, Galantay RV, Hersche O: The pattern of pain produced by irritation of the acromioclavicular joint and the subacromial space, *J Shoulder Elbow Surg* 7(4):352-355, 1998.

48. McLaughlin HL: On the frozen shoulder, *Bull Hosp Jt Dis* 12:383-390, 1951.

49. O'Brien SJ, Pagnani MJ, Fealy S, et al: The active compression test: a new and effective test for diagnosing labral tears and acromioclavicular joint abnormality, *Am J Sports Med* 26(5):610-613, 1998.

50. Walton J, Mahajan S, Paxinos A, et al: Diagnostic values of tests for acromioclavicular joint pain, *J Bone Joint Surg Am* 86A(4):807-812, 2004.

51. Magee DJ: *Orthopedic physical assessment* (chap 5), ed 4, Philadelphia, 2002, Saunders.

52. Jacob AK, Sallay PI: Therapeutic efficacy of corticosteroid injections in the acromioclavicular joint, *Biomed Sci Instrum* 34:380-385, 1997.

53. Chronopoulos E, Kim TK, Park HB, et al: Diagnostic value of physical tests for isolated chronic acromioclavicular lesions, *Am J Sports Med* 32(3):655-661, 2004.

54. Johnson RJ: Acromioclavicular joint injuries, *Phys Sports Med* 29(11):31-35, 2001.

55. Aalders GJ, van Vroonhoven TJ, van der Werken C, et al: An exceptional case of pneumothorax—"a new adventure of the K wire," *Injury* 16(8):564-565, 1985.

56. Zanca P: Shoulder pain: involvement of the acromioclavicular joint (analysis of 1,000 cases), *Am J Roentgenol Radium Ther Nucl Med* 112(3):493-506, 1971.

57. Bannister GC, Wallace WA, Stableforth PG, et al: The management of acute acromioclavicular dislocation. A randomised prospective controlled trial, *J Bone Joint Surg Br* 71(5):848-850, 1989.

58. Bossart PJ, Joyce SM, Manaster BJ, et al: Lack of efficacy of "weighted" radiographs in diagnosing acute acromioclavicular separation, *Ann Emerg Med* 17(1):20-24, 1988.

59. Yap JJ, Curl LA, Kvitne RS, et al: The value of weighted views of the acromioclavicular joint. Results of a survey, *Am J Sports Med* 27(6):806-809, 1999.

60. Ernberg LA, Potter HG: Radiographic evaluation of the acromioclavicular and sternoclavicular joints, *Clin Sports Med* 22(2):255-275, 2003.

61. Schimpf M, Carlos N, McFarland EG: The deceptive nature of clavicle fractures in young patients, *Phys Sports Med* 27(3):119-128, 1999.

62. Bosworth BM: Acromioclavicular separation: new method of repair, *Surg Gynecol Obstet* 73:866-871, 1941.

63. Nuber GW, Bowen BK: Acromioclavicular joint injuries and distal clavicle fractures, *J Am Acad Orthop Surg* 5(1):11-18, 1997.

64. Lemos MJ: The evaluation and treatment of the injured acromioclavicular joint in athletes, *Am J Sports Med* 26(1):137-144, 1998.

65. Bergfeld JA, Andrish JT, Clancy WG: Evaluation of the acromioclavicular joint following first- and second-degree sprains, *Am J Sports Med* 6(4):153-159, 1978.

66. Mumford EB: Acromioclavicular dislocation: a new operative treatment, *J Bone Joint Surg Am* 23:799-802, 1941.

67. Gurd FB: The treatment of complete dislocation of the outer end of the clavicle: an hitherto undescribed operation, *Ann Surg* 113:1094-1098, 1941.

68. Alford W, Bach BR Jr: Open distal clavicle resection, *Oper Tech Sports Med* 12(1):9-17, 2004.

69. Kay SP, Dragoo JL, Lee R: Long-term results of arthroscopic resection of the distal clavicle with concomitant subacromial decompression, *Arthroscopy* 19(8):805-809, 2003.

70. Kay SP, Ellman H, Harris E: Arthroscopic distal clavicle excision. Technique and early results, *Clin Orthop* 301:181-184, 1994.

71. Bigliani LU, Nicholson GP, Flatow EL: Arthroscopic resection of the distal clavicle, *Orthop Clin North Am* 24(1):133-141, 1993.

72. Flatow EL, Cordasco FA, Bigliani LU: Arthroscopic resection of the outer end of the clavicle from a superior approach: a critical, quantitative, radiographic assessment of bone removal, *Arthroscopy* 8(1):55-64, 1992.

73. Flatow EL, Duralde XA, Nicholson GP, et al: Arthroscopic resection of the distal clavicle with a superior approach, *J Shoulder Elbow Surg* 4(1 pt 1):41-50, 1995.

74. Sellards R, Nicholson GP: Arthroscopic distal clavicle resection, *Oper Tech Sports Med* 12(1):18-26, 2004.

75. Nuber GW, Bowen MK: Arthroscopic treatment of acromioclavicular joint injuries and results, *Clin Sports Med* 22(2):301-317, 2003.

76. Clarke HD, McCann PD: Acromioclavicular joint injuries, *Orthop Clin North Am* 31(2):177-187, 2000.

77. Mouhsine E, Garofalo R, Crevoisier X, et al: Grade I and II acromioclavicular dislocations: results of conservative treatment, *J Shoulder Elbow Surg* 12(6):599-602, 2003.

78. Walsh WM, Peterson DA, Shelton G, et al: Shoulder strength following acromioclavicular injury, *Am J Sports Med* 13(3):153-158, 1985.

79. O'Neill DB, Zarins B, Gelberman RH, et al: Compression of the anterior interosseous nerve after use of a sling for dislocation of the acromioclavicular joint. A report of two cases, *J Bone Joint Surg Am* 72(7):1100-1102, 1990.

80. MacDonald PB, Alexander MJ, Frejuk J, et al: Comprehensive functional analysis of shoulders following complete acromioclavicular separation, *Am J Sports Med* 16(5):475-480, 1988.

81. Imatani RJ, Hanlon JJ, Cady GW: Acute, complete acromioclavicular separation, *J Bone Joint Surg Am* 57(3):328-332, 1975.

82. Shamus JL, Shamus EC: A taping technique for the treatment of acromioclavicular joint sprains: a case study, *J Orthop Sports Phys Ther* 25(6):390-394, 1997.

83. Powers JA, Bach PJ: Acromioclavicular separations. Closed or open treatment? *Clin Orthop* 104:213-223, 1974.

84. Cox JS: Current method of treatment of acromioclavicular joint dislocations, *Orthopedics* 15(9):1041-1044, 1992.

85. Phillips AM, Smart C, Groom AF: Acromioclavicular dislocation. Conservative or surgical therapy, *Clin Orthop* 353:10-17, 1998.

86. Bradley JP, Elkousy H: Decision making: operative versus nonoperative treatment of acromioclavicular joint injuries, *Clin Sports Med* 22(2):277-290, 2003.

87. Larsen E, Bjerg-Nielsen A, Christensen P: Conservative or surgical treatment of acromioclavicular dislocation. A prospective, controlled, randomized study, *J Bone Joint Surg Am* 68(4):552-555, 1986.

88. Glick JM, Milburn LJ, Haggerty JF, et al: Dislocated acromioclavicular joint: follow-up study of 35 unreduced acromioclavicular dislocations, *Am J Sports Med* 5(6):264-270, 1977.

89. McFarland EG, Blivin SJ, Doehring CB, et al: Treatment of grade III acromioclavicular separations in professional throwing athletes: results of a survey, *Am J Orthop* 26(11):771-774, 1997.

90. Dumontier C, Sautet A, Man M, et al: Acromioclavicular dislocations: treatment by coracoacromial ligamentoplasty, *J Shoulder Elbow Surg* 4(2):130-134, 1995.

91. Gladstone J, Wilk K, Andrews JR: Nonoperative treatment of AC joint injuries, *Oper Tech Sports Med* 5:78-87, 1997.

92. Weinstein DM, McCann PD, McIlveen SJ, et al: Surgical treatment of complete acromioclavicular dislocations, *Am J Sports Med* 23(3):324-331, 1995.

93. Davies GJ: *A compendium of isokinetic exercise,* ed 4, Onalaska, WI, 1994, S & S Publishing.

94. Dvir Z: *Isokinetics: muscle testing, interpretation and clinical applications,* ed 2, Philadelphia, 2003, Elsevier Science.

95. Tibone J, Sellers R, Tonino P: Strength testing after third-degree acromioclavicular dislocations, *Am J Sports Med* 20(3):328-331, 1992.

96. Goldbeck TG, Davies GJ: Test-retest reliability of the closed kinetic chain upper extremity stability test: a clinical field test, *J Sports Rehabil* 9:35-45, 2000.

97. Davies GJ: Normative data for the closed kinetic chain upper extremity stability test. Personal communication, 2001.

98. Ponce BA, Millett PJ, Warner JP: Acromioclavicular joint instability—reconstruction indications and techniques, *Oper Tech Sports Med* 12(1):35-42, 2004.

99. Kwon YW, Iannotti JP: Operative treatment of acromioclavicular joint injuries and results, *Clin Sports Med* 22(2):291-300, 2003.

100. O'Carroll PF, Sheehan JM: Open reduction and percutaneous Kirschner wire fixation in complete disruption of the acromioclavicular joint, *Injury* 13(4):299-301, 1982.

101. Bargren JH, Erlanger S, Dick HM: Biomechanics and comparison of two operative methods of treatment of complete acromioclavicular separation, *Clin Orthop* 130:267-272, 1978.

102. Sim E, Schwarz N, Hocker K, et al: Repair of complete acromioclavicular separations using the acromioclavicular-hook plate, *Clin Orthop* 314:134-142, 1995.

103. Smith MJ, Stewart MJ: Acute acromioclavicular separations. A 20-year study, *Am J Sports Med* 7(1):62-71, 1979.

104. Habernek H, Weinstabl R, Schmid L, et al: A crook plate for treatment of acromioclavicular joint separation: indication, technique, and results after one year, *J Trauma* 35(6):893-901, 1993.

105. Lizaur A, Marco L, Cebrian R: Acute dislocation of the acromioclavicular joint. Traumatic anatomy and the importance of deltoid and trapezius, *J Bone Joint Surg Br* 76(4):602-606, 1994.

106. Paavolainen P, Bjorkenheim JM, Paukku P, et al: Surgical treatment of acromioclavicular dislocation: a review of 39 patients, *Injury* 14(5):415-420, 1983.

107. Neviaser JS: Acromioclavicular dislocation treated by transference of the coraco-acromial ligament. A long-term follow-up in a series of 112 cases, *Clin Orthop* 58:57-68, 1968.

108. Roper BA, Levack B: The surgical treatment of acromioclavicular dislocations, *J Bone Joint Surg Br* 64(5):597-599, 1982.

109. Lindsey RW, Gutowski WT: The migration of a broken pin following fixation of the acromioclavicular joint. A case report and review of the literature, *Orthopedics* 9(3):413-416, 1986.

110. Sethi GK, Scott SM: Subclavian artery laceration due to migration of a Hagie pin, *Surgery* 80(5):644-646, 1976.

111. Yadav V, Marya KM: Unusual migration of a wire from shoulder to neck, *Indian J Med Sci* 57(3):111-112, 2003.

112. Bailey RW: A dynamic repair for complete acromioclavicular joint dislocation, *J Bone Joint Surg Am* 47:858, 1965 (abstract).

113. Bailey RW, Metten CF, O'Connor GA, et al: A dynamic method of repair for acute and chronic acromioclavicular disruption, *Am J Sports Med* 4(2):58-71, 1976.

114. Berson BL, Gilbert MS, Green S: Acromioclavicular dislocations: treatment by transfer of the conjoined tendon and distal end of the coracoid process to the clavicle, *Clin Orthop* 135:157-164, 1978.

115. Dewar FP, Barrington TW: The treatment of chronic acromioclavicular dislocation, *J Bone Joint Surg Br* 47:32-35, 1965.

116. Brunelli G, Brunelli F: The treatment of acromio-clavicular dislocation by transfer of the short head of biceps, *Int Orthop* 12(2):105-108, 1988.

117. Caspi I, Ezra E, Nerubay J, et al: Musculocutaneous nerve injury after coracoid process transfer for clavicle instability. Report of three cases, *Acta Orthop Scand* 58(3):294-295, 1987.

118. Tsou PM: Percutaneous cannulated screw coracoclavicular fixation for acute acromioclavicular dislocations, *Clin Orthop* 243:112-121, 1989.

119. Harris RI, Wallace AL, Harper GD, et al: Structural properties of the intact and the reconstructed coracoclavicular ligament complex, *Am J Sports Med* 28(1):103-108, 2000.

120. Motamedi AR, Blevins FT, Willis MC, et al: Biomechanics of the coracoclavicular ligament complex and augmentations used in its repair and reconstruction, *Am J Sports Med* 28(3):380-384, 2000.

121. Jari R, Costic RS, Rodosky MW, et al: Biomechanical function of surgical procedures for acromioclavicular joint dislocations, *Arthroscopy* 20(3):237-245, 2004.

122. Fleming RE, Tornberg DN, Kiernan H: An operative repair of acromioclavicular separation, *J Trauma* 18(10):709-712, 1978.

123. Stam L, Dawson I: Complete acromioclavicular dislocations: treatment with a Dacron ligament, *Injury* 22(3):173-176, 1991.

124. Pearsall AW, Hollis JM, Russell GV Jr, et al: Biomechanical comparison of reconstruction techniques for disruption of the acromioclavicular and coracoclavicular ligaments, *J South Orthop Assoc* 11(1):11-17, 2002.

125. Wickham MQ, Wyland DJ, Glisson RR, et al: A biomechanical comparison of suture constructs used for coracoclavicular fixation, *J South Orthop Assoc* 12(3):143-148, 2003.

126. Clayer M, Slavotinek J, Krishnan J: The results of coracoclavicular slings for acromio-clavicular dislocation, *Aust N Z J Surg* 67(6):343-346, 1997.

127. Pfahler M, Krodel A, Refior HJ: Surgical treatment of acromioclavicular dislocation, *Arch Orthop Trauma Surg* 113(6):308-311, 1994.

128. Morrison DS, Lemos MJ: Acromioclavicular separation. Reconstruction using synthetic loop augmentation, *Am J Sports Med* 23(1):105-110, 1995.

129. Stone KR, Carli AD, Day R, et al: Acromioclavicular joint reconstruction using Gore-Tex tape: evaluation of a new surgical technique and rehabilitation protocol. Internet document available at www.stoneclinic.com/acjoint2 (accessed May 5, 2004).

130. Sloan SM, Budoff JE, Hipp JA, et al: Coracoclavicular ligament reconstruction using the lateral half of the conjoined tendon, *J Shoulder Elbow Surg* 13(2):186-190, 2004.

131. Lee SJ, Nicholas SJ, Akizuki KH, et al: Reconstruction of the coracoclavicular ligaments with tendon grafts: a comparative biomechanical study, *Am J Sports Med* 31(5):648-655, 2003.

132. Jones HP, Lemos MJ, Schepsis AA: Salvage of failed acromioclavicular joint reconstruction using autogenous semitendinosus tendon from the knee. Surgical technique and case report, *Am J Sports Med* 29(2):234-237, 2001.

133. Breslow MJ, Jazrawi LM, Bernstein AD, et al: Treatment of acromioclavicular joint separation: suture or suture anchors? *J Shoulder Elbow Surg* 11(3):225-229, 2002.

134. Su EP, Vargas JH, Boynton MD: Using suture anchors for coracoclavicular fixation in treatment of complete acromioclavicular separation, *Am J Orthop* 33(5):256-257, 2004.

135. Baker JE, Nicandri GT, Young DC, et al: A cadaveric study examining acromioclavicular joint congruity after different methods of coracoclavicular loop repair, *J Shoulder Elbow Surg* 12(6):595-598, 2003.

136. Kumar S, Sethi A, Jain AK: Surgical treatment of complete acromioclavicular dislocation using the coracoacromial ligament and coracoclavicular fixation: report of a technique in 14 patients, *J Orthop Trauma* 9(6):507-510, 1995.

137. Pavlik A, Csepai D, Hidas P: Surgical treatment of chronic acromioclavicular joint dislocation by modified Weaver-Dunn procedure, *Knee Surg Sports Traumatol Arthrosc* 9(5):307-312, 2001.

138. Rokito AS, Oh YH, Zuckerman JD: Modified Weaver-Dunn procedure for acromioclavicular joint dislocations, *Orthopedics* 27(1):21-28, 2004.

139. Guy DK, Wirth MA, Griffin JL, et al: Reconstruction of chronic and complete dislocations of the acromioclavicular joint, *Clin Orthop* 347:138-149, 1998.

140. Rolla PR, Surace MF, Murena L: Arthroscopic treatment of acute acromioclavicular joint dislocation, *Arthroscopy* 20(6):662-668, 2004.

141. Wolf EM, Pennington WT: Arthroscopic reconstruction for acromioclavicular joint dislocation, *Arthroscopy* 17(5):558-563, 2001.

142. Wolf EM, Fragomen AT: Arthroscopic reconstruction of the coracoclavicular ligaments for acromioclavicular joint separations, *Oper Tech Sports Med* 12(1):49-55, 2004.

143. Imhoff AB, Chernchujit B: Arthroscopic anatomic stabilization of acromioclavicular joint dislocation, *Oper Tech Sports Med* 12(1):43-48, 2004.

144. Mazzocca AD, Conway JE, Johnson S, et al: The anatomic coracoclavicular ligament reconstruction, *Oper Tech Sports Med* 12(1):56-61, 2004.

Anterior Capsulolabral Reconstruction

Christopher J. Durall, DPT, SCS, ATC, CSCS

Charles Giangarra, MD

C. Scott Humphrey, MD

ANTERIOR CAPSULOLABRAL RECONSTRUCTION

Shoulder pain in the overhead athlete remains a challenging diagnostic problem. In the uninjured shoulder, static and dynamic stabilizers work in unison to maintain the relationship between mobility and stability. However, excessive stress on these structures because of repetitive overhead activities may disrupt this equilibrium secondary to fatigue of the rotator cuff and scapular rotators. This muscle fatigue may lead to anterior glenohumeral translation, and, over the course of time, result in stretching of the anterior capsule. The resultant loose, redundant anterior capsule often develops concurrently with attenuation of the posterior capsulolabral complex, with subsequent instability, internal impingement, and possibly rotator cuff tearing (Figure 27-1). Although some athletes with acquired glenohumeral hyperlaxity or instability will fare well in a comprehensive rehabilitation program, others require surgical stabilization and rehabilitation before returning to competitive play.

Numerous stabilizing approaches have been proposed for the glenohumeral joint, but some of these procedures improve stability at the expense of mobility. For competitive athletes, the loss of full functional motion can be as much of an impediment to successful performance as joint instability. Anterior capsulolabral reconstruction (ACLR) was developed to restore stability to the anterior glenohumeral joint while preserving functional motion in overhead athletes.[1-3] In this chapter we will explain the ACLR procedure and present an evidence-based formulaic postoperative rehabilitation program. Variables such as surgical technique, tissue quality, fixation quality, and associated operative procedures, however, necessitate that the rehabilitation of each patient be somewhat individualized. Such variables also necessitate

regular communication between surgeon and therapist to ensure positive patient outcomes. In keeping with the theme of this book, the rehabilitation protocol that follows was developed specifically for orthopedic sports medicine patients.

SURGICAL PROCEDURE

Anterior capsular shift, or capsulorrhaphy, is an accepted procedure for the correction of anteroinferior instability of the shoulder with an associated capsular redundancy. It has been suggested that capsular redundancy is the major pathologic feature in multidirectional instability.[4] Several variations of the anterior-capsular-shift technique have been espoused.[1-10] These may be divided into three basic categories: a medial-based (glenoid) T-capsular shift (Figure 27-2), a central vertical capsular shift (Figure 27-3), or a lateral-based (humeral) T-capsular shift (Figure 27-4). In this chapter the medial-based glenoid T-capsular shift will be described in detail and then briefly compared with the other two methods.

ACLR is a glenoid-based T-capsular shift.[1,3,5] As described by Jobe and co-workers,[1] it is a modification of the procedure originally described by Bankart[11] and Rowe and Zarins,[12] but with the addition of an inferior capsular shift fashioned on the glenoid side. The surgery is performed as follows.

The shoulder capsule is approached through a surgical incision via the deltopectoral interval. The deltoid muscle and cephalic vein are retracted laterally, and the pectoralis major muscle medially. It is important to leave the cephalic vein attached to the deltoid to minimize postoperative swelling. The conjoined tendon is left intact and is retracted medially. Care must be taken not to retract with too much force, because a musculocutaneous nerve neurapraxia may result.

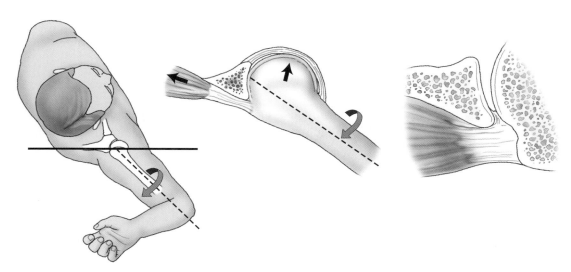

Figure 27-1: Anterior subluxation and resultant anatomic damage with the arm in the coronal plane. Impingement of the rotator cuff on the posterosuperior glenoid labrum occurs during humeral abduction and maximal external rotation. (*From Rockwood CA, Matsen FA: The shoulder, ed 2, Philadelphia, 1998, Saunders.*)

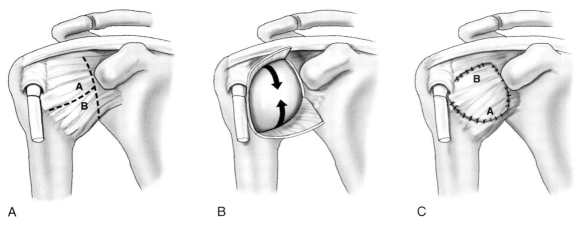

A   B   C

Figure 27-2: Diagrammatic representation of the glenoid-based T-capsular shift described by Jobe and colleagues[1-3] and by Altchek and colleagues.[5] **A,** Capsular incision. **B,** Elevated capsular flaps. Arrows represent the direction each limb is advanced. The inferior flap is shifted first. **C,** Shoulder after suturing. Line A represents sutures from the inferior flap, and line B represents those from the superior flap. (*From Miller M, Larsen K, Luke T, et al: Anterior capsular shift volume reduction: an in vitro comparison of three techniques,* J Shoulder Elbow Surg *12:350-354, 2003.*)

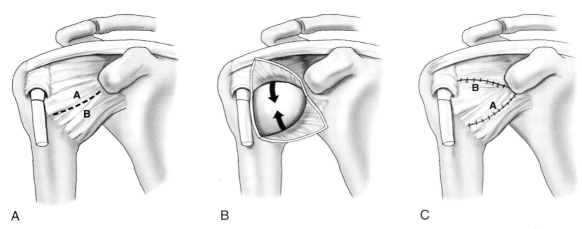

A   B   C

Figure 27-3: Diagrammatic representation of the humeral-based T-capsular shift described by Neer and Foster.[4] **A,** Capsular incisions. **B,** Elevated capsular flaps. Arrows represent the direction in which each flap is advanced. The inferior flap is shifted first. **C,** Shoulder after suturing. Line A represents sutures from the inferior flap, and line B represents those from the superior flap. (*From Miller M, Larsen K, Luke T, et al: Anterior capsular shift volume reduction: an in vitro comparison of three techniques,* J Shoulder Elbow Surg *12:350-354, 2003.*)

The subscapularis muscle is now visible. The exposure of this muscle may be improved by externally rotating the humerus to position the biceps laterally. By means of electrocautery the subscapularis is divided horizontally along the direction of its fibers at the junction of the upper two-thirds and lower third levels, thereby leaving the insertion intact. The glenohumeral joint capsule is then carefully dissected from the overlying subscapularis muscle. The humeral insertion of the subscapularis muscle is left intact with this technique.

The capsule must be palpated for integrity, volume, and ability to buttress the anterior inferior margin. The degree of capsular shift must be tailored to the degree of laxity. A

horizontal capsulotomy is then created at the junction of the upper two thirds and lower third of the capsule. This incision is extended medially beyond the rim of the glenoid, then superiorly and inferiorly over the glenoid, giving the incision its characteristic T shape. The capsular flaps are then dissected from the anterior scapular neck and glenoid rim. More dissection will yield a larger flap, which allows for a greater shift, as may be required for a very unstable shoulder.

The glenoid labrum should be palpated carefully to assess for the presence of a Bankart lesion. If a Bankart lesion is present, it is repaired to the anterior scapular neck by suture fixation or with Mitek bone anchors (Mitek Products, Inc., Westwood, MA).

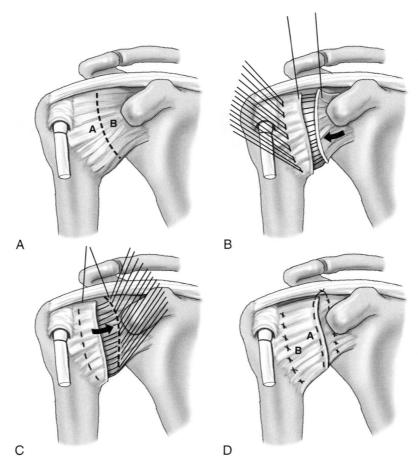

Figure 27-4: Diagrammatic representation of the vertical capsular imbrication described by Wirth and colleagues.[9] **A,** Capsular incision. **B,** Elevated capsular flaps. The arrow demonstrates the medial limb shifting deep to the lateral limb in a superolateral direction. **C,** The lateral limb is then sutured over the medial limb. **D,** Shoulder after suturing. Note that limb *B* has shifted laterally and superiorly. Line *A* represents sutures from the inferior flap, and line B represents those from the superior flap. (*From Miller M, Larsen K, Luke T, et al: Anterior capsular shift volume reduction: an in vitro comparison of three techniques*, J Shoulder Elbow Surg *12:350-354, 2003.*)

Jobe originally described using capsular tissue to buttress the anterior labrum. Shifting the inferior capsule superiorly and suturing it within the margin of the joint to the anterior rim of the glenoid achieved this. With the advent of suture anchors, however, this practice was abandoned, and the capsule is now attached to the anterior scapular neck outside of the joint instead of within it.

After the inferior capsular flap is shifted superiorly, the superior capsular flap is next shifted distally, overlapping the inferior flap. Passive motion of the shoulder is then performed to ensure at least 90 degrees of abduction and 45 degrees of external rotation before tension is noted along the suture lines. The capsule is then closed with interrupted, nonabsorbable sutures, and the subscapularis is reapproximated with absorbable sutures. The arm is splinted postoperatively in a position with an appropriate amount of abduction and external rotation in the scapular plane. The splint is worn full time for 2 to 3 weeks.

Other authors have described a central vertical capsular shift, or capsular imbrication.[9] Briefly, the shoulder capsule is approached through the deltopectoral interval. The proximal two thirds of the subscapularis is divided vertically, thereby detaching it from the capsule. The capsule is incised vertically in the midsubstance, taking care to protect the axillary nerve inferiorly. The anterior aspect of the glenoid is then decorticated, and sutures are passed through drill holes in the glenoid for subsequent repair of the Perthes-Bankart lesion, if present. The medial aspect of the capsule is pulled taut in the lateral direction, and the suture is passed from the glenoid through the capsule. The medial capsular leaflet is shifted superolaterally. The lateral capsule is shifted superomedially, which double-breasts the anterior aspect of the capsule. The subscapularis is then reapproximated, and the wound is closed.

A lateral-based (humeral) T-capsular shift has also been popularized.[4,7,8] As with the other methods of anterior shoulder reconstruction, the surgeon uses an anterior deltopectoral splitting approach. A T-shaped incision is made in the capsule, with one line of the T placed horizontally between the middle and inferior glenohumeral ligaments and the other cut vertically near the anterior capsular insertion of the proximal humerus. The arm is externally rotated as the inferior flap is detached from the inferior part of the humeral neck all the way back to the posterior aspect of the neck. The axillary nerve must be protected during this step. The neck of the humerus is prepared by decorticating the bone to create a bleeding bed. The arm is held in slight flexion and 10 degrees of external rotation on the arm board. The inferior flap is relocated first, and it is pulled forward to tighten the posterior part of the capsule until posterior subluxation no longer occurs and the inferior capsular pouch is eliminated. This flap is then sutured to the stump of the subscapularis tendon and to the part of the capsule remaining on the humerus—the goal being to hold the flap down to the decorticated bony slot. The superior flap (which contains the middle glenohumeral ligament) is then brought down over the inferior flap so that it acts to suspend the humerus and reinforce anteriorly as well. The subscapularis is then repaired in its normal position with nonabsorbable sutures, and the wound is closed.

For the overhead athlete with an especially redundant capsule, a newer variation of the lateral-based T-capsular shift has lead to excellent stability, with patients returning to a highly functional level of athletic performance.[6] This procedure is essentially the same as the humeral-based T-plasty described above, but the subscapularis muscle is split longitudinally in the direction of the fibers, through the midportion (or distal third), allowing its insertion into the humerus to remain intact. The subscapularis muscle fibers are then retracted in the cephalad and caudad directions in order to gain exposure to the capsule. As with Jobe's procedure, this technique allows the surgery to be performed with minimal trauma to the subscapularis muscle. Because the subscapularis tendon and muscle fibers are minimally disrupted, this theoretically allows the patient to achieve athletic performance levels at or near the presurgical level.

Recent literature has focused on comparing the different capsular-shift techniques. Miller and colleagues[13] compared the shoulder joint volume reduction achieved by the humeral-sided T-capsular shift, the glenoid-sided T-capsular shift, and the central vertical capsular shift (Figure 27-5). The humeral-sided T-capsular shift provided the greatest joint volume reduction, followed by the central vertical capsular shift. The glenoid-based T-capsular shift provided the least capsular volume reduction. Deutsch and co-workers compared the biomechanical results of glenoid-based versus humeral-based shift strategies.[14] The authors found no significant difference between two patient groups with respect to restriction of translation in the anterior and inferior directions. The glenoid-based shift caused a significantly greater decrease in posterior translation at 45 and 90 degrees of abduction. The glenoid-based shift also exerted significantly greater restriction on external rotation than the humeral-based shifts. Interpretation of these data is still open to debate, and Deutsch and colleagues acknowledge that long-term clinical studies are necessary to determine whether

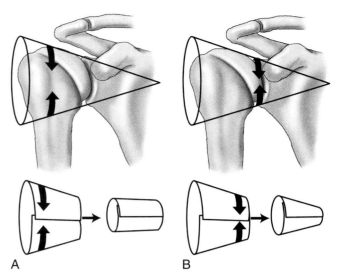

Figure 27-5: Conceptual illustration of the shoulder capsule undergoing shift. The shoulder capsule follows the form of a cone, with its base at the humeral head tapering medially. **A,** Release of the capsule laterally corresponds to the base of the cone and allows a greater arc of capsule to be released for capsulorrhaphy and a greater reduction in volume. **B,** Release more medially provides a shorter arc to shift, which produces a lesser reduction in volume. (*From Miller M, Larsen K, Luke T, et al: Anterior capsular shift volume reduction: an in vitro comparison of three techniques,* J Shoulder Elbow Surg *12:350-354, 2003.*)

restriction of external rotation will predispose the glenohumeral joint to degenerative changes.

In conclusion, the capsular shift techniques discussed here address the fundamental pathology in the refractory overhead athlete who experiences shoulder pain because of instability. These surgical techniques have been developed to address capsular redundancy, which is felt to be the source of instability in this patient population. Early data suggest that performing the capsular-shift surgery with minimal disruption to the subscapularis muscle, as well as basing the T-plasty of the capsule on the humeral side, may lead to stability with better postoperative function and range of motion (ROM) than is possible with other techniques.

OVERVIEW AND GOALS FOR POSTOPERATIVE REHABILITATION

Successful rehabilitation after an ACLR requires an integrated plan of active and passive motion restoration, strengthening, endurance exercise, proprioception enhancement, and improved anticipatory muscle activation. Specific rehabilitation goals after ACLR therefore include restoration of full, pain-free active ROM (AROM) and passive ROM (PROM), optimization of the tension-generating capacity, timing, and synchronization of the shoulder muscles, restoration of proprioception, and ultimately, return to full symptom-free activity. Each of these elements is addressed throughout the rehabilitation process, although one or two of the elements are typically emphasized during each phase of rehabilitation. Successful integration of these elements requires careful program planning and monitoring by the therapist.

The overall goals of the rehabilitation process are a continuation of the ACLR surgical objectives—restoration of glenohumeral stability and full functional ability. An understanding of the mechanisms of glenohumeral joint stability is essential for superior outcomes after rehabilitation for ACLR. Therefore a brief review of glenohumeral stability is presented to provide a rationale for the protocol that follows.

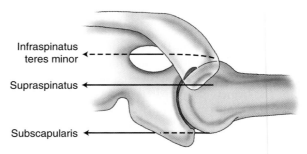

Figure 27-6: Dynamic effect of the rotator cuff causing compression as well as anterior and posterior barrier effect. (*From Kelley MJ, Clark WA: Orthopedic therapy of the shoulder, Philadelphia, 1994, Lippincott.*)

Glenohumeral Joint Stability

Glenohumeral joint stability is dependent on complex interactions among passive and active structures and forces. Stabilizing factors include joint geometry,[15,16] negative intracapsular pressure,[17] adhesion and cohesion of the articular surfaces,[17] the glenoid labrum,[12] and tension in the glenohumeral joint capsule, ligaments, and muscles.[16,18]

The joint capsule and ligaments are lax in the mid ranges of motion to permit adequate joint excursion[17] and tighten at the extremes of motion, causing the humeral head to translate in the opposite direction.[19] Therefore flexion tightens the posterior capsule, pushing the humeral head anteriorly, whereas extension tightens the anterior capsule, pushing the humeral head posteriorly.

Because the capsule and ligaments are effective stabilizers only when taut, several groups of muscles must act to control humeral head movement and therefore assist with stabilization in the mid ranges of motion. Muscles that contribute to glenohumeral joint stability include the biceps brachii (long head), deltoid, latissimus dorsi, pectoralis major, triceps (long head), teres major, the muscles that control scapular movement (rhomboid, levator scapulae, pectoralis minor, trapezius, serratus anterior), and the four rotator cuff muscles—supraspinatus, infraspinatus, teres minor, and subscapularis.[16,20] Muscular "strength" (i.e., torque-generating capacity) is meaningless from a functional perspective unless the muscles can be activated in a timely and appropriate manner. Therefore neuromuscular control and timing must be addressed in addition to strength to prepare the athlete for return to competitive play after surgical stabilization.

Rotator Cuff

The rotator cuff muscles work intimately with the capsuloligamentous system to enhance joint stability by compressing the humeral head in the glenoid fossa[18] and by constraining humeral head movement (Figure 27-6).[21,22] Tension in the rotator cuff and glenohumeral ligaments causes compression of the convex humeral head into the concave glenoid fossa, stabilizing the humeral head against translation. All four portions of the rotator cuff contribute to this joint compres-

sion effect, and loss of tension-generating capacity in any of the four portions significantly reduces compression stabilization.

In addition to the compressive effect, the cuff muscles act with the capsuloligamentous system to create dynamic "slings," which resist humeral head movement away from the center of the glenoid.[21,22] The subscapularis, for example, can act as a barrier or sling to reduce anterior humeral head translation.[23,24] The sling action of the subscapularis is most pronounced in the lower ranges of elevation; with glenohumeral joint elevation, the subscapularis' line of action moves superiorly, reducing its ability to limit anterior humeral translation.[23,24] The deltoid muscle has also been identified as an important anterior stabilizer of the glenohumeral joint when the humerus is abducted and externally rotated.[25]

The conjoined infraspinatus and teres minor tendons are positioned to act as a dynamic sling against posterior humeral head translation and appear to also resist anterior subluxation of the humerus when acting eccentrically.[26] The supraspinatus is well poised to resist inferior humeral subluxation.[27] It is interesting to note that less electromyographic activity has been recorded in the supraspinatus in shoulders with anterior joint instability during abduction and scaption from 30 to 60 degrees.[28] The rotator cuff muscles, therefore, work collaboratively to stabilize the joint against anterior, posterior, or inferior displacement. The "circle concept," often applied to the glenohumeral capsuloligamentous structures, can be applied to the rotator cuff *muscles* as well. Fatigue of the dynamic stabilizers would logically permit greater humeral head translation during overhead activity. Therefore exercises intended to improve the endurance of the cuff muscles have been included in the rehabilitation protocol discussed later. It is important to remember that endurance and strength are mutually exclusive physiologic properties that require disparate training stimuli.

Evidence suggests that tension-sensitive mechanoreceptors embedded within the ligaments, joint capsule, and labrum induce reflex stimulation of the glenohumeral muscles when stimulated.[20] Activation of the glenohumeral muscles increases tension in the capsuloligamentous system via the direct attachment of the cuff tendons to the joint capsule. Increased tension in the capsuloligamentous complex therefore results in reflexive activation of the cuff muscles to further augment joint stability. The capsuloligamentous complex, then, is not merely a static restraint, but a tension-sensitive receptor complex.

The reflex loop formed between the capsuloligamentous mechanoreceptors and the glenohumeral muscles appears to be disrupted in unstable shoulders.[29] Therefore the capsuloligamentous injury that occurs with shoulder instability affects not only mechanical restraint but also sensorimotor function. The result is alteration in muscle firing patterns and impaired proprioception (i.e., position sense), which may contribute to, or exacerbate, glenohumeral instability.[29]

The time required for nerve conduction from the capsuloligamentous mechanoreceptors, through a reflex arc, and back to the muscles again may be too long to activate the muscles to enhance glenohumeral joint stability during *high-speed* movement. However, volitional muscle activation before a perturbation has been shown to significantly reduce the time to onset of stabilizing muscle activity.[30] Therefore efforts to improve volitional muscle activation in positions of injury vulnerability may reduce the risk of injury. Examples of activities intended to improve proprioception and muscular stabilization during perturbations are provided later in this chapter. Davies and Dickoff-Hoffman have also synopsized shoulder neuromuscular testing and rehabilitation.[31] Both surgical stabilization and plyometric training have been shown to restore some normalcy to the sensorimotor system, enhancing proprioception and neuromuscular reactivity.[30,32,33] A sample upper extremity plyometric training program is shown in Box 27-1.

Scapulothoracic Muscles

The scapula contributes significantly to glenohumeral stability by providing a stable articular surface for the humeral head and an attachment for the scapulohumeral muscles (i.e., rotator cuff, deltoid). The muscles that move the scapula must possess adequate length and strength to optimally align

---

BOX 27-1

Sample Upper Extremity Plyometric Program

Medicine Ball with Trampoline Rebounder (e.g., Plyoback)
- Medicine ball step and pass
- Medicine ball chest pass
- Medicine ball soccer throw (overhead pass)
- Medicine ball side throw (trunk rotation)
- Medicine ball backward side-to-side throw
- D1/D2 diagonal toss
- Single arm toss
- Overhead ER deceleration with ER toss or throw
- Overhead ER deceleration with ER toss or throw with T-band on wrist

Ball dribbling
- Frontal plane—dribble medicine ball on wall through arc (10 o'clock to 3 o'clock position on imaginary clock face)
- Frontal plane—dribble medicine ball on wall through arc with T-band on wrist to resist dribble

Tubing
- IR and ER at 0 degrees; at 90 degrees
- Elbow flexion and extension
- Supination and pronation
- Diagonals

Closed kinetic chain
- 45-degree push-up on edge of flat bench
- Push-up
- Push-up on trampoline
- Push-up on T-foam
- Push-up on BAPS
- Push-up on T-ball
- Push-up (boxes)
- Push-up (clappers)
- Drops from box and then push-up back onto box
- Side-to-side walking
- Wheelbarrows (walking)
- Hand walking on stepper
- Horizontal abduction and adduction on slide-board
- Shoulder circles on slide-board

Bosu (half ball)
- IR and ER at 0 degrees with weight in hand
- IR and ER at 90 degrees with weight in hand

Other
- Self-tossing in a supine position
- Throwing motion with weighted ball in hand (no ball release)

the glenoid relative to the joint reaction force and to maintain the optimal length in the rotator cuff and deltoid muscles. The scapula has been likened to a seal trying to balance a ball (humeral head) on its nose (glenoid) (Figure 27-7).[12] Small, frequent adjustments are required to keep the "ball" balanced, or centered on the glenoid fossa. Scapulohumeral "rhythm," then, can be thought of as more than just the ratio of humeral to scapular movement, because there is a delicate "rhythm" or interplay between the scapula and humerus.

Glenohumeral instability has been shown to coincide with diminished electromyographic (EMG) activity in the serratus anterior—more than in any of the other scapulothoracic muscles (rhomboid, levator scapulae, pectoralis minor, and trapezius).[28,34] Specifically, serratus anterior EMG activity has been shown to diminish in a general population with anterior instability,[28] and during pitching in elite pitchers.[34] The consequence of reduced serratus activity is presumably altered scapular mechanics, and consequently aberrant glenohumeral mechanics.

Biceps Brachii (Long Head)

The long head of the biceps brachii, like the rotator cuff, has important stabilizing functions at the glenohumeral joint. The biceps brachii assists with reducing anterior translation when the humerus is internally rotated and posterior translation when the humerus is externally rotated.[35,36] In addition, the biceps is a key anterior stabilizer when the humerus is in neutral rotation.[24] The biceps, like the supraspinatus, is an important active stabilizer preventing inferior glenohumeral joint translation.[27,36]

POSTOPERATIVE REHABILITATION

Motion Restoration

One of the primary objectives of ACLR is preservation of full functional shoulder ROM. Failure to restore full motion postoperatively will impair functional performance and presumably increase the risk of iatrogenic joint degeneration. However, it is unreasonable to expect full pain-free ROM during the initial phase of rehabilitation because of postoperative pain, inflammation, adaptive tissue shortening, and stiffness from immobilization resulting from soft tissue healing constraints. Nor is it appropriate to force motion *at the expense of the surgical repair.* Overaggressive mobilization and/or return to activity before complete healing can easily result in capsular attenuation and recurrent instability. The anterior capsule, in particular, should be stressed cautiously to avoid reversing the stabilizing effect of the repair. A timetable for motion restoration throughout the rehabilitation process is shown in Table 27-1.

Efforts at motion restoration should be consistent, controlled, and appropriately stressful given the surgeon's assessment of tissue quality and fixation quality. Some stress to the healing tissues is necessary to promote the synthesis of mature

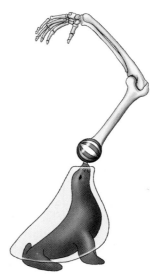

Figure 27-7: Seal balancing a ball on its nose as an analogy for the delicate interplay between the scapula and humerus at the shoulder. (*From Pink M, Jobe FW: Shoulder injuries in athletes,* Clin Manag *11:40, 1991. Used with permission from the American Physical Therapy Association. This material is copyrighted, and any further reproduction or distribution is prohibited.*)

Type I collagen with adequate tensile strength. A concerted effort should be made to restore full active and passive glenohumeral ROM in all planes by the ninth or tenth postoperative week, because collagen maturation will make it more difficult to regain full motion after this time.

Efforts at motion restoration in patients with congenital laxity should be progressed slowly and cautiously. Individuals with congenital laxity tend to form highly compliant nonmineralized connective tissue, which contributes to joint hyperlaxity. It may be prudent, in consultation with the surgeon, to extend the duration of immobilization in patients with congenital laxity.

Again, it is imperative that overhead athletes regain their full ROM. Lack of adequate external rotation, for instance, can easily compromise overhead athletic performance. The glenohumeral joint should be clinically stable yet sufficiently lax to permit functional motion. This balance between functional mobility and joint stability has been described as the "thrower's paradox"[37] but may present a paradoxic rehabilitation challenge for nonthrowing overhead athletes as well. This paradox is manageable with controlled and progressive remobilization.

It is important to address any posterior capsular shortening, because tightness of the posterior capsule causes obligate anterior humeral head migration and subsequent anterior soft tissue compression.[19] Although complaints of anterior shoulder pain are not uncommon after ACLR, the source of the pain should be elucidated to ensure that iatrogenic injury has not occurred.

Phase I: Immediate Postoperative Phase (Day 1 to Week 3)

Rehabilitation after ACLR can begin the day after the procedure, with the surgeon's approval. The objectives of the immediate postoperative phase include decreasing pain and inflammation, increasing pain-free ROM while protecting repair, preserving elbow, wrist, and hand strength and ROM, and preserving or enhancing cardiovascular endurance. "Red flags" or cautionary indicators during this phase include unremitting pain and markedly restricted or excessive glenohumeral joint mobility.

After the repair a postoperative splint or sling is typically used to immobilize the shoulder in slight abduction (depending on tension on the repair) for 1 to 2 weeks. This is worn during all waking hours except for the brief periods of time each day when PROM is performed. In some instances the surgeon may also ask the patient to wear the immobilizer at night.

The shoulder should be moved passively through a comfortable range of elevation in the sagittal and scapular planes one or two times daily. Gentle, pain-free internal and external rotation PROM (preferably in the scapular plane) may be performed with the surgeon's approval. An upper body ergometer may be employed as a means to provide self-PROM or active-assisted ROM (AAROM). Once ROM is adequate, an upper body cycle or rowing machine can also be used to increase core body temperature (thereby improving soft tissue extensibility and neuromuscular function) before exercise or mobilization and/or for cardiovascular fitness. Self-ROM exercises using a wand, golf club, or the contralateral hand may be performed once the splint or sling is removed. It is important to communicate to the patient that combining abduction with external rotation places significant tension on the anterior capsule and therefore should be approached cautiously or completely avoided at this stage.

Depending on the surgeon's preference, gentle, progressive resistance exercise may begin after splint use is discontinued, typically during the third postoperative week. Initially, these exercises should be submaximal and static (i.e., isometric). All of the stabilizers of the glenohumeral joint should be addressed. Isometric exercise efforts should last 5 to 6 seconds for optimal benefit.

Proprioceptive neuromuscular facilitation (PNF) rhythmic stabilization may also be employed by having the patient work to maintain a static position while the therapist attempts to gently perturb the limb from a variety of angles. The scapulothoracic muscles may be challenged via isometric exercise (patient resists efforts by the therapist to displace the scapula from its resting position) with the patient side lying, prone, or seated.

Resistance and duration should be low initially and should be "titrated" in response to the patient's response. Some postexercise discomfort is typical, although not necessarily desirable. Postexercise discomfort that lasts for an extended duration (e.g., 6 to 8 hours) and does not appear to be simply exercise-induced muscle soreness should alert the therapist to significantly adjust the program intensity and duration. Cryotherapy and/or electrical stimulation (e.g., interferential current [IFC], transcutaneous electric nerve stimulation [TENS]) may be used for pain modulation.

Hand-squeezing exercises (e.g., ball squeeze, putty squeeze), active elbow exercise (e.g., flexion and extension with rubber tubing or band), and active wrist exercise (e.g., resisted wrist flexion, extension, radial deviation, ulnar deviation, supination, pronation) can begin on the first postoperative day. Exercising these muscle groups will reduce the undesirable effects of relative disuse during the shoulder immobilization period.

While the shoulder complex and remainder of the upper extremity are emphasized in the therapeutic exercise program, the athlete should continue to strengthen the torso and legs

TABLE 27-1

Weekly Range of Motion Goals after ACLR

	WEEKS 3-4	WEEKS 5-6	WEEKS 7-8	WEEKS 9-10
Flexion	120-140 degrees	160 degrees	165-175 degrees	WNL
Extension	10-25 degrees	30-35 degrees	40-45 degrees	WNL
IR at 45 degrees of scaption	35-45 degrees	—	—	—
ER at 45 degrees of scaption	45-60 degrees	—	—	—
IR at 90 degrees of abduction	—	75 degrees	80-85 degrees (GH and ST)	WNL
ER at 90 degrees of abduction	—	70-75 degrees	80-85 degrees	WNL (>90 degrees for overhead athletes)

Modified from Brotzman SB, Wilk KE: *Clinical orthopedic rehabilitation*, Philadelphia, 2003, Mosby.
ER, External rotation; *GH,* glenohumeral; *IR,* internal rotation; *ST,* scapulothoracic; *WNL,* within normal limits.

throughout the rehabilitation process. Because the torso and legs are significant contributors to torque generation during overhead sports, failure to maintain or improve the strength of the torso and legs will presumably increase stress on the athlete's recovering shoulder when he or she returns to throwing, hitting, and so on. In choosing individual exercises for the torso and legs, the therapist should consider the kinematics and muscular demands of the particular sport as well as identified deficits in the athlete.

Initially, a stationary bike will be the most appropriate device to maintain or improve cardiovascular fitness in patients recovering from ACLR. Once sling or splint use is discontinued, the choice of cardiovascular exercise device should be influenced by the athlete's sport requirements.

Phase II: Intermediate Postoperative Phase (Weeks 3 to 12)

During the second rehabilitation phase, the emphasis in the early portion is on controlled restoration of motion, whereas in the later portion the emphasis shifts toward restoration of functional strength. Goals of this phase include elimination of pain, restoration of full, pain-free ROM (see Table 27-1), enhanced strength of the glenohumeral, scapulothoracic, elbow, wrist, and hand musculature, improved upper extremity hand position sense (proprioception), and enhanced cardiovascular endurance. Causes for concern (i.e., "red flags")

during this phase include lack of full glenohumeral motion by 8 to 10 weeks, excessive joint mobility, and/or significant weakness at week 12.

As in the previous phase, an upper body cycle or rowing machine may be used for the rehabilitation warm-up and/or cool-down. Self-ROM exercises should be performed one or two times daily, assuming the patient is independent with the exercises. Manual joint mobilization techniques may be necessary or advisable, avoiding untoward tension on the anterior capsule.

Adequate extensibility of the posterior cuff or capsule should be obtained (as evidenced by full internal rotation), because a tight posterior cuff or capsule forces the humeral head anteriorly or superiorly during arm elevation, inducing subacromial impingement. This can be accomplished with horizontal adduction (i.e., cross-chest) stretching, and/or side lying glenohumeral internal rotation stretching with the shoulder flexed and abducted to 90 degrees. Adequate extensibility of the pectoralis minor should be obtained to ensure that the subacromial outlet is not compressed as a result of anterior scapular tipping. A stretching maneuver intended to elongate the pectoralis minor while avoiding anterior glenohumeral capsular stress is illustrated in Figure 27-8.

Resistance exercise should be pain free and progressed according to soft tissue healing. Patient response during and after resistance exercise should be observed. Although numbers of repetitions will vary, an exercise set should cease

---

TABLE 27-2

Isokinetic Performance Evaluation of Internal-External Rotation in the Dominant Arm

| | 180 DEG/SEC | | 300 DEG/SEC | | 450 DEG/SEC | |
	ER	IR	ER	IR	ER	IR
Torque/Body Weight						
Exceptional	>20%	>30%	>16%	>28%	>15%	>22%
Excellent	19%-13%	29%-24%	16%-13%	28%-24%	15%-12%	22%-17%
Good	13%-10%	24%-19%	13%-10%	24%-20%	12%-9%	17%-12%
Adequate	10%-7%	19%-14%	10%-7%	20%-16%	9%-6%	12%-8%
Fair	7%-4%	14%-9%	7%-4%	16%-12%	6%-3%	10%-6%
Poor	<4%	<9%	<4%	<12%	<3%	<3%
Average Power (Watts)						
Exceptional	>85	>150	>90	>195	>85	>200
Excellent	84-70	150-120	90-75	195-155	85-66	200-156
Good	70-55	120-90	75-58	150-115	66-48	156-112
Adequate	55-40	90-60	58-42	115-75	48-30	112-69
Fair	40-25	60-30	42-25	75-35	30-12	69-25
Poor	<25	<30	<25	<35	<12	<25

Modified from Newsham KR et al: Isokinetic profile of baseball pitchers' internal/external rotation 180, 300, 450° s⁻¹, *Med Sci Sports Exerc* 30:1489-1495, 1998.

when the patient can no longer maintain strict form or experiences pain in the repair site. Although isometric exercise is commonly used in the early postoperative period, isotonic and isokinetic exercise may be used as well, as long as the resistance and effort are submaximal and the arc of movement is controlled and relatively pain free.

Recommended exercises for the rotator cuff include elevation in the scapular plane (also known as *scaption)* performed with the humerus externally rotated ("full-can" position) to minimize subacromial impingement (Figure 27-9),[38] flexion, press-ups (Figure 27-10), push-ups with a "plus" (i.e., scapular protraction), horizontal abduction with humeral external rotation (limited to the scapular or frontal plane), and internal and external rotation.[39] Internal and external rotation exercise may be initiated with the shoulder adducted and gradually progressed to 90 degrees of elevation in the scapular and/or frontal planes.

Recommended exercises for the scapulothoracic muscles include scaption with humerus externally rotated ("full-can" position), press-ups, push-ups with a "plus," rowing, and horizontal abduction (limited to the scapular or frontal plane).[40] Some postexercise or postactivity soreness is typical, and cryotherapy and/or electrical stimulation may be used in an attempt to modulate this.

Low-intensity plyometric exercise can be incorporated, beginning roughly at week 10. See Box 27-1 for a sample plyometric progression. Isokinetic exercise can be progressed by using slower speeds and greater intensity of patient effort. Strength should be assessed via isokinetic or hand-held dynamometry during weeks 10 to 12 to determine the extent of unilateral deficits. Isokinetic normative tables are shown in Tables 27-3 and 27-4.

Exercises and activities to improve somatosensory function (proprioception and anticipatory or reactive muscle acti-

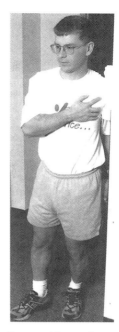

Figure 27-8: Pectoralis stretching technique for clients with anterior glenohumeral hyperlaxity or instability. Rest anterior shoulder to be stretched against corner of wall using towel cushion. Initiate stretch by retracting scapulae and rotating torso away from shoulder. Greater stretch may be obtained by using opposite hand to pull pectoral muscles toward midline of the body. (*From Durall C, Manske RC, Davies GJ: Avoiding shoulder injury from resistance training,* Strength Cond J *23:13, 2001. Copyright © 2004. Reprinted by permission of Alliance Communications Group, a division of Allen Press, Inc.*)

TABLE 27-3

Isokinetic Criteria for Return to Throwing

Bilateral comparison	ER	98%-105%
Bilateral comparison	IR	105%-115%
Bilateral comparison	ABD	98%-103%
Bilateral comparison	ADD	110%-125%
Unilateral ratio	ER/IR	66%-70%
Unilateral ratio	ABD/ADD	78%-85%
Peak torque body weight ratio	ER	18%-22%
Peak torque body weight ratio	IR	28%-32%
Peak torque body weight ratio	ABD	24%-30%
Peak torque body weight ratio	ADD	32%-38%

Modified from Brotzman SB, Wilk K: *Clinical orthopedic rehabilitation,* ed 2, Philadelphia, 2003, Mosby.
*At 180 degrees/second testing velocity.

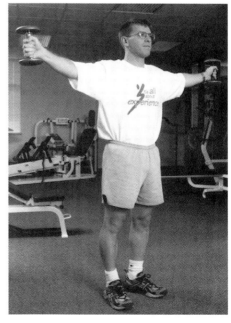

Figure 27-9: Elevation in the scapular plane with humerus externally rotated ("full-can" position). (*From Durall C, Manske RC, Davies GJ: Avoiding shoulder injury from resistance training,* Strength Cond J *23:15, 2001. Copyright © 2004. Reprinted by permission of Alliance Communications Group, a division of Allen Press, Inc.*)

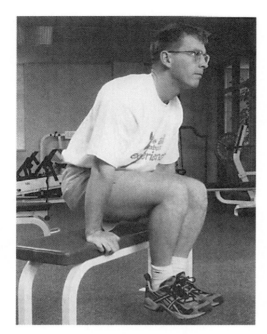

Figure 27-10: Press-up exercise. (*From Durall C, Manske RC, Davies GJ: Avoiding shoulder injury from resistance training,* Strength Cond J *23:16, 2001. Copyright © 2004. Reprinted by permission of Alliance Communications Group, a division of Allen Press, Inc.*)

BOX 27-2

Exercises Intended to Improve Proprioception and Protective Muscular Stabilization

Body Blade through throwing motion with perturbations

Perturbations throughout various arm and shoulder positions (rhythmic stabilization)

Proprioceptive neuromuscular facilitation (PNF) diagonal 1 and diagonal 2 patterns (D1/D2) with perturbations

Internal rotation/external rotation (IR/ER) tubing with perturbations

Push-up on T-foam with perturbations

Push-up on ankle platform with perturbations

Push-up on T-ball with perturbations

Single arm on medicine ball with perturbations

Body Blade through throwing motion

Profitter—side-to-side motion

Step walking on plyoboxes—"wheel barrel"

Push-ups on uneven objects or large exercise ball

---

vation) should be initiated as soon as adequate ROM is available. Somatosensory training is arguably a lower priority during the initial weeks of rehabilitation but becomes increasingly important as the rehabilitation progresses. The accuracy of hand placement or position, which is obviously critical for successful overhand sport performance, can be enhanced via position replication activities and exercises. Examples of position replication activities that may be appropriate during this phase include passively placing the patient's arm at a specific joint angle and then having the patient attempt to replicate the angle from the starting position, or rolling a ball on a wall while attempting to follow a specific path marked on a poster board affixed to the wall.

During this phase, activities and exercises to improve dynamic stabilization during potentially destabilizing activities should be included. The PNF rhythmic stabilization activity discussed in the previous phase is one simple example of this. Examples of additional anticipatory muscle activation exercises and activities can be found in Box 27-2.

The elbow, wrist, and hand muscle groups are challenged during the execution of resistance exercises for the glenohumeral and scapulothoracic joints. However, isolated exercises for the elbow, wrist, and hand should continue if sport demands require. Likewise, sports-specific training of the torso and legs should continue.

An upper body cycle or rowing machine can be employed for aerobic exercise once adequate pain-free ROM is achieved. Upper extremity cycling or rowing exercise will also presumably enhance endurance of many GH and scapulothoracic muscles. Additional low-duration, low-to-moderate intensity exercise is advisable, particularly if the athlete's sport requires prolonged low-moderate intensity exertional efforts. Following the principle of specificity of exercise, these exercises should be tailored as closely as possible to the patient's sport requirements.

TABLE 27-4

ER/IR Peak Torque (PT) Ratios for 125 Professional Baseball Pitchers

RATIO	DOMINANT		NONDOMINANT	
	MEAN	S.D.	MEAN	S.D.
ER/IR 210 degrees PT	66.6%	12.7	73.5%	12.3
ER/IR 300 degrees PT	70.3%	12.3	77.6%	11.9

Modified from Ellenbecker TS, Mattalino AJ: Concentric isokinetic shoulder internal and external rotation strength in professional baseball pitchers, *J Orthop Sports Phys Ther* 25:323-328, 1997.

Phase III: Advanced Strengthening Phase (Weeks 12 to 16)

During the third phase of rehabilitation the athlete will work on increasing functional strength and endurance, enhancing somatosensory function (proprioception and anticipatory muscle activation), and improving cardiovascular endurance. Causes for concern ("red flags") during this phase include pain with resistance training other than acute or delayed-onset muscle soreness, and/or complaints of joint instability.

Before beginning advanced strengthening the athlete should satisfy the following criteria: full, pain-free AROM and PROM; minimal pain with activity or exercise; satisfactory stability as determined by the surgeon; and achievement ≥70% of the strength of the contralateral shoulder in all planes as determined by isokinetic or hand-held dynamometry.[37,41]

Resistance exercises performed during the previous phase are progressed with an emphasis on challenging the muscles in a manner similar to sport requirements. Therefore this phase is a transitional one between general strengthening and performance-specific training and requires thoughtful consideration of the mechanics of the athlete's sport. Plyometric exercises conceivably increase quickness as well as the muscle-tendon unit's tolerance to eccentric stress and therefore should be continued (see Box 27-1). Eccentric exercise should be included to prepare the muscle-tendon unit for high-intensity tensile loading. The posterior shoulder musculature, in particular, should be challenged with eccentric exercise, because these muscles act to decelerate the forward momentum of the arm, thereby protecting the posterior shoulder structures.[42] Ideally, the posterior muscles should be exercised through an arc of motion similar to the deceleration phase of the patient's overhead sport. This may be difficult with free-weights and may require manual resistance imparted by the rehabilitation professional. Eccentric exercise for the biceps brachii is also important because this muscle has dual roles at the elbow and shoulder during the follow-through.[43]

Isokinetic training should continue, with an emphasis on approximating the joint angular velocities used for the target sport. For some sporting activities this is impossible (e.g., pitching), but an effort should be made to match *exercise* velocity with *activity* velocity. Significant correlations have been identified between throwing velocity and glenohumeral internal and external rotation at high angular velocities (240 degrees/sec) but not slower angular velocities (60 degrees/sec) in intercollegiate pitchers.[44,45]

Somatosensory retraining should continue to further enhance position sense and anticipatory muscle activation. Exercises for the elbow, wrist, hand, torso, legs, and cardiovascular system should be progressed to prepare the athlete for the demands of his or her sport.

Phase IV: Return to Activity Phase (Week 16+)

After week 16, the rehabilitation emphasis is on sports-specific training. During this final phase of rehabilitation after an ACLR, the athlete will make the transition from sports-specific training to engaging in the sport itself. Therefore the goal for this final phase is return to full activity. Before making the transition to sports-specific training, patients must have satisfactorily fulfilled criteria of previous phases and have adequate strength as determined by isokinetic or hand-held dynamometry.[37,41,46] Isokinetic testing may be performed during weeks 14 to 16 to determine the athlete's readiness to begin a sports-specific interval-training program. High angular velocities should be used during isokinetic testing to determine readiness to begin throwing.[44,45,47] The external-to-internal rotator torque ratio should be at least 65%, with a range of 66% to 76% reported as "ideal."[37,46,48] Isokinetic normative data for the shoulder are included in Tables 27-2 to 27-4.

Interval programs should be used to return the athlete to preinjury functional status via a stepwise progression. Sample interval throwing, tennis, and golf programs are included in Appendixes A and B. Axe and colleagues[49] (Appendix B) developed interval programs for softball players based on data collected over an entire season.

Many patients become overly eager to rapidly progress to full activity once they start a sports-specific program. The healing muscle-tendon unit continues to be tenuous and prone to injury even after several weeks of high-intensity resistance training, and adequate rest continues to be imperative. Careful guidance by the therapist is crucial to ensure that patients do not overexert themselves. The interval program should be modified and slowly readvanced if the athlete has increased pain. Although the programs in Appendixes A and B do not include simulated games, it is sensible to expose the athlete to stress of the same magnitude and *duration* as the target sporting activity requires before actual game situations are undertaken.

Postactivity soreness is common early in the return-to-sports phase but nonetheless demands attention. The posterior cuff or capsule is under high levels of tensile stress during arm deceleration; this stress can induce tendon or muscle injury. Recovery duration between exercise sessions should be adjusted so the athlete has minimal soreness before the next session. Considerable, lingering pain or complaints of instability with sports-specific training are potentially serious concerns that must be addressed quickly.

A mechanical assessment should be performed to ensure that the athlete's sport mechanics are sound. Therapists with little experience assessing overhead sport mechanics should consult a technique specialist or coach. Mechanical assessment is particularly valuable for younger athletes to ensure that poor technical habits are rectified before they are ingrained.

Home Exercise after Anterior Capsulolabral Reconstruction

Ideally the rehabilitation after an ACLR will occur under the guidance of a knowledgeable therapist in a well-equipped physical therapy center. However, some patients may only be able to attend a limited number of physical therapy appointments because of financial constraints or other issues. In these instances, a thorough home exercise program must be implemented once the patient has been observed to be independent with the exercises and deemed appropriately knowledgeable about the goals of the exercise program. Frequent follow-ups by phone are advisable in these instances to prevent problems from occurring. Patients who have difficulty performing the exercises correctly on a consistent basis may benefit from the use of customized exercise videotapes.

SUMMARY

The shoulder is, by necessity, extremely mobile. The consequence of this extreme mobility is relatively poor intrinsic stability. When subjected to the tremendous forces required for athletic performance, it is not surprising that the glenohumeral joint has a tendency to become unstable.

Stability of the glenohumeral joint is the result of both passive and active stabilizing structures and forces. The anterior capsulolabral reconstruction procedure improves the integrity of the passive elements, so the emphasis in the postoperative rehabilitation program is logically the enhancement of the active stabilizing element—muscle tension–generating ability (i.e., strength) and timing (i.e., neuromuscular control). In addition, careful restoration of motion, restoration of associated joint function, restoration of shoulder proprioception, and guided sports-specific training are necessary to achieve a successful return to high-level overhead sport performance. A distillation of the rehabilitation protocol is provided for quick reference in Box 27-3. Collaboration between surgeon and therapist is essential to ensure that clinical stability is maintained while attempting to maximize functional performance after an anterior capsulolabral reconstruction.

BOX 27-3
Rehabilitation after Anterior-Capsulolabral Reconstruction

General Guidelines

Restoration of shoulder motion is critical for successful athletic performance.

Efforts at motion restoration should be controlled so that the repair is not compromised.

Resisted exercise may begin as early as the third postoperative week, with surgeon approval.

Somatosensory training is important to enhance successful sport performance.

Supervised physical therapy takes 3-6 months.

Activities of Daily Living Progression

Bathing or showering without splint after suture removal

Overhead activities limited until range of motion (ROM) is restored

Phase I: Immediate Postoperative Phase (Day 1-Week 3)

Goals

Decrease pain and inflammation

Increase pain-free ROM *while protecting repair*

Preserve elbow, wrist, and hand strength and ROM

Preserve or enhance cardiovascular endurance

Educate patient

Restrictions

Splint use for 1-2 weeks (waking hours ± sleeping)

Therapeutic Exercises

Pain-free flexion and abduction passive ROM (PROM) one or two times per day

Pain-free internal rotation (IR) and external rotation (ER) in scapular plane with surgeon approval

Upper body cycle for PROM or active-assisted ROM (AAROM)

Rhythmic stabilization for scapular muscles

Submaximal isometrics

    Abduction

    Extension

    Flexion

    IR and ER (in neutral)

    Arm curls

    Arm extensions

    Ball, putty, or sponge squeezes

Resisted wrist flexion, extension, radial deviation, ulnar deviation, supination, pronation

Trunk muscle strengthening (sport-specific if possible)

BOX 27-3

Rehabilitation after Anterior-Capsulolabral Reconstruction—cont'd

Total leg strengthening (sport-specific if possible)

Cardiovascular endurance training (sport-specific if possible)

Concerns

Unremitting pain

Markedly restricted glenohumeral joint mobility

Excessive glenohumeral joint mobility

Phase II: Intermediate Postoperative Phase (Weeks 3-12)

Goals

Eliminate pain

Regain full pain-free ROM *while protecting repair*

Increase strength of glenohumeral (GH) and scapulothoracic (ST) musculature

Improve proprioception

Increase elbow, wrist, and hand strength

Preserve or enhance cardiovascular endurance

Therapeutic Exercises

Upper body cycle or rowing machine warm-up

Pain-free self-ROM (e.g., wand exercises) one or two times per day

Manual joint mobilization techniques as needed (protect anterior capsule)

Posterior cuff stretching (e.g., IR, horizontal adduction)

Pectoralis minor stretching as needed (protect anterior capsule)

Isotonics and isokinetics progressing (per healing and symptoms) from submaximal to maximal effort:

  Flexion

  Scaption ("full-can")

  IR and ER progression from 0-90 degrees of elevation in scapular and/or frontal planes; limit rotation ROM per Table 27-1

  Horizontal abduction (in prone or with reverse-fly machine); limit to scapular or frontal plane

  Rows

  Push-ups with a "plus"

  Press-ups

Plyometrics beginning approximately week 10 (Box 27-1)

Position replication activities (e.g., dart throwing, bean bag toss)

Continue with arm, leg, torso exercise (sport specific)

Sport-specific cardiovascular exercise (e.g., upper body cycle, rowing machine)

Concerns

Lack of full ROM by 8-10 weeks

Excessive joint mobility

Significant weakness by week 12

Phase III: Advanced Strengthening (Weeks 12-16)

Criteria to Advance to Phase III

Full, pain-free AROM and PROM

Minimal pain with activity and exercise

Satisfactory stability (per surgeon)

Strength ≥70% of contralateral side

Goals

Fully eliminate pain

Regain full pain-free ROM

Increase strength of GH and ST musculature

Improve proprioception

Increase elbow, wrist, hand strength

Preserve or enhance cardiovascular endurance

Therapeutic Exercises

Progress intensity per symptoms

Exercise selection should be based on deficits identified via strength testing

Eccentrics for posterior musculature and biceps brachii

Progress plyometrics per Box 27-1

Position replication activities

Anticipatory muscle activation exercises and activities—see Box 27-2

Arm, leg, torso strengthening as needed

Cardiovascular exercise

Concerns

Pain with resistance training other than acute or delayed-onset muscle soreness

Excessive joint mobility

(continued)

BOX 27-3
Rehabilitation after Anterior-Capsulolabral Reconstruction—cont'd

Phase IV: Return to Activity (Week 16+)

Criteria to Advance to Phase IV

Strength ≥85% of contralateral side

Goals

Return to full, pain-free activity, including athletics

Therapeutic Exercise

Sport-specific training

Concerns

Considerable lingering pain or instability with sports-specific training

ACKNOWLEDGMENT

Gratitude is owed to Andrew Newport, PT, DPT, ATC, CSCS for his creative ideas on improving anticipatory muscle activation.

References

1. Jobe F, Giangarra C, Kvitne R, et al: Anterior capsulolabral reconstruction of the shoulder in athletes in overhead sports, *Am J Sports Med* 19:428-434, 1991.

2. Jobe FW, Glousman RE: Anterior capsulolabral reconstruction, *Tech Orthop* 3:29-35, 1989.

3. Jobe F, Schwab D, Brewster C: Anterior capsular reconstruction. In Jobe F, Pink M, Glousman R, editors: *Operative techniques in upper extremity sports injuries,* St. Louis, 1996, Mosby.

4. Neer C, Foster C: Inferior capsular shift for involuntary inferior multidirectional instability of the shoulder, *J Bone Joint Surg Am* 62-A: 897-908, 1980.

5. Altchek D, Warren R, Skyhar M, et al: T-plasty modification of the Bankhart procedure for multidirectional instability of the anterior and inferior types, *J Bone Joint Surg Am* 73-A:105-112, 1991.

6. Giangarra C: Personal communication, 2004.

7. Pollock R, Owens J, Flatow E, et al: Operative results of the inferior capsular shift procedure for multidirectional instability of the shoulder, *J Bone Joint Surg Am* 82-A:919-928, 2000.

8. Ticker J, Warner J: Selective capsular shift technique for anterior and anterior inferior glenohumeral instability, *Clin Sports Med* 19:1-17, 2000.

9. Wirth M, Blatter G, Rockwood C: The capsular imbrication procedure for recurrent anterior instability of the shoulder, *Clin Sports Med* 78-A(2):246-259, 1996.

10. Yamaguchi K, Flatow EL: Management of multidirectional instability, *Clin Sports Med* 14:885-902, 1995.

11. Bankart A: The pathology and treatment of recurrent dislocation of the shoulder-joint, *Br J Surg* 26:23-29, 1938.

12. Rowe CR, Zarins B: Recurrent transient subluxation of the shoulder, *J Bone Joint Surg Am* 63:863-872, 1981.

13. Miller M, Larsen K, Luke T, et al: Anterior capsular shift volume reduction: an in vitro comparison of three techniques, *J Shoulder Elbow Surg* 12:350-354, 2003.

14. Deutsch A, Barber J, Dwight D, et al: Anterior-inferior capsular shift of the shoulder: a biomechanical comparison of glenoid-based versus humeral-based shift strategies, *J Shoulder Elbow Surg* 10: 340-352, 2001.

15. Howell SM, Galinat BJ: The glenoid-labral socket: a constrained articular surface, *Clin Orthop* 243:122-125, 1989.

16. Saha AK: Dynamic stability of the glenohumeral joint, *Acta Orthop Scand* 42:491-505, 1971.

17. Matsen FA, Lippitt SB, Sidles JA, et al: Stability. In Matsen FA, Lippitt SB, Sidles JA, et al, editors: *Practical evaluation and management of the shoulder,* Philadelphia, 1993, Saunders.

18. Lippitt SB, Vanderhooft JE, Harris SL, et al: Glenohumeral stability from concavity-compression: a quantitative analysis, *J Shoulder Elbow Surg* 2:27-35, 1993.

19. Harryman DT, Sidles JA, Clark JM, et al: Translation of the humeral head on the glenoid with passive glenohumeral motion, *J Bone Joint Surg* 72A:1334-1343, 1990.

20. Speer KP, Garrett WE: Muscular control of motion and stability about the pectoral girdle. In Matsen FA, Fu FH, Hawkins RJ, editors: *The shoulder: a balance of mobility and stability.* Rosemont, 1993, American Academy of Orthopaedic Surgeons.

21. Blasier RB, Guldberg RE, Rothman ED: Anterior shoulder stability: contributions of rotator cuff forces and the capsular ligaments in a cadaver model, *J Shoulder Elbow Surg* 1:140-150, 1992.

22. Blasier RB, Soslowsky LJ, Malicky DM, Palmer ML: Posterior glenohumeral subluxation: active and passive stabilization in a biomechanical model, *J Bone Joint Surg Am* 79:433-440, 1997.

23. Malicky DM, Blasier RB, Guldberg RE, et al: Anterior glenohumeral stabilization efficiency in a biomechanical model combining ligamentous and muscular constraints, *Trans Orthop Res Soc* 18:314, 1993.

24. Malicky DM, Soslowsky LJ, Blasier RB, Shyr Y: Anterior glenohumeral stabilization factors: progressive effects in a biomechanical model, *J Orthop Res* 14:282-288, 1996.

25. Kido T, Itoi E, Lee SB, et al: Dynamic stabilizing functions of the deltoid muscle in shoulders with anterior instability, *Am J Sports Med* 31:399-403, 2003.

26. Cain PR, Mutschler TA, Fu FH, Lee SK: Anterior stability of the glenohumeral joint: a dynamic model, *Am J Sports Med* 15:144-148, 1987.

27. Soslowsky LJ, Malicky DM, Blasier RB: Active and passive factors in inferior glenohumeral stabilization: a biomechanical model, *J Shoulder Elbow Surg* 6:371-379, 1997.

28. McMahon PJ, Jobe FW, Pink MM, et al: Comparative electromyographic analysis of shoulder muscles during planar motions: anterior glenohumeral instability versus normal, *J Shoulder Elbow Surg* 5(2 pt 1):118-123, 1996.

29. Lephart SM, Warner JJP, Borsa PA, Fu FH: Proprioception of the shoulder joint in healthy, unstable, and surgically repaired shoulders, *J Shoulder Elbow Surg* 3:371-380, 1994.

30. Myers JB, Riemann BL, Ju YY, et al: Shoulder muscle reflex latencies under various levels of muscle contraction, *Clin Orthop* (407):92-101, 2003.

31. Davies GJ, Dickoff-Hoffman S: Neuromuscular testing and rehabilitation of the shoulder complex, *J Orthop Sports Phys Ther* 18:449-458, 1993.

32. Myers JB, Lephart SM: Sensorimotor deficits contributing to glenohumeral instability, *Clin Orthop* (400):98-104, 2002.

33. Swanik KA, Lephart SM, Swanik CB, et al: The effects of shoulder plyometric training on proprioception and selected muscle performance characteristics, *J Shoulder Elbow Surg* 11:579-586, 2002.

34. Glousman R, Jobe F, Tibone J, et al: Dynamic electromyographic analysis of the throwing shoulder with glenohumeral instability, *J Bone Joint Surg* 70A:220-226, 1988.

35. Pagnani MJ, Warren RF: Stabilizers of the glenohumeral joint, *J Should. Elbow Surg* 3:173-190, 1994.

36. Itoi E, Kuechle DK, Newman SR, et al: Stabilising function of the biceps in stable and unstable shoulders, *J Bone Joint Surg* 75B:546-550, 1993.

37. Wilk KE, Andrews JR, Arrigo C, et al: The strength characteristics of internal and external rotator muscles in professional baseball players, *Am J Sports Med* 1993; 21:61-66.

38. McMahon P, Debski D, Thompson W, et al: Shoulder muscle forces and tendon excursions during scapular plane abduction, *J Shoulder Elbow Surg* 4:199-208, 1993.

39. Townsend H, Jobe FW, Pink M, Perry J: Electromyographic analysis of the glenohumeral muscles during a baseball rehabilitation program, *Am J Sports Med* 19:264-272, 1991.

40. Moseley JB, Jobe FW, Pink M, et al: EMG analysis of the scapular muscles during a shoulder rehabilitation program, *Am J Sports Med* 20:128-134, 1992.

41. Brotzman SB, Wilk K: Clinical orthopedic rehabilitation, ed 2, Philadelphia, 2003, Mosby.

42. Jobe FW, Tibone JE, Perry J, Moynes D: An EMG analysis of the shoulder in throwing and pitching: a preliminary report, *Am J Sports Med* 11:3-5, 1983.

43. Fleisig GS, Andrews JR, Dillman CJ, Escamilla RF: Kinetics of baseball pitching with implications about injury mechanisms, *Am J Sports Med* 23:233-239, 1995.

44. Ellenbecker TS, Mattalino AJ: Concentric isokinetic shoulder internal and external rotation strength in professional baseball pitchers, *J Orthop Sports Phys Ther* 25:323-328, 1997.

45. Pawlowski D, Perrin DH: Relationship between shoulder and elbow isokinetic peak torque, torque acceleration energy, average power, and total work and throwing velocity in intercollegiate pitchers, *Athletic Training* 24:129-132, 1989.

46. Wilk KE, Meister K, Andrews JR: Current concepts in the rehabilitation of the overhead throwing athlete, *Am J Sports Med* 30:136-151, 2002.

47. Newsham KR, Keith CS, Saunders JE, Goffinett AS: Isokinetic profile of baseball pitchers' internal/external rotation 180, 300 450°·s⁻¹, *Med Sci Sports Exerc* 30:1489-1495, 1998.

48. Davies GJ: Compendium of isokinetics in clinical usage, ed 4, Onalaska, 1992, S & S Publishing.

49. Axe MJ, Windley TC, Snyder-Mackler L: Data-based interval throwing programs for collegiate softball players, *J Athl Train* 37:194-203, 2002.

APPENDIX A

Sample Interval Programs for Golf, Tennis, and Baseball

REHABILITATION PROTOCOL

Interval Program for Golfers

This sport-specific protocol is designed to be performed every other day. Each session should begin with the warm-up exercises outlined here. Continue the strengthening, flexibility, and conditioning exercises on the days you are not playing or practicing golf. Advance one stage every 2-4 weeks, depending on the severity of the shoulder problem, as each stage becomes pain free in execution.

Warm-up

Lower extremities: Jog or walk briskly around the practice green area three or four times; stretch the hamstrings, quadriceps, and Achilles tendon.

Upper extremities: Stretch the shoulder (posterior cuff, anterior cuff, rhomboid) and wrist flexors and extensors.

Trunk: Do side bends, extension, and rotation stretching exercises.

Stage 1

Putt	50	3 times/wk
Medium long	0	0 times/wk
Long	0	0 times/wk

Stage 2

Putt	50	3 times/wk
Medium long	20	2 times/wk
Long	0	0 times/wk

Stage 3

Putt	50	3 times/wk
Medium long	40	3 times/wk

Long   0   0 times/wk

Not more than one third of best distance.

Stage 4

Putt	50	3 times/wk
Medium long	50	3 times/wk
Long	10	2 times/wk

Up to one half of best distance.

Stage 5

Putt	50	3 times/wk
Medium long	50	3 times/wk
Long	10	3 times/wk

Stage 6

Putt	50	3 times/wk
Medium long	50	3 times/wk
Long	20	3 times/wk

Play a round of golf in lieu of one practice session per week.

REHABILITATION PROTOCOL

Interval Program for Tennis Players

This tennis protocol is designed to be performed every other day. Each session should begin with the warm-up exercises outlined as follows. Continue with your strengthening, flexibility, and conditioning exercises on the days you are not following the tennis protocol.

Warm-up

Lower Extremity

- Jog four laps around the tennis court.
- Stretches
  1. Gastrocnemius
  2. Achilles tendon
  3. Hamstring
  4. Quadriceps

Upper Extremity

- Shoulder stretches
  1. Posterior cuff
  2. Inferior capsule
  3. Rhomboids
  4. Forearm and wrist stretches
  5. Wrist flexors
  6. Wrist extensors

Trunk

- Side bends
- Extension
- Rotation

Forehand Ground Strokes

Hit toward the fence on the opposite side of the court. Do not worry about getting the ball in the court.

During all of the strokes listed previously, remember these key steps:

- Bend your knees.
- Turn your body.
- Step toward the ball.
- Hit the ball when it is out in front of you.

Avoid hitting with an open stance because this places undue stress on your shoulder. This is especially true during the forehand stroke if you have had anterior instability or impingement problems. This is also true during the backhand stroke if you have had problems with posterior instability.

On the very first day of these sport-specific drills, start with bouncing the ball and hitting it. Try to bounce the ball yourself and hit it at waist level. This will allow for consistency in the following:

- How the ball comes to you
- Approximating your timing between hits
- Hitting toward a target to ensure follow-through and full extension
- Employing the proper mechanics, thereby placing less stress on the anterior shoulder

Week 1

Day 1
- 25 forehand strokes
- 25 backhand strokes

Day 2   If there are no problems after the first-day workout, increase the number of forehand and backhand strokes.
- 50 forehand strokes
- 50 backhand strokes

Day 3
- 50 forehand strokes (waist level)
- 50 backhand strokes (waist level)
- 25 high forehand strokes
- 25 high backhand strokes

Week 2   Progress to having the ball tossed to you in a timely manner, giving you enough time to recover from your deliberate follow-through (i.e., wait until the ball bounces on the other side of the court before tossing another ball). Always aim the ball at a target or at a spot on the court.

If you are working on basic groundstrokes, have someone bounce the ball to you consistently at waist height.

If you are working on high forehand strokes, have the ball bounced to you at shoulder height or higher.

Day 1
- 25 high forehand strokes
- 50 waist-high forehand strokes
- 50 waist-high backhand strokes
- 25 high backhand strokes

Day 2
- 25 high forehand strokes
- 50 waist-high forehand strokes
- 50 waist-high backhand strokes
- 25 high backhand strokes

Day 3 Alternate hitting the cross-court and down the line, using the waist-high and high forehand and backhand strokes.
- 25 high forehand strokes
- 50 waist-high forehand strokes
- 50 waist-high backhand strokes
- 25 high backhand strokes

Week 3 Continue the three-times-per-week schedule. Add regular and high forehand and backhand volleys. At this point, you may begin having someone hit tennis balls to you from a basket of balls. This will allow you to get the feel of the ball as it comes off another tennis racket. Your partner should wait until the ball that you hit has bounced on the other side of the court before hitting another ball to you. This will give you time to emphasize your follow-through and not hurry to return for the next shot. As always, emphasis is placed on proper body mechanics.

Day 1
- 25 high forehand strokes
- 50 waist-high forehand strokes
- 50 waist-high backhand strokes
- 25 high backhand strokes
- 25 low backhand and forehand volleys
- 25 high backhand and forehand volleys

Day 2
- Same as day 1, week 3

Day 3 Same as day 2, week 3, with emphasis on direction (i.e., down-the-line and cross-court). Remember, having good body mechanics is still a must:

- Keep knees bent.
- Hit the ball on the rise.
- Hit the ball in front of you.
- Turn your body.
- Do not hit the ball with an open stance.
- Stay on the balls of your feet.

Week 4
Day 1 Continue having your partner hit tennis balls from a basket to you. Alternate hitting forehand and backhand strokes with lateral movement along the baseline. Again, emphasis is on good mechanics as described previously.

Alternate hitting the ball down-the-line and cross-court. This drill should be done with a full basket of tennis balls (100-150 tennis balls).

Follow this drill with high and low volleys using half a basket of tennis balls (50-75 balls). This drill is also performed with lateral movement and returning to the middle of the court after the ball is hit.

Your partner should continue allowing enough time for you to return to the middle of the court before hitting the next ball. This is to avoid your rushing the stroke and using faulty mechanics.

Day 2 Same drills as day 1, week 4

Day 3 Same drills as day 2, week 4

Week 5
Day 1 Find a partner able to hit consistent ground strokes (able to hit the ball to the same area consistently, e.g., to your forehand with the ball bouncing approximately waist high).

Begin hitting ground strokes, with your partner alternating hitting the ball to your backhand and to your forehand. Rally for approximately 15 min, then add volleys with your partner hitting to you from the baseline. Alternate between backhand and forehand volleys and high and low volleys. Continue volleying another 15 min. You will have rallied for a total of 30-40 min.

At the end of the session, practice a few serves while standing along the baseline. First, warm up by shadowing for 1 to 3 min. Hold the tennis racquet loosely and swing across your body. Do not swing the racquet hard. When you are ready to practice your serves using a ball, be sure to keep your toss out in front of you, get your racquet up and behind you, bend your knees, and hit up on the ball. Forget about how much power you are generating, and forget about hitting the ball between the service lines. Try hitting the ball as if you are hitting it toward the back fence.

Hit approximately 10 serves from each side of the court. Remember, this is the first time you are serving, so do not try to hit at 100% of your effort.

Day 2   Same as day 1, week 5, but now increase the number of times you practice your serve. After working on your ground strokes and volleys, return to the baseline and work on your second serve. Hit up on the ball, bend your knees, follow through, and keep the toss in front of you. This time hit 20 balls from each side of the court (i.e., 20 into the deuce court and 20 into the advantage court).

Day 3   Same as day 2, week 5, with ground strokes, volleys, and serves. Do not add to the serves. Concentrate on the following:

- Bending your knees
- Preparing the racket
- Using footwork
- Hitting the ball out in front of you
- Keeping your eyes on the ball
- Following through
- Getting in position for the next shot
- Keeping the toss in front of you during the serve

The workout should be the same as day 2, but if you emphasize the proper mechanics listed previously, you should feel as though you had a harder workout than on day 2.

Week 6
Day 1   After the usual warm-up program, start with specific ground-stroke drills, with you hitting the ball down the line and your partner on the other side hitting the ball cross-court. This will force you to move quickly on the court. Emphasize good mechanics as mentioned previously.

Perform this drill for 10-15 min before reversing the direction of your strokes. Now have your partner hit down the line while you hit cross-court.

Proceed to the next drill with your partner hitting the ball to you. Return balls using a forehand, then a backhand, then a put-away volley. Repeat this sequence for 10-15 min. End this session by serving 50 balls to the ad court and 50 balls to the deuce court.

Day 2   Same as day 1, week 6, plus returning serves from both sides of the court (deuce and ad court). End with practicing serves, 50 to each court.

Day 3   Perform the following sequence: warm-up; cross-court and down-the-line drills; backhand, forehand, and volley drills; return of serves; and practice serves.

Week 7
Day 1   Perform the warm-up program. Perform drills as before, and practice return of serves. Before practicing serving, work on hitting 10-15 overhead shots. Continue emphasizing good mechanics. Add the approach shot to your drills.

Day 2   Same as day 1, week 7, except double the number of overhead shots (25-30 overheads).

Day 3   Perform warm-up exercises and cross-court drills. Add the overhead shot to the backhand, forehand, and volley drill, making it the backhand, forehand, volley, and overhead drill.

If you are a serious tennis player, you will want to work on other strokes or other parts of your game. Feel free to gradually add them to your practice and workout sessions. Just as with other strokes, the proper mechanics should be applied to drop volley, slice, heavy topspin, drop shots, and lobs, offensive and defensive.

Week 8
Day 1   Warm-up and play a simulated one-set match. Be sure to take rest periods after every third game. Remember, you will have to concentrate harder on using good mechanics.

Day 2   Perform another simulated game but with a two-set match.

Day 3   Perform another simulated game, this time a best-of-three-set match.

If all goes well, you may make plans to return to your regular workout and game schedule. You may also practice or play on consecutive days if your condition allows it.

REHABILITATION PROTOCOL
Interval Throwing Program for Catchers, Infielders, and Outfielders

Note: Perform each step three times. All throws should have an arc or "hump." The maximum distance thrown by infielders and catchers is 120 feet. The maximum distance thrown by outfielders is 200 feet.

Step 1

Toss the ball with no wind-up. Stand with your feet shoulder-width apart, and face the player to whom you are throwing. Concentrate on rotating and staying on top of the ball.

Number of Throws	Distance (ft)
5	20 (warm-up)
10	30
5	20 (cool-down)

Step 2

Stand sideways in relation to the person to whom you are throwing. Feet are shoulder-width apart. Close up and pivot onto your back foot as you throw.

Number of Throws	Distance (ft)
5	30 (warm-up)
5	40
10	50
5	30 (cool-down)

Step 3

Repeat the position in step 2. Step toward the target with your front leg and follow through with your back leg.

Number of Throws	Distance (ft)
5	50 (warm-up)
5	60
10	70
5	50 (cool-down)

Step 4

Assume the pitcher's stance. Lift and stride with your lead leg. Follow through with your back leg.

Number of Throws	Distance (ft)
5	60 (warm-up)
5	70
10	80
5	60 (cool-down)

Step 5

Outfielders: Lead with your glove-side foot forward. Take one step, crow-hop, and throw the ball.

Infielders: Lead with your glove-side foot forward. Take a shuffle step, and throw the ball. Throw the last five throws in a straight line.

Number of Throws	Distance (ft)
5	70 (warm-up)
5	90
10	100
5	80 (cool-down)

Step 6

Use the throwing technique used in step 5. Assume your playing position. Infielders and catchers do not throw farther than 120 feet. Outfielders do not throw farther than 150 feet (mid outfield).

Number of Throws	Infielder's and Catcher's Distance (ft)	Outfielder's Distance (ft)
5	80 (warm-up)	80 (warm-up)
5	80-90	90-100
5	90-100	110-125
5	110-120	130-150
5	80 (cool-down)	80 (cool down)

Step 7

Infielders, catchers, and outfielders all may assume their playing positions.

Number of Throws	Infielder's and Catcher's Distance (ft)	Outfielder's Distance (ft)
5	80 (warm-up)	80-90
5	80-90	110-130
5	90-100	150-175
5	110-120	180-200
5	80 (cool-down)	90

Step 8

Repeat step 7. Use a Fungo bat to hit to the infielders and outfielders while in their normal playing positions.

REHABILITATION PROTOCOL

Interval Throwing Program for Pitchers

Step 1

Toss the ball (no wind-up) against a wall on alternate days. Start with 25-30 throws, build up to 70 throws, and gradually increase the throwing distance.

Number of Throws	Distance (ft)
25	20 (warm-up phase)
25-40	30-40
10	20 (cool-down phase)

Step 2

Toss the ball (playing catch with easy wind-up) on alternate days.

Number of Throws	Distance (ft)
10	20 (warm-up)
10	30-40
30-40	50
10	20-30 (cool-down)

Step 3

Continue increasing the throwing distance while still tossing the ball with an easy wind-up.

Number of Throws	Distance (ft)
10	20 (warm-up)
10	30-40
30-40	50-60
10	30 (cool-down)

Step 4

Increase throwing distance to a maximum of 60 feet. Continue tossing the ball with an occasional throw at no more than half speed.

Number of Throws	Distance
10	30 (warm-up)
10	40-45
30-40	60-70
10	30 (cool-down)

Step 5

During this step, gradually increase the distance to 150 feet maximum.

Phase 5-1

Number of Throws	Distance (ft)
10	40 (warm-up)
10	50-60
15-20	70-80
10	50-60
10	40 (cool-down)

Phase 5-2

Number of Throws	Distance (ft)
10	40(warm-up)
20	50-60
20-30	80-90
20	50-60
10	40 (cool-down)

Phase 5-3

Number of Throws	Distance (ft)
10	40 (warm-up)
10	60
15-20	100-110
20	60
10	40 (cool-down)

Phase 5-4

Number of Throws	Distance (ft)
10	40 (warm-up)
10	60
15-20	120-150
20	60
10	40 (cool-down)

Step 6

Progress to throwing off the mound at one-half to three-fourths speed. Try to use proper body mechanics, especially when throwing off the mound.

- Stay on top of the ball.
- Keep the elbow up.
- Throw over the top.
- Follow through with the arm and trunk.
- Use the legs to push.

Phase 6-1

Number of Throws	Distance (ft)
10	60 (warm-up)
10	120-150 (lobbing)
30	45 (off the mound)
10	60 (off the mound)
10	40 (cool-down)

Phase 6-2

Number of Throws	Distance (ft)
10	50 (warm-up)
10	120-150
20	45 (off the mound)
20	60 (off the mound)
10	40 (cool-down)

Phase 6-3

Number of Throws	Distance (ft)
10	50 (warm-up)
10	60
10	120-150 (lobbing)
10	45 (off the mound)
30	60 (off the mound)
10	40 (cool-down)

Phase 6-4

Number of Throws	Distance (ft)
10	50 (warm-up)
10	120-150 (lobbing)
10	45 (off the mound)
40-50	60 (off the mound)
10	40 (cool-down)

At this time, if the pitcher has successfully completed phase 6-4 without pain or discomfort and is throwing at approximately three-fourths speed, the pitching coach and trainer may allow the pitcher to proceed to step 7: "up-down bullpens." This exercise is used to simulate a game. The pitcher has rest periods during a series of pitches to reproduce the rest period between innings.

Step 7

Up-down bullpens (one-half to three-fourths speed).

Day 1

Number of Throws	Distance (ft)
10 warm-up throws	120-150 (lobbing)
10 warm-up throws	60 (off the mound)
40 pitches	60 (off the mound)
Rest 10 min	
20 pitches	60 (off the mound)

Day 2

Off.

Day 3

Number of Throws	Distance (ft)
10 warm-up throws	120-150 (lobbing)
10 warm-up throws	60 (off the mound)
30 pitches	60 (off the mound)
Rest 10 min	
10 warm-up throws	60 (off the mound)
20 pitches	60 (off the mound)

Rest 10 min	
10 warm up throws	60 (off the mound)
20 pitches	60 (off the mound)

Day 4

Off.

Day 5

Number of Throws	Distance (ft)
10 warm-up throws	120-150 (lobbing)
10 warm-up throws	60 (off the mound)
30 pitches	60 (off the mound)
Rest 8 min	
20 pitches	60 (off the mound)
Rest 8 min	
20 pitches	60 (off the mound)
Rest 8 min	
20 pitches	60 (off the mound)

At this point, the pitcher is ready to begin a normal routine, from throwing batting practice to pitching in the bullpen. This program can and should be adjusted as needed by the trainer or physical therapist. Each step may take more or less time than listed, and the trainer, physical therapist, and physician should monitor the program. The pitcher should remember that it is necessary to work hard but not overdo it.

From Brotzman SB, Wilk K: *Clinical orthopedic rehabilitation*, ed 2, Philadelphia, 2003, Mosby.

Sample Interval Throwing Program for Softball

SOFTBALL PITCHER'S PROGRAM

Phase I: Early Throwing

- All throws are to tolerance to a maximum of 50% effort.
- All long tosses begin with a crow-hop.

Step 1

Warm-up toss to 30 ft (9.14 m)

10 throws @ 30 ft (9.14 m)

Rest 8 min

10 throws @ 30 ft (9.14 m)

10 long tosses to 40 ft (12.19 m)

Step 2

Warm-up toss to 45 ft (13.72 m)
10 throws @ 45 ft (13.72 m)
Rest 8 min
10 throws @ 45 ft (13.72 m)
10 long tosses to 60 ft (18.29 m)

Step 3

Warm-up toss to 60 ft (18.29 m)
10 throws @ 60 ft (18.29 m)
Rest 8 min
10 throws @ 60 ft (18.29 m)
10 long tosses to 75 ft (22.86 m)

Step 4

Warm-up toss to 75 ft (22.86 m)
10 throws @ 75 ft (22.86 m)
Rest 8 min
10 throws @ 75 ft (22.86 m)
10 long tosses to 90 ft (27.43 m)

Step 5

Warm-up toss to 90 ft (27.43 m)
10 throws @ 90 ft (27.43 m)
Rest 8 min
10 throws @ 90 ft (27.43 m)
10 long tosses to 105 ft (32.00 m)

Step 6

Warm-up toss to 105 ft (32.00 m)
10 throws @ 105 ft (32.00 m)
Rest 8 min
10 throws @ 105 ft (32.00 m)
10 long tosses to 120 ft (36.58 m)

Step 7

Warm-up toss to 120 ft (36.58 m)
10 throws @ 60 ft (18.29 m) (75%)
10 pitches @ 20 ft (6.10 m) (50%)
Rest 8 min
10 throws @ 60 ft (18.29 m) (75%)
5 pitches @ 20 ft (6.10 m) (50%)
10 long tosses to 120 ft (36.58 m)

Step 8

Warm-up toss to 120 ft (36.58 m)
10 throws @ 60 ft (18.29 m) (75%)
10 pitches @ 35 ft (10.67 m) (50%)
Rest 8 min
10 throws @ 60 ft (18.29 m) (75%)
10 pitches @ 35 ft (10.67 m) (50%)
10 long tosses to 120 ft (36.58 m)

Step 9

Warm-up toss to 120 ft (36.58 m)
10 throws @ 60 ft (18.29 m) (75%)
10 pitches @ 46 ft (14.02 m) (50%)
Rest 8 min
10 throws @ 60 ft (18.29 m) (75%)
10 pitches @ 46 ft (14.02 m) (50%)
15 long tosses to 120 ft (36.58 m)

Step 10

Warm-up toss to 120 ft (36.58 m)
10 throws @ 60 ft (18.29 m) (75%)
10 pitches @ 46 ft (14.02 m) (50%)
Rest 8 min
10 pitches @ 46 ft (14.02 m) (50%)
Rest 8 min
10 throws @ 60 ft (18.29 m) (75%)
10 pitches @ 46 ft (14.02 m) (50%)
15 long tosses to 120 ft (36.58 m)

Phase II: Initiation of Pitching

- All pitches are fastballs (no off-speed pitches).
- All pitches to tolerance or maximum effort level specified.
- All long tosses begin with a crow-hop.

Phase III: Intensified Pitching

- Pitch sets 11-15 consist of one fastball to one off-speed pitch at the effort level specified.
- Pitch sets 16-21 consist of a percentage of pitches that match the preinjury pitch mix specific to the athlete at the effort level specified.

- Begin each step with warm-up toss to 120 ft (36.58 m).
- End each step with 20 long tosses to 120 ft (36.58 m).

Step 11

Two throws to each base (75%)
15 pitches (50%)*
15 pitches (50%)*
One throw to each base (75%)
15 pitches (50%)*

Step 12

Two throws to each base (75%)
15 pitches (50%)*
15 pitches (50%)*
15 pitches (50%)*
One throw to each base (75%)
15 pitches (50%)*

Step 13

Two throws to each base (75%)
15 pitches (50%)*
15 pitches (75%)*
15 pitches (75%)*
One throw to each base(75%)
15 pitches (50%)*

Step 14

Two throws to each base (75%)
15 pitches (50%)*
15 pitches (75%)*
15 pitches (75%)*
20 pitches (50%)*
One throw to each base (75%)
15 pitches (50%)*

Step 15

Two throws to each base (100%)
15 pitches (75%)*
15 pitches (75%)*
15 pitches (75%)*
15 pitches (75%)*
One throw to each base (75%)
15 pitches (75%)*

Step 16

One throw to each base (100%)
15 pitches (100%)*
20 pitches (75%)*
15 pitches (100%)*
20 pitches (75%)*
One throw to each base (75%)
20 pitches (75%)*

Step 17

One throw to each base (100%)
15 pitches (100%)*
20 pitches (75%)*
15 pitches (100%)*
15 pitches (100%)*
20 pitches (75%)*
One throw to each base (100%)
15 pitches (75%)*

Step 18

One throw to each base (100%)
20 pitches (100%)*
15 pitches (100%)*
20 pitches (100%)*
15 pitches (100%)*
20 pitches (100%)*
One throw to each base (100%)
15 pitches (100%)*

Step 19

One throw to each base (100%)
20 pitches (100%)*
15 pitches (100%)*
20 pitches (100%)*
15 pitches (100%)*
20 pitches (100%)*
15 pitches (100%)*
One throw to each base (100%)
15 pitches (100%)*

Step 20

Batting practice
100-120 pitches
One throw to each base per 25 pitches

---

*Rest 8 min after these sets.

Step 21

Simulated games

Seven innings

18-20 pitches/inning

8 min rest between innings

Preinjury pitch mix

SOFTBALL CATCHER'S PROGRAM

Phase I: Beginning Throwing (Throws to 50% Effort)

- All long tosses begin with a crow-hop.

Step 1

Warm-up toss to 30 ft (9.14 m)

10 throws @ 30 ft (9.14 m)

Rest 8 min

10 throws @ 30 ft (9.14 m)

10 long tosses to 45 ft (13.72 m)

Step 2

Warm-up toss to 45 ft (13.72 m)

10 throws @ 45 ft (13.72 m)

Rest 8 min

10 throws @ 45 ft (13.72 m)

10 long tosses to 60 ft (18.29 m)

Step 3

Warm up toss to 60 ft (18.29 m)

10 throws @ 60 ft (18.29 m)

Rest 8 min

10 throws @ 60 ft (18.29 m)

10 long tosses to 75 ft (22.6 m)

Step 4

Warm-up toss to 75 ft (22.86 m)

10 throws @ 75 ft (22.86 m)

Rest 8 min

10 throws @ 75 ft (22.86 m)

10 long tosses to 90 ft (27.43 m)

*Rest 8 min after these sets.

Phase II: Catching Practice

- Complete warm-up lap around the field before each step.
- All throws completed to tolerance, not to exceed the effort level specified.
- All throws made after squatting 8 sec to simulate receiving a pitch.
- All long tosses begin with a crow-hop.

Step 5

Warm-up toss to 90 ft (27.43 m)

10 throws to pitcher (50%)*

10 throws to pitcher (50%)*

10 throws to pitcher (50%)*

10 long tosses to 120 ft (36.58 m)

Step 6

Warm-up toss to 90 ft (27.43 m)

10 throws to pitcher (50%)*

15 throws to pitcher (50%)*

10 throws to pitcher (50%)*

15 throws to pitcher (50%)*

15 long tosses up to 120 ft (36.58 m)

Step 7

Warm-up toss to 90 ft (27.43 m)

10 throws to pitcher (75%)*

One throw to first and third bases (50%)*

15 throws to pitcher (50%)*

10 throws to pitcher (75%)*

15 throws to pitcher (50%)*

20 long tosses to 120 ft (36.58 m)

Step 8

Warm-up toss to 90 ft (27.43 m)

10 throws to pitcher (75%)*

Two throws to first and third bases (75%)*

15 throws to pitcher (75%)*

10 throws to pitcher (75%)*

15 throws to pitcher (75%)*

20 long tosses to 120 ft (36.58 m)

Step 9

Warm-up toss to 90 ft (27.43 m)

10 throws to pitcher (75%)*

Two throws to first and third bases (75%)*

10 throws to pitcher (75%)

15 throws to pitcher (75%)*

10 throws to pitcher (75%)*

15 throws to pitcher (75%)*

20 long tosses to 120 ft (36.58 m)

Step 10

Warm-up toss to 90 ft (27.43 m)

10 throws to pitcher (75%)*

Two throws to first and third bases (100%)*

10 throws to pitcher (75%)

Three throws to second base (75%)*

15 throws to pitcher (75%)*

10 throws to pitcher (75%)*

15 throws to pitcher (75%)*

20 long tosses to 120 ft (36.58 m)

Step 11

Simulated game

Warm-up toss to 90 ft (27.43 m)

10 throws to pitcher (75%)*

Two throws to first and third bases (100%)*

15 throws to pitcher (75%)*

10 throws to pitcher (75%)*

15 throws to pitcher (75%)*

10 throws to pitcher (75%)

Three throws to second base (100%)*

10 throws to pitcher (75%)*

10 throws to pitcher (75%)*

20 long tosses to 120 ft (36.58 m)

*Complete 60 ft (18.29 m) sprint, then rest 8 min after these sets.

SOFTBALL INFIELDER'S PROGRAM

General Guidelines

- Complete a warm-up lap around the field before each step.
- Complete a 60 ft (18.29 m) sprint before each set of throws.
- Rest 8 min between sets.

- All throws are limited arc.
- All long tosses begin with a crow-hop.

Step 1

Warm-up toss to 45 ft (13.72 m)

15 throws @ 40 ft (12.19 m) (50%)

Field practice (50%)

Five throws @ 35 ft (10.67 m)

Five throws @ 45 ft (13.72 m)

20 long tosses to 60 ft (18.29 m)

Step 2

Warm-up toss to 60 ft (18.29 m)

20 throws @ 45 ft (13.72 m) (50%)

Field practice (50%)

Five throws @ 45 ft (13.72 m)

10 throws @ 60 ft (18.29 m)

20 long tosses to 75 ft (22.86 m)

Step 3

Warm-up toss to 75 ft (22.86 m)

20 throws @ 60 ft (18.29 m) (50%)

Field practice (75%)

Five throws @ 60 ft (18.29 m)

10 throws @ 75 ft (22.86 m)

20 long tosses to 90 ft (27.43 m)

Step 4

Warm-up toss to 90 ft (27.43 m)

20 throws @ 60 ft (18.29 m) (75%)

Field practice (75%)

Five throws @ 60 ft (18.29 m)

Five throws @ 84 ft (25.60 m)

Five throws @ 120 ft (36.58 m)

20 long tosses to 120 ft (36.58 m)

Step 5

Warm-up toss to 120 ft (36.58 m)

20 throws @ 60 ft (18.29 m) (75%)

Field practice (100%)

Five throws @ 60 ft (18.29 m)

Five throws @ 84 ft (25.60 m)

Five throws @ 120 ft (36.58 m)

20 long tosses to 150 ft (45.72 m)

Step 6

Simulated game

Warm-up toss to 120 ft (36.58 m)

20 throws @ 60 ft (18.29 m) (100%)

Field practice (100%)

Five throws @ 60 ft (18.29 m)

Five throws @ 84 ft (25.60 m)

Five throws @ 120 ft (36.58 m)

One throw to each base from position (100%)

20 long tosses to 150 ft (45.72 m)

SOFTBALL OUTFIELDER'S PROGRAM

General Guidelines

- Complete a warm-up lap around the field before each step.
- All tosses with limited arc.
- All long tosses begin with a crow-hop.

Step 1

Warm-up toss to 45 ft (13.72 m)

Catch fly balls or field ground balls and throw to cutoff at 45 ft (13.72 m) (50% effort); repeat five times with 1 min rest between throws

15 tosses to 60 ft (18.29 m)

Step 2

Warm-up toss to 60 ft (18.29 m)

Catch fly balls or field ground balls and throw to cutoff at 60 ft (18.29 m) (50% effort); repeat five times with 1 min rest between throws

15 tosses to 90 ft (27.43 m)

Step 3

Warm-up toss to 90 ft (27.43 m)

Catch fly balls or field ground balls and throw to cutoff at 90 ft (27.43 m) (75% effort); repeat five times with 1 min rest between throws

15 tosses to 120 ft (36.58 m)

Step 4

Warm-up toss to 120 ft (36.58 m)

Field ground balls and throw to cutoff at 90 ft (27.43 m) (75% effort); repeat five times

Catch fly balls and throw to base at 120 ft (36.58 m) (75% effort); repeat five times with 1 min rest between throws

15 tosses to 150 ft (45.72 m)

Step 5

Warm-up toss to 120 ft (36.58 m)

Field ground balls and throw to cutoff at 90 ft (27.43 m) (100% effort); repeat five times

Catch fly balls and throw to base at 120 ft (36.58 m) (75% effort); repeat five times with 1 min rest between throws

20 tosses to 180 ft (54.86 m)

Step 6

Warm-up toss to 150 ft (45.72 m)

Catch fly balls and throw to base at 150 ft (45.72 m) (100% effort); repeat five times with 1 min rest between throws

Field ground balls and throw to cutoff at 90 ft (27.43 m) (100% effort); repeat five times

20 tosses to 180 ft (54.86 m)

Step 7

Simulated game

Warm-up toss to 180 ft (54.86 m)

Field ground balls and throw to cutoff at 120 ft (36.58 m) (100% effort); repeat five times

Catch fly balls and throw to base at 180 ft (54.86 m) (100% effort); repeat five times with 1 min rest between throws

20 tosses to 180 ft (54.86 m)

SOFTBALL PITCHER'S INSTRUCTIONS

General Rules

1. Break a sweat
2. Shoulder stretches
3. Throwing program
4. Rotator cuff strength
5. Shoulder stretches
6. Ice for 20 min

Warm-up

Begin at 20 ft (6.10 m) and advance 20 ft (6.10 m) at a time, throwing three to five times at each distance at 50% effort until reaching the warm-up distance for that workout. Begin all throws with a crow-hop.

Soreness Rules

If sore more than 1 hour after throwing or the next day, take 1 day off and repeat the most recent throwing program workout.

If sore during warm-up but soreness is gone within the first 15 throws, repeat the previous workout. If shoulder becomes sore during this workout, stop and take 2 days off. On return to throwing, drop down one step.

If sore during warm-up and soreness continues through the first 15 throws, stop throwing and take 2 days off. On return to throwing, drop down one step.

If no soreness, advance one step every throwing day.

A. Baseline or preseason

To establish a base for training and conditioning, begin with step 4 and advance one step daily to step 19, following soreness rules.

B. Nonthrowing arm injury

After medical clearance, begin step 4 and advance one step daily to step 21, following soreness rules.

C. Throwing arm

Bruise or bone involvement: after medical clearance, begin with step 1 and advance program as soreness rules allow, throwing every other day.

D. Throwing arm: tendon or ligament injury (mild)

After medical clearance, begin with step 1 and advance program to step 6, throwing every other day as soreness rules allow. Throw every third day on steps 7-10 as soreness rules allow. Return to throwing every other day as soreness rules allow for steps 11-21.

E. Throwing arm: tendon or ligament injury (moderate, severe, or postoperative)

After medical clearance, begin throwing at step 1. For steps 1-6, advance no more than one step every 3 days, with 2 days' active rest (warm-up and long tosses) after each workout.

Steps 7-10: advance no more than one step every 3 days, with 2 days' active rest (warm-up and long tosses) after each workout.

Advance steps 11-21 daily as soreness rules allow.

SOFTBALL CATCHER'S INSTRUCTIONS
General Rules

1. Break a sweat
2. Shoulder stretches
3. Throwing program
4. Rotator cuff strength
5. Shoulder stretches
6. Ice for 20 min

Warm-up

Begin at 20 ft (6.10 m) and advance 20 ft (6.10 m) at a time, throwing three to five times at each distance at 50% effort until reaching the warm-up distance for that workout. Begin all throws with a crow-hop.

Soreness Rules

If sore more than 1 hour after throwing or the next day, take 1 day off and repeat the most recent throwing program workout.

If sore during warm-up but soreness is gone within the first 15 throws, repeat the previous workout. If shoulder becomes sore during this workout, stop and take 2 days off. On return to throwing, drop down one step.

If sore during warm-up and soreness continues through the first 15 throws, stop throwing and take 2 days off. On return to throwing, drop down one step.

If no soreness, advance one step every throwing day.

A. Baseline or preseason

To establish a base for training and conditioning, begin with step 3 and advance one step daily to step 11, following soreness rules.

B. Nonthrowing arm injury

After medical clearance, begin at step 1 and advance one step daily to step 11, following soreness rules.

C. Throwing arm: bruise or bone involvement

After medical clearance, begin with step 1 and advance one step every other day to step 11, following soreness rules.

D. Throwing arm: tendon or ligament injury (mild)

After medical clearance, begin with step 1 and advance program to step 4, throwing every other day as soreness rules allow. Throw every third day for steps 5-8 as soreness rules allow. Return to throwing every other day as soreness rules allow for steps 9-11.

E. Throwing arm: tendon or ligament injury (moderate, severe, or postoperative)

After medical clearance, begin throwing at step 1.

For steps 1-4, advance no more than one step every 3 days, with 1 day of active rest after each workout day. For steps 5-11, advance no more than one step every 3 days, with 2 days of active rest (see below) after each workout day.

Active rest workout: Warm up to 60 ft (18.29 m). Catch five pitches in squat, but do not throw ball to pitcher. Complete 25 easy long tosses to 60-90 ft (18.29-27.43 m); begin each of these throws with a crow-hop. Run 90 ft (27.43 m) sprint after every five long tosses.

From Axe MJ, Windley TC, Snyder-Mackler L: Data-based interval throwing programs for collegiate softball players, *J Athl Train* 37:194-203, 2002.

CHAPTER 28

Capsular Shift Procedures: Neer and Multidirectional Instabilities

Michael Levinson, PT
David Altchek, MD

MULTIDIRECTIONAL INSTABILITY IS DEFINED

as instability that can be a combination of anterior, posterior, and inferior excursion of the humeral head in relation to the glenoid fossa.[1] Rowe first identified that atraumatic instability can occur in more than one direction.[1] However, it was Neer and Foster who first described multidirectional instability in 1980.[2] Multidirectional instability can be a congenital or an acquired enlargement of the glenohumeral joint volume and a very redundant capsule anteriorly, inferiorly, and/or posteroinferiorly.[3] Defects of the posterior humeral head and anterior labral injury are often associated with multidirectional instability.[4,5] Patients often have generalized joint laxity. There is a much lower incidence of trauma associated with multidirectional instability.[6] Patients are often athletic. Repetitive microtrauma from various sports can lead to multidirectional instability by selectively stretching out the shoulder in comparison with other joints.[7] Patients with multidirectional instability commonly complain of generalized pain when carrying light objects or performing overhead activities.[3] Patients often have a positive sulcus sign and may demonstrate a positive apprehension sign.[8]

SURGICAL INTERVENTION

Conservative treatment for multidirectional instability is generally the initial intervention. Even with a plan of surgical intervention, a rehabilitation program is advocated before surgery.[2] At least initially, many patients will respond well to an aggressive shoulder and scapular strengthening program. In addition, a rehabilitation program will assure patient compliance and enable the surgeon to exclude any patients with psychologic problems.

Standard unidirectional procedures have failed in this population, as they do not address all aspects of the instability. Excessive tightness created on one side of the joint can create a subluxation on the opposite side, resulting in early osteoarthritis.[5,9,10] The original "capsular shift procedure" was first presented by Neer and Foster in 1980.[2] This procedure was designed to reduce the joint volume by equally tightening the anterior, posterior, and inferior capsule. It is an open procedure in which the surgeon determines whether to perform an anterior or posterior procedure based on the side causing the most symptoms. The superficial half of the subscapularis tendon (or posterior rotator cuff tendons if posterior) is divided. A T-shaped incision is made in the capsule, with the vertical segment of the T beginning just medial to the lateral attachment of the capsule to the humerus and extending inferiorly and posteriorly. The inferior flap is pulled upward and is reattached to the soft tissue on the lesser tuberosity. The upper flap is pulled downward and sutured to the soft tissue on the humerus.[2] The rotator interval is imbricated if it is torn or incompetent (Figure 28-1). With this procedure, 31 of 32 subjects experienced satisfactory results with no instability.[2] However, the loss of range of motion (ROM) would be questionable by today's standards.[2] Over the years, clinical success and failure rates have varied greatly.[2,11-13]

Many of surgical techniques modified over the years have been derived from this original "capsular shift procedure." For example, Matsen and co-workers have described dividing the capsule all the way down inferiorly, midway between the humerus and the glenoid rim.[14] The medial capsule is advanced superiorly and laterally while the lateral capsule is advanced superiorly and medially.[14] Altchek and his colleagues modified the Bankart procedure with a T-shaped incision in the anterior capsule. The inferior flap is then advanced superiorly while the superior flap is advanced medially.[15] The repair is then buttressed to the glenoid rim (Figure 28-2).

In recent years, arthroscopic procedures have been developed to treat multidirectional instability. Recently, arthroscopic capsular shrinkage procedures have been used. Both lasers and radiofrequency probes are used to deliver thermal energy to a lax glenohumeral capsule. These procedures have the appeal of being relatively easy technically.

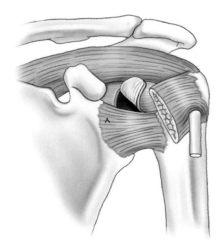
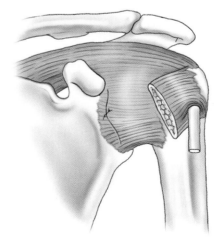

Figure 28-1: Inferior capsular shift. *(From Neer CS, Foster CR: Inferior capsular shift for involuntary inferior and multidirectional instability of the shoulder: a preliminary report, J Bone Joint Surg Am 62A:897-908, 1980.)*

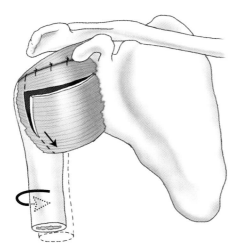

Figure 28-2: Modified Bankart procedure using a T-shaped incision. *(From Altchek DW, Dines DM: The surgical treatment of anterior instability: selective capsular repair, Op Tech Sports Med 1(4):285-292, 1993.)*

They are often done in conjunction with a suture closure of the rotator interval. However, high failure rates have been reported.[16-18] In addition, there is evidence of tissue changes that would create risk for recurrent "stretching out."[19] Other techniques for arthroscopic repairs have been developed over the past 10 years. Currently, suture plication has been advocated for arthroscopic treatment of multidirectional instability and thus far has demonstrated favorable results.[20,21] This technique uses suture hooks to tension the redundant capsule and attach the capsule to the glenoid labrum. The rotator interval is then repaired.[20]

PHASE I: IMMEDIATE POSTOPERATIVE PHASE (WEEKS 1 TO 3)

See Box 28-1. During the immediate postoperative phase of rehabilitation the goals are to begin to gradually restore ROM and avoid the adverse effects of immobilization, while not overstressing the tissue that is healing and remodeling. Also, one wants to promote healing and minimize pain and

---

BOX 28-1
Multidirectional Instability: Capsular Shift Procedures Guidelines

Phase I: Immediate Postoperative Phase (Weeks 1-3)

Goals

Promote healing: reduce pain and inflammation

Forward flexion to 90 degrees

External rotation to 30 degrees

Treatment

Immobilizer

Elbow and wrist active range of motion (ROM)

Gripping exercises

Active assistive ROM: forward flexion (scapular plane)

Active assistive ROM: external rotation

Scapular isometrics

Pain-free, submaximal deltoid isometrics

Modalities as needed

Criteria for Advancement

External rotation to 30 degrees

Forward flexion to 90 degrees

Minimal pain or inflammation

Phase II: Intermediate Phase (Weeks 3-8)

Goals

Continue to promote healing

Begin to restore scapular and rotator cuff strength

Continue to restore forward flexion and external rotation

Treatment

Discharge immobilizer per physician

Wand exercises for forward flexion and external rotation

Pulleys (if 110 degrees forward flexion)

Progress scapula strengthening (begin manual and closed chain)

Week 6-8

Pain-free, submaximal internal and external rotation isometrics

Progress to scapular isotonics

Progress to internal and external rotation isotonics

Initiate latissimus strengthening

Initiate biceps strengthening

Hydrotherapy (if required)

Initiate humeral head control exercises

Initiate scapular plane elevation (with adequate scapular and rotator cuff strength)

Modalities as needed

(continued)

inflammation. Generally the fixation provided by this procedure will allow early, controlled ROM. In addition, with an open procedure there is greater risk of loss of motion, which can be critical depending on the functional demands of the patient. The progression for an arthroscopic procedure is similar; however, generally one will progress ROM more conservatively. As always, a critical goal is to avoid excessive passive stretching of the patient in the latter stages of rehabilitation. Immediate, controlled ROM may also play a role in pain control. There is scientific evidence that motion will stimulate certain mechanoreceptors that will reduce the patient's pain perception.[22,23] In addition, early motion has been demonstrated to have a positive effect on articular cartilage nutrition and collagen fiber remodeling.[24-26]

The patient is instructed to wear the immobilizer at all times other than when performing the home exercise program. The immobilizer will protect against any stressful motion and provide support for the healing tissues. During this phase, passive ROM (PROM) for forward flexion in supine is initiated. Ideally, this should be performed in the plane of the scapula. The plane of the scapula, described by Johnston, which is 30 to 45 degrees anterior to the coronal plane, provides certain advantages.[27,28] First, there is the least amount of torsion to the inferior capsule as the arm is elevated.[27] Secondly, it provides the greatest degree of congruency between the humeral head and the glenoid. This will reduce stress to the capsule and labrum.[28] Wand exercises are initiated for external rotation (Figure 28-3). Forward flexion is limited to 90 degrees and external rotation to 45 degrees if the anterior capsule has been shifted. Patients are instructed to avoid significant pain when performing these ROM exercises, so as to minimize inflammation and delay a normal progression.

Gripping exercises are performed to improve circulation and promote healing. Wrist and elbow ROM exercises are performed to prevent any stiffness or contractures that may

---

BOX 28-1

Multidirectional Instability: Capsular Shift Procedures Guidelines—cont'd

Criteria for Advancement

Minimal pain and inflammation

Forward flexion to 160 degrees

External rotation to 75 degrees

Internal and external rotation strength 5–/5

Phase III: Advanced Strengthening Phase (Weeks 8-12)

Goals

Restore full ROM

Restore normal scapulohumeral rhythm

Upper extremity strength 5/5

Restore normal flexibility

Treatment

Continue active assistive ROM: forward flexion and external rotation

Begin active assistive ROM for internal rotation

Continue aggressive scapula strengthening

Progress strengthening for the rotator cuff, deltoid, biceps, and latissimus (incorporate eccentric training)

Begin proprioceptive neuromuscular training patterns

Progress humeral head control drills

Progress internal and external rotation to "90-90" position if required

Use full upper extremity flexibility program

Begin isokinetic training

Modalities as needed

Criteria for Advancement

Full shoulder ROM

Upper extremity strength 5/5

Normal upper extremity flexibility

No pain or inflammation

Phase IV: Return to Activity Phase (Weeks 12-16)

Goals

Restore normal neuromuscular function

Maintain strength and flexibility to meet the demands of functional activity

Prevent reinjury

Treatment

Isokinetic testing

Continue full upper extremity strengthening and flexibility program

Activity-specific plyometric program

Address trunk and lower extremity needs

Endurance training

Sport- or activity-specific program

Home exercise program

Criteria for Discharge

Pain-free

Independent home exercise program

Independent sport- or activity-specific program

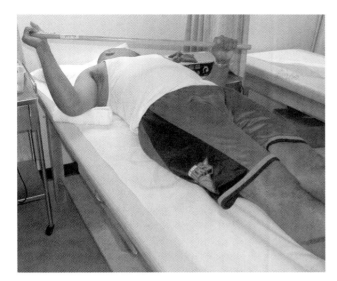

Figure 28-3: Wand exercise for active assistive external rotation.

develop while the patient is in the immobilizer. Scapular isometrics are performed initially to develop proximal musculature and improve posture while in the immobilizer. As pain and inflammation are reduced, submaximal deltoid isometrics are initiated in a modified neutral position. They are initially performed with the elbow flexed to 90 degrees in order to decrease the lever arm and reduce the amount of stress to the glenohumeral joint (Figure 28-4). The patient is again carefully instructed to maintain a pain-free tension so as to minimize inflammation. It is often helpful for the clinician to demonstrate this tension manually to educate the patient. Finally, modalities such as cryotherapy and electric stimulation are used for controlling pain and minimizing inflammation.

PHASE II: INTERMEDIATE PHASE (WEEKS 3 TO 8)

During the intermediate phase, the immobilizer is discharged and the patient will continue to progress ROM. The patient continues wand exercises for forward flexion and external rotation. Precautions are continued to avoid excessive stretch to the capsule and labrum. Active assistive forward flexion can be progressed to pulleys when the patient can achieve approximately 110 degrees in the supine position (Figure 28-5). In addition, the patient should demonstrate humeral head control to avoid any scapular compensation. Active assistive external rotation may be progressed slowly according to the patient's tolerance. The patient's functional demands should be a factor in how quickly external rotation is progressed. The patient who will require greater ROM for overhead activities may need to be progressed more rapidly than a patient whose activity level can sacrifice some mobility for increased stability.

Scapular strengthening is progressed manually in a sidelying position. Wilk advocates performing these exercises

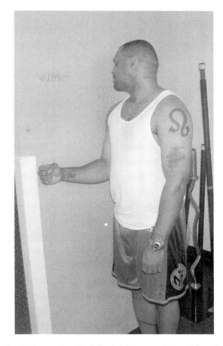

Figure 28-4: Submaximal deltoid isometrics with elbow flexed to 90 degrees.

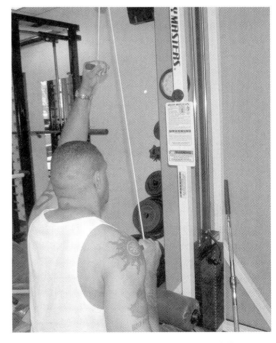

Figure 28-5: Pulleys for active assistive forward flexion.

with the patient's hand fixed to close the kinetic chain and better isolate the scapular muscles.[29] Manual resistance is provided for scapular elevation and depression and protraction and retraction.[29] These "hands-on" techniques can provide tactile feedback to the patient as he or she develops normal scapular control. Early stage closed chain exercises, such as weight shifting or Physioball stabilization exercises,

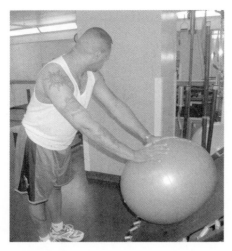

Figure 28-6: Closed chain ball stabilization exercise.

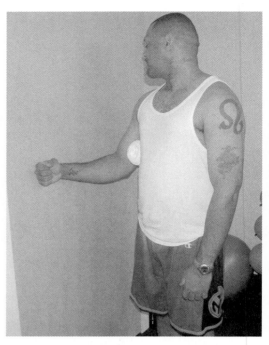

Figure 28-7: Submaximal isometrics for external rotators.

are initiated for scapular strengthening (Figure 28-6). Closed chain exercises, which are performed by fixing the distal end of the limb, provide advantages that are well documented in the lower extremity.[30] However, these principles can also be applied to the upper extremity. By fixing the distal end of the limb, an axial load is created and a compressive force is provided to the joint. This enhances joint stability and decreases stress to the shoulder capsule. In addition, closed chain exercises stimulate the joint mechanoreceptors to facilitate proprioception. Joint proprioception, which is defined as awareness of joint posture, movements, and positional changes, has been found to improve with closed chain exercises.[30,31]

As symptoms and ROM allow, submaximal, pain-free isometrics are initiated for the rotator cuff (Figure 28-7). Before active elevation of the upper extremity is performed, humeral head control must be established. It is well documented that the rotator cuff plays a large role in stabilizing the glenohumeral joint by providing a compressive force to the humeral head.[32,33] With active elevation the rotator cuff centers and steers the humeral head into the glenoid.[34] After surgery the rotator cuff often seems to be reflexively inhibited secondary to pain and inflammation. As mentioned previously, the plane of the scapula is an optimal place to initiate these exercises. This position has been demonstrated to provide the optimal length-tension relationship for the rotator cuff and the deltoid.[27] It has been demonstrated that the lengthened position of these muscles enhances the force generated.[27,35] Again, the patient must be educated to limit the tension of these exercises, to avoid excessive pain and inflammation, as this can result in a reflex inhibition of the rotator cuff, thus reducing humeral head control.[36]

During the 6- to 8-week postoperative period, scapular strengthening is progressed. Restoring scapular strength establishes static proximal stability to provide a stable base of support for glenohumeral movement. Establishing normal scapulothoracic motion provides several advantages. First, it establishes a stable base for glenohumeral rotation. Second,

it maintains the glenoid in position to allow maximal congruency with the humeral head, thus reducing the stress to capsule and labrum. Third, proper scapular positioning creates the proper length-tension relationship of the glenohumeral muscles. Finally, proper elevation of the acromion can reduce the incidence of rotator cuff pathology, such as subacromial impingement.[37,38] Often, rotator cuff pathology may be a result of scapular dysfunction.

When restoring scapular strength, certain principles should be followed. These muscles have a great deal of postural function. Therefore they must be trained for endurance and efficiency. Fatigue is often a cause of scapular dysfunction.[39,40] Additionally, the scapular musculature often functions as force couples and therefore must be trained accordingly. Moseley and co-workers performed an electromyographic (EMG) analysis of 16 shoulder exercises.[41] Based on their analysis and other biomechanical factors, a core group of optimal scapular exercises was established:

- Rowing, emphasizing the rhomboids and middle trapezius (Figure 28-8)
- Push-ups with a plus (maximal protraction), emphasizing the serratus anterior (Figure 28-9)
- Seated press-ups, emphasizing the latissimus and pectoralis minor
- Scaption (elevation in the scapular plane in external rotation), emphasizing the upper and lower trapezius and using the serratus and rhomboids (Figure 28-10)

In addition to this list, shoulder shrugs are performed to strengthen the upper trapezius and levator scapula. Recently, Ekstrom and colleagues have demonstrated that the shoulder shrug exercise produces the greatest EMG activity of the

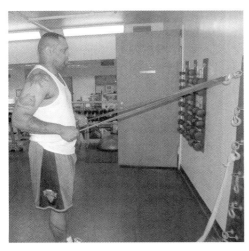

Figure 28-8: Scapula retraction (rowing) with elastic resistance.

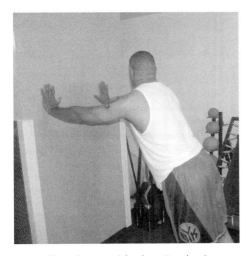

Figure 28-9: Wall push-ups with plus. Emphasis on scapula protraction for the serratus anterior.

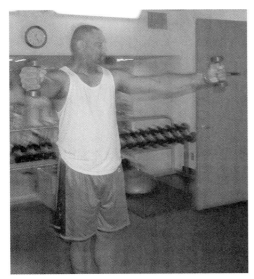

Figure 28-10: Scapula plane elevation using the upper and lower trapezius, rhomboids, and serratus anterior.

upper trapezius muscle[42] (Figure 28-11). The serratus and lower trapezius are also critical in positioning and tilting the scapula for its optimal position. Kibler states that the serratus and lower trapezius appear to be the first muscles involved in inhibition-based muscle dysfunction.[38] Scapular protraction, especially with the scapula upwardly rotated, is also used to strengthen the serratus.[43] Prone elevation of the arm in line with the lower trapezius has been demonstrated to be effective in strengthening that muscle group.[42] However, one must understand that this is a relatively difficult exercise that may not be initiated until later phases.

A final rationale for initiating these scapular exercises early is based on research performed by Hintermeister and colleagues.[44] At times, patients have difficulty performing isolated rotator cuff exercises during the early phases of rehabilitation, secondary to weakness or inflammation. This study demonstrated that certain scapular exercises, such as shrugs, forward punches, rowing, and push-ups with a plus elicit significant rotator cuff activity.[45]

Latissimus strengthening is incorporated into the program. In addition to being a prime extensor of the shoulder and a scapular depressor, the latissimus has been demonstrated to provide a compressive force to the glenohumeral joint, thereby assisting the rotator cuff in controlling the amount of humeral head translation.[45] Strengthening is initiated in a position of 90 degrees of elevation and below until rotator cuff strength has improved (Figure 28-12). Biceps strengthening is initiated. The biceps, which plays a significant role at the elbow, has also been shown to have a stabilizing effect at the glenohumeral joint.[46-48] In addition, Itoi and colleagues have demonstrated a stabilizing function in the abducted and externally rotated position.[46]

If symptoms allow, isotonic internal rotation and external rotation exercises are initiated. As before, shoulder inflammation is monitored carefully when strengthening the rotator

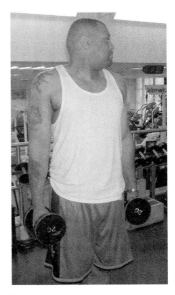

Figure 28-11: Shoulder shrugs emphasizing the upper trapezius.

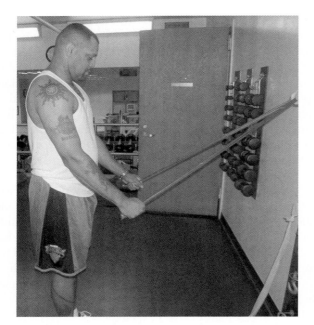

Figure 28-12: Latissimus pull-down with elastic resistance initiated from 90 degrees and below.

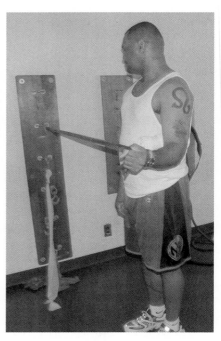

Figure 28-13: External rotation strengthening with elastic resistance.

cuff. Using a small towel roll to move the shoulder into comfortable abduction is preferred to improve circulation (Figure 28-13). Rathburn and MacNab have demonstrated a compromise in the vasculature that supplies the rotator cuff in the adducted position.[49] This position also improves the length-tension relationship of the rotator cuff.[27,35] If scapular and rotator cuff strength are adequate, scapular plane elevation is initiated. Advantages of the scapular plane have been mentioned previously. In addition to those, it should be mentioned that in this plane the deltoid and supraspinatus have a more direct line of pull, thus reducing the chance of subacromial impingement as the arm is elevated.[27,50] The exercise is performed with the thumb in external rotation. The internally rotated or "empty can" position described by Jobe and Moynes, which demonstrates a great deal of supraspinatus activity, is avoided to minimize the chance of subacromial impingement.[51] In addition, Blackburn and co-workers demonstrated greater supraspinatus activity with a prone position with the shoulder horizontally abducted to 100 degrees and externally rotated to 90 degrees.[52] Worrell and colleagues later compared the two positions and found similar results.[53] In addition to strengthening a good portion of the scapular and glenohumeral musculature, this exercise can be a valuable evaluative tool. Throughout the rehabilitation program it can be used to reassess the patient's scapulothoracic function and glenohumeral rhythm.

Patients who are not progressing as well may benefit from hydrotherapy. Speer and colleagues advocated the use of hydrotherapy for those patients having difficulty regaining normal rotator cuff dysfunction.[54] Hydrotherapy requires the use of a pool or water tank and the desire of the patient. One must feel comfortable in the water. The most significant

benefit is using the buoyancy of the water to assist active elevation of the upper extremity. Studies have shown that the arm can weigh up to eight times its original weight at 90 degrees of elevation.[55] In addition, Speer's group hypothesized that the orthostatic pressure may cause a "glove effect," which may stimulate proprioception and send a biofeedback-like response to the patient.[54]

If rotator cuff strength is adequate, humeral head stabilization exercises are initiated. Rhythmic stabilization exercises are initiated. These exercises, which promote muscular co-contraction, are progressed by increasing the challenge to the glenohumeral musculature. For example, one may begin with the elbow in flexion and progress to performing the exercises with the elbow extended. In addition, position of the upper extremity should be progressed to more challenging ranges. Finally, if a good strength base has been established, upper body ergometry can be initiated to begin to restore endurance.

PHASE III: ADVANCED STRENGTHENING PHASE (WEEKS 8 TO 12)

During the advanced strengthening phase, the goals are to restore normal strength, ROM, and flexibility and to begin to restore normal neuromuscular function. This will prepare the patient for the return to activity phase. The patient continues active assistive ROM for forward flexion and external rotation until normal range is restored. The clinician should monitor the patient who is progressing slowly to determine if any capsular restrictions are developing. In such cases the

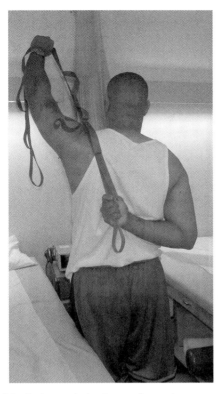

Figure 28-14: Active assistive internal rotation.

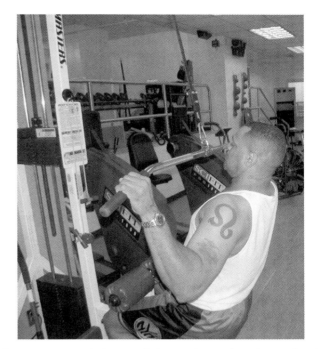

Figure 28-15: Latissimus pull-down advanced to the overhead position.

clinician, after consultation with the surgeon, may need to use various joint mobilization and soft tissue techniques. For example, the patient who is slow to restore forward flexion may have a restriction of the inferior capsule.[56] In addition, the anterior and posterior structures should be assessed. Active assistive internal rotation exercises are performed using either a wand or a strap (Figure 28-14). Scapular mobility should also be assessed to determine if the patient has adequate elevation and protraction. For particularly restricted patients, passive techniques may be necessary. Low-load, long-duration stretches have been shown to be most effective.[57,58] Finally, continuous passive motion is an option. Various continuous passive motion devices allow the patient to work on ROM gradually and slowly.

The patient continues aggressive scapular strengthening for all muscle groups. Emphasis is placed on muscular endurance and efficiency, as these muscles often function posturally. Strengthening is advanced for the latissimus, biceps, rotator cuff, and deltoid. Latissimus strengthening is progressed to the overhead position (Figure 28-15). Strengthening continues to be biased toward the plane of the scapula for reasons mentioned previously. As the patient's strength improves, eccentric strengthening is emphasized (Figure 28-16). Eccentric muscle action is defined as muscular lengthening while resisting a load.[59] Eccentric activity plays a significant role in many high level activities and is best documented in sports activities such as throwing and tennis.[60-62] When incorporating eccentric training the clinician should proceed cautiously, as eccentric exercise has been shown to

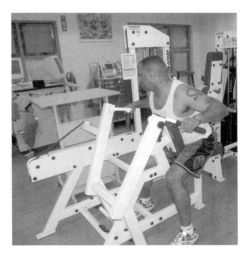

Figure 28-16: Rowing for scapular retraction emphasizing eccentric activity.

be a cause of delayed-onset muscle soreness.[59] Elastic resistance or tubing can be used safely to provide eccentric resistance.

During this phase, proprioceptive training should be advanced. Proprioception, which is defined as the awareness of joint posture, has been demonstrated to become compromised with shoulder instability.[63-66] Vangsness and colleagues found proprioceptive nerve endings in the glenohumeral joint capsular ligaments and free nerve endings in the glenoid labrum.[63] Smith and Brunolti demonstrated proprioceptive

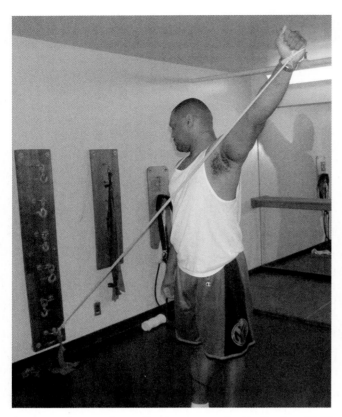

Figure 28-17: Proprioceptive Neuromuscular Facilitation (PNF) D2 flexion pattern with elastic resistance.

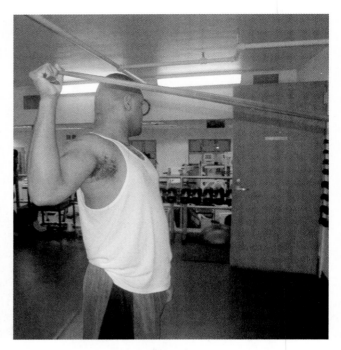

Figure 28-18: Overhead "90-90" position for external rotation strengthening.

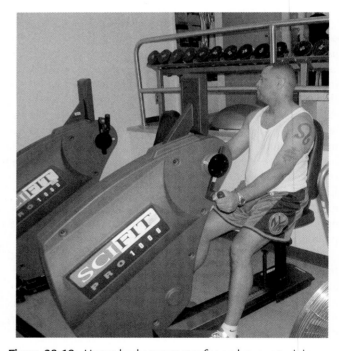

Figure 28-19: Upper body ergometry for endurance training.

deficits after acute glenohumeral dislocations.[64] Lephart and co-workers found abnormal proprioception in subjects with unilateral instability.[65] More recently, two separate studies found proprioceptive deficits in subjects with unstable shoulders that returned to normal after surgery.[65,66] With normal rotator cuff and scapular strength, proprioceptive neuromuscular facilitation patterns are initiated. These patterns are useful in restoring normal movement patterns that are required for all upper extremity activities. The patterns used should be based on the patient's functional demands and deficits. For example, the Diagonal 2 flexion and extension patterns (D2) simulate much of the muscle action that occurs in overhead activities.[67] These patterns are initiated manually. Manual pressure provides the patient with tactile feedback to perform a specific movement pattern correctly. It also allows the clinician greater control of the pattern. As the patient progresses, elastic resistance can be introduced to work both concentrically and eccentrically (Figure 28-17). Along with these patterns, humeral head control exercises are progressed to more challenging positions.

With 5/5 rotator cuff strength and good scapular control, internal rotator (IR) and external rotator (ER) strengthening is advanced to the overhead, abducted, or "90 to 90" position (Figure 28-18). This progression would be based on the functional demands of the patient. If overhead activity is not required, one does not have to follow this progression. This progression must be monitored closely, as this is a challenging position for the rotator cuff.

Endurance training is continued during this phase, using upper body ergometry and various neuromuscular drills while the patient is fatigued (Figure 28-19). Poor musculature endurance can result in a subtle loss of humeral head control that can lead to a loss of stability or rotator cuff pathology. Wickiewicz, using radiographic evaluation, has demonstrated a significant increase in humeral head migration during arm elevation after exhaustive dumbbell training.[68] In addition, Carpenter and co-workers have demonstrated a loss of proprioception with rotator cuff fatigue.[69] Isokinetic training is also incorporated into this phase to enable training at higher speeds and building muscular endurance. In addition, isokinetic testing will provide an objective assessment of shoulder rotator cuff muscle performance, which plays an integral role in the stability of the glenohumeral joint. Isokinetic testing provides specificity with regard to testing the upper extremity at faster, more functional speeds[70] and will allow the clinician to better evaluate when a patient may begin more functional activities.

During this phase, full upper extremity flexibility is restored. Internal rotation and horizontal adduction are addressed. A loss of horizontal adduction may be indicative of a tight posterior capsule, and a loss of internal rotation may be the result of a rotator cuff contracture (Figure 28-20). The clinical significance of this was demonstrated by Harryman and co-workers.[71] They demonstrated that restricted posterior structures can result in an increased anterior and superior humeral head migration as the upper extremity is elevated.[68] This can result in a subacromial impingement or anterior subluxation of the humeral head. Normal upper extremity flexibility is critical for prevention of reinjury as the patient begins more functional activities.

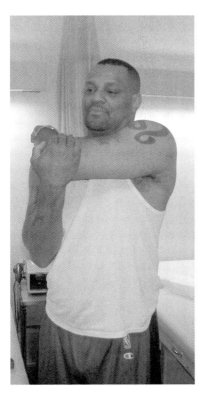

Figure 28-20: Passive horizontal adduction to stretch the posterior capsule.

PHASE IV: RETURN TO ACTIVITY PHASE (WEEKS 12 TO 16)

The return to activity phase allows the patient to transition into the desired sport or functional activity. Normal neuromuscular function should be restored. The requirements of the sport or functional activity must be met. Criteria to enter this phase include normal upper extremity strength, ROM, flexibility, and endurance. Isokinetic testing will provide objective strength data to guide this assessment. For example, in normal patients a 66% external/internal rotation ratio is targeted.[72] However, these ratios will vary according to speed and population. For example, greater internal rotation strength is well documented in overhead athletes.[73,74] This leads to the belief that external rotation strength should be emphasized in these patients.[73,74] In addition, a limb dominance of 5% to 10% is expected for both internal and external rotation in the nonathletic or recreational population.[75] This, at minimum, should be achieved as a criterion for initiating functional activities. Aggressive strengthening and flexibility exercises are performed for the entire upper extremity. In addition, when required in the athletic population, strength and conditioning of the trunk and lower extremities must be addressed.

During this phase neuromuscular drills and proprioceptive training continue to be progressed. As the previously listed criteria are met, a functionally specific plyometric program is initiated. Plyometric training should be used only when required by the demands of the patient. Plyometrics use the stretch reflex of the muscle spindle. An eccentric prestretch of the muscle results in a powerful concentric contraction.[76] Plyometrics are a key component of many athletic activities. The goal of plyometric training is to improve the reactability of the neuromuscular system. Several authors have established guidelines for plyometric exercise.[77,78] First, the training should be activity specific. For example, during the late cocking phase of throwing or serving in tennis, the anterior shoulder musculature is eccentrically prestretched, before a powerful concentric contraction. Second, the quality of work and technique should be emphasized. In addition, the program should be progressive in nature. Upper extremity plyometrics can also incorporate the trunk and lower extremities. The program is progressed from less challenging activities, such as a two-hand chest pass, to activities performed in an overhead position (Figure 28-21). The activities can also be progressed from bilateral to unilateral.

Before returning to activity, a sport- or activity-specific program may be initiated. The patient shall have completed a plyometric program asymptomatically. These programs may range from sport-specific activities such as interval throwing or tennis programs to work hardening activities. Any of these programs should be designed for the patient to progress individually to minimize the chance of reinjury. In addition, the biomechanics of an activity should be assessed to improve performance and reduce the chance of reinjury.

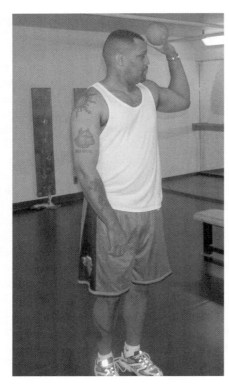

Figure 28-21: Plyometric overhead exercise for advanced training.

Finally, during this phase the patient is instructed regarding a home exercise program that can be performed on a consistent basis. Patients need to maintain a level of strength, flexibility, and endurance as their functional activities increase. The home exercise program should be incorporated into the regular exercise routine, and often modifications are required. For example, continuing to bias the strengthening program toward the plane of the scapula may reduce the chance of reinjury.

SUMMARY

In recent years, improved surgical techniques have allowed shoulder stabilization rehabilitation to progress more rapidly. The advancement from open to arthroscopic procedures has allowed a greater opportunity to restore the patient to the preinjury functional level; however, the principles and functional progressions have not changed greatly. Regardless of surgical technique, the goals are to progress the patient functionally while abiding by the healing constraints of the repaired tissue. A scientific rational progression is critical to avoiding surgical failure or reinjury.

References

1. Rowe CR: Acute and recurrent dislocations of the shoulder, *J Bone Joint Surg Am* 38A:998-1008, 1962.
2. Neer CS, Foster CR: Inferior capsular shift for involuntary inferior and multidirectional instability of the shoulder: a preliminary report, *J Bone Joint Surg Am* 62A:897-908, 1980.
3. McMahon MS, Zarins B: *The athlete's shoulder: multidirectional instability of the shoulder,* New York, 1994, Churchill Livingstone.
4. Altchek DW, Warren RF, Skyhar MJ, et al: T-plasty: a technique for treating multidirectional instability in athletes, *Orthop Trans* 13:569-581,1989.
5. Neer CS: *Shoulder reconstruction,* Philadelphia, 1990, Saunders.
6. Neer CS, Welsh RP: The shoulder in sports, *Orthop Clin North Am* 8-15:583, 1987.
7. Neer CS: Involuntary inferior and multidirectional instability of the shoulder: etiology, recognition and treatment, *Instr Course Lect* 34:232-240, 1985.
8. Yamaguchi K, Flatow EL: Management of multidirectional instability, *Clin Sports Med* 14:885-902, 1995.
9. Hawkins RJ, Angelo RL: Glenohumeral osteoarthrosis, *J Bone Joint Surg Am* 72:1193-1197, 1990.
10. Steinman SR, Flatow EL, Pollock RG, et al: Evaluation and surgical treatment of failed shoulder instability repairs, *Orthop Trans* 16:727-733, 1992.
11. Flatow EL, Warner JI: Instability of the shoulder: Complex problems and failed repairs: part 1. Relevant biomechanics, multidirectional instability and severe glenoid loss, *Instr Course Lect* 47:122-140, 1998.
12. Bak K, Spring BL, Henderson IJP: Inferior capsular shift procedure in athletes with multidirectional instability base on isolated capsular and ligamentous redundancy, *Am J Sports Med* 28:466-471, 2000.
13. Bigliani LU, Kurzweil PR, Schwartzbach CC, et al: Inferior capsular shift procedure for anterior-inferior shoulder instability in athletes, *Am J Sports Med* 22:578-584, 1994.
14. Matsen FA III, Thomas SC, Rockwood CA: Anterior glenohumeral instability. In Rockwood CA, Matsen FA, editors: *The shoulder,* vol 1, ed 2, Philadelphia 1990, Saunders.
15. Altchek DW, Warren RF, Skyhar MJ, et al: T-plasty modification of the Bankart procedure for multidirectional instability of the anterior and inferior types, *J Bone Joint Surg Am* 73A:105-112, 1991.
16. Favorito PJ, Langenderfer MA, Colisimo MJ, et al: Arthroscopic laser-assisted capsular shift in the treatment of patients with multidirectional instability, *Am J Sports Med* 30:322-328, 2002.
17. Joseph TA, Williams JS, Brems JJ: Laser capsulorrhaphy for multidirectional instability of the shoulder, *Am J Sports Med* 31:26-35, 2003.
18. Levy O, Wilson M, Williams H, et al: Thermal capsular shrinkage for shoulder instability. Mid-term longitudinal outcome study, *J Bone Joint Surg Br* 83:640-645, 2001.
19. Wallace AL, Hollinshead RM, Frank CB: Electrothermal shrinkage reduces laxity but alters creep behavior in a lapine ligament model, *J Shoulder Elbow Surg* 10:1-6, 2001.
20. Fischer SP: Arthroscopic treatment of multi-directional instability, *Sports Med Arthrosc Rev* 12:127-134, 2004.
21. Gartsman GM, Roddey TS, Hammerman SM: Arthroscopic treatment of multidirectional glenohumeral instability: 2 to 5-year follow-up, *Arthroscopy* 17:236-243, 2001.
22. Wyke B: The neurology of joints, *Ann Coll Surg Engl* 41:25-40, 1996.
23. Franks C, Akeson W, Woo S, et al: Physiology and therapeutic value of passive joint motion, *Clin Orthop* 185:113, 1995.
24. Akeson WH, Woo SLY, Amiel D: The connective tissue response to immobility: biomechanical changes in periarticular connective tissue of the immobilized rabbit knee, *Clin Orthop* 93:356-362, 1973.

25. Salter RB, Bell RS, Keeley FN: The protective effect of continuous passive motion on living articular cartilage in acute septic arthritis, *Clin Orthop* 159:223-247, 1981.

26. Salter RB, Simmons DC, Malcom BW: The biological effects on continuous passive motion on the healing of full thickness articular cartilage defects, *J Bone Joint Surg Am* 62:1231-1251, 1980.

27. Johnston TB: The movements of the shoulder joint. A plea for the use of the "plane of the scapula" as the plane of reference for movements occurring at the humeri-scapular joint, *Br J Surg* 25:252-260, 1937.

28. Saha AK: Mechanism of shoulder movements and a plea for recognition of the "zero position" of the glenohumeral joint, *Clin Orthop* 173:3-10, 1983.

29. Wilk KE: *The athlete's shoulder: current concepts in the rehabilitation of athletic shoulder injuries,* New York, 1994, Churchill Livingstone.

30. Tippett S: Closed chain exercise, *Orthop Phys Ther Clin North Am* 1:253-268,1992.

31. Wilk KE, Arrigo C, Andrews JA: Closed and open kinetic chain exercise for the upper extremity, *J Sports Rehab* 5:88-102, 1996.

32. Howell SM, Galinat BJ, Renze AJ, et al: Normal and abnormal mechanics of the glenohumeral joint in the horizontal plane, *J Bone Joint Surg Am* 10:227-232, 1988.

33. Warner JP, Deng X, Warren RF: Superoinferior translation in the intact and vented glenohumeral joint, *J Shoulder Elbow Surg* 2:99-105, 1993.

34. Saha AK: Mechanics of elevation of the glenohumeral joint, its application in rehabilitation of flail shoulder in upper brachial plexus injuries and poliomyelitis and in replacement of the upper humerus by prosthesis, *Acta Orthop Scand* 44:688-675, 1973.

35. Poppen NK, Walker PS: Normal and abnormal motion of the shoulder, *J Bone Joint Surg Am* 58:195-201, 1976.

36. Timm K: The isokinetic torque curve of shoulder instability in high school baseball pitchers, *J Orthop Sports Phys Ther* 26:150-154, 1998.

37. Kibler WB: Role of the scapula in the overhead throwing motion, *Contemp Orthop* 22:525-533, 1991.

38. Kibler WB: The role of the scapula in athletic shoulder function, *Am J Sports Med* 26:325-336, 1998.

39. McQuade J, Dawson K, Schmidt G: Scapulothoracic muscle fatigue associated with alterations in scapulohumeral rhythm, *J Orthop Sports Phys Ther* 28:74-80, 1998.

40. Bradley J, Tibone J: Electromyographic analysis of muscle action about the shoulder, *Clin Sports Med* 10:789-795, 1991.

41. Moseley JB, Jobe FW, Pink M: EMG analysis of scapular muscles during a shoulder rehabilitation program, *Am J Sports Med* 20:128-134, 1994.

42. Ekstrom RA, Donnatelli RA, Soderberg GL: Surface electromyographic analysis of exercises for the trapezius and serratus anterior muscles, *J Orthop Sports Phys Ther* 33:247-258, 2003.

43. Decker MJ, Hintermeister RA, Faber KJ, et al: Serratus anterior muscle activity during selected rehabilitation exercises, *Am J Sports Med* 27:784-791, 1999.

44. Hintermeister RA, Lange GW, Schultheis JM, et al: Electromyographic activity and applied load during shoulder rehabilitation exercises using elastic resistance, *Am J Sports Med* 26:210-220, 1998.

45. Bassett R, Browne A, Mosrey B, et al: Glenohumeral muscle force and movement mechanics in a position of shoulder instability, *J Biomech* 23:401-415, 1988.

46. Itoi E, Kuechle DK, Newman SR, et al: Stabilizing function of the biceps in stable and unstable shoulders, *J Bone Joint Surg Am* 75:546-550, 1993.

47. Itoi E, Mutzkin NE, Morrey BF, et al: Stabilizing effect of the long head of the biceps in the hanging arm position, *J Shoulder Elbow Surg* 3:135-142, 1994.

48. Rodosky MW, Harner CD, Fu FH: The role of the long head of the biceps muscle and superior glenoid labrum in anterior stability of the shoulder, *Am J Sports Med* 22:121-130, 1994.

49. Rathbun JB, MacNab I: The microvascular pattern of the rotator cuff, *J Bone Joint Surg Br* 52B:540-553, 1970.

50. Tata GE, Ng L, Kramer JF: Shoulder antagonistic strength ratios during concentric and eccentric muscle actions in the scapular plane, *J Orthop Sports Phys Ther* 18:654-660, 1993.

51. Jobe FW, Moynes DR: Delineation of the diagnostic criteria and a rehabilitation program for rotator cuff injuries, *Am J Sports Med* 10:336-339, 1982.

52. Blackburn TA, Mcleod DW, White B, et al: EMG analysis of posterior rotator cuff exercises, *Athletic Training* 25:40-45, 1990.

53. Worrell TW, Correy BJ, York SL, et al: An analysis of supraspinatus EMG activity and shoulder isometric force development, *Med Sci Sports Exerc* 24:744-748, 1992.

54. Speer KP, Cavanaugh JT, Day L, et al: The role of hydrotherapy in shoulder rehabilitation, *Am J Sports Med* 21:850-853, 1993.

55. Morrey BF, An K: *The shoulder: biomechanics of the shoulder,* Philadelphia, 1990, Saunders.

56. Paris SV: *Extremity dysfunction and mobilization,* Atlanta, 1980, Institute Press.

57. Bonutti PM, Windav JE, Ables BA, et al: Static progressive stretch to reestablish elbow range of motion, *Clin Orthop* 303:128-134, 1994.

58. Nuismer BA, Ekes AM, Holm MB: The use of low load, long stretch devices in rehabilitation programs in the Pacific Northwest, *Am J Occup Ther* 51:538-543, 1997.

59. Bennett JG, Marcus NA: The athlete's shoulder: the decelerator mechanism: eccentric muscular contraction applications at the shoulder, New York, 1994, Churchill Livingstone.

60. DiGiovine MN, Jobe FW, Pink M: An electromyographic analysis of the upper extremity in pitching, *J Shoulder Elbow Surg* 1:15-25, 1992.

61. Pappas AM, Zawacki RM, Sullivan TJ: Biomechanics of baseball pitching: a preliminary report, *Am J Sports Med* 13:216-222, 1985.

62. Ryu RKN, McCormick J, Jobe FW: An EMG analysis of shoulder function in tennis players. *Am J Sports Med* 16:481-485, 1988.

63. Vangsness CT, Ennis M, Taylor JG, et al: Neural anatomy of the glenohumeral ligaments, labrum and subacromial bursa, *Arthroscopy* 11:180-184, 1995.

64. Smith RH, Brunolti J: Shoulder kinesthesia after anterior glenohumeral joint dislocation, *Phys Ther* 69:106-112, 1989.

65. Lephart S, Warner JP, Borsa PA, et al: Proprioception of the shoulder joint in healthy, unstable, and surgically repaired shoulders, *J Shoulder Elbow Surg* 3:371-381, 1994.

66. Zuckerman JD, Gallagher MD, Cuomo F, et al: The effect of instability and subsequent anterior shoulder repair on proprioceptive ability, *J Shoulder Elbow Surg* 6:180-185, 1997.

67. Knott M, Voss D: *Proprioceptive neuromuscular facilitation,* New York, 1968, Harper and Row.

68. Wickiewicz T: Radiographic evaluation of the glenohumeral kinematics—a muscle fatigue model. American Academy of Orthopedic Surgeons Sports Medicine Specialty Meeting, Washington, DC, 1994.

69. Carpenter JE, Blaiser RB, Pellizzon G: The effects of muscle fatigue on shoulder joint position sense, *Am J Sports Med* 26:262-265, 1998.

70. Davies GJ, Wilk KE, Ellenbecker TS: Strength assessment. In Malone TR, Mcpoil T, Nitz AJ, editors: *Orthopedic and sports physical therapy*, ed 3, St. Louis, 1997, Mosby.

71. Harryman DT, Sidles JA, Clark JM, et al: Translation of the humeral head on the glenoid with passive glenohumeral motion, *J Bone Joint Surg Am* 72:1334-1343, 1990.

72. Ivey FM, Calhoun JH, Rusche K, et al: Normal values for isokinetic testing of shoulder strength, *Med Sci Sports Exerc* 16:127-131, 1984.

73. Ellenbecker TS: Shoulder internal and external rotation strength and range of motion of highly skilled junior tennis players, *Isokin Exerc Sci* 2:1-9, 1992.

74. Hinton RY: Isokinetic evaluation of shoulder rotational strength in high school baseball pitchers, *Am J Sports Med* 16:274-279, 1988.

75. Jobe FW, Tibone JE, Perry J, et al: An EMG analysis of the shoulder in pitching. A preliminary report, *Am J Sports Med* 11:3-5, 1983.

76. Chu D: *Jumping into plyometrics,* Champaign, 1992, Leisure Press.

77. Voight M, Draovitch P: *Eccentric muscle training in sports and orthopedics: plyometrics training,* New York, 1991, Churchill Livingstone.

78. Wilk K, Voight M, Keirns M: Stretch shortening drills for the upper extremities: theory and clinical application, *J Orthop Sports Phys Ther* 17:225-239, 1993.

CHAPTER 29

The Bankart Lesion

Timothy F. Tyler, MS, PT, ATC
Stephen J. Nicholas, MD
Aruna M. Seneviratne, MD

CHAPTER OUTLINE

SHOULDER INSTABILITY HAS BEEN REC-OGNIZED since the time of Hippocrates. He treated shoulder dislocations with a variety of reduction maneuvers and in refractory cases used hot irons to cauterize the shoulder capsule.[1,2] The pathophysiology of shoulder instability is extremely complex and is now better understood because of several recent anatomic studies.[3-6] Shoulder instability can be broadly categorized into two main types: those with multidirectional instability, which is responsive to rehabilitation, and those with a traumatic unidirectional dislocation, which leads to recurrent instability. This chapter focuses on one particular lesion that accounts for the majority of shoulder instability: the Bankart lesion, or traumatic avulsion of the capsulolabral complex from the anterior glenoid rim.

On December 15, 1923, A.S. Blundell Bankart published his treatise entitled "Recurrent or Habitual Dislocation of the Shoulder Joint" in the British Medical Journal.[7] In it he describes the mechanism of recurrent dislocations to be "shearing off of the fibrous capsule of the joint from its attachment to the fibrocartilaginous glenoid ligament (labrum)." He also notes that the detachment occurred over practically the entire anterior half of the glenoid rim. He astutely notes that the defect would not heal and therefore would lead to recurrent anterior instability of the shoulder. These observations are now universally accepted, and this shearing off of the capsular labral complex is termed the *Bankart lesion* (Figure 29-1).

The shoulder has the greatest range of motion (ROM) of all joints in the human body, yet normally remains stable. This stability is a result of both the static effects of ligaments and tendons and the dynamic effects of the muscles that surround the shoulder girdle. The scapula also has some contribution to shoulder stability in the manner in which it moves. In general, five mechanisms have been elucidated to provide joint stability: bony joint conformity, negative intraarticular pressure and joint cohesion, the glenoid labrum, the ligamentous and capsular restraints, and the muscular structures surrounding the shoulder girdle, including the rotator cuff, biceps brachii, and scapular rotator muscles. Shoulder stability is dependent on these static and dynamic stabilizers (Table 29-1). The greatest contribution to shoulder stability comes from the labrum and the ligament capsular

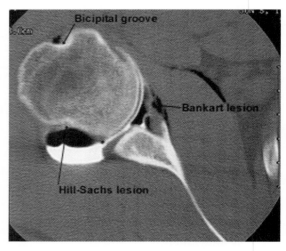

Figure 29-1: Bankart lesion on magnetic resonance imaging scan.

TABLE 29-1

Restraints to Glenohumeral Translations

| TRANSLATION | DYNAMIC RESTRAINTS | | PASSIVE RESTRAINTS |
	PRIMARY RESTRAINTS	SECONDARY RESTRAINTS	
Anterior	Infraspinatus	Deltoid	Anterior Labrum
	Teres minor	Triceps	At 0 degrees ABD—CHL, SGHL, AGHL
			At 45 degrees ABD—MGHL, superior band IGHL
			At 90 degrees ABD—inferior pouch, superior band IGHL
Posterior	Subscapularis	Anterior deltoid	Posterior labrum IGHL posterior band
Inferior	Supraspinatus	Middle deltoid	CHL
		Triceps	IGHL anterior band
Superior	Teres major	Biceps	Posterior inferior capsule
	Latissimus dorsi		

ABD, Abduction; AGHL, anterior glenohumeral ligament; CHL, coracohumeral ligament; IGHL, inferior glenohumeral ligament; MGHL, middle glenohumeral ligament; SGHL, superior glenohumeral ligament.

restraints. Disruption of the labrum from the glenoid rim is inadequate to provide shoulder instability in itself, as described by Speer and colleagues,[6] who concluded that there was additional injury to the capsular structures of the anterior shoulder resulting in stretching that leads to anterior instability.

ANATOMY, HISTOLOGY, AND FUNCTION OF THE CAPSULOLABRAL COMPLEX

Glenohumeral Joint Tissue

The labrum is a fibrous structure that is attached to the glenoid rim throughout its circumference. The superior attachment of the labrum is loose and meniscus-like, and the inferior attachment is firm. Mobility or motion of the labrum above the transverse equator of the glenoid is normal and not pathologic. In contrast, however, inferior mobility is abnormal.[8] The fibers of the biceps tendon intermingle with the superior labrum, and the inferior glenohumeral ligament blends into the inferior labrum. Cooper and Hutchinson studied the gross histologic and vascular anatomy of the glenoid labrum of the human.[3] They found that the arteries that supplied the periphery of the glenoid labrum come from the suprascapular circumflex and posterior circumflex humeral arteries. The superior and anterosuperior parts of the labrum have less vascularity than the posterosuperior and inferior parts, and the vascularity is limited to the periphery of the labrum. Vessels that supply the labrum originate from either the capsular or periosteal vessels and not from the underlying bone. Prodromos and co-workers have noted that the vascularity of the labrum decreases with age.[9]

Ninety percent of the glenohumeral joint capsule is composed of primarily Types I, II, and III collagen. Its composition is similar to that of other joint capsules found in the body.[10] These molecules are arranged in a highly ordered, extended, triple helix to form the ultrastructure of collagen. The remaining portion of this capsuloligamentous structure consists of water, proteoglycans, fibronectin, elastin, and glycoproteins.[10] The specific composition and arrangement of the molecules in individual ligaments provide each with unique functional properties.

Capsular ligamentous structures of the anterior shoulder are mainly composed of distinct thickenings of the anterior capsule. They are the superior glenohumeral ligament (SGHL), the middle glenohumeral ligament (MGHL), and the inferior glenohumeral ligament complex (IGHLC) (Figure 29-2). Of these three structures, the IGHLC is the most important in preventing anterior translation of the humeral head on the glenoid. The IGHLC is actually composed of three functionally separate entities: an anterior band, a posterior band, and an interposed axillary pouch.[11,12]

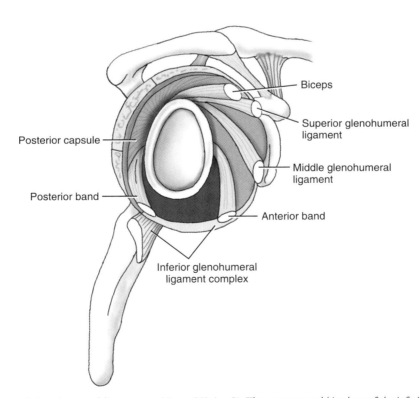

Figure 29-2: Cross section of glenohumeral ligaments. (*From O'Brien SJ: The anatomy and histology of the inferior glenohumeral ligament complex, Am J Sports Med 18:449-456, 1990.*)

Researchers have examined the histology of the IGHLC in 11 fresh-frozen cadaver shoulders. Histologic examination of the joint capsule revealed that the anterior and posterior bands of the IGHLC were readily identifiable as distinct structures, composed of thickened bands of well-organized collagen bundles. The histologic appearance of the axillary pouch revealed that although this area of the capsule appeared to be the thickest, the orientation of the collagen fibers was less organized than in the anterior and posterior bands. They also noted that the IGHLC ran from the glenoid to the humerus and that the humeral attachments took on two configurations. The first was a collarlike attachment where the entire IGHLC attached just inferior to the articular edge of the humeral head; this was observed in six specimens. In the remaining five specimens this attachment was in the shape of a V, with the anterior and posterior bands attaching adjacent to the articular edge of the humeral head and the axillary pouch attaching to the apex of the V, distal to the articular edge.[5] This study provides strong evidence of the value of an intact IGHLC.

The roles of the anterior glenohumeral ligaments in preventing instability are complex and vary with the position of the arm. The IGHL has been recognized to be the primary checkrein against anterior stability with the arm abducted to 90 degrees (Figure 29-3). O'Brien and associates have found that the relative contributions of the components of the IGHL, described previously, change with flexion, extension, and rotation of the arm. With the shoulder in 90 degrees of abduction and 30 degrees of extension, the anterior band of the IGHL becomes the prime stabilizer against both anterior and posterior translation. When the arm is abducted to 90 degrees and is forward flexed to 30 degrees, the posterior band of the IGHLC becomes the prime stabilizer to anterior and posterior translation (see Table 29-1).[11,13-15]

MECHANISM OF INJURY

Indirect force is the most common cause of anterior shoulder dislocation. Falling on the outstretched arm in a position of excessive abduction, external rotation (ER), and extension of the arm is the most common mechanism of injury. Although rare, a direct force from the posterior or posterolateral aspect of the shoulder, which can occur in a fall, can be the cause of anterior dislocation of the shoulder.[16,17]

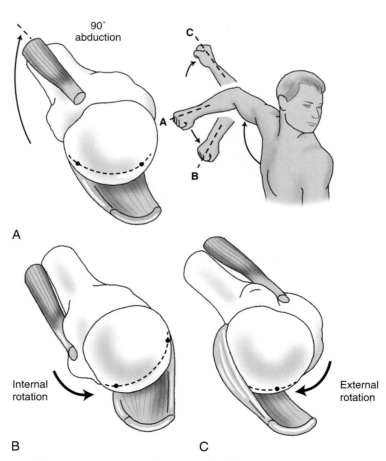

Figure 29-3: Inferior glenohumeral ligament complex at 90 degrees of abduction with internal rotation and external rotation. (*From O'Brien SJ: The anatomy and histology of the inferior glenohumeral ligament complex,* Am J Sports Med *18:449-456, 1990.*)

Stages of Capsuloligamentous Injury and Repair

Once the labrum and its attachments have undergone injury or plastic deformation, they must begin to heal. This is a morphologically complex process that takes place through a continuum of four overlapping phases. Age, tissue quality, nutritional status, degree of injury, mechanical stress, and other factors all influence the healing process.

The initial response is the inflammation phase and begins with the cell's release of histamine, a potent vasodilator. At this point, endothelial buds start to proliferate into the labrum, and the presence of monocytes and macrophages is evident.[18] Biochemical changes, including an increase in water content in the area, take place at the injured tissue. Active collagen synthesis (Type III and Type I) and scar production begin within 4 days.[19]

The second phase is the proliferation phase and is characterized by rapid fibroblast activity. During this phase, immature collagen framework is laid down, elastin production begins, and the water weight is decreased. The healing labrum begins to form an unorganized collagen pattern that seems to increase the tensile strength of the matrix.[20]

The third phase, the remodeling phase, usually begins 6 weeks after injury. During this phase, collagen turnover (synthesis and degradation) is restored to near normal levels. As the labrum matures, the collagen fibers are oriented in line with the tension encountered.[21] Electron microscopic studies reveal that collagen fibrils appear larger in diameter and more densely packed. Type I collagen fibers are more apparent than Type III fibers during this phase.

The final phase, maturation, continues slowly for months and years after injury. During this period, the ligament regains its histologic labrum appearance.[21] The postsurgical Bankart repair will go through this healing process.

CLINICAL EVALUATION

It is important to obtain an accurate history of the mechanism of injury. Some shoulder dislocations are reduced spontaneously, whereas others remain dislocated until physically reduced by a physician. When viewed from the front the dislocated shoulder will have a squared off appearance, and when viewed from the side the distal acromion will appear more prominent and have the appearance of a very large sulcus sign. On presentation to an emergency room, the patient is usually apprehensive, with considerable pain and muscle spasm in the affected shoulder.[22]

Physical examination should focus on accurate assessment of neurovascular status and any associated injuries, such as fractures or brachial plexus injuries. Skin sensation in the distribution of the axillary, lateral, and antebrachial cutaneous nerves should be noted. Initial radiographic evaluation should include a true anteroposterior (AP) view of the shoulder (35 degrees oblique to the body), a transscapular view at right angles to the shoulder, and an axillary view, which usually requires the assistance of a physician. The scapular Y view and the axillary view usually definitively show the direction of dislocation.[23]

There are several techniques for reducing the acutely dislocated shoulder. These methods vary according to physician preference, the timing of patient presentation, and so on. If the dislocation occurs on the field, the team physician should attempt an immediate reduction on the field. This usually consists of a slight abduction and internal rotation (IR) of the affected arm and can be done without excessive traction. If this is unsuccessful, the patient is brought to the locker room for performance of the scapular rotation maneuver. The patient is laid prone on the table, and the injured side is allowed to hang in a dependent position off the edge of the table. The scapula is then manipulated to open the anterior aspect of the joint, so that the congruence of the head and the glenoid is restored, allowing it to slide back into position. If this maneuver proves to be unsuccessful, the patient is transferred to a facility where an intravenous line is placed and a mild sedative and analgesic are administered. This should be performed after obtaining radiographs and with monitoring of vital signs. It is also rather easy to accomplish an intraarticular injection through the large sulcus area. A mixture of lidocaine and bupivacaine 1%, without epinephrine, is injected into the glenohumeral joint, usually without difficulty. This enables the further relief of pain during maneuvers to reduce the shoulder. The next reduction maneuver that is used is the Stimson's technique.[24] The patient is laid prone with the arm hanging off the table, and a weight of approximately 5 lb is applied to provide traction for the arm. After adequate muscle relaxation is achieved, traction is applied to the arm in a straight anterior direction, with compression of the humeral head. If this maneuver fails, the patient is placed supine and the arm is forward elevated. The arm is gently elevated in forward flexion to the upright position, traction is applied in elevation and some abduction, while pressing outward on the humeral head. If the reduction is difficult and if the patient is being evaluated for the first time, it is important to note whether this is indeed an acute dislocation and not a chronic one. If it is a chronic dislocation, further attempts at reduction should be avoided. In general, a mild reduction maneuver should be attempted in dislocations that are less than 3 weeks old. If the dislocation is of longer duration, an open reduction is performed. A final method of attempting to reduce an acutely dislocated shoulder is the Kocher maneuver. The Kocher maneuver uses the double sheet method, where the patient is laid supine. One sheet is placed around the patient's chest and held by an assistant or tied to the table legs, while a second sheet is tied around the physician's waist. This second sheet is also encircled around the patient's forearm, with the elbow flexed at 90 degrees. Traction is then applied by leaning backward in a skiing fashion. Traction is applied in slight abduction while the arm is externally rotated, abducted, then internally rotated. The physician must be fully aware of the fact that undue force may result in damage to the brachial plexus, axillary artery, and soft tissues around the shoulder and in fractures of the proximal humerus. If this technique fails, open reduction is mandated. If reduction is successful, regardless of the technique used, postreduction films are obtained for confirmation of the reduction. These must include an axillary view. On follow-up, special testing should include a sulcus sign test performed at a neutral position and with the shoulder abducted to 90 degrees (Figure 29-4), load and shift test at neutral, apprehension test at 90 degrees of abduction, and the relocation test in order to assess static stability once healing has occurred 6 to 8 weeks posttrauma.

MANAGEMENT

Bankart noted that healing of the capsule to the anterior glenoid did not take place spontaneously, therefore leading to recurrent instability.[25] Nonoperative management has included immobilization of the shoulder in a sling, usually in the internally rotated position. Results of nonoperative treatment, especially in the young athlete with an acute traumatic anterior dislocation, have been uniformly poor.[26,27] In a prospective study, Arciero and colleagues observed that there was an 80% recurrent instability in a nonoperative group, compared with only 14% recurrence in an arthroscopically stabilized group.[28] Recent studies have examined a new method of immobilization after traumatic anterior dislocation of the shoulder. These studies evaluated immobilizing a patient with an acute dislocation with the arm in ER.[29] Magnetic resonance imaging (MRI) suggests that ER increases the amount of coaptation compared with the coaptation achieved with traditional IR immobilization.[30] This study revealed a smaller detached area, opening angle, and length detachment with externally rotated glenohumeral joints after anterior dislocations, as compared with externally rotated shoulders. Based on these MRI observations that the capsulolabral complex reduced to the anterior glenoid rim with ER of the arm, a follow-up study examined the outcomes of externally rotated immobilizations. These same

researchers examined two groups of patients; the first group was treated with the arm in 10 degrees of ER, immobilized for 3 weeks, and the second group with the arm in IR, treated for 3 weeks. They found the recurrence rate to be 30% in the IR group and 0% in the ER group at a mean of 15.5 months follow-up.[31] Based on this research, initial management of acute anterior dislocation should begin with nonoperative treatment, with immobilization of the arm in ER for a minimum of 3 weeks or possibly longer. The length of immobilization remains controversial. Some clinicians have stated that healing takes place in 3 weeks. However, there are no animal or human studies to corroborate this presumption.

If conservative treatment fails, operative intervention should be undertaken. The gold standard for Bankart repair is the open Bankart repair, in which the labrum is anatomically repaired to the anterior glenoid rim (Figure 29-5).[32-34] This is usually accompanied by a shifting of the capsule to restore normal capsular tension. Many techniques have been described to accomplish this goal and are beyond the scope of this chapter. Recurrence rate after open Bankart repair is reported to be approximately 4%.

Arthroscopic capsular shift techniques are now gaining popularity in repair of the Bankart lesion. In the past few years there have been significant technologic advances in implants available to the surgeon for performance of these capsular shifts. Early arthroscopic fixation devices include staples and tacks, which allowed the repair of the labrum to the glenoid. However, they did not allow shifting of the capsule. With the advent of suture anchors, an accurate anatomic repair of the labrum to the glenoid can be performed, and in addition, the capsule can be shifted as in the open procedure.[35-37] Results of arthroscopic Bankart repair with the earlier devices demonstrate that the recurrence rate is fairly high, in the range of 8% to 14%. However, a recent study by Kim and colleagues evaluated the use of suture anchors in the repair of Bankart lesion arthroscopically. At a mean follow-up of 44 months, their recurrence rate was 4%. This rate is comparable to that of the open technique. They found that recurrence was related to an osseous defect

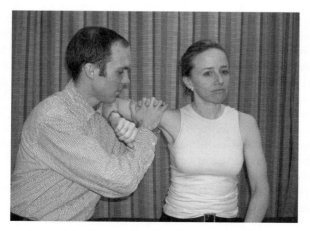

Figure 29-4: Sulcus test at 90 degrees of abduction.

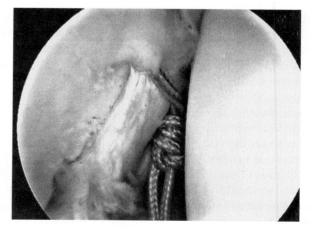

Figure 29-5: Open Bankart repair "gold standard."

greater than 30% of the entire glenoid circumference.[38,39] Therefore, as surgeons become more proficient with arthroscopic techniques and as implants continue to improve, arthroscopic stabilization of the shoulder, specifically for traumatic anterior capsule labral separations, may become the gold standard.

REHABILITATION AND POSTOPERATIVE MANAGEMENT

Phase I: Early Protective Postoperative Phase

Postoperatively the shoulder is placed in a sling without a swathe for 3 to 4 weeks. The position of the arm is in IR slightly anterior to the frontal plane. Because the early arthroscopic fixation strength may be weak, the early rehabilitation program is more conservative than other open stabilization procedures.[40-43] The main focus of the early protective postoperative period (0 to 5 weeks) is to maintain proximal and distal strength and mobility, provide pain relief, and prevent selective hypomobility of sections of the capsule resulting from iatrogenic change from the surgery. During this period elbow ROM and gripping exercises are encouraged. The authors have found that instructing patients to sleep with a pillow under the elbow to support the shoulder may take stress off the anterior joint capsule and reduce discomfort (Figure 29-6). Modalities can be useful tools in providing pain relief. The level of pain, postoperative swelling, and degree of patholaxity that was surgically addressed will determine patient progression. It is recommended that the treating clinician maintain good communication with the surgeon; this is essential to proper care. The specific procedure, concomitant injuries, and tissue quality will also affect the level of progression.

Early mobilization exercises such as pendulums are recommended for pain relief and could prevent adhesion formation.[33,44] Pendulums have been shown to produce very little muscular activity and are considered to be a safe exercise during this period.[45] These researchers even found that increasing the distraction with up to a 3 lb strap weight on the wrist has no greater influence on muscle activation

(Figure 29-7).[45] At this time the mobility of the sternoclavicular joint, acromioclavicular joint, and scapulothoracic joint is addressed, and these joints are mobilized if indicated. Once the milestone of mobility of proximal joints is obtained, manual scapular stabilization is initiated. In the side-lying position, manual resistance can be given to the scapula to resist elevation, depression, protraction, and retraction. Our experience has found that pain can be a limiting factor for starting scapular stabilization and rotator cuff isometrics. However, submaximal pain-free alternating isometrics for IR and ER may begin as early as 7 days after surgery (Figure 29-8). Because there is no splitting or taking down of the shoulder muscles, therapeutic exercise can progress to early stage submaximal rhythmic stabilization exercises in the second half of this early postoperative phase.

Early strengthening of the serratus anterior muscle is encouraged if slightly below 90 degrees of shoulder flexion is maintained and the patient remains pain free. Subsequent atrophy of the serratus anterior muscle, as a result of

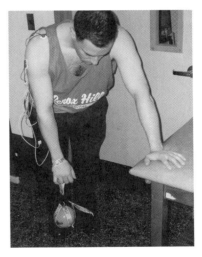

Figure 29-7: Weighted pendulum exercise.

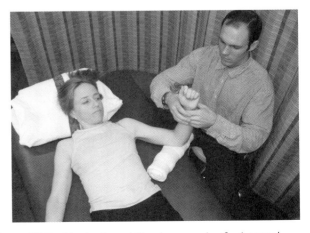

Figure 29-8: Rhythmic stabilization exercise for internal rotation and external rotation below 45 degrees of abduction.

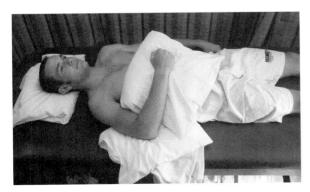

Figure 29-6: Postoperative sleeping position with supported arm.

immobilization, may allow the scapula to rest in a downwardly rotated position, causing inferior border prominence. Decker and colleagues used electromyography (EMG) to determine which exercises consistently elicited the greatest maximum voluntary contraction (MVC) of the serratus anterior.[46] It was revealed that the serratus anterior punch, scaption, dynamic hug (Figure 29-9), knee push-up plus, and push-up plus exercises consistently elicited over 20% of MVC. Most important, it was determined that the push-up plus and the dynamic hug exercises maintained the greatest MVC as well as maintained the scapula in an upwardly rotated position. Although it would be too early in the rehabilitation process to perform these late exercises, Decker and co-workers highlighted the serratus anterior punch as a valuable exercise (Figure 29-10). Performed in a controlled, supervised setting, this is an excellent choice to initiate early serratus anterior neuromuscular reeducation. Progressing to the more challenging serratus anterior strengthening exercises would be considered during the intermediate and

strengthening postoperative phases of the rehabilitation (Figure 29-11).

There is a delicate balance between pushing patients too hard and progressing them as planned. Too often patients may feel better, then worse during this early protective phase, so the laws of tissue healing must be respected. Goals to achieve for progression to the next rehabilitation period are to educate the patient regarding the surgical procedure and expectations during rehabilitation, to provide pain relief so the patient is able to tolerate submaximal isometrics of the rotator cuff muscles at 0 degrees of abduction, and to attain symmetric mobility of the sternoclavicular, acromioclavicular, and scapulothoracic joints and the ability to protract, retract, elevate, and depress the scapula against submaximal manual resistance.

Phase II: Intermediate Postoperative Phase

The fifth through eighth weeks—usually involving two to three visits per week—should focus on the return of scapular stability and glenohumeral ROM. Later in this period, rotator cuff isotonic strengthening is initiated. During this period the patient removes the sling, and active assistive ROM (AAROM) exercises are initiated. These exercises may include the use of a pulley or cane to assist in forward elevation in the plane of the scapula and IR in the scapular plane. Initially, ER stretching is performed in the guarded neutral position with the arm at the side, then progressed into the scapular plane. While progressing through rehabilitation, always consider the patient's morphology, understanding if he or she is hypermobile by nature. Patients with excessive joint laxity or generalized joint hypermobility must be progressed under a watchful eye. Excessively stretching these patients early during their postoperative care may jeopardize the end result. In contrast, not progressing a patient with hypomobility can result in an extreme loss of ROM and limit function.

Stretching and mobilization of the posterior capsule should be emphasized because tightness of the posterior

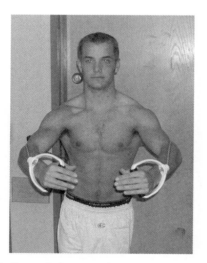

Figure 29-9: Dynamic hug exercise.

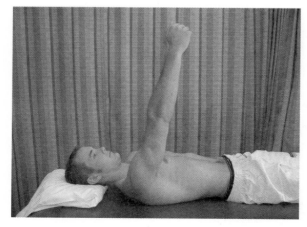

Figure 29-10: Serratus anterior punches below 90 degrees of flexion.

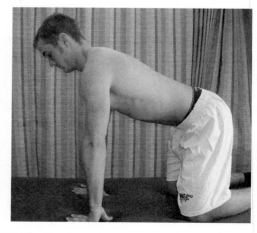

Figure 29-11: Quadruped serratus anterior punches.

shoulder structures has been linked to a loss of IR range of motion.[47] Loss of mobility can potentially limit rehabilitation progress; a tight posterior capsule is thought to cause antero-superior migration of the humeral head with forward elevation of the shoulder, possibly contributing to impingement.[48] An effective method of stretching this area is to stabilize the patient's scapula at the inferior angle manually while the patient provides a cross-chest adduction force in the supine position. Further stretch may be felt by having the patient add slight pressure into IR by pressing inferiorly on the dorsal aspect of the hand or wrist (Figure 29-12). Another effective method of stretching the posterior structures of the shoulder is to have the patient lie on the side with the scapula stabilized, while the arm is horizontally adducted (Figure 29-13). Passive ROM (PROM) of ER and abduction should be limited to 65 and 70 degrees, respectively, so as to not put stress on the healing capsule. Initial ROM goals are to achieve within 10 degrees of full IR and 150 to 165 degrees of passive flexion in the plane of the scapula. Gentle joint mobilizations can help normalize joint arthrokinematics.[49] The goal is to maintain available mobility and prevent excessive scarring. Similar to the practice of Ellenbecker and Mattalino during this time frame, isotonic strengthening exercises are initiated for abduction, scaption, and IR and ER in the scapular plane.[50] In addition, rhythmic stabilization can be performed at this time in the available ROM (Figure 29-14). In order for normal scapulohumeral rhythm to be achieved, dynamic scapular stability of this joint requires restoration. Many authors have examined the EMG activity during scapular strengthening exercises, but when choosing the appropriate exercises clinicians must keep the activity pain free and protect the surgical repair.[44,51,52] The authors often include the bilateral "scapular clock" and rhythmic stabilization of the scapula to emphasize rhomboids and middle and lower trapezius because of the ability to protect the capsule. The scapular clock exercise is a means of aiding the patient in the visualization and awareness of contracting the upper trapezius muscle by movement of the scapula to the 12 o'clock position (Figure 29-15), the

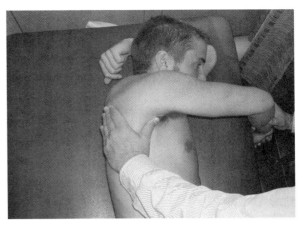

Figure 29-13: Side-lying horizontal adduction posterior shoulder stretch.

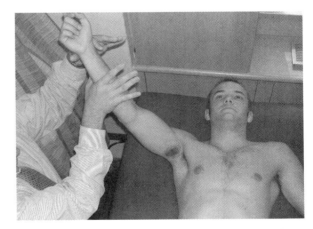

Figure 29-14: Rhythmic stabilization exercise for glenohumeral stability in the scapular plane.

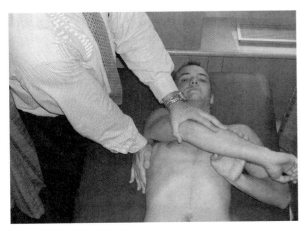

Figure 29-12: Supine posterior capsule stretch.

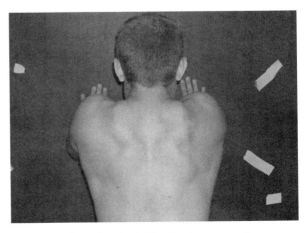

Figure 29-15: Scapular clock 12 o'clock position for upper trapezius.

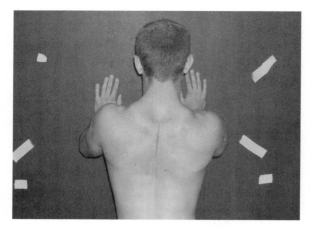

Figure 29-16: Scapular clock 9 o'clock position for rhomboids.

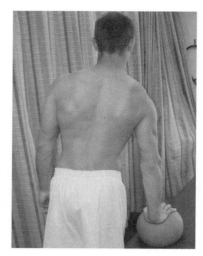

Figure 29-18: Press-up progression into ball.

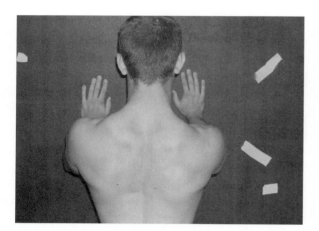

Figure 29-17: Scapular clock 6 o'clock position for middle and lower trapezius.

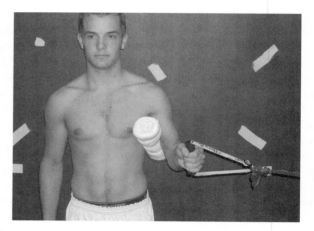

Figure 29-19: Internal rotation with Thera-Band.

rhomboids to the 9 o'clock position (Figure 29-16), and the middle and lower trapezius to between the 6 and 9 o'clock positions (Figure 29-17). Scapular exercises are encouraged in the early phases of rehabilitation to counteract scapulo-humeral dissociation and provide a stable base of support for the AROM to be performed. We also begin a "press-up" exercise progression at this stage to help facilitate the lower trapezius. The patient maintains a straight arm at neutral, with the hand on a pliable ball (we use our plyometric balls) just below waist height, then slowly and with control presses down into the ball, contracting the lower traps to stabilize the scapula (Figure 29-18). This exercise can be progressed by altering balls of various pliability, elevating the table, or performing it bilaterally to gain symmetry. Finally, in the later stages of rehabilitation, the progression can be to bilat-eral, full weight-bearing press-ups.

Strengthening exercises progress to resistance training with elastic bands for shoulder IR, ER, abduction, and extension. Maintaining the glenohumeral joint in the scapular plane (30 to 45 degrees anterior to the frontal plane) will minimize the tensile stress placed on the anterior joint capsule

(Figure 29-19).[53] We have found that giving verbal feedback to lift the chest up and pinch the shoulders back can facilitate scapular stabilization while training the external rotators (Figure 29-20). Hintermeister and colleagues found shoulder elastic resistance training to have a low load on the shoulder and therefore to be safe for postoperative patients.[54]

It is our opinion that free weights should be used with the arm in a dependent position during this period to minimize the potential for detrimental humeral head translation. Side-lying ER is typically initiated during the late portion of this phase. Proper technique, weight, and ROM are important to execute this exercise safely. Stabilizing the humerus to the thorax and not allowing the elbow to drift past the frontal plane of the body will place minimal winding on the anterior capsule. At this phase, minimal weight should be used within the comfortable ROM to prevent ill-advised stress to the healing capsule. It may also be recommended that the patient wait until the end of the intermediate postoperative period

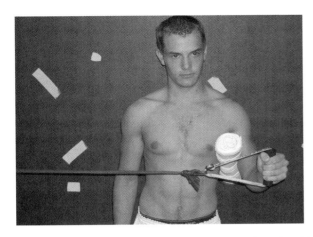

Figure 29-20: External rotation with Thera-Band, maintaining scapular retraction.

to initiate jogging or running for this same reason: the humeral head may be forcibly thrust anteriorly. It is imperative that the therapist maintain supervision of the ROM progression during this period to protect the healing tissue. Clinical milestones required for progression to the next rehabilitation phase include achievement of 150 degrees of flexion in the scapular plane, 65 degrees of ER in the scapular plane, near full IR in the scapular plane, and 110 degrees of abduction; symmetric posterior shoulder flexibility; improved isotonic internal and external strength in available ROM.

Phase III: Strengthening Postoperative Phase

During weeks 8 through 14, rehabilitation continues to work toward full glenohumeral ROM and dynamic stability of the humeral head in the glenoid fossa. Gaining or maintaining full AROM within 10 degrees of flexion in the sagittal plane and ER are to be achieved later during this time phase. At this time regaining ER, abduction, and flexion does not seem to be a limiting factor for recovery. Once the patient has achieved the milestone of 70 to 80 degrees of ER in the plane of the scapula, we begin to acquire ER ROM at 90 degrees of abduction. Although in the past it has been expected that the patient will have full AROM 8 weeks after Bankart repair, for most patients this is an unattainable expectation. In our experience, ER and IR ROM measured in the supine position with the glenohumeral joint abducted 90 degrees typically does not achieve full ROM until 10 to 12 weeks or longer, depending on the patient. This is in agreement with the findings of Ellenbecker and Mattalino, who demonstrated a lack of full return of ROM in 20 patients 12 weeks after Bankart repair and the use of thermal shrinkage. Specifically, forward flexion ROM was returned fully in 50% of the patients. Full abduction ROM was present in 30%, full ER in 20%, and full IR in 25%.[50] In a study of patients with isolated surgically repaired Bankart lesions, Kim and colleagues revealed that these patients had a mean loss of only

2 degrees of ER at 44 months after surgery.[38] In our opinion, the key to a successful rehabilitation of these patients at this phase is finding the balance point between stretching ER and letting the patients naturally regain their range. It has been our experience that the throwing athlete who has symmetric glenohumeral joint accessory motion and ER to at least 90 degrees of ER with total ROM within 20 degrees of the uninvolved upper extremity will achieve ROM with plyometrics and functional activity.

An arm upper body ergometer (UBE) that uses light resistance can be beneficial at this time to facilitate ROM and initiate active muscular control of the shoulder. The axis of rotation of the UBE should remain below the level of the shoulder joint so forward flexion is not forced above 80 degrees. We also stress the retro component of performing the UBE. We hypothesize that by performing retro UBE the patient will be mobilizing the scapula and encouraging proper posture. To avoid stress to the anterior joint capsule the patient should be positioned at a distance from the axis of rotation that does not allow the elbow to move posterior to the frontal plane when performing ergometric revolutions. We do not initiate this exercise earlier because the amount of stress placed on the capsuloligamentous structures during the use of a UBE is unknown. Later in the rehabilitation the UBE can be used as an endurance training tool for the upper extremity.

When designing the strengthening program it is important to match the patient's needs with his or her limitations and goals. A properly designed strengthening program is going to address the patient's needs by attempting to get the most benefit out of each individual exercise. Previous studies have documented which shoulder exercises activate particular muscles and should be considered as the clinician prescribes a program.[51,52,55-58] We have combined many of these programs to address generalized to specific weaknesses. From these studies we have developed the "prone program plus" to address scapular stability and generalized weakness. The prone program plus can be started in this stage of the rehabilitation if the exercises are pain free. The prone program plus includes prone horizontal abduction with glenohumeral IR (thumb down) (Figure 29-21), prone horizontal abduction with glenohumeral ER (thumb up) (Figure 29-22), prone rows, prone shoulder flexion in the scapular plane (Figure 29-23), prone 90/90 glenohumeral ER, push-ups with a plus (initiate exercise in quadruped), and ball press-downs. The prone program has not been put to the test of scientific research, but we believe it targets some of the forgotten scapular muscles during the rehabilitation process. Conversely, Moncrief and colleagues[59] studied a group of exercises that they believed targeted the shoulder rotators. These researchers report that when healthy individuals performed a program of prone ER in 90 degrees of abduction and 90 degrees of flexion, empty can, ER in the side-lying position, horizontal abduction, and prone extension for 20 repetitions over the course of 4 consecutive weeks, there was an increase in isokinetic peak torque and total work of the shoulder internal and external

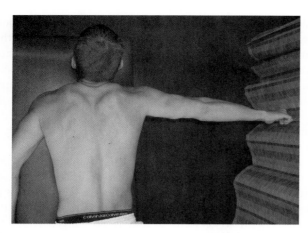

Figure 29-21: Prone program; horizontal abduction with internal rotation.

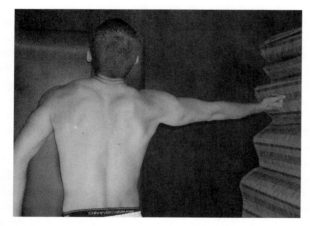

Figure 29-22: Prone program; horizontal abduction with external rotation.

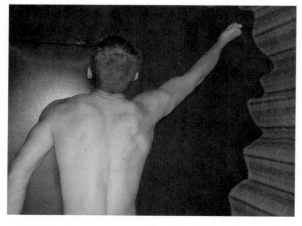

Figure 29-23: Prone program; shoulder flexion in scapular plane with external rotation.

rotators by 8% to 10%. This program may be appropriate for the patient with a Bankart repair and rotator cuff weakness.[59] Patients can easily get into poor habits of performing these exercises with improper form. It is recommended that clinicians educate their patients about these exercises, allowing ample time for them to develop proper form, before prescribing them as part of a home program.

Recent studies have suggested that mechanoreceptors located within the joint capsule may play an integral part in maintaining joint stability.[60] Therefore disruption to an intact glenohumeral joint capsule will compromise the proprioceptive capacity. Lephart and colleagues found that subjects with recurrent instability had both impaired position sense and movement detection when compared with a control group.[61,62] They tested patients with anterior shoulder instability 1 week preoperatively and 6 and 12 months postoperatively for both position sense and detection of motion.[63] By 6 months position sense was significantly different between arms but had improved by 50%, whereas detection of motion was not significantly different. At 1 year, both position sense and detection of motion were equivalent to those in the uninvolved arm. These studies highlight the importance of training proprioception. Although we begin position sense training during the early phase of rehabilitation, we continuously progress with proprioception training throughout the rehabilitation. At this phase, blinded joint position reproduction training plays an integral part in regaining kinesthetic awareness. Furthermore, proprioceptive neuromuscular facilitation (PNF) training will aid in regaining these lost aspects of joint proprioception.

PNF can be described as movements that combine rotation and diagonal components and closely resemble the movement patterns required for sport and work activities. PNF acts to enhance the proprioceptive input and neuromuscular responses while stressing motor relearning in the postoperative phases of rehabilitation. PNF patterns are initiated with the scapula because scapular stability is essential for total function of the shoulder. Scapular patterns are generally performed in the side-lying position with the head and neck in neutral alignment and can be performed in phase I (Figure 29-24). The coupled patterns of anterior elevation and posterior depression and anterior depression and posterior elevation are used, respectively. Trunk rotation should eventually be combined with scapular and extremity PNF patterns to maximize combined muscular movement patterns. Techniques such as hold-relax, slow reversals, and contract-relax are employed specifically to improve motion, whereas rhythmic stabilization, repeated contractions, and combination isotonics are used to enhance concentric and eccentric muscle action. Specifically, the D2 flexion pattern combines flexion, abduction, and ER, emphasizing the posterior rotator cuff and posterior deltoid. These neuromuscular control exercises strive to reestablish scapular positioning and stability of the humeral head in the glenoid.[64]

As the patient progresses through the program, periodic reevaluation of the scapular dyskinesis is highly

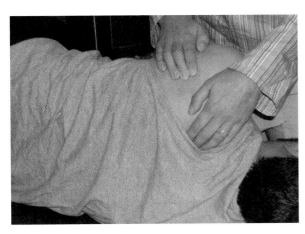

Figure 29-24: Side-lying scapular proprioceptive neuromuscular facilitation (PNF).

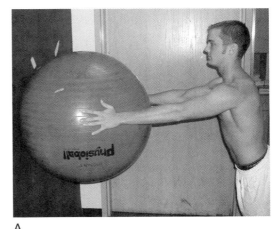

A

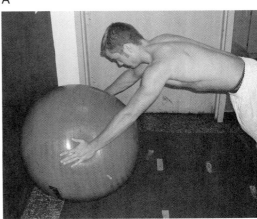

B

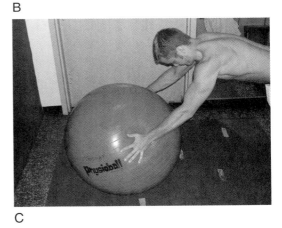

C

Figure 29-25: A, Ball push-up against wall. **B,** Ball push-up with ball wedged against wall. **C,** Ball push-up on flat ground.

recommended. We stress this, especially as the patient gains full ROM and may no longer be inhibited by tight soft tissue structures. The term *scapular dyskinesis,* although indicating that an alteration exists, is a qualitative collective term that does not differentiate among types of scapular positions or motions.[65] Therefore scapular evaluation and categorization is challenging. The most common techniques for objective quantification include visual evaluation, displacement for spine "slide test," and three-dimensional techniques. Kibler and colleagues have recently introduced a new visual technique that may help clinicians standardize categorizations.[65] This dynamic technique categorizes the dyskinesis as belonging to one of four groups. Presenting signs are as follows: type I, inferior angle prominence (horizontal plane movement); type II, medial border prominence dorsally (frontal plane movement); type III, shoulder shrug motion without winging (sagittal plane movement); type IV, bilaterally symmetric movement (normal movement). As with all scapular categorization techniques, issues regarding combined movements, learning curve, and experience exist; however, it does present clinicians with a valuable tool that with practice may enhance our communication. Unfortunately, in our practice the series of initial core scapular stability exercises does not change much based on scapular classification.

We believe that exercises directed toward facilitation of functional muscular firing patterns in both the open and closed chain may provide useful input for return to function after Bankart repair. Lear and Gross demonstrated scapular muscle activity increases with a wall push-up progression (Figure 29-25). However, the strain on the glenohumeral joint capsule is unknown and may be too great for patients after Bankart repair.[66] This exercise should be gradually built up to and advanced with caution. We conclude that clinicians should hold this exercise until the advanced strengthening postoperative phase to protect the healing tissue.

Isotonic exercises emphasizing light resistance and increased repetitions are used for isolated and combined movement patterns of the shoulder. We use a progression from three sets of 10 to two sets of 15 and on to one set of 30 repetitions. If the patient can perform one set of 30 repetitions with good form and no substitution, we progress the patient 1 to 2 lb and back down to three sets of 10 and repeat the cycle. Our rationale is based on lending objectivity to the progression and the tonic nature of the rotator cuff muscles and the scapular stabilizers. Isolated exercises are used to enhance or increase the strength of a particular muscle. Combining isotonic exercises in functional movement

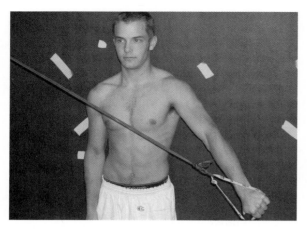

Figure 29-26: D1 extension with resistance.

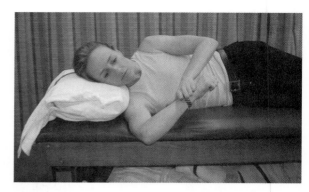

Figure 29-27: Sleeper stretch for gaining internal rotation.

patterns is performed with PNF patterns using elastic resistance or the cable column to enhance coordinated movement. In the case of a swimmer, the D1 pattern with elastic resistance may lead to a carryover to his athletic function (Figure 29-26). Initiation of isokinetic strengthening at this phase may enhance the shoulders' ability to strengthen in a pain-free ROM. It is encouraged that slower speeds are used when strengthening patients with shoulder instability. Isokinetic principles suggest that faster isokinetic speeds create greater translational forces, whereas slower speeds create stronger compressive forces, which would stabilize the shoulder. Milestones that should be met in order to move to the next rehabilitation period include achievement of within 10 degrees of full AROM in flexion, abduction, and IR and ER in the plane of the scapula; normalized scapulothoracic motion and strength; moderate overhead activities without pain; and isometric internal and external strength at least 50% of that on the uninjured side (can be tested with a hand-held dynamometer or isokinetically).

Phase IV: Advanced Strengthening Phase

Approximately 14 weeks after surgery the patient is in the final phase of rehabilitation. Full AROM should be attained by this time. The only restriction on ROM is that ER should not be stretched beyond 90 degrees. It may be preferable to allow the athlete to regain additional degrees of ER over time rather than stress the capsule, potentially stretching the repair. Posterior shoulder stretching is appropriate if full IR has not been achieved yet. Performing the side-lying "sleeper stretch" encourages ROM for IR (Figure 29-27). At the onset of this phase a thorough strength assessment is needed to evaluate the direction of strengthening needed for that particular patient. This assessment may include manual muscle testing, hand-held dynamometry, and/or isokinetic strengthening. Assessment should include the primary shoulder movers, shoulder rotators, and scapular stabilizers. Results of this assessment should be addressed with a well-rounded

strengthening program to include isotonic, concentric, and eccentric loading exercises. When designing these programs consider the everyday demands of each individual. For an overhead-throwing athlete, consider endurance training the posterior cuff eccentrically. If the patient is a manual laborer, consider a functionally challenging isotonic program. Once this phase of rehabilitation is reached, treatment should begin to streamline toward the functional demands of the patient.

Initiation of a properly designed plyometric training program is often the missing link to discharging a high-level patient. Plyometric training for the upper extremity is used to generate rapid and powerful muscular contractions in response to a dynamic stretch-inducing load to a muscle or group of muscles. It is suggested that plyometrics train the entire neuromuscular system, using the principles of stored elastic energy to apply strength as quickly and forcefully as possible. The myotatic stretch reflex develops stored elastic potential. If the exercise movement is slow, such as in weight lifting, the energy is dissipated and nonproductive. However, with rapid movement, this stored elastic energy can be used to generate a force greater than that of the concentric contraction of the muscle alone. Plyometrics employ the principles of progressive loading with the ultimate goal of power development. Using a trampoline will increase the EMG activity and elevate the level of eccentric loading of the shoulder rotators.[67] Therefore a progression from two-handed, side-to-side throws to overhead, then to one-handed overhead throws for throwers is encouraged to maximize the power development of the overhead athlete (Figure 29-28). A well-rounded program will address both the internal and external rotators of the shoulder, together with the core muscles of the trunk. Externally challenging the patient, by permitting stability from a naturally unstable surface, such as a ball, will challenge the entire kinetic chain. Advanced exercises like the Physioball "walk-outs," exemplify this concept (Figure 29-29). As the patient walks out from the ball on his or her hands, core stabilizers as well as glenohumeral stabilizers are challenged. Using the concepts of perturbation training in a closed kinetic chain position for the upper extremities will not only challenge the

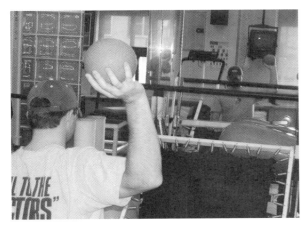

Figure 29-28: Internal rotation plyometric with rebounder.

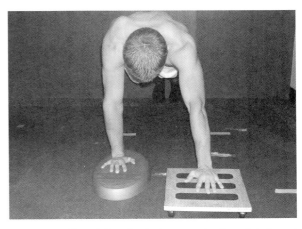

Figure 29-30: Closed kinetic chain perturbation slide board.

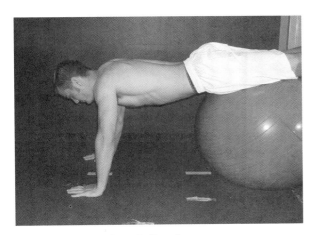

Figure 29-29: Prone Physioball walk-outs.

glenohumeral stability of the advanced patient but will incorporate a full body core workout (Figure 29-30). Milestones to achieve for progression to the final stage of rehabilitation include full pain-free ROM; <20% strength deficits for IR and ER at 90 degrees; and 20% strength deficits throughout. At this point a data-based interval throwing program can begin.

Phase V: Return to Activity Phase

This is the stage of rehabilitation at which very few therapists have the opportunity to discharge their patients. Often patients lose focus, exhaust insurance coverage, or simply disregard the importance of fine-tuning their shoulders before fully returning to their lifestyles. This stage is designed to prepare patients to return, without hesitation, to full participation in all activities. Milestones to mark successful completion of this stage include full pain-free

ROM, isokinetic or hand-held dynamometry showing <10% deficit in all positions, and a normalized closed kinetic chain.[68]

This phase continues to work in functional positions, including the plyometric program, and isokinetic strengthening at 90 degrees of abduction, and a gradual return to sport is permitted once the patient is pain-free and has nearly full ROM in all planes, confidence in the shoulder, and 85% to 90% of the strength of the opposite side on isokinetic testing at 90, 180, and 300 degrees/second for the motions of IR and ER. Confidence is achieved by the ability to achieve pain-free functional movement in that patient's sport. Our experience has demonstrated that the throwing athlete requires 1 to 2 months more to allow the shoulder to accommodate the motion. We are currently using the American Shoulder and Elbow Surgeons' Shoulder Evaluation Form to standardize the documentation of pain, motion, strength, stability, and function. However, we have yet to gather enough data to determine a criterion score for return to sport.

SUMMARY

Considerations must be given if additional procedures are performed for reattachment of labrum, ligaments, or the biceps tendon. However, strong fixation techniques have allowed the rehabilitation to progress more rapidly with these procedures than with the Bankart repair. These guidelines are a continuum of rehabilitation phases based on the effect the surgery has on the tissue and the surrounding structures. Scientific rationale is applied whenever possible, but as surgical procedures evolve, so must the rehabilitation. However, these guidelines are by no means set in stone, nor is every exercise distinct to that phase (Box 29-1). The goals and exercises need to be modified based on the performer, pathology, and performance demands. No exercise prescription should be viewed as protocol, but as a guideline on which to base the rehabilitation.

BOX 29-1

Rehabilitation Guidelines for Bankart Repair

Phase I: Early Protective Phase (0-5 Weeks)

Goals

Protect surgical procedure

Educate patient regarding procedure and therapeutic progression

Regulate pain and control inflammation

Initiate range of motion (ROM) exercises and dynamic stabilization

Perform neuromuscular reeducation of external rotators and scapulothoracic (ST) muscles

Treatment Plan (0-3 Weeks)

Sling immobilization for 2-4 weeks

Gripping exercises

Elbow, wrist, and hand ROM

Pendulum exercises (weighted and unweighted)

Passive ROM (PROM) to active assisted ROM (AAROM)

Internal rotation (IR) and external rotation (ER) proprioception training (controlled range)

Initiate gentle alternating isometrics for IR and ER in 0 degrees of abduction to scapular plane

Initiate passive forward flexion to 90 degrees

Initiate scapular mobility

Treatment Plan (3-5 Weeks)

ROM progression

Forward flexion to 110-130 degrees

ER in scapular plane to 35 degrees (position set at time of surgery)

IR in scapular plane to 60 degrees

Progress submaximal alternating isometrics for IR and ER in scapular plane

Initiate scapular strengthening

Manual scapular retraction

Resisted band retraction

No shoulder extension past trunk

Deltoid isometrics in all directions

Biceps and triceps strengthening

Initiate light band work for IR and ER

Milestones for Progression

Forward flexion to 110 degrees

Abduction to 110 degrees

ER in scapular plane to 35 degrees

IR in scapular plane to 60 degrees

Tolerance of submaximal isometrics

Knowledge of home care and contraindications

Normalized mobility of related joints (acromioclavicular, sternoclavicular, ST)

Phase II: Intermediate Phase (5-8 Weeks)

Goals (General)

Normalize arthrokinematics

Achieve gains in neuromuscular control

Normalize posterior shoulder flexibility

Treatment Plan

ROM progression

Forward flexion to 150-165 degrees

ER in scapular plane to 65 degrees

Full IR in scapular plane

Initiate joint mobilizations as necessary

Initiate posterior capsular stretching

Progress strengthening

IR and ER band in scapular plane

Side-lying ER

Full can (no weight if substitution patterns)

Clockwise/counterclockwise ball against wall

Initiate proprioceptive neuromuscular facilitation (PNF) patterns in available range

Body blade at neutral or rhythmic stabilization

Milestones for Progression

Forward flexion to 150-165 degrees

ER in scapular plane to 65 degrees

Full IR in scapular plane

Symmetric posterior capsule mobility

Progressing isotonic strength with IR and ER in available range

BOX 29-1
Rehabilitation Guidelines for Bankart Repair—cont'd

Phase III: Strengthening Phase (8-14 Weeks)

Goals (General)

Normalize ROM

Progress strength

Normalize scapulothoracic motion and strength

Perform overhead activities without pain

Treatment Plan

ROM progression; initiate stretching IR and ER at 90 degrees of glenohumeral (GH) abduction

Achieve movement within 10 degrees of full AROM in all plans

Progression of scapular retractors and stabilizers

Prone program; lower traps, middle traps, rhomboids

LT; scapular depression

Progress strengthening

Challenging rhythmic stabilization

Upper body ergometer (UBE): forward and retro

Bilateral ball against wall; progress with perturbation

Initiate isokinetic IR and ER in scapular plane

Initiate IR and ER at 90 degrees of GH abduction

Isotonic strengthening; flexion, abduction

Closed kinetic chain (CKC) therapeutic exercise

Milestones for Progression

Within 10 degrees of full AROM in scapular plane

IR and ER <50% deficit

<30% strength deficits; primary shoulder muscles and scapular stabilizers

Phase IV: Advanced Strengthening Phase (14-24 Weeks)

Goals (General)

Achieve pain-free full ROM

Improve muscular endurance

Improve dynamic stability

Treatment Plan

Maintain flexibility

Progress strengthening

Advanced CKC therapeutic exercise

Wall push-ups; with and without ball

Continue with overhead strengthening

Continue with isokinetic IR and ER strengthening at 90 degrees of GH abduction

Advance isotonic strengthening

Advance rhythmic stabilization training in various ranges and positions

Initiate plyometric strengthening

Chest passes

Trunk twists

Overhead passes

90/90 single-arm plyometrics

Milestones for Progression

Strength deficits <20% for IR and ER at 90 degrees of GH abduction

<20% strength deficits throughout

Phase V: Return to Activity Phase (4-6 Months)

Goals (General)

Pain-free full ROM

Normalized strength

Return to sport or activity program

Treatment Plan

Continue isokinetic training

Continue with stability training

Advance plyometric training

Continue with CKC therapeutic exercise

Milestones for Activity

Strength deficits <10% throughout

Normalized CKC testing

Completion of return to sport or activity program

References

1. Weiss KS, Savoie FH III: Recent advances in arthroscopic repair of traumatic anterior glenohumeral instability, *Clin Orthop* 400:117-122, 2002.

2. Sciaroni LN, McMahon PJ, Cheung TG, Lee TQ: Open surgical repair restores joint forces that resist glenohumeral dislocation, *Clin Orthop* 400:58-64, 2002.

3. Cooper ME, Hutchinson MR: The microscopic pathoanatomy of acute anterior shoulder dislocations in a simian model, *Arthroscopy* 18:618-623, 2002.

4. Bigliani LU, Pollock RG, Soslowsky LJ, et al: Tensile properties of the inferior glenohumeral ligament, *J Orthop Res* 10:187-197, 1992.

5. O'Brien SJ, Neves MC, Arnowsky SP, et al: The anatomy and histology of the inferior glenohumeral ligament complex of the shoulder, *Am J Sports Med* 18:449-456, 1990.

6. Speer KP, Deng X, Borrero S, et al: Biomechanical evaluation of a simulated Bankart Lesion, *J Bone Joint Surg Am* 76:1819-1826, 1994.

7. Bankart AS, Cantab MC: Habitual dislocation of the shoulder-joint, 1923, *Clin Orthop* 291:3-6, 1993.

8. Ide J, Maeda S, Takagi K: Normal variations of the glenohumeral ligament complex: an anatomic study for arthroscopic Bankart repair, *Arthroscopy* 20:164-168, 2004.

9. Prodromos CC, Ferry JA, Schiller AL, Zarins B: Histological studies of the glenoid labrum from fetal life to old age, *J Bone Joint Surg* 72:1344-1348, 1990.

10. Kaltsas DS: Comparative study of the properties of the shoulder joint capsule with those of other joint capsules, *Clin Orthop* 173:187-197, 1983.

11. Schwartz R, O'Brien S, Warren RF: Capsular restraints to the anterior-posterior translation of the shoulder. A biomechanical study, *Orthop Trans* 18:409-417, 1987.

12. Urayama M, Itoi E, Hatakeyama Y, et al: Function of the three portions of the inferior glenohumeral ligament: a cadaveric study, *J Shoulder Elbow Surg* 10:589-594, 2001.

13. Steinbeck J, Liljenqvist U, Jerosch J: The anatomy of the glenohumeral ligamentous complex and its contribution to anterior shoulder stability, *J Shoulder Elbow Surg* 7:122-126, 1998.

14. Black KP, Lim TH, McGrady LM, Raasch W: In vitro evaluation of shoulder external rotation after a Bankart reconstruction, *Am J Sports Med* 25:449-453, 1997.

15. Turkel SJ, Panio MW, Marshall JL: Stabilizing mechanisms preventing anterior dislocation of the glenohumeral joint, *J Bone Joint Surg* 63A:1208-1217, 1981.

16. Payne LZ, Altchek DW: The surgical treatment of anterior shoulder instability, *Clin Sports Med* 14:863-883, 1995.

17. Cash JD: Recent advances and perspectives on arthroscopic stabilization of the shoulder, *Clin Sports Med* 10:871-886, 1991.

18. Frank C, Schachar N, Dittrich D: Natural history of healing of the repaired medial collateral, *J Orthop Res* 1:179-188, 1983.

19. Peacock EE: *Wound repair*, ed 3, Philadelphia, 1984, Saunders.

20. Woo SL, Matthews JV, Akeson WH, et al: Connective tissue response to immobility: correlative study of biomechanical measurements of normal and immobilized rabbit knees, *Arthritis Rheum* 18:257-264, 1975.

21. Frank C, Woo SL-Y, Amiei D, et al: Medial collateral ligament healing: a multidisciplinary assessment in rabbits, *Am J Sports Med* 11:379-389, 1983.

22. Burgess B, Sennett BJ: Traumatic shoulder instability. Nonsurgical management versus surgical intervention, *Orthop Nurs* 22:345-350, 2003.

23. Rozing PM, de Bakker HM, Obermann WR: Radiographic views in recurrent anterior shoulder dislocation. Comparison of six methods for identification of typical lesions, *Acta Orthop Scand* 57:328-330, 1986.

24. Stimson LA: An easy method of reducing dislocations of the shoulder and hip, *Med Rec* 57:356-357, 1900.

25. Bankart AS, Cantab MC: Recurrent or habitual dislocation of the shoulder-joint, 1923, *Clin Orthop* 291:3-6, 1993.

26. Rokito AS, Namkoong S, Zuckerman JD, Gallagher MA: Open surgical treatment of anterior glenohumeral instability: an historical perspective and review of the literature. Part I, *Am J Orthop* 27:723-725, 1998.

27. Rokito AS, Namkoong S, Zuckerman JD, Gallagher MA: Open surgical treatment of anterior glenohumeral instability: an historical perspective and review of the literature. Part II, *Am J Orthop* 27:784-790, 1998.

28. Arciero RA, Wheeler JH, Ryan JB, McBride JT: Arthroscopic Bankart repair versus nonoperative treatment for acute, initial anterior shoulder dislocations, *Am J Sports Med* 22:589-594, 1994.

29. Itoi E, Hatakeyama Y, Urayama M, et al: Position of immobilization after dislocation of the shoulder: a cadaveric study, *J Bone Joint Surg Am* 81:385-390, 1999.

30. Itoi E, Sashi R, Minagawa H, et al: Position of immobilization after dislocation of the glenohumeral joint. A study with use of magnetic resonance imaging, *J Bone Joint Surg Am* 83-A:661-667, 2001.

31. Itoi E, Hatakeyama Y, Kido T, et al: A new method of immobilization after traumatic anterior dislocation of the shoulder: a preliminary study, *J Shoulder Elbow Surg* 12:413-415, 2003.

32. Rowe CR, Patel D, Southmayd WW: The Bankart procedure: a long-term end-result study, *J Bone Joint Surg Am* 60:1-16, 1978.

33. Gill TJ, Micheli LJ, Gebhard F, Binder C: Bankart repair for anterior instability of the shoulder. Long-term outcome, *J Bone Joint Surg Am* 79:850-857, 1997.

34. Gill TJ, Zarins B: Open repairs for the treatment of anterior shoulder instability, *Am J Sports Med* 31:142-153, 2003.

35. Tauro JC, Carter FM: Arthroscopic capsular advancement for anterior and anterior-inferior shoulder instability: a preliminary report, *Arthroscopy* 10:513-517, 1994.

36. Tauro JC: Arthroscopic inferior capsular split and advancement for anterior and inferior shoulder instability: technique and results at 2- to 5-year follow-up, *Arthroscopy* 16:451-456, 2000.

37. Marcacci M, Zaffagnini S, Petitto A, et al: Arthroscopic management of recurrent anterior dislocation of the shoulder: analysis of technical modifications on the Caspari procedure, *Arthroscopy* 12:144-149, 1996.

38. Kim SH, Ha KI, Cho YB, et al: Arthroscopic anterior stabilization of the shoulder: two to six-year follow-up, *J Bone Joint Surg Am* 85-A:1511-1518, 2003.

39. Kim SH, Ha KI, Kim SH: Bankart repair in traumatic anterior shoulder instability: open versus arthroscopic technique, *Arthroscopy* 18:755-763, 2002.

40. Benedetto KP, Glotzer W: Arthroscopic Bankart procedure by suture technique: indications, technique, and results, *Arthroscopy* 8:111-115, 1992.

41. Shea KP, O'Keefe RM Jr, Fulkerson JP: Comparison of initial pull-out strength of arthroscopic suture and staple Bankart repair techniques, *Arthroscopy* 8:179-182, 1992.

42. Hecker AT, Shea M, Hayhurst JO, et al: Pull-out strength of suture anchors for rotator cuff and Bankart lesion repairs, *Am J Sports Med* 21:874-879, 1993.

43. McEleney ET, Donovan MJ, Shea KP, Nowak MD: Initial failure strength of open and arthroscopic Bankart repairs, *Arthroscopy* 11:426-431, 1995.

44. McCann P, Wootten M, Kadaba M, Bigliani L: A kinematic and electromyographic study of shoulder rehabilitation exercises, *Clin Orthop* 288:179-187, 1993.

45. Ellsworth AA, Mullaney MJ, Nicholas SJ, et al: Electromyography of selected shoulder musculature during unweighted and weighted pendulum exercises, *J Orthop Sports Phys Ther* 34:A57, 2004.

46. Decker MJ, Hintermeister RA, Faber KJ, Hawkins RJ: Serratus anterior muscle activity during selected rehabilitation exercises, *Am J Sports Med* 27:784-791, 1999.

47. Tyler TF, Roy T, Nicholas SJ, Gleim GW: Reliability and validity of a new method of measuring posterior shoulder tightness, *J Orthop Sports Phys Ther* 29:262-274, 1999.

48. Harryman D, Sidles J, Clark J, et al: Translation of the humeral head on the glenoid with passive glenohumeral motion, *J Bone Joint Surg* 72A:1334-1343, 1990.

49. Conroy DE, Hayes KW: The effect of joint mobilization as a component of comprehensive treatment for primary shoulder impingement syndrome, *J Orthop Sports Phys Ther* 28:3-14, 1999.

50. Ellenbecker TS, Mattalino AJ: Glenohumeral joint range of motion and rotator cuff strength following arthroscopic anterior stabilization with thermal capsulorrhaphy, *J Orthop Sports Phys Ther* 29:160-167, 1999.

51. Moseley JB, Jobe FW, Pink M, et al: ECG analysis of scapular muscles during a shoulder rehabilitation program, *Am J Sports Med* 20:128-134, 1994.

52. McMahon PJ, Jobe FW, Pink MM, et al: Comparative electromyographic analysis of shoulder muscles during planar motions: anterior glenohumeral instability versus normal, *J Shoulder Elbow Surg* 2:118-123, 1996.

53. Johnston TB: The movements of the shoulder-joint: a plea for the use of the 'plane of the scapula' as the plane of reference for movements occurring at the humero-scapular joint, *Brit J Surg* 25:252-260, 1937.

54. Hintermeister RA, Lange GW, Schultheis JM, et al: Electromyographic activity and applied load during shoulder rehabilitation exercises using elastic resistance, *Am J Sports Med* 26:210-232, 1998.

55. Ballantyne B, O'Hare S, Paschall J, et al: Electromyographic activity of selected shoulder muscles in commonly used therapeutic exercises, *Phys Ther* 73:668-682, 1993.

56. Townsend H, Jobe FW, Pink M, Perry J: Electromyographic analysis of the glenohumeral muscles during a baseball rehabilitation program, *Am J Sports Med* 19:264-272, 1991.

57. Takeda Y, Kashiwaguchi S, Endo K, et al: The most effective exercise for strengthening the supraspinatus muscle: evaluation by magnetic resonance imaging, *Am J Sports Med* 30:374-381, 2002.

58. Decker MJ, Tokish JM, Ellis HB, et al: Subscapularis muscle activity during selected rehabilitation exercises, *Am J Sports Med* 31:126-134, 2003.

59. Moncrief SA, Lau JD, Gale JR, Scott SA: Effect of rotator cuff exercise on humeral rotation torque in healthy individuals, *J Strength Cond Res* 16:262-270, 2002.

60. Jerosch J, Steinbeck J, Schroder M, et al: Intraoperative EMG response of the musculature after stimulation of the glenohumeral joint capsule, *Acta Orthop Belg* 63:8-14, 1997.

61. Lephart SM, Pincivero DM, Giraldo JL, Fu FH: The role of proprioception in the management and rehabilitation of athletic injuries, *Am J Sports Med* 25:130-137, 1997.

62. Myers JB, Ju Y-Y, Hwang J-H, et al: Reflexive muscle activation alterations in shoulders with anterior glenohumeral instability, *Am J Sports Med* 32:1013-1021, 2004.

63. Zuckerman JD, Gallagher MA, Cuomo F, Rokito A: The effect of instability and subsequent anterior shoulder repair on proprioceptive ability, *J Shoulder Elbow Surg* 12:105-109, 2003.

64. Kibler WB: Shoulder rehabilitation: principles and practice, *Med Sci Sports Exerc* 4S:40-50, 1998.

65. Kibler WB, Uhl TL, Maddux JWQ, et al: Qualitative clinical evaluation of scapular dysfunction: a reliability study, *J Shoulder Elbow Surg* 11:550-556, 2002.

66. Lear LJ, Gross MT: An electromyographical analysis of the scapular stabilizing synergists during a push-up progression, *J Orthop Sports Phys Ther* 28:146-156, 1998.

67. Cordasco FA, Wolfe IN, Wootten ME, Bigliani LU: An electromyographic analysis of the shoulder during a medicine ball rehabilitation program, *Am J Sports Med* 24:386-392, 1994.

68. Ellenbecker TS, Davies GJ, editors: *Closed kinetic chain exercise: a comprehensive guide to multiple-joint exercise*, Champaign, IL, 2001, Human Kinetics.

CHAPTER 30

Rehabilitation after Thermal-Assisted Capsular Shrinkage of the Glenohumeral Joint

Michael M. Reinold, DPT, PT, ATC, CSCS
Kevin E. Wilk, DPT, PT
Leonard C. Macrina, MSPT, CSCS
Jeffrey R. Dugas, MD
James R. Andrews, MD

INSTABILITY OF THE GLENOHUMERAL

joint is a common pathology observed by clinicians in the orthopedic and sports medicine setting. Shoulder instability encompasses a wide spectrum of conditions ranging from subtle subluxations to gross instability. Some individuals appear to have congenitally increased elasticity of the glenohumeral joint capsule and often have instability in more than one direction (i.e., multidirectional instability). In contrast, overhead athletes tend to exhibit acquired laxity of the shoulder joint capsule caused by the repetitive stresses and excessive motions necessary to perform their overhead sport, which may be superimposed on a small degree of congenital laxity. This acquired laxity can often lead to a variety of symptoms, such as internal impingement, labral lesions, rotator cuff lesions, and instability.[1-5]

Traditional open procedures to correct acquired laxity in the overhead athlete have often resulted in unfavorable failure rates caused by overconstraint (tightness) of the glenohumeral joint capsule.[6-9] Also, the postoperative consequential loss of motion does not allow the athlete's shoulder to generate the rotational torque required to throw at a high level. Recent technologic advances have led to the development of a procedure to arthroscopically apply thermal energy to the joint capsule, selectively shrinking the capsular tissue. Thus the glenohumeral joint capsule may be shrunk in one isolated region, such as the anterior band of the anterior-inferior glenohumeral joint capsule, or the entire capsule. Despite the dramatic increase of knowledge regarding thermal modification of soft tissues over the past several years, no unanimity of opinion regarding the usefulness or appropriateness of this technique exists.[10-18] Furthermore, there appears to be controversy in the postoperative management of these patients.[10,17,18] The purpose of this chapter is to discuss the current knowledge of the treatment of joint instability using thermal-assisted capsular shrinkage (TACS), as well as the postoperative rehabilitation.

BASIC SCIENCE

The use of thermal energy as a surgical procedure dates as far back as the time of Hippocrates.[19] In the early part of the nineteenth century, Cushing and Bovie[20] began using heat as a means of coagulation and removal of tumors in neurosurgery. More recently, Fanton[11] began using thermal energy to arthroscopically shrink collagen fibers through the use of an electrical thermal heat probe (Figure 30-1). These advancements have led to the development of thermal-assisted shrinkage of the soft tissues in unstable shoulders.

Collagen fibers provide the building blocks within the soft tissues of the glenohumeral joint capsule. The collagen molecules are composed of three polypeptide chains arranged in a triple helix orientation. This triple helix is stabilized by heat-sensitive intramolecular cross-links. The collagen molecules themselves are arranged in parallel bundles to form fibrils, which are connected by heat-stable intermolecular cross-links. The application of thermal energy causes a break-

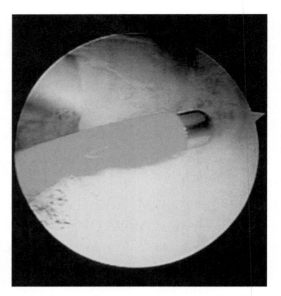

Figure 30-1: The monopolar radiofrequency thermal heat probe. *(From Oretac Interventions, Inc., Menlo Park, CA.)*

age of the intramolecular cross-links. This unwinding of the triple helix causes a transition from a highly organized crystalline structure to a random, gel-like substance.[21,22] Generalized tissue shrinkage occurs as a result of the breakdown of intramolecular bonds while the intermolecular bonds remain stable.

Naseef and colleagues[23] reported maximal shrinkage of bovine tissue to 50% of preoperative length to occur at temperatures of 65 °C or above when exposed to thermal energy for at least 1 minute. Application at lesser temperatures did not result in tissue shrinkage, and exposure at temperatures greater than 80 °C resulted in tissue necrosis. The results of this study and others have established that the effects of thermal energy on collagen tissue tend to vary based on numerous factors. These factors include temperature of application, duration of application, age of the patient, the mechanical stress placed on the tissue at the time of shrinkage, the anatomic location of the tissue, and the type of heat probe used.[11,23-25]

In response to exposure of thermal energy, the affected tissues undergo an inflammatory response, which is soon followed by a period of active tissue repair.[13,21,25-27] By 4 to 6 weeks following exposure, new collagen molecules and small fibrils are present.[13,21,25-27] Hecht and colleagues[21] documented a significant decrease in tissue stiffness for 6 weeks following TACS in the bovine model. At 2 weeks, tissue stiffness was reduced by 65% and at 6 weeks by 20%. Tissue stiffness returned to the preoperative level by 12 weeks after surgery. Similarly, Hecht and colleagues[27] reported a 48% decrease in tissue stiffness immediately following exposure to thermal energy and 26% decrease at 2 weeks postoperatively. This was followed by a gradual improvement of the tissue's mechanical properties by 6 weeks postoperatively and full return of tissue stiffness by 12 weeks. During this time it

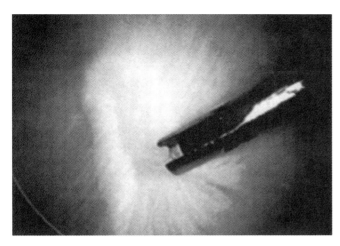

Figure 30-2: Application of thermal energy using the laser energy device.

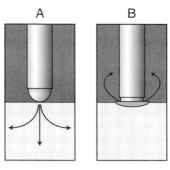

Figure 30-3: Application of thermal energy using the **A,** monopolar and **B,** bipolar radiofrequency devices. Notice the increased depth of tissue penetration by the monopolar device.

appears the collagen tissue is susceptible to "stretch out," or creep due to the decrease in stiffness. Wallace and colleagues[28] demonstrated this creep of the tissues in 3 weeks following shrinkage in rabbit specimens. Schaefer et al[29] noted a 19% decrease in rabbit tendon stiffness at 8 weeks following thermal application. Furthermore, Schaefer et al[29] reported that the resting length of rabbit patellar tendons was 7% longer at 8 weeks postsurgery, compared with their original length before laser energy shrinkage. Thus the rehabilitation specialist should carefully consider this period of decreased tissue stiffness when developing a postoperative rehabilitation program and treating the patient who has undergone TACS.

METHODS OF THERMAL APPLICATION

Currently, thermal energy is applied using both laser energy and radiofrequency energy. Laser energy is delivered in a uniform beam of light that emits radiant heat energy. This energy is transferred to the tissues to produce the desired shrinkage effect (Figure 30-2). Radiofrequency energy involves rapidly oscillating electromagnetic fields within the tissues to cause movement of electrically charged particles. The motion of these particles produces heat. Radiofrequency energy may be applied through either monopolar or bipolar devices. Monopolar devices generate electromagnetic fields by conducting an alternating current between a probe, the tissue, and a grounding plate. Bipolar devices generate electromagnetic fields by directing energy between two points at the end of the probe. The depth of penetration of the monopolar device has been observed to be between 1.0 and 5.0 mm,[11] whereas bipolar technology penetrated between 0.35 and 1.0 mm (Figure 30-3).[21]

Osmond and colleagues[16] compared the effects of laser and monopolar radiofrequency energy in an in vitro bovine model. Results indicated that both methods of application can achieve similar and predictable tissue modification dependent on the temperature settings. Regardless of the type of energy (laser or radiofrequency) or probe (monopolar or bipolar) that is used, the same effects are produced on the treated tissues. The effects on tissue appear to be heat related and not method-of-delivery related. Some clinicians have reported that it is easier to control and maintain a constant temperature using the radiofrequency method versus the laser.[15,18,30]

CLINICAL APPLICATION

The ability of thermal energy to be applied arthroscopically to tighten the capsule appears advantageous for the overhead athlete with acquired shoulder laxity. The potential disadvantages of increased pain, increased scar tissue formation, loss of motion, increased risk of infection, extended hospitalization, and longer recovery times may be minimized. Opening the anterior capsule to perform a capsular shift or tightening procedure may result in significant stiffness and difficulty regaining range of motion (ROM). In addition, using an arthroscopic approach eliminates the need to detach the subscapularis muscle, which acts to eccentrically control external rotation during the throwing motion.[31] With detachment of the subscapularis muscle there is the potential for healing at an abnormal length, anterior tightness, excessive scarring, and the potential for a loss of external rotation, which is necessary to generate torque during the late cocking phase of the overhead throwing motion.

The goal of TACS of the glenohumeral joint is to decrease the volume of the joint capsule and subsequently reduce the amount of translation of the humerus on the glenoid. In most cases, the capsular tissue is shrunk from the level of the posterior band of the inferior glenohumeral ligament complex through the axillary recess and up the anterior side of the shoulder to include the middle glenohumeral ligament. This encompasses the entire inferior glenohumeral ligament complex. Depending on the amount of inferior laxity present, the surgeon may opt to apply thermal energy to the capsule at the rotator cuff interval (between the supraspinatus and subscapularis musculature) and the superior glenohumeral ligament to further stabilize the joint. Conversely, the capsule may be "selectively shrunk," that is, only a predetermined portion is shrunk. The surgical technique will vary based on the type of patient, type of laxity present, and response to the thermal procedure. Rovner and colleagues[32] demonstrated a 30% reduction in volume within the glenohumeral joint capsule in a human cadaveric model. Tibone and colleagues[33] reported, intraoperatively in human glenohumeral joints, a decrease in humeral head anterior translation from 10.9 mm to 6.4 mm and a decrease in posterior translation from 7.2 mm to 4.4 mm following laser TACS. In a subsequent study by Tibone and colleagues,[34] the authors repeated their investigation of glenohumeral translation following TACS with a monopolar radiofrequency probe. Results were similar to laser treatment; anterior translation was decreased from 9.3 mm to 5.8 mm and posterior translation was decreased from 6.8 mm to 4.0 mm. Thus early reports on TACS of the glenohumeral joint capsule appear promising.

Variations exist on the way that the thermal probe may be applied to the shoulder capsule. Currently, two common delivery patterns are the "striping" and "paintbrush" techniques. Striping the capsule has been suggested as a means to preserve as much normal tissue as possible (Figure 30-4). The thermal probe is applied in a linear fashion in multiple parallel sections, similar to a gridlike pattern, leaving an area of viable tissue between the heated tissue lines. The paintbrush method involves applying continuous thermal application in a uniform manner using a side-to-side motion, similar to a paintbrush.

Lu and colleagues[35] compared the two methods of thermal application. Immediately following surgery both techniques were compared. The results indicated similar rates of shrinkage. At 6 weeks following surgery the tissues that received the striping technique had almost completely repaired, but the paintbrush group continued to show signs of some nonvi-

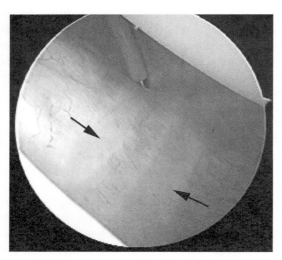

Figure 30-4: The striping method of thermal application. The *arrows* depict the area of capsular tissue modified using the thermal probe. An area of viable tissue is located between the stripes.

able areas of tissue. Furthermore, mechanical testing at 6 weeks indicated that the joint capsule in the striping technique group had better mechanical properties than the capsule in the paintbrush group. This was consistent with Hecht and colleagues,[21,27] who reported a duration of 12 weeks before the tissues recovered their mechanical properties to the preoperative values following the paintbrush method. Thus, although both techniques may initially produce similar amounts of tissue shrinkage, the striping technique may allow quicker tissue healing times and recovery of mechanical properties.[35] The rehabilitation program is similar between the two techniques; however, constant monitoring and a slower progression during the first 4 to 6 weeks postoperatively may be advocated to ensure that excessive capsular tissue elongation does not occur with the paintbrush technique. Further research is required to substantiate or refute these suggestions.

REHABILITATION FOLLOWING THERMAL-ASSISTED CAPSULAR SHRINKAGE (TACS)

Controversy exists regarding the postoperative rehabilitation following TACS, in particular, regarding care during the first 4 to 6 weeks. Some clinicians have advocated immobilization during the first 2 to 4 weeks whereas others have suggested gentle restricted motion.[10,18] Most rehabilitation programs have been based on anecdotal clinical observations and preliminary data. In this section, we begin by discussing previously published rehabilitation programs. We then provide an overview of our basic principles of rehabilitation following TACS, as well as specific programs designed for the overhead athlete. Our rehabilitation program is based on the clinical experience and outcomes observed in over 800 TACS patients treated between 1997 and 2004.[36]

Ellenbecker and Mattalino[10] provided an overview of their surgical approach and rehabilitation program for 20 patients with unidirectional shoulder instability who were treated using thermal capsulorrhaphy (capsular shrinkage). The authors note that arthroscopic Bankart repairs and capsular shifts were performed concomitantly on an undocumented number of patients at the time of surgery. Rehabilitation consisted of 2 weeks of immobilization followed by a gradual progression of ROM and strengthening exercises. ROM assessment and isokinetic strength testing were performed at approximately 12 weeks postoperatively. The results indicated that 10 patients (50%) achieved full shoulder flexion. Only four patients (20%) regained full shoulder external rotation (ER), with a mean loss of 13 degrees. Five patients (25%) were able to achieve full shoulder internal rotation (IR); average loss of IR motion was 8 degrees. Isokinetic testing indicated normal strength of the external rotators and a mean deficit of 4% for the internal rotators.

Tyler and colleagues[18] described their surgical technique and rehabilitation considerations using thermal energy. The authors recommended the shoulder be placed in a sling without a swathe for 3 to 4 weeks. Active-assisted ROM and strengthening exercises were initiated at 4 weeks and gradually progressed as tolerated. At 8 weeks and beyond, isotonic, isokinetic, and plyometric exercises were incorporated. The authors report that, based on their protocol, full ROM is not typically achieved until week 10 to 12 following surgery.

In both published papers the authors advocated a period of immobilization immediately postoperatively (2 and 4 weeks, respectively) to minimize the risk of stretching the healing tissues.[10,18] It has been our clinical experience that some patients who are immobilized for 2 to 4 weeks, especially overhead athletes, have a higher risk of developing a long-term loss of motion and capsular tightness. It is our belief that the rehabilitation program should be individualized based on the patient and type of instability. A brief period of immobilization may be necessary in some patients with congenital laxity but not indicated in patients such as overhead athletes with acquired laxity. The following section illustrates several guidelines used to determine the most appropriate treatment program following TACS.

REHABILITATION GUIDELINES FOLLOWING TACS

Our postoperative rehabilitation program is based on six key factors that determine the type and aggressiveness of the program prescribed (Box 30-1). We briefly discuss these factors as they relate to the rehabilitation program.

BOX 30-1

Six Key Factors to Consider When Designing the Rehabilitation Program following Thermal-Assisted Capsular Shrinkage

1. **Type of instability present (tissue type)**

   Congenital (positive sulcus sign) versus acquired (negative sulcus sign)

2. **Patient's inflammatory reaction and response to surgery**

   Poor healing (soft end feel) versus excessive fibroblastic activity (hard end feel)

3. **Concomitant surgical procedure**

   Adjust to healing constraint of each tissue

4. **Precautions following surgery**

   Caution against early stretching

   Tissues susceptible to elongation

5. **Gradual rate of progression**

6. **Team approach to treatment**

   Communication between physician and rehabilitation specialist

---

The first factor is the type of instability present in the athlete. The rehabilitation programs will differ depending on whether the patient has congenital or acquired laxity. Overhead athletes typically develop acquired laxity as a result of the repetitive and high stresses placed on the glenohumeral joint capsule. The overhead athlete begins restricted passive ROM exercises immediately postoperatively to prevent excessive capsular scarring. The rehabilitation program for the patient with congenital, multidirectional instability is much more conservative and does not involve early ROM to allow healing of the capsule.

Before establishing the rate of progression of the program, a thorough evaluation of the uninvolved shoulder should be conducted. Of particular interest to us is the sulcus test, which we use as a sign of generalized, or congenital, shoulder joint laxity. We consider an inferior displacement of 10 mm or more a positive test. Clinical experience indicates that people with more than 10 mm of inferior displacement usually exhibit significant hypermobility; thus inherent stability is often compromised. In these individuals, ROM exercises are progressed more cautiously than for the patient who does not exhibit significant congenital glenohumeral joint capsular laxity.

Second, the rehabilitation program must be adjusted according to the patient's unique response to surgery. It has been our clinical experience that the healing response after TACS varies greatly among patients. As previously stated, the application of thermal energy causes an inflammatory response in the involved tissues. This response triggers the proliferation of collagen ground tissue and can be present for 8 weeks postoperatively. Some patients exhibit a poor healing response with less revascularization and collagen synthesis. Other patients exhibit a heightened healing response, which requires careful monitoring to prevent excessive scar tissue formation and long-term motion restrictions. Hayashi and colleagues[13] arthroscopically evaluated patients following TACS and reported increased vascularity in some patients, even at 3 to 6 months postoperatively. Forty percent of these patients exhibited motion restriction that required surgical intervention. The rate of progression should be adjusted on a weekly basis and is modified based on the amount of motion, as well as the capsular end feel exhibited by the specific patient. The quality of end feel is assessed by applying slight overpressure into the end-range of the patient's available passive ROM, noting the sensation, or end feel, as the joint reaches the limits of ROM.[37] Thus an overhead athlete with decreased ROM and a hard end feel at 4 weeks postoperatively will have an accelerated rate of regaining motion. Conversely, a patient with excessive ROM and a soft end feel will have his or her ROM progression significantly slowed, potentially using a sling to avoid motion.

The third factor takes into consideration any concomitant procedure performed at the time of the TACS. As described earlier, 95% of the overhead athletes who have undergone TACS have additional procedures performed concomitantly. Certain precautions may exist based on the extent of the surgical intervention such as superior labral lesion (SLAP) repairs or subacromial decompressions. The rehabilitation program must be based on the healing constraints of each concomitant procedure.

The next factor to consider is the surgical precautions following TACS. We recommend that therapists be extremely cautious with stretching and ROM exercise during the first 4 to 6 weeks following thermal application. Several studies discussed earlier have reported a significant decrease in tissue stiffness at 4 to 6 weeks after surgery.[17,29,38] Thus we recommend tissue precautions for 8 to 10 weeks, with extreme caution during the first 4 to 6 weeks when the treated collagen is most susceptible to elongation or creep. This concern does not lead us to immobilize every patient but rather informs us to be prudent in our rehabilitation program regarding ROM and motions during functional activities.

The fifth factor is our preference of a gradual rate of progression throughout rehabilitation rather than speeding up and slowing down the program because of periods of immobilization. It has been our clinical experience that patients who are immobilized for 2 to 4 weeks and then rapidly progressed to restore ROM because of capsular tightness have a poorer outcome than the patient with a planned and steady program. Our program follows a gradual progression based on periodic observations of the patient's ROM and capsular end feel. The patient is assessed at least once per week to ensure a steady progression.

The last factor to ensure a successful outcome following TACS is effective communication between the orthopedic surgeon and the rehabilitation team. Information regarding the amount of tissue shrinkage at the time of surgery, intraoperative ROM, and stability are all critical to the therapist regarding the rate of rehabilitation progression. The therapist must also be aware of any concomitant surgical procedures that were performed.

Rehabilitation following TACS in the Overhead Athlete

Our basic rehabilitation program for TACS performed in overhead athletes consists of four phases (Box 30-2). This program incorporates the basic concepts of rehabilitation following TACS and applies to most TACS procedures. Certain modifications from this program based on specific concomitant surgical procedures are discussed separately. These include TACS for the congenitally unstable patient and TACS performed concomitantly with glenoid labrum procedures and subacromial decompressions. Separate programs are used for these procedures based on the specific surgical procedure and soft tissue healing constraints.

Phase I is initiated on postoperative day 1 with immediate restricted motion. This is to prevent loss of motion and any neurologic complications. The patient is instructed to use a sling during functional activities for the first 7 to 10 days and to sleep in the sling with a swathe for 2 weeks. Elbow and wrist ROM and hand gripping exercises are performed immediately following surgery. Passive and active-assisted ROM exercises for the glenohumeral joint are cautiously performed in a restricted motion. Shoulder rotation is performed in the scapular plane at 30 to 45 degrees of abduction. ER is allowed to neutral and IR to 25 to 30 degrees for the first 5 to 7 days. Cryotherapy is used before and after rehabilitation for the first 7 to 10 days. After 10 days, moist heat is used before and ice after exercise.

ROM is progressed by the end of week 2 to allow 90 degrees of flexion, 25 degrees of ER, and 45 degrees of IR in the scapular plane. The therapist performs passive ROM, and active-assisted ROM is performed by the patient using a cane or bar. From week 3 to the end of week 4, ROM is gradually progressed to allow shoulder flexion to 125 degrees, ER in the scapular plane to 45 degrees, and full IR. During the first 4 weeks, we do not allow excessive external rotation or elevation, and we do not allow shoulder extension. This is to avoid applying excessive stress to the anterior and anterior-inferior portions of the joint capsule.

Our program is based on the theory that immediate motion assists in collagen synthesis, organization, alignment, and enhancement of tensile strength.[39,40] The rehabilitation program should allow for progressive applied loads to stimulate the collagen tissue. However, we are extremely cautious with ROM for the first 4 to 6 weeks although actual time frames vary depending on the patient's progression. We evaluate the patient on a weekly basis to reassess the rate of progression. The patient's ROM and capsular end feel are used to rate our progression. The program must be continuously adjusted based on the patient's response to surgery and rehabilitation.

Patients are instructed on submaximal and subpainful isometric contractions on postoperative day 1 to stimulate muscle training. The movements allowed are ER, IR, abduction, flexion, and extension in mid-ROM with the arm to the side. In addition, starting 1 week after surgery, the therapist performs rhythmic stabilization drills to enhance dynamic stabilization, improve proprioception, and produce rotator cuff co-contractions (Figure 30-5).[18,41-43] Depending on the patient's response, we begin light ER/IR isotonic strengthening exercises using exercise tubing at 7 to 10 days postoperatively. Shoulder rotation strengthening is performed at 0 degrees of abduction. We often have the athlete place a towel between the arm and the body. This has been shown to increase electromyographic activity of the posterior rotator cuff musculature.[44] Scapular strengthening exercises are usually initiated during the second week. Exercises include prone rowing, prone horizontal abduction, and prone extension and are performed in a restricted ROM. At week 4, the patient is allowed to begin active isotonic exercises with 1 lb.

At week 5, active-assisted ER and IR ROM is performed at 90 degrees of shoulder abduction. By the end of week 6, the patient should exhibit 75 degrees of external rotation, 60 to 65 degrees of internal rotation, and 160 degrees of shoulder flexion. We have found through clinical follow-up data that

BOX 30-2

Rehabilitation Program after Thermal-Assisted Capsulorrhaphy for Individuals with Acquired Laxity

I. Phase I—Protection Phase (Day 1 to Week 6)

Goals

Allow soft tissue healing

Diminish pain and inflammation

Initiate protected motion

Retard muscular atrophy

Weeks 0 to 2

- Sling use for 7 to 10 days
- Sleep in sling/brace for 14 days

Exercises:

- Hand gripping exercises
- Elbow and wrist range-of-motion (ROM) exercises
- Active ROM cervical spine
- Passive and active-assisted shoulder ROM exercises
  - Elevation to 75 to 90 degrees (flexion to 70 degrees week 1, flexion to 90 degrees week 2)
  - Internal rotation (IR) in scapular plane at 30 to 45 degrees of abduction (45 degrees by 2 weeks)
  - External rotation (ER) in scapular plane at 30 to 45 degrees of abduction (25 degrees by 2 weeks)
  - NO aggressive stretching
- Rope and pulley (shoulder flexion) active-assisted ROM
- Cryotherapy to control pain (before and after treatment)
- Submaximal isometrics (ER, IR, abduction, flexion, extension)
- Rhythmic stabilization exercises at 7 days
- Proprioception and neuromuscular control drills

Weeks 3 to 4

- Shoulder ROM exercises (passive ROM, active-assisted ROM, active ROM):
  - Elevation to 125 to 135 degrees
  - IR, in scapular plane, full motion (60 to 65 degrees)
  - ER, in scapular plane 45 degrees by week 4
  - At week 4, begin ER/IR at 90 degrees of abduction
  - ER at 90 degrees of abduction to 45 to 50 degrees
  - No extension
  - NO aggressive stretching
- Shoulder strengthening exercises:

- Active ROM program (begin at week 3)
- Initiate LIGHT isotonic program (use 1 lb at week 4)
- ER/IR exercise tubing (0 degrees of abduction)
- Continue dynamic stabilization drills
- Scapular strengthening exercises
- Biceps/triceps strengthening
- Proprioceptive neuromuscular facilitation D2 flexion/extension manual resistance (limited ROM)
- Emphasize ER strengthening and scapular musculature
- Continue use of cryotherapy and modalities to control pain

Weeks 5 to 6

- Continue all exercises listed above
- Progress ROM to the following:
  - Elevation to 160 degrees by week 6
  - ER at 90 degrees of abduction (75 to 80 degrees) by 6 weeks
  - IR at 90 degrees of abduction (60 to 65 degrees) by 6 weeks
- Initiate Thrower's Ten Program (strengthening)
- Continue emphasis on ER and scapular muscles

II. Phase II—Intermediate Phase (Weeks 7 to 12)

Goals

Restore full ROM (week 8)

Restore functional ROM (weeks 10 to 11)

Normalize arthrokinematics

Improve dynamic stability, muscular strength

Weeks 7 to 8

- Progress shoulder ROM to the following:
  - Elevation to 180 degrees
  - ER at 90 degrees of abduction to 90 to 100 degrees by week 8
  - IR at 90 degrees of abduction to 60 to 65 degrees by week 8
- Continue stretching program
  - May become more aggressive with ROM progression and stretching
  - May perform joint mobilization techniques

(continued)

BOX 30-2

Rehabilitation Program after Thermal-Assisted Capsulorrhaphy for Individuals with Acquired Laxity—cont'd

- Strengthening exercises:
  - Continue Thrower's Ten Program
  - Continue manual resistance, dynamic stabilization drills
  - Rhythmic stabilization drills
  - Initiate plyometrics (two-hand drills)

Weeks 9 to 12
- Progress shoulder ROM to the overhead athlete's demands
  - Gradual progression from weeks 9 to 12
  - Continue stretching into ER
  - ER at 90 degrees of abduction to 110 to 115 degrees by weeks 10 to 12
  - Continue stretching program for posterior structures (IR, horizontal adduction)
- Strengthening exercises:
  - Progress isotonic program
  - Continue Thrower's Ten Program
  - May initiate more aggressive strengthening
    - Push-ups
    - Bench press (do NOT allow arm below body)
    - Latissimus pull-downs (IN FRONT of body)
    - Single-hand plyometrics throwing (initiate 14 to 18 days following the introduction of two-hand plyometrics)
    - Plyoball wall drills

III. Phase III—Advanced Activity and Strengthening Phase (Weeks 12 to 20)

Goals

Improve strength, power, and endurance

Enhance neuromuscular control

Functional activities

Criteria to enter phase III:
1. Full ROM
2. No pain or tenderness
3. Muscular strength 80% of contralateral side

Weeks 12 to 16
- Continue all stretching exercises
- Self-performed capsular stretches, active ROM, passive stretching

- Continue all strengthening exercises
  - Thrower's Ten Program
  - Progress isotonics
  - Plyometrics
    - Two-hand drills progress to one-hand drills
    - Throwing into plyoback 1 lb ball (week 13)
    - Neuromuscular control/dynamic stabilization drills

Weeks 16 to 22
- Initiate interval sport program (throwing, tennis, swimming, etc.) week 16
- Progress all exercises listed above
- May resume normal training program
- Continue specific strengthening exercises
- Progress interval program (throwing program to phase II) weeks 22 to 23

Week 22
- Progress to phase II interval throwing program or sport-specific training
- Continue isotonic strengthening
- Continue flexibility and ROM
- Continue plyometrics

IV. Phase IV—Return to Activity Phase (Week 26 and Beyond)

Goals

Gradual return to unrestricted activities

Maintain static and dynamic stability of shoulder joint

Criteria to enter phase IV:
1. Full functional ROM
2. No pain or tenderness
3. Satisfactory muscular strength (isokinetic test)
4. Satisfactory clinical examination

Exercises:
- Continue maintenance for ROM (stretching)
- Continue strengthening exercises (Thrower's Ten Program)
- Gradual return to competition
  - Progress throwing program to game situations—months 6 to 7

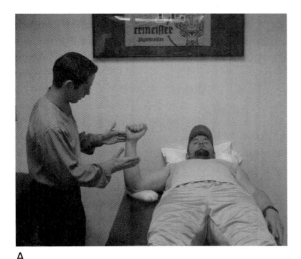

A

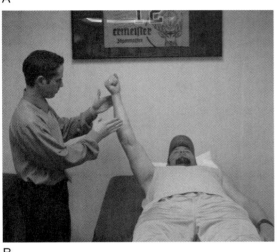

B

Figure 30-5: A, Rhythmic stabilization drills. The patient's arm is positioned in neutral rotation and in the scapular plane at 45 degrees of abduction. The patient is instructed to hold that static position. **B,** The patient's arm is positioned in approximately 100 degrees of flexion with 10 degrees of horizontal abduction.

if the overhead athlete does not fulfill these goals by the end of week 6, long-term motion complications often persist.

The athlete's strengthening program is progressed at weeks 5 to 6 to include our Thrower's Ten Program (Figure 30-6). These exercises have been selected based on our own electromyographic studies, as well as the works of numerous investigators,[41,44-49] and focus on the predominant muscles used during the overhead throwing motion. During this phase, emphasis is placed on the external rotators and the scapular muscles. Our biomechanical laboratory studies have shown high electromyographic activity of the posterior rotator cuff muscles during side-lying ER, prone rowing into ER (Figure 30-7), and standing tubing ER with a towel placed between the arm and the trunk.[44,49] Our goal is for the overhead athlete at week 8 to exhibit an ER/IR muscular ratio of 70% to 72% documented by manual muscle testing

with a handheld dynamometer or through the use of isometric testing on an isokinetic device.

Phase two is the intermediate phase and spans weeks 7 to 12. Goals of this phase include restoring full ROM, enhancing dynamic glenohumeral joint stabilization, and increasing muscular strength. Full "functional" ROM is achieved by week 8 with 180 degrees of flexion, 90 to 100 degrees of ER at 90 degrees of abduction, and 60 to 65 degrees of IR. If motion restrictions do not allow the achievement of these goals by the end of week 8, the program is progressed to include aggressive stretching techniques such as end-range mobilizations and capsular stretching.

From weeks 9 to 12, the overhead athlete is gradually progressed to gain full "thrower's" ROM. The rate of progression is adjusted according to the patient's ROM and end feel. Our program attempts to restore full flexion, IR, and approximately 110 to 115 degrees of ER in the overhead athlete by week 12 (Figure 30-8). Wilk[50] and others have documented that professional baseball pitchers exhibit 129 ± 9 degrees of ER. Thus our goal in rehabilitation is to obtain 110 to 115 degrees of ER through stretching and then allow functional exercise drills, such as plyometrics, to gain the remaining ROM. We believe this allows the athlete to regain neuromuscular control more effectively than stretching the athlete to excessive motions such as 125 to 130 degrees. During this phase, the rehabilitation specialist should continue to stretch the soft tissues of the posterior shoulder through the use of stretches such as supine horizontal adduction or side-lying adduction (Figure 30-9).[51]

We continue to use the Thrower's Ten Program with the addition of dynamic stabilization drills at this time. Drills used that facilitate dynamic stabilization of the glenohumeral joint include rhythmic stabilization with exercise tubing (Figure 30-10), rhythmic stabilization while performing push-ups on a medicine ball (Figure 30-11), and closed chain stabilization drills using a ball against a wall (Figure 30-12).[41] We strongly recommend the integration of these exercise drills.[41]

In addition to the Thrower's Ten Program and manual resistance dynamic stabilization drills, the overhead athlete's strengthening is progressed to include plyometrics and more aggressive isotonic strengthening.[41] We begin incorporating two-hand plyometric drills at weeks 7 to 8. The first plyometric drill we use is the two-hand chest pass; we then progress to two-hand side-to-side throws and side throws.[52,53] If the athlete can perform these drills asymptomatically after 1 week, we progress to two-hand overhead soccer throws. The one-hand plyometric standing baseball throw (Figure 30-13) is begun 14 to 18 days following the initiation of the two-hand drills; this is to ensure a gradual progression without the occurrence of pain or capsular irritability.

Aggressive strengthening performed during this phase includes prone push-ups, bench press, seated rowing, and front latissimus pulldowns on progressive resistance exercise equipment. Exercise equipment is used initially to ensure safe

Text continued on p. 596

The Thrower's Ten Program is designed to exercise the major muscles necessary for throwing. The Program's goal is to be an organized and concise exercise program. In addition, all exercises included are specific to the thrower and are designed to improve strength, power, and endurance of the shoulder complex musculature.

1A. **Diagonal Pattern D2 Extension:** Involved hand will grip tubing handle overhead and out to the side. Pull tubing down and across your body to the opposite side of leg. During the motion, lead with your thumb. Perform _____ sets of _____ repetitions _____ daily.

1B. **Diagonal Pattern D2 Flexion:** Gripping tubing handle in hand of involved arm, begin with arm out from side 45° and palm facing backward. After turning palm forward, proceed to flex elbow and bring arm up and over involved shoulder. Turn palm down and reverse to take arm to starting position. Exercise should be performed _____ sets of _____ repetitions _____ daily.

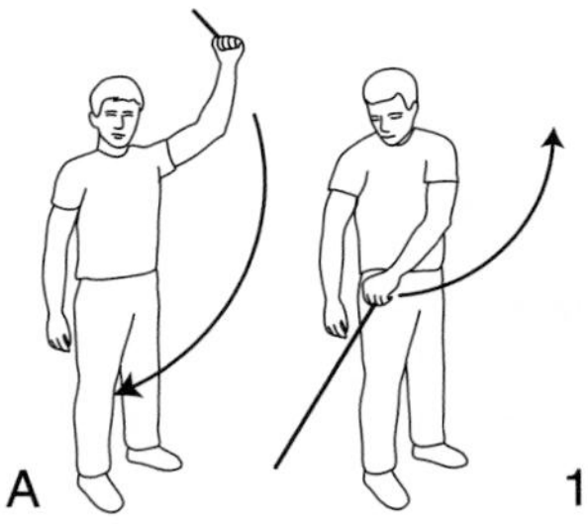

2A. **External Rotation at 0° Abduction:** Stand with involved elbow fixed at side, elbow at 90° and involved arm across front of body. Grip tubing handle while the other end of tubing is fixed. Pull out arm, keeping elbow at side. Return tubing slowly and controlled. Perform _____ sets of _____ repetitions _____ times daily.

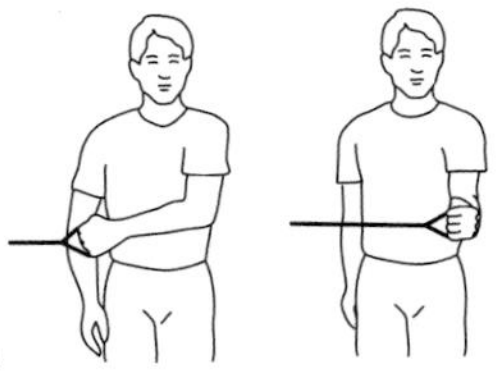

2B. **Internal Rotation at 0° Abduction:** Standing with elbow at side fixed at 90° and shoulder rotated out. Grip tubing handle while other end of tubing is fixed. Pull arm across body keeping elbow at side. Return tubing slowly and controlled. Perform _____ sets of _____ repetitions _____ times daily.

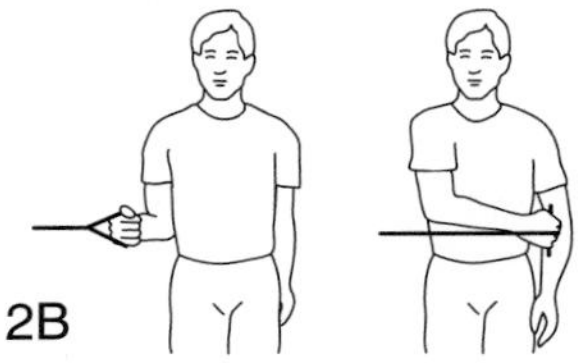

2C. (Optional) **External Rotation at 90° Abduction:** Stand with shoulder abducted 90°. Grip tubing handle while the other end is fixed straight ahead, slightly lower than the shoulder. Keeping shoulder abducted rotate shoulder back keeping elbow at 90°. Return tubing and hand to start position.
I. Slow Speed Sets: (Slow and Controlled) Perform _____ sets of _____ repetitions _____ times daily.
II. Fast Speed Sets: Perform _____ sets of _____ repetitions _____ times daily.

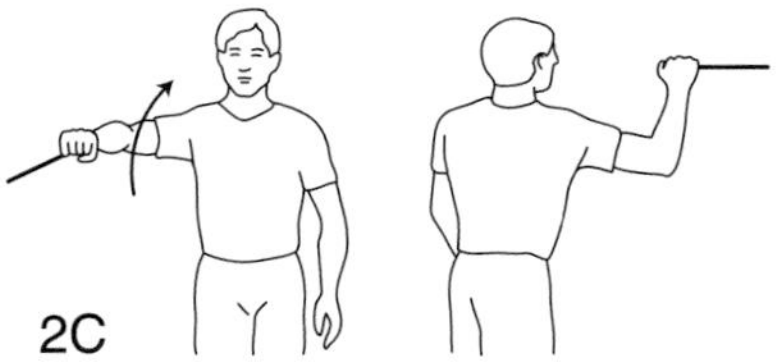

2D. (Optional) **Internal Rotation at 90° Abduction:** Stand with shoulder abducted to 90°, externally rotated 90° and elbow bent to 90°. Keeping shoulder abducted, rotate shoulder forward, keeping elbow bent at 90°. Return tubing and hand to start position.
I. Slow Speed Sets: (Slow and Controlled) Perform _____ sets of _____ repetitions _____ times daily.
II. Fast Speed Sets: Perform _____ sets of _____ repetitions _____ times daily.

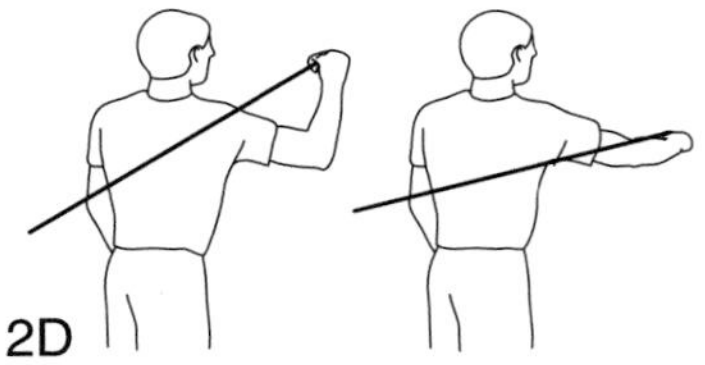

3. **Shoulder Abduction to 90°:** Stand with arm at side, elbow straight, and palm against side. Raise arm to the side, palm down, until arm reaches 90° (shoulder level). Perform _____ sets of _____ repetitions _____ times daily.

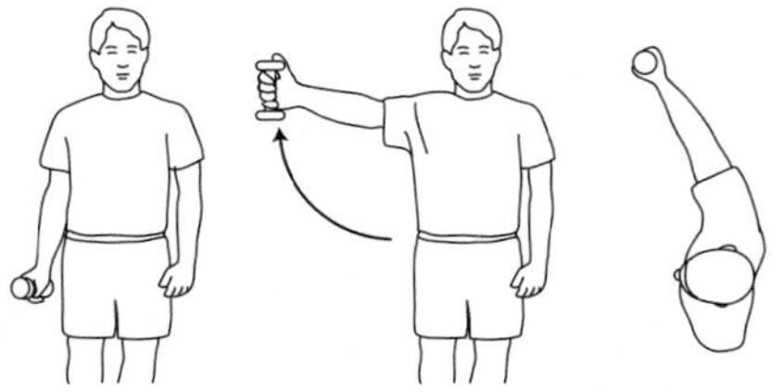

Figure 30-6: Thrower's Ten Program. *(From the Advanced Continuing Education Institute, LLC.)*

4. **Scaption, External Rotation:** Stand with elbow straight and thumb up. Raise arm to shoulder level at 30° angle in front of body. Do not go above shoulder height. Hold 2 seconds and lower slowly. Perform _____ sets of _____ repetitions _____ _____ times daily.

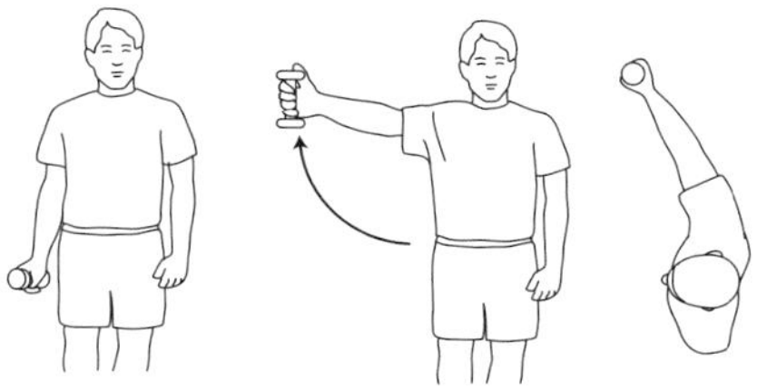

5. **Sidelying External Rotation:** Lie on uninvolved side, with involved arm at side of body and elbow bent to 90°. Keeping the elbow of involved arm fixed to side, raise arm. Hold _____ seconds and lower slowly. Perform _____ sets of _____ repetitions _____ times daily.

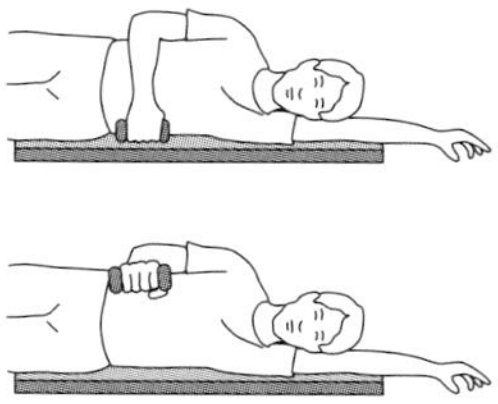

6A. **Prone Horizontal Abduction (Neutral):** Lie on table, face down, with involved arm hanging straight to the floor, and palm facing down. Raise arm out to the side, parallel to the floor. Hold 2 seconds and lower slowly. Perform _____ sets of _____ repetitions _____ times daily.

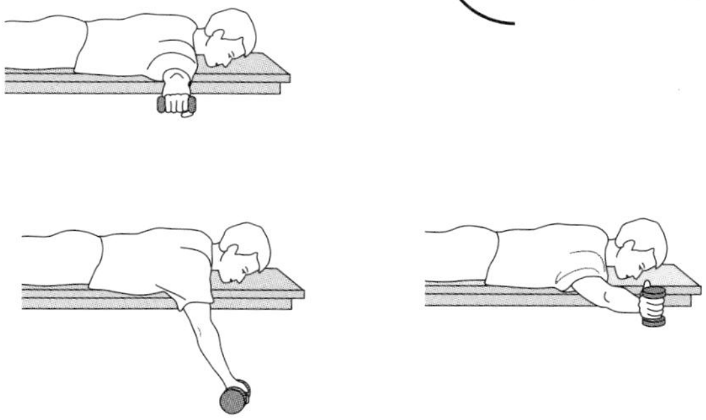

6B. **Prone Horizontal Abduction (Full ER, 100° ABD):** Lie on table face down, with involved arm hanging straight to the floor, and thumb rotated up (hitchhiker). Raise arm out to the side with arm slightly in front of shoulder, parallel to the floor. Hold 2 seconds and lower slowly. Perform _____ sets of _____ repetitions _____ times daily.

6C. **Prone Rowing:** Lying on your stomach with your involved arm handing over the side of the table, dumbbell in hand and elbow straight. Slowly raise arm, bending elbow, and bring dumbbell as high as possible. Hold at the top for 2 seconds, then slowly lower. Perform _____ sets of _____ repetitions _____ times daily.

6D. **Prone Rowing into External Rotation:** Lying on your stomach with your involved arm hanging over the side of the table, dumbbell in hand and elbow straight. Slowly raise arm, bending elbow, up to the level of the table. Pause 1 second. Then rotate shoulder upward until dumbbell is even with the table, keeping elbow at 90°. Hold at the top for 2 seconds, then slowly lower taking 2-3 seconds. Perform _____ sets of _____ repetitions _____ times daily.

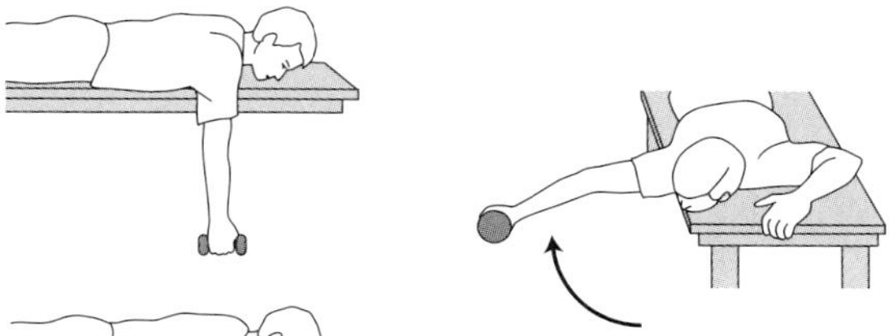

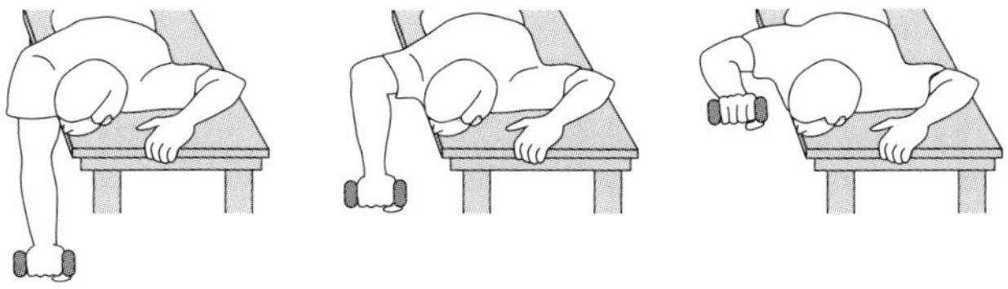

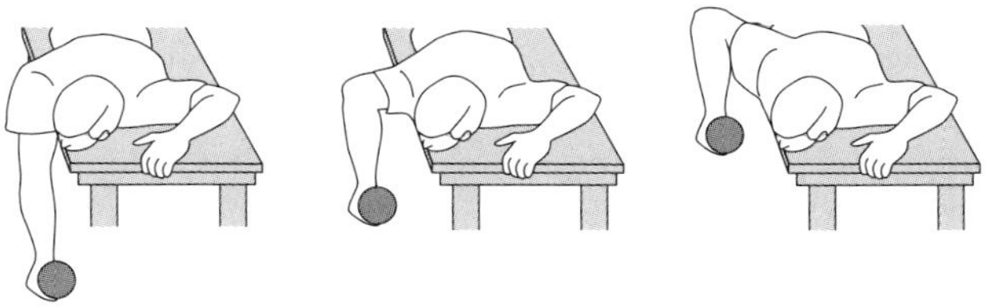

Figure 30-6: continued

7. **Press-ups:** Seated on a chair or table, place both hands firmly on the sides of the chair or table, palm down and fingers pointed outward. Hands should be placed equal with shoulders. Slowly push downward through the hands to elevate your body. Hold the elevated position for 2 seconds and lower body slowly. Perform _____ sets of _____ repetitions ___ _____ times daily.

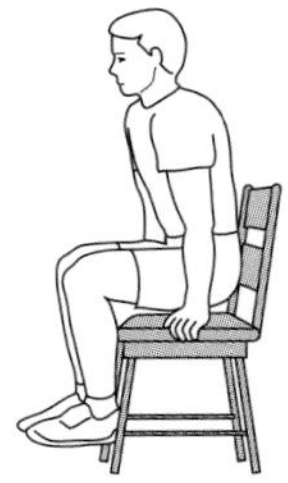

8. **Push-ups:** Start in the down position with arms in a comfortable position. Place hands no more than shoulder width apart. Push up as high as possible, rolling shoulders forward after elbows are straight. Start with a push-up into wall. Gradually progress to table top and eventually to floor as tolerable. Perform _____ sets of _____ repetitions _____ __ times daily.

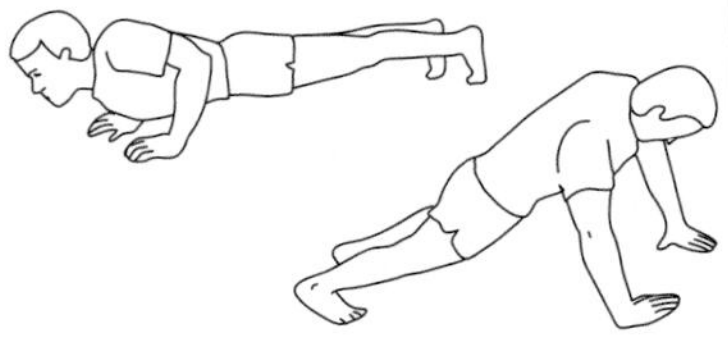

9A. **Elbow Flexion:** Standing with arm against side and palm facing inward, bend elbow upward turning palm up as you progress. Hold 2 seconds and lower slowly. Perform _____ sets of _____ repetitions _____ times daily.

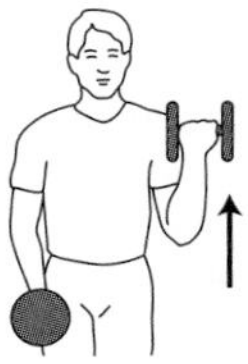

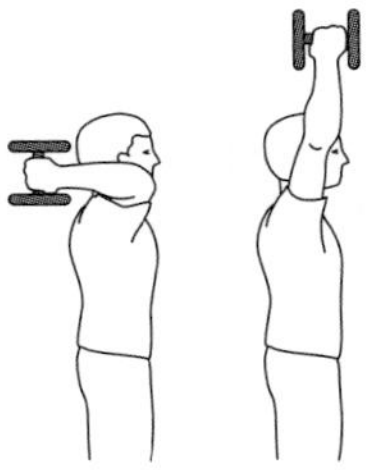

9B. **Elbow Extension (Abduction):** Raise involved arm overhead. Provide support at elbow from uninvolved hand. Straighten arm overhead. Hold 2 seconds and lower slowly. Perform _____ sets of _____ repetitions _____ times daily.

10A. **Wrist Extension:** Supporting the forearm and with palm facing downward, raise weight in hand as far as possible. Hold 2 seconds and lower slowly. Perform _____ sets of _____ repetitions _____ times daily.

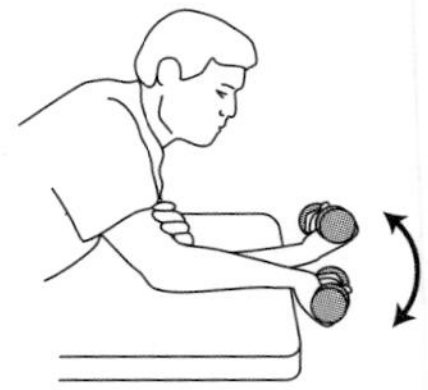

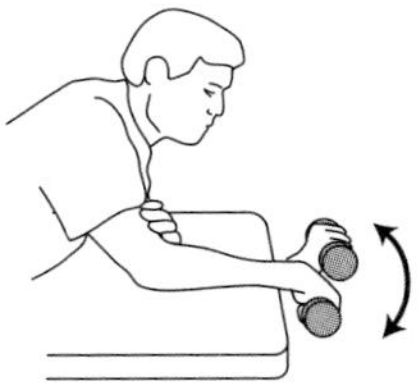

10B. **Wrist Flexion:** Supporting the forearm and with palm facing upward, lower a weight in hand as far as possible and then curl it up as high as possible. Hold for 2 seconds and lower slowly.

10C. **Supination:** Forearm supported on table with wrist in neutral position. Using a weight or hammer, roll wrist taking palm up. Hold for a 2 count and return to starting position. Perform _____ sets of _____ repetitions _____ times daily.

10D. **Pronation:** Forearm should be supported on a table with wrist in neutral position. Using a weight or hammer, roll wrist taking palm down. Hold for a 2 count and return to starting position. Perform _____ sets of _____ repetitions _____ times daily.

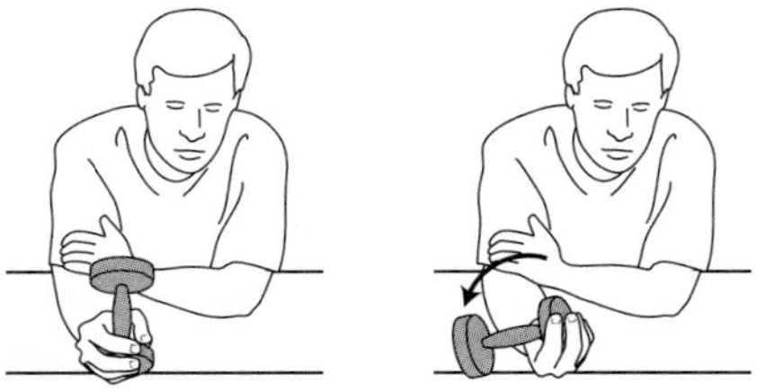

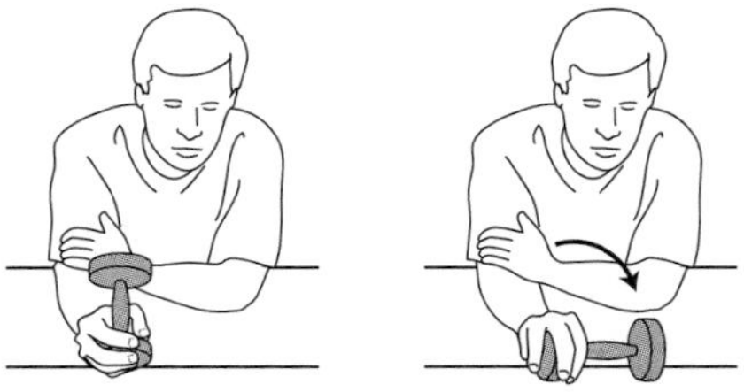

Figure 30-6: continued

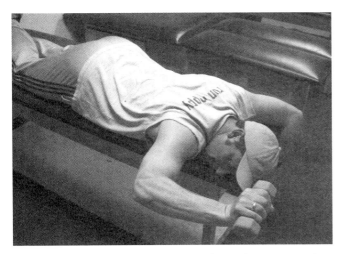

Figure 30-7: Prone rowing into external rotation to strengthen the posterior rotator cuff muscles.

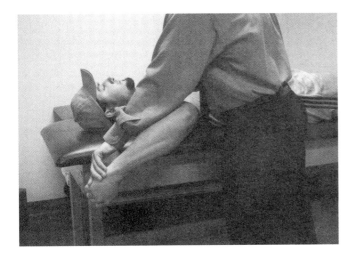

Figure 30-8: Full "thrower's" external rotation ROM.

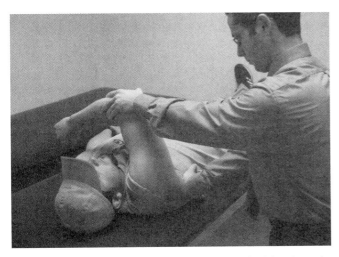

Figure 30-9: Manual stretching into horizontal adduction. The therapist stabilizes the scapula.

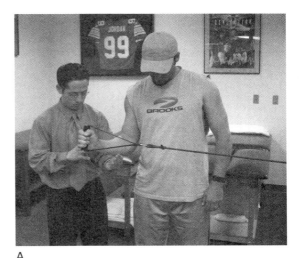

A

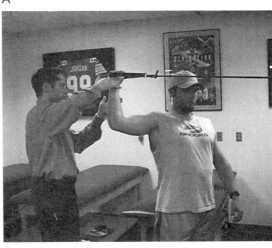

B

Figure 30-10: A, Rhythmic stabilization with exercise tubing to facilitate the dynamic stabilizers of the glenohumeral joint. **B,** The exercise can be further progressed to the 90-degrees abducted shoulder position.

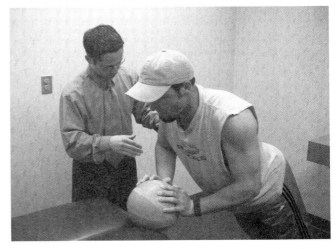

Figure 30-11: Rhythmic stabilization drills while performing a push-up on a medicine ball.

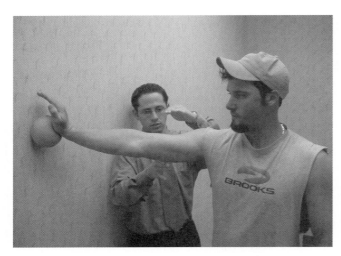

Figure 30-12: Rhythmic stabilization drill: stabilization into a ball against the wall.

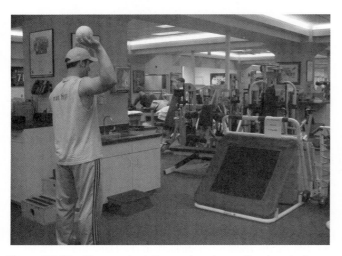

Figure 30-13: Plyometric drill: one-hand standing baseball throw.

movement in a restricted ROM. If the athlete cannot perform these drills asymptomatically, a thorough examination including ROM and strength must be performed to ensure that the program is adjusted accordingly.

Phase III, the advanced activity and strengthening phase, begins at the end of week 12 and progresses to week 20. The goals of this phase are to improve muscular strength, power, and endurance while gradually increasing functional activities. The criteria for the athlete to progress to this phase are full ROM, no pain or tenderness, and muscle strength of at least 80% of the contralateral side. This is documented by an isokinetic strength test at week 12.

We routinely perform a series of isokinetic tests for overhead athletes that we refer to as the Thrower's Series.[54] This consists of testing the strength of the shoulder rotators at 90 degrees of shoulder abduction and of the shoulder abductors/adductors at speeds of 180 and 300 degrees/second.

Normative strength values for isokinetic testing of the overhead throwing athlete have been published in several papers[55,56] and are summarized in Table 30-1. Schexneider and colleagues[57] have documented a 5% to 15% difference in the dominant versus nondominant shoulder musculature in the general population. For the overhead athlete, we suggest relying more heavily on the unilateral muscle ratios (ER/IR and abduction/adduction) and the torque–to–body weight ratios because of the increased emphasis on the dominant upper extremity.

All of the strengthening exercises are progressed during phase III. In addition, the athlete should maintain established motion, thus continuation of stretching exercises is strongly encouraged. Sport-specific drills are initiated at week 12. This includes throwing a 1 lb medicine ball into a bounce-back device for overhead throwers, swinging a light club or stick for golfers, and swinging a racket for swing mechanics in tennis players.

At week 16 we begin a formal interval sport program.[58,59] For the overhead thrower we initiate a long-toss interval throwing program.[58] The athlete throws three times per week with a day off from throwing in between. Each step is performed at least two times on separate days before we allow the athlete to progress to the next step. Throwing should be performed without pain or significant increase in symptoms. If symptoms are experienced at a particular step within the program, the athlete is instructed to regress to the prior step until symptoms subside. We believe it is important for the overhead athlete to perform stretching and an abbreviated strengthening program before and after performing the interval sport program. Typically, our overhead throwers warm up, stretch, and perform one set of their exercise program before throwing, followed by two additional sets of their exercise program after throwing. This provides an adequate warm-up but also ensures maintenance of necessary ROM and flexibility of the shoulder joint.

Usually at week 22 or 23 the patient progresses to phase II of the throwing program, throwing off a mound.[58] In phase II the number of throws, intensity, and type of pitch are progressed to gradually increase stress on the shoulder joint. Specific interval programs for tennis and golf may also be initiated at this time.[58]

The final phase, the return to activity phase, is usually initiated at approximately 26 to 29 weeks and represents a gradual return to sport participation. The criteria to enter phase IV are full ROM, no pain or tenderness, satisfactory strength as measured by isokinetic testing (see Table 30-1), and a satisfactory clinical examination. Usually at 6 to 7 months following surgery, our overhead athletes progress to game situations and begin a return to competition. We instruct the athlete to continue to maintain the desired strength and ROM through stretching and strengthening exercises. Reinold and colleagues[36] report a mean of 8.4 months to return to competition; Andrews and Levitz[1] have reported the time required for a thrower to return to competition following TACS is 9.6 months following surgery.

Rehabilitation following TACS for the Athlete with Congenital Shoulder Instability

The rehabilitation program following TACS for the patient with congenital shoulder instability is dramatically different than for the overhead athlete with acquired laxity (Box 30-3). The rate of progression is much slower, particularly regarding ROM. This is due to reported collagen deficiency,[60] inefficient dynamic stabilization, and poor proprioceptive abilities in that population.[61] Shoulder joint immobilization is usually employed immediately following surgery to allow early healing of the capsular structures; passive ROM is not initiated until approximately 2 to 4 weeks postoperatively. At this time, the patient is assessed and progressed to controlled passive ROM exercises if excessive laxity is not present. Our goal is to gradually progress ROM to about 80% of the preoperative motion by week 12 and then to allow the patient to regain the remaining motion on his or her own through functional activities.

Emphasis of the rehabilitation program is placed on reestablishing proprioception, neuromuscular control, and dynamic stabilization. The ultimate goal of the program is to restore stability and functional mobility. The key to successful rehabilitation is to individualize the program to the patient's tissue status and healing response to surgery.

Rehabilitation following TACS with Glenoid Labrum Procedures

Labral lesions frequently occur in the overhead athlete because of the tremendous amount of force produced at extreme ranges of motion. The specific rehabilitation program following TACS with concomitant surgical intervention involving the glenoid labrum varies depending on the severity of the labral pathology. As previously mentioned, labral debridements are commonly performed at the time of TACS in overhead athletes (67% of the overhead athletes).[36] The rehabilitation program does not change significantly if only a debridement of a frayed labrum is performed. Overhead throwing athletes commonly have a type II SLAP lesion. This lesion involves fraying of the glenoid-labral complex with a detachment of the biceps tendon from the glenoid rim. Most frequently a "peel-back" lesion is present. Intervention involves surgically repairing the detached tendon using suture anchors. Approximately 33% of the overhead athletes with TACS at our center also have a SLAP lesion repair performed concomitantly.

Postoperative rehabilitation is delayed in comparison to the isolated TACS procedure (Box 30-4). Rate of progression of the program is slower to allow healing of the anatomic reattachment of the biceps tendon. No isolated biceps strengthening is allowed for the first 6 to 8 weeks

Text continued on p. 602

TABLE 30-1

Isokinetic Shoulder Strength Criteria for Overhead Athletes

| VELOCITY (DEG/SEC) | BILATERAL COMPARISONS (DOMINANT ARM/NONDOMINANT ARM) | | | |
	EXTERNAL ROTATION (ER)	INTERNAL ROTATION (IR)	ABDUCTION	ADDUCTION
180	98%-105%	110%-120%	98%-105%	110%-128%
300	85%-95%	105%-115%	96%-102%	111%-129%

Unilateral Muscle Ratios

VELOCITY (DEG/SEC)	ER/IR	ABDUCTION/ADDUCTION	ER/ABDUCTION
180	66%-76%	78%-84%	67%-75%
300	61%-71%	88%-94%	60%-70%

Peak Torque-to-Body Weight Ratios

VELOCITY (DEG/SEC)	ER	IR	ABDUCTION	ADDUCTION
180	18%-23%	28%-33%	26%-33%	32%-38%
300	12%-20%	25%-30%	20%-25%	28%-34%

Data published previously in Savoie FH III, Field LD: Thermal versus suture treatment of symptomatic capsular laxity, *Clin Sports Med* 19:63-75, 2000; and Jobe FW, Giangarra CE, Kvitne RS, et al: Anterior capsulolabral reconstruction of the shoulder in athletes in overhand sports, *Am J Sports Med* 19:428-434, 1991.

BOX 30-3

Rehabilitation Program following Thermal-Assisted Capsulorrhaphy for Individuals with Atraumatic Congenital Instability

I. Phase I—Protection Phase (Weeks 0 to 8)

Goals

Allow healing of tightened capsule

Begin early protected motion of the elbow, wrist, and hand

Decrease pain/inflammation

Weeks 0 to 2

Precautions:

- Sleep in immobilizer/sling for 14 days
- No overhead activities for 12 weeks
- Avoid abduction, flexion, and external rotation (ER)

Exercises

- Gripping exercises with putty
- Elbow flexion/extension and pronation/supination
- Active range of motion (ROM) cervical spine
- After 10 days, active abduction may be allowed, but is not to exceed 70 degrees

Weeks 2 to 4

Goals

Gradual increase in range of motion (ROM)

Normalize arthrokinematics

Improve strength

Decrease pain/inflammation

ROM exercises

- Active-assisted exercises (pulley and L-bar)
- Forward flexion to 90 degrees
- Abduction to 90 degrees (plane of scapula)
- ER in scapular plane to neutral
- Internal rotation (IR) to 35 degrees
- No extension

Strengthening exercises

- Isometrics initiated in all planes to tolerance
- Progressive resistive exercises to elbow and wrist
- Scapular strengthening (isometrics)
- Rhythmic stabilization drills (neutral rotation)

Conditioning program for the following:

- Trunk
- Lower extremities
- Cardiovascular

Decrease pain/inflammation:

- Ice, nonsteroidal antiinflammatory drugs, modalities

Weeks 4 to 6

- Gradual increase to full ROM

ROM exercises:

- L-bar active-assisted exercises
- Shoulder flexion to 125 degrees by week 6
- ER scapular plane to 25 degrees by week 6
- IR scapular plane to 45 degrees by week 6

Strengthening exercises:

- Continue with exercises listed above
- Rhythmic stabilization drills into wall
- Scapular strengthening
- Therapeutic tubing initiated (week 5)
- Active ROM exercise

Gentle mobilization to reestablish normal arthrokinematics to the following:

- Scapulothoracic joint
- Glenohumeral joint
- Sternoclavicular joint

II. Phase II—Intermediate Phase (Weeks 6 to 12)

Goals

Full, nonpainful ROM at weeks 10 to 12

Normalize arthrokinematics

Increase strength

Improve neuromuscular control

Weeks 6 to 8

ROM exercises:

- L-bar active-assisted exercises
  - Flexion to 145 degrees by week 8

BOX 30-3

Rehabilitation Program following Thermal-Assisted Capsulorrhaphy for Individuals with Atraumatic Congenital Instability—cont'd

* ER scapular plane to 45 degrees by week 8
* IR scapular plane to 50 degrees by week 8
* Initiate capsular self-stretches
* Continue joint mobilization
* Gradually increase to 80% of full ROM by week 12

Strengthening exercises:
* Continue all exercises listed above
* Initiate isotonic dumbbell and tubing program
  * Side-lying ER
  * Side-lying IR
  * Shoulder abduction
  * Supraspinatus
  * Latissimus dorsi
  * Rhomboids
  * Biceps curl
  * Triceps curl
  * Shoulder shrugs
  * Push-ups (into wall or table)
* Continue neuromuscular control exercises for scapulo-thoracic joint

Weeks 8 to 12
Goals:
80% of full ROM
Continue with all exercises listed above
Continue with joint mobilization and capsular self-stretches

ROM exercises:
* Active-assisted ROM with an L-bar
* Flexion to 160 degrees at weeks 8 to 10
* ER at 90 degrees of abduction to 75 degrees at week 10
* IR at 90 degrees of abduction to 50 to 55 degrees

III. Phase III—Dynamic Strengthening Phase (Weeks 12 to 20)
Goals
Improve strength, power, endurance
Improve neuromuscular control
Prepare the athlete to begin to throw

Criteria to enter phase III:
1. Full, nonpainful ROM (80% of ROM of contralateral shoulder)
2. No pain or tenderness
3. Strength 70% or greater compared with the contralateral side

Emphasis of phase III:
* High-speed, high-energy strengthening exercises
* Eccentric exercises
* Diagonal patterns

Exercises:
* Fundamental shoulder exercises
* Continue tubing exercises for ER/IR
* Tubing for rhomboids
* Tubing for latissimus dorsi
* Tubing for biceps
* Tubing for diagonal patterns D2 extension
* Tubing for diagonal patterns D2 flexion
* Continue dumbbell exercises for supraspinatus and deltoid
* Continue serratus anterior strengthening exercises
* Continue neuromuscular exercises
* Continue capsular self-stretches
* Gradual return to recreational activities

IV. Phase IV—Return to Activity (Weeks 20 to 28)
Goal
Progressively increase activities to prepare patient for full functional return

Criteria to progress to phase IV:
* Full ROM
* No pain or tenderness
* Isokinetic test that fulfills criteria
* Satisfactory clinical examination

Exercises:
* Continue all strengthening
* Emphasize closed kinetic chain
* Initiate recreational sport (weeks 24 to 26)—physician clearance required

BOX 30-4

Rehabilitation Program following Thermal-Assisted Capsulorrhaphy with Type II Superior Labral Lesion (SLAP) Repair

I. Phase I—Immediate Postoperative Phase: "Restrictive Motion" (Day 1 to Week 6)

Goals

Protect the anatomic repair

Prevent negative effects of immobilization

Promote dynamic stability

Diminish pain and inflammation

Weeks 0 to 2

- Sling for 4 weeks
- Sleep in immobilizer for 4 weeks
- Elbow/hand range of motion (ROM)
- Hand gripping exercises
- Passive and gentle active-assisted ROM exercise
  - Week 1: flexion to 75 degrees; week 2: flexion to 90 degrees
  - Elevation in scapular plane to 75 degrees
  - External rotation (ER)/internal rotation (IR) with arm in scapular plane
  - ER to 10 to 15 degrees
  - IR to 45 degrees
  - NO excessive ER or extension or abduction
- Submaximal isometrics for shoulder musculature (all planes—shoulder in neutral, elbow bent 90 degrees)
- Initiate rhythmic stabilization drills (day 5)
- NO isolated biceps contractions
- Cryotherapy, modalities as indicated

Weeks 3 to 4

- Discontinue use of sling at 4 weeks
- Sleep in immobilizer until week 4
- Continue gentle ROM exercises (passive ROM and active-assisted ROM)
  - Flexion to 115 to 120 degrees
  - Abduction to 90 to 100 degrees
  - ER in scapular plane and 35 degrees of abduction to 35 to 45 degrees
  - IR in scapular plane and 35 degrees of abduction to 55 to 60 degrees
  - NOTE: Rate of progression based on evaluation of the patient.

- No excessive ER, extension, or elevation
- Continue rhythmic stabilization drills
- Initiate proprioception training
- Tubing ER/IR at 0 degrees of abduction (week 3)
- Continue isometrics
- Continue use of cryotherapy

Weeks 5 to 6

- Gradually improve ROM
  - Flexion to 155 to 160 degrees
  - ER at 45 degrees of abduction: 55 to 65 degrees
  - IR at 45 degrees of abduction: 55 to 60 degrees
  - At 6 weeks begin light and gradual ER at 90 degrees of abduction—progress to 75 degrees of ER
- May initiate stretching exercises
- May initiate light (easy) ROM at 90 degrees of abduction
- Continue tubing ER/IR (arm at side)
- Proprioceptive neuromuscular facilitation (PNF) manual resistance
- Initiate active shoulder abduction (without resistance)
- Initiate "full can" exercise (weight of arm)
- Initiate prone rowing, prone horizontal abduction
- Progress to Thrower's Ten Program week 6
- NO biceps strengthening

II. Phase II—Intermediate Phase (Weeks 7 to 12)

Goals

Gradually restore full ROM (week 8)

Restore functional ROM (weeks 10 to 12)

Preserve the integrity of the surgical repair

Restore muscular strength and balance

Weeks 7 to 8

- Gradually progress ROM:
  - Flexion to 180 degrees
  - ER at 90 degrees of abduction: 90 to 100 degrees
  - IR at 90 degrees of abduction: 60 to 65 degrees
- Continue to progress isotonic strengthening program
- Continue PNF strengthening
- Initiate active ROM elbow flexion week 8

BOX 30-4

Rehabilitation Program following Thermal-Assisted Capsulorrhaphy with Type II Superior Labral Lesion (SLAP) Repair—cont'd

Weeks 8 to 10
- Gradually increase ROM
  - ER at 90 degrees of abduction to 100 to 105 degrees
  - IR at 90 degrees of abduction to 60 to 65 degrees

Weeks 10 to 12
- May initiate slightly more aggressive strengthening
- May progress isotonic elbow flexion week 12
- Progress ER to thrower's motion from weeks 10 to 12
  - ER at 90 degrees of abduction: 110 to 115 in thrower's (weeks 10 to 12)
- Progress isotonic strengthening exercises
- May begin two-hand plyometrics week 12 (3 to 5 lb)
  - Chest pass
  - Side-to-side throw
  - Overhead soccer throw
- Continue all stretching exercises
- Progress ROM to functional demands (i.e., overhead athlete)
- Progress isotonic strengthening program
- Continue Thrower's Ten Program

III. Phase III—Advanced Activity and Strengthening Phase (Weeks 12 to 22)

Goals

Maintain full ROM

Improve muscular strength, power, and endurance

Gradually initiate functional activities

Enhance neuromuscular control

Progress functional activities

Criteria to enter phase III:
1. Full, nonpainful ROM
2. Satisfactory stability
3. Muscular strength (good grade or better)
4. No pain or tenderness

Weeks 12 to 16
- Continue all stretching exercises (capsular stretches)
- Maintain thrower's motion (especially ER)
- Continue strengthening exercises:
  - Thrower's Ten Program or fundamental exercises
  - PNF manual resistance

- Endurance training
- May initiate more aggressive strengthening
  - Push-ups
  - Bench press (do NOT allow arm below body)
  - Seated row (do NOT allow arm behind body)
  - Lat pulldowns (IN FRONT of body)
- May progress plyometric throwing (14 to 18 days following initiation of two-hand plyometrics)
  - One-hand 90/90 throws (week 14)
  - Wall dribbles
- Restricted sport activities (light swimming, half golf swings)

Weeks 16 to 22
- Continue all exercises listed above
- Continue all stretching
- Continue Thrower's Ten Program
- Continue plyometrics program
- May resume normal training program
- Initiate interval sport program (throwing, etc.) week 16

Week 22
- Continue isotonic strengthening, plyometrics, and flexibility
- Progress to phase II interval throwing or sport-specific training

IV. Phase IV—Return to Activity Phase (Week 26 and Beyond)

Goals

Gradual return to sport activities

Maintain strength, mobility, and dynamic stability

Criteria to enter phase IV:
1. Full functional ROM
2. Muscular performance isokinetic (fulfills criteria)
3. Satisfactory shoulder stability
4. No pain or tenderness

Exercises:
- Gradually progress sport activities to unrestrictive participation
- Continue stretching and strengthening program

postoperatively to allow for adequate healing.[41] The athlete is instructed to sleep in an immobilizer and wear a sling in the daytime for the first 4 weeks. Early motion without stretching is still advocated in a protected ROM below 90 degrees of elevation for the first 2 weeks. By the end of week 4, the athlete should exhibit 115 to 120 degrees of flexion, 35 to 40 degrees of ER, and 55 to 60 degrees of IR in the scapular plane. Submaximal isometrics for the shoulder musculature are performed for the first 4 weeks with the addition of rhythmic stabilization drills by the end of week 1. Light ER/IR isotonic strengthening with the arm at 0 degrees of abduction is initiated with exercise tubing during week 3.

Range of motion is progressed to 155 to 160 degrees of flexion, 55 to 65 degrees of ER at 45 degrees of abduction, and 55 to 60 degrees of IR at 45 degrees of abduction by week 5. Light isotonic exercises with the weight of the arm may be initiated at this time, including shoulder abduction, scaption with external rotation, prone rowing, and prone horizontal abduction. The strengthening program is advanced to include the Thrower's Ten Program at week 6. Active ROM elbow flexion is initiated at week 8.

Full ROM is gradually restored in these athletes by week 8, with a similar progression to full thrower's motion through functional exercises by week 10 to 12. Reestablishment of motion is usually accomplished with little to no difficulty. Advanced strengthening exercises and plyometric drills are incorporated at week 12. The athlete performs two-hand plyometric drills for approximately 14 to 18 days before progressing to incorporate one-hand drills by week 14. The athlete may begin an interval sport program at week 16 and progresses at the same rate as the isolated TACS patient. Andrews and Levitz[1] reported that overhead athletes required 11.2 months to return to competitive sports following TACS and a labral repair.

Rehabilitation following TACS with Subacromial Decompression

Subacromial decompression (SAD) is another common surgical procedure performed at the time of thermal shrinkage. Twenty percent of the TACS of overhead athletes performed at our center also had a SAD at the time of surgery.[36] The surgical treatment of SAD involves the removal of the anterior and undersurface of the acromion, coracoacromial arch, and possibly the distal portion of the clavicle. The athlete who undergoes a combined TACS with SAD is progressed more rapidly in comparison with an isolated TACS. SAD often results in increased irritability, inflammation, and bleeding postoperatively. This rapid healing response tends to inhibit the progression of ROM because of excessive scarring in the subacromial space. Thus the primary complication following combined TACS and SAD procedures is typically loss of motion caused by excessive scar tissue formation. Because of this, we advocate accelerating the rehabilitation program to ensure that full ROM is achieved without

the development of any significant glenohumeral joint adhesions. The overhead athlete is gradually progressed to reach full functional ROM by weeks 4 to 6, in contrast to 8 weeks in an isolated TACS.

Early emphasis is placed on reestablishing proprioception, neuromuscular control, and dynamic stability. Aggressive strengthening exercises, including the Thrower's Ten Program and exercise machine weights, are incorporated by weeks 6 to 8. Two-hand plyometric drills are initiated at week 8 to train the upper extremity musculature to develop and withstand high-load, repetitive forces, as well as facilitate the progression to full thrower's ROM. Two-hand drills are progressed to one-hand drills in 10 to 14 days to ensure proper progression of exercise tolerance. Because of the faster rehabilitation approach, the overhead athlete is allowed to begin an interval sport program to prepare for a return to competition at weeks 12 to 14. Overhead throwers usually begin the interval throwing program by lobbing the ball for 30 feet at this time in preparation for the formal interval throwing program.[58] Rate of progression through the interval sport programs is consistent regardless of the concomitant procedures performed. Clinical observations reveal that athletes who deviate from the program by progressing too fast may exhibit a greater degree of symptomatic complaints while throwing.

CLINICAL OUTCOMES

Use of TACS of the glenohumeral joint capsule to address shoulder instability appears to be declining because of recent studies reporting poor outcomes.[62,63] Toth and colleagues[63] reported the results of TACS in 80 patients with a mean follow-up of 3.3 years. Six surgeons performed TACS using a monopolar device on a variety of patients with various ages, types of instability, dislocation histories, activities, and previous surgeries. The authors noted a 31% failure rate, although the rate of failure increased from 21.7% in patients with concomitant labral repair to 39.2% without a repair. Furthermore, 21.7% of patients with anterior instability failed versus 27.7% with multidirectional instability (MDI) and 80% with posterior instability.

Similarly, Krishnan and colleagues[62] reported the results of 86 patients with a minimal 2-year follow-up undergoing TACS. The authors performed the procedure on a variety of patient populations and noted a mean 39.5% failure rate. The rate of failure increased from 30.4% in patients with anterior instability undergoing concomitant Bankart repairs to 33% without the labral repair. Furthermore, 41.6% of patients with posterior instability and 59% of patients with MDI failed the TACS procedure.

TACS has been performed on a wide variety of patient populations with several different pathologies. The TACS procedure may not be the most ideal surgery for patients with posterior and multidirectional instability because of the increased failure rates reported in these populations.[62,63] Several authors have reported 82% to 93% return to competition following thermal capsular shrinkage procedures in the overhead athlete.[36,64-66]

Savoie and Field[66] compared the outcomes of 30 athletes undergoing an arthroscopic monopolar TACS versus 27 patients with arthroscopic capsular shift procedures at a mean follow-up of 27 months. Eighty-eight percent of athletes undergoing the TACS procedure returned to competition, and 82% of those undergoing the capsular shift returned. Lyons and colleagues[65] performed a 2-year follow-up of 27 patients undergoing TACS using a laser probe. The authors report that 86% of athletes returned to their previous level of competition.

Furthermore, Levitz and colleagues[64] compared two groups of overhead athletes diagnosed with internal impingement. The first group consisted of 51 athletes undergoing traditional rotator cuff debridement, labral debridement, and superior labral (SLAP) lesion repair. The second group consisted of 31 athletes undergoing the same traditional procedure with the addition of TACS. Mean time of follow-up was 2 years. The authors report that 80% of the athletes in group 1 returned to competition at a mean of 7.2 months, and 93% of athletes in group 2 returned to competition at a mean of 8.4 months.

Our center began performing TACS in 1997 and has since treated over 800 patients. During the period spanning from July 1997 to December 1999, 307 TACS procedures were performed. The results of 130 of these athletes were recently analyzed.[36] Only patients classified as overhead athletes were included for follow-up. These included baseball, softball, and tennis players, as well as swimmers and football quarterbacks. Subjects with history of traumatic shoulder dislocation were excluded from follow-up.

Mean (± SD) age of patients at time of surgical intervention was 24 ± 6 years (range 15.3 to 49.1 years). One hundred five (81%) were baseball players, 14 (11%) were softball players, 4 (3%) were tennis players, 4 (3%) were football quarterbacks, and 3 (2%) were swimmers. Eighty of the 105 baseball players (76%) were pitchers. Fifty-four (42%) of patients were professional athletes, 49 (38%) were collegiate athletes, 16 (12%) were high school athletes, and 11 (8%) were recreational athletes.

One hundred twenty-three of the 130 (95%) patients had concomitant procedures performed at the time of thermal heat probe application. Procedures performed at a frequency of greater than 1% are listed in Table 30-2. One hundred nine of the 113 (96%) male overhead athletes underwent a concomitant procedure at the time of TACS whereas only 14 of the 17 (81%) female athletes had concomitant surgeries.

Patients were contacted at a mean (± SD) of 29.3 ± 8.7 months (range 15.4 to 46.6 months). Evaluation consisted of the Modified Athletic Shoulder Outcome Scale as described by Tibone and Bradley[67] and modified by Reinold and colleagues.[36]

One hundred thirteen of 130 (87%) athletes returned to competition at the same level or higher. Mean (± SD) time to return to competition following surgery was 8.4 ± 4.6

months. Mean scores of the Modified Athletic Shoulder Outcome Scale are listed in Table 30-3. Mean (± SD) overall score was 79 ± 14.5 out of a possible 90 points. Seventy-five (66%) athletes reported excellent outcomes, 24 (21%) good, 11 (10%) fair, and 3 (3%) poor.

Comparing outcomes between gender, 89% of males returned to competition with a mean (± SD) outcome score of 80 ± 13.2. In contrast, 71% of females returned to competition with a mean (± SD) score of 70 ± 20.7.

Of the 7 athletes with an isolated TACS procedure, 5 of the 7 (71%) returned to competition with a mean (± SD)

TABLE 30-2

Concomitant Procedures Performed at the Time of Thermal Application

CONCOMITANT PROCEDURE	NUMBER OF PATIENTS (PERCENTAGE OF PROCEDURES)
Labral debridement	90 (69%)
Rotator cuff debridement	84 (65%)
SLAP type II repair*	45 (35%)
Subacromial decompression	22 (17%)
Anterior Bankart repair	10 (8%)
Rotator cuff repair	4 (3%)

*Repair of a superior labral lesion.

TABLE 30-3

Mean (± SD) Outcome Scores for the Modified Athletic Shoulder Outcome Scale

	POINTS
Pain	8.4 ± 2.3/10
Strength and endurance	8.9 ± 1.8/10
Stability	9.0 ± 2.1/10
Intensity	8.9 ± 1.7/10
Performance (total)	43.6 ± 10.7/50
Frequency (percent) with 50/50 point score	74 (57%)
Frequency (percent) with 40/50 point score	21 (16%)
Frequency (percent) with 30/50 point score	6 (5%)
Frequency (percent) with 20/50 point score	9 (7%)
Frequency (percent) with 10/50 point score	3 (2%)
Frequency (percent) with 0/50 point score	0 (0%)
Overall score	**79.1 ± 14.6/90**

Modified from Tibone JE, Bradley JP: Evaluation of treatment outcomes for the athlete's shoulder. In Matsen FA III, Fu FH, Hawkins RJ: *The shoulder: a balance of mobility and stability,* Rosemont, IL, 1993, American Academy of Orthopedic Surgeons.

outcome score of 73 ± 14.1 (good). However, 100% (4 of 4) of male athletes but only 33% (1 of 3) of female athletes with an isolated TACS procedure returned to competition. Comparing outcomes between different concomitant procedures revealed similar results regardless of the procedure performed. Ninety percent of TACS with Bankart repairs returned to competition with a mean (± SD) outcome score of 84 ± 7.2 (excellent); 87% of TACS with labral debridement and rotator cuff debridement returned with a mean (± SD) outcome score of 80 ± 13.1 (excellent); 86% of TACS with subacromial decompressions returned to competition with a mean (± SD) outcome score of 83 ± 10.8 (excellent); and 84% of TACS with SLAP repairs returned to competition with a mean (± SD) outcome score of 79 ± 13.2 (good).

Analyzing the results from year to year (Table 30-4), outcome scores, percent return, and time to return showed similar results each year, although a trend toward the percentage of patients returning to competition steadily rose from 1997 to 1999 whereas the time to return to competition showed a steady decrease.

No adverse effects were noted in any of the 130 subjects. None of the subjects had surgical complications such as neuropathy or recurrent instability. Of the 17 patients who did not return to competition, 42% were diagnosed with MDI and 35% had previous surgical procedures on the shoulder. Eighteen percent of patients reported that their inability to return to competition was not related to shoulder outcome.

The results of our study indicate superior outcomes to those reported using open and arthroscopic stabilization procedures without TACS[68-76] and similar outcomes to those of Savoie and Field,[66] Lyons and colleagues,[65] and Levitz and colleagues[64] using TACS. Eighty-eight percent of patients had good to excellent results, with 87% returning to the same level of competition at a mean of 8.4 months postoperatively.

Based on our clinical experience, the use of TACS may enhance the functional outcomes in overhead athletes, possibly by minimizing the common postoperative complications often associated with open stabilization procedures such as subscapularis scarring, decreased capsular mobility, and decreased ROM.

SUMMARY

Thermal capsular shrinkage of the glenohumeral joint capsule appears to be a promising modality for the surgical treatment of shoulder instability. TACS is predominantly used at our center to treat patients with acquired unidirectional hyperlaxity, such as overhead athletes, with excellent results. Caution should be taken when rehabilitating patients with congenital laxity, posterior instability, or acute dislocations, because results have not been shown to be as good. It appears that TACS is a useful and successful treatment technique based on appropriate patient selection and a carefully designed postoperative rehabilitation program.

TACS does not appear to be used as an isolated procedure in the majority of patients and especially overhead athletes. Rather, various surgical procedures are performed concomitantly to restore function to the glenohumeral joint. The overall functional outcome is greatly dependent on the rehabilitation program. Dynamic stabilization, proprioception, and neuromuscular control all play a vital role in the rehabilitation program. The soft tissue response to thermal energy appears to be highly patient specific. Some patients exhibit an increase in cellular activity and thus significant scarring and stiffness, whereas others exhibit a poor shrinkage response and not as much decrease in ROM. The rehabilitation program must be assessed and adjusted frequently based on the six key factors discussed to ensure a successful outcome. The preliminary outcome of 130 patients at our center undergoing TACS and following this rehabilitation protocol report good to excellent results in 88% of patients at a mean of 29 months postoperatively.[36] Eighty-seven percent of overhead athletes returned to competition.[36] Further studies are required to more effectively assess the utility of this surgical procedure and postoperative rehabilitation regimen. We remain somewhat concerned about the long-term effects of the application of thermal energy to the glenohumeral joint. The concern is regarding the tensile properties of the collagen tissue. Further basic science and clinical studies are

TABLE 30-4

Outcome Trends over Time from 1997 to 1999

	1997 (n = 30)	1998 (n = 56)	1999 (n = 44)	OVERALL MEAN, 1997–1999 (n = 130)
Mean % return to competition	80	87	88	87
Mean time to return to competition (months)	8.9	8.5	8.2	8.4
Overall outcome score (mean points/90)	82.6	76.7	79.6	79

required to adequately determine the short- and long-term effects of thermal energy on the soft tissue.

References

1. Andrews JR, Levitz G: Current concepts: shoulder internal impingement. Presented at 2000 American Orthopaedic Society for Sports Medicine, Sun Valley, ID, June 20, 2000.
2. Burkhart SS, Morgan CO: The peel-back mechanism: its role in producing and extending posterior type II SLAP lesions and its effect on SLAP repair rehabilitation, *Arthroscopy* 14(6):637-640, 1998.
3. Jobe CM: Posterior superior glenoid impingement: expanded spectrum, *Arthroscopy* 11:530-536, 1990.
4. Meister K, Andrews JR: Classification and treatment of rotator cuff injuries in the overhand athlete, *J Orthop Sports Phys Ther* 18(2):413-421, 1993.
5. Walch G, Boileu P, Noel E, et al: Impingement of the deep surface of the supraspinatus tendon on the posteriosuperior glenoid rim: an arthroscopic study, *J Shoulder Elbow Surg* 1:238-245, 1992.
6. Bigliani LU, Kurzweil PR, Schwartzbach CC, et al: Inferior capsular shift procedure for anterior-inferior shoulder instability in athletes, *Am J Sports Med* 22(5):578-584, 1994.
7. Kvitne RS, Jobe FW, Jobe CM: Shoulder instability in the overhead or throwing athlete, *Clin Sports Med* 14:917-935, 1995.
8. Lusardi DA, Wirth MA, Wurtz D, et al: Loss of external rotation following anterior capsulorraphy of the shoulder, *J Bone Joint Surg* 75A:1185-1192, 1993.
9. Protzman RR: Anterior instability of the shoulder, *J Bone Joint Surg* 62A:909-918, 1980.
10. Ellenbecker TS, Mattalino AJ: Glenohumeral joint ROM and rotator cuff strength following arthroscopic anterior stabilization with thermal capsulorraphy, *J Orthop Sports Phys Ther* 29:160-167, 1999.
11. Fanton GS: Arthroscopic electrothermal surgery of the shoulder, *Op Tech Sports Med* 6:139-146, 1998.
12. Foster TE, Elman M: Arthroscopic delivery systems used for thermally induced shoulder capsulorraphy, *Op Tech Sports Med* 6:126-130, 1998.
13. Hayashi K, Thabit G III, Massa KL, et al: The effect of thermal heating on the length and histologic properties of the glenohumeral joint capsule, *Am J Sports Med* 25:107-112, 1997.
14. Karas SG, Noonan TJ, Horan MP, Hawkins RJ: Electrothermal arthroscopic shoulder capsulorraphy: a minimum two year follow-up. Presented at 2000 American Orthopedic Society for Sports Medicine, Sun Valley, ID, June 20, 2000.
15. Obrzut SL, Hecht P, Hayashi K, et al: The effects of radiofrequency on the length and temperature properties of the glenohumeral joint capsule, *Arthroscopy* 14:395-400, 1998.
16. Osmond C, Hecht P, Hayashi K, et al: Comparative effects of laser and radiofrequency energy on joint capsule, *Clin Orthop* 375:286-294, 2000.
17. Schlegel TF: The effect of postoperative immobilization on the healing of radiofrequency heat probe modified tissue. Presented at AOSSM Specialty Day, AAOS annual meeting, Anaheim, CA, February 7, 1999.
18. Tyler TF, Calabrese GJ, Parker RD, Nicholas SP: Electrothermally-assisted capsulorraphy (ETAC): a new surgical method for glenohumeral instability and its rehabilitation consideration, *J Orthop Sports Phys Ther* 30(7):390-399, 2000.

19. Matsen FA, Thomas SC, Rockwood CA, et al: Glenohumeral instability in the shoulder. In Rockwood CA, Matsen FA, editors: *The shoulder,* Philadelphia, 1998, Saunders.
20. Cushing H, Bovie WT: Electro-surgery as an aid to the removal of intracranial tumors, *Surg Gynecol Obst* 47:751-784, 1928.
21. Hecht P, Hayashi K, Cooley AJ, et al: The thermal effect of monopolar radiofrequency energy on the properties of joint capsule, *Am J Sports Med* 26(6):808-814, 1998.
22. Selecky MT, Vangsness CT Jr, Lial WL, et al: The effects of laser induced collagen shortening on the biomechanical properties of the inferior glenohumeral ligament complex, *Am J Sports Med* 27:168-172, 1997.
23. Naseef GS, Foster TE, Trauner K, et al: The thermal properties of bovine joint capsule. The basic science of laser and radiofrequency induced capsular shrinkage, *Am J Sports Med* 25:670-674, 1997.
24. Chvapil M, Jenosvsky L: The shrinkage temperature of collagen fibers isolated from the tail tendons of rats of various ages and from different places of the same tendon, *Gerontologia* 1:18-29, 1963.
25. Le Lous M, Cohen-Sola LL, Allain JC, et al: Age related evolution of stable collagen retinaculation in human skin, *Connect Tissue Res* 13:145-155, 1985.
26. Hayashi K, Nieckarz JA, Thabit G III, et al: Effect of nonablative laser energy on the joint capsule: an in vivo rabbit study using holmium:YAG laser, *Laser Surg Med* 20:164-171, 1997.
27. Hecht P, Hayashi K, Lu Y, et al: Monopolar radiofrequency energy effects on joint capsular tissue: potential treatment for joint instability. An in vivo mechanical, morphological, and biochemical study using an ovine model, *Am J Sports Med* 27(6):761-771, 1999.
28. Wallace AL, Hollinshead RM, Frank CB: Creep behavior of lapine model of ligament laxity after electrothermal shrinkage in vivo. Presented at AOSSM Specialty Day, AAOS annual meeting, Anaheim, CA, February 7, 1999.
29. Schaefer SL, Cicardei MJ, Arnoczky SD, et al: Tissue shrinkage with the holmium:yttrium aluminum garnet laser. A postoperative assessment of tissue length, stiffness, and structure, *Am J Sports Med* 25:841-848, 1997.
30. Lopez MJ, Hayashi K, Fanton GS, et al: The effect of radiofrequency energy on the ultrastructure of joint capsular collagen, *Arthroscopy* 14(5):495-501, 1998.
31. DiGiovine NM, Jobe FW, Pink M, et al: An electromyographic analysis of the upper extremity in pitching, *J Shoulder Elbow Surg* 1:15-24, 1992.
32. Rovner AD, Luke TA, Karas SG: Shoulder capsule volumetric change after open inferior capsular shift versus thermal capsulorrhaphy: a cadaveric model. Presented at annual AOSSM meeting, Sun Valley, ID, June 20, 2000.
33. Tibone UE, McMahon PJ, Shrader TA, et al: Glenohumeral joint translation after arthroscopic nonablative thermal capsuloplasty with a laser, *Am J Sports Med* 26:495-498, 1997.
34. Tibone JE, Lee TQ, Black AD, et al: Glenohumeral translation after arthroscopic thermal capsuloplasty with a radiofrequency probe, *J Shoulder Elbow Surg* 9(6):514-518, 2000.
35. Lu Y, Hayashi K, Edwars RB III, et al: The effect of monopolar radiofrequency treatment pattern on joint capsular healing. In vitro and in vivo studies using an ovine model, *Am J Sports Med* 28(5):711-719, 2000.
36. Reinold MM, Wilk KE, Hooks TR, et al: Thermal assisted capsular shrinkage of glenohumeral joint in overhead athletes: a 15- to 47-month follow-up, *J Orthop Sports Phys* 33(8):455-467, 2003.

37. Magee DJ: *Orthopedic physical assessment,* ed 3, Philadelphia, 1997, Saunders, pp 21-22.

38. Hayashi K, Markel MD, Thabit G: The effect of nonablative laser energy on joint capsular properties. An in vitro mechanical study using a rabbit model, *Am J Sports Med* 23:482-487, 1995.

39. Gelberman R: Tendon. In Woo SL, Buckwalter JA, editors: *Injury and repair of the musculoskeletal soft tissues,* Park Ridge, IL, 1988, American Academy of Orthopedic Surgeons.

40. Tipton CM, Matthes RD, Maynard JA, et al: The influence of physical activity on ligaments and tendons, *Med Sci Sports* 7:165-175, 1975.

41. Wilk KE, Reinold MM, Andrews JR: Postoperative treatment principles in the throwing athlete, *Sports Med Arthrosc Rev* 9:69-95, 2001.

42. Wilk KE: The applied physiology of baseball. In Garrett WR, Kirkendall TR, Squire DL, editors: *Principles and practice of primary care sports medicine,* Philadelphia, 1999, Lippincott Williams & Wilkins.

43. Wilk KE, Arrigo CA: Current concepts in the rehabilitation of the athlete shoulder, *J Orthop Sports Phys Ther* 18:365-378, 1993.

44. Fleisig GS, Jameson GG, Cody K, et al: Muscle activity during shoulder rehabilitation exercises. The 3rd North American Congress on Biomechanics, Waterloo, Ontario, Canada, October 18, 1996.

45. Blackburn TA, McLeod WB, White B: EMG analysis of the posterior rotator cuff exercises, *J Athl Train* 25:40-45, 1990.

46. Moseley JB, Jobe FW, Pink M, et al: EMG analysis of the scapular muscles during a shoulder rehabilitation program, *Am J Sports Med* 20:182-184, 1992.

47. Pappas AM, Zawacki RM: Rehabilitation of the pitching shoulder, *Am J Sports Med* 13:223-231, 1985.

48. Townsend H, Jobe FW, Pink M, et al: EMG analysis of the glenohumeral muscles during a baseball rehabilitation program, *Am J Sports Med* 19:264-269, 1991.

49. Wilk KE, Meister K, Andrews JR: Current concepts in the rehabilitation of the overhead throwing athlete, *Am J Sports Med* 30(1):136-151, 2002.

50. Wilk KE: Rehabilitation of the overhead athlete. Presented at the American Orthopaedic Society Sports Medicine Meeting, Sun Valley, ID, June 18, 2000.

51. Tyler TF, Nicholas SJ, Roy T, et al: Quantification of posterior capsule tightness and motion loss in patients with shoulder impingement, *Am J Sports Med* 28(5):668-673, 2000.

52. Wilk KE: Conditioning and training techniques for the shoulder. In Hawkins RJ, Misamore GW, editors: *Shoulder injuries in the athlete,* New York, 1996, Churchill Livingstone.

53. Wilk KE, Keirns MA, Voight ML, et al: Stretch-shortening drills for the upper extremity: theory and clinical application, *J Orthop Sports Phys Ther* 17:225-239, 1993.

54. Wilk KE, Arrigo CA, Andrews JR: Standardized isokinetic testing protocol for the throwing shoulder: the Thrower's Series, *Isokin Exerc Sci* 1(2):63-71, 1991.

55. Wilk KE, Andrews JR, Arrigo CA, et al: The strength characteristics of the internal and external rotator muscles in professional baseball pitchers, *Am J Sports Med* 21:61-69, 1993.

56. Wilk KE, Arrigo CA, Andrews JR: The abductor and adductor strength characteristics of professional baseball pitchers, *Am J Sports Med* 23(3):307-311, 1995.

57. Schexneider MA, Catlin PA, Davies GJ: An isokinetic estimation of total arm strength, *Isokin Exerc Sci* 1(3):117-121, 1991.

58. Reinold MM, Wilk KE, Reed J, et al: Interval sport programs: guidelines for baseball, tennis, and golf, *J Orthop Sports Phys Ther* 32(6):293-298, 2002.

59. Wilk KE, Andrews JR, Arrigo CA, et al: *Preventive and rehabilitative exercises for the shoulder and elbow,* ed 6, Birmingham, AL, 2001, American Sports Medicine Institute.

60. Hawkins RJ, Misamore GW: Overview of glenohumeral instability. In Hawkins RJ, Mesamore GW, editors: *Shoulder injuries in the athlete,* New York, 1996, Churchill Livingstone.

61. Blasier RB, Carpenter JE, Huston LJ: Shoulder proprioception: effects of joint laxity, joint position and direction of motion, *Orthop Rev* 23:45-50, 1994.

62. Krishnan SG, Hawkins RJ, Karas SG, et al: Electrothermal arthroscopic shoulder capsulorrhaphy: a minimum two year follow-up. Presented at the 2002 Annual Meeting of the American Orthopedic Society for Sports Medicine, Orlando, FL, June 30, 2002.

63. Toth AP, Cordasco FA, Althchek DW, O'Brien SJ: Thermal assisted capsular shrinkage for shoulder instability: minimum two year follow-up. Presented at the 2002 Annual Meeting of the American Orthopedic Society for Sports Medicine, Orlando, FL, June 30, 2002.

64. Levitz CL, Dugas J, Andrews JR: The use of arthroscopic thermal capsulorrhaphy to treat internal impingement in baseball players, *Arthroscopy* 17:573-577, 2001.

65. Lyons TR, Griffith PL, Savoie FH, Field LD: Laser-assisted capsulorrhaphy for multidirectional instability of the shoulder, *Arthroscopy* 17:25-30, 2001.

66. Savoie FH III, Field LD: Thermal versus suture treatment of symptomatic capsular laxity, *Clin Sports Med* 19:63-75, 2000.

67. Tibone JE, Bradley JP: Evaluation of treatment outcomes for the athlete's shoulder. In Matsen FA III, Fu FH, Hawkins RJ: *The shoulder: a balance of mobility and stability,* Rosemont, IL, 1993, American Academy of Orthopedic Surgeons.

68. Bigliani LU, Kurzweil PR, Schwartzbach CC, et al: Inferior capsular shift procedure for anterior-inferior shoulder instability in athletes, *Am J Sports Med* 22(5):578-584, 1994.

69. Jobe FW, Giangarra CE, Kvitne RS, et al: Anterior capsulolabral reconstruction of the shoulder in athletes in overhand sports, *Am J Sports Med* 19:428-434, 1991.

70. Lombardo SJ, Kerlan RK, Jobe FW, et al: The modified Bristow procedure for recurrent dislocations of the shoulder, *J Bone Joint Surg* 58A:256-261, 1976.

71. Montgomery WH, Jobe FW: Functional outcomes in athletes after modified anterior capsulolabral reconstruction, *Am J Sports Med* 22:352-358, 1994.

72. Pagnani MJ, Warren RF, Althchek DW, et al: Arthroscopic shoulder stabilization using transglenoid sutures: a four-year minimum follow-up, *Am J Sports Med* 24:459-467, 1996.

73. Rowe CR, Patel D, Southmayd WW: The Bankart procedure: a long-term end-result study, *J Bone Joint Surg* 60A:1-16, 1978.

74. Rowe CR, Zarins B, Ciullo JV: Recurrent anterior dislocation of the shoulder after surgical repair, *J Bone Joint Surg* 66A:159-168, 1984.

75. Rubenstein DL, Jobe FW, Glousman RE, et al: Anterior capsulolabral reconstruction of the shoulder in athletes, *J Shoulder Elbow Surg* 1:229-237, 1992.

76. Torg JS, Balduini FC, Ronci C, et al: A modified Bristow-Heffet-May procedure for recurrent dislocation and subluxation of the shoulder, *J Bone Joint Surg* 69A:904-913, 1987.

CHAPTER 31

Examination, Surgical Procedures, and Rehabilitation Procedures for Superior Labral Anterior and Posterior (SLAP) Injuries

Jason Jennings, DPT, SCS, ATC, MTC, CSCS

George J. Davies, DPT, MEd, PT, SCS, ATC, LAT, CSCS, FAPTA

Suzanne M. Tanner, MD

Bradley L. Fowler, MD

CHAPTER OUTLINE

ARTHROSCOPY HAS ENHANCED OUR knowledge of superior labral anterior and posterior (SLAP) lesions over the past decade. Despite this increased understanding and appreciation, few detailed rehabilitation programs are described in the literature. Glenoid labral tears confined to the superior aspect of the glenoid rim are receiving more attention as advances in arthroscopy allow for a better understanding of the complex pathophysiology of the shoulder joint. Each type of SLAP lesion requires its own treatment approach. Although numerous studies have presented details of operative techniques and clinical outcomes of patients with SLAP lesions, the rehabilitation programs used after surgery have only received brief mention.[1-7] Before beginning a rehabilitation program it is important to understand the pathology both anatomically and biomechanically. This chapter reviews the anatomy, classification of normal variants, biomechanics, mechanisms of injuries, physical examination, pathologies and classification system, imaging studies, concomitant pathologies, surgical procedures, rehabilitation, and outcome research studies related to SLAP lesions. A specific focus of this chapter is the rehabilitation program for surgical repair of a type II SLAP lesion. The rationale for this approach is that type II SLAP lesions epidemiologically are the most common type requiring surgical repair. Indications for various progressions vary depending on associated pathologies (e.g., rotator cuff tears, glenohumeral instability, etc.). The rehabilitation program provides evidence-based guidelines integrated with empirically based procedures. The protocol is divided into four phases:

- Phase I—protective phase (weeks 0 to 6)
- Phase II—guarded protection/normalize arthrokinematics/develop neuromuscular control phase (weeks 6 to 12)
- Phase III—dynamic power and neuromuscular reactive training phase (weeks 12 to 18)
- Phase IV—functional specificity and return to activity phase (weeks 18 to 24)

ANATOMY

The anterior, inferior, and posterior labra are firmly attached to the glenoid, and separation from the glenoid is pathologic. The labrum is usually a circumferential ovoid rim of primarily fibrous tissue located at the periphery of the glenoid articular surface.[8] There may also be an occasional thin zone of fibrocartilage in conjunction with the fibrous tissue. The labrum is approximately 3 mm high and 4 mm wide. The biceps tendon and the superior glenohumeral ligament are continuous with the superior labrum.[8] Distinction between the biceps and the labrum may be difficult because they blend together over the glenoid.[9] The biceps also has an attachment to the supraglenoid tubercle (also referred to as the biceps anchor). Via cadaveric dissections, Detrisac and Johnson[8] defined "normal" glenoid labra and divided them into five separate types. Later this classification was simplified by

Williams and colleagues[10] into two distinct types: a labrum attached to the glenoid at its periphery through a fibrocartilaginous transitional zone and a labrum secured to the glenoid both peripherally and centrally.

CLASSIFICATION OF NORMAL VARIANTS

Two normal anatomic variants have been described. A sublabral recess, or sublabral foramen, is a physiologic detachment of the superior labrum that has been observed in several studies involving normal shoulders.[11,12] The Buford complex, which is less common, involves the absence of the anterosuperior labrum.[10,12] Both of these variants have been described to have a cordlike middle glenohumeral ligament.[12] Recent findings reveal that these variants may have a higher association with superior labral pathology and may be more common than previously described.[12]

BIOMECHANICS

The long head of the biceps has been shown to be an important glenohumeral stabilizer, and it loses much of its effect after sectioning of its origin.[13-15] Cadaveric biomechanical models have shown that the biceps anchor is the primary restraint of the long head of the biceps and the superior labrum is a secondary restraint to linear stiffness. However, disruption of both restraints is required to produce the laxity typically seen in a type II SLAP lesion.[13]

Evidence from electromyographic studies has shown that high biceps activity occurs during the cocking phase of throwing.[16-18] Data from a cadaveric biomechanical model suggest that biceps superior labral lesions can be created in the late cocking and early deceleration positions in the overhead athlete; however, these lesions occur at a greater rate and require significantly less force to produce the "peel-back injury" in the late cocking position.[19]

MECHANISMS OF INJURIES

The incidence and etiology of SLAP lesions remain uncertain. Proposed mechanisms of injuries include the following:

- A fall on an outstretched arm, with the shoulder positioned in abduction and slight forward flexion at the time of impact.[7]
- An eccentric deceleration mechanism in throwers as the biceps contracts to slow down the rapidly extending elbow in the follow-through phase of pitching.[9]
- Repetitive overhead activity.[7,9]
- Traction injury either as a result of a sudden pull on the arm,[7] or as a result of repetitive trauma.[9]
- "Posterior-dominant" biceps attachment undergoes a torsional peel-back of the posterosuperior labrum for type II SLAP lesions.[3] This injury is described as a tor-

sional force that "peels back" the biceps and posterior labrum as the shoulder goes into extreme abduction and external rotation during the cocking phase of throwing. Once the lesion is initiated in the thrower, the torsional peel-back is repeated every time the arm is brought into the cocked position, causing progressive failure over time, with enlargement of the lesion.

- Internal impingement is the process by which the articular surface of the rotator cuff can become diseased secondary to direct abutment against the glenoid rim and labrum.[19,20]

PHYSICAL EXAMINATION

The diagnosis of the SLAP lesion is challenging and difficult. The cluster of signs and symptoms may mimic or occur in conjunction with other shoulder pathologies. Often a definitive diagnosis is only accomplished through arthroscopy. Although numerous tests have been described with good sensitivity and specificity by the original authors, repeated studies of these tests do not show the same reliability.[21,22] In patients with a suspected SLAP lesion, an accurate diagnosis is made by relying on the cluster of signs and symptoms, corroborative special tests, and imaging studies, rather than one individual test.

History: Chief Complaint

Symptoms may make it difficult to differentiate SLAP lesions from other painful shoulder pathologies. Several authors have suggested "clinical pearls" that may help with examination. Patients may complain of pain in the shoulder that is usually greater with overhead activities.[7,9] Sensations of locking, clicking, or popping with activity may also be reported.[4,7,15,23-26] The pain may be described as "deep within the shoulder joint."[4,26] Although there may be concomitant instability associated with the SLAP lesions, most patients have a chief complaint of pain, not instability.[6,7,9] The patient may also experience loss of range of motion and strength, plus tenderness in the bicipital groove area.

Special Tests

A variety of special tests have been described with varying sensitivity and specificity. No tests have repeatedly been shown to be the definitive clinical test for the diagnosis of SLAP lesions. There is still controversy among clinicians as to which special test is the most useful diagnostic tool. The special tests include the following:

- Biceps tension test[7]
- Compression-rotation test[7]
- O'Brien's active compression test (Figure 31-1)[26]
- Crank test[25]
- Speed's test (Figure 31-2)[27]
- Biceps load test I[23]

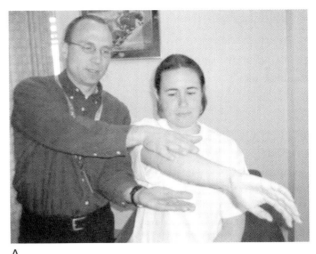

A

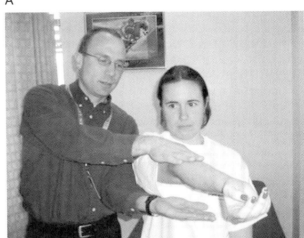

B

Figure 31-1: A, O'Brien's active compression test—part 1. **B,** O'Brien's active compression test—part 2.

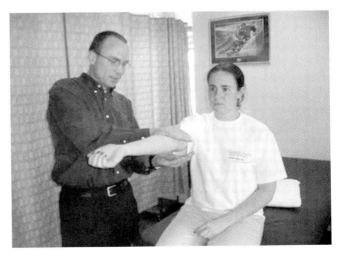

Figure 31-2: Speed's test.

- Biceps load test II[24]
- Anterior slide test[28]
- "SLAP prehension" test[29]
- Clunk test[30]
- Jobe relocation test[2]

PATHOLOGIES AND CLASSIFICATION SYSTEM

Andrews and colleagues[9] were the first to report superior labral lesions associated with the long head of the biceps origin. Snyder and colleagues,[7] in their landmark 1990 article, coined the term *SLAP lesion* and classified these lesions into four distinct types (Figure 31-3).

In type I SLAP lesions, the superior labrum had marked fraying with a degenerative appearance, but the peripheral labral edge remained firmly attached to the glenoid, and the attachment of the biceps tendon to the labrum was intact.

In type II SLAP lesions, fraying and degenerative changes were similar in appearance to those of type I. In addition, the superior labrum and attached biceps tendon were stripped off the underlying glenoid, with the result that the biceps-labral anchor was unstable and arched away from the glenoid.

Morgan and colleagues[5] later classified type II SLAP lesions into three distinct subtypes. They also concluded from this study that lesions caused by trauma more often involve the anterosuperior labrum, whereas those lesions involved with the overhead throwing athlete involve the posterior or combined variety.

- Anterior SLAP lesion (anterosuperior labrum)
- Posterior SLAP lesion (posterosuperior labrum)
- Combined SLAP lesion (combined anterior and posterior labrum)

In type III SLAP lesions, a bucket-handle tear is noted in the superior labrum. The central portion of the tear is displaceable into the joint, and the peripheral portion of the labrum remains firmly attached to the underlying glenoid and to the biceps tendon, which is also intact.

In type IV SLAP lesions, there are bucket-handle tears of the superior labrum similar to those of type III, but in addition, the tear extends into the biceps tendon creating a grade II strain or partial tear of the biceps tendon.

Maffet and colleagues[31] later expanded Snyder's original classification to include three additional types of lesions. A type V SLAP lesion consists of an anteroinferior Bankart lesion that continues superiorly to include separation of the biceps tendon (type II SLAP lesion). A type VI SLAP lesion involves a type II biceps tendon separation and an unstable flap tear of the superior labrum. In a type VII SLAP lesion, the biceps tendon–superior labrum separation extends anteriorly to involve the middle glenohumeral ligament.

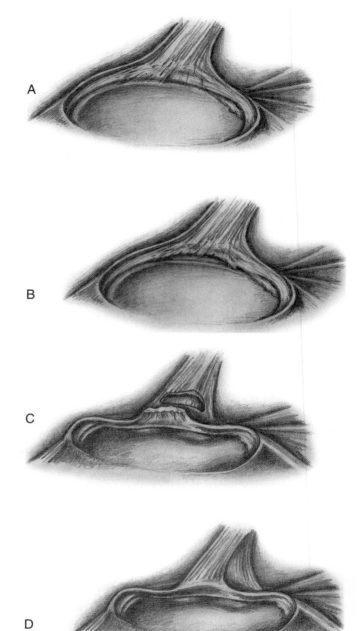

Figure 31-3: A, Type I SLAP lesion; **B,** type II SLAP lesion; **C,** type III SLAP lesion; **D,** type IV SLAP lesion.

IMAGING STUDIES

Conventional radiographs (anteroposterior, supraspinatus outlet, and axillary views) are recommended as the initial imaging studies in the workup of any painful shoulder, but they are of little help with making the diagnosis of a SLAP lesion. Imaging modalities that have shown at least some effectiveness in detecting SLAP lesions include computed tomography (CT) arthrography, magnetic resonance imaging (MRI), and magnetic resonance (MR) arthrography.

Double-contrast CT arthrography has been shown in several studies to be a reasonably effective tool for diagnosing SLAP tears, but it has several limitations.[32,33] It is very difficult to evaluate the labrum in the presence of a full-thickness rotator cuff tear, it is difficult to determine the type of SLAP lesion, and there is no way of diagnosing partial rotator cuff tears.[6] For these reasons, as well as the fact that MRI gives much better resolution to the soft tissues about the shoulder than does CT, CT arthrography is rarely used today in the workup of SLAP tears.

Although conventional MRI has been shown to be better than CT arthrography for detecting SLAP tears, several early studies showed some limitations with plain MR as well.[34-36] In an effort to improve MRI of labral injuries and partial rotator cuff tears, MR arthrography has gained widespread use. Several authors have shown that by distending the joint with saline or gadolinium (Figure 31-4), the accuracy of detecting labral tears may be improved. Studies with MR arthrography have demonstrated sensitivities of up to 96%, specificities of up to 92%, and accuracy of up to 90% in diagnosing SLAP tears.[37-41] Interestingly, Connell and colleagues[42] have reported on 102 cases of arthroscopically confirmed SLAP lesions in which they had 98% sensitivity, 89.5% specificity, and 95.7% accuracy with noncontrast MRI. It is clear that MRI is the modality of choice for evaluating SLAP tears, but whether the addition of contrast is essential or not remains debatable.

Magnetic resonance findings that may indicate a SLAP lesion include high signal intensity in the labral-biceps anchor, high signal intensity between the superior glenoid and the labrum, and deformity or displacement of the superior labrum.[40] These findings are usually best seen on the oblique coronal T1-weighted views. There is a great deal of anatomic variability at the superior glenoid-labral attachment, so differentiating normal from pathologic findings is always a challenge. A sublabral recess, which may look very much like a type II SLAP lesion, has been shown to be present in 71% of normal shoulders.[43] Other normal variants, such as a sublabral hole or a Buford complex, may also make the superior labral complex appear falsely abnormal or injured.[10]

Another MR finding that is closely associated with SLAP lesions is the presence of a supraglenoid ganglion cyst.[44,45] A ganglion cyst near the superior glenoid and cysts that extend into either the suprascapular or the spinoglenoid notch are nearly always associated with SLAP lesions.[45] Ganglion cysts that extend into the spinoglenoid or suprascapular notches may compress the suprascapular nerve and cause a suprascapular nerve palsy. Therefore, when a ganglion cyst is seen on MRI, particularly if it is in association with a suprascapular nerve palsy, there must be a very high index of suspicion of an underlying SLAP lesion.

Despite continued advances and diagnostic imaging, making the diagnosis of a SLAP tear before arthroscopy remains a significant challenge. At this time, diagnostic glenohumeral arthroscopy remains the only definitive way to diagnose a SLAP lesion.

CONCOMITANT PATHOLOGIES

A high incidence of associated pathology has been described in patients with SLAP lesions. Commonly associated shoulder pathologies include, but are not limited to, rotator cuff pathology,* glenohumeral instability,† acromioclavicular joint arthritis,[7] and ganglionic cysts within the spinoglenoid notch and occasionally in the suprascapular notch.[44,45,47]

Kim and colleagues[46] reported the presence of other associated intraarticular lesions in 123 of 139 patients (88%) who had superior labral pathology confirmed with arthroscopy. The results of this study suggest that isolated SLAP lesions with no other associated pathologic findings are uncommon.

NONOPERATIVE MANAGEMENT

The benefit of nonoperative treatment for SLAP lesions is difficult to determine because definitive diagnosis requires arthroscopic evaluation. Nonoperative treatment options include activity modifications and strengthening of scapular

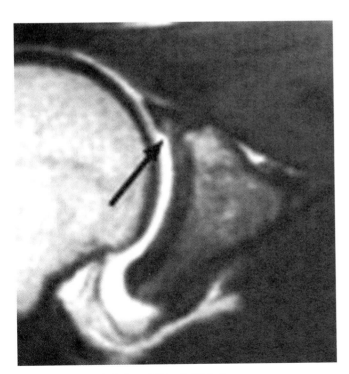

Figure 31-4: Gadolinium MRI—SLAP lesion.

---

*References 1, 4, 5, 7, 23, 28, and 46.
†References 1, 4, 5, 7, 9, 23, 28, and 46.

stabilizers, glenohumeral musculature, and rotator cuff musculature. Exercises such as shoulder press, bench press, and latissimus dorsi pulldowns (behind the neck) should be avoided because of increased stress to the superior labrum and anterior glenohumeral joint capsule.[48] Most SLAP lesions in overhead throwing athletes are type II and may not be amenable to nonsurgical treatment.[48]

SURGICAL PROCEDURES

Surgical Indications

Operative treatment is indicated for symptomatic patients with a suspected SLAP tear who fail nonoperative management for approximately 4 to 6 weeks. Occasionally, the diagnosis is not suspected preoperatively and is detected during arthroscopy for other conditions.

Operative Treatment

For all SLAP lesions, it is critical to perform examination under anesthesia to detect associated pathologies that also require treatment, such as instability, a Bankart lesion, or rotator cuff tears. As previously discussed, Kim and colleagues[46] found that SLAP lesions rarely exist in isolation.

During shoulder arthroscopy, the superior labrum and biceps anchor are visualized and assessed with probing. SLAP lesions must be differentiated from normal anatomic variants. These variants include the following:

- Normal sublabral hole at the 2 o'clock position
- Meniscoid appearance of the superior labrum
- Labral fibers attached medial to the glenoid articular surface[48]
- Buford complex (reattachment of the middle glenohumeral ligaments) (if a SLAP lesion, it can result in marked restriction of rotation)[40,49]

Arthroscopic findings suggestive of type II SLAP lesions include the following[50]:

- A space between the edge of the glenoid articular cartilage and the attachment of the biceps anchor
- A sublabral sulcus greater than 5 mm in depth
- Arching of the biceps-labral complex greater than 3 to 4 mm away from the glenoid when traction is applied to the biceps tendon

Nam and Snyder[51] recommend treatment of type I SLAP lesions with "conservative debridement" of the frayed labrum. Gartsman and Hammerman,[4] conversely, do not regard minor fraying at the free edge of the labrum as an abnormality, so they do not perform debridement. Arthroscopic evaluation is imperative to check for an associated supraspinatus tear[46] or instability.[52]

Long-term results of simple debridement for unstable SLAP lesions, such as type II lesions, have been poor. Management, therefore, includes repair.[40,52] The site of repair depends on the subtype (anterior, posterior, or combined). Burkhart and Morgan[1] report that anterior type II SLAP lesions are characterized by two arthroscopic findings:

1. "Uncovered" glenoid for 5 mm or more medial to the corner of the glenoid under the biceps root
2. "Displacement vertex" of the biceps root, indicating an unstable biceps anchor

They report that posterior type II SLAP lesions display the following arthroscopic features:

- "Uncovered" glenoid for 5 mm or more medial to the corner of the glenoid
- Positive "peel-back" sign with the shoulder in 60 degrees of abduction and full external rotation
- Positive "drive-through" sign in which the scope sheath can be passed superior to inferior

Combined anterior-posterior type II SLAP lesions have findings of both anterior and posterior lesions.[1] The technique for arthroscopic repair of type II lesions includes decorticating the sublabral bone[4,48] and stabilizing the biceps-labral complex, often with a single-anchor, double-suture technique.[51] Fixation options include suture anchors with arthroscopically tied knots, bioabsorbable tacks, and transosseous sutures. Advantages of suture anchors include stable fixation[53] and superior results compared with absorbable tack.[48]

An absorbable tack can be used by skewering the superior labrum immediately adjacent to the biceps tendon with a cannulated drill bit, and then placing a tack over the guide wire. Although placement of tacks may be technically easier than use of suture anchors, risks include synovitis, bone erosion around the tack, tack fragmentation, and foreign body reaction.[54] Disadvantages include fear that impingement of the head of the tack and the greater tuberosity of the humerus may occur in the late cocking phase of pitching (in effect creating resistance to peel-back)[53] and the recommendation that strict immobilization be continued until 4 weeks postoperatively.[55] Exposure is difficult for placement of the transosseous sutures.[40] They are seldom used today.

Recommendations for treatment of type III lesions vary. Higgins and Warner[52] suggest excising the bucket-handle component with no attempt to repair this lesion.[52] Gartsman and Hammerman[4] recommend excising the bucket-handle labral tear if it is less than one third the width of the labrum. They repair the major portion of the superior labrum to the glenoid. If the bucket-handle tear is one third or more of the width of the labrum, the detached portion is repaired.

Higgins and Warner[52] and Gartsman and Hammerman[4] agree on treatment for type IV lesions. If the longitudinal tear in the long head of the bicep tendon is less than one third the diameter of the tendon, they excise the torn fragment. If the fragment is one third or more the diameter of the tendon, they repair the torn fragment to the major portion of the biceps tendon and the superior labrum is also repaired. Another option for treatment of degenerative biceps tendon in a young, active patient is a tenodesis,[51] which is discussed in detail in Chapter 34.

Suprascapular neuropathy secondary to compression by a cyst in the spinoglenoid notch may occur in association with SLAP tears. Arthroscopic techniques may be used for both cyst excision and repair of labral pathology[56] (Table 31-1).

Results

Accurate determination of treatment results of SLAP lesions is hampered by inability to accurately diagnose the condition by physical examination or imaging tests, uncertain results of nonoperative management, unknown natural history, variability of the anatomy of the biceps-labral anchor, the rarity of type III and IV lesions, and the frequent association of SLAP lesions with other pathology.[46] Surgical results are strongly influenced by stability of the shoulder. In unstable shoulders, the prognosis for labral resection and biceps anchor stabilization remains poor unless concomitant anterior or multidirectional instability is also corrected.[48]

To avoid obscuring results of treatment of SLAP lesions from other pathology, Stetson and colleagues[57] evaluated a subset of 23 patients with isolated SLAP lesions. Type I, II, III, and IV lesions were treated surgically. Follow-up was an average of 3.8 years with a minimum of 14 months. Eighty-two percent of patients had good or excellent results. Some failures were attributed to persistent associated shoulder instability.

TABLE 31-1

Surgical Treatment of SLAP Lesions Types I to VII

TYPE OF SLAP LESION	TREATMENT
I	Débridement
II	Biceps anchor stabilization
III	Excision of bucket-handle tear
IV	Excision of bucket-handle tear, biceps tenodesis, or labral repair (depends on patient's age and biceps tendon involvement)
V	Bankart repair and biceps anchor stabilization
VI	Flap débridement and biceps anchor stabilization
VII	Biceps anchor stabilization and repair of middle glenohumeral ligament

SLAP = Superior labrum anterior and posterior.
From Musgrave DS, Rodosky MW: SLAP lesions: current concepts. *Am J Orthop* 2001; 29-38.

Field and Savoie[58] repaired 15 type II SLAP tears and 5 type IV SLAP tears with transosseous suture fixation. At follow-up after 12 to 42 months, all of the 20 patients had good or excellent results. All athletes were able to return to their previous sports with no limitations.[58] Kim and colleagues[59] reported on 43 patients with isolated SLAP lesions treated with arthroscopic repair with suture anchors. Mean follow-up was 33 months. Ninety-four percent had satisfactory results, but inferior results were found in overhead throwing athletes.

Complications of operative intervention include recurrence, articular cartilage damage, laceration of the long head of the biceps tendon, stiffness, and pain.[55]

REHABILITATION

Arthroscopy has enhanced our knowledge of the SLAP lesion over the past decade. Despite this wealth of information, no detailed rehabilitation program has been described. The rehabilitation program described in this chapter is for a type II SLAP lesion because this accounts for many superior labral pathologies and because this is the primary SLAP lesion that is surgically repaired. The purpose of this section is to provide guidelines (Box 31-1) and rehabilitation procedures based on the current literature and empirically based treatment recommendations. Indications for various progressions may vary pending on other comorbidities (e.g., rotator cuff tears, instabilities).

Phase I: Protective Phase (Weeks 0 to 6)

Goals

- Protect the surgical repair
- Decrease pain and inflammation
- Restore arthrokinematics and prevent capsular secondary hypomobility and adaptive flexibility deficits
- Active range of motion
- Prevent reflex inhibition and muscle atrophy
- Shoulder complex kinetic chain rehabilitation
- Develop neuromuscular control of shoulder complex
- Leg exercises and core stability

Protect the Surgical Repair

Initially the operated extremity is placed at the side in a sling (or with a small bolster to prevent the "wringing-out" effect), which is worn for immobilization at all times the first week postsurgically.[1,2,4,5] Codman's exercises, passive range of motion (PROM) to 90 degrees of flexion and abduction, are begun at weeks 2 to 3.[1,2,5] It is critical that patients with posterior SLAP lesion repairs be protected against external rotation past 0 degrees for 3 weeks because this is where the peel-back phenomenon has been observed, even with no abduction (that is, peel-back occurs with external rotation

BOX 31-1

Gundersen Lutheran Sports Medicine Rehabilitation Protocol for SLAP Type II Repairs

Phase I (Weeks 1 to 6)

Sling

- 24 hr/day for the first week
- Weeks 2 to 3 may have extremity out of sling for ROM exercises
- Discharge sling weeks 3 to 4 (per physician approval)

Passive Range of Motion

- Weeks 2 to 3
  - Begin Codman's pendulum exercises
  - Forward flexion to 90 degrees
  - External rotation limited to 0 degrees (at neutral and 90/90 to avoid "peel-back")
- Weeks 3 to 6
  - Gradually increase PROM in all planes as tolerated by the patient

Active Range of Motion

- Week 4 to 6
  - 0 to 90 degrees of shoulder flexion and scaption

Strengthening

- Week 3
  - Modified scapulothoracic
- Weeks 4 to 6
  - Submaximal, multiple-angle isometrics
  - Short-arc, submaximal exercises

Vocational

- Weeks 4 to 6
  - Return to light duty work

Phase II (Weeks 6 to 12)

Passive Range of Motion

- Progress as tolerated, full ROM achieved at weeks 8 to 10

Active Range of Motion

- Progress as tolerated, full ROM achieved at weeks 10 to 12

Strengthening (Lower Intensity, High Repetitions [Isotonics, Isokinetics])

- Week 6: Progressive resistance exercises (PREs) initiated (except biceps)
- Week 8: Begin submaximal PREs for biceps
- Week 10: Strengthening above 90 degrees (submaximal)

Proprioception

- OKC rhythmic stabilizations at week 6
- CKC rhythmic stabilizations at weeks 10 to 12
- Progressions
  - Submaximal → maximal
  - Slow speeds → fast speeds
  - Known patterns → random patterns
  - Eyes open → eyes closed
  - OKC → CKC

Vocational

- Weeks 8 to 12: return to moderately strenuous work

Phase III (Weeks 12 to 18)

Range of Motion

- Maintain full ROM

Strengthening

- Continue phase II and use principles of progression and overload
- Higher intensity, lower repetitions
- Strengthening above 90 degrees (submaximal → maximal)

Proprioception

Progressions per phase II

- Nonprovocative positions → provocative positions (i.e., 90 degrees of shoulder flexion to 90/90 abduction and external rotation)
- CKC exercises from stable surface → unstable surface
- CKC exercises from two-arm support → one-arm support

only).[3] Sling use is continued during this period when not performing the range-of-motion (ROM) regimen.[1,2,4,5] Sling use is discontinued while performing activities of daily living (ADLs) during weeks 3 to 4.[1,2,4,5] The operative extremity may be used for ADLs requiring minimal stress to the biceps-labral complex.[1,2] To protect the surgical repair, avoid activities that stress the biceps because they may create excessive stress on the surgical site. Elbow flexion, supination activities, and using the biceps as an additional lever to help with shoulder flexion must be avoided. During weeks 3 to 6, PROM is progressively increased in all planes as tolerated.[1,2,5]

Decrease Pain and Inflammation

Various medications to decrease the pain and inflammation can be used to help prevent the reflex inhibition that may occur as a result of postoperative morbidity. Several physical therapy modalities may be used to decrease the pain and inflammation, such as interferential electrical stimulation and cryotherapy.

Restore Arthrokinematics and Prevent Capsular Secondary Hypomobility and Adaptive Flexibility Deficits

Often following surgical procedures, capsular limitations may be present leading to obligate translations of the humeral head in the direction opposite the tight tissue constraints.[60,61] It has been suggested that there are selective hypomobilities of the inferior or posterior capsule of the shoulder joint.[7] In these cases, via obligate translational forces, the humeral head would migrate into a superior and anterior direction, which could lead to compromise of the surgical repair of the SLAP lesion.

For patients with selective hypomobilities (beginning as early as week 3) the total end-range time (TERT) stretching formula[62-64] can be applied. Obviously, the positioning of the patient to stretch the noncontractile tissue must be careful to protect the healing surgical site. The TERT formula is used to create plastic deformation of the noncontractile tissue.[62] This formula is based on intensity times duration times frequency. The intensity is the maximal stretch intensity the patient can tolerate based on comfort. Research indicates that 20 minutes is probably the optimum duration of the stretch.[63] However, we have found that 10-minute duration is ideal for patient tolerance and clinical efficiency. The optimal frequency is three times per day. The first and second TERTs can usually be performed by the passive warm-up at the start of the treatment program and by stretching again at the completion of the session. The patient needs to complete the third TERT as part of the home exercise program (HEP). This formula can be used on any joint in the body with noncontractile tissue limitations. The following example shows how this concept can be efficiently applied in the clinic setting:

- Active warm-up: exercises that can be used include upper body ergometry; this may necessitate short-arc motions, active-assistive range of motion (AAROM), and so on
- Heat in a stretched position—first TERT (Figure 31-5)
- Mobilizations/ROM:
  - Physiologic mobilizations
  - Accessory movements (Figure 31-6)
  - PROM/AAROM per restrictions
- Therapeutic exercises (as described later)
- Ice in a stretched position; second TERT is applied at the completion of the physical therapy treatment session
- The patient performs a third TERT via HEP

BOX 31-1

Gundersen Lutheran Sports Medicine Rehabilitation Protocol for SLAP Type II Repairs—cont'd

Functional and Sport Specific
- Month 4: begin plyometrics training (two-arm throws)
- Month 4: may begin modified interval throwing program

Phase IV (Weeks 18 and Beyond)

Functional and Sport Specific
- Isokinetic testing (IR/ER) at weeks 18 to 20 (if overhead athlete or laborer)

- Week 20: plyometric training (one-arm throws)
- Month 6: may begin throwing at full velocity
  - Months 7 to 8: pitchers are allowed full-velocity throwing from the mound
- Return to full sporting activities at approximately month 6 (see criteria discussed in phase IV)

Vocational
- Months 5 to 6: return to strenuous work

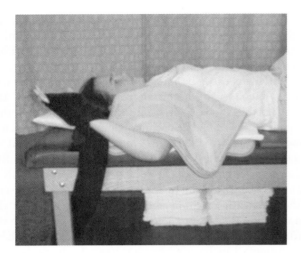

Figure 31-5: First TERT—heat in a stretched position.

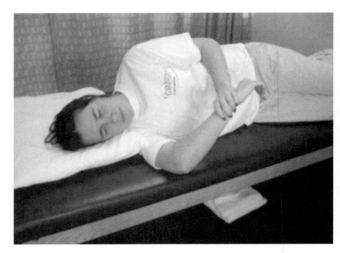

Figure 31-7: "Sleeper stretch" for stretching the posterior musculotendinous structures (infraspinatus and teres minor).

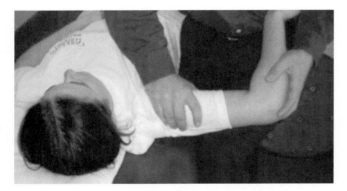

Figure 31-6: Glenohumeral posterior glide accessory mobilizations.

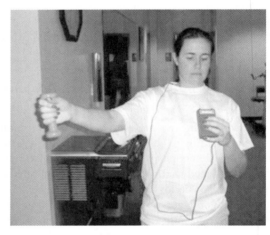

Figure 31-8: Biofeedback inhibition training to the upper trapezius muscle to prevent the compensatory shoulder shrug sign.

If there are additional concerns that the contractile tissue (musculotendinous unit) is involved as a limiting factor, static positional stretching (Figure 31-7) or proprioceptive neuromuscular facilitation (PNF) contract-relax techniques are used. The static portion of the stretches should be held for 30 seconds for younger patients.[65-67] If the patient is older than 60, the stretched position should be maintained for 60 seconds.[68]

Active Range of Motion: Develop Neuromuscular Control of Shoulder Complex

At weeks 4 to 6, active shoulder flexion and scaption (0 to 90 degrees) with the thumb in the neutral position to protect the repair (avoid external rotation of the shoulder) and to prevent iatrogenically creating an impingement syndrome (avoid internal rotation of the shoulder) can be initiated. The patient may initially begin with short arcs from 0 to 60 or 0 to 90 degrees of scaption to minimize stresses to the healing tissues. If the patient demonstrates a compensatory shoulder shrug, biofeedback inhibition training (Figure 31-8) is used

to decrease the upper trapezius compensatory movements that create the shrug motion.

Prevent Reflex Inhibition and Muscle Atrophy

With most type II SLAP repairs, around weeks 4 to 6, submaximal, pain-free, multiple-angle isometrics of the rotator cuff muscles are initiated to prevent reflex inhibition and muscular atrophy. Exercises are performed in a supportive position in the scapular plane to prevent any dependent traction on the surgical repair site.

Shoulder Complex Kinetic Chain Rehabilitation

Proximal stability (scapular stabilization) for distal functional mobility forms the philosophy of the kinetic chain rehabilitation of the shoulder complex. A modified version of the "core scapular exercises" described by Moseley and colleagues[69] for dynamic stabilization of the scapulothoracic area is initiated at this time: elevations for the upper trapezius, retraction exercises for the middle trapezius and rhomboids, and the plus maneuver of the "push-up plus" for the serratus anterior recruitment for scapular protraction. The press-down exercise to recruit the latissimus, lower trapezius, and teres major muscles is delayed until approximately 6 to 8 weeks to protect against superior glenohumeral shear forces to the healing area.

Leg Exercises and Core Stability

Rehabilitation of the shoulder complex involves rehabilitation of the entire kinetic chain. Consequently, leg exercises and core stability training are also incorporated into the rehabilitation program as the symptoms and soft tissue healing constraints permit.

Phase II: Guarded Protection, Normalizing Arthrokinematics, and Neuromuscular Control (Weeks 6 to 12)

Goals

- Protect the surgical repair
- Normalize arthrokinematics by increasing passive and active range of motion to full
- Improve neuromuscular proactive control of the shoulder complex
- Increase shoulder complex strength, power, and endurance

Protect the Surgical Repair

Exercises that stress the biceps–labral complex repair (e.g., heavy loading of biceps curls, supination, glenohumeral flexion with the palm up, which recruits the long head of the biceps as an accessory shoulder flexor) are avoided early and progressively increased as the soft tissue healing process occurs. Typically, submaximal isotonic or isokinetic strengthening exercises begin at weeks 6 to 8.

Normalizing Arthrokinematics by Increasing Passive and Active Range of Motion to Full

All stretching, mobilization, and flexibility programs are continued as in phase I. Active range of motion (AROM) in all planes with no restrictions may be performed.[1,2,4,5] Continue with the TERT formula stretching applications if there are any indications that the patient continues to demonstrate any selective hypomobilities. As previously indicated, selective hypomobilities may compromise the surgery because of the obligate translations and shear forces on the surgical site.

Moreover, selective hypomobilities may cause pain due to the superior translation of the humeral head causing compromise of the subacromial space, leading to an impingement syndrome. Restoration of the normal joint arthrokinematics and full ROM is a primary focus during this phase to prevent any long-term sequelae. Full PROM should be achieved by 8 to 10 weeks. Full AROM should be accomplished by 10 to 12 weeks.

Improve Neuromuscular Proactive Control of the Shoulder Complex

The importance of proprioception and shoulder function in normal shoulders has previously been described.[70] Proprioception of the shoulder is diminished in the shoulder following pathology and surgery.[70-72]

PNF exercises from submaximal to maximal intensity are excellent exercises to begin the resistive training of the patient because the clinician can "feel" the patient's efforts and adjust the resistance to customize the appropriate forces.

Proprioceptive/kinesthetic exercises, such as angular joint replication training and end-ROM replication training, recruit the joint mechanoreceptors and promote shoulder joint control. These exercises are *proactive* exercises, meaning the patient is in control and knows when and where to create the forces and where to stop in the ROM.

Rhythmic stabilization (perturbation training) guidelines[61] for open kinetic chain (OKC) exercises, beginning at week 6, include the following:

- Submaximal effort to maximal effort
- Slow speed to faster speed
- Known pattern to random pattern

The increases in the force production are self-explanatory, applying the principles of progression and overload. Moving from slow to faster speeds is important for the development of neuromuscular training. Most functional activities, particularly those in sports activities, occur at high angular velocities. Another important guideline is to vary the perturbations from a known to a random pattern. In the known pattern, the patient can "preset" the muscles readying for the load. This is "proactive training." It is important to progress to random pattern perturbations in order to enhance the "reactive" neuromuscular system. This is more functional for many ADLs and sports performance activities.

As the program progresses toward more advanced exercises to regain muscular strength, power, and endurance, extensive "hands-on" perturbation training is incorporated. To progress beyond the basic guidelines previously described for facilitating neuromuscular activation and control, the empirical progressions to increase the intensity include the following:

- Eyes open to eyes closed
- Nonprovocative shoulder positions (90 degrees of shoulder flexion) to provocative shoulder positions

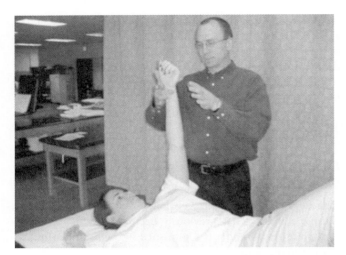

Figure 31-9: Perturbation training with the shoulder in a nonprovocative position (glenohumeral flexion of 90 degrees).

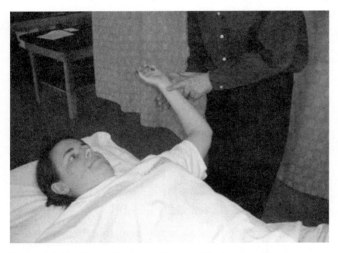

Figure 31-10: Perturbation training with the shoulder in a provocative position (glenohumeral 90 degrees of abduction and 90 degrees of external rotation).

(90/90 degrees of abduction/external rotation) (Figures 31-9 and 31-10)
- OKC to closed kinetic chain (CKC) (weeks 8 to 10)
- CKC exercises from a stable surface (wall, floor) to an unstable surface (tilt board, etc.)
- CKC exercises from bilateral to unilateral arm support

Increase Shoulder Complex Strength, Power, and Endurance

As a general guideline, performing 3 sets of 10 repetitions with gradual weight increases applies the principles of progression and overload. Super-sets with alternating agonist and antagonist muscle groups are used. Progression from larger muscle groups to smaller muscle groups also allows for

a better-quality workout at this stage of the rehabilitation program. Progressive resistive strengthening (isotonic and isokinetic) is initiated at weeks 6 to 8 for the rotator cuff and glenohumeral joint.[1,2,4,5]

The exercises we recommend are the "core scapulothoracic" exercises (Figure 31-11) by Moseley and colleagues.[69] The "glenohumeral core" exercises described by Townsend and colleagues[73] are also incorporated into the rehabilitation program at this time (Figure 31-12).

The design of the therapeutic exercise program follows the exercise progression continuum advocated by Davies.[74] The exercise progression continuum uses the following sequence of exercises and progression:
- Multiple-angle isometrics—submaximal intensity
- Multiple-angle isometrics—maximal intensity
- Short-arc exercises—submaximal intensity
- Short-arc exercises—maximal intensity
- Full ROM—submaximal intensity
- Full ROM—maximal intensity

Using this progression has allowed us to accelerate rehabilitation in a progressive manner while continuing to respect soft tissue healing constraints.

Phase III: Dynamic Power and Neuromuscular Reactive Training (Weeks 12 to 18)

Goals
- Maintain full ROM
- Increase muscular strength, power, and endurance
- Improve neuromuscular dynamic stability
- Develop neuromuscular proactive training
- Develop functional specificity simulations

Maintain Full Range of Motion

All flexibility, stretching, and strengthening exercises are continued as described in phase II.

Increase Muscular Strength, Power, and Endurance

Continue per phases I and II with emphasis focused on increased intensity (weight) with 3 sets of 10 repetitions as the training response occurs in the muscles.

Improve Neuromuscular Dynamic Stability

Many of the aforementioned principles are applied to the rhythmic stabilization exercises, and the guidelines are implemented to continually increase the intensity of the exercises, increase the reactive responses, and progress to a more provocative position.

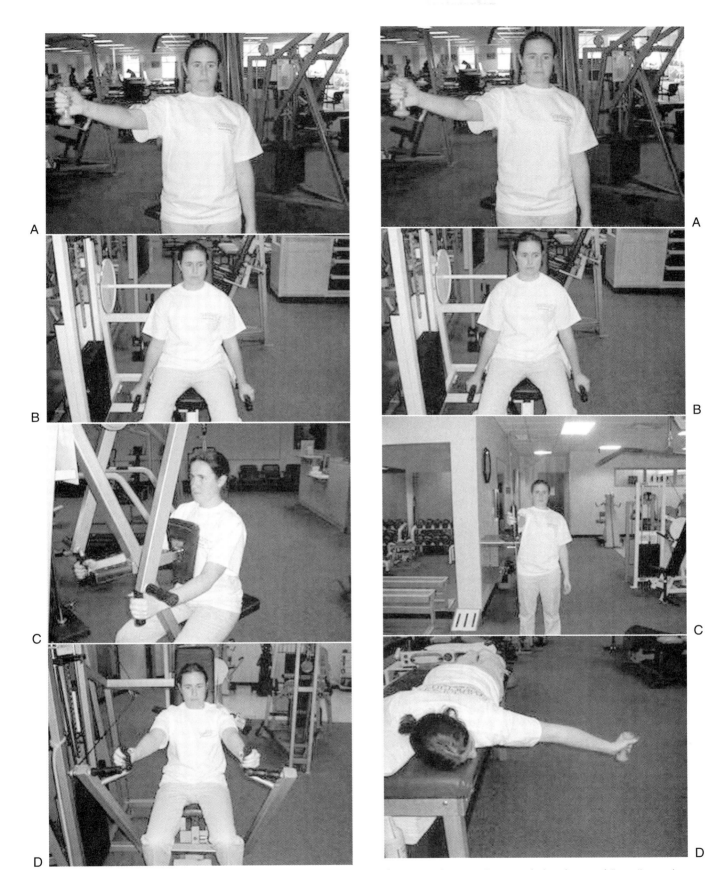

Figure 31-11: Four Moseley scapulothoracic "core" exercises.
A, Scaption with thumb up (superset) with **B,** press-down.
C, Rowing with neutral grip (superset) with **D,** decline press
with neutral grip.

Figure 31-12: Four Townsend glenohumeral "core" exercises.
A, Scaption with thumb up (superset) with **B,** press-down.
C, Flexion with thumb up—body blade (superset) with
D, external rotation with horizontal extension.

Develop Neuromuscular Proactive Training

Plyometric exercises are incorporated at approximately the fourth month postoperatively. Plyometric training progressions follow a logical sequence as with other rehabilitation progressions. Plyometrics can safely be started with two-hand core stability trunk exercises. Progression continues from two-arm chest plyometrics, to two-arm trunk rotational exercises, followed by two-arm overhead throws. The patient progresses to single-arm throwing for isolated glenohumeral plyometrics starting at the side (Figure 31-13). From a practical standpoint, this is accomplished most effectively with a Plyoback System (Exertools, Novato, CA). The patient then uses the Shoulder Horn (Power Systems, Knoxville, TN) (Figure 31-14) to progress from the side to the 90/90 degree position with support. This can be performed in a free toss format (with someone else) or with a Plyoback System. Then the Shoulder Horn is removed and the patient performs the plyometric drills in the 90/90-degree position at a submaximal intensity (Figure 31-15).

Develop Functional Specificity Simulations

This is individualized based on the patient's particular activities. As an example, at 4 months, the athlete who is returning to an overhead throwing sport may begin a submaximal interval throwing program[1,2,4,5] (Table 31-2). Throwing should begin with low-velocity, short-distance throwing with the athlete concentrating on proper throwing mechanics.[4]

Phase IV: Functional Specificity and Return To Activities (Weeks 18 to 24)

Goals

- Develop neuromuscular dynamic stability
- Develop neuromuscular reactive training
- Develop plyometric power
- Develop functional specificity performance
- Initiate interval throwing program

Develop Neuromuscular Dynamic Stability

Progression of the isotonic and isokinetic resistive training programs increases to maximal intensity based on the functional activities of the patient. Total body conditioning continues, including cardiorespiratory training, lower extremity training, core (trunk) training, scapulothoracic training, glenohumeral training, and total arm strength.

Develop Neuromuscular Reactive Training

The primary change that occurs at this phase is the switch from proactive to reactive training. Reactive training more closely simulates many functional situations. One example

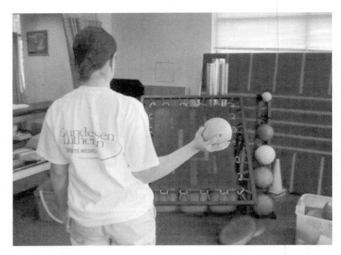

Figure 31-13: One-arm plyometrics with the arm at the side.

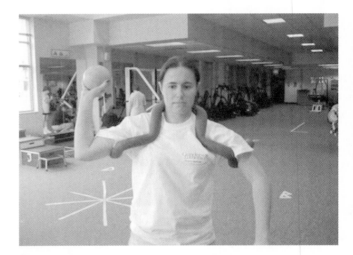

Figure 31-14: Plyometrics at 90 degrees of abduction and 90 degrees of external rotation with the use of the Shoulder Horn.

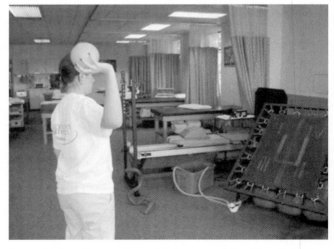

Figure 31-15: Plyometrics at 90 degrees of shoulder abduction and 90 degrees of shoulder external rotation.

would be the progression from proactive (known pattern) to reactive (unknown pattern) perturbation training. Knowing the exact location of the plyometric ball, such as Rebounder throwing, illustrates the concept of proactive training. Plyometric drills in which the clinician throws the plyometric ball in different positions and locations stress the reactions to the stimulus (i.e., neuromuscular reactive training).

Develop Plyometric Power

Plyometric exercises are increased in intensity by manipulating the speed, repetitions, sets, and so on. Moreover, a progression to isolated single-arm exercises (week 20) progresses to the functional activity position for the patient. As an example, with the overhead throwing athlete the 90/90 degree position would be used. Because of the high electromyographic activity in the posterior rotator cuff muscles during the eccentric deceleration phase of throwing, "retroplyos" (Figure 31-16) can also be included as part of the training and conditioning program.[75]

Develop Functional Specificity Performance

Specificity training for the particular activity that the patient is returning to becomes the focus of the program in the return to activities phase. For example, if the patient is returning to throwing, specific activities that mimic the sport are incorporated into the program. If the patient is a tennis player, the activities would simulate the different stokes used in playing the game.

Interval Throwing Program

An interval throwing program is initiated and at approximately 6 months, athletes may begin throwing at full speed, while at 7 to 8 months pitchers are allowed full-velocity throwing from the mound[1,2,4,5] (Table 31-3).

PARAMETERS FOR RETURN TO ACTIVITY—FUNCTIONAL TESTING ALGORITHM

A functional testing algorithm (FTA), which is a progressive, step-by-step process, is used to evaluate and progress a patient through the rehabilitation program. The details and specific criteria are described by Davies and Zilmer.[76] The FTA progresses through a series of stages, with each stage becoming progressively more difficult. The patient must pass through each stage in a systematic process in order to progress to higher levels of functional activities. If the patient fails a test of the FTA, the rehabilitation program is then focused on that area until the deficit is adequately addressed.

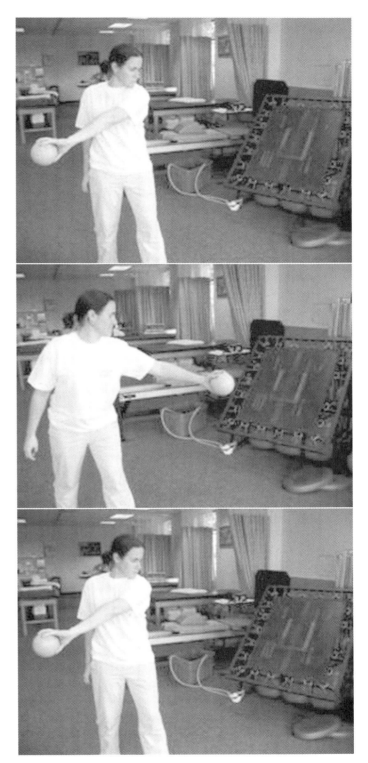

Figure 31-16: "Retro-plyos" for posterior shoulder and arm power development.

TABLE 31-2

Interval Throwing Program for Baseball Players: Phase I

45' PHASE

Step 1: A) Warm-up Throwing
B) 45' (25 Throws)
C) Rest 5-10 min.
D) Warm-up Throwing
E) 45' (25 Throws)

Step 2: A) Warm-up Throwing
B) 45' (25 Throws)
C) Rest 5-10 min.
D) Warm-up Throwing
E) 45' (25 Throws)
F) Rest 5-10 min.
G) Warm-up Throwing
H) 45' (25 Throws)

60' PHASE

Step 3: A) Warm-up Throwing
B) 60' (25 Throws)
C) Rest 5-10 min.
D) Warm-up Throwing
E) 60' (25 Throws)

Step 4: A) Warm-up Throwing
B) 60' (25 Throws)
C) Rest 5-10 min.
D) Warm-up Throwing
E) 60' (25 Throws)
F) Rest 5-10 min.
G) Warm-up Throwing
H) 60' (25 Throws)

90' PHASE

Step 5: A) Warm-up Throwing
B) 90' (25 Throws)
C) Rest 5-10 min.
D) Warm-up Throwing
E) 90' (25 Throws)

Step 6: A) Warm-up Throwing
B) 90' (25 Throws)
C) Rest 5-10 min.
D) Warm-up Throwing
E) 90' (25 Throws)
F) Rest 5-10 min.
G) Warm-up Throwing
H) 90' (25 Throws)

120' PHASE

Step 7: A) Warm-up Throwing
B) 120' (25 Throws)
C) Rest 5-10 min.
D) Warm-up Throwing
E) 120' (25 Throws)

Step 8: A) Warm-up Throwing
B) 120' (25 Throws)
C) Rest 5-10 min.
D) Warm-up Throwing
E) 120' (25 Throws)
F) Rest 5-10 min.
G) Warm-up throwing
H) 120' (25 Throws)

150' PHASE

Step 9: A) Warm-up Throwing
B) 150' (25 Throws)
C) Rest 5-10 min.
D) Warm-up Throwing
E) 150' (25 Throws)

Step 10: A) Warm-up Throwing
B) 150' (25 Throws)
C) Rest 5-10 min.
D) Warm-up Throwing
E) 150' (25 Throws)
F) Rest 5-10 min.
G) Warm-up Throwing
H) 150' (25 Throws)

180' PHASE

Step 11: A) Warm-up Throwing
B) 180' (25 Throws)
C) Rest 5-10 min.
D) Warm-up Throwing
E) 180' (25 Throws)

Step 12: A) Warm-up Throwing
B) 180' (25 Throws)
C) Rest 5-10 min.
D) Warm-up Throwing
E) 180' (25 Throws)
F) Rest 5-10 min.
G) Warm-up Throwing
H) 180' (25 Throws)

Step 13: A) Warm-up Throwing
B) 180' (25 Throws)
C) Rest 5-10 min.
D) Warm-up Throwing
E) 180' (25 Throws)
F) Rest 5-10 min.
G) Warm-up Throwing
H) 180' (20 Throws)
I) Rest 5-10 min.
J) Warm-up Throwing
K) 15 throws progressing from 120 → 90'

Step 14: Return to respective position or progress to step 14 below.

All throws should be on an arc with a crow-hop

Warm-up throws consist of 10-20 throws at approximately 30 feet

Throwing Program should be performed every other day, 3 times per week unless otherwise specified by your physician or rehabilitation specialist.

Perform each step ___ times before progressing to next step.

Flat Ground Throwing for Baseball Pitchers

Step 14:

A) Warm-up Throwing

B) Throw 60 ft. (10-15 throws)

C) Throw 90 ft. (10 throws)

D) Throw 120 ft. (10 throws)

E) Throw 60 ft. (flat ground) using pitching mechanics (20-30 throws)

Progress to Phase II—Throwing Off the Mound

45 feet = 13.7 meters

60 feet = 18.3 meters

90 feet = 27.4 meters

120 feet = 36.6 meters

150 feet = 45.7 meters

Step 15:

A) Warm-up Throwing

B) Throw 60 ft. (10-15 throws)

C) Throw 90 ft. (10 throws)

D) Throw 120 ft. (10 throws)

E) Throw 60 ft. (flat ground) using pitching mechanics (20-30 throws)

F) Throw 60-90 ft. (10-15 throws)

G) Throw 60 ft. (flat ground) using pitching mechanics (20 throws)

From American Sports Medicine Institute, Birmingham, AL. *Preventive & Rehabilitative Exercises for the Shoulder and Elbow*, 6th Ed, 2001, Kevin Wilk, Ed.

TABLE 31-3

Interval Throwing Program: Phase II—Throwing Off the Mound

STAGE ONE: FASTBALLS ONLY

Step 1: Interval Throwing
15 Throws off mound 50%*

Step 2: Interval Throwing
30 Throws off mound 50%

Step 3: Interval Throwing
45 Throws off mound 50%

Step 4: Interval Throwing
60 Throws off mound 50%

Step 5: Interval Throwing
70 Throws off mound 50%

Step 6: 45 Throws off mound 50%
30 Throws off mound 75%

Step 7: 30 Throws off mound 50%
45 Throws off mound 75%

Step 8: 10 Throws off mound 50%
65 Throws off mound 75%

STAGE TWO: FASTBALLS ONLY

Step 9: 60 Throws off mound 75%
15 Throws in Batting Practice

Step 10: 50-60 Throws off mound 75%
30 Throws in Batting Practice

Step 11: 45-50 Throws off mound 75%
45 Throws in Batting Practice

STAGE THREE

Step 12: 30 Throws off mound 75% warm-up
15 Throws off mound 50% BEGIN BREAKING BALLS
45-60 Throws in Batting Practice (fastball only)

Step 13: 30 Throws off mound 75%
30 Breaking Balls 75%
30 Throws in Batting Practice

Step 14: 30 throws off mound 75%
60-90 Throws in Batting Practice (Gradually increase breaking balls)

Step 15: SIMULATED GAME: PROGRESSING BY 15 THROWS PER WORKOUT (Pitch Count)

ALL THROWING OFF THE MOUND SHOULD BE DONE IN THE PRESENCE OF YOUR PITCHING COACH OR SPORT BIOMECHANIST TO STRESS PROPER THROWING MECHANICS

(Use speed gun to aid in effort control)

Use Interval Throwing 120 ft (36.6 m) Phase as warm-up

*Percentage effort.
From American Sports Medicine Institute, Birmingham, AL. *Preventive & Rehabilitative Exercises for the Shoulder and Elbow,* 6th Ed, 2001, Kevin Wilk, Ed.

Stages of the FTA include the following:

- Medical approval
- Soft tissue healing times—satisfactory
- Visual Analog Pain Scale:
  - Rest—ideally 0/10
  - Activities of Daily Living—ideally 0/10
  - Higher levels of activity—less than 3/10
- AROM/PROM goniometric measurements—bilateral comparison—within 10%
- Manual muscle testing normal and pain free in all planes of motion
- Isokinetic testing (if applicable)—bilateral comparison—within 10% (if isokinetic testing is not applicable, may use handheld dynamometer comparisons of selective muscles within 10%)
  - Peak torque/body weight (BW)—within normative data for age, gender, sport, and so on[74]
- Isokinetic testing of unilateral strength ratios—external rotators (ERs) at 65% to 75% of the internal rotators (IRs)[77]
- Isokinetic testing demonstrates that the IRs are approximately 30%, 25%, and 20% of BW at 60, 180, and 300 degrees per second, respectively[74]
- Isokinetic testing demonstrates that the ERs are approximately 20%, 17%, and 15% of BW at 60, 180, and 300 degrees per second, respectively[74]
- CKC upper extremity functional test—within 10% of the normative data for gender (norms: males—21 touches; females—23 touches)[78]
- Pain free with clinical simulations of the activity
- If returning to overhead throwing, volleyball, or tennis, scores are within 10% of the Functional Throwing Performance Index (FTPI) normative data[73] (norms: males—47%; females—29%)
- Ability to complete the entire interval throwing program without pain and with normal mechanics

The FTA provides a progressive and efficient method to use test results along with clinical judgment to progress and discharge a patient safely back into activity.

SUMMARY

This chapter reviews the anatomy, classification of normal variants, biomechanics, mechanisms of injuries, pathologies and classification system, physical examination, imaging studies, concomitant pathologies, surgical procedures, rehabilitation, and outcome research studies related to SLAP lesions. A specific focus of this chapter is to outline details of a rehabilitation program after surgical repair of a type II SLAP lesion.

References

1. Burkhart SS, Morgan C: SLAP lesions in the overhead throwing athlete, *Orthop Clin North Am* 32(3):431-441, 2001.
2. Burkhart SS, Morgan CD, Kibler WB: The disabled throwing shoulder: spectrum of pathology part II: evaluation and treatment of SLAP lesions in throwers, *Arthroscopy* 19(5):531-539, 2003.
3. Burkhart SS, Morgan CD: The peel-back mechanism: its role in producing and extending posterior type II SLAP lesions and its effect on SLAP repair rehabilitation, *Arthroscopy* 14(6):637-640, 1998.
4. Gartsman GM, Hammerman SM: Superior labrum anterior and posterior lesions, *Clin Sports Med* 19(1):115-124, 2000.
5. Morgan CD, Burkhart SS, Palmeri M, et al: Type II SLAP lesions: three subtypes and their relationships to superior instability and rotator cuff tears, *Arthroscopy* 14(6):553-565, 1998.
6. Musgrave DS, Rodosky MW: SLAP lesions: current concepts, *Am J Orthop,* Jan 2001, pp 29-38.
7. Snyder SJ, Karzel RP, Del Pizzo W: SLAP lesions of the shoulder, *Arthroscopy* 6(4):274-279, 1990.
8. Detrisac DA, Johnson LL: Glenoid labrum. In *Arthroscopic shoulder anatomy: pathologic and surgical implications,* Thorofare, NJ, 1986, Slack, pp 21-30, 69-89.
9. Andrews JR, Carson WG, Mcleod WD: Glenoid labrum tears related to the long head of the biceps, *Am J Sports Med* 13(5):337-341, 1985.
10. Williams MM, Snyder SJ, Buford D: The Buford complex—the "cord-like" middle glenohumeral ligament and absent anterosuperior labrum complex: a normal anatomic capsulolabral variant, *Arthroscopy* 10:241-247, 1994.
11. Cooper DE, Arnoczky SP, O'Brien SJ, et al: Anatomy, histology and vascularity of the glenoid labrum, *J Bone Joint Surg Am* 74: 46-52, 1992.
12. Ilahi OM, Labbe MR, Cosculluela P: Variants of the anterosuperior glenoid labrum and associated pathology, *Arthroscopy* 18(8):882-886, 2002.
13. Healey JH, Barton S, Noble P, et al: Biomechanical evaluation of the origin of the long head of the bicep tendon, *Arthroscopy* 17(4):378-382, 2001.
14. Pagnani MJ, Deng XH, Warren RF, et al: Effect of lesions of the superior portion of the glenoid labrum on the glenohumeral translation, *J Bone Joint Surg Am* 77:1003-1010, 1995.
15. Rodosky MW, Harner CD, Fu FH: The role of the long head of the biceps muscle and superior glenoid labrum in anterior instability of the shoulder, *Am J Sports Med* 22:121-130, 1994.
16. DiGiovine NM, Jobe FW, Pink M, et al: An electromyographic analysis of the upper extremity in pitching. EMG and motion analysis, *J Shoulder Elbow Surg* 1:15-25, 1992.
17. Gowan ID, Jobe FW, Tibone JE, et al: A comparative electromyographic analysis of the shoulder during pitching: professional versus amateur pitchers, *Am J Sports Med* 15:586-590, 1987.
18. Jobe FW, Moynes DR, Tibone JE, et al: An EMG analysis of the shoulder in pitching: a second report, *Am J Sports Med* 12:218-220, 1984.
19. Davidson PA, Elattrache NS, Jobe CM, et al: Rotator cuff and posterior-superior glenoid labrum injury associated with increased glenohumeral motion: a new site of impingement, *J Shoulder Elbow Surg* 4:384-390, 1995.
20. Meister K: Internal impingement in the shoulder of the overhead athlete: pathophysiology, diagnosis, and treatment, *Am J Orthop* 29:433-439, 2000.

21. Bennett WF: Specificity of the Speed's test: arthroscopic technique for evaluating the biceps tendon at the level of the bicipital groove, *Arthroscopy* 14(8):789-796, 1998.

22. Guanche CA, Jones DC: Clinical testing for tears of the glenoid labrum, *Arthroscopy* 19(5):517-523, 2003.

23. Kim SH, Ha K, Han K: Biceps load test: a clinical test for superior labrum anterior and posterior lesions in shoulders with recurrent anterior dislocation, *Am J Sports Med* 27(3):300-303, 1999.

24. Kim SH, Ha K, Ahn J, et al: Biceps load test II: a clinical test for SLAP lesions of the shoulder, *Arthroscopy* 17(2):160-164, 2001.

25. Liu SH, Henry MH, Nuccin SL: A prospective evaluation of a new physical examination in predicting glenoid labral tears, *Am J Sports Med* 24(6):721-725, 1996.

26. O'Brien SJ, Pagnani MJ, Fealy S, et al: The active compression test: a new and effective test for diagnosing labral tears and acromio-clavicular joint abnormality, *Am J Sports Med* 26(5):610-613, 1998.

27. Crenshaw AH, Kilgore WE: Surgical treatment of bicipital tenosynovitis, *J Bone Joint Surg Am* 48A:1496-1502, 1966.

28. Kibler WB: Specificity and sensitivity of the anterior slide test in throwing athletes with superior glenoid labral tears, *Arthroscopy* 11(3):296-300, 1995.

29. Berg EE, Ciullo JV: A clinical test for superior glenoid labral or "SLAP" lesion, *Clin J Sports Med* 8:121-123, 1998.

30. Andrews JR: Physical exam of the shoulder. In Zarins B, editor: *Injuries to the throwing arm,* Philadelphia, 1985, Saunders.

31. Maffet MW, Gartzman GM, Moseley JB: Superior labrum–biceps tendon complex lesions of the shoulder, *Am J Sports Med* 23:93-98, 1995.

32. Hunter JC, Blatz DJ, Escobedo EM: SLAP lesions of the glenoid labrum: CT arthrographic and arthroscopic correlation, *Radiology* 184(2):513-518, 1992.

33. Callaghan JJ, McNeish LM, Dehavan JP, et al: Perspective comparison study of double contrast computed tomography arthrography and arthroscopy of the shoulder, *Am J Sports Med* 16:13-19, 1998.

34. Hodler J, Kursunoglu-Brahme S, Flannigan B, et al: Injuries of the superior portion of the glenoid labrum involving the insertion of the biceps tendon: MR imaging findings in nine cases, *Am J Roentgenol* 159:565-568, 1992.

35. Cartland JP, Crues JV III, Stauffer A, et al: MR imaging in the evaluation of SLAP injuries of the shoulder: findings in 10 patients, *Am J Radiol* 159:787-792, 1992.

36. Smith AM, McCauley TR, Jokl P: SLAP lesions of the glenoid labrum diagnosed with MR imaging, *Skeletal Radiol* 22:507-510, 1993.

37. Kreitner KF, Botchen K, Rude J, et al: Superior labrum and labral-bicipital complex: MR imaging with pathologic-anatomic and histologic correlation, *Am J Roentgenol* 170:599-605, 1998.

38. Chandnani VP, Yeaher TD, DeBarardino T, et al: Glenoid labral tears: prospective evaluation with MR imaging, MR arthrography, and CT arthrography, *Am J Roentgenol* 161:1229-1235, 1993.

39. Jee WH, McCauley TR, Katz LD, et al: Superior labral anterior posterior (SLAP) lesions of the glenoid labrum: reliability and accuracy of MR arthrography for diagnosis, *Radiology* 218: 127-132, 2001.

40. Mileski RA, Snyder SJ: Superior labral lesions in the shoulder: patho-anatomy and surgical management, *J Am Acad Orthop Surg* 6:121-131, 1998.

41. Bencardio JT, Beltran J, Rosenberg ZS, et al: Superior labrum anterior-posterior lesions: diagnosis with MR arthrography of the shoulder, *Radiology* 214:267-271, 2000.

42. Connell DA, Potter HG, Wickiewicz TL, et al: Noncontrast magnetic resonance imaging of superior labral lesions: 102 cases confirmed at arthroscopic surgery, *Am J Sports Med* 27:208-213, 1999.

43. Smith TK, Chopp TM, Aufdemorte TB, et al: Sublabral recess of the superior glenoid labrum: study of cadavers with conventional nonenhanced MR imaging, MR arthrography, anatomic dissection, and limited histologic examination, *Radiology* 201:251-256, 1996.

44. Ferrick MR, Marzo JM: Suprascapular entrapment neuropathy and ganglionic cysts about the shoulder, *Orthopedics* 22(4): 430-435, 1999.

45. Moore TP, Fritts HM, Quick DC, et al: Suprascapular nerve entrapment caused by supraglenoid cyst compression, *J Shoulder Elbow Surg* 6:455-462, 1997.

46. Kim TK, Queale WS, Cosgarea AJ, et al: Clinical features of the different types of SLAP lesions, *J Bone Joint Surg Am* 85A(1):66-71, 2003.

47. Ferrick MR, Marzo JM: Ganglion cyst of the shoulder associated with a glenoid labral tear and symptomatic glenohumeral instability: a case report, *Am J Sports Med* 25:717-719, 1997.

48. Jazrawi LM, McCluskey GM, Andrews JR: Superior labral anterior and posterior lesions and internal impingement in the overhead athlete, *AAOS Instr Course Lect* 52:43-63, 2003.

49. Snyder SJ: *Shoulder arthroscopy,* New York, 1994, McGraw-Hill.

50. Getelman MH, Snyder SJ: Arthroscopic management of SLAP lesions and biceps tendon injuries. In Chow JCY, editor: *Advanced arthroscopy,* New York, 2001, Springer-Verlag.

51. Nam EK, Snyder SJ: The diagnosis and treatment of superior labrum, and anterior and posterior (SLAP) lesions, *Am J Sports Med* 31(5):798-810, 2003.

52. Higgins LD, Warner JP: Superior labral lesions: anatomy, pathology and treatment, *Clin Orthop* 390:73-82, 2001.

53. Burkhart SS, Parten PM: Dead arm syndrome: torsional SLAP lesions versus internal impingement, *Tech Shoulder Elbow Surg* 2:74-84, 2001.

54. Burkhart A, Imhoff AB, Roscher E: Foreign-body reaction to the bioabsorable Suretac device, *Arthroscopy* 16:91-95, 2000.

55. Miller MD, Howard RF, Plancher KD: Superior labral anterior to posterior (SLAP) repair. In *Surgical atlas of sports medicine,* Philadelphia, 2003, Saunders.

56. Chen AL, Ong BC, Rose DJ: Arthroscopic management of spinoglenoid cysts associated with SLAP lesions and suprascapular neuropathy, *Arthroscopy* 19(6):1-7, 2003.

57. Stetson WB, Snyder SJ, Karzel RP, et al: Long-term clinical follow-up of isolated SLAP lesions of the shoulder. Presented at the 65th annual meeting of the American Academy of Orthopaedic Surgeons, March 1998.

58. Field LD, Savoie FH III: Arthroscopic suture repair of superior labral detachment lesions of the shoulder, *Am J Sports Med* 21:783-790, 1993.

59. Kim SH, Ha KL, Kim SH, et al: Results of arthroscopic treatment of superior labral lesions, *J Bone Joint Surg Am* 84A:981-985, 2002.

60. Harryman DT, Sidles JA, Clark JM, et al: Translation of the humeral head on the glenoid with passive glenohumeral motion, *J Bone Joint Surg Am* 72A:1334-1343, 1990.

61. Karduna AR, Williams GR, Williams JL, et al: Kinematics of the glenohumeral joint: influences of muscle forces, ligamentous constraints and articular geometry, *J Orthop Res* 14:986-993, 1996.

62. Davies GJ, Ellenbecker TS: Focused exercise aids shoulder hypomobility, *Biomechanics,* Nov 1999, pp 77-81.

63. McClure PW, Blackburn LG, Dusold C: The use of splints in the treatment of joint stiffness: biological rationale and algorithm for making clinical decisions, *Phys Ther* 74:1101-1107, 1994.

64. Sapega AA, Quedenfeld TC: Biophysical factors in range of motion exercises, *Phys Sports Med* 9:57-65, 1981.

65. Bandy WD, Irion JM: The effect of time of static stretching on the flexibility of the hamstring muscles, *Phys Ther* 74:845-850, 1994.

66. Bandy WD, Irion JM, Briggler M: The effect of time and frequency of static stretch on flexibility of the hamstring muscles, *Phys Ther* 77:1090-1096, 1997.

67. Bandy WD, Irion JM, Briggler M: The effect of static stretch and dynamic range of motion on the flexibility of the hamstring muscles, *J Orthop Sports Phys Ther* 27:295-300, 1998.

68. Feland JB, Myrer JW, Schulthies SS, et al: The effect of duration of stretching on the hamstring muscle group for increased range of motion in people aged 65 years and older, *Phys Ther* 81(5):1110-1117, 2001.

69. Moseley JB, Jobe FW, Pink M, et al: EMG analysis of the scapular muscles during a shoulder rehabilitation program, *Am J Sports Med* 20:128-134, 1992.

70. Lephart SM, Warner JP, Borsa PA, et al: Proprioception of the shoulder in normal, unstable, and post-surgical individuals, *J Shoulder Elbow Surg* 3:371-380, 1994.

71. Lephart SM, Henry TJ: The physiological bases for open and closed kinetic chain rehabilitation for the upper extremity, *J Sports Rehabil* 5:71-87, 1996.

72. Lephart SM, Pincivero DM, Giraldo JL, et al: The role of proprioception in the management and rehabilitation of athletic injuries, *Am J Sports Med* 25:130-137, 1997.

73. Townsend H, Jobe FW, Pink M, et al: Electromyographic analysis of glenohumeral muscles during a baseball rehabilitation program, *Am J Sports Med* 19(3):264-272, 1991.

74. Davies GJ: *A compendium of isokinetics in clinical usage,* ed 4, Onalaska, WI, 1992, S & S Publishers.

75. Schulte-Edelmann JA, Davies GJ, Kernozek TW, et al: The effects of plyometric training of the posterior shoulder and elbow, *J Strength Cond Res* 19:129-134, 2004.

76. Davies GJ, Zilmer DA: Functional progression of exercise during rehabilitation. In Ellenbecker TS, editor: *Knee ligament rehabilitation,* ed 2, Philadelphia, 2000, Churchill Livingstone.

77. Davies GJ, Hoffman SD: Neuromuscular testing and rehabilitation of the shoulder complex, *J Orthop Sports Phys Ther* 18(2):449-458, 1993.

78. Goldbeck TG, Davies GJ: Test-retest reliability of the closed kinetic chain upper extremity stability test: a clinical field test, *J Sports Rehabil* 9(1):35-45, 2000.

CHAPTER 32

Subacromial Impingement, Acromioplasty, and Subacromial Decompression

Robert A. Schulte, PT, DSc, SCS, ACSM-ES, MBA
Darin T. Leetun, MD
Cory D. Warner, MPT, CSCS

CHAPTER OUTLINE

Photographs courtesy Katherine C. Schulte.

THE EARLY CONCEPTS OF SUBACROMIAL

impingement were first introduced by Meyer almost 70 years ago.[1,2] His thoughts at that time were that mechanical attrition under the acromion was the cause of both cuff degeneration and biceps tendon rupture. Neer later proposed in the early 1970s that the difference in size and shape of the structures of the acromial arch led to impingement and cuff pathology.[3,4] Dr. Neer identified the anterior third of the undersurface of the acromion, the coracoacromial ligament, and the acromioclavicular joint as the sources of compression and injury to the rotator cuff.

Pressure studies of the subacromial space have demonstrated that lifting a 1 kg weight can increase subacromial contact pressure enough to block circulation.[5] An association between the change in acromial morphology and incidence of cuff tears has been presented by Bigliani and associates.[6] They identified three types of acromion: type I acromion, or flat acromion, with an incidence of 17%; type II acromion, or curved acromion, with an incidence of 43%; and type III acromion, or hooked acromion, with an incidence of 40% (Figure 32-1). A significant increase in full-thickness rotator cuff tears was seen with the type III acromion, acromion with anterior spurs, and acromion with greater angle of anterior slope. Morrison and Bigliani[7] later presented information indicating that 80% of patients with positive arthrograms had an associated type III acromion. In looking further at the idea of impingement, Wuh and Snyder[8] proposed a modification to the Bigliani classification looking at acromial thickness, as well as acromial shape. Acromial thickness was measured at the anterior to middle third of the acromion and classified into three types: type A, less than 8 mm thickness; type B, 8 to 12 mm thickness; and type C, greater than 12 mm thickness. Edelson and Taitz[9] found that a more horizontal acromion was associated with greater degenerative changes and that the degenerative changes increased with increased length of the acromion. Gartsman[10] proposed that an increased angle of inclination narrows the supraspinatus outlet, resulting in a type I acromion associated with impingement. Banas and colleagues[11] described a "lateral acromial angle." As lateral acromial angle decreased, a statistically significant increase in cuff disease was seen. Although association of unfused acromial epiphyses has been made with rotator cuff tears, little evidence to suggest that this predisposes the shoulder to development of cuff tears has been brought forth.[9,12,13] It has been noted that spurs, which are essentially osteophytes that form on the anterior one third of the acromion at the insertion of the coracoacromial ligament, tend to decrease the volume available for the supraspinatus tendon excursion.[14-16] Aoki and associates[17] noted in lateral radiographs that acromions with spur formation had a flatter slope with increasing pitting on the surface of greater tuberosity. Flattening of the slope of the acromion may produce impingement of the rotator cuff between the acromion and the superior surface of the tuberosity. A comparison of asymptomatic patients with individuals having stage II impingement revealed that the latter group had a statistically flatter acromial slope. Burns and Whipple[18] have noted that contact by the anterior tip of the acromion on the supraspinatus tendon and the greater tuberosity is greatest in the middle ranges of humeral elevation from 60 to 120 degrees. Dye compression studies and pressure-sensitive film have also confirmed these findings.[19,20] Studies using optical stereophotogrammetric techniques assessing subacromial contact have shown that the acromion comes closest to the cuff tendons between 60 and 120 degrees of elevation, with contact focused on the supraspinatus insertion.[21] With internal rotation of 20 degrees, more contact was noted than in neutral rotation. It was also noted that increased contact was observed with shoulders having type III acromions versus other types. Caspari and Thal[22] studied impingement, defining *impingement* as focused acromial contact compressing the supraspinatus insertion. They were able to show that 50% of this

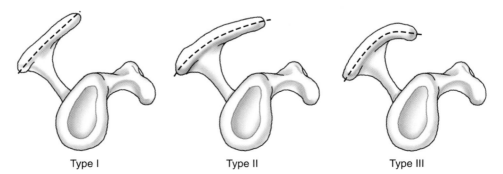

| Type I | Type II | Type III |

Figure 32-1: Acromion morphology classification types. *(From Jobe FW, editor: Operative techniques in upper extremity sports injuries, St Louis, 1996, Mosby.)*

contact could be eliminated just by removing anterior ridges of the acromion, that being the bony spurs. Total flattening of the anterior one third of the acromion successfully removed impingement in 100% of specimens. They also looked at *total flattening*, that is, making the entire acromion flush with the posterior acromion, and found that this did not necessarily eliminate impingement. In fact, this often destroyed the broad pattern of subacromial contact over the cuff tendons and humeral head (termed *buffering*). Buffering is thought to be a passive stabilizing effect on humeral head ascent.

SUBACROMIAL IMPINGEMENT ANATOMY, BIOMECHANICS, AND KINEMATICS

Looking at impingement, an understanding of superior shoulder anatomy is vital. The coracoacromial arch makes important contributions to impingement. The coracoacromial arch consists of the bony acromion, the coracoacromial ligament, and the coracoid process. This forms the roof of the space known as the supraspinatus outlet through which the supraspinatus tendon passes. The arch is implicated in impingement and rotator cuff pathology (Figure 32-2). The acromion itself can play a role because os acromiale can be seen in the general population and has an overall incidence of 1.4%, with 62% being bilateral.[23,24]

Classification of the os acromiale is broken into three types: meso-acromion, meta-acromion, and basi-acromion.[25] Dynamic os acromiale motion can play a role in impingement. The coracoacromial ligament is a triangular structure running from the lateral aspect of the coracoid to the anterior-inferior acromion.[26-28] Anterior-inferior spurs tend to develop by ossification of the coracoacromial ligament.[29] Understanding subacromial impingement, one must keep in mind the biomechanics and kinematics of the shoulder and shoulder girdle. Twenty-six muscles control the shoulder girdle, four of which make up the rotator cuff. Equally important is the makeup of the rotator cuff itself. The cuff is a five-layer structure.[30] Layer four contains collagen fibers running perpendicular to the primary orientation of the cuff tendons. This layer likely assists in distribution of forces between the different tendons and may explain why normal kinematics can be maintained in the presence of tendon defects. Along this same line, Gohlke and associates[31] speculated that fiber variation and orientation, as well as the distinct layers within the capsular complex, leads to significant shear stress in the rotator cuff. Along with this, intratendinous interdigitations and variations in cuff structure are important in cuff pathology. Another important aspect of the cuff has to do with blood supply. Blood reaches the rotator cuff from the posterior humeral circumflex artery, as well as the suprascapular arteries, forming an intralattice arcade over

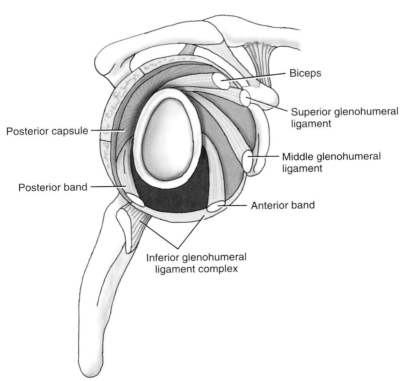

Figure 32-2: Coracoacromial arch. *(From O'Brien SJ, Neves MC, Arnoczky SP, et al: The anatomy and histology of the anterior glenohumeral ligament complex of the shoulder, Am J Sports Med 18:449-456, 1990.)*

the posterior cuff and making the major blood supply to the teres minor and the infraspinatus.[32] The anterior circumflex humeral artery supplies portions of the anterior superior cuff in conjunction with the thoracoacromial artery along with a variable distal branch called the suprahumeral artery.[33] The acromial branch of the thoracoacromial artery usually supplies the supraspinatus.

Rotator cuff kinematics are also important for overall function of the shoulder. The primarily function of the rotator cuff is to act as a humeral head depressor and dynamic stabilizer. It also serves as the fulcrum that the deltoid uses to elevate the arm.[34] The subscapularis is an internal rotator, as well as a dynamic barrier to anterior displacement of the humeral head.[35] The supraspinatus provides 50% of the torque output for shoulder elevation.[36] Infraspinatus and teres minor have been classically described as the primary external rotators of the arm, providing 80% of the external rotation force.[37] Obviously, the moment arms of the muscles change with differential position of the shoulder. The subscapularis is an internal rotator with an adductor moment arm greatest for the superior portion of the subscapularis. External rotation increases the ability of the superior portion of the subscapularis to elevate the arm. The adductor moment arm of the anterior portion of the supraspinatus decreases with internal rotation, whereas the posterior portion of the supraspinatus decreases with external rotation.[38-42] Internal rotation markedly enhances the effectiveness of superior torsion of the infraspinatus as an abductor.

IMPINGEMENT ETIOLOGY/SOFT TISSUE INJURY

Impingement is multifactorial in nature with many implicating factors, including tension overload, repetitive stress, and intrinsic factors related to the cuff (e.g., poor vascularity, alterations in material properties of the cuff, alteration in matrix composition of the cuff, and aging).[43-48] Multiple initial events could lead to possibility of impingement. Rotator cuff shutdown resulting from injury can alter the biomechanics of the rotator cuff and the humeral head depressive effect. Deutsch and associates[49] were able to show significant superior humeral head migration on the glenoid in stage I and II impingement patients compared with a group of normal controls. Progressive cuff shutdown can be related to injury or repetitive microtrauma. Also related to this idea of impingement is the potential of internal rotation deficits, which alter the biomechanics of the shoulder. Multiple authors have noted obligate humeral translation during motion.[50-52] The rotator cuff, despite normal function, may be unable to keep the humeral head depressed if an internal rotation deficit causes obligatory superior migration of the humeral head with motion. It is speculated that anterior-superior humeral migration occurs with overhead activities in the presence of a tight posterior capsule. Another cause of impingement would be a loss of the normal stability of the shoulder. Several authors have reported secondary impinge-

ment in association with glenohumeral instability.[53-56] The labrum works as a static ring allowing capsular attachment for good stability of the shoulder. The labrum also works as a mechanical bumper, almost like a chock block underneath a car tire. With stability of the labrum lost, a secondary loss of the normal stabilizing effect of the capsule, as well as the labrum bumper, can lead to superior migration of the humeral head and impingement. Repetitive capsular strain can lead to instability and secondary impingement. Jobe[57] has been attributed as the first to bring this idea of instability impingement to the forefront. Another potential source for impingement is the idea that degenerative changes occur within the rotator cuff with microtrauma. Nirschl[58] has proposed that a primary degenerative tendinopathy occurs in cuffs similar to that seen in lateral epicondylitis or Achilles tendon ruptures. This can lead to cuff shutdown with secondary impingement, due to cuff dysfunction. Primary impingement related to acromial morphology is a culprit in the whole pathologic spectrum of impingement in the shoulder. Jobe also describes the concept of posterior-superior glenoid impingement, which has been termed *internal impingement*.[59-62] Internal impingement is a clinical entity commonly present in overhead athletes. Structural pathology most commonly involves a partial-thickness injury to the articular surface of the rotator cuff and injury to the superior glenoid labrum. Underlying laxity in the anterior glenohumeral capsule is a common comorbidity that accompanies internal impingement. Pathomechanical impairments in this condition involve abnormal humeral translation or abnormal scapular protraction. Anterior microinstability may commonly be due to anterior capsular injury, a Bankart lesion, a biceps/superior labrum injury, or reduced dynamic stability caused by posterior rotator cuff weakness. Abnormal scapular protraction can result from loss of muscular control of the normal scapulothoracic (ST) force couple and corresponding glenoid position. The effect of the pathomechanical impairments and structural pathology produce a dysfunctional physiologic position involving humeral hyperangulation and excessive external rotation. Symptoms and signs include sharp pain, clicking or grinding on rotation, and feelings of instability or looseness. Although the majority of the symptoms are created in cocking or acceleration involving dynamic overhead throwing, static positioning of shoulder abduction and external rotation has been observed in our practice to create internal impingement in nonthrowing patients as well (Figure 32-3). Clinical examination findings include decreased glenohumeral (GH) internal rotation, tenderness along the posterior-superior joint line, anterior instability, and a positive Jobe subluxation relocation test that causes posterior joint line pain with external rotation and abduction. Impingement is a multifactorial issue with mechanical reasons (spurs, outlet morphology, cuff dysvascularity), cuff aging (tendon primary degeneration, increasing stiffness, cuff vascular changes), glenohumeral instability, scapula dyskinesia, and total body kinetic chain factors that can all play a part in the impingement process (Table 32-1).

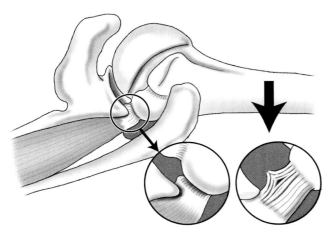

Figure 32-3: Schematic representation of posterior-superior (internal) impingement. *(From Walch G, Borleau P, Noel E, Donell T: Impingement of the deep surface of the supraspinatus tendon on the posterior glenoid rim: an arthroscopic study,* J Shoulder Elbow Surg *1:239, 1992.)*

SHOULDER IMPINGEMENT CLASSIFICATION

Impingement patients typically experience insidious onset of shoulder pain with overhead activities. Patients may be awakened at night with pain and may have difficulties lying on the affected shoulder. Pain is typically located in the lateral aspect of the humerus. Generally, patients do not complain of loss of motion, although physical examination will find subtle internal rotation deficits in a number of patients that need to be addressed. Patients frequently complain of a painful arc of motion between 70 and 120 degrees of elevation. Some atrophy of the shoulder girdle musculature may be seen if it has been a chronic condition. Areas of tenderness may be localized to the region of the subacromial bursa, the anterior acromion, the coracoacromial ligaments, or the area of the greater tuberosity at the supraspinatus insertion. Hypertrophy and scarring of the subacromial bursa can lead to noticeable subacromial crepitus on physical examination. Patients will typically limit their active range of motion (AROM) in abduction and forward flexion secondary to pain associated with reaching above the horizontal plane. Typically, active forward elevation and abduction is more

---

TABLE 32-1

Functional and Structural Impairments Contributing to Impingement

PRIMARY IMPINGEMENT	SECONDARY IMPINGEMENT	INTERNAL IMPINGEMENT (POSTERIOR)	INTERNAL IMPINGEMENT (ANTERIOR)
Acromion morphology	Glenohumeral force couple muscle imbalance	Anterior humeral ligament laxity	Posterior humeral ligament laxity
Acromioclavicular arthrosis	Eccentric tensile overload of long head of bicep	Posterior rotator cuff weakness	Anterior rotator cuff weakness
Coracoacromial ligament hypertrophy	Multidirectional glenohumeral ligament laxity	Excessive scapular protraction	Excessive humeral internal rotation
Coracoid impingement	Glenoid labral lesion	Excessive humeral external rotation	
Subacromial bursal fibrosis	Scapular dyskinesia	Increased thoracic kyphosis	
Prominent humeral greater tuberosity	Posterior capsular tightness		
Overhead activity	Scapulothoracic force couple imbalance		

uncomfortable than passive range of motion (PROM) because of the presence of tendon injury and irritation. Many examination schemes have been proposed to aid in the diagnosis of neuromusculoskeletal conditions. Although the allopathic approach uses special tests to identify a pathology-based diagnosis, an impairment-based diagnosis may be more appropriate when classifying impingement syndrome of the shoulder. The biopsychosocial model used in physical therapy attempts to determine the cause, nature, and extent of the problem on the "whole" person, whereas the medical diagnosis simply identifies the pathologic entity.[63] Schulte and Davies[64] describe an algorithm-based shoulder examination scheme that uses practice patterns, or categories of diagnosis that are based on the similarities in impairments and functional limitations that impingement syndrome causes. The shoulder algorithm's sequential and selective use of special tests to help differentiate the impairment-based diagnosis makes it an effective examination scheme in diagnosing impingement syndrome because it considers both structural and functional factors that may be contributing to subacromial impingement.

The overhead thrower with supraspinatus impingement syndrome serves as an excellent example of why we attempt to ascertain the underlying cause of the pain and dysfunction. As previously discussed, primary impingement is a mechanical impingement of the rotator cuff beneath the coracoacromial arch and typically results from subacromial overcrowding. Secondary impingement is a relative decrease in the subacromial space caused by microinstability of the GH joint or scapulothoracic dyskinesia. In the authors' opinion, an athlete younger than 30 years of age is doubtful to have a true primary impingement without an underlying instability. Neer and Poppen[65] have categorized stages of impingement related to patient age, clinical course, and physical signs (Table 32-2). If the athlete has a primary impingement, he or she usually has selective hypomobility of various portions of the shoulder capsule. Heating and stretching, mobilizations, and other manual therapy techniques would be indicated in treating this patient to normalize his or her capsular mobility and range of motion (ROM). However, if this athlete with similar signs and symptoms actually has a secondary impingement caused by underlying microinstability, heating and stretching would be contraindicated for specific parts of the shoulder. Therefore, before one begins an intervention program, the differential examination to establish a precise impairment-based diagnosis must be performed. Schulte and Davies[64] propose beginning every shoulder examination by performing the sulcus sign/inferior test to determine the status of GH stability (Figures 32-4 to 32-6). The importance of establishing a basis of shoulder

---

TABLE 32-2

Neer and Hawkins Progressive Stages of Impingement

	STAGE I: EDEMA AND INFLAMMATION	STAGE II: FIBROSIS AND TENDONITIS	STAGE III: BONE SPURS AND TENDON RUPTURES
Age	Younger than 25 years, but may occur at any age	25–40 years	Greater than 40 years
Clinical course	Reversible lesion	Not reversible by modification of activity	Not reversible
Physical signs	Tenderness to palpation over the greater tuberosity of the humerus	Stage I signs plus the following:	Stage I and II signs plus the following:
	Tenderness along anterior ridge or acromion	Greater degree of soft tissue crepitus may be felt because of scarring in subacromial space	Limitation of range of motion, more pronounced with active motion
	Painful arc of abduction between 60 and 120 degrees, increased with resistance at 90 degrees	Catching sensation with lowering of arm at approximately 100 degrees	Weakness of shoulder abduction and external rotation
	Positive impingement signs	Limitation of active and passive range of motion	Infraspinatus atrophy
	Shoulder range of motion may be restricted with significant subacromial inflammation		Biceps tendon and acromioclavicular joint tenderness

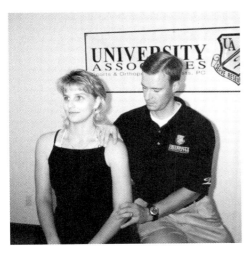

Figure 32-4: Sulcus sign at 0 degrees.

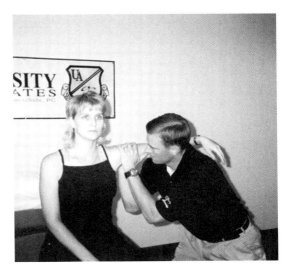

Figure 32-5: Sulcus sign at 90 degrees.

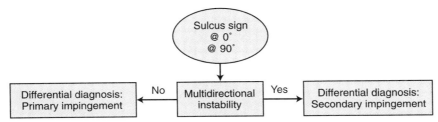

Figure 32-6: Algorithm-based shoulder examination sequence to determine if underlying instability exists in the glenohumeral joint.

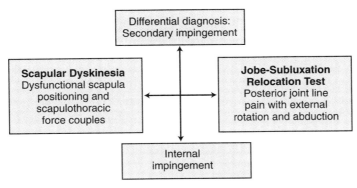

Figure 32-7: Algorithm-based shoulder examination sequence to identify potential internal impingement dysfunction.

stability in every patient examination, even when there is no history of trauma, is essential. This concept is supported when considering that the incidence of trauma as a causative factor in patients who have multidirectional instability (MDI) is much lower than in patients who have recurrent anterior shoulder dislocations.[66] Essentially, all patients should be assessed for instability regardless of their history. Results of this portion of the examination sequence help determine whether the patient has MDI or the first half of bidirectional instability. For example, if later in the examination sequence we find that the patient has positive impingement syndrome tests, we know it may be a secondary impingement syndrome because of the underlying instability (Figure 32-7). Although the scope of this chapter is not to provide an extensive review of the complete shoulder examination process, the impingement examination sequence of the shoulder algorithm is helpful to differentiate a primary, a secondary, and an internal impingement (Figure 32-8). Therefore, before one begins an intervention program, a differential examination to establish a precise impairment-based diagnosis must be performed.

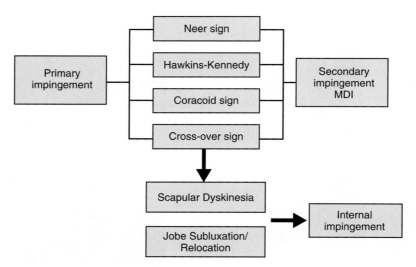

Figure 32-8: Impingement classifications and the algorithm-based shoulder examination sequence of special tests.

Impingement intervention programs, which are presented later in this chapter, are predicated on the initial examination and ability to distinguish impingement classification and stage of progression.

NONOPERATIVE REHABILITATION PROTOCOL PHILOSOPHY

Most impingement protocols are classified into two types of impingement: primary and secondary. This system designates a broad causative classification of impingement but is not specific to the underlying impairment(s), which can advance to dysfunction and potential disability. Whereas most protocols use an exhaustive list of various modalities to treat the condition in various phases, specific impairment-based criteria are not identified. Another limitation with some intervention protocols is the lack of consideration as to the stage of disease progression and dysfunction present in an affected individual. Considering the clinical course involving Neer's progressive stages of impingement (see Table 32-2), the impairments and goals of a person who is classified with stage I primary impingement should be different than if that same person was classified with stage III primary impingement. Whereas the patient with stage I primary impingement has the potential to reverse tissue morbidity, the patient with stage III primary impingement is likely to have an acute exacerbation involving a chronic condition that has limited potential to resolve. A study by Morrison[67] identified that although 91% of patients with a type I acromion achieved successful outcomes from physical therapy, only 66% had positive outcomes with a type II or type III acromion. The study was limited in that it did not classify patients into progressive stages of impingement, and the long-term outcomes are unknown because patients were not followed longitudinally. Traditionally, surgery for rotator

cuff impingement (subacromial decompression) has been advocated when symptoms have persisted despite conservative treatment for more than 1 year. In our opinion, earlier subacromial decompression/distal clavicle resection should be given serious consideration after only 6 weeks if supervised conservative intervention fails to alleviate symptoms in patients with type II or type III primary impingement. The rationale is based on (1) addressing the structural impairment that will not resolve and (2) preventing stage II and III disease progression caused by the primary impingement. One study assessed the progression of impingement syndrome to a rotator cuff tear following an open acromioplasty.[68] The initial outcomes demonstrated that 69% of patients had good to excellent results; however, acromioplasty did not prevent a significant proportion of patients from progressing to a cuff tear. Of the 96 patients, 12 developed complete rotator cuff tears and 7 developed partial rotator cuff tears. Outcomes involving arthroscopic subacromial decompression are unknown.

SUBACROMIAL CORTICOSTEROID INJECTIONS

Although subacromial corticosteroid injections with lidocaine may be diagnostic and therapeutic as an adjunct to acute impingement rehabilitation, it is important to consider potential catabolic effects on healing tissue. There exists some controversy on subacromial injection during the subacute to chronic phase, when antiinflammatory measures are applied without regard for adequate cellular matrix adaptation. Even application of corticosteroids during the acute stage can have a negative effect on connective tissue because the strong antiinflammatory effect may abort the natural healing process.[69] On an anecdotal note, the effectiveness of cortisone injections as an antiinflammatory may indirectly interfere with impingement. When pain resolves, a patient may feel that everything is normal and not make efforts to correct impingement impairments that can be causing progressive staging of impingement and rotator cuff disease. The importance of properly training, conditioning, and correcting structural or functional impairments should be the foundation for successful outcomes involving subacromial impingement. Effective and ineffective uses of corticosteroids are identified in Table 32-3.[69]

CONSERVATIVE IMPINGEMENT PROTOCOLS

Primary Impingement

Phase I interventions for nonoperative primary impingement are integrated with Neer and Poppen[65] progressive stages of impingement to emphasize the importance of considering age, chronicity or severity of the condition, comorbidity, and level of participation. The examiner should consider the possibility that selective hypomobility of the posterior capsule can contribute to superior head migration and subacromial impingement. Finally, the examiner must consider that primary impingement can develop into a secondary impingement over time (Figure 32-9).

Secondary Impingement

Phase I to phase IV interventions for nonoperative secondary impingement involve criteria-based functional progression. Because secondary impingement involves many of the same structural impairments that are involved in primary impingement, phase I primary impingement intervention goals and strategies are considered within all phases of secondary impingement.

Text continued on p. 650

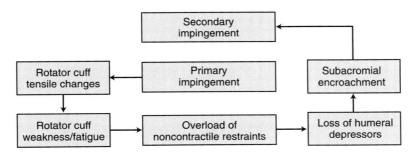

Figure 32-9: Proposed multifactorial etiology for the development of primary into secondary impingement.

TABLE 32-3

Effective and Ineffective Uses of Corticosteroids

EFFECTIVE USE OF CORTICOSTEROIDS	INEFFECTIVE USE OF CORTICOSTEROIDS
6-week preinjection trial of rest, adjusted level of play, conditioning	Administered during acute trauma
Discrete, palpable site of pain	Intratendinous injection
Peritendinous of inflammatory target tissue	Multiple injections (more than three)
Limit of three injections	Injection immediately before competition
Relative rest post injection (2-6 weeks)	Joint instability
Correct mechanical cause of injury	Undefined diagnosis

From Leadbetter WB: An introduction to sports-induced soft-tissue inflammation. In Leadbetter WB, Buckwalter JA, Gordon SL, editors: *Sports-induced inflammation: clinical and basic science concepts,* Park Ridge, IL, 1990, American Academy of Orthopaedic Surgeons, p 78.

Nonoperative Primary Impingement Protocol—Progressive Stage I Considerations (Schulte & Leetun)

Nonoperative Primary Impingement Stage I: Edema & Inflammation Phase I: Immediate Management **IMPAIRMENTS**	Intervention Goals & Strategies Stage I Phase I **INTERVENTION & GOALS**
Impaired joint mobility, motor function, muscle performance, and ROM associated with localized inflammation. • Supraspinatus • Subacromial bursa • Long-head biceps tendon • Acromioclavicular ligament **Test & Measures** • *Analog Scales* • *Description Index* • *Diagnostic Ultrasound* Impaired joint mobility, motor function, muscle performance, and ROM associated with connective tissue dysfunction. • Type II or III acromion • Coracoacromial ligament hypertrophy • Prominent humeral greater tuberosity **Test & Measures** • *Analog Scales* • *Description Index* • *Diagnostic Ultrasound*	GOAL: Decrease inflammation Modalities • Cryotherapy • Phonophoresis • Iontophoresis (dexamethasone) • Oral pharmacologics (NSAIDs) • Subacromial injection (10 ml 1% lidocaine) GOAL: Decrease dysfunctional movement pattern that is causing insult to respective tissue Activity modification • Relative rest: Avoid overhead activities that increase symptoms • Utilize biofeedback to increase neuromuscular control of the scapula musculature (Figure 32-10) • Retrain functional movement patterns GOAL: Increase joint arthrokinematics to improve osteo-kinematic overhead function Manual therapy (Grades 2, 3, 4) • Posterior glide of GH joint (Figure 32-11) • Anterior/inferior glide of sternoclavicular joint (Figure 32-12)

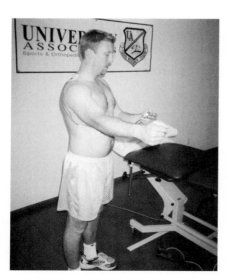

Figure 32-10: Upper trapezius inhibition with biofeedback.

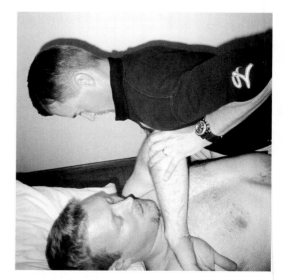

Figure 32-11: Posterior glide of the glenohumeral joint.

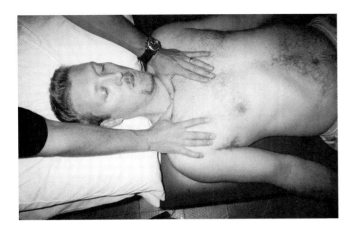

Figure 32-12: Anterior-inferior glide of the sternoclavicular joint.

Nonoperative Primary Impingement Protocol—Progressive Stage II Considerations (Schulte & Leetun)

Nonoperative Primary Impingement
Stage II: Fibrosis & Tendonitis
Phase I: Immediate Management

The structural impairments identified in Stage I are more severe in Stage II. The progressive nature of the tissue injury is sometimes not reversible by modification of activity alone. Additional impairments contributing to primary impingement may include the following

IMPAIRMENTS

Impaired posture
- Forward head
- Anterior tilted and downward rotated scapula
- Thoracic kyphosis
  Test & Measures
  - *Analog Scales*
  - *Description Index*
  - *Diagnostic Ultrasound*

Impaired muscle performance
- Reduced muscular extensibility in scapular downward rotators
- Reduced muscular extensibility of GH external rotators
- Reduced ST upward rotation and GH force couple
  Test & Measures
  - *Muscle Length Tests*
  - *Scapular Assist Test*

Intervention Goals & Strategies
Stage II
Phase I

Stage I Intervention Goals and Strategies may be included. Consideration involving the severity of tissue morbidity and healing potential should be considered to identify relevant goals and outcome expectations. Additional impairments contributing to primary impingement may include the following.

INTERVENTION

GOAL: Increase posture awareness and enhance body mechanics for improved postural stabilization.

Positional training
- Head nods

Scapular taping (Figures 32-13 & 32-14)
- Tape scapula into posterior tilt
- Tape scapula into upward rotation

Manual therapy (Grades 2, 3, 4)
- Thoracic extension mobilizations (Figure 32-15)
- Pectoralis stretch

GOAL: Increase length-tension characteristics of GH and ST force couples

Stretching
- Posterior cuff stretching (Figure 32-16)
- Rhomboid stretching
- Latissimus dorsi stretching

Nonoperative Primary Impingement Protocol—Progressive Stage III Considerations (Schulte & Leetun)

Nonoperative Primary Impingement
Stage III: Bone Spur & Tendon Rupture
Phase I: Immediate Management

The structural impairments identified in Stage III are not reversible and are significantly more debilitating considering the irreversible nature of chronic microtrauma and potential of complete tissue failure. At this stage impairments can contribute to a functional limitation. Functional limitations are measured by testing the performance of the patient's physical level.

FUNCTIONAL LIMITATION

Limited ability to perform vocational and avocational activities of daily living (ADLs) that are specific to the individual.

Test & Measures

• *DASH Questionaire*[73]

When the functional limitations cannot be remedied and the condition is progressing toward disability, appropriate surgical consultation is warranted to consider subacromial decompression and/or partial rotator cuff debridement (see arthroscopic subacromial decompression protocols)

Intervention Goals & Strategies
Stage III
Phase I

Functional limitation occurs when impairments result in restriction of the ability to perform a physical action, task, or activity in an efficient, typically expected, or competent manner. In Stage III, many of the impairments cannot be remedied by physical therapy intervention and an enablement strategy should be implemented to prevent disability.

INTERVENTION & GOALS

GOAL: Decrease compensatory strategies by using other abilities to accomplish the intended goal

Utilize contralateral extremity

• Neuromuscular re-education

• Active–assisted positioning

GOAL: Modify the task or environment to allow the patient to perform the activity within the restrictions that the patient's condition imposes

Utilize assistive devices

• Step ladder

• Ergonomic overhead friendly environment

It is essential that the correct diagnosis be made in order to properly select the appropriate surgical procedure that will counter the impairments and dysfunction.

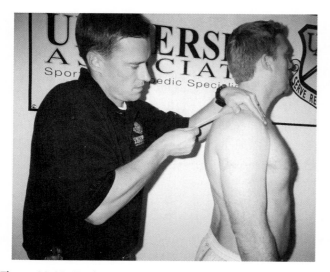

Figure 32-13: Taping to correct anterior scapular tilt.

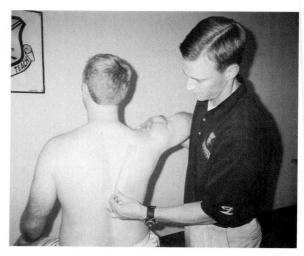

Figure 32-14: Taping to assist upward scapular rotation.

Nonoperative Secondary Impingement
Phase I: Preparation & Protection

The structural tissue injures and localized inflammation identified in primary impingement is also typically present in secondary impingement. The impairments, however, are caused more from functional characteristics than structural morphology.

IMPAIRMENTS

Impaired muscle performance (scapular weakness)

- Rhomboids
- Middle trapezius
- Lower trapezius
- Serratus anterior

  Test & Measures
  - *Manual Muscle Test*
  - *Lateral Scapular Slide Test*

Impaired posture (lumbopelvic control)

- Crossed pelvis syndrome

  Test & Measures
  - *Thomas Test*
  - *Hip Extension Muscle Activation Sequencing*

Impaired muscle performance (distal kinetic chain strength)

- Wrist flexors and extensor weakness

  Test & Measures
  - *Dynamoneter Testing*

Intervention Goals & Strategies
Tissue Preparation & Protection

Stage I Intervention Goals and Strategies for managing Primary Impingement inflammatory tissues are included. Special consideration of the underlying impairment of the secondary impingement (functional) is the early focus of this phase of the intervention.

INTERVENTION & GOALS

GOAL: Increase strength and endurance strengthening (below 90 degrees elevation)

- Manual scapular resistance (Figure 32-17)
- Scapular rhythmic stabilization
- Press-up (Figure 32-18)
- Chest press (+) (Figure 32-19)
- Rowing
- Scapular plane punch "full can" (Figure 32-20)

GOAL: Increase core strength and control

- Increase erector spinae and iliopsoas flexibility (Figure 32-21)
- Increase tranverse abdominus and gluteal maximus / medius facilitation (Figure 32-22)

GOAL: Increase total arm strength (TAS)

- Forearm WorkOut (WOW)
  - Flexion and extension (Figure 32-23)

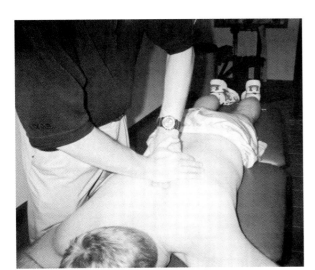

Figure 32-15: Thoracic mobilization to increase extension.

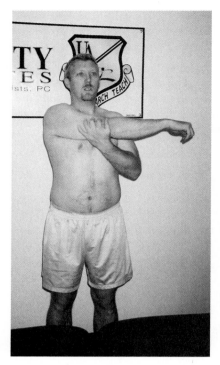

Figure 32-16: Posterior cuff stretching.

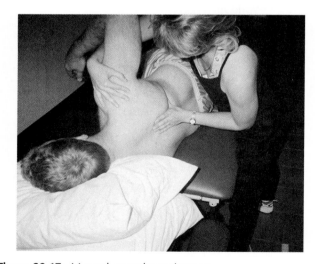

Figure 32-17: Manual scapular resistance.

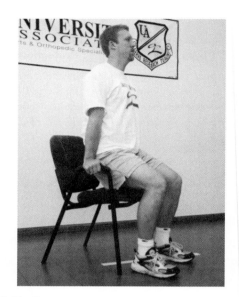

Figure 32-18: Press-up.

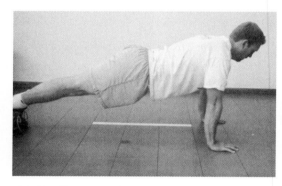

Figure 32-19: Chest-press (+).

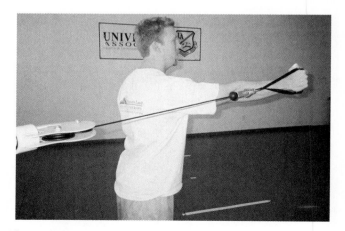

Figure 32-20: Scaption punch, "full can."

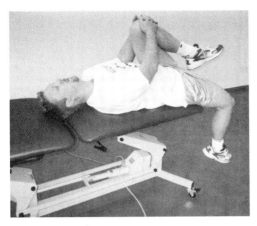

Figure 32-21: Iliopsoas stretch.

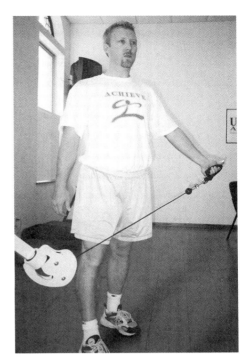

Figure 32-24: Deltoid pulley exercises.

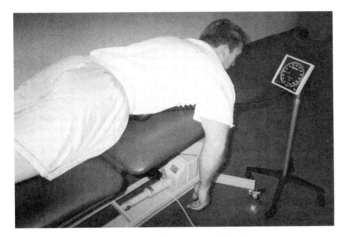

Figure 32-22: Transverse abdominus facilitation.

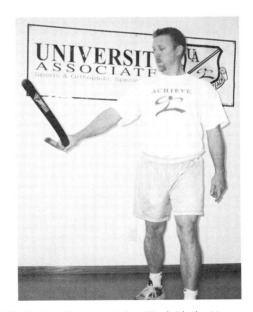

Figure 32-25: Oscillatory training (BodyBlade, Hymanson, Playa del Rey, CA) for deltoid.

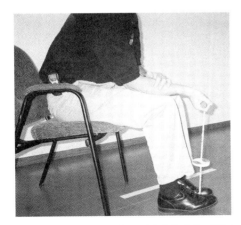

Figure 32-23: Oscillatory training with WorkOutWhizzer (WOW, Wilson J. Innovative Fitness, Green Bay, WI) for total arm strengthening.

Nonoperative Secondary Impingement Protocol—Rehabilitation Phase II
(Schulte & Leetun)

Nonoperative Secondary Impingement
Stage II: Intermediate Phase

Criteria for progression to Phase II.
- *The localized inflammation in associated tissues should be controlled or significantly diminished.*
- *Improved scapular muscle function.*
- *Patient is able to control exacerbation of symptoms*

IMPAIRMENTS

Impaired muscle performance (GH force couple)
- Deltoid
- Supraspinatus
- Subscapularis
- Teres minor and infraspinatus
  Test & Measures
  - *Electroneuromyography*
  - *Manual Muscle Testing*

Impaired muscle performance (ST force couple)
- Upper trapezius
- Lower trapezius
- Serratus anterior
  Test & Measures
  - *Manual Muscle Test*
  - *Videoanalysis*

Intervention Goals & Strategies
Proximal Stability for Distal Mobility

Phase II Intervention Goals include enhancing the scapular platform control and initiating strengthening involving distal force couples (GH and ST). Closed-kinetic chain exercises are integrated to stimulate co-contraction and promote scapulohumeral control and stability.

INTERVENTION & GOALS

GOAL: Increase strength and endurance strengthening (below 90 degrees elevation)
Deltoid concentric/eccentrics (30-60 degrees)
- Standing pulley (Figure 32-24)
- Standing bodyblade (Figure 32-25)

Rotator cuff/Swiss ball
- Seated "full can" pulley (scaption) (Figure 32-26)
- Seated Diagonal I and Diagonal II PNF pulley (Figure 32-27)
- Seated WOWs (internal and external rotation [IR and ER] modified neutral) (Figure 32-28)

GOAL: Increase ST neuromuscular control
Biofeedback: neuromuscular re-education
- Upper trapezius inhibition (see Figure 32-10)
- Mirror motion
- 90-degree scaption "laser show" (Figure 32-29)

Closed kinetic chain
Swiss ball
- Prone on elbows (Figure 32-30)
- Prone on elbows (Figure 32-30)
- Scapular walk-out (Figure 32-31)
- Balance board (Figure 32-32)

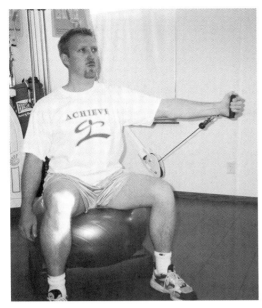

Figure 32-26: Dynamic seated "full can" pulleys (scaption) for rotator cuff strengthening.

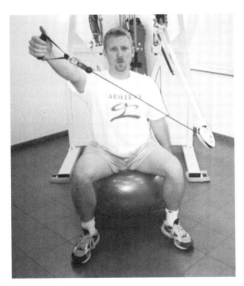

Figure 32-27: Dynamic seated diagonal pulleys (proprioceptive neuromuscular facilitation) for rotator cuff strengthening.

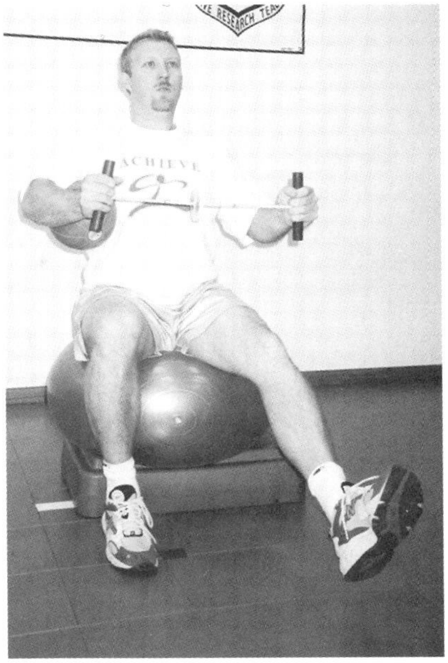

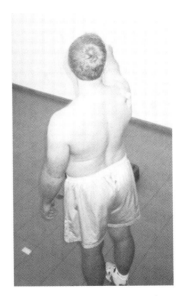

Figure 32-28: Dynamic seated oscillatory training (WOW, Wilson J. Innovative Fitness, Green Bay, WI) for rotator cuff strengthening.

Figure 32-29: Scapulothoracic neuromuscular reeducation with laser pointers.

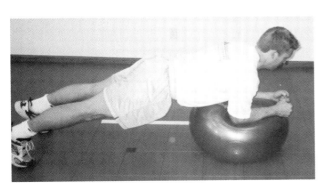

Figure 32-30: Scapulothoracic closed kinetic chain prone on elbow.

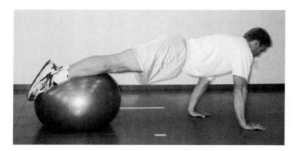

Figure 32-31: Scapulothoracic closed kinetic chain scapular walk-out.

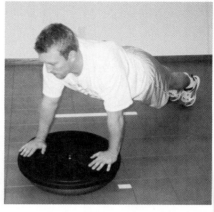

Figure 32-32: Scapulothoracic closed kinetic chain balance board training.

Nonoperative Secondary Impingement Protocol—Rehabilitation Phase III (Schulte & Leetun)

Nonoperative Secondary Impingement Phase III: Advanced Strengthening

Criteria for progression to Phase III.
- *Improved GH strength.*
- *Improved ST endurance.*
- *Normal active assisted ROM.*

IMPAIRMENTS

Impaired muscle performance (humeral head depressors)
- Long head of the bicep
- Rotator cuff

Test & Measures
- *Palpation*
- *Electroneuromyography*
- *Manual Muscle Testing*

Impaired motor function and muscle performance (proprioceptive and kinesthesia deficiency)
- Upper extremity
- Trunk
- Lower extremity

Intervention Goals & Strategies Integrated Force Couple Control

Phase III intervention goals include enhancing integrated GH and ST movement patterns and creating a posterior dominant shoulder (ER / IR to 3:4)

INTERVENTION & GOALS

GOAL: Increase depressor functions of the long head of bicep mechanism to decrease humeral head superior migration

Proprioceptive neuromuscular facilitation (PNF) / Lunge position

Diagonal I (DI) pain-free range (bicep/subscapularis)
- 30-degree WOW progressions (Figure 32-33)
- Bodyblade

Diagonal II (DII) pain-free range (posterior cuff)
- 30-degree WOW progressions
- Bodyblade (Figure 32-34)

Rotator cuff concentric/eccentric pulleys
- Shoulder horn (Figure 32-35)

GOAL: Increase quality and quantity of movement between and across body segments

PNF / rhythmic stabilization
- Multiple direction
- Slow → fast
- Isometric → dynamic

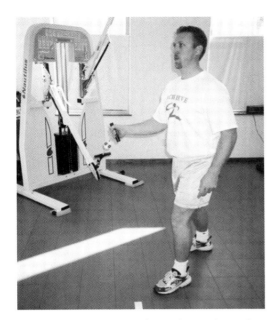

Figure 32-33: Dynamic Diagonal 1 (DI) proprioceptive neuromuscular facilitation oscillatory training (WOW).

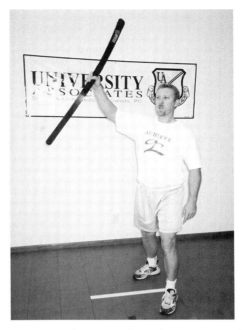

Figure 32-34: Dynamic DI proprioceptive neuromuscular facilitation oscillatory training (BodyBlade, Hymanson, Playa del Rey, CA).

Nonoperative Secondary Impingement Protocol—Rehabilitation Phase III (Schulte & Leetun)—cont'd

Test & Measures

- *K.A.T System*
- *Timed test*
- *Videoanalysis*

Impaired muscle performance (150-180 degrees)

Serratus anterior

- Lower fibers (isometric control)
- Upper fibers (eccentric control)
- Lower trapezius (concentric control)

    Test & Measures

    - *Palpation*
    - *Electroneuromyography*
    - *Manual Muscle Testing*

Joint position replication training

- Static scaption targeting
- Dynamic scaption targeting
    - Unilateral standing
    - Trampoline
    - BOSU (Figure 32-36)

GOAL: Increase serratus neuromuscular (150-180 degrees) control at provocative positions.

Overhead ball compressions (10 second hold) (Figure 32-37)

Overhead pulley pulls 1 count concentric / 2 count eccentric (Figure 32-38)

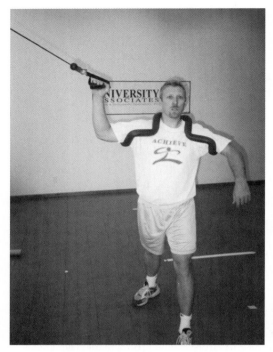

Figure 32-35: Dynamic concentric/eccentric pulleys with Shoulder Horn (Final Designs, Highlands Ranch, CO).

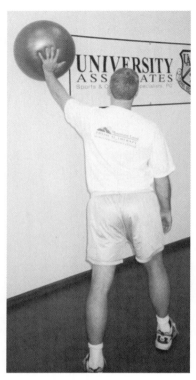

Figure 32-37: Serratus overhead ball compression.

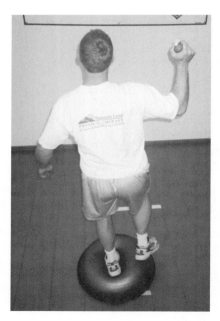

Figure 32-36: Dynamic joint position replication training on Both Sides Up (BOSU) Balance Trainer (DW Fitness, Canton, OH).

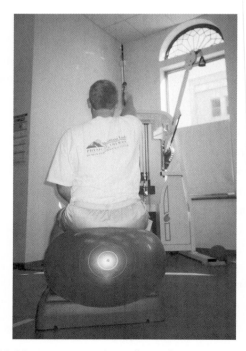

Figure 32-38: Lower trapezius pulley pulls.

Nonoperative Secondary Impingement Protocol—Rehabilitation Phase IV
(Schulte & Leetun)

Nonoperative Secondary Impingement
Phase IV: Return to Activity

Criteria for progression to Phase IV.
- *GH & ST functional neuromuscular control*
- *Posterior dominant shoulder*
- *Posterior capsule mobility*
- *Nonprovocative special tests*
- *Full, nonpainful ROM*

OBJECTIVE TESTING CRITERIA

Isokinetic / manual dynamometer testing

Increased unilateral ER/IR relationship by 10% to 76%

AROM

Isolated GH IR demonstrates appropriate ROM. (60-70 degrees)

SportsRAC (Sports Rehabilitation And Coordination)

Achievement of level 6-7 with excellent GH control and synchrony achievement scores

Nonprovocative special tests of impingement

Neers

Hawkins Kennedy

Coracoid

Crossover

Functional Test & Measures

- *Functional Throwing Performance Index*
- *Pitch Velocity (radar gun)*
- *Biomechanical Video Analysis*

Intervention Goals & Strategies
Performance Enhancement

Phase IV Intervention Goals include enhancing strength and conditioning parameters that improve power and performance related to the activity. Integration of interval programs that include throwing, racquet, and hitting activities should be included.

PERFORMANCE ENHANCEMENT

GOAL: Increase power and speed

Plyometrics

Core exercises
- Two-handed throw with trunk rot
- Two-handed throw with sit-up (Figure 32-39)

Rotator cuff plyoback
- Shoulder horn
- Retro throwing (Figure 32-40)
- Isolated GH plyometrics 90°/90°

GOAL: Increase quality and quantity of movement between and across body segments

Lower extremity
- Lunges
- Single leg hop
- Cross over hop

Swiss ball (TBS)

Prone alternate arm / leg lift with lumbopelvic stabilization
- Prone middle trap (Figure 32-41)
- Prone lower trap (Figure 32-42)

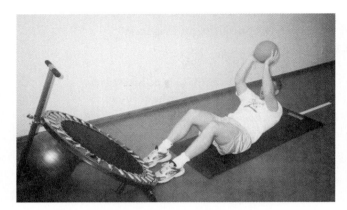

Figure 32-39: Plyometric two-hand throw with sit-up.

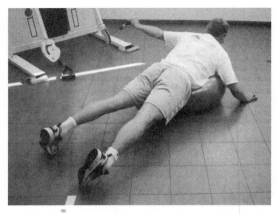

Figure 32-41: Dynamic middle trapezius strengthening on Swiss ball.

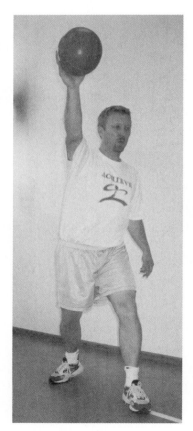

Figure 32-40: Plyometric retro throwing for posterior cuff deceleration.

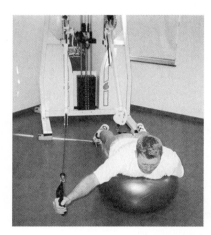

Figure 32-42: Dynamic lower trapezius strengthening on Swiss ball.

ARTHROSCOPIC SUBACROMIAL DECOMPRESSION

The emphasis of decompression addresses the anterior one third of the acromion. Studies by Caspari and Thal[22] have indicated that flattening of the anterior third of the acromion successfully improves impingement. Neer's original technique of anterior acromioplasty involves detachment of a small segment of the deltoid origin anteriorly to allow subacromial access.[44] He indicated the need to remove a wedge-shaped portion of bone from the anterior acromion tapered anterior to posterior approximately 2 cm. Ellman[70] initially described arthroscopic acromioplasty. With arthroscopic acromioplasty, the acromion is initially dealt with from the lateral portal by resecting any spurring that would occur on the acromion anterior to the clavicle itself. Release by complete resection of the coracoacromial ligament is not carried out at this time. With the scope placed in the lateral portal, a burr is brought in from posterior and, using a cutting block technique, the acromion is turned into a type I acromion for the anterior one third of the acromion. Attention is then returned to visualizing posterior with bringing the burr in laterally, trying to remove the lateral tilt of the acromion. This also allows a 90/90 view of the acromion to ensure that a flat surface is obtained viewing laterally as well as posteriorly. A benefit of arthroscopic subacromial decompression is elimination of any deltoid detachment, allowing for active early rehabilitation because protection of a deltoid repair is not required. This postoperative protocol can be more aggressive, with early elimination of sling protection and early aggressive restoration of ROM and strengthening therapeutic exercises.

OPERATIVE CONSIDERATIONS AND REHABILITATION PHILOSOPHY

Successful outcomes involving subacromial decompression are based on correctly diagnosing the cause of the underlying impairment. Performing arthroscopic subacromial decompression will not necessarily alleviate impingement when the cause is from capsular laxity or GH instability. An improper diagnosis can lead to an inappropriate surgical procedure and potentially set a course for failure involving rehabilitation. If subacromial decompression is determined to be the best course of management, an anterior acromioplasty is the recommended procedure because this region is primarily responsible for rotator cuff impingement. Consideration involving complete acromioplasty resection should be implemented cautiously. This procedure involves a posterior acromioplasty that disrupts the deltoid attachment and undermines the deltoid supraspinatus force couple. This can unnecessarily complicate the rehabilitation process and lead to less than optimal outcomes. Finally, many cases involving arthroscopic subacromial impingement may have combined surgical procedures. After arthroscopic subacromial decompression with partial rotator cuff debridement, rehabilitation providers must consider a variety of tissue healing characteristics that will drive rehabilitation progression. Contractile tissue healing dynamics involving rotator cuff repair will often supercede the arthroscopic subacromial decompression progression when performed as a combination surgical procedure. Information related to postoperative rehabilitation involving rotator cuff repair is discussed in Chapter 33.

ARTHROSCOPIC SUBACROMIAL DECOMPRESSION WITH DISTAL CLAVICLE RESECTION

The rehabilitation protocol must consider the bony and soft tissue trauma that is associated with impaired joint mobility, motor function, muscle performance, and ROM. Important functional impairments that must be addressed include total body strength, GH and ST force couples, neuromuscular control, and correction of biomechanical faults. Utilization of early neuromuscular and fine motor control technologies during the early phases of healing is useful to counter the detrimental effects of immobilization. The protocol also uses a variety of oscillatory training devices that have demonstrated increased proprioceptive training in subjects.[71] Utilization of nonoperative phase protocol techniques identified in this chapter (taping, modalities, and adjunctive techniques) can be readily implemented in arthroscopic subacromial decompression to address identified impairments. It should be remembered that the protocols are not strictly prescriptive, but rather guidelines that offer impairment-based strategies. Empirical observations have identified that clinical exacerbation of symptoms spike during the start of postoperative phase II subacromial decompression with clavicle resection. Davies[72] postulates two possible reasons for pain recurrence and exacerbation during phase II:

1. The patient's shoulder feels significantly better than it had during the progressive preoperative impingement period; therefore the patient begins to move the shoulder more, increasing pain.

2. The progressive nature of therapeutic exercise demands during rehabilitation increase pain.

During the end of phase II (6 to 8 weeks), patients start to have decreased pain with overhead activities. A reason for the improvement may be related to the synovialization that occurs over the bare denuded exposed bone and exposed free nerve endings. During this period a pseudomembrane develops over the denuded bone and symptoms decrease significantly. The ability of the provider to anticipate the potential for symptom variances and prognostic indicators may help prepare patients for some of the expectations and challenges that they may experience as they progress rehabilitation. Anticipating these variances may decrease patient anxiety and frustrations during rehabilitation. Ultimately, modification, progression, and deviation of the protocol should always be considered and driven by individual circumstances that should be continually evaluated and assessed.

Text continued on p. 660

Arthroscopic Subacromial Decompression—With Distal Clavicle Resection Phase I
(Schulte & Leetun)

Phase I: Immediate Postoperative
Weeks: 0-3

Contraindications / Instructions

Range of motion:
- *Flexion < 120°*
- *ER < 45°*
- *Abduction < 45°*
- *Horizontal adduction*

Resistance exercises:
- *Avoid rotation exercises with unsupported modified neutral position of the shoulder (30°/30°/30°)*
- *Motions should be active assisted*

Immobilization:
- *Discontinuance of a sling should be encouraged within 10 days*
- *Use for protection / deterrent if there is risk for physical contact in public (crowded mall, etc.)*

IMPAIRMENTS

Impaired joint mobility, motor function, muscle performance, and ROM associated with bony or soft tissue surgery

Pain

Test & Measures
- *Analog Scales*
- *Description Index*
- *Questionnaire*

Decreased ROM
- Impaired joint mobility
  - ST
  - Sternoclavicular
  - GH

Phase I: Immediate Postoperative
Weeks: 0-3

Phase I Intervention
Goals and Strategies

The primary goal for managing postoperative subacromial decompression during Phase I is to reduce the effects of immobilization, control inflammation, and promote early neuromuscular control of the shoulder. TAS initiatives should be facilitated immediately including scapular, forearm, and hand musculature. Home instruction should focus primarily on posterior capsular stretching exercises and self-applied therapeutic modalities for pain control (cryotherapy / moist heat).

INTERVENTION & GOALS

GOAL: Decrease pain quality and quantity

Therapeutic modalities
- Iontophoresis
- Microcurrent
- Interferential current
- Ultrasound
- Cryotherapy
- TENS

Medications
- Dexamethasone (iontophoresis)
- Narcotics (decrease dependency after 2 weeks)
- NSAIDs (persistent pain)

GOAL: Increase ROM

ST (side-lying supported scaption)
- Scapular mobilization
- Thoracic anterior/posterior glides

Arthroscopic Subacromial Decompression—With Distal Clavicle Resection Phase I (Schulte & Leetun)—cont'd

Test & Measures
- *End-feel*
- *Goniometry*
- *Impingement Tests*
- *Videographics*

Decreased strength and endurance due to inactivity
- TAS weakness

  Test & Measures
  - *Electroneuromyography*
  - *Dynamometer*
  - *Manual Muscle Test*
  - *Videographics*

Decreased neuromuscular control
- Impaired joint kinesthesia
  - Upper extremity kinetic chain

  Test & Measures
  - *Joint Replication Scores*
  - *Coordination & Synchrony Proficiency Scores (SportsRac)*
  - *Videographics*

Limited independence in activities of daily living
- Impaired ability to dress without exacerbating shoulder symptoms
- Impaired ability to reach overhead for personal items

Test & Measures
- *Observation*
- *Interview*
- *ADL Scales*

Sternoclavicular (supine supported scaption)
- Anterior/inferior glides

GH (supine supported scaption)
- GH distraction
- Posterior glide
- Inferior glide

Lateral rotator and postcapsule stretch (Figure 32-43A and B)
- S^4 positions (supine and side-lying supported scaption)

GOAL: Increase TAS

Scapula (side-lying supported scaption)
- Scapular squeeze
- Scapular clocks (Figure 32-44)
- Manual scapular resistance

Forearm and hand
- WOWs (flexion and extension)
- Grip strength

GOAL: Improve fine motor control and coordinated muscle function in the shoulder or forearm while managing the inflammatory process

SportsRac
- Progress setting that is one setting less than pain-free abduction
- Challenge total body kinetic chain

GOAL: Improved ability to perform physical actions and tasks related to self care and home management

Donning/doffing clothes
- Suggested button down shirt, sweater, and jacket vs. pullover type

Ergonomic modification
- Modify cupboard height by utilizing step ladder to avoid excessive overhead activism during the acute phase of rehabilitation

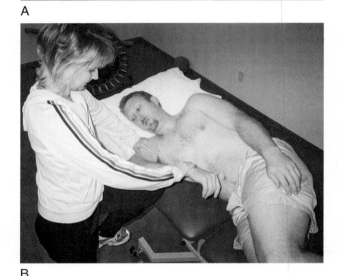

A

B

Figure 32-43: **A,** S⁴ lateral rotator and posterior capsule stretch (supine). **B,** S⁴ lateral rotator and posterior capsule stretch (side lying).

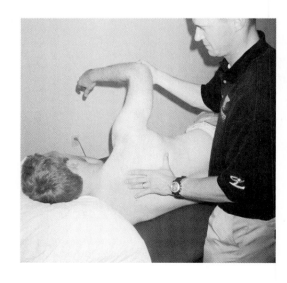

Figure 32-44: Scapular clocks.

Arthroscopic Subacromial Decompression—With Distal Clavicle Resection Phase II (Schulte & Leetun)

Phase II: Intermediate Postoperative
Weeks: 3-6

Criteria for Progression to Phase II

- *Resolving pain & controlled nonreactive inflammation*
- *120-degree flexion; 45-degree ER and abduction*
- *Adequate joint arthrokinematics*
- *Good ST control*

Contraindications/Instructions

Range of Motion:

- *Flexion < 150 degrees*
- *ER < 60 degrees*
- *Abduction < 90 degrees*
- *IR < 45 degrees*
- *Horizontal adduction*

Resistance exercises:

- *Perform all rotation exercises with the shoulder in modified neutral position (30°/30°/30°)*
- *Activities should progress from isometric to isotonic controlled motion exercises*

IMPAIRMENTS

Impaired joint mobility, motor function, muscle performance, and ROM associated with bony of soft tissue surgery

Pain

Test & Measures

- *Analog Scales*
- *Description Index*
- *Questionnaire*

Impaired muscle performance

- GH force couple
  - ▪ Teres minor and infraspinatus
  - ▪ Subscapularis
  - ▪ Supraspinatus
- ST force couple
  - ▪ Upper trapezius
  - ▪ Lower trapezius
  - ▪ Serratus anterior

Phase II: Intermediate Postoperative
Weeks: 3-6

Phase II Intervention

Goals and Strategies

The primary goal for managing postoperative subacromial decompression during Phase II is to eliminate residual pain, enhance proximal control, and promote GH and ST force couples. Closed-kinetic chain exercises are integrated to stimulate co-contraction and promote scapulohumeral control and stability. Utilization of oscillatory training devices is implemented to advance neuromuscular control and kinesthesia. Activities should be performed in positions that challenge total body control. Close monitoring of activity tolerance is essential to ensure progression

INTERVENTION & GOALS

Resistance exercises should focus on quality not quantity. A limit of 20 reps per each exercise is initially recommended. Progress patient's speed/resistance before repetitions.

GOAL: Decrease pain quality and quantity

Therapeutic modalities

- Heat before / cryotherapy after treatment
- Discontinue as appropriate

Medications

- Decrease NSAID dependency

Subacromial injection (see remarks)

GOAL: Increase strength and endurance

Closed-kinetic chain rotator cuff isometrics

- Joint approximation with Swiss ball (IR/ER/scaption) (Figure 32-45)

Closed-kinetic chain scapular stabilization

- Prone on elbows (Figure 32-46)

(continued)

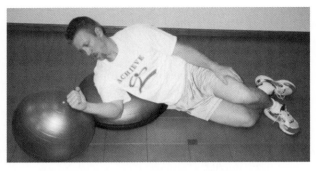

Figure 32-45: Closed kinetic chain Swiss ball approximations.

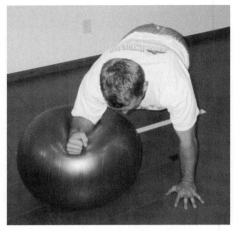

Figure 32-46: Closed kinetic chain Swiss ball prone on elbows.

Arthroscopic Subacromial Decompression—With Distal Clavicle Resection Phase II (Schulte & Leetun)—cont'd

Test & Measures
- *Palpation*
- *Electroneuromyography*
- *Manual Muscle Test*
- *Videographics*

Decreased neuromuscular control
- Impaired joint kinesthesia
  - Upper extremity kinetic chain

Test & Measures
- *Joint Replication Scores*
- *Coordination & Synchrony Proficiency Scores (SportsRac)*
- *Videographics*

- Tripod position
- Modified pull-up (Figure 32-47)
- Progress to phase II nonoperative neuromuscular control exercise protocol

Open kinetic chain rotator cuff isotonics (Scaption)
- BodyBlade
- WorkOutWhizzer
- BOING (Figure 32-48)
- Progress to phase II nonoperative rotator cuff Swiss ball exercise protocol

GOAL: Normalize fine motor control and coordinated muscle function in the shoulder or forearm while in functional positions

SportsRac
- Progress setting through level six
- Challenge total body kinetic chain

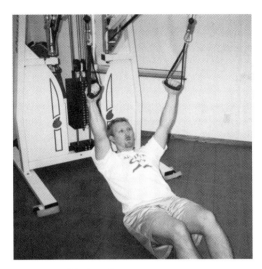

Figure 32-47: Modified pull-up.

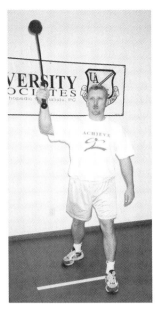

Figure 32-48: Body Oscillation Integrates Neuromuscular Gain (BOING) (OPTP Orthopedic Physical Therapy Products, Minneapolis, MN) rotator cuff training in scaption.

Arthroscopic Subacromial Decompression—With Distal Clavicle Resection Phase III (Schulte & Leetun)

Phase III: Advanced Strengthening
Weeks: 6-10

Criteria for Progression to Phase III

- *Pain-free ROM*
- *No positive signs for impingement*
- *Strength deficits < 30% of contralateral shoulder*
- *Excellent ST control in functional positions*

Contraindications / Instructions

- *Begin horizontal adduction movements as tolerated*
- *Prevent loss of IR motion*

Resistance exercises:

- *Perform exercises with the shoulder in sport/occupation required functional positions*
- *Activities should progress from isotonic to plyometric / power facilitated functional exercises*
- *Consider isokinetics but emphasize functional speed mechanics*

Phase III: Advanced Strengthening
Weeks: 6-10

Phase III Intervention

Goals and Strategies

The primary goal for managing postoperative subacromial decompression during Phase III is to improve endurance and power characteristics and prepare for progressive return to functional activities. Plyometric exercises are integrated to simulate repeated stretch-shortening cycles involved in functional movement patterns. Utilization of advanced PNF diagonals are integrated with oscillatory training devices to advance neuromuscular control and total body kinetics. Close monitoring of activity performance is essential to ensure proper mechanics and safety.

(continued)

Arthroscopic Subacromial Decompression—With Distal Clavicle Resection Phase III (Schulte & Leetun)—cont'd

IMPAIRMENTS	INTERVENTION & GOALS

Impaired joint mobility, motor function, muscle performance, and ROM associated with bony or soft tissue surgery

Decreased neuromuscular control
- Impaired functional overhead position joint kinesthesia

Test & Measures
- *High Speed Video*
- *Coordination & Synchrony Proficiency Scores (SportsRac)*

Impaired muscle performance (eccentric/decelerate loading)
- Scapula
  - Rhomboids
  - Pectoralis minor
  - Serratus anterior
- Rotator cuff
  - Infraspinatus and teres minor
  - Subscapularis

Test & Measures
- *Palpation*
- *Electroneuromyography*
- *Manual Muscle Test*
- *Isokinetic Testing*

Advanced strengthening is emphasized; however maintaining an aggressive stretching program in selective hypomobility (especially IR) is essential.

GOAL: Increase quality and quantity of movement between and across body segments

PNF / pulleys in functional position
- DI: functional range
- DII: functional range

Oscillatory training devices in functional position (Figure 32-49)
- DI: functional range
- DII: functional range

GOAL: Increase control of proximal to distal deceleration stresses

Plyometrics
- Rhythmic stabilization functional position (quick stretch)
- See Phase III plyometric nonoperative secondary impingement protocol

Open and closed kinetic chain scapular stabilization
- Upper extremity closed kinetic chain stability test UECKCST (Figure 32-50)
- Stairmaster upper extremity
- Scapular decelerations (Figure 32-51)
- Progress to Phase II nonoperative neuromuscular control exercise protocol

Resistance should be increased with appropriate recovery time between workouts to prevent overtraining and reactive inflammation

TBS should focus on core and lower extremity strength and endurance (see Phase II nonoperative secondary impingement)

Advance sport specific biomechanics into regimen at 50%-75% intensity

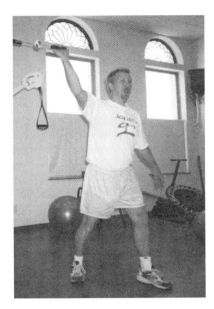

Figure 32-49: Oscillatory training involving activity-specific functional range.

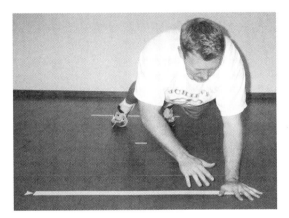

Figure 32-50: Upper extremity closed kinetic chain stability training.

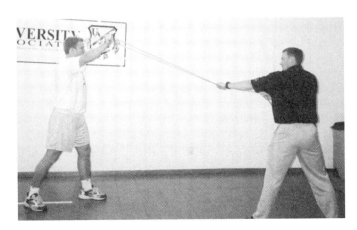

Figure 32-51: Surgical tubing scapular decelerations.

Arthroscopic Subacromial Decompression—With Distal Clavicle Resection Phase IV (Schulte & Leetun)

Phase IV: Return to Activity
Weeks: 10-14

Criteria for Progression to Phase IV
- *Pain-free ROM*
- *No positive signs for impingement*
- *Strength deficits < 10% of contralateral shoulder*
- *Patient efficacy with maintenance program and recurrence prevention*

Contraindications / instructions
- *Dysfunctional kinetic chain compensations*
- *Perform foundational shoulder exercises ("Magnificent 7")*
  - *ER/IR rotation stretch*
  - *ER/IR strength exercise (emphasize posterior dominant shoulder)*
  - *Full cans*
  - *Pectoralis door stretch*
  - *Prone middle and lower trapezius exercises*
  - *Serratus punch*
  - *Bicep curls*

DISCHARGE CRITERIA

Achievement of anticipated goals and expected outcomes

Structural and functional impairments have been remedied in order to improve function and prevent disability

Test & Measures
- **Athletic Shoulder Outcome Rating Scale Tibone & Bradley[74]**

Phase IV: Return to Activity
Weeks: 10-14

Phase IV Intervention
Goals and Strategies

The primary goal for managing postoperative subacromial decompression during Phase IV is unrestricted return to functional activities and independent maintenance for injury prevention.

Progressive interval program for overhead sports should be implemented and advanced as outlined
- *Throwing athlete*
- *Tennis player*
- *Golf athlete*

Optimize specific sport / occupational biomechanics to increase performance and decrease injury recurrences

Isolated acromioplasty is likely to improve two times faster then an acromioplasty with a distal clavicle resection. (It is advised that horizontal adduction isn't started after 8 weeks in most cases involving clavicle resection.)

OUTCOMES

Improved GH and ST force couples and neuromuscular control needed to depress humeral head with overhead activities. Resolved structural (primary) and functional (secondary) impingement impairments.

GOAL: Increase adherence to preventative strategies and reduce risks that may undermine future health-related quality of life factors.

SUMMARY

Functional requirements of the shoulder have evolved over time with varying demands of occupations and sport-specific movements. The shoulder is an inherently unstable joint based on the anatomic relationship of the glenoid and the humeral head. The shoulder complex is actually composed of the ST, sternoclavicular, GH, and acromioclavicular joints working together in a synergistic manner to produce a functional outcome. Evaluation and treatment of shoulder injuries should focus on pathology and dysfunction related to impaired ST and GH force couples, acromioclavicular osteokinematics, and resulting subacromial space impingement. Impairment-based diagnosis, etiology, and impingement classifications should be used when one treats these conditions. Intervention of subacromial impingement includes conservative, nonoperative, operative, therapeutic exercise, neuromuscular reeducation, and other evidence-based rehabilitation protocols (Box 32-1).

BOX 32-1

Rehabilitation Program Following Subacromial Decompression/Distal Clavicle Resection: Protocol Outline (Schulte and Leetun)

I. Phase I—Immediate Postoperative Phase: "Controlled Motion" (Weeks 0 to 3)

Goals

Protect the anatomic repair

Prevent negative effects of immobilization; progress passive to active ROM; goals:

- 100 degrees of flexion as tolerated
- 45 degrees of ER
- 45 degrees of abduction as tolerated

Promote TAS

Diminish pain and inflammation

Weeks 0 to 3

- Sling worn for comfort: 1 week
- Discontinue sling: week 2
- Elbow/hand ROM
- Scapular squeeze
- Scapular clocks
- Manual scapular resistance
- Hand gripping exercises
- Pulleys/T-bar
- Scapular mobilization
- Thoracic anterior-posterior glides
- Passive and gentle active-assisted ROM exercise: NO resisted motions during first 2 weeks
  - Week 1: flexion to 80 degrees
  - Week 2: flexion to 100 degrees
  - Elevation in scapular plane to 80 degrees
  - ER to 45 degrees
  - IR to 20 degrees
- Submaximal isometrics for shoulder musculature at 2 weeks
- Cryotherapy, modalities as indicated

II. Phase II—Intermediate Phase (Weeks 3 to 6)

Goals

Increase ROM as tolerated; ROM goals:

- 120 degrees of flexion
- 60 degrees of ER and abduction
- 45 degrees of IR

Perform all rotation exercises with the shoulder in modified neutral position (30°/30°/30°)

Activities should progress from isometric to isotonic controlled motion exercises

Closed kinetic chain exercises are integrated to stimulate co-contraction and promote scapulohumeral control and stability

Utilization of oscillatory training devices is implemented to advance neuromuscular control and kinesthesia

Weeks 3 to 5

- Closed kinetic chain exercises are integrated to stimulate co-contraction and promote scapulohumeral control and stability
  - Prone on elbows
  - Tripod position
  - Modified pull-up

Weeks 5 to 6

- Open kinetic chain rotator cuff isotonics (scaption)
  - BodyBlade
  - WorkOutWhizzer
  - BOING
  - Progress to phase II nonoperative rotator cuff Swiss ball exercise protocol

III. Phase III—Advanced Strengthening Phase (Weeks 6 to 10)

Criteria to Enter Phase III

- Pain-free ROM
- No positive signs of impingement
- Strength deficits less than 30% of contralateral shoulder
- Excellent ST control in functional positions
- Progress to functional activities

Weeks 6 to 8

- Proprioceptive neuromuscular facilitation/pulleys in functional position
  - DI functional range
  - DII functional range

(continued)

BOX 32-1

Rehabilitation Program Following Subacromial Decompression/Distal Clavicle Resection: Protocol Outline (Schulte and Leetun)—cont'd

- Oscillatory training devices in functional position
  - DI functional range
  - DII functional range

Weeks 8 to 10
- Plyometrics
  - Rhythmic stabilization functional position (quick stretch)
  - See phase III plyometric nonoperative secondary impingement protocol
- Open kinetic chain and closed kinetic chain scapular stabilization
  - UECKCST
  - Stairmaster upper extremity
  - Scapular decelerations
- Progress to phase II nonoperative neuromuscular control exercise protocol
- Resistance should be increased with appropriate recovery time between workouts to prevent overtraining and reactive inflammation
- TBS should focus on core and lower extremity strength and endurance; advance sport-specific biomechanics into regimen at 50% to 75 % intensity

IV. Phase IV—Return to Activity Phase (Weeks 10 to 14)

Criteria for progression to Phase IV
- Pain-free ROM
- No positive signs of impingement
- Strength deficits less than 10% of contralateral shoulder
- Patient efficacy with maintenance program and recurrence prevention

Contraindications/Instructions
- Dysfunctional kinetic chain compensations

Perform Foundational Shoulder Exercises
- "Magnificent 7"
- ER/IR stretch
- ER/IR strength exercises (emphasize posterior dominant shoulder)
- Full cans
- Pectoralis door stretch
- Prone middle and lower trapezius exercises
- Serratus punch
- Bicep curls

Weeks 12 to 14
- The primary goal for managing postoperative subacromial decompression during phase IV is unrestricted return to functional activities and independent maintenance for injury prevention
- Progressive interval program for overhead sports should be implemented and advanced as outlined
  - Throwing athlete
  - Tennis player
  - Golf athlete
- Optimize specific sport/occupational biomechanics to performance and injury recurrences
- Isolated acromioplasty is likely to improve twice as fast as an acromioplasty with a distal clavicle resection (horizontal adduction is not started until after 8 weeks in most cases involving clavicle resection)

Maintenance Program
- Advance activities to unrestrictive participation
- Maintain consistency with stretching and strengthening program

References

1. Meyer AW: The minute anatomy of attrition lesions, *J Bone Joint Surg* 13:341-348, 1931.

2. Meyer AW: Chronic functional lesions of the shoulder, *Arch Surg* 35:646-674, 1937.

3. Neer CS II: Anterior acromioplasty for chronic impingement in the shoulder: a preliminary report, *J Bone Joint Surg* 54A:41-50, 1972.

4. Neer CS II: Cuff tears, biceps lesions, and impingement. In Neer CS II, editor: *Shoulder reconstruction,* Philadelphia, 1990, Saunders, pp 41-142.

5. Sigholm G, Styf J, Korner L, et al: Pressure recordings in the subacromial bursa, *J Orthop Res* 6:123-128, 1988.

6. Bigliani LU, Morrison DS, April EW: The morphology of the acromion and its relationship to rotator cuff tears, *Orthop Trans* 10:228, 1986.

7. Morrison DS, Bigliani LU: The clinical significance of variations in acromial morphology, *Orthop Trans* 11:234, 1987.

8. Wuh HCK, Snyder SJ: A modified classification of the supraspinatus outlet view based on configuration and the anatomic thickness of the acromion, *Orthop Trans* 16:767, 1992.

9. Edelson JG, Taitz C: Anatomy of the coracoacromial arch: relationship to the degeneration of the acromion, *J Bone Joint Surg* 74B:589-594, 1992.

10. Gartsman GM: Arthroscopic acromioplasty for lesions of the rotator cuff, *J Bone Joint Surg* 72A:169, 1990.

11. Banas MP, Miller RJ, Totterman S: Relationship between the lateral acromial angle and rotator cuff disease, *J Shoulder Elbow Surg* 4:454-461, 1995.

12. Bigliani LU, Norris TR, Fischer J, et al: The relationship between the unfused acromial epiphysis and the subacromial lesions, *Orthop Trans* 7:138, 1983.

13. Mudge MK, Fryman CK, Wood VE: Rotator cuff tears associated with os acromiale, *J Bone Joint Surg* 66A:427-429, 1984.

14. Kessel L, Watson M: The painful arc syndrome; clinical classification as a guide to management, *J Bone Joint Surg* 59B:166-172, 1977.

15. Petersson CJ, Gentz CF: Ruptures of the supraspinatus tendon; the significance of distally pointing acromioclavicular osteophytes, *Clin Orthop* 174:143-148, 1983.

16. Rockwood CA, Lyons FR: Shoulder impingement syndrome; diagnosis, radiographic evaluation, and treatment with a modified Neer acromioplasty, *J Bone Joint Surg* 75A:409-424, 1993.

17. Aoki M, Ishiti S, Usui M: The slope of the acromion and rotator cuff impingement, *Orthop Trans* 10:228, 1986.

18. Burns WC II, Whipple TL: Anatomic relationships in the shoulder impingement syndrome, *Clin Orthop* 294:96-102, 1993.

19. Jerosch J, Castro WH, Sons JU, et al: Etiology of subacromial impingement syndrome; a biomechanical study, *Beitr Orthop Traumatol* 36:411-418, 1989.

20. Nasca RJ, Salter EG, Well CE: Contact areas of the "subacromial" joint. In Bateman JE, Welsh RP, editors: *Surgery of the shoulder,* Philadelphia, 1984, BC Decker.

21. Flatow EL, Soslowsky LJ, Ticker JB, et al: Excursion of the rotator cuff under the acromion: patterns of subacromial contact, *Am J Sports Med* 22:779-788, 1994.

22. Caspari RB, Thal R: Arthroscopic subacromial decompression: technical considerations, *Tech Orthop* 9:102-107, 1994.

23. Liberson F: Os acromiale: a contested anomaly, *J Bone Joint Surg* 19:683-689, 1937.

24. Edelson JG, Zuckerman J, Hershkovitz I: Os acromiale: anatomy and surgical implications, *J Bone Joint Surg* 75B:551-555, 1993.

25. Folliasson A: Un cas d'os acromial, *Rev d' Orthop* 20:533-538, 1933.

26. Sakar K, Taine W, Uhthoff HK: The ultrastructure of the coracoacromial ligament in patients with chronic impingement syndrome, *Clin Orthop* 330:40-44, 1990.

27. Soslowsky LJ, An CH, DeBano CM, et al: The coracoacromial ligament: in situ load and viscoelastic properties in rotator cuff disease, *Clin Orthop* 330:40-44, 1996.

28. Soslowsky LJ, An CH, Johnston SP, et al: Geometric and mechanical properties of the coracoacromial ligament and their relationship to rotator cuff disease, *Clin Orthop* 304:10-17, 1994.

29. Flatow EL, Fealy S, April EW, et al: The coracoacromial ligament: anatomy morphology and a study of acromial enthesopathy, *J Shoulder Elbow Surg* 5:S60, 1996 (abstract).

30. Clark JM, Harryman DT II: Tendons, ligaments and capsule of the rotator cuffs: gross and microscopic anatomy, *J Bone Joint Surg* 74A:713-725, 1992.

31. Gohlke F, Daum P, Eulert J: The stabilizing function of the capsule of the glenohumeral joint and the corresponding role of the coracoacromial arch, *J Shoulder Elbow Surg* 3:S24, 1994 (abstract).

32. Gerber C, Schneeberger AG, Vinh TS: The arterial vascularization of the humeral head: an anatomical study, *J Bone Joint Surg* 72A:1486-1494, 1990.

33. Rothman RH, Parke WW: The vascular anatomy of the rotator cuff, *Clin Orthop* 41:176-186, 1965.

34. Inman VT, Saunders JB, Abbott LC: Observations on the functions of the shoulder joint, *J Bone Joint Surg* 26:1-30, 1944.

35. Turkel SJ, Panio MW, Marshall JL, et al: Stabilizing mechanisms preventing anterior dislocation of the glenohumeral joint, *J Bone Joint Surg* 63A:1208-1217, 1981.

36. Howell SM, Imobersteg AM, Seger DH, et al: Clarification of the role of the supraspinatus muscle in shoulder function, *J Bone Joint Surg* 68A:398-404, 1985.

37. Iannotti JB, editor: *Rotator cuff disorders: evaluation and treatment,* Park Ridge, IL, 1991, American Academy of Orthopaedic Surgeons.

38. Hughes RE, An KN: Force analysis of rotator cuff muscles, *Clin Orthop* 330:75-83, 1996.

39. Kronberg M, Nemeth G, Brostrom LA: Muscle activity and coordination in the normal shoulder: an electromyographic study, *Clin Orthop* 257:76-85, 1990.

40. McCann PD, Wooten ME, Kadaba MP, et al: A kinematic and electromyographic study of shoulder rehabilitation exercises, *Clin Orthop* 288:179-188, 1993.

41. Sigholm G, Herberts P, Almstrom C, et al: Electromyographic analysis of shoulder muscle load, *J Orthop Res* 1:379-386, 1984.

42. Townsend H, Jobe FW, Pink M, et al: Electromyographic analysis of the glenohumeral muscles during a baseball rehabilitation program, *Am J Sports Med* 19:264-272, 1991.

43. Blevins FT, Djurasovic M, Flatow EL, et al: Biology of the rotator cuff tendon, *Orthop Clin North Am* 28:1-16, 1997.

44. Cofield RH: Rotator cuff disease of the shoulder, *J Bone Joint Surg* 67A:974-979, 1985.

45. Fu FH, Harner CD, Klein AH: Shoulder impingement syndrome: a critical review, *Clin Orthop* 269:162-173, 1991.

46. Soslowsky LJ, Carpenter JE, Bucchieri JS, et al: Biomechanics of the rotator cuff, *Orthop Clin North Am* 28:17-30, 1997.

47. Uhthoff HK, Drummond DI, Sakar K, et al: The role of impingement syndrome: a clinical, radiological and histological study, *Int Orthop* 12:97, 1988.

48. Uhthoff HJ, Sana S: Pathology of failure of the rotator cuff tendon, *Orthop Clin North Am* 28:31-41, 1997.

49. Deutsch A, Altchek D, Schwartz E, et al: Radiologic measurement of superior displacement of the humeral head in the impingement syndrome, *J Shoulder Elbow Joint Surg* 5:186, 1996.

50. Harryman DT, Sidles JA, Clark JM, et al: Translation of the humeral head on the glenoid with passive glenohumeral motion, *J Bone Joint Surg Am* 72:1334-1343, 1990.

51. Howell SM, Galinat BJ, Renzi AJ, et al: Normal and abnormal mechanics of the glenohumeral joint in the horizontal plane, *J Bone Joint Surg Am* 70:227-232, 1988.

52. Wuelker N, Schmotzer H, Thren K, et al: Translation of the glenohumeral joint with simulated active elevation, *Clin Orthop* 309:193-200, 1994.

53. Hawkins RJ, Kennedy JC: Impingement syndrome in athletes, *Am J Sports Med* 8:151-158, 1980.

54. Jobe FW, Kvitne RS: Shoulder pain in the overhand or throwing athlete: the relationship of anterior instability and rotator cuff impingement, *Orthop Rev* 18:963-975, 1989.

55. Jobe FW: Impingement problems in the athlete, *Instr Course Lect* 38:205-209, 1989.

56. Nirschl RP: Rotator cuff tendonitis: basic concepts of pathoetiology, *Instr Course Lect* 38:439-445, 1989.m

57. Jobe FW: Impingement problems in the athlete. In Barr JS Jr, editor: *Instructional course lectures,* XXXVIII, Park Ridge, IL, 1989, American Academy of Orthopaedic Surgeons.

58. Nirschl RP: Rotator cuff surgery. In Barr JS Jr, editor: *Instructional course lectures,* XXXVIII, Park Ridge, IL, 1989, American Academy of Orthopaedic Surgeons.

59. Jobe CM: Posterior superior glenoid impingement, *J Shoulder Elbow Surg* 1195:530-536, 1995.

60. Hawkins RJ, Kennedy JC: Impingement syndrome in athletes, *Am J Sports Med* 8:151, 1980.

61. Kibler WB, Uhl TL, Maddox JW, et al: Qualitative clinical evaluation of scapular dysfunction: a reliability study, *J Shoulder Elbow Surg* 11:550-556, 2002.

62. Kibler WB: The role of the scapula in athletic shoulder function, *Am J Sports Med* 26:325-337, 1998.

63. Cocchiarella L, Andersson GBJ, editors: *Guides to the evaluation of permanent impairment,* ed 5, Chicago, 2001, American Medical Association.

64. Schulte RA, Davies GJ: Examination and management of shoulder pain in an adolescent pitcher, *Phys Ther Case Rep* 4(3):1-18, 2001.

65. Neer CS, Poppen NK: Supraspinatus outlet. Presented at the meeting of the American Shoulder and Elbow Society, San Francisco, January 1987.

66. Neer CS, Welsh RP: The shoulder in sports, *Orthop Clin North Am* 8:583-591, 1977.

67. Morrison DS: Conservative management for subacromial impingement of the shoulder. Presented at the meeting of the American Shoulder and Elbow Society, San Francisco, January 1993.

68. Hyvovnen P, Lohi S, Jalovaara P: Open acromioplasty does not prevent the progression of an impingement syndrome to a tear, *J Bone Joint Surg* 80B(5):813-816, 1998.

69. Leadbetter WB, Buckwalter JA, Gordon SL, editors: *Sports-induced inflammation: clinical and basic science concepts,* Park Ridge, IL, 1990, American Academy of Orthopaedic Surgeons, p 78.

70. Ellman H: Arthroscopic subacromial decompression: analysis of one- to three-year results, *Arthroscopy* 3:173-181, 1987.

71. Schulte RA, Warner CD: Oscillatory devices accelerate proprioception training, *Biomechanics,* May 2001, pp 85-90.

72. Davies GD: Advances in examination and treatment of the shoulder complex. Advanced Concepts in Examination and Treatment of the Shoulder. North Dakota Physical Therapy Association Meeting and Workshop, Spearfish, SD, October 15, 2003.

CHAPTER 33

Rehabilitation after Mini-Open and Arthroscopic Repair of the Rotator Cuff

Todd S. Ellenbecker, PT, DPT, MS, SCS, OCS, CSCS
David S. Bailie, MD
W. Benjamin Kibler, MD, FACSM

CHAPTER OUTLINE

REHABILITATION OF THE PATIENT AFTER

a rotator cuff repair requires a detailed understanding of the underlying cause of the tear and the pathophysiology of the rotator cuff, in addition to the basic science and surgical procedures used to repair the rotator cuff and associated pathology. The purpose of this chapter is to provide basic scientific information about the rotator cuff, as well as to give brief overviews of the surgical techniques currently used to repair rotator cuff tears. Finally, a detailed description of a rehabilitation protocol highlighting the techniques used to restore normal joint arthrokinematics and rotator cuff and scapular strength will be presented.

PATHOPHYSIOLOGY OF ROTATOR CUFF DYSFUNCTION

As a broad generalization, tears of the rotator cuff can be caused by an underlying impingement progression or an instability progression. It is beyond the scope of this chapter to completely review these progressions; however, understanding the pathomechanical factors leading to rotator cuff tears will lead to a greater understanding of the type of rotator cuff tear (bursal or articular side tear) as well as allow the clinician to design a complete rehabilitation program based on these underlying factors.

Neer[1] pioneered the concept of primary compressive disease or impingement occurring as a direct result of compression of the rotator cuff tendons between the humeral head and the overlying anterior third of the acromion, coracoacromial ligament, coracoid, or acromial-clavicular joint.[1,2] The subacromial space has been measured using anteroposterior radiographs and found to be 7 to 13 mm in patients with shoulder pain[3] and 6 to 14 mm in patients with normal shoulders.[4] Biomechanical analysis of the shoulder has produced theoretic estimates of the compressive forces against the acromion with elevation of the shoulder, which can provide an understanding of the pathomechanics of impingement that leads to a rotator cuff tear.[5-7] Poppen and Walker[5] calculated this force at 0.42 times body weight, with Lucas[6] estimating this force at 10.2 times the weight of the arm. Peak forces against the acromion were measured between 85 degrees and 136 degrees of elevation, a position inherent in sport-specific movements and movement patterns used in activities of daily living.[7]

Neer[1,2] outlined three stages of primary impingement as it relates to rotator cuff pathology. Stage I, edema and hemorrhage, results from the mechanical irritation of the tendon from the impingement incurred with overhead activity. This is characteristically observed in younger patients who are more athletic and is described as a reversible condition with conservative physical therapy. The second stage of compressive disease outlined by Neer is termed *fibrosis* and *tendinitis*. This occurs from repeated episodes of mechanical inflammation and can include thickening or fibrosis of the subacromial bursae. The typical age range for this stage of injury is 25 to 40 years. Neer's stage III impingement lesion is termed

bone spurs and *tendon rupture* and is the result of continued mechanical compression of the rotator cuff tendons. Full-thickness tears of the rotator cuff, partial-thickness tears of the rotator cuff, biceps tendon lesions, and bony alteration of the acromion and acromioclavicular (AC) joint may be associated with this stage.[1,2] In addition to bony alterations that are acquired with repetitive stress to the shoulder, the native shape of the acromion is of clinical relevance. The specific shape of the overlying acromion process, termed *acromial architecture,* has been studied in relation to full-thickness tears of the rotator cuff.[8,9] Bigliani and colleagues[8] described three types of acromions: type I (flat), type II (curved), and type III (hooked). A type III or hooked acromion was found in 70% of cadaveric shoulders with a full-thickness rotator cuff tear, whereas a type I acromion had only a 3% incidence.[8] In a series of 200 clinically evaluated patients, 80% with a positive arthrogram had a type III acromion.[9]

In addition to the impingement-based progression, stresses caused by tendon overload caused by glenohumeral joint instability can lead to a rotator cuff tear. One example is the repetitive tensile overload imparted to the rotator cuff tendons during the deceleration and follow-through phases of overhead sport activities.[10] The tensile stresses incurred by the rotator cuff during the arm deceleration phase of the throwing motion to resist joint distraction, horizontal adduction, and internal rotation are reported to be as high as 1090 N with biomechanical study of highly skilled pitchers.[11] The presence of either acquired or congenital capsular laxity, as well as labral insufficiency, can greatly increase the tensile stresses to the rotator cuff muscle tendon units.[12,13] Because of the increased humeral head translation, the rotator cuff can become impinged secondary to the ensuing instability.[12,13] A progressive loss of glenohumeral joint stability is created when the dynamic stabilizing functions of the rotator cuff are diminished because of fatigue and tendon injury.[13] The effects of secondary impingement can lead to rotator cuff tears as the instability and impingement continue.

CLASSIFICATION OF ROTATOR CUFF TEARS

One of the factors that affect the progression of resistive exercise and range of motion (ROM) is tear type. The degree of rotator cuff tear—partial or full thickness—and tear size are important determinants of rehabilitative progression.

Partial versus Full-Thickness Tears

There are several primary types of rotator cuff tears commonly described in the literature. Full-thickness tears in the rotator cuff consist of tears that involve the entire thickness (from top to bottom) of the rotator cuff tendon or tendons. Full-thickness tears are often initiated in the critical zone of the supraspinatus tendon and can extend to include the infraspinatus, teres minor, and subscapularis tendons.[14] Often associated with a tear in the subscapularis tendon is subluxation of the biceps long head tendon from the intertubercular groove, or either partial or complete tears of the biceps tendon. Histologically, full-thickness rotator cuff tears show a variety of findings ranging from almost entirely acellular and avascular margins to neovascularization with cellular infiltrate.[14]

The effects of a full-thickness rotator cuff tear on glenohumeral joint stability were studied by Loehr and colleagues.[15] Changes in stability of the glenohumeral joint were assessed with selective division of the supraspinatus and/or infraspinatus tendons. The findings indicated that a one-tendon lesion of either the supraspinatus or the infraspinatus did not influence the movement patterns of the glenohumeral joint, whereas a two-tendon lesion induced significant changes compatible with instability of the glenohumeral joint. Therefore patients with full-thickness rotator cuff tears may have additional stress and dependence placed on the dynamic stabilizing function of the remaining rotator cuff tendons because of increased humeral head translation and ensuing instability.

Additional research on full-thickness rotator cuff tears has significant clinical ramifications. One hundred consecutive patients with full-thickness tears of the rotator cuff were prospectively evaluated to determine the incidence of associated intraarticular pathology by Miller and Savoie.[16] Of 100 patients, 74 had one or more coexisting intraarticular abnormalities, with anterior labral tears occurring in 62 and biceps tendon tears in 16. The results of this study clearly indicate the importance of a thorough clinical examination of the patient with rotator cuff pathology.

A second type of rotator cuff tear is an incomplete or partial-thickness tear. Partial-thickness tears can occur on the superior surface (bursal side) or undersurface (articular side) of the rotator cuff. Although both bursal and articular side tears are partial-thickness tears of the rotator cuff, significant differences in etiology are proposed for each.[13]

Neer[1,2] and Fukuda and co-workers[17] have both emphasized that superior surface (bursal side) tears in the rotator cuff are the result of subacromial impingement. In the classification scheme listed earlier in this chapter, tears on the superior or bursal side of the rotator cuff are generally associated with both primary and secondary compressive disease as well as macrotraumatic tendon failure. The progression of the mechanical irritation on the superior surface can produce a partial-thickness tear that can ultimately progress to a full-thickness tear.[1,2,13]

Partial-thickness tears on the undersurface or articular side of the rotator cuff are generally associated with tensile loads and glenohumeral joint instability.[13,18] Undersurface tears are commonly found in overhead-throwing athletes, where anterior instability, capsular and labral insufficiency, and dynamic muscular imbalances are often reported. To further understand the differing etiologies of rotator cuff tears, Nakajima and colleagues[18] performed a histologic and biomechanical study of the rotator cuff tendons. With regard to biomechanics, their results showed greater deformation

and tensile strength of the bursal side of the supraspinatus tendon. The bursal side of the supraspinatus tendon was composed of a group of longitudinal tendon bundles that could disperse a tensile load and generate greater resistance to elongation than the articular or undersurface of the tendon. These authors found the articular surface to be composed of a tendon, ligament, and joint capsule complex that elongated poorly and tore more easily,[18] further reinforcing the proposal that tensile stresses produce undersurface rotator cuff tears.

Classification of Tear Size

One of the factors that predicates the rate at which a patient can be rehabilitated after a rotator cuff repair is tear size.[19] Full-thickness rotator cuff tears can be classified by the actual size of the tear, with small tears measuring less than 1 cm across the full-thickness defect, medium tears ranging from 1 to 3 cm, large tears ranging from 3 to 5 cm, and massive tears being larger than 5 cm. Inspection of the patient's operative report will most often provide an estimate of tear size, which can be used to estimate the amount of tissue repair, mobilization, and subsequent damage found at the time of surgery. These factors all have implications when designing a rehabilitation program, starting with the amount of immobilization (larger tears typically are immobilized for a longer period of time than smaller tears) and ultimately influencing the rate at which ROM and strength are progressed. Knowledge of this classification system will assist the clinician in understanding the operative report and communicating with the patient and physician regarding the size of the rotator cuff tear and subsequent repair.

INDICATIONS FOR OPERATIVE MANAGEMENT OF ROTATOR CUFF TEARS

Indications and principles for operative treatment of partial and complete rotator cuff tears continue to evolve. This is mainly because of the lack of precise knowledge of the pathoetiology and natural history of rotator cuff injuries.

There are imprecise indications for surgery, even in the face of documented rotator cuff tears. It is a well-established fact that a relatively high percentage of rotator cuff tears are functionally asymptomatic. Even in the presence of symptoms, prospective studies have shown that pain relief and increased ROM can be achieved in up to 50% of cases with nonoperative treatment. Strength is not significantly changed, however, and improvement in total functional capability is variable. Poor prognostic factors for pain relief or predictable functional improvement include pain that interrupts sleep, tears greater than 1 cm, the presence of symptoms for more than 1 year, and severe weakness of abduction or external rotation on initial examination.[20]

At this point in time, both arthroscopic and mini-open surgical techniques have been demonstrated to be effective in relieving symptoms of pain, improving strength, and increasing function in terms of functional outcomes measures in all types of tears, from partial-thickness to moderate-sized complete tears. There continues to be much debate and a lack of consensus regarding many other aspects of rotator cuff surgery. These include whether to take down a partial rotator cuff tear entirely or repair it through the cuff; the role of anterior and posterior releases in mobilizing for repair; optimum suture configuration—simple, mattress, or Mason-Allen type; and fixation geometry—single or double row anchor, bone tunnels, or a combination.

The literature does suggest several techniques that can help in surgical decision making and surgical treatment.[20] Complete probing and evaluation from intraarticular and bursal sides will help determine the size, depth, and location of partial-thickness tears. Most recommendations continue to emphasize that symptomatic partial tears that involve more than 50% of the width of the tendon should be treated with repair techniques. Evaluation of the width of the rotator cuff footprint can give an estimation of the degree of articular-sided partial tearing. More than 6 mm of footprint exposure suggests 50% full-thickness loss. Reconstitution of the total footprint contact area is thought to be optimal. In partial-thickness tears, this appears to be best accomplished by complete tear take-down and suture anchor repair.

There is a small subset of articular-sided partial rotator cuff tears in which the injury is in the substance of the tendon, with a flap configuration and an intact footprint. These can be repaired by arthroscopic through-and-through suture repairs, with the passing instruments, usually spinal needles, being introduced from the subacromial space through the tear and the stitches being passed from an anterior intraarticular portal through the needles into the subacromial space and being tied there.

Bursal-sided partial tears have less healing capability and require treatment like complete tears for relief of symptoms. They are more frequently associated with subacromial impingement.

ROLE OF ACROMIOPLASTY

Acromioplasty (subacromial decompression [SAD]) has been classically done in conjunction with rotator cuff repair. This has been thought to remove the offending bone spur or acromial hook and to lower the rate of recurrent pain and tears. However, the rationale for this was based on Neer's original work demonstrating a "type III" acromion to be present with most tears.[1,2]

Recent understanding of tear types has raised questions as to whether an SAD needs to be performed routinely. The current thinking in the United States is that rotator cuff repairs in the presence of classic primary "outlet" impingement should also include an SAD. Tensile overload tears in younger patients without primary impingement need not have an SAD for a good result. Their impingement symptoms are secondary from either primary or dynamic instability. However, if the

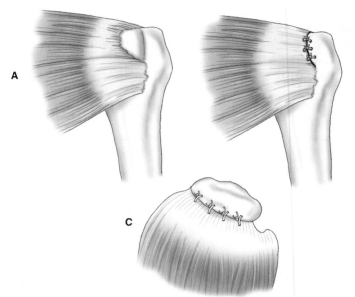

Figure 33-1: A, Crescent-shaped rotator cuff tear without much retraction can be repaired directly to bone with minimal tension. **B** and **C,** repair of crescent-shaped rotator cuff tear: **B,** posterior view; **C,** superior view. (*From Burkhart SS: A stepwise approach to arthroscopic rotator cuff repair based on biomechanical principles,* Arthroscopy *16:82-90, 2000.*)

coracoacromial ligament shows hypertrophic wear, then a limited decompression can be helpful.

PRINCIPLES OF OPERATIVE MANAGEMENT OF FULL-THICKNESS ROTATOR CUFF TEARS

Efficacious operative treatment of complete rotator cuff tears is based on several principles: tear pattern recognition, secure fixation, and restoration of the footprint. Proper tear pattern recognition is crucial. Many repairs fail because of a lack of proper recognition, such that a nonanatomic repair is attempted, with increased tension and poor restoration of anatomy.[21]

Tear Pattern Recognition

Complete tear patterns can be broadly divided into two types: crescent shaped and U shaped (with several variations). Crescent-shaped tears do not usually retract far from the greater tuberosity and can usually be directly repaired back to the greater tuberosity (Figure 33-1). The crescent-shaped tear's greatest extent is most frequently in a transverse direction to the longitudinal axis of the tendon. The surgeon should always check the anterior and posterior attachments of the crescent-shaped tear, because these tissues are usually plastically deformed and are not normal. They must be debrided to allow high-quality tissue attachment. Adhesions on both surfaces will need to be removed to allow complete mobilization, resulting in decreased tension on the repair.

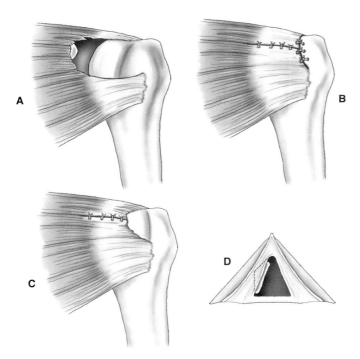

Figure 33-2: A, Large U-shaped cuff tear extending to glenoid. **B,** Repair of U-shaped cuff tears begins with side-to-side sutures that converge the free margin of the cuff toward the bone bed (margin convergence). **C,** After side-to-side sutures are placed, the free margin of the cuff is repaired to bone with suture anchors. **D,** Closing an L-shaped or U-shaped tear is much like closing a tent flap. (*From Burkhart SS: A stepwise approach to arthroscopic rotator cuff repair based on biomechanical principles,* Arthroscopy 16:82-90, 2000.)

U-shaped tears frequently have their greatest extent in a longitudinal direction to the tendon (Figure 33-2). The medial point of the tear does not represent retraction, but represents the configuration that an L- or T-shaped tear assumes with muscle contraction. Mobilization of the two tendon leaves by release of the subacromial and intraarticular adhesions will allow better recognition of the tear pattern. The longitudinal component can be repaired by margin convergence, and the transverse component, now a crescent-shaped tear, can then be repaired to the bone. This can be conceptualized as a "U to T" or a "U to L" repair.

Margin convergence by longitudinal side-to-side closure of the tear leaves will progressively decrease the strain on the lateral margins of the tear, so that the resulting strain on the lateral transverse margin is within repair tolerance.[21] It is usually easiest to place the transverse fixation anchors in the bone and the stitches in the lateral part of the tendon first, without tying them. They can then be used as traction sutures to place the longitudinal side-to-side stitches in order from lateral to medial. Each successive suture becomes the next stay suture. The sutures are then tied from medial to lateral, "zipping up" the repair.

Secure fixation can be optimized by emphasizing minimal shear on the repair, proper suture placement in the tendon, and proper fixation placement.

Minimal shear can be obtained by repair of the tear according to the tear pattern, by proper anterior and posterior releases, and by mobilization of the cuff from the subacromial and intraarticular adhesions.[21] If these adhesions are not removed, they may act as proximal tethers, increasing shear at the distal repair site as motion is regained and muscle activation force is applied.

Fixation Methods in Rotator Cuff Repair

Suture placement in the tendon is the subject of much study.[22,23] The types of suture placement may be categorized as simple, mattress, or combination (modified Mason-Allen). Although there is literature favoring each type of suture placement, it is probably more important how securely the sutures are tied (proper loop security of tendon to bone and knot security within the throws of the knot) and how much load is carried across each suture. Cyclic biomechanical testing has demonstrated that knot security is enhanced by using braided sutures, alternating post limbs of the sutures, and past-pointing to minimize slack within the stitch. Double loading each suture anchor increases the number of fixation points, thereby decreasing the load on each individual suture.[23]

Fixation placement should result in proper position of the cuff to bone and optimum pull-out strength of the fixation device or construct. Suture anchors should be placed at a 45-degree angle to increase the anchor's resistance to pull-out. For single-row repairs, anchors are placed within 4 to 5 mm of the articular margin. Biomechanical testing under cyclic loading indicates that these constructs are stronger than fixation by transosseous tunnels. However, in osteopenic bone, tunnels may be the fixation type of choice. The entrance to the tunnels should also be close to the articular margin, and the exits on the humerus should be placed far enough apart to allow a good bony buttress.

Lately, double-row repairs have been advocated to maximize suture placement and load per suture and maximize fixation placement. The rows consist of either medial suture anchors and lateral bone tunnels or medial and lateral suture anchors.[23] Clinical reports demonstrate good results from either of these techniques. The double-row repairs also appear to result in the closest reapproximation of the total geometry of the rotator cuff footprint. Most repairs replicate the width, but not the size, of the original insertion. By allowing a larger, more physiologic area of contact, these double-row repairs have a theoretic ability to increase healing potential and ultimate tensile strength of the repair construct.

Role of Diagnostic Arthroscopy

Historically, rotator cuff repairs have been performed using an anterolateral approach. With the initial development of arthroscopic surgery, many other associated lesions were found to coexist with rotator cuff disease. The role of arthroscopy, even if the surgeon plans on doing an "open" repair, remains important.

Diagnostic arthroscopy is helpful for several reasons. First, it helps the surgeon classify the tear type: size, tendon involvement, pattern, and tissue quality. This information will allow better intraoperative planning regarding which strategies to use to accomplish a tension-free repair.

Second, arthroscopy allows for the identification of associated pathology that may be missed with an entirely open surgery. This includes labral tears, glenohumeral chondral injury, loose bodies, lesions of the biceps, capsular injury, and lesions of the subscapularis. It allows treatment of these entities, which, if left untreated, may lead to persistent pain and functional deficits.

Arthroscopy also assists in the identification of subacromial anatomy in order to plan proper levels of decompression, if indicated. Sloping of the acromion and spur size and location are more readily discernible. Significant AC joint pathology can also be delineated and treated.

The presence of labral tears is an important consideration when treatment is planned. Failure to address this pathology will result in less-than-satisfactory outcomes. This includes debridement of partial or nonrepairable lesions or formal suture repair, if indicated.

We have found that rehabilitation must be more aggressive, in terms of ROM, when dealing with combined rotator cuff and labral repairs. Younger patients will more likely have labral tears that require repair. Older patients with degenerative tears rarely need repairs, as they will often lead to a stiff shoulder.

STRATEGIES FOR IRREPARABLE ROTATOR CUFF TEARS

There is much controversy in the literature regarding the treatment of massive irreparable rotator cuff tears. Specific techniques include arthroscopic debridement, tuberoplasty, aggressive mobilization with complete repair, partial repair, tendon transfer, and reverse prostheses. The detailed discussion of these is beyond the scope of this chapter, but the clinician should be aware of their use.

The most common way to address irreparable rotator cuff tears in the general orthopedic community is debridement. In theory, pain is improved, with less predictable gains in ROM and function. This involves removal of all debris and debridement of the necrotic rotator cuff edges and flaps with limited SAD and preservation of the coracoacromial arch. Failure to do the latter may result in anterosuperior instability, a debilitating problem.

Tuberoplasty has been described as a pain-relieving procedure for rotator cuff arthropathy. Its use is not widely accepted. It involves the arthroscopic reshaping of the greater tuberosity to allow for a smooth articulation between this and the acromion.

With newer techniques and better understanding of their pattern, larger tears that were once thought to be irreparable can be mobilized and repaired. If a complete repair can be done, it must not have any excess tension or failure will occur. If a complete repair cannot be done, partial repair to restore the normal force couples has been effective. Even if a superior opening is left, restoration of anterior and posterior force couples will allow near-normal function. As often used in Europe, muscle transposition or a reverse prosthesis can be used to restore function. However, these techniques often lead to only fair results, with potentially catastrophic outcomes with failures. Examples of these techniques include superior subscapular transposition for deficient supraspinatus, superior infraspinatus transposition, pectoralis major transfer for irreparable subscapularis tears, deltoid transfer for irreparable supraspinatus tears, and latissimus dorsi transfer for supraspinatus tears.

Finally, reverse ball-in-socket prostheses have been popularized in Europe and are currently being investigated in the United States by the Food and Drug Administration. These devices place the "socket" component in the humerus and a "ball" in the glenoid, which shifts the center of rotation inferiorly and laterally, allowing the deltoid to become more effective.

REPAIR OF THE ROTATOR CUFF USING THE MINI-OPEN DELTOID SPLITTING TECHNIQUE

The use of a mini-open rotator cuff repair has been favored over the last few years. It uses a small (3 cm or less) deltoid splitting incision at the lateral aspect of the shoulder at the level of the tear.[20] A true mini-open repair preserves all deltoid attachment to the acromion and requires advanced knowledge of the tear pattern, because of limited visibility. Most of the "work" is done arthroscopically, including decompression, labral debridement or repair, rotator cuff debridement and mobilization, and tuberosity preparation.[20] Suture anchors can also be placed arthroscopically. The lateral arthroscopic portal is then enlarged slightly, to allow suture passage and tendon repair.

The arm can be rotated to access all areas of the cuff. This includes the upper third of the subscapularis, the entire supraspinatus, and the upper half of the infraspinatus. The primary pitfall of this technique is limited access, need for extensive shoulder surgery experience, and risk of inadvertent deltoid detachment.

Postoperatively, aggressive rehabilitation can be instituted, because of a small sound cuff repair and preservation of the acromial attachment of the deltoid. One of us allows immediate passive motion, with use of a sling for 4 weeks. This may be reduced to 2 to 3 weeks for smaller tears. Other factors should be conveyed to the therapist, including tear size, tissue quality, and other associated pathologies. Patients typically progress through rehabilitation at a rapid pace, assuming no interfering circumstances.

REHABILITATION AFTER MINI-OPEN ROTATOR CUFF REPAIR

The initial step in the rehabilitation process of the patient after rotator cuff repair is the postoperative evaluation. Although many of the detailed special tests inherent in the preoperative evaluation of a patient with shoulder dysfunction are not indicated, critical details regarding the patient's ROM, posture, and underlying mobility status should be obtained.

Postoperative Evaluation

It is beyond the scope of this chapter to outline all aspects of the postoperative examination; however, several critical aspects are mentioned here. Obtaining information regarding the nature of the injury and, if known, the mechanism of injury, as well as additional information regarding the time periods from injury to surgery and from surgery to the start of postoperative therapy is necessary and provides insight into the possible degree of atrophy and disuse, as well as the time period for healing.

After the subjective evaluation, observation of the patient's posture provides critical information regarding muscular atrophy and scapular dysfunction. Evaluation of the patient's shoulder heights, noting that when the injured dominant shoulder is held higher than the contralateral nondominant shoulder, often indicates a protective mechanism and periscapular muscle guarding. Viewing the patient from the posterior aspect can reveal atrophy over the supraspinous and infraspinous fossae, as well as prominence of the scapula caused by weakness of the lower trapezius and serratus anterior muscles.[24] Noting where the scapulas are most prominent (inferior border or medial border) can indicate the type of scapular pathology present.[25]

Finally, assessment of both the accessory and physiologic mobility of the patient's shoulder is indicated. Careful goniometric evaluation of passive ROM (PROM) in the patterns of flexion, coronal plane abduction, and internal and external rotation with 45 degrees of abduction is recommended. Stabilization of the scapula is recommended during measurement of humeral rotation to prevent substitution.[26] In addition, the underlying mobility profile of the patient should be assessed. Evaluation of the anterior, posterior, and inferior translation of the humeral head relative to the glenoid should be bilaterally performed using manual anterior and posterior translation tests as well as the multidirectional instability (MDI) sulcus sign.

The key areas mentioned previously provide the clinician with important information regarding the underlying mobility status of the patient, initial baseline ROM, and scapular characteristics without jeopardizing patient comfort or stressing the rotator cuff repair.

Early Postoperative Phase (Weeks 0 to 4 through 6)

After the initial evaluation, treatment is commenced with a primary goal of increasing PROM, initiating scapular stabilization, and turning on the rotator cuff via protected active ROM (AROM) (Box 33-1). Passive ROM is started in all planes unless surgical complications were encountered or alternative procedures such as capsular plication and thermal capsulorrhaphy were performed, which would require protected motion for an initial period during postoperative rehabilitation.

Hatakeyama and colleagues[27] studied the effects of passive ranges of humeral internal and external rotation on cadaveric rotator cuff repairs in 30 degrees of elevation in the scapular, coronal, and sagittal planes. Results showed that in the coronal and scapular planes, tension on the repaired supraspinatus tendon increased in both 30 and 60 degrees of internal rotation. In contrast, 30 and 60 degrees of external rotation in the scapular and coronal planes actually decreased stress on the repaired tendon. Use of the sagittal plane for rotational ROM produced tensions greater than during internal and external rotation in the frontal or scapular plane. Therefore, based on these results, humeral rotation in the early phase after rotator cuff repair is recommended in the scapular and coronal planes with up to 30 to 60 degrees of external rotation unless otherwise limited by surgical repair of an anterior-based rotator cuff lesion.[27]

Additional recommendations for early PROM include the progression of glenohumeral joint abduction during external rotation physiologic mobilization. For patient comfort, the initial abduction position for physiologic ROM ranges between 30 and 45 degrees (Figure 33-3). Based on the orientation of the rotator cuff's insertion into the greater tuberosity (Figure 33-4), progression of the patient's glenohumeral abduction range during external rotation stretching to 80 to 90 degrees of abduction (Figure 33-5) when tolerated is recommended to reduce stress to the tendon caused by the orientation and wring-out type phenomenon created by the adducted position.[28] This 80- to 90-degree abducted position is used to increase external rotation ROM through this early stage of rehabilitation, with a final progression recommended to eventual adducted external rotation stretching later in the rehabilitation sequence when tendon healing is more pronounced.

In addition to the physiologic ROM performed in this initial rehabilitation phase, accessory mobilization is recommended based on the assessment performed on the initial visit. Reductions in anterior, posterior, or caudal glides compared with the contralateral side should be addressed through the use of graded peripheral joint mobilization along the lines

BOX 33-1

Postoperative Rehabilitation Protocol for Mini-Open Rotator Cuff Repair Using Deltoid Splitting Approach (Medium-Size Tear)

General Guidelines

Progression of resistive exercise and range of motion (ROM) is dependent on patient tolerance.

Resistance exercise should not be performed with specific shoulder joint pain or pain over the incision site.

A sling is provided to the patient for support as needed with daily activities and to wear at night. The patient is weaned from the sling as tolerated.

Early home exercises prescribed for the patient after surgery include stomach rubs, sawing, and gripping activity.

Progression to active ROM (AROM) against gravity and duration of sling use is predicated both on the size of the rotator cuff tear and on quality of the tissue and is guided by the referring physician.

Postoperative Weeks 1 and 2

1. Early passive ROM (PROM) to patient tolerance during the first 4-6 weeks
   a. flexion
   b. scapular and coronal plane abduction
   c. internal rotation (IR) and external rotation (ER) with 90 to 45 degrees of abduction
2. Submaximal isometric IR and ER, flexion and extension, and adduction
3. Mobilization of the glenohumeral joint and scapulothoracic joint; passive stretching of elbow, forearm, and wrist to terminal ranges
4. Side-lying scapular protraction and retraction resistance to encourage early serratus anterior and lower trapezius activation and endurance
5. Home exercise instruction
   a. instruction in PROM and active assisted range of motion (AAROM) home exercises with T-bar, pulleys, or opposite arm assistance in supine position using ROM to patient tolerance
   b. weight-bearing (closed chain) Codman's exercise instruction over a ball, countertop, or table
   c. therapeutic exercise for grip strength maintenance

Postoperative Week 3

1. Continue shoulder ROM exercises from previous weeks and isometric strength program to patient tolerance; progress patient to active assistive ROM
2. Add upper body ergometer (UBE) if available

3. Begin active scapular strengthening exercises, and continue side-lying manual scapular stabilization exercises:
   a. scapular retraction
   b. scapular retraction with depression
4. Begin resistive exercise for total arm strength using positions with glenohumeral joint completely supported, including:
   a. bicep curls
   b. tricep curls
   c. wrist curls—flexors, extensors, radial and ulnar deviators
5. Begin submaximal rhythmic stabilization using the balance point position (90-100 degrees of elevation) in supine position to initiate dynamic stabilization

Postoperative Weeks 5-7

1. Initiate isotonic resistance exercise focusing on the following movements:
   a. side-lying ER
   b. prone extension
   c. prone horizontal abduction (limited range to 45 degrees)
   d. supine IR
   e. flexion to 90 degrees

   A low-resistance, high-repetition (e.g., 30 reps) format is recommended, using no resistance initially (i.e., weight of the arm).
2. Progression to full PROM and AROM in all planes including ER and IR in neutral adduction progressing from the 90-degree abducted position used initially postoperatively
3. External rotation oscillation (resisted ER with towel roll under axilla and oscillation device)
4. Home exercise program for strengthening the rotator cuff and scapular musculature with isotonic weights and/or elastic tubing (Thera-Band)

Postoperative Week 8

1. Begin closed chain step-ups and quadruped rhythmic stabilization exercise
2. Initiate upper extremity plyometric chest passes and functional two-hand rotation tennis groundstroke or golf swing simulation using small exercise ball progressing to light medicine ball as tolerated

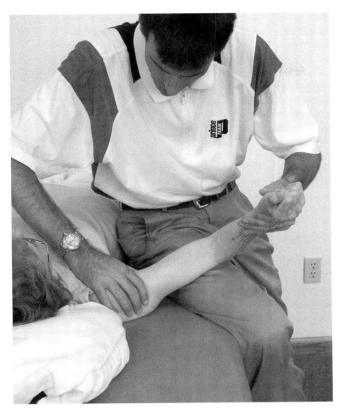

Figure 33-3: Technique used in early postoperative phase to gain external rotation using 45 to 60 degrees of glenohumeral joint abduction.

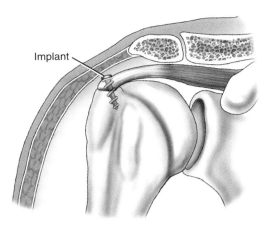

Figure 33-4: Anterior view of the glenohumeral joint depicting rotator cuff insertion and degree of wrap-around of the supraspinatus tendon on the top of the humeral head with insertion into the greater tuberosity. Note: Adducting the shoulder increases this wrap-around effect for the rotator cuff; therefore adduction is not a position recommended for early rotational range-of-motion work after rotator cuff repair.

BOX 33-1

Postoperative Rehabilitation Protocol—cont'd

Postoperative Week 10

1. Initiation of submaximal isokinetic exercise for IR and ER in the modified neutral position

   Criterion for progression to isokinetic exercise:

   a. patient has IR and ER ROM greater than that used during the isokinetic exercise

   b. patient can complete isotonic exercise program without pain with a 2-3 lb weight or medium-resistance surgical tubing or Thera-Band

2. Progression to 90-degree abducted rotational training in patients returning to overhead work or sport activity

   a. prone external rotation

   b. standing external and internal rotation with 90 degrees of abduction in the scapular plane

   c. statue of liberty (external rotation oscillation)

Postoperative Week 12 (3 Months)

1. Progression to maximal isokinetics in IR and ER and isokinetic testing to assess strength in modified base

30/30/30 position; formal documentation of AROM, PROM, and administration of shoulder rating scales

2. Begin interval return programs if the following criteria have been met:

   a. IR and ER strength minimum of 85% of contralateral extremity

   b. ER and IR ratio of 60% or higher

   c. Pain-free ROM

   d. Negative impingement and instability signs during clinical exam

Postoperative Week 16 (4 Months)

1. Isokinetic reevaluation, documentation of AROM, PROM, and shoulder rating scales

2. Progression continues for return to full upper extremity sport activity (e.g., throwing, serving in tennis)

3. Preparation for discharge from formal physical therapy to home program phase

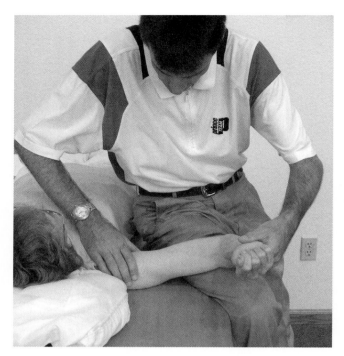

Figure 33-5: Progression to the 90-degree abducted position as soon as the patient is able to increase external rotation range of motion.

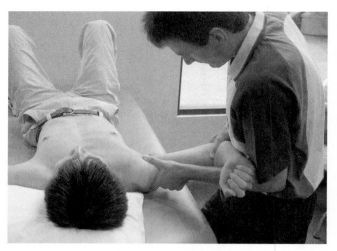

Figure 33-6: Combination mobilization technique combining the caudal glide with slight anterior glide with the humerus in external rotation to increase stress on the anterior capsule and address limitations in external rotation range of motion.

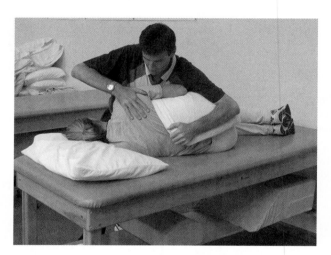

Figure 33-7: Scapular stabilization exercise. The clinician resists protraction and retraction via manual hand contacts.

of the glenohumeral joint.[29,30] It is important to remember that the anterior angulation of the glenoid and humeral retrotorsion necessitate that true anterior and posterior glide mobilizations be performed on a 30-degree angle to accommodate this articular geometry. Use of the scapular plane as a reference point for the anterior or posterior glide is recommended. Finally, the use of the caudal glide accessory mobilization to facilitate elevation is part of the manual treatment after rotator cuff repair. Combining the caudally directed force with a slightly anteriorly directed force (approximately 30 degrees) as well as placing the glenohumeral joint in external rotation can be used to stress the anterior band of the inferior glenohumeral ligament when external rotation limitations are present (Figure 33-6). Likewise, the addition of a slight posterior direction (approximately 30 degrees) to the caudal glide can be used to address the posterior band of the inferior glenohumeral ligament. Performing the caudal glides as described can be further intensified to improve rotational ROM by increasing the resting capsular tension by externally rotating the glenohumeral joint to near end range during the caudal anterior force application, and internally rotating the glenohumeral joint during the caudal-posterior glide to address internal rotation deficiency.[31]

In addition to the early PROM, scapular stabilization exercise is started because of the important role proper upward rotation plays in normal humeral elevation.[32] Figure 33-7 shows a manual scapular stabilization technique used to work the rhomboids and middle and lower trapezius throughout rehabilitation. Use of this manual technique allows for direct

scapular contact and bypasses the glenohumeral joint, allowing for immediate use of the technique after a surgical procedure. The intensity and repetitions of this technique are steadily increased throughout postoperative rehabilitation.

Initiation of active assistive ROM (AAROM) and AROM is recommended during this time period using the supine position. Use of the 90 degrees of shoulder flexion in supine allows the patient to use the extremity in a function length-tension arc with minimal effects of gravity during this early rehabilitation stage. Small controlled movements by the patient from the 90-degree reference position coupled with very submaximal rhythmic stabilization can be used to stimulate early co-contraction of the scapular stabilizers and rotator cuff muscle-tendon units. Active assistive exercises using a wand, cane, or upright pulleys are indicated in this position for enhancing humeral elevation and have been

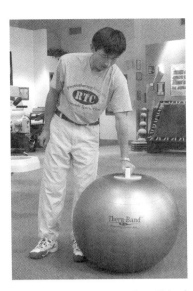

Figure 33-8: Ball approximation exercise. This closed chain exercise creating muscular co-contraction is used early in rehabilitation.

shown to induce very low levels of safe muscular activity, documented using electromyography (EMG) by McCann and colleagues.[33] Gentle closed kinetic chain exercise over an exercise ball (Figure 33-8) or rocker platform provides early stimulation of the rotator cuff and scapular muscles,[34] with joint compression inherent in the closed chain exercise minimizing humeral shear during execution of these exercises.[35]

Progression during the later stages of this phase to submaximal multiple angle isometrics for internal and external rotation as well as side-lying external rotation and prone shoulder extension to neutral with an externally rotated humeral position are used to prepare the muscle tendon unit for resistive exercise in the next phase.[36] In addition, repetitive motion exercise such as use of the upper body ergometer is initiated during this phase, with both frontward and backward movement indicated.

Total Arm Strength Phase (Weeks 6 to 12)

Progression to terminal ROM in both active and passive modes in addition to progressive resistive exercise for the rotator cuff and scapular muscles characterize the second phase of postoperative rotator cuff rehabilitation. Use of the exercise movement patterns that are characterized by high levels of rotator cuff activation, and use of positions that do not create impingement and minimize stress to the repair, are recommended. Electromyographic research provides the necessary rationale for the selection of these exercises, which include: side-lying external rotation, prone extension with externally rotated humeral position, and prone horizontal abduction with externally rotated humeral position.[36-39] Use of these exercises has been shown to increase isokinetically measured internal and external rotation strength after 4 weeks of thrice-weekly training.[40] A very low resistance and

higher repetition base are used (e.g., three to four sets of 15 to 20 repetitions to foster local muscle endurance).[41] Use of elastic resistance for internal and external rotation in 20 to 30 degrees of glenohumeral joint abduction in the scapular plane is also recommended.[42]

Rationale for the use of submaximal resistance levels during this stage as well as the gradual progression from AAROM and AROM during the first 4 to 6 weeks postoperatively can be found in a study by Burkhart and co-workers.[43] In this study, cadaveric rotator cuff repairs of medium size using transosseous tunnel fixation were subjected to repeated cyclic loads of 180 N or approximately 40 lb. A 5 mm gap occurred after 25 cycles of repetitive loading, which corresponded to a 50% failure of the rotator cuff repair. A complete 10 mm failure of the tendon repair was found after just 188 cycles. In a similar study using Mitek RC suture anchors (Mitek Products, Westwood, MA), Burkhart and colleagues[44] used cyclic loading patterns and found a 50% failure of the repair after a mean of 61 cycles, and complete 10 mm failure after 285 cycles. Repetitive loading after rotator cuff repair can ultimately result in the re-mergence of the rotator cuff defect regardless of whether transosseous tunnels or suture anchors are used. Clinician and patient alike should be cautioned against heavy resistive loading in the early postoperative phase.

Progression of scapular exercise to include patterns such as external rotation with retraction,[45] serratus punches in the supine position, and quadruped rhythmic stabilization progressively challenge the serratus anterior and lower trapezius force couple for the provision of scapular stabilization.

Copious use of rotational exercise to increase strength of the subscapularis (internal rotation) and infraspinatus and teres minor (external rotation) is supported in the basic science literature by Otis and co-workers,[46] who outlined the important role of the subscapularis, infraspinatus, and teres minor during arm elevation. The use of rotational strengthening to improve anti-gravity elevation is a key benefit expected from the rotationally biased exercise program described in this postoperative rotator cuff rehabilitation program. This rotational exercise is preferred over attempts at resistive elevation either with resistance or simply against gravity, which often produce shoulder hiking (type III Kibler scapular dysfunction) during arm elevation in patients with significant scapular and rotator cuff weakness after rotator cuff repair.

An additional exercise used throughout rehabilitation to assist with regaining active elevation through the promotion of rotator cuff and scapular strength is the closed chain clock and closed chain rhythmic stabilization exercise (Figure 33-9). This exercise uses the scapular plane with 80 to 90 degrees of humeral elevation and an exercise ball to allow the patient to perform active and resistive exercise for the rotator cuff and scapular muscles using angle-specific length-tension relationships. The use of the closed chain environment afforded by the exercise ball permits the patient to use this exercise position before he or she would be able to

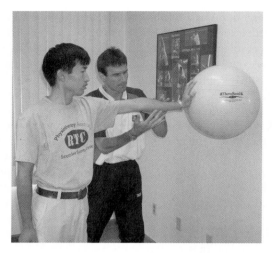

Figure 33-9: Closed chain exercise with the glenohumeral joint abducted 80 to 90 degrees in the scapular plane, with manual contacts applied by the therapist to challenge the patient's scapular stabilizers and promote co-contraction while working in a functionally specific length-tension position.

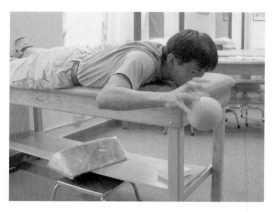

Figure 33-10: Prone plyometric catches with the glenohumeral joint in the 90/90 position.

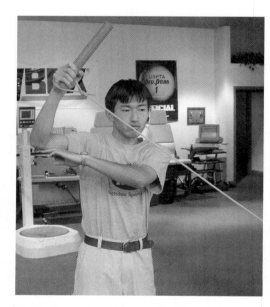

Figure 33-11: External rotation oscillation exercise using the scapular plane and 90 degrees of elevation.

independently and actively assume this position without severe scapular compensation as a result of postsurgical weakness. The use of rhythmic stabilization provided by the clinician further challenges the patient.

Progression of the resistive exercise to include isokinetic exercise in the modified base position for internal and external rotation occurs typically between weeks 10 and 12 postoperatively. The accommodative resistance inherent with isokinetics provides optimal resistance through the ROM in addition to allowing for the measurement of bilateral strength comparisons and muscular balance via unilateral strength ratios.[47,48] Contractile velocities ranging between 120 and 240 degrees per second are used for most patients, with faster velocities between 210 and 360 degrees per second reserved for more elite athletes and for patients later in the rehabilitation progression. Again, multiple sets (four to seven) through the velocity spectrum using 15 to 20 repetitions per set are recommended to foster local muscular endurance.

Return to Activity Phase (Weeks 12 to 16)

Objective measurement at 12 weeks postoperatively is followed and includes an isokinetic assessment of internal and external rotation strength in the modified base position, as well as careful documentation of AROM of flexion, abduction, and internal and external rotation with 90 degrees of abduction with scapular stabilization. Reevaluation of the patient using manual clinical techniques such as impingement and instability tests is also done at this time. Coupled with completion of subjective rating scales such as that of the American Shoulder and Elbow Surgeons[49,50] these objective and clinical tests provide guidance for the clinician regarding progression of the patient to functional activity simulation exercises and eventually interval sport return programming.

The presence of significant deficits in internal and external rotation strength and especially decreases in the unilateral strength balance, such as external/internal rotation ratios well below the desired 66% to 75% level, preclude the patient's progression to interval return programs at this time postoperatively.

Sport simulation exercises include the use of the 90/90 (abduction/external rotation) position during exercise either with isotonic weights (i.e., prone external rotation), prone plyometric ball catches (Figure 33-10) or external rotation at 90 degrees of abduction using the scapular plane and oscillation devices such as the body blade (Hymanson, TX) or Thera-Band resistance bar (Hygienic Corporation, Akron, OH) (Figure 33-11).

Continued training of the posterior rotator cuff to achieve optimal balance between the external and internal rotators as well as in the scapular stabilizers is recommended. Gradual progression to interval sport return programs for throwing, tennis, golf, and swimming is eventually started based on the repeated evaluation of muscular strength and balance, ROM, and clinical examination. Patients continue with home exercises after discharge from physical therapy with a core group of exercises emphasizing rotator cuff and scapular activation.

INDICATIONS FOR ARTHROSCOPIC REPAIR OF THE ROTATOR CUFF

The indications for arthroscopic rotator repair are continuing to evolve. As orthopedic surgeons have become more skillful with the arthroscope, more and more surgeons have been performing arthroscopic rotator cuff repair. Principles of and indications for arthroscopic repair remain the same as for open repairs. The surgeon must recognize the tear pattern, correctly and adequately mobilize the tissue, achieve tension-free approximation of the rotator cuff to the greater tuberosity, and finally achieve a secure repair to the tuberosity. Arthroscopic techniques and instruments have improved such that, from the standpoint of both the surgeon and patient, arthroscopic rotator cuff repair is a viable and attractive alternative to open rotator cuff repair. By repairing the rotator cuff through arthroscopic portals and cannulas, the deltoid is further protected from injury, and patients often have less pain as there is less surgical dissection to expose the rotator cuff. In addition, the rotator cuff can be assessed from multiple viewing angles through different portals to allow a better assessment of the rotator cuff.

The inability to obtain a secure anatomic repair would be a contraindication to arthroscopic repair and indicate the need for the surgeon to abort the arthroscopic repair and convert to an open repair. The efficacy of arthroscopic repair remains somewhat controversial. Multiple authors have shown equivalent results to open repair,[21,51,52] whereas others have shown good functional results with apparent failure of the arthroscopic repair on follow-up imaging of the rotator cuff.[53]

TECHNIQUE OF ARTHROSCOPIC ROTATOR CUFF REPAIR

Arthroscopic rotator cuff repair uses a preparatory arthroscopic evaluation including glenohumeral inspection and any required intraarticular surgery and the SAD components of bursectomy and/or acromioplasty. On completion of SAD, the rotator cuff is evaluated for repair through arthroscopic cannulas. One of the technical challenges of all-arthroscopic repair is fully appreciating the tear pattern and reapproximating the tear in the correct anatomic orientation to the greater tuberosity. It is more difficult to manipulate the torn tendon edge and determine the correct placement of the tendon to the bone. This is dependent on correct portal placement and ability to correctly identify the tear pattern. It is often

much easier to pull the tendon edge to the bone at different angles and configuration of repair through a small open incision than it is through arthroscopic portals. For this reason, ample experience at repairing rotator cuffs through open techniques is often a prerequisite to understanding tear patterns and achieving anatomic reapproximation of the rotator cuff tear.

Patients may be positioned for arthroscopic rotator cuff repairs in either in a lateral decubitus position with an overhead traction device or a beach-chair position with an assistant providing distal distraction or positioning the arm at varying angles of elevation and rotation for optimal visualization of the rotator cuff. Arthroscopic repairs may be performed with an arthroscopic pump system maintaining distention of the subacromial space and providing pressure for diminishing bleeding, both of which are very important for visualizing the rotator cuff. The fluid pressure and duration, however, may ultimately determine the length of surgery, as the soft tissues become edematous from the fluid and ultimately obscure the visualization for the repair. Therefore all of the operative components of the arthroscopic procedure must generally be performed within 2 hours. This includes the diagnostic arthroscopy, any operative procedure within the glenohumeral joint such as labral repair, debridement or loose body removal and the SAD, and mobilization and repair of the rotator cuff. If the tissues become too edematous to complete the repair arthroscopically then the procedure must be converted to an open procedure. Arthroscopic cannulas minimize fluid extravasation into the soft tissues. Care must be taken to ensure that the cannulas do not partially extrude from the subacromial space, allowing more rapid egress of the fluid into the deltoid muscle.

Arthroscopic rotator cuff repair is generally performed through at least three working portals. A standard posterior portal is used for arthroscopic visualization of the subacromial space. A standard anterior portal is used for suture management. An anterolateral portal is used for SAD and repair of the rotator cuff. Accessory portals may also be used as necessary. An accessory posterolateral portal may be used for more direct visualization of the rotator cuff during repair. This portal is generally anterior and lateral to the posterolateral corner of the acromion. The posterolateral viewing portal provides a more optimum orientation of the arthroscope to the torn edge of the tendon and does not crowd the anterolateral portal or compromise the deltoid by having the portals too close together. An accessory anterolateral portal may be necessary for suture anchor placement. This portal is often made through a small stab incision that does not compromise the deltoid. Because the only device that passes through this portal is the anchor inserter, the portal is not any larger than the core diameter of the anchor and its inserter. Arthroscopic cannulas are necessary to allow passage of suture and instruments through a single defect in the deltoid. Multiple passes of the cannula or instruments through the deltoid may compromise the deltoid and therefore negate the beneficial effects of the all-arthroscopic repair.

Two additional portals may be used by the surgeon for the passage of sutures through the rotator cuff.[54] These are the subclavian and modified Neviaser portals. The subclavian portal is placed anterior and inferior to the distal clavicle, with passage of suture passing instrument inferior and parallel to the undersurface of the clavicle into the subacromial space. This portal is very useful for repair of anterior supraspinatus tears, as there is a straight path to penetrate the rotator cuff for retrieval of the suture from the suture anchor. Similarly the modified Neviaser portal is used for a direct pathway for suture retrieval through the posterior supraspinatus and infraspinatus tendons. The modified Neviaser portal is placed in the soft spot posterior to the AC joint and is angled laterally beneath the posterior acromion into the subacromial space. The subclavian and modified Neviaser portals are used without arthroscopic cannulas because the portals are made through small stab incisions.

On completion of the SAD, the rotator cuff tear is assessed for size, orientation, mobility, and quality of tendinous tissue. Subacromial and capsulolabral adhesions are released with a blunt elevator. Care must be taken when elevating the posterior superior capsule from the labrum, as the suprascapular nerve lies approximately 2 cm medial to the superior labrum in the spinoglenoid notch. Therefore the capsulolabral dissection should not extend more than 1 to 1.5 cm medial to the labrum. Traction sutures placed through the margin of the rotator cuff tear will provide countertraction for the release of the adhesions and will confirm that adequate release has been performed when the tendon edge is pulled to the anticipated repair site. Excessive tension on the traction sutures to reapproximate the tendon indicates inadequate release or failure to recognize the tear pattern. Nonanatomic repair of an L-shaped tear to a crescent-shaped repair will result in either excessive tension on the repair and early failure or postoperative loss of ROM.[55,56] In large to massive tears the configuration of the tear may require side-to-side margin convergence repair of the anterior and posterior leaves of the tear. This diminishes the strain on the rotator cuff and allows tension-free repair of the lateral margin of the tear to the greater tuberosity.[57] Occasionally, massive rotator cuff tears may require additional releases to achieve adequate mobility of the tendon to allow repair.[58] A rotator interval slide may be performed by releasing the supraspinatus from the coracohumeral ligament. A posterior interval slide is performed by releasing the interval between the supraspinatus and infraspinatus tendons to the level of the acromial spine. Massive rotator cuff tears are often easier to repair via these arthroscopic techniques than traditional open techniques. The arthroscope allows increased visualization to perform the releases and allows better access to the medial margin of the tear for repair via margin convergence.

After the tendon is mobilized and the repair orientation is determined, the greater tuberosity is prepared by abrading the cortical bone of the anchor site lateral to articular margin. Placements of the anchors are generally in the area of the abraded tuberosity. More lateral placement of the anchors allows the tendon to be brought over the anatomic footprint of the rotator cuff insertion. However, more lateral placement may also increase the tension on the repair, and care must be taken to adequately mobilize the tendon before passage of sutures from a laterally placed anchor.

Arthroscopic rotator cuff repairs use suture anchors placed in the greater tuberosity rather than in the traditional transosseous tunnels. Biomechanical evaluation of suture anchors has shown that rotator cuff fixation with anchors is superior to transosseous tunnels.[44] Many surgeons who continue to perform open rotator cuff repairs now use suture anchors rather than bone tunnels because the anchor fixation is stronger, quicker, and easier to achieve. One limitation of arthroscopic repair is the difficulty in passing sutures through the tendon for repair, as compared with passing sutures with open techniques. It is much more difficult to place a tendon-grasping suture such as with a modified Mason-Allen suture technique arthroscopically. Much stronger fixation of the tendon may be accomplished with a double-loaded suture anchor, such that one pair of sutures is placed in horizontal mattress fashion and the second suture pair is passed in simple suture fashion.[59] The suture tail of the simple suture is passed behind the anticipated loop of the horizontal mattress suture. The horizontal mattress suture is then tied and the simple suture is tied such that it grasps not only the tendon it encompasses, but also the tendon fixed by the horizontal mattress suture. Another modification of this technique is to place a suture that is not attached to an anchor in horizontal mattress fashion through the tendon and tying it around the tendon. This suture loop then acts as the grasping suture for a subsequent simple suture from a suture anchor.

Passage of the sutures and suture management are often the most demanding aspects of arthroscopic rotator cuff repair. As the technique of arthroscopic rotator cuff repair has continue to evolve, multiple suture-passing devices and techniques have been commercially developed. Fundamentally, the most efficient suture-passing techniques require a direct line of sight between the anchor and the anticipated point of suture passage through the tendon. Suture passage may be performed by direct technique via arthroscopic suture-passage needles, or suture retrievers. Suture passage may also be performed by an indirect technique via a shuttling system that first passes a suture loop through the tendon. The suture loop is then used to pull the anchor suture through the tendon. Often a combination of techniques is required to pass the sutures, depending on the location in the tendon where suture will pass. Side-to-side margin convergence sutures are placed by direct hand-off of a suture from a penetrating suture retriever through one leaf of the tendon to another penetrating retriever through the other leaf of the tendon. On passage of each set of sutures, the sutures must be separated from adjacent suture pairs and identified as a pair with a tagging hemostat. Larger and more complex tears require more sutures for repair, and often suture management becomes a serious problem. Great care must be taken during the passage and tying of sutures to prevent entanglement of sutures with adjacent sutures. Commercially available suture straws are helpful in identifying and separating sutures to prevent suture entanglement. These are usually unnecessary if the surgeon has a clear plan for passage of the sutures. All the sutures are passed first and then tied sequentially such that tying a suture pair does not obscure visualization for tying the remaining sets. Margin convergence sutures are passed and tied first to allow identification of the lateral margin of the tear for repair to the greater tuberosity with a suture anchor. Margin convergence sutures are passed and tied sequentially in a medial-to-lateral direction to converge the rotator cuff repair to the greater tuberosity.

Multiple knot tying techniques have been developed and espoused by various authors. Fundamentally, successful arthroscopic rotator cuff repair requires loop and knot security.[22] The arthroscopic knot must reapproximate the tendon to the bone without gapping of the repair that occurs when there is slack in the loop (loop integrity). The knot must also hold itself via friction within the suture to prevent knot slippage. Horizontal mattress sutures generally will not slide through the tendon and must be tied with reversing half-hitch sutures. Reversing the suture post and the orientation of the suture throw increases the friction of the knot and thereby increases the knot integrity. It can be difficult to maintain tension on the first half hitch, and therefore loop integrity may be lost, with excessive slack in the suture loop. Sliding knots and sliding locking knots have been developed that prevent the knot from backing off from the tendon as it is being repaired. It is important to note but sometimes difficult to appreciate the degree of tension placed on the rotator cuff by the sutures. Adequate mobilization of the tendon before suturing the tendon will help prevent repair failures. Despite all the care taken to mobilize and repair the tendon with tension-free repair and good loop and knot integrity, the ultimate outcome of the repair is most often dependent on the quality of the tendon itself. Most rotator cuff failures occur because the suture pulls through the tendon. Use of grasping sutures such as arthroscopic Mason-Allen sutures will help to prevent sutures from pulling through the tendon.

After the sutures have been tied and cut, the integrity of the repair is assessed. The shoulder is taken through a full ROM to ensure there is no gapping of the repaired tissue and no loss of motion resulting from excessive tension of the repair. Clearance of the knot beneath the acromion is also evaluated during ROM of the shoulder. Generally if there has been adequate visualization of subacromial space to allow arthroscopic repair, an adequate acromioplasty has been performed and there will be no impingement of the sutures on the undersurface of the acromion. The repair is tested with an arthroscopic probe to be sure the tendon is closely approximated to the bone. The intraoperative findings of ROM and integrity of the repair will dictate the postoperative rehabilitation regimen.

RAMIFICATIONS OF SURGICAL TECHNIQUE FOR POSTOPERATIVE REHABILITATION AND POSTOPERATIVE PROTECTION

Similar to the surgical approach inherent in the deltoid splitting approach, the fact that the all-arthroscopic rotator cuff repair does not violate the integrity of the overlying deltoid muscle in any way permits immediate progression of PROM and AAROM and eventual AROM. Because similar healing constraints are ultimately needed for the rotator cuff, postoperative protection principles including sling use and immobilization are presently similar. With specific reference to rehabilitation after arthroscopic rotator cuff repair, the reader is directed to the postoperative protocol for mini-open rotator cuff repair, because at this time, rehabilitation of the all-arthroscopic rotator cuff repair follows similar sequences and procedures.

REHABILITATION AFTER ARTHROSCOPIC ROTATOR CUFF REPAIR

A recent survey conducted by Wilk[60] polled leading fellowship-trained orthopedic surgeons regarding rotator cuff repair. The results of the poll indicated that 85% of the surgeons have performed all-arthroscopic rotator cuff repairs, with 15% saying they have not. Factors used to determine whether the all-arthroscopic technique was performed included tear size, mobility of the tissue, and tissue quality, as well as the age and activity level of the patient. Furthermore, the survey asked about the direction of postoperative rehabilitation after the all-arthroscopic procedure as compared with the mini-open procedure. Twelve percent of surgeons surveyed said they progressed rehabilitation at a faster rate with the all-arthroscopic procedure, whereas 12% stated they actually slowed the rate of rehabilitation progression. Seventy-six percent said they guided rehabilitation at the same rate as for the mini-open procedure. Clearly, no objective standards have as yet been established that provide rationale for altering the progression of rehabilitation, as neither the mini-open nor the all-arthroscopic procedure alters the deltoid origin. Further research and development of objectively based rehabilitation protocols are needed to advance the understanding of clinical rehabilitation that follows the all-arthroscopic rotator cuff repair.

OUTCOMES AFTER MINI-OPEN AND ARTHROSCOPIC ROTATOR CUFF REPAIR

Objective outcomes after arthroscopically assisted mini-open rotator cuff repair were retrospectively collected on 59 patients with a mean age of 58 years by Ellenbecker and co-workers.[61] ROM measured at 6 and 12 weeks postoperatively, as well as isokinetic internal and external rotation strength obtained in 30 degrees of elevation in the scapular plane (modified base position), were analyzed. In addition, the self-report section of the modified American Shoulder and Elbow Surgeons rating scale was used at 12 weeks postoperatively and measured 38 out of 45 possible points. To summarize these data, patients by 12 weeks postoperatively achieved a level at which 4- to 9-degree deficits in cardinal plane active motion were present, and 8% to 10% deficits in isokinetic external shoulder rotation strength were measured. Internal rotation was equal between extremities. Unilateral strength ratios (external rotators [ER]/internal rotators [IR]) ranged between 41% and 62% on the involved extremity at 12 weeks postoperatively. The desired goal or standard for the unilateral ER/IR ratio is 66% to 75%, indicating proper development of the posterior rotator cuff.[47,48] This information shows that by 12 weeks postoperatively, patients have minimal deficits in motion and only mild deficiencies in posterior rotator cuff strength (ER).

Evaluation of strength at 6 months and 1 year after open rotator cuff repair using an open deltopectoral approach with detachment (15 subjects) and mini-open deltoid splitting approach (10 subjects) using a Cybex isokinetic dynamometer was performed by Kirschenbaum and colleagues.[62] Testing was performed bilaterally at 90 degrees/second, with deficits in external rotation at 6 months postoperatively measured at 24%. By 1 year postoperatively the involved extremity had achieved a level of strength 42% greater than in the uninjured extremity for external rotation. Internal rotation was not measured. This study shows significant deficits in external rotation strength 6 months after rotator cuff repair and highlights the potential complications of deltoid detachment and delayed strengthening, which is required with the more extensive approaches used in open rotator cuff repair.

ADDITIONAL OUTCOME STUDIES AFTER ROTATOR CUFF REPAIR

Blevins and co-workers[63] performed a follow-up of 78 patients after mini-open rotator cuff repair. Average follow-up was 29.2 months postoperatively. Active elevation improved from 129 degrees preoperatively to 166 degrees postoperatively, with weakness measurable during clinical evaluation using manual muscle testing (MMT) in 83% of patients preoperatively and only 22% postoperatively. Eighty-nine percent were satisfied with their results, and the researchers found no statistical correlation between tear size and the Hospital for Special Surgery shoulder score.

Burkhart and colleagues[21] reported on 62 patients who had all-arthroscopic rotator cuff repairs, of which 59 were available for follow-up. Tears were categorized by tear size as well as tear shape. Crescent-shaped tears were repaired in a direct tendon-to-bone fashion, and U-shaped tears were repaired by a margin convergence technique as described earlier in this chapter. Good and excellent results were reported in 95% of all cases, with the large and massive tears fairing equally as well as the small and medium tears. U-shaped tears repaired via margin convergence were equal in ultimate result to the crescent-shaped tears repaired directly to bone.

COMPARISON BETWEEN MINI-OPEN AND ARTHROSCOPIC ROTATOR CUFF REPAIRS

Kim and co-workers[64] performed 76 rotator cuff repairs of full-thickness tears, with 42 being performed solely using arthroscopy and the remaining 34 repairs being salvaged using the mini-open technique. They report improved shoulder function in both groups, with no significant difference between the two groups in postoperative ROM, strength, or functional scores. Their data analysis revealed that the ultimate outcome after surgery was related more to tear size than to the method of repair.

Severud and colleagues[65] reported the results of 64 rotator cuff repairs by the same surgeon at a mean follow-up of 44 months. This study included 35 repairs performed arthroscopically and 29 performed using the mini-open deltoid splitting approach. Severud and co-workers[65] found no significant difference in postoperative UCLA rating scales between groups; however, one important finding relates to the recovery of postoperative ROM. The authors report the development of fibrous ankylosis in four of 29 cases in the mini-open group (14%) and in 0 of 35 cases in the all-arthroscopic group (0%). This trend for better ROM in the all-arthroscopic group will likely be an area of future study in prospective studies evaluating the potential outcomes after rotator cuff repair.

In a large series of arthroscopic rotator cuff repairs by Wolf and co-workers,[52] 94% reported good and excellent results at a follow-up at 4 to 10 years. One hundred and five patients underwent all-arthroscopic rotator cuff repair and were evaluated at a mean of 75 months postoperatively using the modified UCLA rating scale. Ninety-six percent of the patients stated that they were satisfied with their results, and only four patients rated the surgery as unsuccessful. The results from this study compare favorably with the published reports that followed open rotator cuff repair, in which good and excellent results were reported in 71% to 92% of patients, and in 77% to 88% of patients who underwent SAD alone without repair.[52]

Finally, a recent study by Galatz and colleagues[53] evaluated the outcome and integrity of the rotator cuff after arthroscopic repair of large and massive rotator cuff tears. Eighteen all-arthroscopic tears were evaluated 1 and 2 years postoperatively. Preoperative functional rating scales were measured at 48.3 and increased to 84.6 at 1 year postoperatively. Between the first and second years, however, the functional rating score decreased to a mean of 79.9. Patients similarly showed improved active elevation ROM between preoperative measures, where eight of 18 had less than 95 degrees, to a mean at 1 year postoperatively of 152 degrees, but decreased to 142 degrees at 2 years postoperatively.

Galatz and co-workers[53] also found recurrent defects in the repaired rotator cuff tendon in 17 of 18 patients at 1 year postoperatively when evaluated with ultrasound. They concluded that a large percentage of patients who undergo all-arthroscopic rotator cuff repair appear to have recurrent defects, and that decline in function occurs between the first and second year after surgery. Gaziely and colleagues[66] studied the anatomic results of 98 patients at an average 4-year follow-up after mini-open deltoid splitting rotator cuff repair and found 11% of repaired rotator cuffs to be "thinned" but fully intact, and 65% of repairs to be fully intact. The functional results obtained via a Constant's functional score correlated more closely with the anatomic status of the rotator cuff at follow-up viewed with ultrasonography than with preoperative tear size. Further study examining both the objective functional outcome and tendon integrity after rotator cuff repair will provide further guidance to rehabilitation professionals.

SUMMARY

The basic scientific information and surgical overviews provided in this chapter are meant to instill a greater understanding of the anatomic and biomechanical demands on the rotator cuff and the surgical procedures applied to restore the anatomy and biomechanics. The postoperative rehabilitation protocol that progressively increases the intensity of ROM and strength training based on many principles from the basic science literature is presented as a guide to assist clinicians in rehabilitation after rotator cuff repair. Further research will assist clinicians in the development of optimal rehabilitation progressions as more information becomes available.

References

1. Neer CS: Anterior acromioplasty for the chronic impingement syndrome in the shoulder. A preliminary report, *J Bone Joint Surg* 54A:41, 1972.
2. Neer CS: Impingement lesions, *Clin Orthop* 173:70, 1983.
3. Golding FC: The shoulder: the forgotten joint, *Br J Radiol* 35:149, 1962.
4. Cotton RE, Rideout DF: Tears of the humeral rotator cuff: a radiological and pathological necropsy survey, *J Bone Joint Surg* 46B:314, 1964.
5. Poppen NK, Walker PS: Forces at the glenohumeral joint in abduction, *Clin Orthop* 135:165, 1978.
6. Lucas DB: Biomechanics of the shoulder joint, *Arch Surg* 107:425, 1973.
7. Wuelker N, Plitz W, Roetman B: Biomechanical data concerning the shoulder impingement syndrome, *Clin Orthop* 303:242, 1994.
8. Bigliani LU, Ticker JB, Flatow EL, et al: The relationship of acromial architecture to rotator cuff disease, *Clin Sports Med* 10:823, 1991.
9. Zuckerman JD, Kummer FJ, Cuomo F, et al: The influence of coracoacromial arch anatomy on rotator cuff tears, *J Shoulder Elbow Surg* 1:4, 1992.
10. Nirschl RP: Shoulder tendonitis. In Pettrone FP, editor: *Upper extremity injuries in athletes. American Academy of Orthopaedic Surgeons Symposium*, St. Louis, 1988, Mosby.
11. Fleisig GS, Andrews JR, Dillman CJ, Escamilla RF: Kinetics of baseball pitching with implications about injury mechanisms, *Am J Sports Med* 23:233, 1995.
12. Jobe FW, Kivitne RS: Shoulder pain in the overhand or throwing athlete: the relationship of anterior instability and rotator cuff impingement, *Orthop Rev* 28:963, 1989.
13. Andrews JR, Alexander EJ: Rotator cuff injury in throwing and racquet sports, *Sports Med Arthroscop Rev* 3:30, 1995.
14. Iannotti JP: Lesions of the rotator cuff: pathology and pathogenesis. In Matsen FA, Fu FH, Hawkins RJ, editors: *The shoulder: a balance of mobility and stability*, Rosemont, IL, 1993, American Academy of Orthopaedic Surgeons.
15. Loehr JF, Helmig P, Sojbjerg JO, Jung A: Shoulder instability caused by rotator cuff lesions: an in vitro study, *Clin Orthop* 303:84, 1994.
16. Miller C, Savoie FH: Glenohumeral abnormalities associated with full-thickness tears of the rotator cuff, *Orthop Rev* 23:159, 1994.
17. Fukuda H, Hamada K, Yamanaka K: Pathology and pathogenesis of bursal side rotator cuff tears viewed from en bloc histologic sections, *Clin Orthop* 254:75, 1990.
18. Nakajima T, Rokumma N, Kazutoshi H, et al: Histologic and biomechanical characteristics of the supraspinatus tendon: reference to rotator cuff tearing, *J Shoulder Elbow Surgery* 3:79, 1994.
19. Timmerman LA, Andrews JR, Wilk KE: Mini Open repair of the rotator cuff. In Andrews JR, Wilk KE, editors: *The athletes shoulder*, Philadelphia, 1994, Churchill Livingstone.
20. Itoi E, Tabata S: Conservative treatment of rotator cuff tears, *Clin Orthop* 275:165, 1992.
21. Burkhart SS, Danaceau SM, Pearce CE Jr: Arthroscopic rotator cuff repair: analysis of results by tear size and by repair technique—margin convergence versus direct tendon-to-bone repair, *Arthroscopy* 17:905-912, 2001.
22. Burkhart SS: A stepwise approach to arthroscopic rotator cuff repair based on biomechanical principles, *Arthroscopy* 16:82-90, 2000.
23. Fealy S, Kingham P, Altchek DW: Mini-open rotator cuff repair using a 2 row fixation technique. Outcomes analysis in patients with small, moderate, and large rotator cuff tears, *Arthroscopy* 18:665-670, 2002.
24. Kibler WB: The role of the scapula in athletic shoulder function, *Am J Sports Med* 26:325-337, 1998.
25. Kibler WB, Uhl TL, Maddux JWQ, et al: Qualitative clinical evaluation of scapular dysfunction: a reliability study, *J Shoulder Elbow Surgery* 11:550-556, 2002.
26. Ellenbecker TS, Roetert EP, Piorkowski PA, Schulz DA: Glenohumeral joint internal and external rotation range of motion in elite junior tennis players, *J Orthop Sports Phys Ther* 24:336-341, 1996.
27. Hatakeyama Y, Itoi E, Urayama M, et al: Effect of superior capsule and coracohumeral ligament release on strain in the repaired rotator cuff tendon, *Am J Sports Medicine* 29:633-640, 2001.
28. Rathburn JB, MacNab I: The microvascular pattern of the rotator cuff, *J Bone Joint Surg* 52B:540, 1970.
29. Maitland GD: *Peripheral manipulation*, London, 1970, Butterworth.
30. McMahon TJ, Donatelli RA: Manual therapy techniques. In Donatelli RA, editor: *Physical therapy of the shoulder*, ed 4, Philadelphia, 2004, Churchill Livingstone.

31. Gerber C, Werner CML, Macy JC, et al: Effect of selective capsulorrhaphy on the passive range of motion of the glenohumeral joint, *J Bone Joint Surgery* 85-A:48-55, 2003.

32. Bagg SD, Forrest WJ: A biomechanical analysis of scapular rotation during arm abduction in the scapular plane, *Arch Phys Med Rehabil* 238-245, 1988.

33. McCann PD, Wooten ME, Kadaba MP, Bigliani LU: A kinematic and electromyographic study of shoulder rehabilitation exercises, *Clin Orthop* 288:178-189, 1993.

34. Kibler WB, Livingston B, Bruce R: Current concepts in shoulder rehabilitation. In: *Advances in operative orthopaedics,* vol 3, St Louis, 1995, Mosby.

35. Warner JPP, Bowen MK, Deng X, et al: Effect of joint compression on inferior stability of the glenohumeral joint, *J Shoulder Elbow Surgery* 8:31-36, 1999.

36. Townsend H, Jobe FW, Pink M, et al: Electromyographic analysis of the glenohumeral muscles during a baseball rehabilitation program, *Am J Sports Med* 19:264, 1991.

37. Ballantyne BT, O'Hare SJ, Paschall JL, et al: Electromyographic activity of selected shoulder muscles in commonly used therapeutic exercises, *Phys Ther* 73:668, 1993.

38. Blackburn TA, McLeod WD, White B, et al: EMG analysis of posterior rotator cuff exercises, *Athletic Training* 25:40, 1990.

39. Reinhold MM, Wilk KE, Fleisig GS, et al: Electromyographic analysis of the rotator cuff and deltoid musculature during common shoulder external rotation exercises, *J Orthop Sports Phys Ther* 34:385-394.

40. Moncrief SA, Lau JD, Gale JR, Scott SA: Effect of rotator cuff exercise on humeral rotation torque in healthy individuals, *J Strength Cond Res* 16:262-270, 2002.

41. Ellenbecker TS: Rehabilitation of shoulder and elbow injuries in tennis players, *Clin Sports Med* 14:87-109, 1995.

42. Page P, Ellenbecker TS: *The scientific and clinical application of elastic resistance,* Champaign, IL, 2003, Human Kinetics.

43. Burkhart SS, Johnson TC, Wirth MA, Athanasiou KA: Cyclic loading of transosseous rotator cuff repairs: tension overload as a possible cause of failure, *Arthroscopy* 13:172-176, 1997a.

44. Burkhart SS, Pagan JLD, Wirth MA, Athanasiou KA: Cyclic loading of anchor-based rotator cuff repairs: confirmation of the tension overload phenomenon and comparison of suture anchor fixation with transosseous fixation, *Arthroscopy* 13:720-724, 1997b.

45. MaCabe RA, Tyler TF, Nicholas SJ, McHugh MP: Selective activation of the lower trapezius muscle in patients with shoulder impingement, *J Orthop Sports Phys Ther* 31:A-45, 2001 (abstract).

46. Otis JC, Jiang CC, Wickiewicz TL, et al: Changes in moment arms of the rotator cuff and deltoid muscles with abduction and rotation, *J Bone Joint Surgery* 76-A:667-676, 1994.

47. Ellenbecker TS, Davies GJ: The application of isokinetics in testing and rehabilitation of the shoulder complex, *J Athl Train* 35:338-350, 2000.

48. Davies GJ: *A compendium of isokinetic in clinical usage,* LaCrosse, WI, 1992, S & S Publishers.

49. Beaton D, Richards RR: Assessing the reliability and responsiveness of 5 shoulder questionnaires, *J Shoulder Elbow Surgery* 7:565-572, 1998.

50. Richards RR, An KN, Bigliani LU, et al: A standardized method for the assessment of shoulder function, *J Shoulder Elbow Surgery* 3:347-352, 1994.

51. Bennett WF: Arthroscopic repair of full-thickness supraspinatus tears (small-to-medium): a prospective study with 2- to 4-year follow-up, *Arthroscopy* 19:249-256, 2003.

52. Wolf EM, Pennington WT, Agrawal V: Arthroscopic rotator cuff repair: 4- to 10-year results, *Arthroscopy* 20:5-12, 2004.

53. Galatz LM, Ball CM, Teefey SA, et al: The outcome and repair integrity of completely arthroscopically repaired large and massive rotator cuff tears, *J Bone Joint Surg Am* 86-A:219-224, 2004.

54. Nord KD, Mauck BM: The new subclavian portal and modified Neviaser portal for arthroscopic rotator cuff repair, *Arthroscopy* 19:1030-1034, 2003.

55. Lo IK, Burkhart SS: Current concepts in arthroscopic rotator cuff repair, *Am J Sports Med* 31:308-324, 2003.

56. Kibler WB, Dome DC: Chronic shoulder injuries. In Garrick J, editor: *Orthopedic knowledge update: sports medicine,* Rosemont, 2004, American Academy of Orthopaedic Surgery.

57. Burkhart SS, Athanasiou KA, Wirth MA: Margin convergence: a method of reducing strain in massive rotator cuff tears, *Arthroscopy* 12:335-338, 1996.

58. Tauro JC: Arthroscopic repair of large rotator cuff tears using the interval slide technique, *Arthroscopy* 20:13-21, 2004.

59. Scheibel MT, Habermeyer P: A modified Mason-Allen technique for rotator cuff repair using suture anchors, *Arthroscopy* 19:330-333, 2003.

60. Wilk KE: Unpublished Survey. Arthroscopic Rotator Cuff Repair. Presented at APTA National Symposium, Washington DC, June 2003.

61. Ellenbecker TS, Elmore EE, Bailie DS: Glenohumeral joint range of motion and rotational strength following rotator cuff repair using a mini-open deltoid splitting technique. Accepted for publication in *J Orthop Sports Phys Therapy,* 2006.

62. Kirschenbaum D, Coyle MP, Leddy JP, et al: Shoulder strength with rotator cuff tears. Pre and postoperative analysis, *Clin Orthop* 288:174-178, 1993.

63. Blevins FT, Warren RF, Cavo C, et al: Arthroscopic assisted rotator cuff repair: Results using a mini-open deltoid splitting approach, *Arthroscopy* 12:50-59, 1996.

64. Kim SH, Ha KI, Park JH, et al: Arthroscopic versus mini-open salvage repair of the rotator cuff tear: outcome analysis at 2 to 6 years' follow-up, *Arthroscopy* 19:746-754, 2003.

65. Severud EL, Ruotolo C, Abbott DD, Nottage WM: All-arthroscopic versus mini-open rotator cuff repair: a long term retrospective outcome comparison, *Arthroscopy* 19:234-238, 2003.

66. Gazielly DF, Gleyze P, Montagnon C: Functional and anatomical results after rotator cuff repair, *Clin Orthop* 304:43-53, 1994.

CHAPTER 34

Rehabilitation after Surgical Treatment of the Long-Head Biceps Tendon

Todd S. Ellenbecker, PT, DPT, MS, SCS, OCS, CSCS
David S. Bailie, MD

THE IMPORTANT ROLE OF THE BICEPS

in upper extremity function has more recently been investigated. In addition, the increased focus on injury identification and ultimately on treatment of superior labral anterior to posterior (SLAP) injury has also created interest in understanding the role and function of the long head of the biceps tendon (LHBT). The close relationship of the LHBT to the superior labrum, subscapularis, rotator interval, and coracohumeral ligament has created an increased interest in the functional anatomy, biomechanics, and evaluation methods of the LHBT in the literature.[1] The purpose of this chapter is to review the anatomy and biomechanics of the LHBT as well as to discuss the proposed mechanisms of LHBT injury and give an overview of surgical treatment (both open and arthroscopic) and postoperative rehabilitation strategies.

ANATOMY AND BIOMECHANICS OF THE LONG HEAD BICEPS TENDON

The LHBT originates within the glenohumeral joint and after coursing through the bicipital groove between the greater and lesser tuberosities joins the short head of the biceps at the level of the deltoid tubercle. Habermeyer and colleagues,[2] in an anatomic study, found the LHBT to originate from the posterior superior labrum in 48% of specimens examined and from the supraglenoid tubercle in 20%. Twenty-eight percent had an origin of the LHBT in both sites.[2] Within the glenohumeral joint, the tendon is intraarticular but extrasynovial, ensheathed by a continuation of the synovial lining of the articular capsule.[3]

The function of the LHBT is controversial. Kumar and co-workers[4] reported upward migration of the humeral head in 15 cadavers with intraarticular release of the LHBT. Dynamic depression of the humeral head was demonstrated by Warner and McMahon,[5] who also showed superior migration of the humeral head relative to the contralateral or control shoulder in seven patients with loss of the LHBT. Several studies[6-8] have identified the function of the LHBT as a stabilizer against anterior humeral head translation. The torsional rigidity of the anterior capsule is reportedly increased, and forces transmitted to the inferior glenohumeral ligament complex are decreased, during simulated contraction of the biceps in experimental studies.[6] Detachment of the biceps anchor at the superior labrum has been shown to increase the strain on the inferior glenohumeral ligament complex up to 120%.[9] These studies show the important role the biceps and superior labrum play in the stabilization of the human glenohumeral joint.

Dynamic muscular activity of the biceps has been measured using electromyography (EMG) during both planar motions and functional activities.[10,11] Yamaguchi and colleagues[11] studied the EMG activity of the biceps in 40 subjects who had their elbows locked in a brace to prohibit elbow movement and isolate shoulder function. Planar shoulder motions were performed, including internal and external rotation and scapular elevation. EMG activity of the biceps ranged from 1.7% to 3.6% of maximal activation levels. In addition, no difference was found in the study by Yamaguchi and co-workers[11] between subjects with full-thickness rotator cuff tears and normal subjects. The conclusion drawn by the researchers was that, given the EMG results of the investigation, the function of the biceps during isolated glenohumeral motion does not include active contraction of the biceps. Levy and colleagues,[12] using similar methodology, also found limited EMG activity of the LHBT during shoulder motion and concluded that "any hypothesis on biceps function at the shoulder must be a passive role of the tendon or tension in association with elbow and forearm activity."

Glousman and co-workers[10] compared the EMG activity among throwing athletes diagnosed with glenohumeral joint instability and in normal throwing athletes. Increases in biceps EMG activity were found during the acceleration phase of the throwing motion in the group of athletes with glenohumeral joint instability. This increased activity in the biceps was thought to improve glenohumeral joint stabilization.

In summary, despite the exact origin of the LHBT and the common finding of some function of humeral head depression by the LHBT, controversy exists regarding the exact function of the LHBT at the shoulder. Further research will likely delineate whether this role is passive or involves an active contractile function. Clinicians, however, can be confident that the low levels of muscular activity found during glenohumeral movements in the LHBT indicate that shoulder movement will not provide significant contractile tension and stress to labral repair or biceps stabilization procedures.

INJURY MECHANISMS

Injury to the biceps tendon can occur as an isolated entity; however, in most cases problems with this structure occur in conjunction with glenohumeral joint impingement or instability.[1]

The specific pathomechanics that lead to injury in the LHBT typically focus around impingement or compression of the tendon in the suprahumeral space. According the Neer,[13] in most patients with LHBT pathology the primary source of the pain is glenohumeral impingement, with biceps tendonitis being secondary. "Both Charles Neer and Charles Rockwood have stressed the fact that 95% to 98% of patients with the diagnosis of biceps tendonitis have in reality a primary diagnosis of impingement syndrome."[14,15]

In addition to impingement as the primary pathomechanical factor in biceps tendonitis, Eakin and colleagues[1] have described the close association between glenohumeral joint instability and biceps involvement. Forces generated, particularly during overhead shoulder motions in sports, on a repetitive basis eventually exceed the capability of the anterior static restraints of the shoulder. Eventually, progressive attenuation of these restraints can cause a traction injury to both the rotator cuff and the biceps tendon. This attenuation can lead to secondary impingement against the coracoacromial arch by the biceps tendon, creating further injury.[1]

In addition, primary tendinosis has been described as being a factor in the pathogenesis of LHBT injury. Factors leading to degenerative tendinosis include hypovascularity[16] and fiber failure, as well as mechanical irritation within the intertubercular groove.[1] Kraushaar and Nirschl[17] have described the degenerative response of tendon injury and highlighted the lack of inflammatory cells and high concentration of fibroblasts and vascular hyperplasia in histologic study of injured tendons. This tendon degeneration can lead to failure and tendon rupture. Studies of pathologic LHBTs have defined specific areas in which the inflammation tends to occur. A cadaveric study looking at the LHBT showed that the inflammation of the tendon occurred primarily at the supraglenoid tubercle origin or at the distal extent of the bicipital groove.[18] In a study of patients with primary bicipital tenosynovitis, Post and Benca[19] stated that all the inflammation observed occurred in the bicipital groove and never in the intracapsular portion of the tendon. They also observed inflammatory changes in the walls of the bicipital groove.

Finally, LHBT instability has been described as another form of biceps pathology at the glenohumeral joint. Although rare, this condition was thought to be primarily a result of tearing of the transverse ligament, which overlies the bicipital groove of the humerus.[1] Cadaveric study, however, has shown that even with transection of the transverse humeral ligament over the groove, the LHBT did not subluxate medially.[20] Walch and co-workers[21] have highlighted the importance of the rotator interval lesion and the critical function of the coracohumeral ligament and superior glenohumeral ligament as stabilizers of the LHBT.

In summary, Table 34-1 lists the classification of biceps tendon pathology at the glenohumeral joint based on the descriptions of Curtis and Snyder.[3] The close association of other glenohumeral joint abnormalities such as rotator cuff impingement and glenohumeral joint instability emphasizes the importance of performing a comprehensive examination of the patient with suspected LHBT involvement.

CLINICAL DIAGNOSIS OF BICEPS TENDON PATHOLOGY

Two clinical tests that have been widely used in orthopedic evaluation of the patient with anterior shoulder pain are Speed's and Yergason's tests. Both involve manual resistance applied to the patient to reproduce pain in the bicipital groove of the proximal humerus. A recent study by Holtby and Razmjou[22] evaluated 152 patients with complaints of anterior shoulder pain to determine the validity of Yergason's and Speed's test results by comparing them with the findings of surgery. Fifty subjects from the original pool of 152 patients met the criteria for surgery and were evaluated against the clinical findings of positive Speed's and Yergason's test results. Of the 50 subjects, two were found to have bicipital tendonitis secondary to rotator cuff pathology, 10 biceps partial

tears, and two complete ruptures. Fifteen patients had a type I SLAP lesion, 12 had type II SLAP lesions, and one patient had a type IV SLAP lesion. The authors reported sensitivity values of 79% for Yergason's test and 32% for Speed's test, as well as specificity of 60% for Yergason's test and 75% for Speed's test. The authors conclude that although these two biceps tests have moderate levels of specificity, their outcome is unlikely to cause a change in the pretest diagnosis. No alternative tests were provided by the authors to more accurately assess biceps tendon pathology clinically. It is important for the clinician to recognize the wide spectrum of surgically confirmed anatomic findings that are commonly associated with positive clinical Speed's and Yergason's test results and the importance of a comprehensive clinical examination in orthopedics and sports medicine.

TREATMENT OF BICEPS TENDON PATHOLOGY

Treatment of LHBT pathology begins with standard nonoperative measures, including physical therapy.[23,24] Corticosteroid injections may be beneficial, but care must be taken to avoid injection into the tendon substance.[25] When nonoperative therapy fails, surgical treatment has generally centered around tenodesis of the LHBT. This treatment, however, has not shown lasting benefit in long-term follow up.[26,27] The lack of long-term efficacy has been suggested to result from a loss of function of the LHBT as a humeral head depressor.[13,27] In this chapter, arthroscopic debridement of the LHBT, biceps tenodesis, and tenotomy are all discussed, followed by a discussion of rehabilitation guidelines after surgical treatment of the LHBT.

Arthroscopic Debridement of the Biceps Long Head Tendon

Arthroscopic visualization of the 3 to 4 cm of intraarticular LHBT is part of standard shoulder arthroscopy. However,

---

TABLE 34-1

Classification of Biceps Pathology

Secondary biceps tendonitis	Occurs secondary to either rotator cuff impingement or glenohumeral joint instability
Primary biceps tendonitis	Caused by eccentric overload, hypovascularity, and abnormalities within the bicipital groove leading to attrition of the tendon
Biceps tendon instability	Occurs infrequently, but may occur with rotator interval lesions or rotator cuff tears
Biceps tendon rupture	Can be acute or chronic; actual tendon rupture can be the end stage of any of the disorders listed in this table

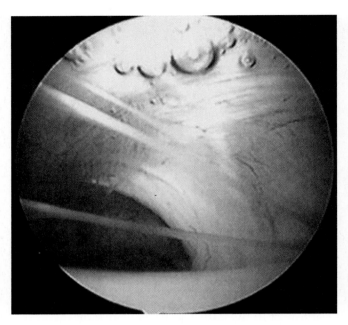

Figure 34-1: Biceps adhesions and tenosynovitis.

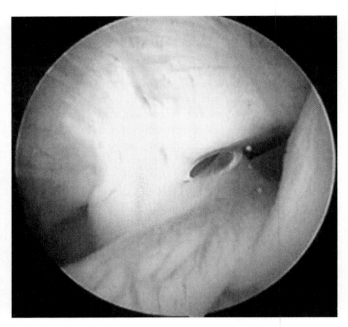

Figure 34-2: Spinal needle introduced during arthroscopy.

visualization of the remainder of the tendon within the bicipital groove is difficult.[28] Given this difficulty and the fact that tenodesis of the LHBT may not be the optimal treatment of the severely inflamed tendon in some cases, an arthroscopic portal has been developed to address LHBT tenosynovitis.

When significant LHBT tenosynovitis was observed during routine arthroscopic evaluation of the shoulder, the LHBT portal was used. This included inflamed tenosynovium or adhesions along the LHBT (Figure 34-1). With the standard posterolateral portal used for viewing, a spinal needle is passed from the anterior lateral shoulder over the LHBT tendon (Figure 34-2). The spinal needle is then oriented from lateral to medial, so as to pass into the joint through the bicipital groove proximal to the transverse humeral ligament. After localization, the needle is removed and a 4 mm skin incision is made. A 3.5 mm arthroscopic cannula, with blunt obturator, is introduced into the joint at the desired location. The LHBT is then retracted into the joint using a probe from the anterior portal. The camera is oriented to look down into the bicipital groove. A 70-degree arthroscope can be used to aid in visualization. In the presence of significant inflammation or adhesions, debridement is performed through the LHBT portal using a shaver or a radiofrequency device (Figure 34-3).

Rehabilitation after Arthroscopic Debridement of the Long Head Biceps Tendon

Rehabilitation commences in the first week postoperatively with full shoulder flexion, abduction, and internal and external rotation to patient tolerance. Shoulder extension is limited

to neutral with no hyperextension performed to minimize stress to the biceps postoperatively. No limitation in elbow range of motion is typically encountered; however, aggressive elbow extension stretching is not indicated to minimize the passive tension at the proximal end of the biceps. Immediate postoperative goals are for the reattainment of full active and passive range of motion equal to that on the contralateral side unless other procedures are performed along with the biceps debridement, such as capsular plications, labral repairs, or selective thermal capsulorrhaphy. Such procedures may require limitations in external rotation to protect the anterior capsule for the treatment of anterior glenohumeral joint instability.[29]

Limitation in shoulder flexion active range of motion is not warranted because of the finding of very low levels of biceps activity during shoulder flexion movement patterns.[11,12] However, limited elbow flexion activity is recommended both in therapeutic environments as well as with activities of daily living (ADLs) to minimize stress to the newly debrided tendon.

Early scapular stabilization and submaximal rotator cuff activation using patterns with high levels of rotator cuff activity were confirmed via EMG research,[30-32] which include side-lying external rotation, prone extension to neutral only, and limited-range prone horizontal abduction with an externally rotated humeral position. Low-resistance, high-repetition formats are used to foster local muscular endurance.

Progression to more-aggressive activity, including isokinetic internal and external rotation training and upper extremity plyometric exercises with medicine balls, is indicated after 6 to 8 weeks postoperatively when initial rotator cuff and scapular resistive exercise are well-tolerated and

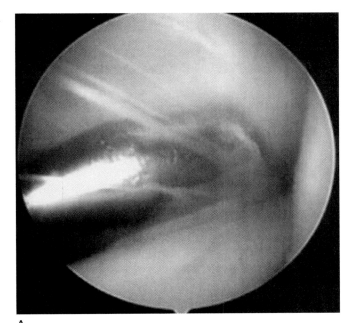

A

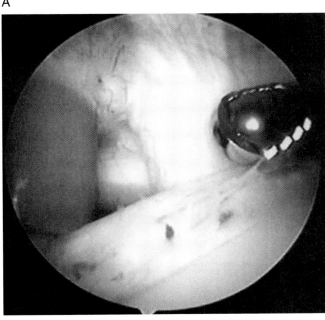

B

Figure 34-3: Debridement of the biceps long head tendon with **A,** a radiofrequency device or **B,** a shaver.

progressing. In addition, isolated biceps (elbow flexion) exercise is initiated at this time based on patient tolerance. Discharge to a home exercise program and interval sport return program is predicated on return of rotator cuff strength, return of full range of motion, and an unremarkable clinical examination including no provocation of symptoms with Speed's, Yergason's, or the impingement test in the postoperative extremity.

Outcome after Arthroscopic Debridement of the Long Head Biceps Tendon

In a retrospective study by the authors of this chapter, 11 patients with an average age of 31.2 years underwent LHBT debridement using the technique described in this chapter. As part of the surgical procedure, a full diagnostic arthroscopic evaluation was performed, at which time 10 of the patients had simultaneous procedures for additional pathology. Inclusion in the study required observation of significant inflammation of the LHBT at the time of arthroscopy, requiring debridement. In addition, all patients had a preoperative clinical diagnosis of LHBT tenosynovitis, as determined by the presence of tenderness over the LHBT and positive Speed's or Yergason's test results. Nine patients had a positive response to injection of lidocaine into the LHBT sheath, and all patients underwent formal physical therapy postoperatively, based on the primary pathology, to achieve full range of motion and rotator cuff and scapular strength. Patients were then progressed to a home exercise program.

All 11 patients in whom the LHBT portal was used were available for follow-up and had preoperative and postoperative American Shoulder and Elbow Surgeons (ASES) and Single Assessment Numeric Evaluation (SANE) scores recorded.[33,34] At a mean follow-up time of 23 months (range 15 to 30), ASES scores significantly improved from 43.5 preoperatively (±3.5) to 94.2 (±1.5) postoperatively. This was significant at the $P < .001$ level. The average SANE score improved from 36.4 (±3.6) preoperatively to a postoperative score of 95.0 (±1.7) (Tables 34-2 and 34-3). All patients (11 of 11) had a clinical resolution of the LHBT symptoms within the first 6 weeks after surgery. Statistically significant improvements in postoperative ASES and SANE scores have been obtained in patients who underwent shoulder arthroscopy using an LHBT arthroscopic portal. The use of this portal is advocated to allow a more complete arthroscopic evaluation in patients with LHBT pathology. Further research including long-term follow-up is needed to better evaluate the effectiveness of this surgical technique.

Surgical Technique of Biceps Tenodesis

The first report of biceps tenodesis was published in 1926 by Gilchrest[35] and involved tenodesis of the biceps tendon to the coracoid process. Figure 34-4 demonstrates several different approaches to biceps tenodesis that have been used historically. Lippman[36] published a technique that involved tenodesis of the LHBT to the lesser tuberosity using sutures (see Figure 34-4, A). Hitchcock[37] tenodesed the biceps long head in the bicipital groove using an osteal periosteal flap (see Figure 34-4, B). Froimson[38] pioneered a keyhole technique pictured in Figure 34-4, C, which is similar to the technique developed by Post[19] that incorporated transosseous suturing (see Figure 34-4, D). Each of these techniques uses an open technique or surgical exposure that now is most commonly performed using an anterior deltoid splitting approach.[39] During the open exposure the deltoid is split, along with the rotator interval, to gain exposure to the underlying LHBT. The bicipital groove is opened medially to avoid the laterally based vasculature and a traction suture is placed on the biceps tendon just proximal to where the tendon enters the bicipital groove. The biceps proximal attachment is released while longitudinal traction is maintained.[39] The intraarticular portion of the now released biceps tendon is excised.

The preferred open method used by Edwards and Walch[39] involves the use of a 7 mm diameter unicortical hole placed approximately 1 cm distal to the proximal aspect of the bicipital groove created in the floor of the groove. The transected end of the biceps tendon is then grasped and, with the shoulder and elbow flexed, the proximal end of the tendon is inserted into the newly created hole. A 9 mm bioabsorbable interference screw is then inserted and secured until it is flush with the humeral cortex.[39] We favor a similar technique, using the Biotenodesis system (Arthrex, Naples, FL).

The biceps long head tenodesis can be performed arthroscopically as an alternative to the open technique variations described previously. Complete assessment of the biceps tendon can be accomplished by pulling the intertubercular portion of the biceps tendon intraarticularly. After adequate debridement of the tendon and diagnostic arthroscopy, an anterolateral portal is created approximately 2 to 3 cm

---

TABLE 34-2

Associated Pathologies in Patients with Long Head Biceps Tenosynovitis

PATIENT NUMBER	ASSOCIATED PROCEDURE	ASES PREOPERATIVE	ASES POSTOPERATIVE	SANE PREOPERATIVE	SANE POSTOPERATIVE
1	Bankart repair	24	95	25	100
2	Subacromial bursectomy	38	98	40	95
3	Rotator interval and SGHL repair	60	91	40	90
4	SGHL repair	51	94	50	100
5	None	32	90	35	90
6	Rotator cuff and reverse Bankart	62	100	50	100
7	SAD, DCE	44	100	40	95
8	Bankart repair	36	92	35	100
9	SAD, DCE	50	100	50	100
10	Subacromial bursectomy	38	84	20	85
11	Rotator cuff repair	43	92	15	90
	Mean ± (P < .001)	43.5 ± 3.5	94.2 ± 1.5	36.4 ± 3.6	95 ± 1.7

ASES, American Shoulder and Elbow Surgeons score; *DCE*, distal clavicle excision; *SAD*, subacromial decompression; *SANE*, Single Assessment Numeric Evaluation score; *SGHL*, superior glenohumeral ligament.

TABLE 34-3

Average Preoperative and Postoperative ASES and SANE Scores

ASES PREOPERATIVE	ASES POSTOPERATIVE	SANE PREOPERATIVE	SANE POSTOPERATIVE
43.5	94.2*	36.4	95*

*Statistically significant difference, P < .001.

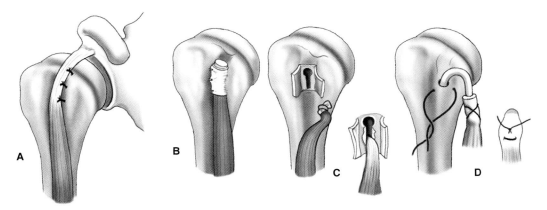

Figure 34-4: Different techniques for biceps tenodesis. **A,** Lippman's suture tenodesis. **B,** Hitchcock's osteal periosteal tenodesis. **C,** Froimson's keyhole technique. **D,** Post's technique for biceps tenodesis. (*From Edwards TB, Walch G: Biceps tenodesis: indications and techniques,* Op Tech Sports Med *10:99-104, 2002.*)

anterior and lateral to the anterolateral corner of the acromion. Using traction sutures to stabilize the biceps tendon, electrocautery is introduced and the biceps tendon is released close to its insertion on the superior labrum. The residual stump on the superior labrum is debrided to a stable and smooth margin. Similar to the method used in the open procedure, a hole is made in the proximal portion of the bicipital groove and a screw is introduced and secured until it is flush with the bottom of the groove. Various screw and drill sizes are available to accommodate variable tendon sizes.

Another method used by one of the authors is to fixate the resected LHBT to bone using a suture anchor. This can be done through a mini-open deltoid splitting incision or arthroscopically. The tendon is released arthroscopically and retrieved at the entry point into the joint. A locking stitch is placed in the free end after excising the intraarticular portion. The site of fixation is debrided to create a bleeding bone bed for healing. The anchor is then seated, and the attached sutures are used to secure the LHBT bone. The free ends of the locking suture are then used to reinforce the tenodesis by sewing to the rotator interval capsule or to the tissue overlying the bicipital groove.

Alternatively, a soft tissue tenodesis can be performed in the same manner as the anchor technique. The tendon is secured using the locking suture but without anchoring it to bone.

Rehabilitation after Biceps Tenodesis or Tenotomy

Rehabilitation after either tenodesis or tenotomy of the LHBT is often predicated on the additional procedures performed concomitantly with the biceps procedure. Use of passive and active assistive range of motion and protection of certain ranges of motion may be necessary because of repair of the rotator cuff or capsular procedures that warrant specific limitations in range of motion. For example, if a biceps tenodesis is performed with a subscapularis repair, external

rotation is limited for the first 6 weeks postoperatively to protect the subscapularis repair.[40]

Protection Phase

Isolated biceps tenodesis or tenotomy rehabilitation commences with early passive, active assistive, and active shoulder range of motion to patient tolerance. A sling may be used to limit elbow active and resistive movements with ADLs, especially when outside the home or at work for the initial 4 or even 6 weeks.[40,41] Limitation of shoulder extension to avoid hyperextension beyond the plane of the body is maintained in addition to limitation of terminal elbow extension to limit tension on the tenodesis and to limit distal migratory stress of the released biceps tendon.[40] Some authors also impose additional limitations in glenohumeral joint motion, such as Richards and colleagues,[40] who recommend abstaining from overhead stretching for the initial 6 weeks postoperatively, as well. Elbow extension often is not painful to the patient, but limiting terminal motion is indicated to allow early scarring of the released biceps tendon as well as to minimize stress to the tenodesis.

Scapular strengthening is initiated in the first few weeks postoperatively with the arm at the side, with progression to submaximal rotator cuff strengthening using the movement of internal and external rotation at the side. Progression to a full rotator cuff strengthening program occurs by 6 weeks postoperatively because of low levels of stress on the biceps musculature during exercises focusing on high levels of rotator cuff activation.[30-32] Delaying active forceful concentric and eccentric elbow flexion exercise as well as shoulder flexion with the forearm supinated and elbow extended until at least 6 weeks postoperatively is nearly globally recommended.[40,42] Some question as to the degree of protection from active and active assistive exercises in forward flexion is raised by the basic science investigations of Yamaguchi and colleagues[11] and Levy,[12] who showed minimal activation of the LHBT with glenohumeral joint flexion, as well as other motions of the glenohumeral joint, including internal and external rotation and scapular plane elevation. Edwards and Walch[43] do advise that no heavy manual labor or activity, in particular eccentric-type overload muscular contractions of the biceps, be performed after biceps tenotomy for 6 to 12 weeks to allow for scarring of the tendon in the bicipital groove. This scarring in the bicipital groove minimizes the chance for development of a poor cosmetic result because of distal migration.

Total Arm Strength Phase

After 6 weeks postoperatively, most authors[40-42] support the use of rotator cuff and scapular strengthening as well as a gradual progression to submaximal biceps contractions, such as in resistive elbow flexion activity. Progressive increases in rotator cuff and scapular activation as well as the addition of functional exercises such as upper extremity plyometrics[44] and isokinetics[45] using the modified base position for internal and external rotation are followed by 8 to 10 weeks postoperatively. Discharge parameters after biceps tenotomy and tenodesis are similar to those used after rehabilitation of mini-open rotator cuff repairs and include return of antigravity elevation equal to the contralateral extremity, rotational strength return equal to the contralateral extremity documented with dynamometry, and successful levels of patient satisfaction on subjective rating scales.[33,34]

OUTCOMES AFTER BICEPS TENODESIS AND TENOTOMY

For the severely degenerated LHBT, even when rotator cuff pathology is present and treated, the treatment of choice has been tenodesis or resection.[23,24,26,27] Short-term (6 to 12 months) follow-up of biceps tenodesis has shown good or excellent results in 74% to 94% of patients.[26,27] However, these results have been shown to decline with long-term follow-up. Berlemann and Bayley showed 67% good or excellent results at 7 years, and Becker and Cofield showed only 50% good or excellent results at 13 years.[25,26] This decline has been postulated to be the result of loss of the humeral head depression effect of the LHBT. Gill and colleagues[46] reported on the results of 30 arthroscopic biceps tendon releases at follow-up at an average of 19 months. The mean postoperative ASES shoulder score was 81.8, with a significant reduction in pain and improvement in function noted after the procedure. In addition, 90% of the patients in this series returned to sport activity at the same level as or better than preoperatively, and 96.7% of patients returned to work at the same status as preoperatively as well. In all, four shoulders were rated as poor in this series. There was no unifying factor among these four shoulders; two patients simply reported continued pain, one experienced impingement, and one patient did have a cosmetic deformity. This complication rate of 12%[46] in this study is less than a reported complication rate with tenodesis of 33%.[46]

In addition to functional loss, one great concern for many patients is the inherent cosmetic defect that may be caused by undergoing a tenolysis versus undergoing an actual stabilization of the proximal biceps in a tenodesis. In a retrospective study, Osbahr and co-workers[47] performed a follow-up of 80 patients who underwent biceps tenotomy and 80 patients who underwent biceps tenodesis over a 5-year period. Patients were evaluated for the presence of anterior shoulder pain, muscular spasms in the biceps, and cosmetic deformity of the biceps. No statistical difference was found between the population of patients who underwent biceps tenodesis and those who underwent tenotomy in any of the three main parameters studied. In addition, no differences were found between men and women between the groups. The authors conclude that no difference in cosmetic appearance, recurrent muscular spasm, or anterior shoulder pain was present in a large sample of patients who underwent biceps tenotomy and tenodesis.

SUMMARY

This chapter outlines the biomechanical and anatomic characteristics of the normal and pathologic LHBT. In addition, surgical techniques ranging from arthroscopic debridement and tenotomy to mini-open tenodesis of the long head of the biceps are presented with rehabilitative guidelines based on the basic science literature available at this time. Because isolated biceps pathology is often rare, proper and comprehensive rehabilitation of the patient after operative management of biceps pathology requires a complete understanding of the status of the rotator cuff and other intraarticular structures.

References

1. Eakin CL, Faber KJ, Hawkins RJ, Hovis D: Biceps tendon disorders in athletes. *J Am Acad Orthop Surg* 7:300-310, 1999.

2. Habermeyer P, Kaiser E, Knappe M, et al: Functional anatomy and biomechanics of the long biceps tendon, *Unfallchirurg* 90:319-329, 1987.

3. Curtis AS, Snyder SJ: Evaluation and treatment of biceps tendon pathology, *Orthop Clin North Am* 24:33-43, 1993.

4. Kumar VP, Satku K, Balasubramaniam P: The role of the long head of the biceps brachii in the stabilization of the head of the humerus, *Clin Orthop* 244:172-175, 1989.

5. Warner JJP, McMahon PJ: The role of the long head of the biceps brachii in superior stability of the glenohumeral joint, *J Bone Joint Surgery* 77-A:366-373, 1995.

6. Rodosky MW, Harner CD, Fu F: The role of the long head of the biceps muscle and superior glenoid labrum in anterior stability of the shoulder, *Am J Sports Med* 22:121-130, 1994.

7. Pagnani MJ, Deng XH, Warren RF, et al: Role of the long head of the biceps brachii in glenohumeral stability. A biomechanical study in cadavera, *J Shoulder Elbow Surg* 5:255-262, 1996.

8. Itoi E, Kuechle DK, Newman SR, et al: Stabilising function of the biceps in stable and unstable shoulders, *J Bone Joint Surg Br* 75:546-550, 1993.

9. Cheng J, Karzel R: Superior labrum anterior posterior lesions of the shoulder: operative techniques of management, *Op Tech Sports Med* 5:249-256, 1997.

10. Glousman RE, Barron J, Jobe FW, et al: An electromyographic analysis of the elbow in normal and injured pitchers with medial collateral ligament insufficiency, *Am J Sports Med* 20:311-317, 1992.

11. Yamaguchi K, Riew KD, Galatz LM, Syme JA, Neviaser RJ: Biceps activity during shoulder motion: an EMG analysis, *Clin Orthop* 336:122-129, 1997.

12. Levy AS, Kelly BT, Lintner SA, et al: Function of the long head of the biceps at the shoulder: electromyographic analysis, *J Shoulder Elbow Surg* 10:250-255, 2001.

13. Neer CS: Anterior acromioplasty for the chronic impingement syndrome in the shoulder, *J Bone Joint Surg Am* 54A:41-50, 1972.

14. Burkhead WZ: The biceps tendon. In: Rockwood CA Jr, Matsen III FA, editors: *The shoulder*, Philadelphia, 1990, Saunders.

15. Burkhead WZ Jr, Arcand MA, Zeman C, et al: The biceps tendon. In Rockwood CA, Matsen FA, editors, *The shoulder*, ed 2, Philadelphia, 1998, Saunders.

16. Rathburn JB, MacNab I: The microvascular pattern of the rotator cuff, *J Bone Joint Surg* 52B:540, 1970.

17. Kraushaar BS, Nirschl RP: Tendonosis of the elbow (tennis elbow): clinical features and findings of histological, immunohistochemical, and electron microscopy studies, *J Bone Joint Surg* 81-A:259-278, 1999.

18. Depalma AF, Callery GE: Bicipital tenosynovitis, *Clin Orthop* 3:69-85, 1955.

19. Post M, Benca P: Primary tendinitis of the long head of the biceps, *Clin Orthop* 246:117-125, 1989.

20. Paavolainen P, Bjorkenheim JM, Slatis P, Paukku P: Operative treatment of severe proximal humeral fractures, *Acta Orthop Scand* 54:374-379, 1983.

21. Walch G, Nove-Josserand L, Levigne C, Renaud E: Tears of the supraspinatus tendon associated with "hidden" lesions of the rotator interval, *J Shoulder Elbow Surg* 3:353-360, 1994.

22. Holtby R, Razmjou H: Accuracy of the Speed's and Yergason's tests in detecting biceps pathology and SLAP lesions: comparison with arthroscopic findings, *Arthroscopy* 20:231-236, 2004.

23. Neviaser RJ: Lesions of the biceps and tendinitis of the shoulder, *Orthop Clin North Am* 11:343-348, 1980.

24. Warren RF: Lesions of the long head of the biceps tendon, *Instr Course Lect* 34:204-209, 1985.

25. Becker DA, Cofield RH: Tenodesis of the long head of the biceps brachii for chronic bicipital tendinitis, *J Bone Joint Surg Am* 71A:376-380, 1989.

26. Berlemann U, Bayley I: Tenodesis of the long head of the biceps brachii in the painful shoulder: improving results in the long term, *J Shoulder Elbow Surg* 4:429-435, 1995.

27. Refior HJ, Sowa D: Long tendon of the biceps brachii: site of predilection for degenerative lesions, *J Shoulder Elbow Surg* 4:436-440, 1995.

28. Favorito PJ, Harding III WG, Heidt RS: Complete arthroscopic examination of the long head of the biceps tendon, *Arthroscopy* 17:430-432, 2001.

29. Black KP, Lim TH, McGrady LM, Raasch W: In vitro evaluation of shoulder external rotation after a Bankart reconstruction, *Am J Sports Med* 25:449-453, 1997.

30. Blackburn TA, McLeod WD, White B, et al: EMG analysis of posterior rotator cuff exercises, *Athletic Training* 25:40, 1990.

31. Ballantyne BT, O'Hare SJ, Paschall JL, et al: Electromyographic activity of selected shoulder muscles in commonly used therapeutic exercises, *Phys Ther* 73:668, 1993.

32. Townsend H, Jobe FW, Pink M, et al: Electromyographic analysis of the glenohumeral muscles during a baseball rehabilitation program, *Am J Sports Med* 19:264, 1991.

33. Beaton D, Richards RR: Assessing the reliability and responsiveness of 5 shoulder questionnaires, *J Shoulder Elbow Surg* 7:565-572, 1998.

34. Williams GN, Gangel TJ, Arciero RA, et al: Comparison of the single assessment numeric evaluation method and two shoulder rating scales, *Am J Sports Med* 27:882-890, 1999.

35. Gilchrest EL: Two cases of spontaneous rupture of the long head of the biceps flexor cubiti, *Surg Clin North Am* 6:539-554, 1926.

36. Lippman RK: Frozen shoulder, periarthritis, bicipital tendosynovitis, *Arch Surg* 47:283-296, 1943.

37. Hitchcock HH, Bechtol CO: Painful shoulder: observations on the role of the tendon of the long head of the biceps brachii in its causation, *J Bone Joint Surg Am* 30:263-273, 1948.

38. Froimson AI, Oh I: Keyhole tenodesis of the biceps origin at the shoulder, *Clin Orthop* 112:245-249, 1974.

39. Edwards TB, Walch G: Biceps tenodesis: indications and techniques, *Op Tech Sports Med* 10:99-104, 2002.

40. Richards DP, Burkart SS, Lo IKY: Arthroscopic biceps tenodesis with interference screw fixation: the lateral decubitus position, *Op Tech Sports Med* 11:15-23, 2003.

41. Mazzocca AD, Nordelinger MA, Romeo AA: Mini open and sub pectoral biceps tenodesis, *Op Tech Sports Med* 11:24-31, 2003.

42. Mazzocca AD, Romeo AA: Arthroscopic biceps tenodesis in the beach chair position, *Op Tech Sports Med* 11:6-14, 2003.

43. Edwards TB, Walch G: Biceps tendonitis: classification and treatment with tenotomy, *Op Tech Sports Med* 11:2-5, 2003.

44. Cordasco FA, Wolfe IN, Wooten ME, Bigliani LU: *Am J Sports Med* 24:386-392, 1996.

45. Ellenbecker TS, Davies GJ: The application of isokinetics in testing and rehabilitation of the shoulder complex, *J Athl Train* 35:338-350, 2000.

46. Gill TJ, McIrivin E, Mair SD, Hawkins RJ: Results of tenotomy for treatment of pathology of the long head of the biceps brachii, *J Shoulder Elbow Surg* 10:247-249, 2001.

47. Osbahr DC, Diamond AB, Speer KP: The cosmetic appearance of the biceps muscle after long-head tenotomy versus tenodesis, *Arthroscopy* 18:483-487, 2002.

Index